Manual of
Clinical Oncology

T0200212

Manual of
Clinical Oncology

8TH EDITION

Editors

Bartosz Chmielowski, MD, PhD
Associate Clinical Professor
Jonsson Comprehensive Cancer Center
Division of Hematology and Oncology
University of California, Los Angeles
Los Angeles, California

Mary Territo, MD
Emeritus Professor of Medicine
Division of Hematology and Oncology
David Geffen School of Medicine
University of California, Los Angeles
Los Angeles, California

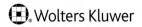 Wolters Kluwer

Philadelphia • Baltimore • New York • London
Buenos Aires • Hong Kong • Sydney • Tokyo

Executive Editor: Rebecca Gaertner
Acquisitions Editor: Ryan Shaw
Editorial Coordinator: Emily Buccieri and Emilie Moyer
Marketing Manager: Rachel Mante Leung
Senior Production Project Manager: Alicia Jackson
Design Coordinator: Terry Mallon
Manufacturing Coordinator: Beth Welsh
Prepress Vendor: SPi Global

8th edition

Library of Congress Cataloging-in-Publication Data
Names: Chmielowski, Bartosz, editor. | Territo, Mary C., editor.
Title: Manual of clinical oncology / editors, Bartosz Chmielowski, Mary Territo.
Other titles: Manual of clinical oncology (Casciato)
Description: Eighth edition. | Philadelphia : Wolters Kluwer, [2017] | Includes bibliographical references and index.
Identifiers: LCCN 2016044205 | ISBN 9781496349576
Subjects: | MESH: Neoplasms—diagnosis | Neoplasms—therapy | Medical Oncology—methods | Handbooks
Classification: LCC RC262.5 | NLM QZ 39 | DDC 616.99/4—dc23 LC record available at https://lccn.loc.gov/2016044205

CCS0721

Contributors

Russell K. Brynes, MD
Professor of Clinical Pathology
Chief, Hematopathology Service
Department of Pathology
Keck School of Medicine
University of Southern California
Los Angeles, California

Pranatharthi H. Chandrasekar,
MD, FACP, FIDSA
Professor, Internal Medicine and Infectious
 Diseases
Chief, Division of Infectious Diseases
Wayne State University
Chief, Infectious Diseases
Karmanos Cancer Institute
Detroit, Michigan

Howard A. Chansky, MD
Professor and Chair
Department of Orthopaedics and Sports Medicine
University of Washington School of Medicine
Seattle, Washington

Bartosz Chmielowski, MD, PhD
Associate Clinical Professor
Jonsson Comprehensive Cancer Center
Division of Hematology and Oncology
University of California, Los Angeles
Los Angeles, California

Darin J. Davidson, MD, MHSc, FRCSC
Assistant Professor
Musculoskeletal Oncology Service
Program Director, Musculoskeletal Oncology
 Fellowship
Department of Orthopaedics and Sports
 Medicine
University of Washington School of Medicine
Seattle, Washington

Lisa M. DeAngelis, MD
Professor of Neurology
Weill Cornell Medical College
Chair, Department of Neurology
Memorial Sloan Kettering Cancer Center
New York, New York

Chaitanya R. Divgi, MD
Professor of Radiology
Executive Vice-Chair, Research
Chief of Nuclear Medicine and Molecular
 Imaging
Department of Radiology
Columbia University
New York, New York

Alexandra Drakaki, MD, PhD
Assistant Professor of Medicine and Urology
Director—Genitourinary Medical Oncology
 Program
Division of Hematology and Oncology
Institute of Urologic Oncology
University of California, Los Angeles
Los Angeles, California

Martin J. Edelman, MD, FACP
Professor of Medicine
Head, Section of Solid Tumor Oncology
Associate Director, Division of Hematology and
 Oncology
University of Maryland Greenebaum Cancer
 Center
University of Maryland School of Medicine
Baltimore, Maryland

Lawrence H. Einhorn, MD
Distinguished Professor of Medicine
Department of Medicine—Hematology/Oncology
Indiana University
Indianapolis, Indiana

Herbert Eradat, MD, MS
Assistant Clinical Professor of Medicine
UCLA Lymphoma Program
Division of Hematology and Oncology
David Geffen School of Medicine at UCLA
Los Angeles, California

Robert A. Figlin, MD, FACP
Steven Spielberg Family Chair in Hematology
 Oncology
Professor of Medicine and Biomedical Sciences
Director, Division of Hematology and Oncology
Deputy Director
Samuel Oschin Comprehensive Cancer Institute
Cedars-Sinai Medical Center
Los Angeles, California

Charles A. Forscher, MD
Medical Director, Sarcoma Program
Samuel Oschin Cancer Center
Cedars-Sinai Medical Center
Assistant Clinical Professor
David Geffen School of Medicine at UCLA
Los Angeles, California

David R. Gandara, MD
Professor of Medicine
Director, Thoracic Oncology Program
Senior Advisor to the Director
UC Davis Comprehensive Cancer Center
Sacramento, California

Patricia A. Ganz, MD
Distinguished Professor Health Policy and Management and Medicine
UCLA Fielding School of Public Health
David Geffen School of Medicine at UCLA
Director, Cancer Prevention and Control Research
Jonsson Comprehensive Cancer Center
Los Angeles, California

Axel Grothey, MD
Professor of Oncology
Department of Oncology
Mayo Clinic College of Medicine
Rochester, Minnesota

Shireen N. Heidari, MD
Fellow in Palliative Medicine
UCLA Department of Medicine, Palliative Care Service
Los Angeles, California

Siwen Hu-Lieskovan, MD, PhD
Assistant Clinical Professor
Division of Hematology and Oncology
Department of Medicine
David Geffen School of Medicine at UCLA
Los Angeles, California

Carole G. H. Hurvitz, MD
Emeritus Director Pediatric Hematology Oncology
Cedars Sinai Medical Center
Samuel Oschin Comprehensive Cancer Institute
Emeritus Professor of Pediatrics
David Geffen School of Medicine
University of California, Los Angeles
Los Angeles, California

Amy A. Jacobson, RN, NP-BC
Clinical Research Nurse, Nurse Practitioner
UCLA-LIVESTRONG^TM Survivorship Center of Excellence
Jonsson Comprehensive Cancer Center
Los Angeles, California

Pashtoon Murtaza Kasi, MD
Assistant Professor
College of Medicine/Oncology
Mayo Clinic, Florida
Jacksonville, Florida

Hyung L. Kim, MD
Medallion Chair in Urology
Director, Academic Programs, Urology
Co-director, Urologic Oncology
Associate Director, Samuel Oschin Comprehensive Cancer Center
Cedars Sinai Medical Center
Los Angeles, California

Mira Kistler, MD
Fellow in Hematology Oncology
Division of Hematology and Oncology
David Geffen School of Medicine at UCLA
Los Angeles, California

Rekha A. Kumbla, MD
Division of Hematology and Oncology
Olive View–UCLA Medical Center and Cedars Sinai Medical Center
Los Angeles, California

Sarah M. Larson, MD
Assistant Professor
Division of Hematology and Oncology
Department of Medicine
University of California, Los Angeles
Los Angeles, California

Steve P. Lee, MD, PhD
Professor of Clinical Radiation Oncology
Department of Radiation Oncology
David Geffen School of Medicine at UCLA
Los Angeles, California

Margaret I. Liang, MD
Gynecologic Oncology Fellow
Division of Gynecologic Oncology
Department of Obstetrics and Gynecology
University of California, Los Angeles
Los Angeles, California

Sandy T. Liu, MD
Hematology/Oncology Fellow
Division of Hematology and Oncology
David Geffen School of Medicine at UCLA
Los Angeles, California

Alison W. Loren, MD, MS, FACP
Director, Hematology/Oncology Fellowship
Associate Professor of Medicine
Division of Hematology and Oncology
Perelman School of Medicine of the University of Pennsylvania
Perelman Center for Advanced Medicine
Philadelphia, Pennsylvania

Sonia Mahajan, MD
Visiting Scientist
Department of Radiology
Columbia University
New York, New York

Carolyn Maxwell, MD
Assistant Professor of Medicine
Stony Brook University School of Medicine
Division of Endocrinology
Department of Medicine
Stony Brook Medicine
Stony Brook, New York

Sanaz Memarzadeh, MD, PhD
Professor
UCLA Division of Gynecologic Oncology
Department of Obstetrics and Gynecology
Department of Biological Chemistry
David Geffen School of Medicine
Los Angeles, California

Ronald T. Mitsuyasu, MD
Professor of Medicine
Director, UCLA Center for Clinical AIDS
Research and Education
David Geffen School of Medicine at UCLA
University of California, Los Angeles
Los Angeles, California

Theodore B. Moore, MD, MS
Professor and Chief
Division of Pediatric Hematology/Oncology
Department of Pediatrics
David Geffen School of Medicine at UCLA
Los Angeles, California

Bhagyashri Navalkele, MBBS, MD
Infectious Diseases Fellow
Division of Infectious Diseases
Department of Internal Medicine
Wayne State University School of Medicine
Detroit, Michigan

Andrew Huy Cao Nguyen, MD
Clinical Research Assistant
UCLA Department of Family Medicine
University of California, Los Angeles
Los Angeles, California

Ronald L. Paquette, MD
Blood and Marrow Transplant Program
Cedars-Sinai Medical Center
Samuel Oschin Comprehensive Cancer
Institute
Los Angeles, California

Mark D. Pegram, MD
Director of Breast Oncology Program
Medical Oncology
Stanford University
Stanford, California

Lauren C. Pinter-Brown, MD, FACP
Health Sciences Professor of Medicine
Chao Family Comprehensive Cancer Center
University of California, Irvine
Irvine, California

Antoni Ribas, MD, PhD
Professor of Medicine
Professor of Surgery
Professor of Molecular and Medical
Pharmacology
Director, Tumor Immunology Program, Jonsson
Comprehensive Cancer Center (JCCC)
David Geffen School of Medicine
Chair, Melanoma Committee at SWOG
University of California, Los Angeles (UCLA)
Los Angeles, California

Kathryn J. Ruddy, MD, MPH
Associate Professor of Oncology
Mayo Clinic
Rochester, Minnesota

Jordan E. Rullo, PhD, ABPP
Assistant Professor
Board Certified Clinical Health Psychologist
Department of Psychology and Psychiatry and
Division of General Internal Medicine
Mayo Clinic
Rochester, Minnesota

Gary Schiller, MD
Professor of Medicine
Director, Aramont Program for Clinical
Translational Research in Human
Malignancies
Hematological Malignancy/Stem Cell
Transplantation Unit
David Geffen School of Medicine at UCLA
Los Angeles, California

Mary E. Sehl, MD, PhD
Assistant Professor
Division of Hematology and Oncology
Department of Medicine
Department of Biomathematics
David Geffen School of Medicine
University of California, Los Angeles
Los Angeles, California

Maie A. St. John, MD, PhD
Associate Professor-in-Residence
Samuel and Della Pearlman Chair in Head
and Neck Surgery
Co-Director, UCLA Head and Neck Cancer
Program
Department of Head and Neck Surgery
University of California, Los Angeles
Los Angeles, California

Mary Territo, MD
Emeritus Professor of Medicine
Division of Hematology and Oncology
David Geffen School of Medicine
University of California, Los Angeles
Los Angeles, California

Yoshie Umemura, MD
Fellow
Department of Neurology
Memorial Sloan Kettering Cancer Center
New York, New York

Maria E. Vergara-Lluri, MD
Assistant Professor of Clinical Pathology
Hematopathology Service
Department of Pathology
Keck School of Medicine
University of Southern California
Los Angeles, California

Richard F. Wagner, Jr., MD
E.B. Smith Professor of Dermatology
Director of Mohs Surgery and Cutaneous
  Oncology
The University of Texas Medical Branch
Galveston, Texas

David Wallenstein, MD
UCLA Department of Family Medicine
UCLA Family Medicine Ambulatory Palliative
  Care and Pain Clinic
UCLA Palliative Care Service
Medical Director
Skirball Hospice Program, Los Angeles Jewish
  Home
Los Angeles, California

Deborah J. Wong, MD, PhD
Assistant Clinical Professor of Medicine
Division of Hematology and Oncology
Department of Medicine
David Geffen School of Medicine
University of California, Los Angeles
Los Angeles, California

Rodolfo Zamora, MD
Acting Instructor
Department of Orthopaedics and Sports
  Medicine
University of Washington School of
  Medicine
Fellow, Orthopaedic Oncology
University of Washington
Seattle, Washington

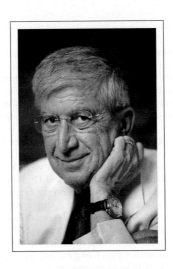

In Memoriam
Dennis Casciato, MD
May 7, 1939–December 6, 2013

This edition of the *Manual of Clinical Oncology* is being dedicated to
Dr. Dennis Casciato who passed away in 2013.

Dennis received his bachelor degree in Biophysics from UC Berkley in
1960 and his MD in 1964 from UC San Francisco. He began his training in
Internal Medicine at Orange County Medical Center (1964–1966). He then
served as a Major in the US Army from 1966–1969. Following his tour in the
Army, he returned to complete his residency and undertake his Hematology
Fellowship at UCLA–Wadsworth Veterans Association Medical Center
(1969–1971). He then continued at the Wadsworth VA hospital where he
was a research associate in Hematology and Infectious Diseases (1972–1974),
Chief of Postgraduate Training from 1974–1977 and Chief of Hematology
from 1978–1983. He was a member of the UCLA School of Medicine faculty
from 1973–2012. In 1983, he transitioned into private practice and continued
as Chief of Medicine at hospitals in the San Fernando Valley in California
where he lived with his wife, Joy, and raised his sons, Frank and Andrew.

The *Manual of Clinical Oncology* was a labor of love for Dr. Casciato, and
through the years, he was devoted to maintaining the *Manual of Clinical
Oncology* as a quality resource for the oncologic community. Dennis was a
consummate clinician/teacher and a major champion for the importance of
the humanistic aspects of medicine.

Preface

The *Manual of Bedside Oncology* was first published in 1983 as a concise guide to the bedside management of cancer patients. It was collaboration between Drs. Dennis Casciato and Barry Lowitz who were the primary authors of all of the chapters. Because of its popularity, a second edition was produced in 1988 with a change of name to *Manual of Clinical Oncology* in order to more accurately reflect the content. Drs. Casciato and Lowitz continued to collaborate and edit editions 3 and 4, and with the increasing complexity of oncology, began inviting experts in various areas to help with the writing of certain chapters. Dr. Casciato was the sole editor of the fifth edition and then invited Dr. Mary Territo to serve as associate editor on editions 6 and 7 in the area of hematologic malignancies. Dr. Casciato began organizing the eighth edition, but when he realized he had a serious illness and would not be able to proceed, he recruited Dr. Bartosz Chmielowski to serve as coeditor with Dr. Territo. Dr. Chmielowski is on the faculty of the UCLA School of Medicine and had contributed to editions 6 and 7 with his expertise in melanoma and sarcomas and has a well-known broad-based knowledge and experience in solid tumors.

Over the years, the Manual has grown to encompass the developments and advances in oncology that have occurred. For this eighth edition, we have tried to incorporate the major achievements in immunotherapies, biologics, and targeted therapies that have been developed. At the same time, we strive to continue the main goals that Dr. Casciato has had for the Manual since its inception, to present a comprehensive, concise, and current reference for the treatment of cancer patients and to reaffirm the unique relationship between the cancer patients and their doctors.

Bartosz Chmielowski
Mary Territo

Contents

Appendices

General Aspects

Biology of Cancer and Implications for Clinical Oncology

Bartosz Chmielowski

I. HALLMARKS OF CANCER

All cancers originate from normal cells of the host. Hence, a normal cell must undergo a series of changes in order to become tumorigenic and finally malignant. The tumor is not only composed of malignant cells but also contains a number of normal cells that were recruited; they are required for tumor growth. The understanding of cancer biology must not be limited only to studying malignant cells but also must include analysis of its environment.

Several distinct capabilities have been described that characterize the processes of achieving the growth advantage by cancerous cell and of tumorigenesis.

A. **Sustaining proliferative signaling.** The growth of normal cells is in homeostasis, assuring the maintenance of the integrity of organs. Malignant cells have an ability to proliferate uncontrollably. Cancers use multiple mechanisms to sustain their proliferation:

1. Tumors may produce growth factors for which they have receptors in an autocrine fashion.

2. Tumors may stimulate surrounding normal tissues and these normal tissues provide growth factors for the tumor.

3. Tumor may become hypersensitive to growth factors through up-regulation of growth receptors or alterations of the structure of these receptors.

4. Finally, they may become independent of growth factors by the presence of somatic mutations activating downstream pathways, for example, BRAF mutations activating the mitogen-activated protein kinase (MAPK) pathway, or mutations in phosphoinositide-3-kinase (PI3K) leading to activation of the PI3K/Akt/mTOR pathway, or by altering the negative feedback loops.

5. Tumors may stimulate surrounding normal tissues, and these normal tissues provide growth factors for growth.

B. **Evading growth suppressors.** Normal cells use multiple mechanisms to regulate negatively cell proliferation; most of these processes occur through the products of activation of tumor suppressor genes. Loss of function of these gene products allows tumor cells to evade the inhibitory mechanisms. Multiple genes have been implicated, but most of their products act as a part of the network of processes, and fortunately the cells can frequently compensate for the loss of function of a single gene; that is, loss of the function of a single tumor suppressor is not sufficient to induce oncogenesis.

1. The **RB** protein is responsible for the control of the cell cycle and the switch from resting state to cell division, mainly in response to the stimuli outside of the cell. The cells that lack the RB protein do not have this control mechanism. The retinoblastoma gene (RB1) was the first of these abnormal genes to be discovered. Subsequently, a number of other suppressor gene

abnormalities have been found, particularly in uncommon or rare hereditary diseases. Examples include Wilms tumor (WT1), familial polyposis (APC), familial melanoma (CDKN20), and familial breast and ovarian cancers (BRCA-1 and BRCA-2).

2. The **p53** protein (TP53) is also a cell cycle control protein, but it responds mainly to the intracellular stressors, and it can stop cell cycle until the abnormal processes have been corrected. It can detect DNA abnormalities, such as nucleotide mismatches and DNA strand breaks, including those caused by radiation and chemotherapy. The function of p53 is thought to be critical in preserving the integrity of the cellular genome.

   a. When DNA lesions are detected, the p53 protein arrests cells in the quiescent G_1 and G_2 phases of the cell cycle, preventing cells from entering the DNA synthetic (S) phase of the cell cycle. The p53 protein can then induce repair mechanism proteins or trigger proteins, which cause apoptosis.

   b. In the absence of intact apoptosis, cancer cells can continue through sequential cell divisions and accumulate nucleotide mismatches and progressive DNA mutations.

   c. *In vitro* studies have shown that chemotherapy and radiation kill cancer cells through DNA damage, which triggers p53 protein–induced apoptosis. In contrast, p53 protein–deficient mouse thymocytes and resting lymphocytes remain viable after irradiation.

   d. Many human cancers are found to have mutant p53 suppressor genes. Mutant p53 is characteristic of Li-Fraumeni syndrome, a hereditary autosomal dominant syndrome of both soft tissue and epithelial cancers at multiple sites starting at an early age.

3. The *NF2* gene and its product **Merlin**. Merlin is responsible for maintaining of contact inhibition through E-cadherins. Normal cells stop proliferating when a desired density of cells is achieved. This process is dysregulated in cancer (loss of contact inhibition).

4. The **LKB1** epithelial polarity protein is responsible for maintaining tissue integrity and contributes to the contact inhibition phenomenon. The functional LKB1 can even overcome signals originating from strong oncogenes such as *Myc*.

5. Tumor growth factor-β (**TGF-β**) functions as a suppressor of tumor growth, but in the advanced malignancies its function may change and it may lead to increased aggressiveness of cancer through promotion of the epithelial-to-mesenchymal transformation.

C. Resisting cell death.

   1. **Apoptosis.** Under normal conditions, cells that get damaged undergo programmed cell death in the process of apoptosis. Cancer cells have ability to avoid this process despite apoptosis-inducing stressors such as DNA damage or oncogene hypersignaling. Apoptosis is balanced by activity of antiapoptotic molecules from the Bcl-2 family (Bcl-2, Bcl-x_L, Bcl-w, Mcl-1, A1) and of proapoptotic molecules Bax and Bak. Cancer cells may express higher levels of the antiapoptotic or lower levels of proapoptotic molecules. TP53 is able to induce apoptosis; cancer cells that lack this oncogene can escape it.

      a. **Apoptosis occurs in normal tissue reabsorption**. Apoptosis also results in the disappearance during embryogenesis of webs between fingers of primates, allowing the formation of individual digits. Apoptosis results in the elimination of normal senescent cells when they become old and useless and of thymic T cells that recognize "self" and thereby prevent immune attack by these cells on the host.

b. **Apoptosis eliminates cells with abnormal DNA** caused either by irreparable DNA damage or by inaccurate, incomplete, or redundant transcription of DNA. This is a major mechanism for maintaining chromosome number in cells of a particular species and in preventing aneuploidy. The process ensures that only cells that have fully and accurately replicated their entire DNA can enter mitosis.

c. **Apoptotic cells can be recognized microscopically.** Apoptotic cells show clumps of intracellular organelles in the absence of necrosis. The nuclei are condensed and fragmented; intracellular structures are degenerated and compartmentalized. As the cell falls apart, phagocytes take up the fragments. Unlike the process of cell necrosis, apoptosis does not cause an inflammatory response. Apoptosis requires synthesis of specific proteins that have been highly conserved throughout evolution.

d. **Caspases.** The final stage of the various death pathways is mediated through activation of the caspases, which represent a family of cysteine proteases. The activation of caspases is determined by the intrinsic and extrinsic pathways of apoptosis. The intrinsic pathway is a mitochondrial-dependent pathway mediated by the Bcl-2 family of proteins. Exposure to cytotoxic stress results in disruption of the mitochondrial membrane, which then leads to release of protease activators. Caspase-9 is subsequently activated, setting off a cascade of events that commit the cell to undergo apoptosis. The extrinsic pathway is mediated by ligand binding to the tumor necrosis factor (TNF) family of receptors, which includes TNF-related apoptosis-inducing ligand and others, and certain essential adaptor proteins. These adaptor proteins recruit various proteases that cleave the N-terminal domain of caspase-8, which leads to activation of the caspase cascade.

2. **Autophagy** is a natural process that allows cells to break down intracellular organelles upon exposure to stressors with help of lysosomes and recycle nutrients. It is also a protective process in case of neoplastic transformation. This process is regulated by PI3-kinase, AKT, and mTOR pathway and by protein Beclin-1. Cancer cells may use autophagy to recycle their nutrients and escape damaging agents.

3. **Necrosis** is another process of cell death in which cells increase in size and break, releasing multiple proinflammatory cytokines. Immune cells are attracted to the areas of necrosis to eliminate the remnants of cells. Cancer can use this process to induce an inflammatory proneoplastic environment, stimulate angiogenesis, and even use these cytokines to stimulate its own growth.

D. **Enabling replicative immortality.** Normal cells are able to undergo only a limited number of divisions before they undergo one of two processes: **senescence** (the cells remain dormant, nondividing, but their state can be possibly reversed) or **crisis/apoptosis** (irreversible process leading to cell death). This process is governed by the presence of telomeres on the ends of chromosomes. In physiologic conditions, telomeres shorten with each division and hence make cells more susceptible to apoptosis/senescence. Shortening of telomeres is also a natural defense mechanism against development of cancer: potentially neoplastic cells divide and lose parts of telomeres with every division until their DNA is unprotected and they enter into the state of crisis. The cells that are able to maintain the activity of telomerase, an enzyme that is responsible for lengthening of telomeres, can potentially proliferate uncontrollably and turn into cancer.

In some cases, precancerous cells have actually a low level of telomerase and become more vulnerable to apoptosis, but at the same time, in the presence of other prooncogenic events, their DNA is more susceptible to breakage and formation of multiple new fusion products, which will eventually give growth advantage to these cells and assure neoplastic transformation.

E. **Inducing angiogenesis.** The growth of cells can occur only when required nutrients are delivered and waste metabolites are removed from the cell environment. This process requires the presence of blood vessels. It is possible that microscopic lesions rely on osmosis for delivery of nutrients, but it has been shown that early in carcinogenesis, the "angiogenic switch" occurs that promotes new blood vessel formation. Vascular endothelial growth factor-A (VEGF-A) is the main protein responsible for neoangiogenesis. Its action is counterbalanced by the activity of thrombospondin-1 (TSP-1). Interestingly, tumor vasculature is not normal appearing; blood vessels are distorted, branched, and leaky and areas of hemorrhage are observed. Different cancers rely on neovascularization to a different degree; for example, renal cell carcinoma is highly vascularized, but pancreatic adenocarcinoma may have a paucity of new blood vessels. Not only cancer cells but also the cells of tumor environment such as infiltrating immune cells (macrophages, mast cells, neutrophils, myeloid progenitors) and bone marrow–derived vascular progenitor cells induce angiogenesis.

1. VEGF induces receptors for itself on mature and nonproliferating blood vessel endothelial cells. These normal, resting endothelial cells do not have the receptor until they are exposed to VEGF.

2. VEGF induces the production and activity of multiple other growth factors that contribute to blood vessel formation.

3. VEGF can be induced by *c-ras* and by other oncogenes and growth factors, which then induce further production of VEGF.

4. VEGF appears to prevent apoptosis in induced endothelial cells.

F. **Activating invasion and metastasis.** Cancer cells are characterized by a unique ability of local invasion and formation of distant metastasis. E-cadherin is one of most important cell surface adhesion molecules responsible for maintaining tissue integrity. Multiple cancers express E-cadherin at a low level and express molecules implicated in cell migration such as N-cadherin at higher levels.

Formation of distant metastasis is a multistep process and it consists of the following:

1. Local invasion
2. Migration into lymphatic and blood vessels
3. Spread of cancer cells through vasculature
4. Extravasation of cancer cells into tissue of remote organs
5. Growth of cancer cells in the new environment to form macroscopic tumors

Molecular events occurring during the process of formation metastasis resemble steps of embryonic morphogenesis. The process by itself has been named **epithelial–mesenchymal transition** (EMT) and involves genes playing a physiologic role in embryogenesis such as *Snail, Slug, Twist,* and *Zeb1/2*. These genes are regulated by the intracellular oncogenic events, but they can be also influenced by microenvironmental stimuli. Invasive and metastatic potential of cancer is strongly dependent on the cross talk between neoplastic cells and the stroma.

Some cancers are characterized more by the ability of local invasion rather than formation of distant metastasis. They can invade into the adjacent tissue ("collective invasion"), which is frequently seen in squamous cell carcinomas of the head and neck area, and cause significant morbidity. Other cancers can spread through spaces in the extracellular matrix ("amoeboid invasion").

Tissue invasion and formation of distant metastasis are two different processes. When macroscopic metastases are seen, it implicates that cancer cells were able to adapt to the new tissue environment that is very different from the environment of the primary site. Most probably, metastasis uses the same hallmarks for its growth and survival as the primary site. It is a random process, and therefore we frequently see that metastases may be diagnosed many years after the treatment of the primary tumor. The difficulty with adaptation to the new tissue environment also explains why not all patients with circulating tumor cells end up with metastatic disease.

G. **Reprogramming energy metabolism.** In normal conditions, the cell metabolism depends mainly on aerobic glycolysis, in which glucose is metabolized into pyruvate in the cytoplasm and finally into carbon dioxide in the mitochondria. Cancer cells switch their metabolism from aerobic to anaerobic glycolysis, which is a less efficient way of producing of ATP. Cancer cells compensate by an increased use of glucose to achieve the same level of ATP. It is frequently achieved by up-regulation of glucose transporters such as GLUT1. Hypoxic conditions in the tumor environment further accentuate the process. Glycolytic intermediate processes are used by cancer cells for generation of nucleosides and amino acids that are essential for tumor proliferation and growth. In addition, some cancers have actually a mixed population of cells: some rely on glucose-dependent metabolism and some use lactate. Lactate is produced during anaerobic glycolysis and it can provide the fuel for neighboring cells. Gliomas and other cancers were found to contain activating mutations in the isocitrate dehydrogenase 1/2 (IDH) gene; the clones that contain these mutations have a growth advantage through altered metabolism.

H. **Evading immune destruction.** The function of the immune system in the control of growth of abnormal cells is insurmountable. The immune cells continue surveying the body and eliminate pathogens and potentially cancerous cells. For cancer cells to survive, they have to evade this surveillance and they can achieve it by disabling components of the immune system. The detailed discussion on the tumor–immune system interactions can be found in Chapter 5.

II. ENABLING CANCER CHARACTERISTICS

Hallmarks of cancer are a set of features that allow malignant cells to proliferate, survive, and metastasize. These abilities are acquired through the development of various enabling characteristics.

A. **Genomic instability and mutation.** The process of progression from a normal cell to a premalignant cell and finally to a malignant cell is achieved because of the instability of the genome: proliferating cells generate new mutations in a stochastic way and only the clones that acquired features allowing them to evade the defense mechanisms can survive. This observation implies that premalignant cells would contain fewer mutations than metastatic lesions, and this has been shown to be true in most cancers. Not all changes must be elicited by mutational changes; the epigenetic changes such as DNA methylation or histone modification can change the expression of oncogenes too.

Under normal conditions, the mechanisms responsible for genome stability (repair mechanisms) assure that any randomly created mutations are repaired or an abnormal cell is eliminated. In the presence of external mutagens or heritable susceptibility factors such as mutations in tumor suppressor genes, the repair mechanisms malfunction and allow abnormal cells to survive.

The genes involved in the supervision of these processes have been named "**caretaker genes**." They are responsible for

1. Detecting DNA damage and activating the repair mechanisms
2. Repairing damaged DNA directly
3. Inactivating mutagenic factors

Inactivation of caretaker genes leads to an increased mutation rate and increased genome instability.

The **gatekeeper genes** are responsible for inhibiting tumor growth or promoting death. A mutation in such a gene may promote the development of cancer by decreasing the DNA repair window from G_1 to S phase (see Section III).

B. **Tumor-promoting inflammation.** It has been recognized that tumors consist not only of neoplastic cells but also of a variety of cells of the innate and adaptive immune systems. The density of immune cells and their localization within the tumor are different among different malignancies. Initially it was postulated that the presence of these cells reflected an attempt of eradication of a tumor by the immune system. Currently we know that these inflammatory infiltrates can actually promote tumorigenesis and cancer growth by providing cytokines and growth and survival factors for the tumor, by stimulating angiogenesis, and by facilitating invasion and metastasis. Inflammation can ignite the transition from a premalignant state to full malignancy, for example, by release of reactive oxygen species that have mutagenic capabilities.

III. PRINCIPLES OF CANCER CELL GROWTH
A. **Normal cell reproduction**
  1. **The cell cycle** is depicted in Figure 1-1. Cell replication proceeds through a number of phases that are biochemically initiated by external stimuli and modulated by both external and internal growth controls. Certain oncogenes and cell cycle–specific proteins are activated and deactivated synchronously as the cell progresses through the phases of the cell cycle. Most cells must enter the cell cycle to be killed by chemotherapy or radiation therapy. Many cytotoxic agents act at more than one phase of the cell cycle, including those classified as *phase specific.*
     a. In the **G_0 phase** (gap 0 or resting phase), cells are generally programmed to perform specialized functions. An example of drugs that are active in this phase is glucocorticoids for mature lymphocytes.
     b. In the **G_1 phase** (gap 1 or interphase), proteins and RNA are synthesized for specialized cell functions. In late G_1, a burst of RNA synthesis occurs, and many of the enzymes necessary for DNA synthesis are manufactured. An example of drugs that are active in this phase is L-asparaginase.

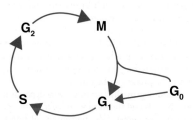

Figure 1-1 Phases of cell growth.

    c. In the **S phase** (DNA synthesis), the cellular content of DNA doubles. Examples of drugs that are active in this phase are procarbazine and antimetabolites.

    d. In the **G_2 phase** (gap 2), DNA synthesis ceases, protein and RNA syntheses continue, and the microtubular precursors of the mitotic spindle are produced. Examples of drugs that are active in this phase are bleomycin and plant alkaloids.

    e. In the **M phase** (mitosis), the rates of protein and RNA synthesis diminish abruptly, while the genetic material is segregated into daughter cells. After completion of mitosis, the new cells enter either the G_0 or the G_1 phase. Examples of drugs that are active in this phase are plant alkaloids.

2. Cyclins activate the various phases of the cell cycle. Most normal cells capable of reproduction proliferate in response to external stimuli, such as growth factors, certain hormones, and antigen–histocompatibility complexes, which affect cell surface receptors. These receptors then transduce the signal that results in cell division. Tyrosine kinases (TKs) are an essential part of the cascade of proliferative signals, from extracellular growth factors to the nucleus. Cyclins combine with, activate, and direct the action of special TKs, called cyclin-dependent kinases.

3. Cell cycle *checkpoints*. Cells that are capable of reproducing are normally stopped at specific phases of the cell cycle called *checkpoints*. The most important of these are immediately preceding the initiation of DNA synthesis and immediately preceding the act of mitosis. These histologically quiescent periods are probably mediated by decreased activity of cyclin-associated kinases and tumor suppressor proteins. In fact, the cells in these phases are biochemically active as they prepare proteins to enter the next phase of the cell cycle and correct any genetic defects before going on to reproduce.

    a. Normal cells have mechanisms that detect abnormalities in DNA sequences. When DNA is damaged, a number of repair mechanisms replace damaged nucleotides with normal molecules. These mechanisms are most important during cellular reproduction to ensure that new genetic material in daughter cells is an exact copy of the parent cell.

    b. The first checkpoint occurs in the late G_1 phase, just before cells enter the S phase. Even if the proper extracellular signals are received and all of the machinery is in place for DNA synthesis, the DNA must be in an acceptable state, with no lesions, before the cell can leave G_1. If lesions are detected, either they are repaired or the cell is made to undergo apoptosis. This stopping point is one of the actions of the p53 protein.

    c. The second checkpoint occurs just before the cell enters the M phase; the cell cycle inhibitors stop the cell until it is determined whether the new progenies are worthy successors with accurate genetic copies of the parent. A cell that has not completely and accurately replicated all of its DNA or that does not have the full complement of proteins, spindle materials, and other substances to complete mitosis is arrested at this checkpoint until everything is in order and before the M phase can begin.

4. Kinetics of tumor growth. Tumor growth depends on the size of the proliferating pool of cells and the number of cells dying spontaneously. The larger the tumor mass, the greater the percentage of nondividing and dying cells and the longer it takes for the average cell to divide.

a. **The lag phase.** During the earliest phase of tumor development, a small mass of a tumor does not enlarge very much. The working hypothesis about this lag phase is that the "precancer" cells are dividing, but the rate of birth of new cells is offset by cell death. During this phase, the dividing cells are accumulating various mutations. These mutations help the surviving cells improve their adaptivity to the supply of nutrients, increase the rate at which the mutated cells divide, decrease the rate of apoptosis sensitivity, provide them with invasive properties, make the mutated cells more responsiveness to host factors, and produce angiogenesis factors. Before the angiogenesis factors are expressed, the small tumor does not have its own blood supply and is dependent on local factors to get all the necessary nutrients. Animal models suggested that these tiny cancers may remain unchanged in size and undetectable for many years before they enter the logarithmic phase and are large enough to be detectable.

b. **The log phase.** The tumor now shows rapid exponential growth of the tumor mass. There is a relatively high proportion of cells undergoing division, with rapidly declining rates of cell death, and the *growth fraction* (ratio of dividing to total cells) is high. This rapid growth also reflects the adaptivity of the cells and the production by the tumor cells of angiogenesis factors that induce the surrounding tissues to form new blood vessels that "feed" the tumor mass. When the tumor's growth fraction is at its highest level, it is still clinically undetectable. Although the reduction in cell number is small, the fractional cell kill from a dose of effective chemotherapy would be significantly higher than later in the course of the tumor.

c. **The plateau phase.** Tumor growth slows down as the percentage of dividing cells decreases, and a larger percentage of cells are dying. The hypotheses are that growth rates eventually plateau because of restrictions of space and nutrient availability, of limitation of blood supply, and of genetic mutations, which cause a higher death rate of cells. The curve becomes asymptotic with some maximum.

IV. THE TUMOR ENVIRONMENT

As discussed before, the tumor consists not only of cancer cells but also of a myriad of cells that are important in cancer growth and survival. The supportive cells interact with cancer cells, but they also interact with each other, assuring the growth advantage for the tumor. This reciprocal interaction remains essential for tumorigenesis. Tumor environment is not a stable structure: it changes as cells progress from potentially cancerous cells to invasive cancers; different populations of noncancerous cells are found at different stages of cancer. Different cells of the tumor environment are a potential target for anticancer therapies.

A. **Cancer cells** are obviously the most important part of any tumor and they are ultimately responsible for damage caused to the host.

B. **Cancer stem cells (CSCs).** The presence of CSCs is still a controversial notion, and it differs from tumor to tumor. They make a small percentage of all cancer cells, and they are characterized by the ability to reproduce and self-renew and are responsible for generation of a new progeny of cancer cells. They are believed to be more resistant to standard therapies and they are the source of tumor recurrence after achieving initial remission. CSCs are closely related to normal stem cells and share many of the behaviors and features of those normal stem cells. Some theories suggest that CSCs may originate from normal tissue stem cells, other state that they are formed by transdifferentiation of malignant cells. The fact that some tumors may remain dormant for many years after the initial surgery or radiotherapy may be explained by the presence of CSCs. CSCs were first described in hematologic malignancies.

C. **Endothelial cells** are the cells that form tumor-related vasculature. In the presence of VEGF, angiopoietin, and FGF, they are able to enter the tumor and form new blood vessels that are crucial for delivery of nutrients needed for tumor growth. Tumor-associated endothelial cells may have different surface markers from normal endothelial cells and they are a potential target for the therapeutic agents.

D. **Pericytes** are mesenchymal cells that are an essential part of blood vessels; they provide structural and paracrine support. They are a source of Ang-1 that can slow down new blood vessel formation. Possibly tumors with a lower pericyte density have a higher propensity to invade and disseminate.

E. **Immune cells** can play a dual function in the tumor environment: some of them are a part of antitumor response by the immune system, and some actually promote tumor growth by causing chronic inflammation. Various immune cells were implicated in tumorigenesis, including mast cells, macrophages, neutrophils, and even T and B lymphocytes. They can promote angiogenesis, tumor invasion, and metastatic dissemination. In addition, there is a subgroup of bone marrow–derived cells (myeloid derived suppressor cells) and a subgroup of T lymphocytes, named T regulatory cells, that have ability to suppress host immune responses against cancer.

F. **Fibroblasts** are the main cells that form tumor stroma. A subgroup of fibroblasts—myofibroblasts—enhance cancer proliferation, angiogenesis, invasion, and metastasis.

G. **Stromal cells** are frequently recruited from surrounding normal tissues. Bone marrow is a source of many mesenchymal cancer stromal cells.

H. **Metastatic niche** is a term used to describe a permissive environment for cancer cells that disseminate via blood vessels. If such a niche is present, cancer cells do not have to induce the stromal support, but they use preexisting, natural normal tissue stroma. Cancer can promote creation of these niches by secreting cytokines into the blood stream.

V. MOLECULAR AND GENETIC TESTING

Multiple molecular and genetic techniques are currently used in cancer research and in clinical oncology. They are helpful in the discovery process, diagnosis, and prognostic or response assessments and frequently allow physicians to select appropriate patients for appropriate therapy.

A. **Detection of mutations.** This is normally a targeted testing, and the goal is to detect an expected mutation based on the clinical presentation. Mutations may involve one or multiple genes.

1. **Polymerase chain reaction (PCR)** is probably the most important molecular tool in research and in clinical molecular testing. It allows for rapid amplification of even trace amounts of DNA. Two primers must be designed in such a way that they can flank the sequence of interest to allow amplification to occur. This technique is not only rapid but also very sensitive (DNA can be amplified from a single cell), specific (even one nucleotide variation can be detected), robust (even DNA of substandard quality can be used), and inexpensive. PCR has a wide clinical utility:

    a. Genotyping in particular genomic location allows for detection of point mutations, insertions, deletion, single nucleotide polymorphism (SNP), and some structural variants. It can be used to detect genetic predisposition to cancer, for example, mutations in BRCA1 gene in women with familial breast cancer, or mutations in mismatch repair genes in Lynch syndrome.

    b. Detection of rare sequences, for example, detection of herpes virus 8 sequence in samples of Kaposi sarcoma.

    c. Quantifying the amount of nucleic acid sequence may be important for monitoring for the presence of residual disease for example, monitoring of the level of bcr-abl in patients with chronic myelogenous leukemia on therapy with imatinib.

    d. Gene expression profiles are used for prognostic tests for recurrence of the disease in patients with breast cancer, prostate cancer, and uveal melanoma.

    e. Measurement of viral DNA or RNA in patients infected with HIV, hepatitis B or C, or other viruses.

  2. Restriction enzyme digestion is a method that uses bacterial enzymes that are able to cleave a very specific sequence of DNA. If a mutation alters DNA sequence, the digestion would not occur and parts of DNA obtained after digestion would vary in their size. This method cannot be used for disorders characterized by multiple mutations or when mutations occur in the sites not recognized by restriction enzymes. It is used less frequently in clinical oncology.

  3. Amplification refractory mutation system (ARMS) is a PCR-based method in which two sets of primers are included in one test tube. The test primers are designed in such a way that they bind or do not bind to DNA containing a mutation of interest. The second set of primers is an internal control for the quality of PCR. It can be used in detection of point mutations such as V600E BRAF mutation in melanoma, lung cancer, or colon cancer. It is a fast method and multiple samples can be tested at the same time, but it is not used in cancers with multiple mutations, and unique primers must be designed for each mutation even if it is in the same location, that is, for detection of V600E versus V600K BRAF mutation.

  4. Allele-specific oligonucleotide (ASO) hybridization is a PCR-based method that uses two membranes on which a PCR product is applied and hybridized with labeled probes that are specific to a mutation on the first membrane and to normal DNA sequence on the second membrane. A panel of mutations for a single patient can be analyzed, but one can detect only one mutation, so it can be used in analysis of tumors with a small number of mutations only.

  5. Genotyping microarrays can be used to test multiple mutations in one patient or one mutation in multiple patient samples at the same time. This is an automated high-throughput technique with an automated sample analysis; it is expensive and not suitable for testing of a small number of samples in the experimental setting (see Section V).

B. Cytogenetic studies are helpful in cancers that are not characterized by point mutations or short deletions, but rather by larger structural changes of chromosomes such as translocations, duplications, and isochromosomes (see Appendix A).

  1. Chromosomal analysis. The cells are arrested in metaphase of their division and individual chromosomes are identified based on their size and banding.

It can identify abnormalities in the number of chromosomes and larger structural abnormalities, but it does not detect small losses or gains of DNA.

2. **Fluorescence in situ hybridization (FISH)** can detect large chromosome abnormalities, but probes can be also designed to detect smaller microdeletions or duplications. The probes connected with a fluorescent dye hybridize with a DNA sequence of interest and appear under the microscope as a fluorescent dot. When normal chromosomes are present, two dots should be seen for each pair of chromosomes. If only one is seen, it is equal to a chromosome loss; if more than two are present it shows additional chromosomes. FISH can be used to detect translocations, for example, EWSR-FLI1 in Ewing sarcoma. Probes of two different colors are used: one for each gene of interest. Normally they should be on two different chromosomes. If translocation is present, these dots will overlap. FISH can be used to detect a wide range of structural abnormalities for diagnostic purposes, to serve as a tool for detection of residual disease after therapy.

3. **Spectral karyotyping (SKY)** is a technique based on FISH in which probes of multiple colors are used at the same time to mark all 22 pairs of autosomes and chromosomes X and Y. The readout is computerized. The technique is very expensive, and it cannot detect changes within a single chromosome and small rearrangements.

4. **Comparative genomic hybridization (CGH)** is able to detect amplifications and deletions of smaller DNA regions throughout the whole genome. The tested DNA is compared to the normal one to identify the areas of DNA gains and losses. SNP array is a form of targeted CGH that can help with detection of absence or loss of heterozygosity. The method is not able to detect balanced translocations, inversions, or insertions because they are not associated with a change in copy number.

C. **Genotypic tests** are used when no target mutations are selected before the test is performed. They encompass a larger part of the genome and allow for discovery of unknown or unpredictable variations.

1. **Heteroduplex analysis** and **single-strand conformation analysis (SSCA) are methods** used to detect the presence of point mutations on one strand of DNA, but they cannot detect their location.

2. **Automated sequencing** method uses fluorescently labeled primers or chain terminators to detect the exact sequence of DNA. It can be used to identify precisely not only known or expected mutations but also unknown mutations.

3. **Whole-genome sequencing** does not require identification of a region of interest. The whole DNA sequence is analyzed. Although the method is the most comprehensive, it identifies an increasing number of mutations that are possibly not pathogenic, so-called variants of unknown significance (VUSs). The differentiation between VUSs and mutations responsible for pathogenesis may be challenging.

4. **Southern blotting** is a technique that uses different restriction enzymes to digest DNA into fragments of different length, which are transferred on a membrane and hybridized with a radioactive probe. The location of bands on the membrane corresponds to their size. It can detect a wide range of mutations, but a large amount of DNA is required.

D. **Next-generation sequencing (NGS).** The improvement in technologies led to the development of NGS, in which multiple small fragments of DNA are sequenced in parallel; it expedites the process and decreases its cost. Patient's purified DNA must be amplified and then fragmented so sequencing can occur.

Next, the data are analyzed by computers and aligned against reference DNA, so the whole sequence can be restored from fragments. Third-generation sequencing uses the same concept, but with a single DNA molecule as a template in attempt to reduce the frequency of errors introduced by amplification. NGS can be applied to the whole genome (coding and noncoding DNA), exomes (only DNA encoding proteins is included, 85% of mutations are included in these regions), or even targeted areas of a limited number of genes (10 to 300 genes). Targeted sequencing is faster, is less expensive, and decreases the chance for identification of VUSs.

The clinical applicability of the results of sequencing must be approached with caution: a significant number of nonpathogenic genes are identified and they must be skillfully differentiated from pathogenic genes. The results are frequently compared to the results available in mutation databases, but currently available databases are not comprehensive enough. An increasing number of medical institutions have molecular tumor boards that attempt to interpret the sequencing results in the context of available knowledge. NGS is the most advanced molecular testing used in the clinic, but ordering of these tests is not always appropriate, especially when the results are unlikely to change the diagnostic or treatment paradigm and when a simpler diagnostic test will lead to the same result.

E. **Gene expression profiling.** The processes of transcription, in which RNA is created on the DNA template, and translation, in which proteins are made based on the code of the messenger RNA (mRNA), are responsible for transferring the information encoded in cancer DNA into proteins, the effector molecules. The molecular analysis of gene expression has been more and more frequently used for disease classification, diagnosis, prognostication, and selection of the treatment. Most of gene expression tests are based on the measurement of mRNA that bridges between DNA and proteins, and they use the microarray technology. Gene expression profile gives information mainly on higher and lower level of gene expression, but it does not give information about mutations or structural changes.

1. **Microarrays (oligonucleotide arrays)** use slides that have short probes synthesized directly on the glass. Patient's mRNA is isolated, reversely transcribed into cDNA, amplified by PCR, transcribed into biotin-labeled cRNA, and hybridized with probes on the glass. Next, fluorophores are applied and scanned by a computerized laser scanner. It allows for obtaining information on a relative level of expression of thousands of genes at the same time; the genes can be identified by their location on the glass.

2. **Transcriptome sequencing** is another method of gene expression profile using the direct sequencing of RNA on the glass.

3. **Clinical applicability.** Currently several gene expression tests are used in the clinic. The 21-gene recurrence score (RS—Oncotype Dx) in patients with breast cancer may identify patients who are most and least likely to derive benefit from adjuvant chemotherapy. Also in breast cancer, other prognostic assays (EndoPredict, Predictor Analysis of Microarray 50 PAM 50, Breast Cancer Index) can be used. Similar RS tests are also available for patients with stage II and III colon cancer and for patients with prostate cancer. The gene expression–based tests predicting the risk of distant metastasis are also available for patients with uveal melanoma and stage I and II cutaneous melanoma. The number of available tests will continue to grow, but they should be prescribed only if they have been validated and if their result will change the patient management. Assays must be analyzed with an equal scrutiny as the new medications before they are wildly accepted in the clinic.

VI. PRECISION MEDICINE

Precision medicine (also known as personalized medicine) is an emerging approach for disease treatment and prevention that takes into account individual variability in genes, environment, and lifestyle for each person. Launched with a $215 million investment in the President Obama's 2016 Budget, the Precision Medicine Initiative will pioneer a new model of patient-powered research that promises to accelerate biomedical discoveries and provide clinicians with new tools, knowledge, and therapies to select which treatments will work best for which patients. This concept is based on the assumption that better insights into the biologic, environmental, and behavioral influences can lead to better therapeutic options.

A. **Why is the precision medicine such a new idea?** When one hears about precision medicine, it is possible to believe that, in the past, physicians did not recognize that not every tumor was the same and not every patient was the same. It is obviously not true. We do not treat lung cancer and breast cancer the same. We recognize that estrogen receptor–positive and Her-2/neu-amplified breast cancers are different diseases and we offer different treatments. Physicians and scientists have attempted to be as precise as the current state of knowledge allowed them. The precision medicine initiative brings something new, with the following goals:

1. New technologies were developed, and therefore the testing of cancer is more detailed and more comprehensive.
2. Environmental and genetic factors are included in the selection of the treatment
3. The access to FDA-approved and unapproved medications is supposed to be facilitated. It may require regulatory modernization.
4. The data on the efficacy of medications will be accessible and shared with other investigators. It will assure a success through collaboration.
5. Patients will be more involved in decision making and it will increase their satisfaction.
6. It will possibly reduce health care costs, because patients will not be treated with drugs of questionable benefit.

B. **Principles of protecting privacy and building trust.** As an enormous exchange of information, including possible private health information, is anticipated, the set of core values and responsible strategies for sustaining public trust and for maximizing the benefits of precision medicine must be established.

1. **Governance.** The set of rules to assure program oversight, design, implementation, and evaluation, including regular reassessment of participants, methods, and outcomes. The privacy of participants will need to be protected, and the whole process must be in agreement with the current laws.
2. **Transparency.** Participants are informed about all steps, benefits, and risks associated with the process.
3. **Respect for participant's preferences.** Participants decide on the level at which the information is shared, and they may withdraw the consent at any time.
4. **Empowerment through access to information.** Innovative, responsible, and consumer-friendly ways of sharing research data with participants should be developed.
5. **Assurance of responsible data sharing, access, and use.** Only authorized people will be able to access information.
6. **High data quality and integrity.** Standards of accuracy, relevance, and completeness should be maintained and up to date.

C. **Creation of a voluntary national research cohort.** It is anticipated that more than 1 million Americans will contribute information on their health, life style, environmental factors, and other variables to the database. They will also undergo extensive characterization of biologic specimens (cell populations, proteins, metabolites, RNA, and DNA, whole-genome sequencing). The database will be available to researchers.

D. **New clinical trial designs.** The "basket" clinical trials are characterized by a use of a single drug in patients with a variety of cancers that share the same molecular abnormality. The "umbrella" clinical trials are designed to test the impact of different drugs on different mutations in a single type of cancer. An example is the NCI-MATCH clinical trial that enrolls patients with any cancer histology as long as it contains one of the following mutations: ALK rearrangement, ROS1 translocation, V600 BRAF mutation, EGFR mutation, HER2 mutations or amplification, NF1 mutations, NF2 loss, cKIT mutations, PTEN mutations or deletions, SMO mutations, and PIK3CA mutation or amplification. Depending on the mutations, patients are treated with crizotinib, trametinib +/– dabrafenib, afatinib, osimertinib, ado-trastuzumab emtansine, defactinib, sunitinib, taselisib, or vismodegib. This is the largest trial to date that attempts to determine whether treating cancers according to their molecular abnormalities is effective.

E. **Possible limitations:**
   1. The tests used to identify molecular abnormalities must be reliable and valid to decrease the chance of false-positive or false-negative results.
   2. It may be difficult to differentiate between driver mutations (responsible for cancer growth) and bystander mutations.
   3. The access to medications may remain difficult because of laws and regulations despite attempts to facilitate it.
   4. It is possible that no medications are available for detected mutations.
   5. The clinical meaning of the identified mutations in one cancer may be different from another cancer. BRAF inhibitors are breakthrough drugs in the treatment of BRAF-mutated melanoma, but they have a limited activity in BRAF-mutated colorectal cancer. The early clinical trial in which the treatment was selected based on the sequencing results—the SHIVA trial—showed that only 40% of patients had cancers containing mutations against which treatments were available and they did not have any clinical benefit when treated with molecularly selected agents compared to standard therapy.
   6. Currently physicians do not have enough knowledge of genetics and molecular biology to be able to routinely apply the results in the clinical practice.

VII. PHILOSOPHY OF MEDICAL PRACTICE OF CLINICAL ONCOLOGY

Both Dr. Dennis Casciato and Dr. Barry Lowitz, the cofounders of the *Manual of Clinical Oncology*, paid special attention to philosophical aspects of medical care. They embraced the newest achievements in oncology but never forgot to discuss the limitations and the human aspect of care. These are my principles of philosophy of practice of clinical oncology.

A. **See a person in your patient.** We obviously know that we provide medical care to human beings, but we also know that that our daily practice is busy and demanding, and it does not consist only of interactions with patients but also of interactions with colleagues, supervisors, administration, insurance companies, and public. Physicians may become so occupied with these interactions that they start treating patients more mechanistically and forget that patients have their own feelings and the diagnosis of cancer and the treatment they go through are significant stressors. Recognize that you may get trapped in the craziness of daily practice, and when you enter the exam room to see your patient, you should leave it behind and devote yourself to this patient.

You should apply the standard bioethical principles to your practice:

1. **Autonomy** (*Voluntas aegroti suprema lex*). Patients can make their own decisions without coercion after understanding risk and benefits associated with the treatment. They have the right to choose or refuse the treatment.
2. **Justice** (*Iustitia*). The benefits of the treatment should be equally distributed among all societal groups. This principle cannot be applied without consideration of distribution of scarce resources, competing needs, rights, and laws.
3. **Beneficence** (*Salus aegroti suprema lex*). The treatment is provided with the intent of doing good for patients. It requires that health care providers maintain skills and knowledge to apply this principle.
4. **Nonmaleficence** (*Primum non nocere*). The treatment should not harm the patient and other members of society.

B. **Strive to learn.** The field of medicine is constantly changing. It is our duty to advance scientific knowledge and make relevant information available to patients. I believe the medical profession is one of the best professions: it combines a scientific pursuit with service for people.

C. **Provide care that is most efficacious but weigh the benefits against the possibility of side effects.** When we make decisions on the choice of the treatment, we must always recognize the priorities of the patient who will receive it; for example, a 5% improvement in overall survival may be considered meaningful for one patient but not as important for another especially when the treatment is associated with side effects.

In addition, we have to be able to interpret the clinical meaning of medical advances. Very often clinical trials show a statistically significant improvement, but it may not translate to a clinical benefit. Is a statistically significant median 2-week improvement in overall survival meaningful for patients? On the other hand, we have to realize that these statistical benefits reflect a hypothetical average patient. Very frequently, there are subgroups of patients who may benefit much more and subgroups who do not benefit at all, but we are not able to identify these subgroups before the treatment is started.

We have another responsibility of not providing treatments that are not likely to benefit a patient. When you tell your patient of another line of chemotherapy that has a 2% chance to shrink the tumor, the patient does not hear that the treatment has a 98% chance of providing no benefit. It is our responsibility to offer supportive care alone if the next line of chemotherapy would not offer a meaningful clinical benefit and we should not regard this decision as a personal failure.

D. **Recognize cultural and social differences among your patients.** We live in more and more diverse society and we treat patients of different cultural and social backgrounds. Our upbringing and personal development shape our own set of values and priorities, and they might be very different from your patient's. In many countries, cancer is still considered a stigma, and these patients might not be so open to share their symptoms and to engage family members in their care. These patients may also opt not to seek preventive care. We tend to notify our patients about their diagnosis and prognosis. Depending on the cultural background, patients may prefer not to know their diagnosis and outcome and designate a family member or even a physician to make decisions on their behalf. Successful communication between the health care provider is also dependent on the availability to understand the language. We must recognize that the use of family members to interpret for the patient, although very convenient, may result in loss of important information, and professional medical interpreters might be a better choice. In addition, we treat patients of different social backgrounds. We should be able to recognize the needs of lesbian–gay–bisexual–transgender (LGBT) patients with cancer, of adolescents and young adults, of the elderly, of pregnant women, and of others. Although they may have similar malignancies, their social environment would influence the care.

E. **Respect your colleagues.** We provide the medical care not alone but with the group of our colleagues, nurse practitioners, nurses, medical assistants, and administrative staff. They all strive to provide excellent care and we must interact with them with a high degree of professionalism and must recognize their values and needs.

F. **Take care of yourself and avoid burnout.** US physicians suffer more burnout than other American workers. It is commonly defined as loss of enthusiasm for work, feelings of cynicism, and a low sense of personal accomplishment. First, we must personally recognize that we all are at risk for burnout and that it can influence the patient care negatively. It can originate from an increased number of work hours, increased number of bureaucratic tasks, insufficient income, changes in the health care policies, and even increased computerization. The switch to the use of electronic health records had a significant impact on lowering the quality of life of physicians; the tasks that were previously the responsibility of other personnel have become the responsibility of physicians. Next, we must employ techniques to decrease the risk of burnout. Living a generally healthy lifestyle, including weight control and regular exercise; having a strong social report (family, partners, friends); engagement in activities outside of the workplace; working on organizational skills; and mental training that enables one to attend to aspects of experience in a nonjudgmental, nonreactive way, which in turn helps cultivate clear thinking, equanimity, compassion, and open-heartedness, are helpful.

G. **Consider costs of medical care.** It is important to think about the different types of costs related to the cancer care and the burden associated with them on the patient and society. Patients should be made aware that the cost of care is not only related to the cost of medications, scans, laboratory tests, and doctor visits, but the treatment of their cancer will be associated with increased costs of transportation, a possible need for a caregiver or long-term care facility, a possible loss of employment, and increased expenses for family members. The decision on the choice of therapy should not exclude the financial burden; for example, patients may opt to get the treatment that is given every 3 weeks instead of 2 weeks, or receive the treatment in a facility closer to their home.

The cost of cancer care has been rising quickly. In 2014, Americans spent $374 billion on prescriptions; 9% of this money ($32.6 billion) was spent on oncology drugs. Additional $11.1 billion was spent on supportive care treatments. It is certainly accompanied by the improvement in the length and quality of life of cancer patients. Can we do anything to minimize costs and not to jeopardize quality? Oncologists can apply the treatment pathways/algorithms that would help them to use the treatments of the highest benefit and not to offer treatments of negligible benefit. They can reduce the use of supportive care. Different chemotherapy drugs have a different emetogenic potential, and not every patient requires antinausea medications with every infusion. Not every chemotherapy causes severe neutropenia, and therefore, in many cases, growth factors can be omitted. It has recently been shown that bisphosphonates used every 3 months in patients with bone metastasis reduce the frequency of skeletal events to the same degree as when they are given monthly. Frequent imaging, especially in patients who are in remission, does not prolong their life, and moreover, popular PET-CT scans are more expensive than are standard CT scans, but they rarely add advantage to the patient care. Physicians tend to order excessive blood tests, although they do not intend to use the results to change the management. Scans and laboratory tests should be ordered judiciously. These are only examples of actions that can decrease the cost and keep the quality of care.

ACKNOWLEDGMENT

The author would like to acknowledge Drs. Dennis A. Casciato and Barry B. Lowitz, who significantly contributed to earlier versions of this chapter.

Suggested Readings

Collins FS, Varmus H. A new initiative on precision medicine. *N Engl J Med* 2015;372:793.

Coote JH, Joyner MJ. Is precision medicine the route to a healthy world? *Lancet* 2015;385:1617.

Easton DF, Pharoah PD, Antoniou AC, et al. Gene-panel sequencing and the prediction of breast-cancer risk. *N Engl J Med* 2015;372:2243.

Evan GI, Vousden KH. Proliferation, cell cycle and apoptosis in cancer. *Nature* 2001;411:342.

Hanahan D, Weinberg RA. Hallmarks of cancer: the next generation. *Cell* 2011;144 (5):646.

Moore PS, Chang Y. Detection of herpesvirus-like DNA sequences in Kaposi's sarcoma in patients with and without HIV infection. *N Engl J Med* 1995;332:1181.

Waddell N, Pajic M, Patch AM, et al. Whole genomes redefine the mutational landscape of pancreatic cancer. *Nature* 2015;518:495.

2

Nuclear Medicine

Sonia Mahajan and Chaitanya R. Divgi

I. DEFINITIONS

A. **Nuclear medicine** is the use of radioactive tracers in the form of unsealed radiopharmaceuticals for the diagnosis, therapy, and laboratory testing of human diseases. Common radionuclides used in nuclear medicine are listed in Table 2-1; common radiopharmaceuticals for diagnostic imaging and for therapy are listed in Table 2-2.

B. **Radioactivity, radioisotopes, and radionuclides.** The nucleus contains a variety of subatomic particles, such as protons and neutrons, which are held together by incredibly strong short-range forces. The **atomic number** (Z) of an atom is the number of protons in the nucleus and is characteristic of a particular element. The **mass number** of an atom is the sum of the protons and the neutrons (A); it is this number that we refer to in this section unless otherwise specified. Radioactive elements occur when the balance of subatomic particles in the nucleus is inherently unstable.

1. **The half-life** ($t_{1/2}$) is the time required for one-half of the atoms to undergo radioactive decay. The half-life of most clinically relevant radioisotopes is short, and they do not exist in nature. Some naturally occurring elements are radioactive; for example, ^{40}K accounts for 0.1% of the potassium found within the human body and has a half-life of 1.26×10^9 years. All elements with atomic weights greater than ^{209}Bi are radioactive. The transuranium elements may also have half-lives of 10,000 years or more.

2. **Forms of radioactive emissions**

   a. **Gamma rays:** Photoelectric energy that is capable of penetrating a meter or more through human tissue

   b. **Beta rays:** Particulate emissions with the mass of an electron and a negative charge that are capable of penetrating from a few millimeters to about a centimeter in tissue

   c. **Positrons:** Particulate emissions with the mass of an electron and a positive charge that travel for a few millimeters in tissue and then interact with an electron, forming annihilation radiation

   d. **Annihilation radiation:** Two gamma photons of 511-keV energy traveling at 180 degrees from each other that are created when an electron and a positron combine

   e. **Alpha particles:** Two neutrons and two protons (a helium nucleus) that are capable of traveling for about 10 to 20 cell diameters in tissues

   f. **X-rays:** Result from rearrangement of electrons in orbit around the nucleus

   g. **Auger electrons:** Low-energy electrons that are emitted from the orbits around the nucleus and travel only a few microns in tissue

   h. **Applications.** Gamma rays and annihilation radiation in particular are useful for various diagnostic imaging applications. The shorter range particles, such as alpha particles, beta rays, and Auger electrons, are used for therapeutic applications.

TABLE 2-1	**Nuclides used in Nuclear Medicine**		
C	Carbon (^{11}C)	P	Phosphorus (^{32}P)
F	Fluorine (^{18}F)	Ra	Radium (^{223}Ra)
Ga	Gallium (^{67}Ga)	Rb	Rubidium (^{82}Rb)
I	Iodine (^{123}I, ^{124}I, ^{125}I, ^{131}I)	S	Sulfur (^{35}S)
In	Indium (^{111}In)	Sr	Strontium (^{89}Sr)
Kr	Krypton (^{81}Kr)	Tc	Technetium (^{99m}Tc); m = metastable
Lu	Lutetium (^{177}Lu)	Tl	Thallium (^{201}Tl)
Mo	Molybdenum (^{99}Mo)	U	Uranium (^{235}U, ^{238}U)
N	Nitrogen (^{13}N)	Xe	Xenon (^{127}Xe, ^{133}Xe)
O	Oxygen (^{15}O)	Y	Yttrium (^{90}Y)

3. **Quantity of radioactivity**
   a. **Becquerel (Bq).** One disintegration per second (dps) is defined as 1 Bq of radioactivity, in honor of the discoverer of radioactivity, Henri Becquerel. Typical doses used for imaging are in the milliCurie (mCi) range, 1 mCi being 37 MegaBecquerels (MBq). A Curie (Ci), also in honor of a discoverer of radioactivity, Marie Curie, is 37 GigaBecquerels.
   b. **Curies (Ci).** The Curie unit is based on the amount of radioactivity in 1 g of radium or 3.7×10^{10} dps. Typical diagnostic doses range from 1 mCi (37 MBq) to 30 mCi (1,110 MBq).

4. **Quantity of absorbed radiation**
   a. **Rads.** When radioactive emissions interact with matter, a fraction of the total energy is absorbed. The rad is equivalent to 1 erg of energy absorbed per gram of tissue.
   b. **Gray (Gy).** One Gray is 100 rad; 1 centiGray (cGy) is 1 rad.
   c. **Rem** (R), or roentgen equivalent man, was introduced because not all radiation emitted has equivalent biologic potency for a given amount of radiation dose absorbed. For gamma photons and x-rays, the rad dose and the rem dose are the same. For larger particles (e.g., the alpha particle), the rem is the rad dose times a "quality factor." For alpha particles, the quality factor is much higher, so that for a given rad dose, the rem for alpha-particle exposure is much greater than that for gamma exposure: The exact value is under debate but is typically assumed to be at least 20-fold higher.
   d. **Sieverts** (Sv). One Sv is 100 Rem.

C. **How much radiation exposure is safe?** The answer is the ALARA principle, which means "as low as reasonably achievable."
   1. **In the workplace,** a maximum of 5,000 milliRem (mRem) per year is permitted; 25% of this dose (1,250 mRem) is sought. Directives for pregnant workers permit 5 milliSv (mSv) per 9-month gestational period.
   2. **The general public** in the United States receives an average of 2.9 mSv/yr from naturally occurring radiation. The mandated level for the general public is now set at 1 mSv/yr.
   3. **Diagnostic exposure** for the purpose of patient management has no limits because the doses involved are relatively low, and it is generally believed that the benefits outweigh the risks associated with indicated studies.
   4. **Therapeutic radioisotopes** sometimes require admission to the hospital. In the United States, the Nuclear Regulatory Commission has established guidelines such that therapy may be administered on an outpatient basis provided the radiation dose to the general public is within acceptable limits (see above), usually calculated based on the amount and effective residence

TABLE 2-2 Some Diagnostic and Therapeutic Radiopharmaceuticals

Nuclide	Pharmaceutical	Pharmacology	Dosage	Patient Preparation	Use
11C	Choline	Cell membrane phospholipid	8–10 mCi	None	Prostate cancer recurrence
18F	FDG	Glycolysis	10 mCi	Fasting	Tumor viability
18F	Sodium fluoride	Bone mineralization	10 mCi	None	Bone diseases
67Ga	Citrate	TF receptor	10 mCi	Laxatives	Lymphoma, inflammation
131I	Sodium iodide	Thyroid hormone	5–10 μCi RAIU	Off thyroid hormone, iodine	Thyroid dysfunction, thyroid cancer
131I	MIBG	Catecholamine uptake	0.5 mCi	Off α-, β-agonists, labetalol, TCA, reserpine, CCB, cocaine	Neuroendocrine tumor
123I	Sodium iodide	Thyroid hormone	25 μCi	Off thyroid hormone, iodides	Thyroid dysfunction
111In	Leukocytes	Target inflammation	5 mCi	None	Phlegmon
111In	Pentetreotide	Somatostatin receptors	5 mCi	Off steroids; laxatives	Endocrine malignancy
111In	ProstaScint	Anti-PSMA MoAb	6 mCi	Laxatives, enema	Prostate cancer recurrence
223Ra	Dichloride	Bone mineralization	1.3 μCi/kg	None	Castration-resistant prostate cancer
153Sm	Samarium lexidronam	Hydroxyapatite	1 mCi/kg	Positive bone scan	Bone pain in prostate, breast, lung cancers
89Sr	Strontium-89	Bone mineralization	4 mCi/70 kg	Positive bone scan	Bone pain in prostate cancer
99mTc	Phosphonates	Bone mineralization	25 mCi	None	Bone disease
99mTc	Sulfur colloid	Lymphatic clearance	0.2–0.5 mCi	None	Identify sentinel node
99mTc	Albumin	Lymphatic clearance	1 mCi	None	Lymphatic drainage
99mTc	Aggregated albumin	Capillary blockade	5 mCi	None	Pulmonary emboli
99mTc	Erythrocytes	Vascular markers	30 mCi	Off β-blockers	Measure LVEF
99mTc	Pertechnetates	NIS induced thyroid trap	10 mCi	Off thyroxine, iodine, recent radiographic contrast, antithyroid drugs	Thyroid nodule
99mTc	MIBI	Lipophilicity and intracellular binding	20 mCi	Fasting; stop xanthines	Tumor viability, cardiac perfusion, hyper-functioning parathyroid tissue/nodule
99mTc	CEA scan	Anti-CEA MoAb	20–30 mCi	Laxatives	Colorectal cancer
201Tl	Chloride	Na+–K+ pump	5 mCi	None	Tumor viability
90Y	Ibritumomab	Anti-CD20 MoAb	0.3–0.4 mCi/kg	See text	Refractory lymphoma

Key: CEA, carcinoembryonic antigen; FDG, fluorodeoxyglucose; LVEF, left ventricular ejection fraction; MIBG, metaiodobenzylguanidine; MIBI, methoxyisobutyl isonitrile; MoAb, monoclonal antibody; PSMA, prostate-specific membrane antigen; TF, transferrin; WB, whole-body dose; TCA, Tricyclic antidepressants; CCB, Calcium channel blockers; NPO, Nil per oral; HMPAO, Hexamethylpropyleneamine oxime.

time of the administered radioactivity; if data are not available for such determination to be made, hospitalization with radiation isolation precautions needs to be carried out until the radiation levels fall to 5 to 7 mR/hr at 1 m from the treated subject. After that point, the patient is not subjected to special precautions.

D. Instrumentation

1. **Well counters.** A radiation-sensitive crystal (usually sodium iodide) is fashioned so that a small test tube containing a body fluid can be placed in its well. For each decay, the energy from the emitted radiation is deposited in the crystal, and the crystal is induced to emit a pulse of light. This light pulse is converted to a weak electrical signal by a photoelectric tube (PhotoMultiplier Tube or PMT). Further amplification results in a signal that can be read as an individual "count." The amount of radiotracer present is proportional to the total amount (cpm) detected. By reference to standards of known activity, the absolute amount of activity can be detected.

2. **Gamma camera devices** are the most commonly used imaging device for the widely available radiopharmaceuticals, such as ^{99m}Tc, ^{111}In, and ^{131}I. The gamma camera detects photons via a sodium iodide crystal, encased in a lead shield and directly coupled to PMTs. A collimator (a thick lead shield with holes) acts as a lens to focus the radiation. Gamma rays emitted by the radiotracer given to the patient travel through the holes in the collimator to strike the radiation-sensitive crystal. A light pulse is thus created in the crystal and amplified by the PMTs. A computer calculates where the photon hit the crystal, with the strongest signal being nearest the site where the photon struck the detector. Resolution is about 1 cm or so for most planar gamma cameras.

3. **Single photon emission computerized tomography (SPECT).** Tomographic gamma camera images are acquired by rotating the camera around the patient (increasingly using two or more cameras on the same gantry); the data are reconstructed into tomographic images in three planes—transaxial, coronal and sagittal. SPECT is being increasingly used to provide better delineation especially of deep lesions; newer hybrid devices incorporate CT (SPECT/CT).

4. **Positron emission tomography** (PET) has the highest resolution and is the most sensitive imaging device available for nuclear medicine. For reasons related to the physics of positron emission decay, the image can be converted into an accurate, quantitative three-dimensional distribution of radioactivity with a resolution of about 3 to 5 mm in depth within the body. The most commonly used PET radiotracer in the clinic is ^{18}F, typically as ^{18}F-fludeoxyglucose or FDG. ^{13}N-labeled ammonia (^{13}NH$_3$) is approved for clinical use to assess myocardial perfusion. ^{11}C-labeled compounds are more frequently used for research; radioactive carbon can substitute for stable carbon in a molecule and thus not alter its chemical or biologic properties. These elements may be readily incorporated into biologic molecules. Carbon-11 and nitrogen-13, given their short half-lives (20 and 10 minutes, respectively) need to be produced in a cyclotron situated in close proximity to the PET camera. The 108-minute half-life of ^{18}F has spurred the development of commercial radiopharmaceutical manufacturers that are able to produce radiopharmaceutical in bulk and ship to imaging centers that are in relative proximity (about 2 hours travel time).

Other positron emitters with longer half-lives are also being studied. Radioiodine has been the hallmark of nuclear medicine; iodine-124 is a positron emitter with a 4.2-day half-life that makes it an ideal surrogate for ^{131}I; it has been both studied as the iodide in thyroid cancer and labeled with antibodies that target tumor-associated antigens. Zirconium-89 (^{89}Zr) is a radiometal that has similarly been used with antigen-binding proteins of interest in cancer.

5. **Hybrid devices**

   a. **SPECT/CT.** Addition of CT to a SPECT device enables the use of CT to calculate attenuation of the photon with resultant improvement in accurate anatomic localization of the radioactive signal as well as, potentially, the ability to quantify the signal. Most commercial SPECT units are thus now available with a CT.

   b. **PET/CT.** The number of PET/CT devices has mushroomed in the 21st century, and most PET instruments commercially available are PET/CT. Advances in PET/CT devices have enabled increasingly improved morphologic correlates (by improvements in the CT component, typically by increasing the number of CT detectors); at the same time, improvements in PET technology, most notably time-of-flight (ToF) imaging, have improved both quantification and image contrast.

   c. **PET/MR.** The success of PET/CT spurred exploration of combining PET with MRI. There are currently a limited number of hybrid PET/MR devices being used; their cost as well as the lack of demonstration of a clear INCREMENTAL clinical advantage to PET/CT has limited their increased utilization (as have current constraints in reimbursement).

6. **Production of radioactivity**

   a. **Cyclotron.** The cyclotron accelerates subatomic particles (e.g., protons, deuterons, helium nuclei, alpha particles) to speeds approaching the speed of light. Single photon emitting radionuclides approved by the FDA of relevance to oncologic imaging include the iodine isotopes ^{123}I and ^{131}I and the radiometals ^{67}Ga and ^{111}In. Currently FDA-approved positron-emitting radiopharmaceuticals of relevance in oncologic imaging include ^{18}F-labeled sodium fluoride (Na^{18}F) for bone imaging, deoxyglucose (^{18}FDG, fludeoxyglucose) for tumor imaging, and ^{11}C-labeled choline for imaging prostate cancer.

   b. **Reactors.** The reactor is fueled by heavy elements, such as ^{238}U and ^{235}U, which undergo spontaneous fission. Neutrons are emitted from the nucleus and, when present in sufficient quantities, "split" the uranium atoms, with the consequent release of large amounts of energy. An entire cascade of radioactive elements is produced in this process; these elements, called *fission products,* include ^{99}Mo (from which ^{99m}Tc is derived), ^{131}I, ^{125}I, ^{32}P, and ^{35}S. In some cases, a target element is bombarded with neutrons to produce the radioactive element used in medicine (e.g., ^{89}Sr). In other cases, fission products are separated to obtain the radioisotope (^{131}I, ^{125}I).

II. TUMOR IMAGING STUDIES

A. **Bone scanning**

   1. **Indications** for bone scanning are to determine the presence and extent of primary and metastatic tumor involving bone (especially in prostate and breast cancer). Some cancers that metastasize to bone do not provoke increased hydroxyapatite turnover, and bone scans are not very useful in these cancers (multiple myeloma, thyroid cancer, some hormone receptor–negative breast cancers).

E. **Lymphoscintigraphy: sentinel node detection**

 1. **Indication:** Detection of the sentinel lymph node in patients scheduled to undergo surgical resection of primary breast carcinoma or melanoma

 2. **Radiopharmaceutical:** ^{99m}Tc sulfur colloid (in many cases, particularly for melanoma, passed through a 0.22-micron filter to decrease particle size). When filtered radiopharmaceutical is used, lymphatic channels are seen more frequently, and sentinel nodes are seen earlier. Several groups in the United States use unfiltered ^{99m}Tc sulfur colloid; this may permit greater flexibility from injection time to intraoperative detection, but may result in a lower proportion of sentinel nodes being visualized by imaging up to 2 hours after injection, though detection at surgery by intraoperative gamma probes remains feasible.

 3. **Procedural notes.** After perilesional intradermal injection (or other site optimized for delineation of draining nodes) of the radiocolloid, serial gamma camera imaging (anterior and lateral views) is carried out to determine the lymphatic drainage and identify the first node that concentrates tracer. This is usually supplemented by intraoperative detection of nodal radioactivity using a gamma probe.

 4. **Interpretation.** Serial images permit detection of the first node to concentrate radioactivity. It has been proposed that disease status of this node is representative of overall nodal status.

F. **Metaiodobenzylguanidine (MIBG) imaging of norepinephrine transporter**

 1. **Indication:** To identify metastatic and primary tumor sites for pheochromocytoma/paraganglioma, and neuroblastoma

 2. **Radiopharmaceutical:** Iobenguane sulfate, ^{131}I-(MIBG sulfate), or ^{123}I-(MIBG sulfate)

 3. **Principle.** MIBG is normally concentrated by adrenergic tissues in cytoplasmic storage granules that also contain other catecholamines. Anything that blocks uptake or promotes release of these storage granules can potentially lead to false-negative results (see Section II.F.6).

 4. **Procedural notes**

 a. **The typical imaging dose** for an adult is 0.5 mCi of ^{131}I and 10 mCi of ^{123}I. For children under 18 years of age, a body surface area adjustment is made assuming the adult dose is for a 1.7-m^2 individual. Patients are pretreated with stable iodide (for adults, 10 drops daily of a 1 g/mL solution starting just before injection and continuing until the last day of imaging).

 b. **Technique:** The patient is imaged with the whole-body camera at 24 hours, and at 48 hours (when ^{131}I is administered) if necessary, with special attention to the retroperitoneum and adrenal region. SPECT of regions of interest is possible in most instances the day after ^{123}I-MIBG injection.

 c. **Warning.** Hypertensive crises in patients with pheochromocytoma are rare after injection of a diagnostic dose of MIBG. Pregnancy is not an absolute contraindication, but the potential risk to the fetus should be carefully assessed.

 5. **Interpretation.** MIBG is cleared by glomerular filtration from the plasma and is rapidly taken up in catecholamine storage granules in tissue sites containing sympathetic nerves or adrenergic storage sites. Thus, uptake occurs in the heart, kidneys, liver, and adrenals at most imaging times. Tumors show up as areas of increased uptake.

6. **Drug interactions.** The following drugs have the potential to interfere with the uptake of MIBG by neuroblastoma and pheochromocytoma and should be stopped a few days to weeks before beginning the imaging, depending on the pharmacology of the drug.
   a. Antihypertensives: Labetalol, reserpine, calcium channel blockers
   b. Amitriptyline, imipramine, and derivatives
   c. Doxepin
   d. Sympathetic amines
   e. Cocaine

7. **MIBG as treatment.** Several groups have used ^{131}I-MIBG as therapy for the neuroendocrine tumors. Typical doses range up to 200 mCi ^{131}I. Dose-limiting toxicity is hematopoietic; most patients recover their blood counts completely and are eligible to be retreated, in the absence of disease progression, at 3- to 6-month intervals. For therapy studies, saturation with saturated solution of potassium iodide (SSKI) is carried out typically for a week after therapy.

G. **Pentetreotide (octreotide) imaging**
   1. **Indication:** For diagnostic workup of neuroendocrine tumors that bear somatostatin receptors
   2. **Radiopharmaceutical.** Pentetreotide is a diethylenetriaminepentaacetic acid (DTPA) chelate conjugate of octreotide, which is a long-acting analog of human somatostatin. ^{111}In is bound to the chelate.
   3. **Principle.** ^{111}In-pentetreotide binds to somatostatin receptors (SSTR), particularly SSTR subtype 2, throughout the body. Neuroendocrine tumors highly express these receptors and thus concentrate sufficient amounts of the radioactive agent to be seen by scintigraphy.
   4. **Procedural notes.** The patient undergoes daily planar and SPECT imaging until it is determined whether the agent is helpful. Typical imaging times are 4, 24, and 48 hours after injection. Because the agent is excreted into the bowel, the patient should be given a mild laxative the evening before the 24- and 48-hour imaging times.
      a. **False-negative results** may occur in patients who are concurrently taking octreotide acetate for control of symptoms related to neuroendocrine tumors.
   5. **Interpretation.** The normal pituitary gland, thyroid gland, and liver are seen. Uptake in tumors bearing somatostatin receptors is apparent beginning at 4 hours, with the 24- and 48-hour images showing the greatest tissue contrast. The sensitivity for detecting tumor types depends on the frequency of somatostatin receptor. Those patients with positive scans are most likely to benefit from treatment with octreotide acetate.
      a. **New lesions that were previously occult,** despite extensive workup, were identified in nearly 30% of patients studied with ^{111}In-pentetreotide. Carcinoid tumors, neuroblastomas, pheochromocytoma, paragangliomas, small cell lung cancer, and meningiomas were detected in about 90% of cases.
      b. **Granulomatous lesions** and other inflammatory lesions, including tuberculosis, sarcoidosis, rheumatoid arthritis, and Graves ophthalmopathy, may also be positive.

H. **ProstaScint for prostate tumor imaging**
   1. **Indications:** Detection of prostate cancer outside the prostatic bed or recurrent prostate cancer in the prostatic bed. This test is rarely used, having been supplanted by MRI.

2. **Radiopharmaceutical.** ^{111}In-capromab pendetide (ProstaScint) consists of a monoclonal antibody, to which ^{111}In is attached by a chelate, against the prostate-specific membrane antigen (PSMA).

3. **Principle.** The antibody reacts with an antigen specifically found in prostate cancer cells. After intravenous administration, the antibody is gradually cleared from the circulation while localizing in tumor tissue.

4. **Procedural notes.** Anterior and posterior whole-body images followed by SPECT (preferably SPECT/CT) of the infrahepatic abdomen and pelvis are obtained typically 4 days after injection. Because the radioactivity may be concentrated in the liver and is usually excreted through the bowel, it is important to prepare the bowel with an oral laxative the night before.

5. **Interpretation.** Areas of increased uptake in abdominopelvic nodal basins, as well in the prostate bed, are sought. SPECT is important for the region of the prostate bed and the obturator nodes. Early (soon after tracer administration) and delayed image sets were compared to ensure that abnormal uptake in the delayed image is not in a vascular region. Some groups do not carry out the early image sets and instead carry out "dual-isotope" imaging using ^{99m}Tc-labeled red cells to delineate the vascular structures. Increasingly, groups are beginning to use SPECT/CT so that the CT component can provide anatomic localization of radioactivity distribution. In such instances, the early images are not necessary. It is also important to ensure that the patient voids urine as completely as possible before imaging.

I. **Tumor viability imaging: ^{201}Tl chloride and ^{99m}Tc sestaMIBI**

1. **Indications.** FDG PET/CT is increasingly used in place of these agents, particularly in areas outside the brain.
   a. Differential diagnosis of breast masses
   b. Viability assessment of primary bone tumors after chemotherapy
   c. Monitoring viability of well-differentiated thyroid cancer
   d. Imaging of parathyroid adenomas
   e. Imaging of brain tumors (SPECT)

2. **Radiopharmaceutical**
   a. **^{99m}Tc methoxyisobutyl isonitrile** (MIBI) is a monovalent cationic form of ^{99m}Tc that is highly lipid soluble. The agent is formed as a central ^{99m}Tc atom surrounded by six isobutyl nitrile molecules; for this reason, it is sometimes referred to as *sestaMIBI*.
   b. **^{201}Tl (thallous) chloride** is a radioisotope of thallium, which is in the actinide series of elements and behaves *in vivo* as an analog of potassium.

3. **Principle.** ^{201}Tl chloride is a widely used cardiac perfusion agent that is taken up by most viable cells as a potassium analog and transported by the Na$^+$–K$^+$ pump. **^{99m}Tc sestaMIBI** is also used to monitor cardiac perfusion. In addition, when taken up into the cell by a different mechanism, it can be used as a marker for cellular viability. After introduction into the bloodstream, both of these agents are rapidly cleared from the circulation in proportion to cardiac output.

4. **Procedural notes.** The tracer is injected intravenously, and imaging is begun over the region of interest within 20 minutes of injection, frequently at an early and a late time after injection (e.g., 5 and 60 minutes after injection). For breast imaging, a special breast apparatus permits planar lateral views of the breast in the prone position. This appears to be a technical advance. For brain and other imaging, SPECT scanning is performed.

5. **Interpretation**
    a. **Breast masses.** About 25% of patients who are subjected to screening mammography have "dense" breasts that obfuscate interpretation. If these patients also have palpable breast masses, there may be a clinical dilemma in regard to biopsy of these lesions. It has been reported that uptake of ^{201}Tl is negative in fibrocystic disease and positive in 96% of breast cancer nodules. Similar results have been observed in patients with breast masses imaged with MIBI. The negative predictive value for breast cancer with these studies is likely to improve the specificity of breast mammography and is applicable to both dense breasts and normal breasts.
    b. **Primary bone tumors** are frequently treated with chemotherapy before surgery. ^{201}Tl and ^{99m}Tc sestaMIBI are both taken up with high sensitivity into primary bone tumors and extremity sarcomas. Chondrosarcoma is an exception. MIBI uptake is lost in tumors responding to chemotherapy and has also been shown to correlate well with response to therapy.
    c. **Brain tumors.** ^{201}Tl chloride appears to be the agent of choice for evaluating supratentorial primary brain tumors when FDG PET is not available. SPECT imaging is accurate for assessing the viability of brain tumors. In our experience, ^{201}Tl is preferred over ^{99m}Tc sestaMIBI because uptake in the choroid plexus is not as marked.
    d. **Thyroid cancer imaging.** ^{201}Tl whole-body imaging is a good way to monitor the activity of well-differentiated thyroid cancer during the interval when the patient is fully suppressed on thyroid hormone. The total uptake, as a percentage of the total-body uptake, is a monitor of the cellular viability of the tumor and can be used to assess the effectiveness of primary cancer treatment.
    e. **Parathyroid imaging.** With careful comparisons of ^{201}Tl or ^{99m}Tc sestaMIBI imaging, it is sometimes possible to detect parathyroid adenomas in the neck or upper mediastinum when other modalities are negative. Still, the sensitivity of these techniques is disappointingly low (about 50%) in patients with intact parathyroid glands and considerably higher (about 80%) for the detection of recurrence. FDG PET has not been found to be useful for parathyroid imaging.

III. OTHER IMAGING STUDIES USED IN ONCOLOGY

A. **Cardiac functional studies.** Equilibrium (gated) blood pool imaging is used to evaluate possible cardiac **failure** and to monitor changes after **treatment** with cardiotoxic drugs.
    1. **Radiopharmaceutical.** Stannous pyrophosphate (1 mg) is administered 20 minutes before injecting ^{99m}Tc pertechnetate. The stannous pyrophosphate enters and is trapped in the RBCs. The ^{99m}Tc pertechnetate diffuses into the RBCs and is bound to hemoglobin. About 75% of the dose is labeled to the RBCs.
    2. **Interpretation.** Images obtained during rest are interpreted qualitatively to determine areas of abnormal wall motion, size of cardiac chambers, presence of intrinsic or extrinsic compression of the cardiac contour, and size and shape of the outflow tracts. Images are interpreted quantitatively for a physiologic assessment of the quantity of blood ejected from the left ventricle with each beat (the left ventricular ejection fraction [LVEF]).
B. **Vascular flow and bleeding** studies can be used to detect the patency of venous access in the upper extremities (e.g., postsubclavian catheter-placement swelling, superior vena cava syndrome), to assess for the presence of hemangioma as a space-occupying lesion, or to determine a site for bleeding. ^{99m}Tc pertechnetate

or ^{99m}Tc sulfur colloid can be used as transient labels of the vasculature. *In vivo* labeling of RBCs with ^{99m}Tc may be used as more long-term vascular labels (see Section III.A.1).

C. **^{99m}Tc-macroaggregated albumin for lung perfusion** can be used to evaluate patients suspected of having pulmonary embolism and to determine the lung function capacity before pulmonary resection. ^{99m}Tc-labeled macroaggregates of albumin (30 to 60 micron in diameter) are injected **intravenously** and are trapped in the prearteriolar bed during first pass through the pulmonary circulation. The distribution of radioactivity is proportional to pulmonary blood flow.

D. **Studies of pulmonary ventilation** can be used to determine whether a ventilation–perfusion "mismatch" exists as an aid in the differential diagnosis of pulmonary embolism and to assess the ventilatory capacity of the human lung. ^{133}Xe gas, ^{127}Xe gas, ^{81m}Kr, and ^{99m}Tc-DTPA aerosol imaging is used as a surrogate for inspiratory air. As the patient breathes, a gamma camera obtains an image of the distribution of radioactivity. Several minutes of breathing is required to achieve equilibrium with bullae and fistulous tracts.

E. **Infection imaging**
   1. **^{67}Ga citrate appears to be taken up by the cells near the region of the infection.** ^{67}Ga imaging requires several days to complete, and normal physiologic uptake (especially in the abdomen) interferes with interpretation. ^{67}Ga citrate imaging is sensitive for making the diagnosis of *Pneumocystis carinii* pneumonia at a relatively early stage.
   2. **Radiolabeled (^{111}In or ^{99m}Tc) WBCs** progressively accumulate at the site of infection. The labeled WBC method requires external manipulation and labeling of the patient's blood. WBC imaging with ^{111}In shows uptake in the liver, spleen, and bone marrow, but not in other sites within the abdomen. Sensitivity for acute infection approaches 90%.
   3. **FDG PET** has a high sensitivity rate for detection of infection. Its utility in patients with cancer is limited by its comparable sensitivity for viable cancer detection, with consequent inability to differentiate infection from recurrent cancer.

IV. THERAPEUTIC RADIOISOTOPES

A. **^{131}I for well-differentiated thyroid cancer**
   1. **Radiopharmaceutical:** Sodium iodide (^{131}I), oral solution
   2. **Patient selection** Patients considered for radioactive ^{131}I are those at high risk for recurrence of well-differentiated thyroid cancer, either papillary or follicular (see Chapter 16).
   3. **Procedural notes.**
      a. Some experts simply treat all high-risk patients after surgery with >100 mCi of ^{131}I. A thyroid remnant, if present, is ablated with administered doses sufficient to deliver at least 300 Gy to the normal thyroid.
      b. In most situations, some form of testing is performed for the ability of the tumor to concentrate radioactive iodine, and patients are treated if there is residual ^{131}I-concentrating tissue in the neck. At the time of testing, patients are expected to be hypothyroid (thyroid-stimulating hormone level >30 IU/mL) and to have a low serum iodine concentration (<5 μg/dL). Patients are prepared by being off thyroid hormone (thyroxine for 6 weeks and tri-iodothyronine for 3 weeks) and on a low-iodide diet (for 3 weeks before treatment).
      c. The approval of recombinant thyrotropin (rhTSH) has enabled evaluation and treatment of patients in the euthyroid state. The recommended dose of rhTSH is 0.9 mg IM daily for 2 days. Typically, ^{131}I for therapy is given on the third day.

4. **Dose selection:** 150 mCi to treat uptake in lymph nodes in the neck and mediastinum, 150 to 200 mCi for patients with pulmonary metastases, 200 mCi for patients with skeletal or other distant metastatic disease

5. **Treatment response.** Patients respond best to treatment when the tumor is small (total tumor burden <200 g) and confined to local or regional areas of the body.

6. **Follow-up.** Patients are normally evaluated at yearly intervals. Consideration for retreatment required taking the patient off thyroid hormone, allowing hypothyroidism to develop, and treating with high-dose ^{131}I until no appreciable ^{131}I tissue is present ("clean slate"). This has been considerably simplified by rhTSH administration. As stated above, 0.9 mg rhTSH is given intramuscularly daily for 2 days. A diagnostic dose of radioiodine (5 to 10 mCi ^{123}I or 1 to 2 mCi ^{131}I) is then given either 4 hours after the second injection or the next day. Elevation of thyroglobulin levels (measured in the hypothyroid state or 3 days after the second injection of rhTSH) indicates a high likelihood of recurrence of thyroid cancer in patients with well-differentiated thyroid cancer. In patients with unusually aggressive thyroid cancers, retreatment at a shorter interval can be considered (usually at about 6 months).

7. **Treatment complications.** The most common complication of high-dose ^{131}I treatment is sialadenitis, which occurs in about 20% of patients at doses >200 mCi; a few patients develop chronic sialadenitis. ^{131}I does not significantly increase the risk for leukemia. However, the possibility of leukemia or myelodysplastic syndrome must always be borne in mind when large doses of therapeutic radioactivity are given to patients with relatively indolent cancers.

B. **Metastatic bone pain palliation with radioisotopes**

1. **Radiopharmaceuticals:** ^{89}Sr chloride, 4 mCi; or ^{153}Sm-EDTMP, 1 mCi/kg. ^{153}Sm emits gamma rays and thus can be evaluated for radioactivity distribution.

2. **Principle.** Various human tumors produce a strong osteoblastic reaction that results in the deposition of bone-seeking radionuclides in the hydroxyapatite crystal in the region of the tumor. When given in sufficient quantity, the radionuclide radiates the active bony regions near the metastases sufficiently to relieve pain. It is unclear whether the benefits of treatment are due to the irradiation of the bone or of the tumor itself. The usual dose is thought to be about 7 to 10 Gy.

3. **Procedural notes.** Patients should have platelet counts >60,000/μL and WBC counts >2,500/μL, and painful bone lesions should be demonstrated as being positive on bone scan preferably carried out within 3 weeks of the treatment. Patients should not be treated with ^{89}Sr unless their life expectancy is at least 3 months. Patients with platelet counts >150,000/μL may be treated at the recommended dose; those with lower platelet counts should be treated at lower doses and monitored carefully for hematopoietic toxicity.

   a. Complete blood counts should be repeated every 2 weeks for 4 months. Platelet and WBC counts are typically decreased by about 30%, and the nadir counts occur 12 to 16 weeks after injection.

   b. Because the radioactivity is primarily excreted in the urine, the patient should be continent or catheterized to minimize contamination of clothing and the patient's home environment.

4. **Treatment response.** Patients with cancers of the prostate, breast, and lung have been treated with these radiopharmaceuticals, but, in principle, any tumor with an osteoblastic component on bone scan could be treated.

The usual onset of pain relief occurs within 7 to 21 days after administration (earlier for ^{153}Sm-EDTMP). Patients should be counseled about the possibility of a "flare response," in which pain is increased for a period of days to weeks after the treatment. A significant proportion of patients (75% to 80%) do get significant pain relief, and the typical duration of response is 3 to 4 months.

5. **Contraindications and precautions.** Pregnancy is an absolute contraindication, and women of childbearing age should have a pregnancy test the day before administration of a radiopharmaceutical. Patients may be considered for retreatment, usually after 90 days, if they have responded well to initial therapy and provided that hematopoietic toxicity was not excessively severe. Most patients tolerate multiple injections without major side effects.

C. **Treatment of metastatic castration-resistant prostate cancer with ^{223}RaCl$_3$.**

1. **Radiopharmaceutical:** ^{223}Ra-chloride, 50 KBq/Kg (or 1.3 microCi/Kg) every 4 weeks for six administrations.

2. **Principle.** Metastatic prostate cancer is a bone-tropic malignancy, and the osseous metastases usually elicit a strong osteoblastic reaction that results in the deposition of bone-seeking radionuclides in the hydroxyapatite crystal in the region of the tumor. The high linear energy transfer, short-distance alpha emissions of ^{223}Ra putatively target cancer cells adjacent to the cortex while largely sparing normal marrow cells. The agent was found to significantly increase survival in patients with castration-resistant prostate cancer (CRPC), and is FDA approved for this condition.

3. **Procedural notes.** Patients should have bone-predominant disease (defined as symptomatic bone metastases and no visceral disease), and no bulky (>3 cm) lymphadenopathy; platelet counts should be >60,000/μL and WBC counts >2,400/μL; and painful bone lesions should be demonstrated as being positive on bone scan. Patients should not be treated unless their life expectancy is at least 6 months (duration of therapy).

   a. Complete blood counts should be repeated every 4 weeks. This is a surprisingly safe therapy, with myelosuppression mild and reversible.

   b. Because the agent is an alpha emitter, the treatment can be given in the outpatient setting with Universal Precautions alone being observed.

4. **Treatment response.** Response evaluation is difficult in these patients, and most practitioners use patient symptomatology as the basis for continuance of therapy. PSA levels in particular can be misleading. CT scans are encouraged by some groups midway (3 months) through therapy, primarily to rule out progressive visceral disease. Some data suggest that changes in alkaline phosphatase levels may be a useful surrogate for response.

   Patients should be counseled about the possibility of a "flare response," in which pain is increased for a period of days to weeks after treatment. Diarrhea is invariable, starting about 3 days after therapy and persisting for 3 to 5 days. Nausea is less common and temporally similar to the diarrhea. A variable proportion of patients (50% to 80%) have significant pain relief.

5. **Contraindications and precautions.** Bulky lymphadenopathy, parenchymal metastases, and a life expectancy <6 months are absolute contraindications. Most patients tolerate the multiple injections without major side effects.

D. **Colloidal ^{32}P for malignant effusions**

1. **Radiopharmaceutical:** Chromic ^{32}P-phosphate colloidal suspension

2. **Dosage.** In a 70-kg patient, 6 to 12 mCi is used for intrapleural administration and 10 to 20 mCi for intraperitoneal administration. Great care should

be taken to ensure that all radioactivity is deposited in the intended body cavity. Large tumor masses or loculation of fluid is a relative contraindication to treatment.

3. **Treatment response.** Most patients receive some benefit from treatment in terms of control of effusions. There is a growing interest in the use of ^{32}P in the treatment of low-volume ovarian cancer.

E. **^{90}Y-labeled anti-CD20 antibody for lymphoma**

1. **Radiopharmaceutical:** ^{90}Y-labeled ibritumomab tiuxetan

2. **Indications.** ^{90}Y-labeled ibritumomab tiuxetan, is indicated for the treatment of patients with relapsed or refractory low-grade follicular or transformed B-cell NHL, including patients with rituximab-refractory follicular NHL.

3. **Dosage.** Ibritumomab is a murine antibody that reacts with CD20, a cell-surface receptor found on most B-cell lymphomas. Tiuxetan is a proprietary chelate that binds radioactive metals to antibody. The dose of ibritumomab tiuxetan in patients with platelet counts >150,000/μL is 0.4 mCi/kg body weight, and in patients with platelets between 100,000 and 149,000/μL is 0.3 mCi/kg. In both instances, the maximum administered dose should not exceed 32 mCi ^{90}Y. Patients with >25% lymphomatous involvement of marrow should not be treated with this agent.

   a. **Assessing biodistribution.** The patient initially receives 250 mg/m^2 of rituximab, anti-CD20 antibody. The rituximab is followed by 5 mCi ^{111}In-labeled ibritumomab tiuxetan. Whole-body ^{111}In images are then carried out 2 to 24 hours and 48 to 72 hours after injection to assess biodistribution. Visual assessment of favorable biodistribution is defined by tumor uptake of radioactivity: easily detectable uptake in blood pool on the first-day image, decreasing subsequently, and moderate uptake in normal liver and spleen with low uptake in normal kidneys and normal bowel.

   b. **Treatment** is carried out in an identical manner to the diagnostic infusion. The patient is treated between 7 and 9 days after this first infusion. The patient receives 250 mg/m^2 of rituximab. This is followed by ^{90}Y-labeled ibritumomab tiuxetan at a dose of 0.3 to 0.4 mCi/kg body weight (to a maximum of 32 mCi), usually given over 10 minutes.

4. **Toxicity.** Acute side effects are rare. Grade 3 or greater hematologic toxicity occurs in almost half of all treated patients and requires support (granulocyte-colony stimulating factor [G-CSF] for neutropenia, transfusions for thrombocytopenia) in about 10% to 30%. Toxicity nadirs occur between 7 and 9 weeks after treatment and last for about 3 weeks. Patients should be monitored closely for hematologic toxicity for at least 8 weeks or until recovery (usually 12 weeks).

5. **Efficacy.** Ibritumomab tiuxetan in combination with rituximab gives significantly higher overall response rates compared with rituximab alone (80% vs. 56%). The complete response rate with ibritumomab tiuxetan is also higher than with rituximab alone (30% to 34% vs. 16% to 20%). The secondary end points, duration of response and time to progression, are not significantly different between the two treatment arms; however, there is a trend toward longer time to progression in patients with follicular NHL (15 months in the ibritumomab tiuxetan arm vs. 10 months in the rituximab arm) and in patients who have achieved a complete response (25 months vs. 13 months, respectively).

3 Radiation Oncology

Steve P. Lee

I. INTRODUCTION

A. **Radiation oncology** is a medical discipline specializing in the utilization of radiation for therapeutic purposes. **Radiation therapy** (RT) is a treatment modality in which ionizing radiation is used for patients with cancers and other diseases. Among the main cancer treatment modalities, RT and surgery aim to provide local–regional tumor control, while chemotherapy addresses systemic metastases in addition to serving frequently as a radiation-sensitizing agent.

B. **A radiation oncologist** analyzes and discusses the benefits and risks of RT, designs and controls the treatment process, cares for the patient's treatment-induced side effects, and continuously monitors the patient's disease status. The delivery of RT necessitates the efforts of other health care professionals.

1. **Medical physicists** ensure the proper functioning of radiation-producing machines and maintain treatment planning hardware and software.

2. **Dosimetrists** and physicists perform treatment planning for individual patients to the specifications of radiation oncologists.

3. **Radiation therapists** operate treatment machines to irradiate patients according to specific treatment plans.

4. **Collaborators:** Radiation oncologists also collaborate closely with diagnostic radiologists, pathologists, surgeons, medical oncologists, and other supporting specialists including nurses, dieticians, dentists, physical therapists, geneticists, psychiatrists or clinical psychologists, social workers, administrative assistants, and so on.

II. PHYSICAL, CHEMICAL, AND BIOLOGIC BASIS OF RADIATION ACTION

A. **Ionizing radiation.** Radiation in the energy range used for RT can cause the ejection of orbital electrons and result in the *ionization* of atoms or molecules. The amount of energy deposited within a certain amount of tissue is defined as the *absorbed dose* with a unit of **gray** (Gy; 1 Gy = 1 J/kg). The older unit of **rad** is equivalent to 1 centigray (cGy; 1 rad = 1 cGy). The types of radiation commonly used clinically are as follows:

1. **Photons** are identical to *electromagnetic waves*. The energy range used for RT pertains to either **x-rays**, which are commonly produced by a *linear accelerator* (LINAC), or **γ-rays**, which are emitted from radioactive isotopes. Photons of different energies interact with matters differently: from low to high energy, the absorption mechanism ranges from *photoelectric effect*, *Compton effect*, to *pair production*. Modern therapeutic machines produce photon beams with energy of *megavoltage* (or *million electron volt*, MeV) range, rather than *kilovoltage* (*kilo-electron volt*, keV) as used in diagnostic radiology. In general, the higher the photon energy, the greater the depth of penetration into the body and the more "skin-sparing" effect with less radiation-induced dermatitis.

2. **Electrons** dissipate their energy rapidly as they enter tissue. Thus, they have a relatively short depth of penetration and generally are used to treat superficial lesions. Their effective range in tissue also depends on their energy.

3. **Other radiation particles** used for RT include **protons**, **neutrons**, and **heavy ions** such as carbon anions. These particles are characterized by the so-called **linear energy transfer (LET)**, a quantity measuring the rate of energy loss per length of path traversed. Heavy ions have high LET and thus are "densely ionizing," compared to the low-LET photons and electrons, which are "sparsely ionizing."

   a. **Relative biologic effectiveness (RBE)** is defined as the ratio of doses needed to produce the same biologic endpoint between a standard low-LET photon beam (by convention 250 keV x-ray) and another radiation of different LET. In general, higher-LET particles have higher RBE up to a certain level (approximately 100 keV/μ), beyond which RBE actually declines due to "wastage" of further energy transfer.

   b. Another factor that depends on LET is the efficiency of oxygen molecules to enhance radiation cell killing (mediated by oxygen radical formation). Lower-LET radiation tends to depend more on the presence of oxygen to effect cellular damage and thus have a higher **oxygen enhancement ratio (OER**, defined as the ratio of doses needed for a particular radiation to produce the same cell survival between anoxic and oxic environments) compared to higher-LET particles.

   c. **Protons** have a level of LET or RBE similar to photons and thus have no significant biologic advantage over high-energy photons or electrons. A proton beam, however, has a special physical property of releasing very little energy as it traverses into tissue until a fixed depth is reached where almost all the dose is deposited (called a "Bragg peak"). The depth of this peak can be manipulated electronically to coincide with the target by varying the incident energy of the protons. Thus, proton radiation has a dosimetric advantage when treating a deep-seated tumor next to a critical normal structure.

   d. **Neutrons** do not possess the dosimetric advantage of protons since they do not have the depth–dose characteristic of a Bragg peak. Nevertheless, neutrons have high LET and low OER; that is, their cell-killing function does not depend significantly on the presence of oxygen. Thus, neutrons have the biologic advantage of treating tumors that are relatively resistant to photons due to the presence of significant hypoxia (see Section III.C.1).

   e. **Heavy ions** have high LET and low OER, as well as the presence of a Bragg peak. Thus, if used properly, they possess both the biologic and physical advantages seen in neutrons and protons, respectively.

B. **Mechanism of damage to cellular targets.** Where water is abundant, short-lived (10^{-10} to 10^{-12} seconds) hydroxyl radicals can be formed by ionizing radiation (via a process called *radiolysis*) and impact on a nearby (~100 Å) macromolecule such as DNA to damage its chemical bonds (**indirect action**). Alternatively, such chemical bond damage can result readily from the direct deposition of radiation energy (**direct action**). Evidence suggests DNA to be the main target of radiation action in cells. The "elementary lesions" include *base damages, cross-links, single-strand breaks,* and *double-strand breaks.* Studies have shown that "complex clustered damages" or "multiply damaged sites" are created upon irradiation, each of which consists of multiple elementary lesions spanning a few nanometers, or about 20 base pairs, of DNA. These damages can remain unrepaired and lead to eventual cell "lethality," which is defined operationally as the *loss of reproductive integrity* (i.e., inability to maintain clonogenicity). Such mode of *mitotic death* is considered a predominant mechanism of radiation killing, but other process such as *interphase death* and *apoptosis* (programmed cell death) also play important roles.

C. **Cellular and tissue response to radiation damage.** Many molecular mechanisms have been identified to govern a cell's response to radiation damage, with an intricate network of signal transduction pathways leading to either cell death or survival. The ultimate outcome is a result of complex chain events dictated not only by the biophysical interaction between radiation particles and DNA but also by molecular and genetic determinants such as oncogenes, tumor suppressor genes, and cell cycle regulation. In addition, extracellular and tissue conditions such as hypoxia, cell–cell interaction, and extracellular matrix can also modify the final expression of radiation effects on cells and tissues.

III. BIOLOGIC BASIS FOR RADIATION THERAPY

A. **Target cell hypothesis.** A biophysical interpretation of the radiation mechanism can be made between a given dose, *D*, and the observed fraction of surviving clonogenic cells (*surviving fraction, SF*). The basic assumption is that critical targets exist within each cell; when ionizing radiation particles hit these targets, loss of cellular clonogenicity may result. This is the essence of the so-called "target cell hypothesis" or "hit theory."

B. **Cell survival curves.** When plotted as a semilog graph of $\log_e SF$ versus *D*, almost all mammalian radiation survival curves reveal a very similar shape with a "curvy shoulder" at the low-dose region, in contiguity with a relatively linear tail toward the high-dose region. This suggests that at least *two* biophysical mechanisms seem to be operating simultaneously to produce such a result (termed "two-component theory"):

1. The **linear component** signifies that radiation action on the critical target within a cell is a *random* (specifically, *Poisson*) process, resulting in *logarithmic* decrease in survival such that equal dose increments cause a constant logarithmic proportion of cell deaths. It is commonly described as a "single-hit" killing, which results in nonrepairable damage, leading directly to cell death.

2. The **curvy shoulder**, however, reflects a much more complex situation whereby interactions of more than one target lesion are at work to result in eventual cell lethality (thus described as "multitarget" killing). Before subsequent interacting events can take place, the initial lesion may be repaired. Thus, the ultimate expression of this mode of cell killing depends on the kinetics and efficiency of the repair process (see Section III.C.3).

3. **Quantitative models.** The above-mentioned dual processes, which characterize the observed survival curve, have been formulated as the **single-hit, multitarget (SHMT) model**. However, its mathematic expression is rather too cumbersome to be used for routine clinical applications. Another mechanistically oriented theory, the **linear–quadratic (LQ) model**, has become widely popular due to its relatively simple mathematics. Based on this model, the SF after a single treatment of radiation dose *D* can be characterized by the following equation:

$$SF = exp\left(-\alpha D - \beta D^2\right)$$

where α and β are tissue-specific parameters governing intrinsic radiation sensitivity. The LQ model can be used to explain the differential sensitivities of malignant tumors *versus* normal tissues to *fractionation* radiotherapy (i.e., dividing the overall therapy into numerous fractions of small-dose irradiation). The **α/β ratio** (with a unit of dose, Gy) is used clinically to characterize how various tissues respond to fractionation treatment.

    a. Acute-responding tissues, such as most cancers and fast-dividing normal cells, typically have high α/β (approximately 8 to 10 Gy) and, upon irradiation, will express **acute effects** (e.g., tumor shrinkage, dermatitis, mucositis).

    b. Late-responding tissues (normal cells that rarely proliferate but can express **late effects** such as fibrosis and vascular and nerve damage) have low α/β (approximately 2 to 5 Gy).

    c. On a typical survival curve, the LQ model seems to predict well the observed survival result at the low-dose range, up to about 6 to 8 Gy. At a much higher dose, the LQ model seems to overestimate cell lethality, whereas the SF is seen to be better fit by the SHMT model (see Section V.F.7).

    d. Upon fractionation using small dose per fraction repeatedly, an effectively linear survival curve results from the repetition of the initial curvy shoulder primarily due to repair of cellular damages (see Section III.C.3). Ultimately, it is seen that acute-responding cells are killed predominantly, while the late-responding tissues are relatively spared due to their higher capacity to repair.

C. Fractionation radiobiology. The biologic processes occurring in between the treatment fractions have been summarized as the "*4 Rs of fractionation radiobiology*":

    1. Reoxygenation. The damage of tissues by radiation depends largely on the formation of hydroxyl radicals, which in turn depend on the availability of oxygen molecules in close proximity. Fractionation allows oxygen to diffuse into the usually hypoxic center of an expanding tumor during the interval between fractions and thus enables more tumor cell killing during the subsequent treatment.

    2. Repopulation. During a fractionated radiotherapy course, surviving tumor and normal tissue progenitor cells can continue to repopulate by mitotic growth. Additionally, in acute-responding cells **accelerated repopulation** can be stimulated iatrogenically by cytotoxic intervention such as radiation. Thus, to maximize the chance of tumor control, unnecessary protraction of the *overall treatment time* should be avoided (see Section III.E.2).

    3. Repair. Repair machinery within cells can reverse initial partial damages caused by a relatively small amount of radiation dose. Cells would die if such damages fail to be repaired sufficiently while being accumulated by further radiation insults. Such repair mechanism is called **sublethal damage (SLD) repair**. As the dose per fraction decreases and interfractional time interval remains enough to allow for complete SLD repair, the total dose required to achieve a certain level of cell death would be increased. Thus, fractionation helps spare cells from radiation killing compared to single-dose irradiation. Furthermore, late-responding tissues tend to show higher SLD repair capacity and thus can be spared relatively more than acute-responding malignant cells, which might lack adequate repair mechanisms.

    4. Redistribution. Cells exhibit differential sensitivities toward radiation at different phases of the cell cycle. Most mammalian cells are more sensitive at the junction between G2 and M phases. After an initial fraction of dose, the cells at a more resistant (e.g., late S phase may survive but then progress eventually to the sensitive phases in time, allowing more efficient killing during the next fraction. Thus, fast cycling cells (like epithelial or mucosal cells and most cancers) are more prone to radiation killing than slow or dormant ones (such as connective tissue cells).

D. **Dose rate effect.** The biologic effect of a given radiation dose also depends on the rate it is delivered. With decreasing dose rate, the cell survival increases due to SLD repair. Cell survival is also enhanced due to repopulation as the treatment course gets further protracted until a limit (characterized by non-repairable single-hit killing) is reached. Beyond this limit further decrease of dose rate will in fact give rise to more cell death (*inverse dose rate effect*) due to cell cycle arrest at G_2 phase, where cells are most vulnerable to radiation killing.

   1. Once-daily fractionated RT typically utilizes a dose rate above 1 Gy/min.
   2. For continuous **low–dose rate (LDR) brachytherapy** (or *implant*; see Section V.A.4), radioactive seeds are typically inserted into a patient's body for a long period of time, with radiation dose emitting at a rate on the order of about 1 cGy/min.
   3. **High–dose rate (HDR) brachytherapy** has gained wide popularity, using a dose rate on the order of about 1 Gy/min, similar to external beam *teletherapy*.

E. **Altered fractionation.** The fractionation scheme used in conventional RT usually utilizes 1.8 to 2 Gy per fraction to a total dose that is required for a particular malignancy (e.g., about 70 Gy for gross epithelial cancers, or substantially less for more radiosensitive tumors such as lymphomas). However, by exploiting the radiobiologic principles as listed above, therapeutic benefit can be increased via *altered fractionation* regimens.

   1. Since fractionation preferentially spares late-responding normal tissues, a strategy of **hyperfractionation** can be used to enhance tumor cell killing while maintaining the same degree of late normal tissue damage. More fractions are delivered (usually twice daily) using a smaller dose per fraction but culminating in a higher total dose, while keeping the time of overall treatment course about the same as conventional fractionation.
   2. In order to overcome the potential bottleneck for tumor control due to accelerated repopulation (see Section III.C.2) of cancer cells, a strategy of **accelerated fractionation** can be used to deliver a conventional level of total dose, while shortening the time of overall treatment course with more intensely fractionated patterns. A lower dose per fraction is delivered two or three times daily.
   3. Based on the LQ model, a quantity termed **biologically effective dose (BED)** has proven convenient in quantifying radiobiologic effects and has enabled comparisons among various clinical trials using different fractionation schemes. For late-responding tissues,

   $$BED = D \cdot \left\{ 1 + \left[d/(\alpha/\beta) \right] \right\}$$

   where D is the total dose and d is the dose per fraction. BED is versatile since it is "linearly additive"; that is, one can sum up directly all BED values for partial treatments with various fractionation regimens or special techniques, such as brachytherapy, in order to predict the net biologic effect to a tissue characterized by a specific α/β.

   4. The biologic impact of fractionation may be neglected on the conventional treatment plans based on physical dosimetry alone (see Section IV.B.2). The problem is known as the "**double-trouble**" effect: the first trouble comes from the difference between physical dose prescribed and actual dose received at any anatomic point, and the second trouble results from

the variation of biologic effects with different dose per fraction ("the hot gets hotter, the cold gets colder"). Clinicians armed with only physical dose dosimetry plans will often estimate biologic effects qualitatively. A more sophisticated quantitative guideline based on "biologic optimization" using BED might be helpful.

5. Despite the therapeutic advantage of increasing fractionation (smaller dose per fraction over higher number of fractions) that is supported by decades of clinical observations, **single-dose** treatments as well as **hypofractionation** (larger dose per fraction over fewer number of fractions) have gained popularity in recent years due to advancing physics and technology in facilitating ultraprecision-oriented irradiation techniques (see Sections V.A to V.F).

F. **Dose response curves.** The terms **tumor control probability (TCP)** and **normal tissue complication probability (NTCP)** can be used to assess clinical consequences of RT quantitatively as functions of dose.

1. TCP is defined via Poisson statistics as the probability of killing all tumor cells so that none can survive:

$$TCP = exp\,(-M \cdot SF)$$

where M denotes the number of clonogenic cells, and SF is an explicit function of dose as discussed in Section III.B.3.

2. Similarly, NTCP can be formulated if a complication is assumed to arise due to the radiation-induced depletion of the so-called **functional subunits** (**FSUs**; i.e., the structural units that give rise to a particular physiologic function of the normal tissue). Thus,

$$NTCP = exp\,(-N \cdot SF)$$

where N denotes the number of FSUs. In reality, complexity in the structural organization of these FSUs may determine the ultimate clinical outcome (see Sections III.G and III.H below).

3. As probability curves, both TCP and NTCP exhibit rising sigmoid shapes from 0% to 100% when plotted linearly against increasing dose. The higher the number of cells or FSUs, the more either dose–response curve shifts to the right (higher-dose region).

4. Only when the NTCP curve is sufficiently situated to the right of the TCP is it warranted clinically to irradiate. Almost all innovations in clinical radiation oncology have been based on attempts to separate these two curves.

5. With a sharply rising sigmoid shape, TCP dictates that once a certain dose is deemed necessary to achieve adequate tumor control, the treatment should not be terminated prematurely since almost no therapeutic gain would be expected until the whole course is near completion (i.e., "all-or-nothing" response).

6. For a given malignancy or normal tissue, factors that may "flatten" (i.e., decrease slope of) the respective sigmoid TCP or NTCP curves include the wide variation of radiation sensitivity in a patient population.

7. For the prophylactic control of subclinical metastases in a target organ (e.g., brain) by radiation, the dose–response curve may be flattened due to random distribution of metastatic tumor burdens. Thus, a moderate amount of dose can still be beneficial, in contrast to the substantially larger dose required for the control of bulky tumors.

G. **Tissue organization.** The structural organization of the FSUs in a normal tissue may be critical in determining the kinetics of its damage expression as well as the effect of heterogeneous dose distribution across its volume.

  1. Based on physiologic and cellular kinetics reasoning, most normal tissues can be separated structurally into **type-H (hierarchical)** or **type-F (flexible)** tissues.

    a. **Type-H** tissues (e.g., bone marrow, skin, and gastrointestinal tract) contain stem cells that are destined to mature into functional cells. As they lose clonogenicity in the process, functional cells become radioresistant because only the mitotically active stem cells are likely to be sensitive to radiation killing.

    b. **Type-F** tissues (e.g., lung, liver, and kidney) contain cells that can maintain their proliferation capacity (thus are radiosensitive) and serve their normal physiologic function simultaneously.

    c. Upon irradiation, type-F tissues can exhibit a dose-dependent kinetics of damage expression—the higher the dose, the earlier the time of expression. In contrast, the kinetics of damage for type-H tissues is relatively independent of the dose.

  2. The spatial orientation of normal tissue can also be separated into **parallel** and **series** structures. Parallel structures are typified by the kidney, liver, lung, and tumors, while series structures include the GI tract and spinal cord. Most normal tissues have mixed characteristics of both; thus, a concept of *relative seriality* has been proposed based on the perceived organization of FSUs.

H. **Heterogeneous dose distribution.** Clinicians have been trained to be familiar with the overall radiation effect (e.g., NTCP) of a normal tissue or "**organ at risk**" (**OAR**) being irradiated with *uniform* dose distribution. However, modern treatment techniques using inverse planning and IMRT (see Section V.A.2) often result in *heterogeneous* dose distribution.

  1. The cumulative biologic effects of partial-volume irradiations that might not amount to the effect predicted based on the same total physical dose assumed to be uniformly deposited for the whole organ is called the "**volume effect.**"

  2. The degree of dose heterogeneity across an entire OAR volume can be displayed via its **dose–volume histogram (DVH).** Such cumulative histogram takes a shape of a monotonically decreasing stepwise curve on a fractional volume *versus* dose plot.

  3. Tissues *in parallel* have been modeled along the so-called "critical volume" argument. Irradiating a significant volume in tissues such as lungs or liver, even if with moderate doses, can be more detrimental than giving an extremely high dose to only a small volume of the organ.

  4. Tissues *in series* have "critical elements" arranged in chains upon which irradiating even a small volume of the structure might incur a complication. The prime example would be spinal cord, which needs only a hot spot at a given segment to manifest transverse myelitis.

  5. **Equivalent uniform dose (EUD)** has been conceptualized to convert an originally heterogeneous dose distribution into a dose quantity that, if distributed uniformly across the entire volume, gives rise to the same biologic effect.

IV. CLINICAL PRACTICE OF RADIATION THERAPY

A. **Consultation.** Based on the patient's oncologic history, diagnostic data, and physical examination, the radiation oncologist determines and presents to the patient the indications for RT as well as its potential short- and long-term side effects.

1. **Indications.** RT can be used alone or in combination with other methods as the major component of treatment or as an adjuvant modality (see Section V).

   a. Properly used, the intent of RT for most cancer patients is *curative*, that is, aiming for survival extension. It usually uses higher doses; thus, the risks of negative sequelae are greater than for palliative treatment.

   b. For others deemed incurable by any current method of treatment, *palliative* treatment by RT can sustain or improve their quality of life. Examples include relief of pain or prevent pathologic fracture from bone metastases, relief of neurologic dysfunction from intracranial or vertebral metastases, and relief of obstruction of the major vessel, airway, or GI tract.

2. **Negative side effects.** Most normal tissue effects of RT are related to cell killing and are expected to occur only within the irradiated volume. Some effects, such as nausea, vomiting, fatigue, and somnolence, remain unexplained, although there may be a relationship to radiation-induced cytokines. For convenience, time-related side effects of RT can be arbitrarily divided into the following:

   a. **Acute toxicities** that appear usually within 2 to 3 weeks after treatment commences, such as mucositis and diarrhea, are secondary to the depletion of stem cells (esp. for type-H tissues, see Section III.G.1) and are expected to subside gradually as the surviving cells mature into functional cells.

   b. **Subacute toxicities**, such as *Lhermitte syndrome* (electric shock–like sensation down the periphery upon sudden flexion of neck—presumably due to demyelination) or *somnolent syndrome*, occur after several months and are nearly always transient.

   c. **Late toxicities** are secondary to the depletion of slowly proliferating cells or FSUs and are nearly always permanent. These are usually the critical structures that limit the dose prescribed by the radiation oncologists.

B. **Treatment preparation and delivery**

   1. **Simulation** is required in order to determine how to aim the beams of RT according to the patient's anatomic locations of the target lesions and the OARs. The patient is placed on a *simulator* couch with certain *immobilization* measures, since the positioning must be reproducible for subsequent daily treatments. Diagnostic radiographs are then obtained to form the basis of subsequent three-dimensional (3-D)-oriented treatment planning.

   2. **Treatment planning.** The process requires the integrated efforts of radiation oncologists, medical physicists, and dosimetrists.

      a. The first step is the identification of essential anatomic structures relevant to the goal of the treatment. The 3-D extent of each structure of interest can be traced in contoured forms, section by section, on its tomographic images.

      b. Conceptually the treatment target volumes incorporate the **gross tumor volume (GTV),** which represents the detectable extent of the tumor target, the **clinical target volume (CTV),** which includes microscopic tumor extensions, and the **planning target volume (PTV),** which includes margins around the CTV to allow for positional uncertainty.

      c. Normal structures of interest are also identified, contoured, and designated as OARs. The doses to these structures are to be minimized without compromising the coverage for the target volumes. Published DVH constraints are available only as guidelines, since each clinical case may warrant exception based on individualized risk–benefit assessment.

   d. The physicists or dosimetrists perform the treatment planning dosimetry based on the general principle of delivering the physician-prescribed dosages to CTVs while minimizing doses to the OARs as identified.

3. **Treatment delivery.** The actual treatment is delivered by radiation therapists who are proficient in operating each treatment machine. Meticulous quality assurance measures are conducted by physicists at regular intervals to ensure proper functioning of the treatment hardware. Patients are monitored in the clinic by nursing and physician staff in case of excessive side effects or any other medical issues.

4. **Posttreatment follow-up** assessments are essential, both for monitoring cancer control status and management of any lasting or newly appeared treatment sequelae.

V. MODERN TECHNIQUES OF RADIATION THERAPY

A. **Precision oriented RT.** Computerized treatment planning and delivery technology now allow for ultraprecision-oriented RT.

   1. **Conformal RT (CRT).** Traditionally customized metal alloy blocks have been designed and fabricated, using rather rudimentary treatment planning process with 2-D dosimetry, to tailor radiation field over structures of interest that are often irregular in shape. CRT was developed for dose coverage to conform tightly to the target volume in a truly 3-D fashion.

      a. CRT was feasible after 3-D rendering of anatomic structures—based on cross-sectional CT/MRI images—became available. The initially laborious process was greatly alleviated through digital technology.

      b. More recently, treatment machines are equipped with a motorized beam-shaping device called **multileaf collimator (MLC)**, which divides a metal block into an array of inline thin leaves each being driven swiftly via electronic automation to shield radiation outside the target volume boundary.

   2. **Intensity modulated radiation therapy (IMRT)** is a modern technique that allows photon beam intensity to be modulated, in order to deliver specific doses to irregular-shaped target volumes while sparing nearby OARs. The beam modulation can be achieved by combining a group of small field segments, each shaped by MLC and with a different radiation dose delivered.

      a. The essence of IMRT is **inverse planning**, such that the treatment result could be *optimized*. The physicist or dosimetrist feeds in the anatomic information of tumors and OARs as delineated by the radiation oncologist, arranges the beam approaching directions, specifies the desired dosimetric outcome and its priority for each structure of interest (usually in terms of specific DVH parameters), and then lets the computer search for the best beam intensity pattern over the treatment fields (called "fluence map") to achieve such goal.

      b. IMRT plan allows for even tighter dose conformation around the irregular target border, thus can deliver higher target dose while sparing the adjacent normal tissues.

      c. Higher doses can be given via IMRT as a "boost" to the primary tumor bed *sequentially* after an initial treatment field that aims at a broader coverage of the anatomic region. This follows the traditional practice of the **shrinking-field technique,** with the prescribed dosages of various structures (including the tumor) achieved at different time points.

d. IMRT is now often used from the very beginning of the treatment course with the so-called **simultaneous integrated boost (SIB)** technique. For each fraction, the subclinical spread of cancer cells in a broader area is treated to a relatively lower dose, while the primary tumor is irradiated *simultaneously* with a higher dose. Radiobiologic issues arisen due to differential fractionation schemes need to be considered (see Sections III.B to III.E).

e. IMRT has the potential of introducing *dose heterogeneity* within a specific structure because of intensity modulation (see Section III.H). The biologic consequence remains poorly understood despite collective efforts to propose treatment planning guidelines such as **QUANTEC** (**Qu**antitative **A**nalysis of **N**ormal **T**issue **E**ffects in the **C**linic) for many OARs. For tumor targets, partial volume underdose ("cold spot") represents a far more critical issue in limiting TCP rather than what overdose ("hot spot"), or "dose painting," might enhance.

f. Another potential pitfall for IMRT is slightly excessive "integral dose"— the sum of total body dose resulting from undesirable deposits of radiation dose outside the intended treatment volumes—that may be of concern for possibly causing second malignancy for patients cured of his/her original cancer.

g. Traditional IMRT technique uses "**fixed-field**" approach which employs limited number of beam angles for the optimization process. Another option is to acquire a treatment system capable of **volumetric modulated arc therapy (VMAT)** which generates isocentric arcs of radiation beam and can provide more degrees of freedom for IMRT planning optimization. Furthermore, by needing less beam modulation, VMAT can deliver the treatment significantly faster than a typical fixed-field technique.

3. Particle therapy. Treatment planning for charged particles (*protons* and *heavy ions*; see Section II.A.3) may be done in an inverse manner, with intensity modulation tantamount to "dose painting." This may represent the most complicated form of precision-oriented RT, aiming for nearly zero fall-off dose beyond the distal edge of the target volume along the beam path (due to the phenomenon of "Bragg peak"; see Section II.A.3.c). In addition, heavy ions and *neutrons* have the biologic characteristic of significantly higher RBE (Section II.A.3.a) and OER (Section II.A.3.b) which could be exploited for therapeutic gains.

a. Clinical cases which are especially advantageous if treated by charged particle therapy include ocular tumors and pediatric malignancies adjacent to critical tissues such as spinal cord.

b. The main disadvantage of particle therapy has been its extremely high cost of production and operation, requiring intense physics and engineering supports.

c. Due to continuing advances in technology, proton therapy has become more accessible in recent years as many new treatment facilities are established worldwide.

4. Brachytherapy (implant) is another form of precision irradiation.

a. Radioactive sources manufactured as tiny metal seeds are inserted within the tumor bearing area, either via *interstitial* (e.g., soft tissue embedded with tumor cells), *intraluminal* (e.g., esophagus, trachea, or rectum) or *intracavitary* (e.g., vaginal vault) route.

  b. Typical radioisotopes used are iridium (Ir-192), iodine (I-125), palladium (Pd-103), cesium (Cs-137), and strontium (Sr-90). Cobalt (Co-60) and gold (Au-198) are occasionally used. Radium (Ra-226) sources are of historic interest. Each radioisotope is characterized by its specific decay constant (or "half-life"), the kinds and energies of radiation particles it emits (photons, electrons or α-particles), and its initial activity upon insertion.

  c. Depending on the rate of dose delivery (see Section III.D), two general types of brachytherapy are available: **low dose rate (LDR)** and **high dose rate (HDR)**.

  d. The LDR source seeds can be inserted manually via a needle instrument for **permanent implant**, with their radioactivity allowed to decay spontaneously in time. The precise dosimetry is done based on the actual radiographic position of each seed.

  e. For **temporary implant** using the so-called afterloading technique, single or multiple hollow catheters or special apparatus is positioned within the body site first, which allows for preimplant dosimetry planning and optimization. The source seeds are then loaded according to the intended plan for short-term irradiation, usually manually in the case of LDR treatment.

  f. As a temporary implant exclusively, HDR treatment is done via afterloading technique using an electronically controlled unit that houses a single highly radioactive source seed within a shielded container.

  g. Because of the rapid "fall off" of dose in distance from any seed source, the main advantage of brachytherapy is the relatively low integral dose as compared to external beam irradiation. Its disadvantages mainly involve the operative risks associated with invasive (especially interstitial) catheter insertions and the need to observe radiation precautions for clinical personnel and patients.

  h. Following comparable radiobiologic arguments favoring increasing fractionation, LDR treatment could be considered more beneficial than HDR theoretically (see Section III.D). However, the prolonged irradiation time is a relative deterrence for LDR temporary implants. HDR is usually done through a hypofractionated scheme, a practice still considered safe due to the limited volume irradiated (see similar discussion in Section V.B.3.d).

B. Stereotactic irradiation. Precision-oriented treatment planning loses its meaning if the positions of the target and OARs are deviated during actual treatment because of setup uncertainty or motion. Patient immobilization is thus crucial, especially for tumors in the brain and the head and neck.

  1. Stereotactic radiosurgery (SRS). For relatively few and small tumors, *ablating* each lesion precisely with exceptionally high level of radiation dose using the so-called SRS technique may be indicated.

  a. Originally developed by neurosurgeons to locate brain lesions with pinpoint accuracy using a 3-D coordinate system in reference to a rigid frame attached to the patient's skull, stereotactic localization technique is utilized when high-dose radiation is used to substitute invasive surgical resection.

  b. Several different ways of producing radiation for SRS are commercially available. For systems such as the Gamma Knife®, about 200 ^{60}Cobalt radioisotope sources emitting γ-rays are oriented in a hemispherical fashion or other similar geometrical construct, to focus all the beams on a central point called the *isocenter*. Alternatively, such focused radiation can be produced via a LINAC that generates an x-ray beam from a single source rotating around the isocenter.

c. Feasible SRS targets must be small (usually 3 cm or less in diameter), and the number of lesions to be treated should be relatively few.

d. SRS has gained wide popularity to treat central nervous system (CNS) tumors (both benign and malignant) and, at times, neurophysiologic disorders such as trigeminal neuralgia.

e. Extra-CNS tumors (such as in the lung or liver) are also being explored for SRS treatment as long as single or few fractions of large-dose irradiation is deemed appropriate and the problem of motion uncertainty can be resolved (e.g., with technical innovation to compensate respiratory motion for lesions in the trunk; see Sections V.D.3 and V.F).

2. **Stereotactic radiotherapy (SRT).** For many malignancies, the size of primary tumor is typically larger than what SRS can accommodate, and more importantly its edges are often mingled with normal tissues. In such cases, stereotactic technique can be combined with the biologic advantages of *conventional fractionation* (i.e., about 2 Gy per fraction) to provide SRT (since it is a bona fide biologic therapy like ordinary RT, and not emulating physical ablation) as a treatment option.

3. **Selection of SRS versus SRT** (guidelines):

   a. SRT will in general have a theoretical biologic advantage over SRS for most malignancies. SRS is often favored for logistic reasons rather than biologic considerations *per se*, or with a goal to ablate the target lesion when appropriate.

   b. Whenever an aggressive tumor is found located in close proximity to a critical normal tissue, SRT would probably be more beneficial than SRS since the biologic advantage of fractionation can be exploited.

   c. If there is not much radiobiologic difference between tumor (e.g., a benign or low-grade lesion) and the surrounding normal tissue, it may be legitimate to offer SRS treatment as an ablative tool.

   d. Perhaps due to the wide acceptance of SRS, or because SRT is simply a more tedious procedure, there is a pervasive desire to minimize the number of fractions (i.e., *hypofractionation*, with fractional dose significantly higher than 2 Gy) for patient treatment (see Section V.F). However, only with precision-oriented radiation technique is it safe to do so.

C. **Functional image–guided RT.** The development of functional imaging studies like *positron emission tomography* (PET) or *magnetic resonance spectroscopy* (MRS) has allowed physicians to contemplate whether dose escalation to metabolically active or radiation-resistant spots within a tumor might help raise the local tumor control rate. These sophisticated imaging techniques may unite modern molecular biology to clinical radiation oncology using IMRT or particle beams for dose-painting purpose.

D. **Image guided radiation therapy (IGRT).** IGRT is preoccupied with precise tracing of the radiation target in order to compensate for daily setup and motion uncertainties, both in-between (*inter-*) and during (*intra-*) fractionated treatment sessions. Radiographic images are regularly obtained to fine-tune positioning. A more general application of IGRT nowadays is for any target lesion that moves from day to day through the long course of RT.

1. Special imaging devices such as a perpendicular pair of diagnostic x-ray systems ("on-board imager," OBI) or "cone-beam CT (CBCT)" can be added

to currently existing LINACs for the purpose of IGRT. Commercially available ultrasound systems (suitable for imaging soft tissue structures) can also be used for daily image guidance.

2. For relatively fixed targets, internal bony landmarks can be used readily for x-ray positioning. For soft tissue structures which ordinarily will escape radiographic detection, they can be illuminated by other means. For example, metal seeds could be inserted into the target volume as "fiducial markers" to be detected via x-ray imaging.

3. In order to account for the intrafractional motion, *respiratory gating* for tumors in the trunk can be done by synchronizing the treatment field coverage precisely over a target that moves with respiration. Sophisticated devices used include infrared signal to pick up surface motion or radiofrequency wave to track real-time movement of a previously inserted beacon transponder.

E. **Adaptive radiation therapy (ART).** Initially bulky tumors can often shrink readily during the long course of radiation and chemotherapy treatment. The anatomic uncertainty is thus introduced not because of patient motion or setup error, but the significant anatomic deviations of relevant internal structures due to the progressive change of the tumor bulk (or the patient's significant weight loss). ART aims to keep track of this dynamic situation and issue appropriate countermeasures as frequently as possible. The goal is to modify sequentially the treatment plan based on the initial simulation scan and the subsequent daily image verifications, using a sophisticated mathematical image morphing and mapping technique ("deformable algorithm") to mitigate the geometrical incongruities and variations, without actually repeating the laborious simulation and treatment planning processes.

F. **Stereotactic body radiation therapy (SBRT).**

1. While SRS and SRT remain valid terminologies for radiation treatment of CNS tumors, SBRT pertains to treatment for cancers outside the brain and spine.

2. The hallmarks for SBRT are image guidance via stereotactic localization, fine beam collimation accessories, and **hypofractionation** (specifically with five or fewer number of fractions).

3. With highly accurate target volume irradiation, dose escalation becomes feasible without the cost of intolerable normal tissue complications. Like SRS, the biologically equivalent dose delivered with the hypofractionation schemes of SBRT typically exceeds that of conventional fractionated regimen.

4. Since the therapeutic aim of SBRT seems to be tumor ablation in nature, another term has been proposed as a substitute: **stereotactic ablative body radiotherapy (SABR).**

5. So far, SBRT has been applicable mainly for tumors of the trunk (lungs and liver), as well as for prostate cancer. Other anatomic sites have been treated likewise or are currently under clinical investigations.

6. With the favorable therapeutic outcomes of SBRT but the apparent contradiction of hypofractionation to the traditional radiobiologic preference toward more fractionation (see Sections III.C and III.E), new biologic explanations have been proposed. For example, vascular endothelial damage has been postulated as a significant mechanism in addition to mitotic or other modes of cell death. Other hypothesized radiation-induced sequelae beyond the traditional tenet of cellular radiobiology have included immunomodulation or inflammatory responses, as well as genetic effects or molecular signal transduction.

7. New quantitative models have also been proposed to explain the apparent success of hypofractionated RT not predicted by the popular LQ model.

   a. Most investigators acknowledge the inadequacy of the LQ model to predict single-dose cell survival at the high dose region (see Section III.B.3.d).

   b. Some new models have been proposed as a "hybrid" between the LQ and the SHMT models—i.e., constructed to preserve the applicability of the LQ model (with its mathematic simplicity) at the low dose region, while adding a modified version for the high-dose region as predicted by the SHMT model. The BED formulation based on the LQ theory (see Section III.E.3) likewise has been revised.

   c. Some authors have modified the hypothesized mechanism behind the "curvy shoulder" of the cell survival curve (see Section III.B.2) in their proposed models. Higher mathematic complexity often accompanies these new models, which makes their routine applications in clinical settings difficult.

VI. THE ROLE OF RADIATION THERAPY IN OVERALL CANCER MANAGEMENT

A. **Some basic oncologic principles warrant reiteration here:**

   1. Cancer is characterized by a common pathogenic process: starting with neo-plastic transformation of single cells to tumor aggregates which can invade and extent locally, to metastatic shedding and eventual clonogenic establishments at distant sites.

   2. The hallmark of most common malignancies is thus the *spatial* expansion of tumor cell population throughout the host body, in a process which progresses in *time*.

   3. Even when a tumor is diagnosed at a clinically "localized" stage, *subclinical* or *micro*metastasis might have occurred—since the limiting resolution of detecting a tumor remains on the order of 1 cc, which represents a billion (10^9) cells.

   4. Cure of cancer at a late, metastatic stage is often much more difficult to achieve than when it is at the early, localized stage.

   5. Despite the importance of systemic control of all cancer cells, local control of the primary tumor remains a *sine qua non* (i.e., indispensable) condition for cure.

B. **Role of surgical resection**

   1. Malignant tumors can often infiltrate or invade locally, with indistinct borders.

   2. Any tumor resection should aim for eradication of *all* tumor cells, that is, leaving no residual tumor grossly and achieving negative resection margins microscopically. Thus *radical* or *en bloc* resection is often the procedure of choice for cancer surgery.

   3. Theoretically a "90% resection" still leaves behind 100 million (10^8) cells for a 1 cc tumor. Thus, for curative purpose, "partial resection" or "debulking" of tumors should be followed by additional "adjuvant" therapy.

   4. Unfortunately, radical resection can often result in undesirable sequelae: for example, sacrifice of organs, compromise of physiologic functions or unacceptable cosmetic defects.

C. **Role of RT**

   1. For localized tumor embedded within or surrounded by critical normal tissues or organs, RT has the *biologic* advantage (especially via *fractionation*; see Section III.C) of preserving these structures while aiming for eradication of *all* cancer cells within the targeted volume.

2. A typical 1 cc (10^9 cells) epithelial tumor requires about 70 Gy in 7 weeks to achieve a TCP (i.e., the probability of killing *all* cancer cells to none survived; see Section III.F.1) of 90% or above. Such goal of eradicating up to 10+ *logs* of tumor cell is routinely achieved through conventional RT.

3. RT is often used to supplement surgery by mitigating the limitation factors of resection for malignant tumors.

   a. *Primary* RT aims to substitute surgical resection all together.

   b. *Adjuvant* RT aims to supplement the surgical resection (whether radical or conservative) to further eradicate residual disease.

   c. *Neoadjuvant* RT aims to "shrink" the extent of tumor before a planned surgery and enhance the chance of a successful resection (e.g., achieving clear margin). It may attempt to either convert an otherwise unresectable tumor to a resectable one or enable organ-preserving surgery rather than a radical procedure.

4. RT +/– limited surgery is often used as an "organ-preservation" alternative to radical resection. This should be done in principle without compromising the cancer control rate achieved by radical surgery alone. Examples include the following:

   a. Breast cancer: modified radical mastectomy *versus* lumpectomy + RT

   b. Advanced laryngeal cancer: total laryngectomy *versus* primary RT + chemo

   c. Anal canal cancer: abdominal–perineal resection with end colostomy *versus* primary RT + chemo

   d. Muscle invading bladder cancer: radical cystectomy with urinary diversion *versus* transurethral tumor resection + primary RT + chemo

   e. Esophageal cancer: esophagectomy *versus* primary RT + chemo

   f. Ocular melanoma: enucleation *versus* primary RT (brachytherapy or particle therapy)

   g. Soft tissue sarcoma of the extremity: amputation *versus* limb-salvage resection + RT

5. For "regional" spread of cancer along the draining lymphatic chains, RT can likewise either substitute or supplement surgical nodal dissection.

6. As precision-oriented RT (see Section V.A) emulates the ablative role of cancer surgery; it would face the same limitation of the latter: that is, uncertainty of the "ablation" margin. However, such primary RT would be depleted of the critical information otherwise available through postoperative pathologic assessment. Thus, its routine use needs to be judiciously done, especially if utilized alone without supplemental wide-field RT.

D. Role of chemotherapy

1. Chemotherapy aims primarily for the control of systemic spread of cancer cells (i.e., metastasis). Due to toxicity that could limit its applicable dosage, most chemotherapy regimens for epithelial cancers could eliminate only a few *logs* of tumor cell numbers. It is thus feasible for controlling mostly subclinical diseases (each harboring a range of 1 to 10^9 cells), but may be insufficient for controlling gross or bulky tumors.

2. Some primary malignancies, especially originated from hematopoietic cell lines such as leukemia and lymphomas or certain germ cell tumors, are highly sensitive to selected chemotherapeutic agents. Thus they are treated predominantly by such drugs even if the disease presents at a localized stage.

3. Some chemotherapy agents such as cisplatin or 5-fluorouracil may generate synergistic effects if combined with RT. These "radiosensitizing" drugs are invaluable in helping RT further achieve its intended goal of locoregional tumor control as well as facilitating organ conservation approaches (see Section VI.C.4).

4. Other systemic agents such as anthracylines are known to be "radiomimmetic": when given *after* the completion of RT, these drugs may bring back the once acute RT side effects such as dermatitis or mucositis, described as the "recall" phenomenon. Thus, the full course of such drugs is usually completed *before* initiating the planned RT.

Suggested Readings

Alpen EL. Theories and models for cell survival. In: Alpen EL, ed. *Radiation Biophysics*. 2nd ed. San Diego, CA: Academic Press, 1998:132.

Ang KK, Thames HD, Peters LJ. Altered fractionation schedules. In: Perez CA, Brady LW, eds. *Principles and Practice of Radiation Oncology*. 3rd ed. Philadelphia, PA: Lippincott, 1998:119.

Brahme A. Optimized radiation therapy based on radiobiological objectives. *Semin Radiat Oncol* 1999;9:35.

Emami B, Lyman J, Brown A, et al. Tolerance of normal tissue to therapeutic irradiation. *Int J Radiat Oncol Biol Phys* 1991;21:109.

Fowler JF. The linear-quadratic formula and progress in fractionated radiotherapy. *Br J Radiol* 1989;62:679.

Fowler JF. Intercomparisons of new and old schedules in fractionated radiotherapy. *Semin Radiat Oncol* 1992;2:67.

Lee SP. Fractionation in radiobiology: classical concepts and recent development. In: De Salles AAF, et al., eds. *Shaped Beam Radiosurgery*. Berlin/Heidelberg: Springer, 2011:61.

Lee SP, Withers HR, Fowler JF. Radiobiological considerations. In: Slotman BJ, Solberg T, Wurm R, eds. *Extracranial Stereotactic Radiotherapy and Radiosurgery*. New York: Taylor & Francis, 2006:131.

Wheldon TE, Michalowski A, Kirk J. The effect of irradiation on function in self-renewing normal tissues with differing proliferative organisation. *Br J Radiol* 1982;55:759.

Withers HR. The 4R's of radiotherapy. In: Lett JT, Alder H, eds. *Advances in Radiation Biology*. Vol. 5. New York: Academic, 1975:241.

Withers HR, Peters LJ. Biological aspects of radiation therapy. In: Fletcher GH, ed. *Textbook of Radiotherapy*. 3rd ed. Philadelphia, PA: Lea and Febiger, 1980:103.

Withers HR, Taylor JMG, Maciejewski B. Treatment volume and tissue tolerance. *Int J Radiat Oncol Biol Phys* 1988;14:751.

4 Systemic Therapy Agents

Bartosz Chmielowski

I. Alkylating agents

A.	Altretamine	F.	Dacarbazine	K.	Lomustine	P.	Cisplatin
B.	Bendamustine	G.	Ifosfamide	L.	Procarbazine	Q.	Carboplatin
C.	Busulfan	H.	Melphalan	M.	Streptozocin	R.	Oxaliplatin
D.	Chlorambucil	I.	Nitrogen mustard	N.	Temozolomide	S.	Trabectedin
E.	Cyclophosphamide	J.	Carmustine	O.	Thiotepa		

II. Antitumor antibiotics and topoisomerase inhibitors

A.	Actinomycin D	E.	Doxorubicin,	H.	Mitomycin	L.	Irinotecan, liposome
B.	Bleomycin		liposomal	I.	Mitoxantrone	M.	Teniposide
C.	Daunorubicin	F.	Epirubicin	J.	Etoposide	N.	Topotecan
D.	Doxorubicin	G.	Idarubicin	K.	Irinotecan		

III. Antimetabolites

A.	Azacitidine	F.	Fludarabine	K.	6-Mercaptopurine	P.	Pralatrexate
B.	Cladribine	G.	5-Fluorouracil	L.	Methotrexate	Q.	6-Thioguanine
C.	Clofarabine	H.	Capecitabine	M.	Nelarabine	R.	Trifluridine/tipiracil
D.	Cytarabine	I.	Gemcitabine	N.	Pemetrexed		
E.	Decitabine	J.	Hydroxyurea	O.	Pentostatin		

IV. Mitotic spindle agents

A.	Paclitaxel	D.	Docetaxel	H.	Vinblastine	K.	Vindesine
B.	Paclitaxel, protein	E.	Eribulin	I.	Vincristine	L.	Vinorelbine
	bound	F.	Estramustine	J.	Vincristine,		
C.	Cabazitaxel	G.	Ixabepilone		liposomal		

V. Other chemotherapy

A.	Asparaginase	B.	Asparaginase	C.	Asparaginase,	D.	Omacetaxine
	(Elspar)		(Oncaspar)		*Erwinia chrysanthemi*		mepesuccinate

VI. Molecularly Targeted Agents

A.	Alectinib	L.	Trametinib	W.	Vorinostat	HH.	Vismodegib
B.	Ceritinib	M.	Vemurafenib	X.	Lapatinib	II.	Axitinib
C.	Crizotinib	N.	Ibrutinib	Y.	Ruxolitinib	JJ.	Cabozantinib
D.	Venetoclax	O.	Palbociclib	Z.	Everolimus	KK.	Lenvatinib
E.	Bosutinib	P.	Afatinib	AA.	Temsirolimus	LL.	Pazopanib
F.	Dasatinib	Q.	Erlotinib	BB.	Olaparib	MM.	Regorafenib
G.	Imatinib	R.	Gefitinib	CC.	Idelalisib	NN.	Sorafenib
H.	Nilotinib	S.	Osimertinib	DD.	Bortezomib	OO.	Sunitinib
I.	Ponatinib	T.	Belinostat	EE.	Carfilzomib	PP.	Vandetanib
J.	Cobimetinib	U.	Panobinostat	FF.	Ixazomib		
K.	Dabrafenib	V.	Romidepsin	GG.	Sonidegib		

VII. Monoclonal antibodies

A.	Ado-trastuzumab	F.	Brentuximab vedotin	L.	Necitumumab	R.	Pertuzumab
	emtansine	G.	Cetuximab	M.	Nivolumab	S.	Ramucirumab
B.	Alemtuzumab	H.	Daratumumab	N.	Obinutuzumab	T.	Rituximab
C.	Atezolizumab	I.	Dinutuximab	O.	Ofatumumab	U.	Siltuximab
D.	Bevacizumab	J.	Elotuzumab	P.	Panitumumab	V.	Trastuzumab
E.	Blinatumomab	K.	Ipilimumab	Q.	Pembrolizumab		

VIII. Miscellaneous agents

A.	Aldesleukin	E.	Denileukin diftitox
B.	Anagrelide	F.	Interferon alpha
C.	Arsenic trioxide	G.	Lenalidomide
D.	Bexarotene	H.	Lanreotide

I.	Pomalidomide
J.	Sipuleucel-T
K.	Talimogene laherparepvec

L.	Thalidomide
M.	Tretinoin
N.	Ziv-aflibercept

IX. Hormonal agents

A.	Glucocorticoids	D.	Antiandrogens	G.	Aromatase inhibitors
B.	Adrenal inhibitors	E.	Estrogens	H.	LHRH agonists
C.	Androgens	F.	Antiestrogens	I.	Progestins

I. ALKYLATING AGENTS

A. **General pharmacology of alkylating agents.** Alkylating agents work through their reactive intermediates that are able to bind covalently to DNA. They are cell cycle–phase nonspecific.

1. Alkylating agents impair cell function by transferring alkyl groups to amino, carboxyl, sulfhydryl, or phosphate groups of biologically important molecules. Most importantly, nucleic acids (DNA and RNA) and proteins are alkylated. The number 7 (N-7) position of guanine in DNA and RNA is the most actively alkylated site; the O-6 group of guanine is alkylated by nitrosoureas. Alkylation of guanine results in abnormal nucleotide sequences, miscoding of messenger RNA, cross-linked DNA strands that cannot replicate, breakage of DNA strands, and other damage to the transcription and translation of genetic material.

2. The primary mode of action for most alkylating agents is by means of cross-linking of DNA strands or the appearance of breaks in DNA. Such abnormal DNA is not able to complete the replication cycle, and it leads to cytotoxicity.

3. Tumor resistance to these drugs appears to be related to the capacity of cells to repair nucleic acid damage and to inactivate the drugs by conjugation with glutathione.

B. **Altretamine** (hexamethylmelamine, Hexalen)

1. **Indication.** Recurrent ovarian carcinoma

2. **Pharmacology**

   a. **Mechanism is unknown.** It structurally resembles an alkylating agent, but the exact mechanism of its activity is unknown.

   b. **Metabolism.** Rapidly demethylated and hydroxylated in the liver by the microsomal P450 system. Excreted in urine and hepatobiliary tract as metabolites

3. **Toxicity**

   a. **Dose limiting.** Nausea and vomiting, which may worsen with continued therapy

   b. **Common.** Neurotoxicity (25%), including paresthesias, hypoesthesia, hyperreflexia, motor weakness, agitation, confusion, hallucinations, lethargy, depression, coma; myelosuppression (mild) with nadir blood cell counts occurring 3 to 4 weeks after starting treatment; nausea and vomiting

   c. **Occasional.** Abnormal LFTs, flulike syndrome; abdominal cramps, diarrhea

   d. **Rare.** Alopecia, skin rashes, cystitis

C. **Bendamustine** (Treanda, Bendeka)

1. **Indications.** Chronic lymphocytic leukemia (CLL), low-grade B-cell non-Hodgkin lymphoma (NHL) that has progressed within 6 months of treatment with a rituximab-containing regimen

    2. **Pharmacology.** Bendamustine is a bifunctional mechlorethamine derivative containing a purine-like benzimidazole ring. About 90% of the drug is excreted in the feces.

    3. **Toxicity**

      a. **Dose limiting.** Hematosuppression

      b. **Common.** Nausea, vomiting, diarrhea, fever, fatigue, headache, stomatitis, rash, infusion reactions (consider administering an antihistamine, acetaminophen, and corticosteroids prophylactically)

      c. **Occasional.** Anaphylactic reactions, severe skin reactions, acute renal failure; peripheral edema, tachycardia, hypotension, dizziness; myelodysplasia; dysgeusia

D. Busulfan (Myleran, Busulfex)

    1. **Indications.** Part of conditioning regimen for bone marrow transplantation, chronic myelogenous leukemia (CML) palliation

    2. **Pharmacology.** Acts directly; catabolized to inactive products that are excreted in the urine

    3. **Toxicity**

      a. **Dose limiting.** Reversible and irreversible myelosuppression with slow recovery; blood cell counts fall for about 2 weeks after discontinuation of drug

      b. **Common.** Gastrointestinal (GI) upset (mild), sterility

      c. **Occasional.** Skin hyperpigmentation, alopecia, rash; gynecomastia, cataracts, LFT abnormalities; seizures

      d. **Rare.** Pulmonary fibrosis ("busulfan lung"; see Chapter 30), retroperitoneal fibrosis, endocardial fibrosis; addisonian-like asthenia (without biochemical evidence of adrenal insufficiency); hypotension, impotence, hemorrhagic cystitis, secondary neoplasms

E. Chlorambucil (Leukeran)

    1. **Indications.** CLL, Waldenström macroglobulinemia, lymphomas

    2. **Pharmacology.** It acts directly; spontaneously hydrolyzed to inactive and active products (e.g., phenylacetic acid mustard); also is extensively metabolized by the hepatic P450 microsomal system. The drug and metabolic products are excreted in urine.

    3. **Toxicity.** Least toxic alkylating agent

      a. **Dose limiting.** Myelosuppression

      b. **Occasional.** GI upset (minimal or absent at usual doses), mild LFT abnormalities, sterility, rash

      c. **Rare.** Rash, alopecia, fever; cachexia, pulmonary fibrosis, neurologic or ocular toxicity, cystitis; acute leukemia

F. Cyclophosphamide (Cytoxan)

    1. **Indications.** Used in a wide variety of conditions: Hodgkin disease, lymphocytic lymphoma, mixed cell–type lymphoma, histiocytic lymphoma, Burkitt lymphoma; multiple myeloma, leukemias, mycosis fungoides, neuroblastoma, adenocarcinoma of ovary, retinoblastoma, breast carcinoma, conditioning regimen for bone marrow transplant

    2. **Pharmacology.** Native drug is inactive and requires activation by liver P450 microsomal oxidase system to form an aldehyde that decomposes in plasma and peripheral tissues to yield acrolein and an alkylating metabolite (e.g., phosphoramide mustard). The P450 system also metabolizes metabolites to inactive compounds. Active and inactive metabolites are excreted in urine.

3. Toxicity
  a. Dose limiting
   (1) Myelosuppression. Leukopenia develops 8 to 14 days after administration. Thrombocytopenia occurs but is rarely significant.
   (2) Effects on urinary bladder. Degradative products are responsible for hemorrhagic cystitis, which can be prevented by maintaining a high urine output. Hemorrhagic cystitis is more common and can be severe when massive doses are used (e.g., for bone marrow transplantation); under these circumstances, the use of mesna can be preventative. Urinary bladder fibrosis with telangiectasia of the mucosa can occur (usually after long-term oral therapy) without episodes of cystitis. Bladder carcinoma has occurred.
  b. Side effects
   (1) Common. Alopecia, stomatitis, aspermia, amenorrhea; headache (fast onset, short duration). Nausea and vomiting are common after doses of 700 mg/m^2 or more.
   (2) Occasional. Skin or fingernail hyperpigmentation; metallic taste during injection; sneezing or a cold sensation in the nose after injection; abnormal LFTs, dizziness; allergy, fever
   (3) Rare. Transient syndrome of inappropriate secretion of antidiuretic hormone (SIADH, especially if given with a large volume of fluid), hypothyroidism, cataracts, jaundice, pulmonary fibrosis; cardiac necrosis and acute myopericarditis (with high doses); secondary neoplasms (acute leukemia, bladder carcinoma)
G. Dacarbazine [dimethyl-triazeno-imidazole-carboxamide (DTIC, DIC), imidazole carboxamide]
 1. Indications. Hodgkin lymphoma, malignant melanoma, sarcomas, neuroblastoma
 2. Pharmacology
  a. Mechanisms. Dacarbazine acts as a purine analog and inhibits DNA synthesis; it is an alkylating agent and it interacts with SH groups.
  b. Metabolism. It is activated in the liver by oxidative N-methylation by the hepatic P450 microsomal system. Excreted in urine predominantly (50% of the drug is unchanged); minor hepatobiliary and pulmonary excretion
 3. Toxicity
  a. Dose limiting. Myelosuppression, usually mild, but it occurs late, 2 to 4 weeks after treatment
  b. Common. Nausea and vomiting (often severe), anorexia; pain along the injection site
  c. Occasional. Alopecia, facial flushing, photosensitivity, abnormal LFTs. Flulike syndrome (malaise, myalgia, chills, and fever) developing 1 week after treatment and lasting several days
  d. Rare. Diarrhea, stomatitis; cerebral dysfunction; hepatic necrosis; azotemia; anaphylaxis
H. Ifosfamide (Ifex)
 1. Indications. Lymphomas, sarcomas, relapsed testicular tumors, and various carcinomas
 2. Pharmacology
  a. Mechanisms. It produces phosphotriesters as the predominant reaction products.
   The treatment of intact cell nuclei may also result in the formation of DNA–DNA cross-links.

b. **Metabolism.** Ifosfamide is activated by metabolism in the liver by the mixed-function oxidase system of the smooth endoplasmic reticulum. The drug undergoes hepatic activation to an aldehyde form that decomposes in plasma and peripheral tissues to yield acrolein and its alkylating metabolite. Acrolein is highly toxic to urothelial mucosa. The chloroacetaldehyde metabolite may be responsible for much of the neurotoxic effects, particularly in patients with renal dysfunction. Drug and metabolites are excreted in urine.

3. **Toxicity**
   a. **Dose limiting.** Myelosuppression, hemorrhagic cystitis, encephalopathy
   b. **Common.** Alopecia; anorexia, constipation, nausea, and vomiting; amenorrhea, oligospermia, and infertility
   c. **Neurotoxicity** (especially with hepatic or renal dysfunction, hypoalbuminemia, low bicarbonate levels, or with rapid infusion): Somnolence, confusion, depression, hallucinations, dizziness, cranial nerve dysfunction, and ataxia. These effects usually resolve within 3 days of discontinuation of drug.
   d. **Occasional.** Salivation, stomatitis, diarrhea; urticaria, hyperpigmentation, nail ridging; abnormal LFTs, phlebitis, fever; hypotension, hypertension, hypokalemia; renal tubular acidosis (at high doses); SIADH
   e. **Rare.** Coma; renal tubular acidosis, or Fanconi-like syndrome

I. **Melphalan** (Alkeran)
   1. **Indications.** Multiple myeloma. The injection form is used in bone marrow transplantation.
   2. **Pharmacology**
      a. **Mechanism.** A phenylalanine derivative of nitrogen mustard, a bifunctional alkylating agent
      b. **Metabolism.** Acts directly. Ninety percent of the drug is bound to plasma proteins and undergoes rapid hydrolysis in the bloodstream to inert products. Melphalan is excreted in the urine (about 30%) as unchanged drug and metabolites, and the remainder is cleared in feces.
   3. **Toxicity**
      a. **Dose limiting.** Myelosuppression may be cumulative, and recovery may be prolonged.
      b. **Occasional.** Anorexia, nausea, vomiting, mucositis, sterility
      c. **Rare.** Alopecia, pruritus, rash, hypersensitivity; secondary malignancies (acute leukemia); pulmonary fibrosis, vasculitis, cataracts

J. **Nitrogen mustard** (mechlorethamine, Mustargen)
   1. **Indication.** Hodgkin lymphoma; topical use for T-cell lymphoma
   2. **Pharmacology**
      a. **Mechanism.** A prototype of the alkylating agents
      b. **Metabolism.** In water or body fluids, mechlorethamine undergoes rapid chemical transformation and combines with water or reactive compounds of cells, so that the drug is no longer present in active form a few minutes after administration. Metabolites are mostly excreted in urine.
   3. **Toxicity**
      a. **Dose limiting.** Myelosuppression
      b. **Common.** Severe nausea and vomiting beginning 1 hour after administration; skin necrosis if extravasated (sodium thiosulfate may be tried);

burning at IV injection site and facial flushing; metallic taste; discoloration of the infused vein; abnormal LFTs within 1 week of therapy (up to 90% of patients)

    c. Occasional. Alopecia, sterility, diarrhea, thrombophlebitis, gynecomastia

    d. Rare. Neurotoxicity (including hearing loss), angioedema, secondary neoplasms

K. Carmustine [BCNU, bischlorethyl nitrosourea (BiCNU)]

  1. Indications. Brain tumors, myeloma, and Hodgkin and non-Hodgkin lymphoma. In high doses for bone marrow transplantation. In the form of implantable wafers: glioblastoma multiforme

  2. Pharmacology

    a. Mechanism. Forms interstrand cross-links in DNA preventing DNA replication and transcription. Also binds to and modifies (carbamoylates) many proteins.

    b. Metabolism. Highly lipid-soluble drug that enters the brain. Rapid spontaneous decomposition to active and inert product. Most of the intact drug and metabolic products are excreted in urine.

  3. Toxicity

    a. Dose limiting. Myelosuppression is prolonged, cumulative, and substantially aggravated by concurrent radiation therapy.

    b. Common. Nausea and vomiting may last 8 to 24 hours. BCNU causes local pain during injection or hypotension during a too rapid or concentrated injection.

    c. Occasional. Stomatitis, esophagitis, diarrhea, LFT abnormalities; alopecia, facial flushing, brown discoloration of skin; interstitial lung disease with pulmonary fibrosis (with prolonged therapy and higher doses, especially with cumulative doses >1,400 mg/m^2); dizziness, optic neuritis, ataxia, organic brain syndrome; renal insufficiency

    d. Rare. Secondary malignancies

L. Lomustine [CCNU, cyclohexyl chlorethyl nitrosourea]

  1. Indications. Brain tumors and Hodgkin disease

  2. Pharmacology (as carmustine, see Section K)

M. Procarbazine (*N*-methylhydrazine, Matulane, Natulan)

  1. Indications. Hodgkin lymphoma

  2. Pharmacology

    a. Mechanism. Procarbazine inhibits transmethylation of methyl groups of methionine into t-RNA. As the result, it causes cessation of protein synthesis. It may also damage DNA directly.

    b. Metabolism. Rapidly and extensively in the liver and possibly tumor cells to a variety of free radical and alkylating species. Metabolic activation of the drug is required. Readily enters the cerebrospinal fluid. Degraded in the liver to inactive compounds, which are excreted in urine (70%). Less than 10% of the drug is excreted in unchanged form.

  3. Toxicity

    a. Dose limiting. Myelosuppression, which is most pronounced 4 weeks after starting treatment

    b. Common. Nausea and vomiting, which decrease with continued use; flu-like syndrome (usually with initial therapy); sensitizes tissues to radiation; amenorrhea and azoospermia, sterility

    c. Occasional. Dermatitis, hyperpigmentation, photosensitivity; stomatitis, dysphagia, diarrhea; hypotension, tachycardia; urinary frequency, hematuria; gynecomastia

    d. Neurologic. Procarbazine results in disorders of consciousness or mild peripheral neuropathies in about 10% of cases. These abnormalities are reversible and rarely serious enough to alter drug dosage. Manifestations of toxicity include sedation, depression, agitation, psychosis, decreased deep tendon reflexes, paresthesias, myalgias, and ataxia.

    e. Rare. Xerostomia, retinal hemorrhage, photophobia, papilledema; hypersensitivity pneumonitis, secondary malignancy

N. Streptozocin (streptozotocin, Zanosar)

  1. Indications. Islet cell cancer of the pancreas, carcinoid tumors

  2. Pharmacology

    a. Mechanism. Alkylating agent. A cell cycle–nonspecific nitrosourea analog. Inhibits DNA synthesis and the DNA repair enzyme, guanine-O^6-methyltransferase; affects pyrimidine nucleotide metabolism and inhibits enzymes involved in gluconeogenesis. Selectively targets pancreatic β cells, presumably due to the glucose moiety on the molecule.

    b. Metabolism. Drug is a type of nitrosourea that is extensively metabolized by the liver to active metabolites and has a short plasma half-life (<1 hour). Crosses the blood–brain barrier. Excreted in urine as metabolites and unchanged drug

  3. Toxicity

    a. Dose limiting. Nephrotoxicity initially appears as proteinuria and progresses to glycosuria, aminoaciduria, proximal renal tubular acidosis, nephrogenic diabetes insipidus, and renal failure if the drug is continued.

    b. Common. Nausea and vomiting (often severe), myelosuppression (mild, but may be cumulative), hypoglycemia after infusion, vein irritation during infusion, altered glucose metabolism with either hypoglycemia or hyperglycemia

    c. Occasional. Diarrhea, abdominal cramps, LFT abnormalities

    d. Rare. Central nervous system toxicity, fever, secondary malignancies

O. Temozolomide (Temodar, Temodal)

  1. Indications. Brain tumors; metastatic melanoma

  2. Pharmacology. Structurally and functionally similar to dacarbazine

    a. Mechanisms. Activated to the reactive compound (MTIC) by nonenzymatic hydrolysis in tumors. The drug methylates guanine residues in DNA and inhibits DNA, RNA, and protein synthesis but does not cross-link DNA strands. Nonclassic alkylating agent, cell cycle nonspecific.

    b. Metabolism. Excreted predominantly by the renal tubules. Because the drug is lipophilic, it crosses the blood–brain barrier.

  3. Toxicity

    a. Dose limiting. Myelosuppression

    b. Common. Mild to moderately severe nausea and vomiting, diarrhea, headache, fatigue, mild transaminase elevation

    c. Occasional. Photosensitivity, myalgias, fever

    d. Rare. Prolonged cytopenia, myelodysplastic syndrome (MDS)

P. Thiotepa (triethylenethiophosphoramide, Thioplex)

  1. Indications. Intracavitary for malignant effusions, intravesicular for urinary bladder, and intrathecal use for meningeal metastasis; severe thrombocytosis. Also can be used for breast and ovarian cancers and for hematopoietic stem cell transplantation

  2. Pharmacology. Ethylenimine analog, chemically related to nitrogen mustard

    a. Mechanism. Alkylates the N-7 position of guanine, which severs the linkage between the purine base and the sugar and liberates alkylated guanines.

    b. **Metabolism.** Rapidly decomposed in plasma and excreted in urine. Extensively metabolized by the hepatic P450 microsomal system to active and inactive metabolites

3. Toxicity

    a. **Dose limiting.** Myelosuppression, which may be cumulative

    b. **Common** (for intravesicular administration). Chemical cystitis, abdominal pain, hematuria, dysuria, frequency, urgency, ureteral obstruction; nausea and vomiting 6 hours after treatment

    c. **Occasional.** GI upset, abnormal LFTs, rash, hives; hypersensitivity

    d. **Rare.** Alopecia, fever, angioedema, secondary malignancies

Q. Cisplatin [*cis*-diamminedichloroplatinum (CDDP), Platinol]

1. Indications. A wide variety of malignancies

2. Pharmacology

    a. **Mechanism.** A heavy metal alkylator of DNA. Covalently bonds to proteins, RNA, and especially DNA, forming platinum-based cross-links. The transisomer has virtually no antitumor activity. Acquired resistance to cisplatin involves alterations in transmembrane transport of drugs, intracellular levels of glutathione (GSH) or sulfhydryl-containing proteins, and the capacity to repair cisplatin DNA lesions.

    b. **Metabolism.** Widely distributed in the body, except for the CNS. Long half-life in plasma (up to 3 days); may remain bound in tissues for months. Biliary excretion accounts for <10% of the total drug excretion. Approximately 15% of drug is excreted in the urine unchanged, and 10% to 40% of the remainder is excreted in the urine within 24 hours.

3. Toxicity

    a. **Dose limiting**

        (1) **Cumulative renal insufficiency.** The incidence of renal insufficiency is about 5% with adequate hydration measures and 25% to 45% without hydration measures.

        (2) **Peripheral sensory neuropathy** develops after the administration of 200 mg/m^2 and can become dose limiting when the cumulative cisplatin dose exceeds 400 mg/m^2. Symptoms may progress after treatment is discontinued and include loss of proprioception and vibratory senses, hyporeflexia, and the Lhermitte sign. Symptoms may resolve slowly after many months.

        (3) **Ototoxicity** with tinnitus and high-frequency hearing loss occurs in 5% of patients. Ototoxicity occurs more commonly in patients receiving doses of >100 mg/m^2 by rapid infusion or high cumulative doses.

    b. **Common.** Severe nausea and vomiting (both acute and delayed) occur in all treated patients; preventative antiemetic regimens are required. Hypokalemia, hypomagnesemia (occasionally difficult to correct), and mild myelosuppression occur very frequently; anorexia and metallic taste of foods; alopecia; azoospermia, sterility, impotence.

    c. **Occasional.** Alopecia, loss of taste, vein irritation, transiently abnormal LFTs, SIADH, hypophosphatemia, myalgia, fever; optic neuritis

    d. **Rare.** Altered color perception and reversible focal encephalopathy that often causes cortical blindness. Raynaud phenomenon, bradycardia, bundle-branch block, congestive heart failure; anaphylaxis, tetany

R. Carboplatin (Paraplatin)

1. **Indications.** A wide variety of malignancies
2. **Pharmacology**
   a. **Mechanisms.** Heavy metal alkylating-like agent with mechanisms very similar to cisplatin, but with different toxicity profile
   b. **Metabolism.** Plasma half-life of only 2 to 3 hours. Excreted in urine as unchanged drug (70%) and metabolites
3. **Toxicity**
   a. **Dose limiting.** Myelosuppression is significant and cumulative, especially thrombocytopenia. Median nadir hematosuppression at 21 days; increased myelosuppression in patients who have reduced creatinine clearance levels or who have received prior chemotherapy.
   b. **Common.** Nausea, vomiting, myalgias, weakness, and nephrotoxicity (but less severe and less common than with cisplatin); pain at injection site; cation electrolyte imbalance
   c. **Occasional.** Reversible abnormal LFTs, azotemia; peripheral neuropathy (5%), visual disturbance; hypersensitivity reactions; amenorrhea, azoospermia, impotence, and sterility
   d. **Rare.** Alopecia, rash, flulike syndrome, hematuria, hyperamylasemia; hearing loss, optic neuritis; alopecia

S. Oxaliplatin (diaminocyclohexane platinum, Eloxatin)

1. **Indications.** Colorectal, pancreatic, and gastric cancers
2. **Pharmacology**
   a. **Mechanisms.** Binds covalently to DNA with preferential binding to the N-7 position of guanine and adenine; intrastrand and interstrand cross-links.
   b. **Metabolism.** Undergoes extensive nonenzymatic conversion to its active cytotoxic species; >50% of the drug is cleared through the kidneys. Only 2% of the drug is excreted in feces.
3. **Toxicity**
   a. **Dose limiting**
      (1) **Acute dysesthesias** in the hands, feet, perioral area, or throat develop within hours or up to 2 days after dosing and may be precipitated or exacerbated by exposure to cold (cold air or beverages); usually resolves within 2 weeks; frequently recurs with further dosing and may be ameliorated by prolonging the infusion to 6 hours. Dysphagia, dyspnea without stridor or wheezing, jaw spasms, dysarthria, voice changes, or chest pressure may occur. In contrast to cisplatin, ototoxicity occurs rarely.
      (2) **Persistent peripheral sensory neuropathy** usually characterized by paresthesias, dysesthesias, and hypesthesia, including deficits in proprioception, which is usually reversible within 4 months of discontinuing oxaliplatin.
   b. **Common.** Anorexia, nausea, vomiting, constipation, diarrhea, abdominal pain; fever, fatigue; mild to moderate myelosuppression; mild to moderate LFT abnormalities
   c. **Occasional.** Allergic reactions, mild nephrotoxicity, headache, stomatitis, taste alteration; back pain, arthralgias
   d. **Rare.** Pulmonary fibrosis

T. Trabectedin (Yondelis)

1. **Indications.** Liposarcoma or leiomyosarcoma after an anthracycline-containing regimen

2. **Pharmacology**
   a. **Mechanism.** It binds guanine residues in the minor groove of DNA, forming adducts and resulting in a bending of the DNA helix toward the major groove. It affects binding of transcription factors and DNA repair.
   b. **Metabolism.** It is metabolized in the liver, and only negligible amount is excreted in urine. The drug is delivered as a 24-hour continuous infusion.
3. **Toxicity**
   a. **Dose limiting.** Rhabdomyolysis (monitor the level of creatinine phosphokinase before each dose), severe and fatal cardiomyopathy (obtain baseline echocardiogram and then every 2 to 3 months while on therapy), severe neutropenia (40%), febrile neutropenia (5%)
   b. **Common.** Elevation of liver enzymes, thrombocytopenia, anemia, nausea, fatigue, vomiting, constipation, decreased appetite, diarrhea, peripheral edema, dyspnea, and headache
   c. **Rare.** Liver failure, peripheral neuropathy

II. ANTITUMOR ANTIBIOTICS AND TOPOISOMERASE INHIBITORS
A. **General pharmacology**
   1. **Antitumor antibiotics** generally are drugs derived from bacteria and in nature provide defense against other hostile microorganisms. They act by a variety of mechanisms. Several of these drugs interfere with DNA through intercalation, a reaction whereby the drug inserts itself between DNA base pairs. Intercalation with DNA prevents DNA replication and messenger RNA production, or both. Other drugs have other actions.
   2. **Topoisomerase inhibitors** are natural or semisynthetic products. DNA topoisomerases are enzymes that alter DNA topology by causing and resealing DNA strand breaks. Topoisomerases bind to DNA domains, forming a "cleavable complex," which allows DNA to unwind in preparation for cell division. Topoisomerase I relaxes supercoiled DNA for a variety of crucial cellular processes. Topoisomerase II catalyzes the double-stranded breaking and resealing of DNA, thereby allowing the passage of one double helical segment of DNA through another. They relax superhelical turns, interconvert knotted rings, and intertwist complementary viral sequences into DNA. Topoisomerases are essential for such events as transcription, replication, and mitosis.
B. **Actinomycin D** (dactinomycin, Cosmegen)
   1. **Indications.** Trophoblastic neoplasms, sarcomas, testicular carcinoma, Wilms tumor
   2. **Pharmacology**
      a. **Mechanism.** Intercalates between DNA base pairs and prevents synthesis of messenger RNA; inhibits topoisomerase II
      b. **Metabolism.** It extensively binds to tissues, resulting in long half-life in plasma and tissue. Excreted in bile and urine as unchanged drug
   3. **Toxicity**
      a. **Dose limiting.** Myelosuppression
      b. **Common.** Nausea and vomiting (often worsening after successive daily doses and lasting several hours), alopecia, acne, erythema, desquamation, hyperpigmentation; radiation-recall reaction. Drug is a vesicant that can cause necrosis if extravasated.
      c. **Occasional.** Stomatitis, cheilitis, glossitis, proctitis, diarrhea; vitamin K antagonism, elevation of LFTs.
      d. **Rare.** Hepatitis, anaphylaxis, hypocalcemia, lethargy

C. **Bleomycin** (Blenoxane)
1. **Indications.** Lymphomas, squamous cell carcinomas, testicular carcinoma, malignant effusions
2. **Pharmacology**
   a. **Mechanism.** It is a mixture of glycopeptides that bind to DNA and form complexes with Fe^{2+}. Oxidation of Fe^{2+} leads to creation of superoxide and hydroxyl radicals.
   b. **Metabolism.** Activated by microsomal reduction; bound to tissues but not to plasma proteins; extensive degradation by hydrolysis in nearly all tissues. Both free drug and metabolic products are excreted into the urine.
3. **Toxicity**
   a. **Dose limiting.** Bleomycin pneumonitis with dyspnea, dry cough, fine moist rales, interstitial radiographic changes, reduced diffusing capacity, hypoxia, and hypocapnia may be lethal. Pulmonary fibrosis and insufficiency occur in 1% of patients receiving cumulative doses of <200 U/m^2 and in 10% of patients receiving larger doses. Advanced age, underlying pulmonary disease, prior or concomitant radiotherapy to the chest, and prior exposure to bleomycin predispose patients to pulmonary toxicity. Patients are monitored with pulmonary function tests and a decline in DL_{CO} is the earliest indicator of toxicity.
   b. **Common**
      (1) Hypersensitivity reactions with mild to severe shaking chills and febrile reactions are common (25% of patients), frequently occurring within 4 to 10 hours of injection. However, they decrease in incidence and severity with subsequent administrations.
      (2) Sensitizes tumor and normal tissues to radiation
      (3) Dermatologic (50% of patients): hyperpigmentation of skin stretch areas (e.g., knuckles, elbows), hyperpigmented striae; hardening, tenderness, or loss of fingernails; hyperkeratosis of palms and fingers, scleroderma-like changes; skin tenderness, pruritus, urticaria, erythroderma, desquamation, alopecia
      (4) Anorexia, mucositis; a rancid smell ("like old gym socks") beginning about 10 seconds after injection
   c. **Occasional.** Nausea, vomiting, unusual tastes; mild reversible myelosuppression, Raynaud phenomenon, phlebitis, pain at injection site
   d. **Rare**
      (1) Hepatotoxicity, pleuropericarditis, arteritis.
      (2) Anaphylaxis-like reaction manifests as confusion, faintness, fever, chills, and wheezing that can progress to hypotension, renal failure, and cardiovascular collapse.
D. **Daunorubicin hydrochloride** (daunomycin). Liposomal daunomycin citrate (DaunoXome) is also available.
1. **Indication.** Acute leukemias, Kaposi sarcoma
2. **Pharmacology.** Anthracycline antitumor antibiotic. It is rapidly and widely distributed in tissues, with highest levels in the heart, kidneys, liver, lungs, and spleen. It does not cross the blood–brain barrier but appears to cross the placenta. Excreted through the hepatobiliary system, with renal clearance accounting for <20% of drug elimination.
3. **Toxicity.** Same as doxorubicin. Daunorubicin may also cause precipitous fatal cardiomyopathy months after therapy has stopped; incidence becomes unacceptable after a cumulative dose above 550 mg/m^2.

E. **Doxorubicin** (hydroxydaunorubicin, Adriamycin)
   1. Indications. Effective in a large variety of tumors
   2. Pharmacology
     a. Mechanism. Anthracycline antitumor antibiotic. Intercalates between DNA base pairs, forms free radicals, alters cell membranes, induces topoisomerase II–dependent DNA damage, inhibits preribosomal DNA and RNA
     b. Metabolism. About 70% of the drug is bound to plasma proteins. Rapidly metabolized by the liver. The release rate from tissue-binding sites is slow compared with the capacity of the liver for metabolism; this results in relatively prolonged plasma levels of drug and metabolites.
     c. Excretion. Metabolites and free drug are extensively excreted in the bile; however, known elimination accounts for only half of the drug.
   3. Toxicity
     a. Dose limiting
       (1) Myelosuppression, particularly leukopenia
       (2) Cardiomyopathy with congestive heart failure, which may become refractory (see Chapter 30, Section VII.D, for further details). Monitor the left ventricular ejection fraction with radionuclide angiography before initiation of treatment, particularly when the cumulative dose exceeds 300 mg/m^2, and periodically thereafter. Risks and benefits should be considered at total cumulative doses of 550 mg/m^2 (400 mg/m^2 with a history of mediastinal irradiation) or for electrocardiographic changes (voltage reduction, significant arrhythmias, ST–T wave changes). Dexrazoxane, a cardioprotectant, can be considered when the cumulative dose exceeds 300 mg/m^2.
     b. Common
       (1) Alopecia; nausea and vomiting (mild to severe); stomatitis
       (2) Doxorubicin is a vesicant; extravasation of the drug results in severe ulceration and necrosis.
       (3) Previously irradiated skin sites may become erythematous and desquamate when the drug is started; this *radiation-recall reaction* can occur years after radiation was given.
     c. Occasional. Diarrhea; hyperpigmentation of nail beds and dermal creases, facial flush, flush along injected vein, skin rash; conjunctivitis, lacrimation; red-colored urine
     d. Rare. Activation of fibrinolysis, interstitial pneumonitis, muscle weakness, fever, chills, anaphylaxis

F. **Doxorubicin, liposomal** (Doxil)
   1. Indications. Kaposi sarcoma, ovarian carcinoma, myeloma
   2. Pharmacology. Doxorubicin is encapsulated in long-circulating liposomes (microscopic vesicles composed of a phospholipid bilayer). The plasma clearance is slower than standard doxorubicin.
   3. Toxicity
     a. Dose limiting. Hematosuppression
     b. Common. Fatigue; mucositis, diarrhea, nausea, vomiting; alopecia; infusion reactions (7%; chills, facial swelling, headache, hypotension, shortness of breath), which resolve on interruption of infusion and which do not preclude continued treatment; palmar–plantar erythrodysesthesia (ulceration, erythema, and desquamation on the hands and feet with pain and inflammation)

  c. Occasional. Cardiomyopathy at cumulative doxorubicin doses above 550 mg/m^2, pain at injection site, radiation-recall reaction; asthenia, pain, fever; red-orange discoloration of urine

  d. Rare. Allergic reaction, hyperglycemia, jaundice, optic neuropathy

G. Epirubicin (4′-epidoxorubicin, pidorubicin, Ellence) is the 4′-epimer of doxorubicin and is a semisynthetic derivative of daunorubicin.

  1. Indication. Breast and gastric cancers

  2. Pharmacology. For mechanisms and metabolism, see *doxorubicin*.

  3. Toxicity. Same as doxorubicin, but with more nausea and vomiting. The risk of developing cardiomyopathy increases substantially after a total dose of 900 mg/m^2 (without mediastinal radiation or treatment with other anthracyclines).

H. Idarubicin (4-demethoxydaunorubicin, Idamycin)

  1. Indication. Acute leukemia

  2. Pharmacology. Anthracycline antitumor antibiotic; an analog of daunorubicin. More lipophilic and better cell uptake than other anthracycline antibiotics; otherwise similar to doxorubicin

  3. Toxicity. Similar to doxorubicin. Myelosuppression is expected. Although idarubicin is less cardiotoxic than doxorubicin and daunorubicin, the same monitoring criteria apply.

I. Mitomycin (mitomycin C, Mutamycin)

  1. Indications. Adenocarcinomas of the stomach or pancreas

  2. Pharmacology

   a. Mechanism. Antitumor antibiotic. After intracellular activation, functions as an alkylating agent; DNA cross-linking, DNA depolymerization, and free-radical formation

   b. Metabolism. Metabolized predominantly in the liver by the P450 system and DT-diaphorase. Excreted mainly through the hepatobiliary system

  3. Toxicity

   a. Dose limiting. Cumulative myelosuppression, which may be severe and prolonged (particularly thrombocytopenia)

   b. Common. Mild nausea and vomiting, anorexia; alopecia, desquamation; a vesicant drug that can cause necrosis if injected subcutaneously (skin erythema and ulceration can occur weeks to months after administration and may appear at a site distant from the site of injection)

   c. Occasional. Alopecia, stomatitis, skin rashes, photosensitivity, pain at site of injection, phlebitis; congestive heart failure; hemolytic–uremic–like syndrome (HUS)

   d. HUS usually occurs after 6 months of therapy or cumulative doses of at least 60 mg. The course may be chronic or fulminant. Blood transfusions may worsen symptoms. Plasmapheresis may be indicated for treatment. (See Chapter 35, Section V.C.)

   e. Rare. Hepatic and renal (cumulative) dysfunction, paresthesias, blurred vision, fever; acute interstitial pneumonitis

J. Mitoxantrone (Novantrone, dihydroxyanthracenedione)

  1. Indications. Breast and prostate cancer, lymphoma, acute leukemia

  2. Pharmacology. Mitoxantrone is synthetic and belongs to the anthracenedione class of compounds, which are analogs to the anthracyclines. Its mechanism of action and routes of metabolism are similar but not identical to doxorubicin.

   a. Mechanism. DNA intercalation, single- and double-strand DNA breakage, inhibition of topoisomerase II

   b. Metabolism. Metabolized by the liver's P450 system; <1% of the drug is excreted in the urine.

3. Toxicity. Compared with the anthracyclines, mitoxantrone is associated with less cardiotoxicity, less nausea and vomiting, and decreased potential for extravasation injury.

    a. Dose limiting. Myelosuppression (nadir at 10 to 14 days)

    b. Common. Mild nausea and vomiting, mucositis; alopecia (usually mild); edema, fatigue; blue discoloration of urine, sclerae, fingernails, and over venous site of injection that may last 48 hours.

    c. Occasional. Cardiomyopathy (most well defined for patients who have previously received other anthracyclines, cyclophosphamide, or mediastinal radiation or have preexisting cardiovascular disease); appears to be less cardiotoxic than doxorubicin. Pruritus, LFT abnormalities, allergic reactions

    d. Rare. Jaundice, seizures, pulmonary toxicity, anaphylaxis

K. Etoposide (VP-16, VePesid, Toposar; oral form is etoposide phosphate [Etopophos])

    1. Indications. Testicular carcinoma, small cell lung cancer, lymphoma, and other malignancies

    2. Pharmacology. An epipodophyllotoxin extracted from the *Podophyllum peltatum* mandrake plant

        a. Mechanisms. A topoisomerase II inhibitor. It causes a prominent G_2 arrest.

        b. Metabolism. Highly bound to plasma proteins (mainly albumin); decreased albumin levels result in potentially greater host toxicity. Metabolized by the liver via glucuronidation to less active metabolites. Excreted in urine (40%) as intact and degraded drug; excretion of the remaining 60% is uncertain.

    3. Toxicity

        a. Dose limiting. Myelosuppression

        b. Common. Nausea and vomiting (with oral dosing, but uncommon with intravenous dosing); alopecia (usually mild); hypotension if rapidly infused; malaise, metallic taste during drug infusion

        c. Occasional. Anemia, thrombocytopenia, pain at injection site, phlebitis, abnormal LFTs, diarrhea, chills, fever

        d. Rare. Stomatitis, dysphagia, diarrhea, constipation, parotitis, rash, radiation-recall reaction, hyperpigmentation; anaphylaxis, transient hypertension, arrhythmias; somnolence, vertigo, transient cortical blindness; peripheral neuropathy, anaphylactoid reaction

L. Irinotecan (Camptosar)

    1. Indications. Colorectal cancer, lung cancer

    2. Pharmacology. A water-soluble analog of camptothecin that is a relatively inactive prodrug, which is converted to the active agent. Camptothecin was originally isolated from extracts of a Chinese tree.

        a. Mechanisms. Inhibits topoisomerase I; cell cycle–phase specific

        b. Metabolism. Conversion to the active metabolite, SN-38, occurs mainly in the liver but also in the plasma and intestinal mucosa. The major route of elimination is the bile and feces, with renal clearance playing only a minor role.

            (1) The active form of the drug is metabolized by the polymorphic enzyme UGT1A1. Approximately 10% of the North American population is homozygous for the UGT1A1*28 allele and have reduced UGT1A1 activity and are at increased risk of experiencing grade 4 neutropenia.

  3. Toxicity
   a. Dose limiting. Profuse diarrhea (especially in patients 65 years of age and older) and myelosuppression
   b. Common. Neutropenia; mild nausea, vomiting, abdominal cramps; flushing during administration; mild alopecia; weakness, sweating
   c. Occasional. LFT abnormalities, headache, fever, dyspnea, back pain
   d. Rare. Anaphylactoid reaction, acute renal failure

M. Irinotecan, liposomal (Onivyde)
  1. Indications. Adenocarcinoma of the pancreas
  2. Pharmacology. Liposome-encapsulated irinotecan
   a. Mechanisms. Inhibits topoisomerase I; cell cycle–phase specific.
   b. Metabolism. See *irinotecan*.
  3. Toxicity. See *irinotecan*.

N. Teniposide (VM-26, Vumon)
  1. Indication. Acute lymphoblastic leukemia (ALL)
  2. Pharmacology
   a. Mechanism. A semisynthetic derivative of podophyllotoxin; topoisomerase II inhibitor
   b. Metabolism. Virtually all of the drug is bound to protein. Systemic metabolism is significant, but metabolites have not been identified. Renal excretion is only a small fraction of its clearance.
  3. Toxicity
   a. Dose limiting. Neutropenia
   b. Common. Thrombocytopenia, hypotension with too rapid an infusion
   c. Occasional. Nausea and vomiting, alopecia, abnormal LFTs, phlebitis
   d. Rare. Diarrhea, stomatitis; rash, anaphylaxis; azotemia; fever; paresthesias, seizures

O. Topotecan (Hycamtin)
  1. Indications. Ovarian cancer after failure to respond to previous (cisplatin-based) therapies; cervical cancer in combination with cisplatin; relapsed small cell lung cancer
  2. Pharmacology
   a. Mechanisms. A derivative of camptothecin, it inhibits topoisomerase I activity; cell cycle–phase specific
   b. Metabolism. Rapid conversion in plasma to the active lactone form. About 60% of the drug is excreted in urine.
  3. Toxicity
   a. Dose limiting. Myelosuppression
   b. Common. Nausea and vomiting; diarrhea, constipation, abdominal pain; alopecia; headache, fatigue, fever; arthralgias and myalgias
   c. Occasional. Transient elevation of LFTs; paresthesia; rash; microscopic hematuria (30%)

III. ANTIMETABOLITES
A. General pharmacology of antimetabolites
  1. These agents produce antitumor effect because their structure resembles purine or pyrimidine precursors or because they interfere with purine or pyrimidine synthesis. Their activity, therefore, is greatest in the S phase of the cell cycle. In general, these agents have been most effective when cell proliferation is rapid.
  2. The pharmacokinetics of these drugs is characterized by nonlinear dose–response curves; after a certain dose, no more are killed with increasing doses (fluorouracil is an exception). Because of the entry of new cells into

the cycle, the length of time that the cells are exposed to the drug is directly proportional to the killing potential.

B. **Azacitidine** (5-azacitidine, Vidaza)

1. **Indication.** Myelodysplastic syndromes (MDS)

2. **Pharmacology**

a. **Mechanism.** Antimetabolite (cytidine analog). Rapidly phosphorylated and incorporated into DNA and RNA, thereby inhibiting protein synthesis; also inhibits pyrimidine synthesis and DNA methylation.

b. **Metabolism.** Activated by phosphorylation and deactivated by deamination; similar to cytarabine. Excreted in urine (20% as unchanged drug)

3. **Toxicity**

a. **Dose limiting.** Myelosuppression; nausea and vomiting.

b. **Common.** Hepatic dysfunction, fatigue, headache, diarrhea, alopecia, fever, injection site erythema

c. **Occasional.** Neurotoxicity (dizziness, restlessness, confusion), azotemia (transient), arthralgias, hypophosphatemia with myalgia, stomatitis, phlebitis, rash

d. **Rare.** Progressive lethargy and coma, renal tubular acidosis, rhabdomyolysis, hypotension

C. **Cladribine** [2-chlordeoxyadenosine (2-CdA), Leustatin]

1. **Indications.** Hairy cell leukemia

2. **Pharmacology.** An analog of the purine deoxyadenosine

a. **Mechanism.** Antimetabolite. The analog accumulates in cells (particularly lymphocytes), blocks adenosine deaminase, and inhibits RNA and DNA synthesis. Inhibits ribonucleotide reductase. Depletes ATP. Induces apoptosis. Active against both dividing and resting cells

b. **Metabolism.** Rapidly metabolized and eliminated through the kidneys

3. **Toxicity.** Patients are at increased risk for opportunistic infections.

a. **Dose limiting.** Myelosuppression

b. **Common.** Immunosuppression with decreases in CD4+ and CD8+ cells; nausea, skin reactions at injection site; fever in 50% (most likely due to tumor's releasing pyrogens and cytokines), chills, flulike syndrome

c. **Occasional.** Neurotoxicity (headache, dizziness), hypersensitivity reactions, fatigue

d. **Rare.** Severe neurotoxicity, pancreatitis

D. **Clofarabine** (2-chloro-2′-fluorodeoxy-9-beta-D-arabinofurosyladenine, Clolar)

1. **Indications.** Relapsed or refractory ALL

2. **Pharmacology.** Purine antimetabolite

3. **Toxicity**

a. **Dose limiting.**

(1) Capillary leak syndrome (CLS)/systemic inflammatory response syndrome (SIRS) is a development following cytokine release and manifested by hypotension, tachycardia, tachypnea, and pulmonary edema.

(2) Hematosuppression (90%)

(3) Hepatotoxicity and nephrotoxicity

b. **Common.** Tachycardia, hypotension, flushing; headache, fever, chills, fatigue; pruritus, rash; nausea, vomiting, diarrhea; abnormal LFTs (80%); increased creatinine (50%), limb pain

c. **Occasional.** Hypertension, edema, dyspnea, pleural, or pericardial effusion; mucositis; myalgia, arthralgia; irritability, somnolence, agitation; cecitis; CLS (4%), SIRS (2%)

    d. Rare. Hepatic venoocclusive disease, Stevens-Johnson syndrome, hallucination

E. Cytarabine (cytosine arabinoside, Cytosar, ara-C)
1. **Indications.** Acute leukemia, lymphoma, meningeal involvement with tumor
2. **Pharmacology.** An analog of deoxycytidine
   a. **Mechanism.** Antimetabolite. Requires intracellular activation to its phosphorylated derivative (ara-CTP), which inhibits DNA polymerases that are involved in the conversion of cytidine to deoxycytidine; some are incorporated into DNA. Ara-CTP inhibits ribonucleotide reductase, which results in decreased levels of deoxyribonucleotides for DNA synthesis and function.
   b. **Metabolism.** Requires activation to ara-CTP by kinase; deactivated by deaminase; ara-C is rapidly and completely deaminated in liver, plasma, and peripheral tissues; ara-C antitumor activity depends on relative amounts of kinase and deaminase in cells. In patients with renal insufficiency, one metabolite (uracil arabinoside) has the ability to produce high concentrations of ara-CTP, which may result in CNS toxicity. Excreted in urine as inactive metabolites
3. **Toxicity**
   a. **Dose limiting.** Myelosuppression
   b. **Common.** Nausea, vomiting, mucositis, diarrhea (potentiated by the addition of an anthracycline); conjunctivitis (usually within the first 3 days of high-dose regimens, but reduced with prophylactic glucocorticoids eye drops); hydradenitis, arachnoiditis with intrathecal administration
   c. **Neurotoxicity** (cerebellar ataxia, lethargy, confusion) begins on the fourth or fifth day of infusion and usually resolves within 7 days. The incidence and severity of toxicity are related to the dose given (especially with total dose of >48 g/m^2), the rate of infusion (least incidence for continuous infusions), age (particularly older than 60 years), sex (especially male), and the degree of hepatic or renal dysfunction (particularly with creatinine clearance of <60 mL/min). In some cases, it is irreversible or fatal.
   d. **Occasional.** Alopecia, stomatitis, metallic taste, esophagitis, hepatic dysfunction (mild and reversible), pancreatitis, severe GI ulceration; thrombophlebitis; headache; rash, transient skin erythema without exfoliation. *Ara-C syndrome*, described in pediatric patients, is an allergic reaction manifested by fever, flulike syndrome, myalgias, bone pain, maculopapular rash, conjunctivitis, and occasional chest pain (corticosteroids are effective).
   e. **Rare.** Sudden respiratory distress rapidly progressing to noncardiogenic pulmonary edema; pericarditis, cardiomegaly, tamponade; urinary retention

F. Decitabine (5-aza-2′-deoxycytidine, Dacogen)
1. **Indications.** Myelodysplastic syndrome
2. **Pharmacology.** Decitabine is an analogue of the natural nucleoside 2′-decoxycytidine.
   a. **Mechanisms.** Decitabine inhibits DNA methyltransferase, causing hypomethylation of DNA and cellular differentiation or apoptosis.
   b. **Metabolism.** Deamination by cytidine deaminase found principally in the liver but also in granulocytes, intestinal epithelium, and whole blood

3. **Toxicity**
    a. **Dose limiting.** Hematosuppression (nadir at 35 days, recovery at 35 to 50 days)
    b. **Common.** Hematosuppression, fatigue, fever; nausea, constipation (35%), diarrhea; headache, arthralgias, rigors, edema, cough; hyperglycemia, hypokalemia, hypomagnesemia

G. **Fludarabine** (2-fluoroadenine arabinoside-5-phosphate, Fludara)
 1. **Indications.** CLL, low-grade lymphomas
 2. **Pharmacology.** The 5′-monophosphate analog of ara-A (arabinofuranosyladenosine). The 2-fluoro group on the adenosine ring renders this drug resistant to breakdown by adenosine deaminase (compare with cytarabine).
    a. **Mechanism.** Antimetabolite with high specificity for lymphoid cells. Its active metabolite, 2-fluoro-ara-A, appears to act by inhibiting DNA chain extension, DNA polymerase-α, and ribonucleotide reductase. It has activity against both dividing and resting cells and induces apoptosis.
    b. **Metabolism.** Metabolites and unchanged drug (25%) are excreted primarily in urine.
 3. **Toxicity**
    a. **Dose limiting.** Myelosuppression, which may be cumulative; severe autoimmune hemolytic anemia (AIHA) that may or may not be responsive to corticosteroids
    b. **Common.** Immunosuppression with decreases in CD4+ and CD8+ T cells in most patients and associated with increased risk for opportunistic infections (recovery may take more than a year); mild nausea and vomiting; fever with associated flulike syndrome (25%); cough, weakness, arthralgia/myalgias
    c. **Occasional.** Alopecia (mild), abnormal LFTs, tumor lysis syndrome
    d. **Rare.**
        (1) Stomatitis, diarrhea; dermatitis; chest pain, hypotension, interstitial pneumonitis (especially when combined with pentostatin)
        (2) Immune-mediated hematologic effects (AIHA, immunologic thrombocytopenic purpura, acquired hemophilia, transfusion-associated graft vs. host disease)
        (3) Severe neurologic effects, including blindness, coma, and death (especially in patients treated with very high doses)

H. **5-Fluorouracil** (5-FU, Adrucil)
 1. **Indications.** GI, breast, pancreatic, and head and neck carcinomas
 2. **Pharmacology.** A fluoropyrimidine analog
    a. **Mechanism.** Antimetabolite. Requires activation to cytotoxic metabolite forms. Interferes with DNA synthesis by blocking thymidylate synthetase (TS), an enzyme involved in the conversion of deoxyuridylic acid to thymidylic acid. Metabolites (e.g., FUTP) are incorporated into several RNA species, which thereby interfere with RNA function and protein synthesis. Incorporation of another metabolite (FdUTP) into DNA results in inhibition of DNA synthesis and function. It is cell–cycle S-phase specific but acts in other cell cycle phases as well and is unique in having a log linear cell–killing action.
    b. **Metabolism.** 5-FU rapidly enters all tissues, including spinal fluid and malignant effusions. The drug undergoes extensive intracellular activation by a series of phosphorylating enzymes and phosphoribosyl transferase, particularly dihydropyrimidine dehydrogenase. Most of the drug degradation occurs in the liver. Responsive tumors appear to lack degradation enzymes. Metabolism eliminates 90% of 5-FU. Inactive

metabolites are excreted in urine, bile, and breath (as carbon dioxide). The elimination half-life is short, ranging from 10 to 20 minutes.

   3. **Toxicity** is more common and more severe in patients with dihydropyrimidine dehydrogenase deficiency.

      a. **Dose limiting.** Myelosuppression (less common with continuous infusion); mucositis (more common with 5-day infusion); diarrhea

      b. **Common.** Nasal discharge; eye irritation and excessive lacrimation due to dacryocystitis and lacrimal duct stenosis; dry skin, photosensitivity, and pigmentation of the infused vein

      c. **Neurologic.** Reversible cerebellar dysfunction, somnolence, confusion, or seizures occurs in about 1% of patients. Symptoms usually disappear 1 to 6 weeks after the drug is discontinued, but they abate after the dose is reduced or even if the same dose is maintained.

      d. **Occasional.** Esophagitis; hand–foot syndrome with protracted infusion (paresthesia, erythema, and swelling of the palms and soles); coronary vasospasm (particularly in patients with a prior history of myocardial ischemia); thrombophlebitis; nausea, vomiting

      e. **Rare.** Alopecia, dermatitis, loss of nails, dark bands on nails; blurred vision, "black hairy tongue" (hypertrophy of filiform papillae), anaphylaxis, fever

 I. Capecitabine (Xeloda)

   1. **Indications.** Carcinomas of the breast or colon

   2. **Pharmacology.** Capecitabine is a fluoropyrimidine carbamate that is a systemic prodrug of 5′-deoxy-5-fluorouridine (5′-DFUR), which is converted *in vivo* to 5-FU.

      a. **Mechanism.** See *fluorouracil.*

      b. **Metabolism.** Hepatic. Catabolism predominantly via dihydropyrimidine dehydrogenase, which is present in liver, leukocytes, kidney, and other extrahepatic tissues. More than 90% is cleared in the urine (see *5-fluorouracil*).

   3. **Toxicity.** Similar to 5-FU

      a. **Dose limiting.** Diarrhea (50%), hand–foot syndrome

      b. **Common.** Hand–foot syndrome (palmar–plantar erythrodysesthesia or chemotherapy-induced acral erythema) occurs in 15% to 50% of patients; nausea, vomiting, hematosuppression; fatigue

      c. **Occasional.** Abnormal LFTs, neurotoxicity; cardiac ischemia in patients with a prior history of coronary artery disease; tear duct stenosis, conjunctivitis, blepharitis; confusion, cerebellar ataxia

 J. Gemcitabine (Gemzar)

   1. **Indications.** Carcinoma of pancreas, bladder, lung, ovary; soft tissue sarcomas

   2. **Pharmacology.** A fluorine-substituted deoxycytidine analog

      a. **Mechanisms.** Cell-phase specific, primarily killing cells in S phase and also blocking the progression of cells through the G_1 phase to S-phase boundary. Metabolized intracellularly to the active diphosphate and triphosphate. Inhibits ribonucleotide reductase; competes with deoxycytidine triphosphate (dCTP) for incorporation into DNA

      b. **Metabolism.** Undergoes extensive metabolism by deamination in the liver, plasma, and peripheral tissues. Nearly entirely excreted in urine as active drug and metabolites

   3. **Toxicity**

      a. **Dose limiting.** Myelosuppression

b. **Common.** Nausea, vomiting, diarrhea, stomatitis; fever with flulike symptoms (40%); macular or maculopapular rash; transient LFT elevations; mild proteinuria and hematuria

c. **Occasional.** Hair loss, rash, edema

d. **Rare.** Hemolytic–uremic syndrome; pulmonary drug toxicity; hypersensitivity reactions; alopecia

K. **Hydroxyurea** (hydroxycarbamide, Hydrea, Droxia)

1. **Indications.** Myeloproliferative disorders, refractory ovarian cancer, sickle cell disease

2. **Pharmacology.** An analog of urea

   a. **Mechanism.** Antimetabolite. Inhibits DNA synthesis by inhibiting nucleotide reductase, the enzyme that converts ribonucleosides to deoxyribonucleosides. Inhibits DNA repair and thymidine incorporation into DNA. Cell cycle S-phase specific but acts in other phases as well

   b. **Metabolism.** Crosses the blood–brain barrier. Half of the drug is rapidly degraded into inactive compounds by the liver. Inactive products and unchanged drug (50%) are excreted in urine.

3. **Toxicity**

   a. **Dose limiting.** Myelosuppression, which recovers rapidly when treatment is stopped (prominent megaloblastosis)

   b. **Occasional.** Nausea, vomiting, diarrhea; skin rash, facial erythema, hyperpigmentation; azotemia, proteinuria; transient LFT abnormalities; radiation recall phenomenon

   c. **Rare.** Alopecia, mucositis, diarrhea, constipation; neurologic events; pulmonary edema; flulike syndrome; painful perimalleolar ulcers; possible acute leukemia in myeloproliferative disorders

L. **6-Mercaptopurine** (6-MP, Purinethol)

1. **Indication.** Acute lymphoblastic leukemia (maintenance therapy)

2. **Pharmacology**

   a. **Mechanism.** Purine analog that inhibits *de novo* purine synthesis by inhibiting 5-phosphoribosyl-1-pyrophosphate. The parent drug is inactive. Requires intracellular phosphorylation by hypoxanthine–guanine phosphoribosyltransferase (HGPRT) to the monophosphate form, which is eventually metabolized to the triphosphate metabolite. Competes with ribotides for enzymes responsible for conversion of inosinic acid to adenine and xanthine ribotides. Its incorporation into DNA or RNA is of uncertain significance.

   b. **Metabolism.** Mercaptopurine is slowly degraded in the liver, largely by xanthine oxidase. Allopurinol, a xanthine oxidase inhibitor, causes marked increase in its toxicity. Clearance is primarily hepatic with conventional doses.

3. **Toxicity**

   a. **Dose limiting.** Myelosuppression

   b. **Common.** Mild nausea, vomiting, anorexia (25%); usually reversible cholestasis (30%); dry skin, photosensitivity; immunosuppression

   c. **Rare.** Stomatitis, diarrhea, dermatitis, fever, hematuria, Budd-Chiari–like syndrome, hepatic necrosis

M. **Methotrexate** (amethopterin, MTX)

1. **Indications.** A wide variety of conditions

2. **Pharmacology**

   a. **Mechanism.** MTX blocks the enzyme dihydrofolate reductase, preventing formation of reduced (tetrahydro-) folic acid; tetrahydrofolic acid is crucial to the transfer of carbon units in a variety of biochemical reactions. MTX thus blocks formation of thymidylate from deoxyuridylate and prevents synthesis of DNA. The drug also inhibits RNA and protein synthesis and prevents cells from entering the S phase of the cell cycle.

   b. Metabolism. MTX is minimally metabolized by the human species. It is converted in the liver and other cells to higher polyglutamate forms. The drug is distributed to body water; patients with significant effusions eliminate the drug much more slowly. Because 50% to 70% of the drug is bound to plasma proteins, displacement by other drugs (e.g., aspirin, sulfonamides) may result in an increase in toxic effects. About 20% of the drug is eliminated in the bile. It is excreted in urine as unchanged drug (80% to 90% within 24 hours). Renal dysfunction results in dangerous blood levels of MTX and possible further renal damage. The half-life of the drug is 8 to 10 hours.

3. **Toxicity.** Leucovorin can reverse the immediate cytotoxic effects of MTX; generally, 1 mg of leucovorin is given for each 1 mg of MTX.

   a. Dose limiting. Myelosuppression, stomatitis, renal dysfunction

   b. High-dose regimens. Nausea, vomiting, renal tubular necrosis, cortical blindness

   c. Previously irradiated areas. Skin erythema, pulmonary fibrosis, transverse myelitis, cerebritis

   d. Chronic therapy. Liver cirrhosis (reversible hepatic dysfunction occurs with short-term intermittent therapy); osteoporosis (in children)

   e. Neurotoxicity. MTX neurotoxicity depends on dose and route of administration. Within a few hours after intrathecal administration, MTX can produce acute aseptic meningitis that is usually self-limited. A subacute encephalopathy and myelopathy can also occur after intrathecal administration.

   High-dose systemic administration can cause a reversible encephalopathy of rapid onset and resolution that lasts from minutes to hours (stroke-like episodes). Chronic intrathecal combined with high-dose systemic administration can produce a more serious and irreversible leukoencephalopathy that develops months after treatment, is more likely to occur after brain irradiation, and causes dementia, seizures, spasticity, and ataxia.

   f. Occasional. Nausea, vomiting, diarrhea (GI ulceration, hemorrhage, and perforation can occur if therapy is continued after the onset of diarrhea); dermatitis, photosensitivity, altered pigmentation, furunculosis; conjunctivitis, photophobia, excessive lacrimation, cataracts; fever, reversible oligospermia, flank pain (with rapid intravenous infusion)

   g. Rare. Alopecia, MTX pneumonitis (see Chapter 29, Section IV.A)

N. **Nelarabine** (Arranon)

1. **Indications.** Relapsed or refractory T-cell ALL and T-cell lymphoblastic lymphoma

2. **Pharmacology**

   a. Mechanisms. A prodrug of ara-G, nelarabine is demethylated by adenosine deaminase to ara-G and then converted to ara-GTP, which is incorporated into the DNA of the leukemic blasts, leading to inhibition of DNA synthesis and inducing apoptosis. Ara-GTP accumulates at higher levels in T cells, which correlates to clinical response.

   b. Metabolism. Demethylated and hydrolyzed; drug and metabolites are excreted in the urine.

3. **Toxicity**

   a. Dose limiting. Severe neurotoxicity that may not return to baseline after treatment cessation (discontinue drug for grade ≥ 2)

     b. Common. Neurologic (70%; somnolence, confusion, dizziness, ataxia, tremor, peripheral neuropathy; severe neurotoxicity is reported including coma, demyelination, seizures, etc.); hematosuppression; fever, fatigue; nausea, vomiting, constipation; cough, edema

     c. Occasional. Myalgia/arthralgia, abdominal pain, limb pain; stomatitis, dyspnea, cough; elevated transaminases or creatinine, hyper-/hypoglycemia

O. Pemetrexed (Alimta)

    1. Indications. Mesothelioma (with cisplatin) and non–small cell lung cancer (NSCLC)

    2. Pharmacology

     a. Mechanisms. Pyrrolopyrimidine antifolate analog with activity in the S phase of the cell cycle. Inhibition of the folate-dependent enzyme TS is the main site of action. It also inhibits dihydrofolate reductase and two formyltransferases.

     b. Metabolism. Metabolized intracellularly to polyglutamates, which are much more potent than the parent monoglutamate. Principally cleared by the kidneys. About 90% of the drug is excreted unchanged in the urine within 24 hours.

    3. Toxicity. Patients with insufficient folate intake may be at increased risk for host toxicity. A baseline homocysteine level >10 predicts for the development of grade 3 to 4 toxicity.

     a. Dose limiting. Myelosuppression. All patients are given 350 μg/d PO of folic acid and 1,000 mg of vitamin B_{12} SC every 3 weeks to reduce drug toxicity.

     b. Common. Skin rash (usually as the hand–foot syndrome), mucositis, nausea, vomiting, diarrhea; mild dyspnea, fatigue; transient elevation of LFTs

     c. Occasional. Myalgia/arthralgia, fever

P. Pentostatin [2′-deoxycoformycin (dCF), Nipent]

    1. Indications. CLL, hairy cell leukemia, and cutaneous T-cell lymphoma

    2. Pharmacology. A fermentation product of *Streptomyces antibioticus*

     a. Mechanism. Antimetabolite. Both cell cycle specific and cell cycle nonspecific. Inhibitor of adenine deaminase, an enzyme that is important for the metabolism of purine nucleosides. Also inhibits ribonucleotide reductase (resulting in inhibition of DNA synthesis and function) and *S*-adenosyl-L-homocysteine hydrolase (resulting in inhibition of one-carbon–dependent methylation reactions)

     b. Metabolism. Most dCF is excreted unchanged in urine.

    3. Toxicity

     a. Dose limiting. Myelosuppression

     b. Common. Immunosuppression; mild nausea and vomiting, diarrhea, altered taste; fatigue, fever; erythematous, papular, vesiculobullous rashes

     c. Occasional. Chills, myalgia, arthralgia; abnormal LFTs; keratoconjunctivitis, photophobia; cough, renal failure

     d. Rare. Hepatitis; pulmonary infiltrates and insufficiency

Q. Pralatrexate (Folotyn)

    1. Indications. Relapsed or refractory peripheral T-cell lymphoma

    2. Pharmacology: An antineoplastic folate analog

     a. Mechanisms. Competitively inhibits dihydrofolate reductase and polyglutamylation by the enzyme folylpolyglutamyl synthetase

     b. Metabolism. Approximately 33% of the drug is excreted unchanged in the urine.

   3. **Toxicity**
      a. **Dose limiting.** Thrombocytopenia, neutropenia, and mucositis
      b. **Common.** Anorexia, nausea, vomiting, diarrhea, constipation; fatigue, fever, edema; rash
   R. **6-Thioguanine** (6-TG, 6-thioguanine, aminopurine-6-thiol-hemihydrate)
      1. **Indication.** Acute myelogenous leukemia
      2. **Pharmacology**
         a. **Mechanism.** Purine analog with cell cycle–specific activity in the S phase. The drug requires intracellular phosphorylation by HGPRT to the cytotoxic monophosphate form, which is eventually metabolized to the triphosphate metabolite (see *mercaptopurine*). The drug is incorporated extensively into DNA, resulting in miscoding of transcription and DNA replication, and into RNA.
         b. **Metabolism.** Thioguanine is not degraded by xanthine oxidase and, unlike mercaptopurine, can be given in full doses with allopurinol. Clearance of the drug is primarily hepatic, but also renal.
      3. **Toxicity**
         a. **Dose limiting.** Myelosuppression
         b. **Common.** Stomatitis, diarrhea
         c. **Occasional.** Nausea and vomiting, hepatic dysfunction, hepatic veno-occlusive disease; decreased vibratory sensation, unsteady gait
   S. **Trifluridine/tipiracil** (Lonsurf)
      1. **Indications.** Colorectal cancer
      2. **Pharmacology**
         a. **Mechanisms.** A combination of trifluridine, a nucleoside metabolic inhibitor, and tipiracil, a thymidine phosphorylase inhibitor. Inclusion of tipiracil increases trifluridine exposure by inhibiting its metabolism by thymidine phosphorylase.
         b. **Metabolism.** Trifluridine and tipiracil are not metabolized by cytochrome P450 (CYP) enzymes. Trifluridine is mainly eliminated by metabolism via thymidine phosphorylase to form an inactive metabolite. Excreted in urine
      3. **Toxicity**
         a. **Dose limiting.** Myelosuppression
         b. **Common.** Anemia, neutropenia, asthenia/fatigue, nausea, thrombocytopenia, decreased appetite, diarrhea, vomiting, abdominal pain, and pyrexia

IV. MITOTIC SPINDLE AGENTS

   A. **General pharmacology of mitotic spindle agents.** Mitotic spindle is formed by the assembly of microtubules that are composed of multimers of α and β tubulin. Vinca alkaloids (e.g., vincristine) bind to the tubulin dimer, thus inhibiting microtubule assembly (M phase of the cell cycle) and resulting in dissolution of the mitotic spindle structure. Taxanes (e.g., paclitaxel, docetaxel) not only bind to microtubules but also promote microtubule assembly and resistance to depolymerization, resulting in the production of nonfunctional microtubules.
   B. **Paclitaxel** (Taxol)
      1. **Indications.** Carcinomas of the breast, ovary, lung, esophagus, and other sites; Kaposi sarcoma
      2. **Pharmacology.** Isolated from the bark of the Pacific yew tree, *Taxus brevifolia*
         a. **Mechanism.** It stabilizes microtubules; see Section IV.A.
         b. **Metabolism.** Extensively metabolized by the hepatic P450 microsomal system. More than 75% of the drug is excreted in the feces.

3. **Toxicity**
   a. **Dose limiting**
      (1) **Neutropenia.** Carboplatin, cisplatin, and cyclophosphamide decrease paclitaxel's clearance and thus increase myelosuppression; they should be administered after paclitaxel.
      (2) **Hypersensitivity** (up to 40%) is manifested by cutaneous flushing, hypotension, bronchospasm, urticaria, diaphoresis, pain, or angioedema. Reactions usually develop within 10 minutes of starting the treatment; 90% of hypersensitivity reactions develop after the first or second dose. Premedication with corticosteroids is advised. Anaphylaxis occurs in about 3% of patients. Reactions may be caused by Cremophor EL or by the drug itself.
      (3) **Peripheral neuropathy,** particularly in the higher dosage schedules and in patients with concomitant etiologies for peripheral neuropathy. Neurotoxicity occurs less frequently when infused over 24 hours (5%) than when infused over 3 hours (25% to 75%). The distribution typically is "stocking glove" and consists of dysesthesias, paresthesias, and loss of proprioception, which usually resolve within a few months.
   b. **Common.** Alopecia (90%; usually total and sudden, within 3 weeks of treatment); thrombocytopenia (usually not severe); transient arthralgias and myalgias within 3 days of treatment and lasting for about 1 week (ameliorated by nonsteroidal anti-inflammatory agents and prednisone); diarrhea, transient bradycardia (usually asymptomatic)
   c. **Occasional.** Nausea, vomiting, taste changes, mucositis (cumulative), diarrhea; atrioventricular conduction defects, ventricular tachycardia, cardiac angina; necrosis when extravasated; intoxication when infused over 1 hour (because of high alcohol content in the preparation); onycholysis, elevated LFTs
   d. **Rare.** Paralytic ileus, generalized weakness, seizures; myocardial infarction, interstitial pneumonia
C. **Paclitaxel, protein bound** (nab-paclitaxel, albumin-bound paclitaxel, Abraxane)
   1. **Indications.** Metastatic breast cancer, pancreatic cancer, NSCLC
   2. **Pharmacology.** This injectable suspension contains paclitaxel protein-bound particles.
      a. **Mechanisms.** See *paclitaxel.*
      b. **Metabolism.** See *paclitaxel.*
   3. **Toxicity**
      a. **Dose limiting.** Neutropenia
      b. **Common.** Hematosuppression, sensory neuropathy, arthralgias/myalgia (usually transient), GI disturbances, alopecia, fatigue
      c. **Occasional.** Abnormal liver function tests, fluid retention. Premedication with corticosteroids to prevent hypersensitivity reactions is not required for Abraxane.
D. **Cabazitaxel** (Jevtana)
   1. **Indications.** Hormone-refractory prostate cancer previously treated with a docetaxel-containing regimen
   2. **Pharmacology**
      a. **Mechanisms.** A microtubule inhibitor, it binds to tubulin and promotes its assembly into microtubules, while simultaneously inhibiting disassembly, resulting in the inhibition of mitotic and interphase cellular functions.

    b. Metabolism. Extensively metabolized in the liver, mainly by the CYP3A4/5 isoenzyme. Excreted mainly in the feces as numerous metabolites (renal excretion is <5%)

  3. Toxicity

    a. Dose limiting. Severe hypersensitivity reactions (do not give to patients with a history of hypersensitivity reactions to other drugs formulated with polysorbate 80), severe neutropenia

    b. Common. Pancytopenia (>90%); diarrhea, nausea, vomiting, abdominal pain; peripheral neuropathy, dysgeusia; fever, fatigue, alopecia (10%), dyspnea, arthralgia

    c. Occasional. Renal failure, arrhythmia, mucositis

E. Docetaxel (Taxotere)

  1. Indications. Cancers of the breast, lung, stomach, esophagus, and head and neck; hormone-refractory prostate cancer

  2. Pharmacology. The drug is prepared by semisynthesis beginning with a precursor extracted from the needles of the European yew tree.

    a. Mechanisms. Inhibitor of microtubular depolymerization. The binding of docetaxel to microtubules does not alter the number of protofilaments in the bound microtubules, which differs from most spindle poisons currently in clinical use.

    b. Metabolism. Extensively metabolized by the hepatic P450 microsomal system. More than 75% is excreted in feces and a small percentage in urine.

  3. Toxicity

    a. Dose limiting. Myelosuppression

    b. Common. Alopecia (80% except with the weekly schedule), maculopapular rash and dry itchy skin, discoloration of finger nails; mucositis, diarrhea; fatigue, fever

    c. Occasional

      (1) Severe hypersensitivity reactions (<5%) despite premedications. Give dexamethasone, 4 mg PO b.i.d. on the day before, the day of, and the day after docetaxel administration

      (2) Fluid retention that is cumulative in incidence and severity (especially after a cumulative dose of 705 mg/m^2) is reversible (usually within 8 months); the fluid retention usually affects the lower extremities but can also result in ascites or pleural or pericardial effusions.

      (3) GI upset, severe nail reactions; hypotension; transiently elevated liver function tests

      (4) Peripheral neuropathy, which is less common than with paclitaxel, is mainly sensory, but motor or autonomic neuropathy and CNS effects are also seen.

    d. Rare. Cardiac events

F. Eribulin (Halaven)

  1. Indications. Metastatic breast cancer and liposarcoma

  2. Pharmacology

    a. Mechanisms. A nontaxane microtubule inhibitor that is a halichondrin B analog. It inhibits formation of mitotic spindles causing arrest of the cell cycle at the G2/M phase; suppresses microtubule polymerization without affecting depolymerization.

    b. Metabolism. Negligible; more than 80% excreted in the feces as unchanged drug

  3. Toxicity

    a. Dose limiting. Hematosuppression; peripheral neuropathy

    b. Common. Neutropenia (>80%), anemia; nausea, vomiting, stomatitis, constipation, diarrhea, ALT elevation; alopecia (45%); fatigue, fever, headache; peripheral neuropathy that may be prolonged (35%), arthralgia/myalgias, bone pain, limb pain; QT interval prolongation

    c. Occasional. Rash, lacrimation, dysgeusia

    d. Rare. Pharyngolaryngeal pain

G. Estramustine (Emcyt, Estracyt)

  1. Indication. Progressive prostate cancer

  2. Pharmacology. Structurally, estramustine is a combination of estradiol phosphate and nornitrogen mustard.

    a. Mechanism. Cell cycle–specific agent with activity in the mitosis (M) phase by binding to microtubule-associated proteins

    b. Metabolism. Rapidly dephosphorylated in GI tract and metabolized primarily in the liver. About 20% of the drug is excreted in the urine.

  3. Toxicity. Similar to estrogens

    a. Dose limiting. Thromboembolism. Contraindicated in patients with active thrombophlebitis or thromboembolic disorders

    b. Common. Diarrhea; nausea and vomiting (usually mild); skin rash. Gynecomastia in up to 50% of patients (can be prevented by prophylactic irradiation)

    c. Rare. Myelosuppression, cardiovascular complications

H. Ixabepilone (Ixempra)

  1. Indications. Refractory locally advanced or metastatic breast cancer either as monotherapy or in combination (e.g., with capecitabine)

  2. Pharmacology. The drug is an epothilone B analog.

    a. Mechanisms. Binds to the β-tubulin subunit of the microtubule, thus arresting the cell cycle at the G_2/M phase and inducing apoptosis

    b. Metabolism. Extensive hepatic metabolism via CYP3A4 into inactive metabolites. Excreted mostly in the feces, <10% as unchanged drug. The drug has minimal renal excretion.

  3. Toxicity. Cognitive impairment (due to ethanol content of diluent) or hypersensitivity reactions (related to the Cremophor in the diluent) may occur.

    a. Dose limiting. Myelosuppression (particularly neutropenia; grade 4 in 15% to 25%) and peripheral neuropathy (60%)

    b. Common. Alopecia (50%), headache, fatigue, mucositis, GI disturbance, myalgia/arthralgia (50%)

    c. Occasional. Edema, fever, dizziness, palmar–plantar dysesthesia (hand–foot syndrome), skin and nail disorders, hyperpigmentation, motor neuropathy, dysgeusia, increased lacrimation, dyspnea

I. Vinblastine (vinca leukoblastine, Velban)

  1. Indications. Lymphomas, testicular carcinoma, Kaposi sarcoma

  2. Pharmacology

    a. Mechanism. Periwinkle plant alkaloid. Binds to microtubular proteins. Inhibits RNA synthesis by affecting DNA-dependent RNA polymerases. Cell cycle–phase specific; it arrests cells at the G_2-phase and M-phase interface.

    b. Metabolism. Highly bound to plasma proteins and to formed blood elements, especially platelets. Metabolized by the hepatic P450 microsomal system to active and inactive metabolites. Predominantly excreted in bile. Minimal free drug is recovered in urine.

  3. Toxicity

    a. Dose limiting. Neutropenia

      b. Common. Cramps or severe pain in jaw, pharynx, back, or limbs after injection

      c. Occasional. Thrombocytopenia, anemia, alopecia (10%); SIADH, hypertension, Raynaud phenomena, neuropathy

      d. Rare. Nausea, vomiting, diarrhea, mucositis, abdominal cramps, GI hemorrhage; acute interstitial pneumonitis (especially when administered with mitomycin C); ischemic cardiotoxicity

J. Vincristine (leurocristine, Oncovin)

  1. Indications. A wide variety of malignancies

  2. Pharmacology

    a. Mechanism. Same as vinblastine

    b. Metabolism. Same as vinblastine

  3. Toxicity

    a. A dose-dependent peripheral neuropathy universally develops. Cranial nerves and the autonomic system may also be involved. The neuropathies usually reverse within several months. Jaw, throat, or anterior thigh pain occurring within hours of injection disappears within days and usually does not recur.

      (1) Dose limiting. Severe paresthesias, ataxia, footdrop (slapping gait), muscle-wasting cranial nerve palsies, paralytic ileus, obstipation, abdominal pain, optic atrophy, cortical blindness, seizures

      (2) Not dose limiting. Mild hypoesthesia, mild paresthesias, transient jaw pain (and similar syndromes), loss of deep tendon reflexes, constipation

    b. Common. Alopecia (20% to 50%)

    c. Occasional. Mild leukopenia (does not have significant effect on erythrocytes or platelets), rash; polyuria, urinary retention; acute jaw or joint pain, optic nerve atrophy

    d. Rare. Nausea, vomiting, pancreatitis, fever, SIADH

K. Vincristine liposomal (Marqibo)

  1. Indications. Acute lymphoblastic leukemia

  2. Pharmacology. The same as vincristine

  3. Toxicity

    a. A dose-dependent peripheral neuropathy as vincristine

    b. Common. Myelosuppression

    c. Occasional. Constipation, bowel obstruction, and/or paralytic ileus, fatigue, tumor lysis syndrome, pyrexia

    d. Rare. Hepatotoxicity, cardiac arrest

L. Vindesine (desacetylvinblastine amide sulfate, Eldisine)

  1. Indications. Acute lymphocytic leukemia, lung carcinomas, breast cancer, CML, colorectal cancer

  2. Pharmacology. Same as vinblastine

  3. Toxicity. Same as vinblastine, but alopecia is more common with vindesine. Neurotoxicity is same as for vincristine but is generally less severe.

M. Vinorelbine (Navelbine)

  1. Indications. NSCLC, ovarian cancer, breast cancer, and lymphoma

  2. Pharmacology. A semisynthetic alkaloid derived from vinblastine

    a. Mechanisms. Inhibits tubular polymerization, disrupting formation of tubules during mitosis

    b. Metabolism. The majority of the drug is metabolized in the liver by the CYP microsomal system. Drug and metabolites are excreted in bile.

3. **Toxicity**
   a. **Dose limiting.** Myelosuppression, especially neutropenia
   b. **Common.** Fatigue; mild to moderate peripheral neuropathy; nausea, vomiting, constipation, diarrhea
   c. **Occasional.** Stomatitis; jaw pain, myalgias/arthralgias; allergic-type pulmonary reactions; nausea, vomiting, transient abnormalities in LFTs
   d. **Rare.** Thrombocytopenia; hemorrhagic cystitis, SIADH, interstitial pneumonia

V. OTHER CYTOTOXIC CHEMOTHERAPY AGENTS

A. **Asparaginase** (L-asparaginase, Elspar)
   1. **Indication.** Acute lymphoblastic leukemia
   2. **Pharmacology.** The drug is purified from *Escherichia coli* and/or *Erwinia chrysanthemi.*
      a. **Mechanism.** This enzyme hydrolyzes asparagine into aspartic acid and, to a lesser extent, glutamine into glutamic acid. Leads to inhibition of protein synthesis. Kills cells that cannot synthesize asparagine by destroying extracellular asparagine stores. Cell cycle specific for postmitotic G_1 phase
      b. **Metabolism.** Plasma half-life (8 to 30 hours) is independent of dose. Metabolism is independent of hepatic and renal function. Only trace amounts are recovered in urine.
   3. **Toxicity**
      a. **Dose limiting.**
         (1) **Allergic reactions** (including chills, urticaria, skin rashes, fever, laryngeal constriction, asthma, and anaphylactic shock) are the most frequent. Allergic reactions develop within 1 hour of dosing and are most likely to occur after several doses are given, particularly if the last dose was given more than 1 month previously and if the drug is administered intravenously rather than intramuscularly. Patients who respond to *E. coli* asparaginase but develop allergic reactions may be treated relatively safely with another source of the enzyme (e.g., pegaspargase, *Erwinia* source).
         (2) **Coagulation defects** associated with decreased synthesis of fibrinogen, factor V, factor VIII, protein C, antithrombin III, and variably factors VII and IX. Manifestations are usually subclinical but may result in overt CNS thrombosis or pulmonary embolism.
         (3) **Acute pancreatitis** (15%)
      b. **Common**
         (1) **Immediate effects** (50% to 60%): Fever, chills, nausea, vomiting, abdominal cramps
         (2) **Encephalopathy** in 25% to 50% of patients. Lethargy, somnolence, and confusion tend to occur within the first few days of therapy, reverse after completion of therapy, and are rarely a cause for discontinuing treatment. Hemorrhagic and thrombotic CNS events occur later and are associated with induced imbalances in the coagulation and fibrinolytic systems.
         (3) **Hepatitis:** Abnormal LFTs in more than 50% of treated patients but is rarely severe
         (4) **Prerenal azotemia** (65%); a rise in blood urea nitrogen and blood ammonia levels not evidence of toxicity
         (5) **Hyperglycemia**
         (6) Interferes with **thyroid function tests** for up to 1 month, probably due to marked reduction of thyroxine-binding globulin
      c. **Rare.** Mild to moderate myelosuppression, diarrhea, severe renal failure, hyperthermia, Parkinsonian symptoms, serum ammonia increase

B. Asparaginase, pegylated (PEG-L-asparaginase, polyethylene glycol-L-asparaginase, pegaspargase, Oncaspar)

1. **Indications.** Acute lymphoblastic leukemia (particularly in patients who have had hypersensitivity reactions to native asparaginase). Pegaspargase is *contraindicated* in patients with a history of any of the following with prior L-asparaginase treatment: pancreatitis, serious hemorrhagic events, serious thrombosis.

2. **Pharmacology.** See asparaginase above. The drug is purified from *E. coli*.

3. **Toxicity.** IV administration is associated with higher incidences of adverse effects than IM administration.
   a. **Dose limiting.** Allergic reactions (particularly when given IV), 1% to 10% with no prior asparaginase hypersensitivity; 32% with prior asparaginase hypersensitivity
   b. **Common.** Edema, fever, malaise, rash; coagulopathy (7%); increased transaminases (10%)
   c. **Occasional (1% to 5%).** Hypotension, tachycardia, thrombosis; GI upset, pancreatitis (1% to 2%); headache, seizure, CNS thrombosis or hemorrhage (3%), paresthesias; hyperglycemia, hypoglycemia; arthralgias, myalgias

C. Asparaginase, Erwinia chrysanthemi (Erwinaze)

1. **Indications.** ALL in patients who have developed hypersensitivity to *E. coli*-derived asparaginase

2. **Pharmacology.** See asparaginase above.

3. **Toxicity.**
   a. **Dose limiting.** Serious hypersensitivity reactions, including anaphylaxis
   b. **Common** (>1%). Pancreatitis, abnormal transaminases, coagulation abnormalities including thrombosis and hemorrhage, nausea and vomiting, and hyperglycemia

D. Omacetaxine mepesuccinate (Synribo)

1. **Indication.** Chronic- or accelerated-phase chronic myeloid leukemia (CML) with resistance and/or intolerance to two or more tyrosine kinase inhibitors

2. **Pharmacology.**
   a. **Mechanism.** It inhibits protein translation. It interacts with the ribosomal A-site and prevents the correct positioning of amino acid side chains of incoming aminoacyl-tRNAs.
   b. **Metabolism.** Primarily hydrolyzed by plasma esterases with little hepatic metabolism. The major route of elimination is unknown; small amount is secreted in urine.

3. **Toxicity**
   a. **Dose limiting.** Myelosuppression: severe and fatal thrombocytopenia. Fatal cerebral hemorrhage and severe, nonfatal GI hemorrhage occurred in thrombocytopenic patients.
   b. **Common.** Anemia, neutropenia, diarrhea, nausea, fatigue, asthenia, injection site reaction, pyrexia, infection, hyperglycemia, and lymphopenia
   c. **Rare.** Increased lacrimation, bone pain, myalgia, pharyngolaryngeal pain, nasal congestion, dysphonia

VI. MOLECULARLY TARGETED AGENTS

ALK (Anaplastic lymphoma kinase) inhibitors

A. Alectinib (Alecensa)

1. **Indications.** Metastatic or locally advanced ALK-positive NSCLC that progressed on crizotinib

2. **Pharmacology**
   a. **Mechanisms.** A tyrosine kinase inhibitor that targets ALK and RET, and it has activity even against tumors that are resistant to crizotinib.
   b. **Metabolism.** Metabolized in the liver via CYP3A4 and 98% is excreted in the feces.
3. **Toxicity**
   a. **Dose limiting.** Pneumonitis/interstitial lung disease (0.4%), severe myalgia, and creatine phosphokinase (CPK) elevation
   b. **Common.** Fatigue, constipation, edema, and myalgia
   c. **Occasional.** Hepatotoxicity, bradycardia, including symptomatic bradycardia
   d. **Rare.** Visual disturbances
B. **Ceritinib** (Zykadia)
   1. **Indications.** Metastatic or locally advanced ALK-positive NSCLC that progressed on crizotinib. Lung cancer with ROS1 mutation may also respond to therapy.
   2. **Pharmacology**
      a. **Mechanisms.** A tyrosine kinase inhibitor that targets ALK, insulinlike growth factor 1 receptor (IGF-1R), insulin receptor (InsR), and ROS1, and it has activity even against tumors that are resistant to crizotinib.
      b. **Metabolism.** Metabolized in the liver via CYP3A and 93% is excreted in the feces.
   3. **Toxicity**
      a. **Dose limiting.** Pneumonitis/interstitial lung disease (4%), hepatotoxicity, symptomatic bradycardia
      b. **Common.** Diarrhea, nausea, vomiting, abdominal pain, elevation of LFTs, hyperglycemia, elevation of amylase, lipase, neuropathy, visual disturbances
      c. **Occasional.** QTc prolongation, bradycardia
      d. **Rare.** Pancreatitis
C. **Crizotinib** (Xalkori)
   1. **Indications.** Metastatic or locally advanced ALK-positive NSCLC
   2. **Pharmacology**
      a. **Mechanisms.** TK receptor inhibitor, which inhibits anaplastic lymphoma kinase (ALK), hepatocyte growth factor receptor (HGFR, c-MET), and Recepteur d'Origine Nantais (RON). ALK gene abnormalities may result in expression of oncogenic fusion proteins (e.g., ALK fusion protein). Approximately 5% of patients with NSCLC have the abnormal echinoderm microtubule-associated protein-like 4, or EML4-ALK, gene. This gene has a higher prevalence in patients with adenocarcinoma and in never-smokers or light smokers. Crizotinib selectively inhibits ALK TK and reduces proliferation of cells expressing the genetic alteration. Lung cancer with ROS1 mutation may also respond to crizotinib.
      b. **Metabolism.** Metabolized in the liver via CYP3A4/5
   3. **Toxicity**
      a. **Dose limiting.** Hematosuppression
      b. **Common.** Visual disturbances (60%); nausea, vomiting, diarrhea, constipation, esophageal disorders; lymphocytopenia, abnormal LFTs; edema, fatigue, dizziness, neuropathy
      c. **Occasional.** Neutropenia, bradycardia, headache, rash (10%), arthralgia, cough
      d. **Rare.** Thrombocytopenia, QT_c prolongation

BCL2 inhibitors

D. Venetoclax (Venclexta)

1. **Indications.** CLL with 17p deletion
2. **Pharmacology**
   a. **Mechanisms.** It inhibits BCL-2, an antiapoptotic protein. Overexpression of BCL-2 has been demonstrated in CLL cells where it mediates tumor cell survival and has been associated with resistance to chemotherapeutics.
   b. **Metabolism.** Metabolized in the liver by CYP3A4/5 and eliminated in feces
3. **Toxicity**
   a. **Dose limiting.** Neutropenia
   b. **Common.** Neutropenia, diarrhea, nausea, anemia, upper respiratory tract infection, thrombocytopenia, and fatigue
   c. **Occasional.** Pneumonia, febrile neutropenia, pyrexia, AIHA, anemia, hypokalemia, peripheral edema, headache, cough
   d. **Rare.** Tumor lysis syndrome (premedicate with antihyperuricemics and ensure adequate hydration)

BCR-ABL inhibitors

E. Bosutinib (Bosulif)

1. **Indications.** Chronic, accelerated, or blast-phase Ph+ CML with resistance or intolerance to prior therapy
2. **Pharmacology**
   a. **Mechanisms.** It inhibits the BCR-ABL kinase; it is also an inhibitor of SRC family kinases including Src, Lyn, and Hck.
   b. **Metabolism.** Metabolized in the liver by CYP3A4 and eliminated mainly in feces
3. **Toxicity**
   a. **Dose limiting.** Myelosuppression
   b. **Common.** Diarrhea, nausea, vomiting, abdominal pain, rash, fatigue, thrombocytopenia, anemia, and neutropenia
   c. **Occasional.** Elevation of LFTs, fluid retention (pericardial effusion, pleural effusion, pulmonary edema, and/or peripheral edema)

F. Dasatinib (Sprycel)

1. **Indications.** Chronic, accelerated, or blast phase of CML, Philadelphia-chromosome+ ALL
2. **Pharmacology**
   a. **Mechanisms.** An inhibitor of multiple TKs, including BCR-ABL, SRC family (SRC, LCK, YES, FYN), c-KIT, EPHA2, and PDGFRβ. Based on modeling studies, dasatinib is predicted to bind to multiple conformations of the ABL kinase.
   b. **Metabolism.** Metabolized in the liver and excreted in the feces
3. **Toxicity**
   a. **Dose limiting.** Hematosuppression; bleeding events related to thrombocytopenia but also possibly to drug-induced platelet dysfunction
   b. **Common.** Dose-related fluid retention (which can be severe) especially pleural effusions, diarrhea, various dermatoses, headache, fatigue, rash, dyspnea; hypocalcemia, hypophosphatemia
   c. **Occasional.** Neurologic and muscular disorders, prolongation of QT interval, fever, arthralgia/myalgia

G. Imatinib (Gleevec)

1. **Indications.** CML; GI stromal tumors (GIST) expressing *c-kit* TK; consider use in other conditions expressing *c-kit* or platelet-derived growth

factor receptor-β (PDGFR-β) activation. Imatinib is also approved by treatment of dermatofibrosarcoma protuberans (DFSP), myelodysplastic/myeloproliferative diseases (MDS/MPD), aggressive systemic mastocytosis (ASM), hypereosinophilic syndrome/chronic eosinophilic leukemia (HES/CEL), and relapsed/refractory Philadelphia chromosome–positive ALLs (Ph+ ALL).

2. **Pharmacology**
   a. **Mechanisms.** BCR-ABL encodes a protein, P_{210}BCR-ABL. Imatinib occupies the ATP-binding site of the BCR-ABL protein and other related TKs and thus results in subsequent inhibition of substrate phosphorylation. Imatinib is a potent selective inhibitor of the P_{210}BCR-ABL TK, resulting in inhibition of clonogenicity and tumorigenicity and induction of apoptosis of BCR-ABL and Ph+ cells. It also inhibits other activated ABL TKs (including P_{185}BCR-ABL) and other receptor TKs for PDGFR, stem cell factor (SCF), and *c-kit*.
   b. **Metabolism.** Eliminated mainly in feces. The half-life of the parent drug is 18 hours and of the main metabolites is 40 hours.

3. **Toxicity**
   a. **Dose limiting.** Myelosuppression
   b. **Common.** Transient ankle and periorbital edema that is usually mild to moderate; nausea, vomiting (especially when not taken with food), diarrhea; fatigue, headache, rash, musculoskeletal pain, fever
   c. **Occasional.** Fluid retention with pleural effusion, pulmonary edema, ascites (especially in older patients); night sweats, abnormal LFTs, cough
   d. **Rare.** Severe dermatologic reactions

H. **Nilotinib** (Tasigna)
   1. **Indications.** Chronic, accelerated, or blast phase of CML
   2. **Pharmacology**
      a. **Mechanisms.** It is an inhibitor of BCR-ABL, but it has also activity against PDGFR, c-KIT, CSF-1R, and DDR1.
      b. **Metabolism.** Metabolized extensively in the liver by CYP3A4 and P-glycoprotein and excreted in the feces
   3. **Toxicity.** Electrocardiograms should be obtained to monitor the QTc at baseline, 7 days after initiation of therapy, and periodically thereafter, as well as following any dose adjustment. Electrolytes, divalent cations, and other chemistries as suggested below should be followed periodically.
      a. **Dose limiting.** Myelosuppression. Prolongation of the QT interval, which can result in a type of ventricular tachycardia called *torsades de pointes*, which may result in syncope, seizure, or sudden death.
      b. **Common.** Prolongation of QT interval; rash, pruritus; fatigue, headache; musculoskeletal pain; nausea, vomiting, constipation, diarrhea; insomnia, dizziness; hypomagnesemia, hyperkalemia, hyperglycemia; abnormal LFTs; elevated serum lipase/amylase
      c. **Occasional.** Hypophosphatemia, hypokalemia, hyponatremia, hypocalcemia; hyperthyroidism; interstitial lung disease; pancreatitis; urinary urgency; gynecomastia

I. **Ponatinib** (Iclusig)
   1. **Indications.** Chronic, accelerated, or blast phase Ph+ CML with resistance or intolerance to prior therapy. Philadelphia chromosome–positive ALL (Ph+ALL) that is resistant or intolerant to prior tyrosine kinase inhibitor therapy

   2. Pharmacology

      a. Mechanisms. It inhibits the BCR-ABL kinase, including T315I-mutant ABL; it is also an inhibitor of VEGFR, PDGFR, FGFR, EPH receptors and SRC families of kinases, and KIT, RET, TIE2, and FLT3.

      b. Metabolism. Metabolized in the liver by CYP3A4 and eliminated mainly in feces. It is also metabolized by esterases and/or amidases.

   3. Toxicity

      a. Dose limiting. Cardiovascular, cerebrovascular, and peripheral vascular thrombosis, including fatal myocardial infarction and stroke, hepatotoxicity

      b. Common. Hypertension, pancreatitis, rash, abdominal pain, fatigue, headache, dry skin, constipation, arthralgia, nausea, and pyrexia

      c. Occasional. Congestive heart failure (4%), tumor lysis syndrome, GI perforation, hemorrhage, compromised wound healing

BRAF, MEK inhibitors

J. Cobimetinib (Cotellic)

   1. Indications. Melanoma with a BRAF V600E or V600K mutation, in combination with vemurafenib

   2. Pharmacology

      a. Mechanisms. A reversible inhibitor of mitogen-activated protein kinase (MAPK)/extracellular signal–regulated kinase 1 (MEK1) and MEK2

      b. Metabolism. Metabolized in the liver by CYP3A oxidation and UGT2B7 glucuronidation; eliminated mainly in feces and in 18% in urine

   3. Toxicity

      a. Dose limiting. Cardiomyopathy and serous retinopathy and retinal vein occlusion

      b. Common. Liver laboratory abnormalities, elevation of CPK, diarrhea, photosensitivity reaction, nausea, rash, pyrexia, and vomiting

      c. Occasional. Development of new malignancy, hemorrhage, rhabdomyolysis

K. Dabrafenib (Tafinlar)

   1. Indications. Melanoma with a BRAF V600E mutation

   2. Pharmacology

      a. Mechanisms. An inhibitor of some mutated forms of BRAF kinases: BRAF V600E, BRAF V600K, and BRAF V600D enzymes. Dabrafenib also inhibits wild-type BRAF and CRAF kinases and other kinases such as SIK1, NEK11, and LIMK1.

      b. Metabolism. Metabolized in the liver by CYP2C8 and CYP3A4 and eliminated mainly in feces

   3. Toxicity

      a. Dose limiting. Serious febrile reactions, uveitis, iritis

      b. Common. Hyperkeratosis, headache, pyrexia, arthralgia, papilloma, alopecia, and palmar–plantar erythrodysesthesia syndrome

      c. Occasional. Development of new malignancy, hyperglycemia, nephritis, pancreatitis

      d. Rare. *In vitro*, it increased cell proliferation in BRAF wild-type cells. It may cause hemolytic anemia in patients with glucose-6-phosphate dehydrogenase (G6PD) deficiency

L. Trametinib (Mekinist)

   1. Indications. Melanoma with a BRAF V600E or V600K mutation

2. Pharmacology

    a. Mechanisms. An inhibitor of mitogen-activated protein kinase (MAPK)/ extracellular signal–regulated kinase 1 (MEK1) and MEK2

    b. Metabolism. Metabolized via deacetylation alone or with mono-oxygenation or in combination with glucuronidation. Deacetylation is mediated by hydrolytic enzymes.

3. Toxicity

    a. Dose limiting. Cardiomyopathy and retinal vein occlusion, retinal pigment epithelial detachment

    b. Common. Rash, dermatitis, acneiform rash, palmar–plantar erythrodysesthesia syndrome, erythema

    c. Occasional. Diarrhea, renal failure, rhabdomyolysis, xerostomia, dysgeusia, dizziness

    d. Rare. Interstitial lung disease (1.8%)

M. Vemurafenib (Zelboraf)

  1. Indications. Melanoma with a BRAF V600E mutation

  2. Pharmacology

    a. Mechanisms. An inhibitor of BRAF V600E. It has also activity against CRAF, ARAF, wild-type BRAF, SRMS, ACK1, MAP4K5, and FGR.

    b. Metabolism. Metabolized in the liver by CYP3A4, CYP1A2, or CYP2D6 and eliminated mainly in feces

  3. Toxicity

    a. Dose limiting. Uveitis, iritis

    b. Common. Photosensitivity, liver enzyme elevation, arthralgia, rash, alopecia, fatigue, nausea, pruritus, skin papilloma, palmar–plantar erythrodysesthesia syndrome, keratosis pilaris

    c. Occasional. QTc prolongation

    d. Rare. New primary malignant melanomas

BTK (Bruton tyrosine kinase) inhibitors

N. Ibrutinib (Imbruvica)

  1. Indications. Mantle cell lymphoma (MCL) who have received at least one priortherapy, CLL, Waldenström macroglobulinemia (WM)

  2. Pharmacology

    a. Mechanisms. It forms a covalent bond with a cysteine residue in the BTK active site, leading to inhibition of BTK enzymatic activity. BTK is a signaling molecule of the B-cell antigen receptor (BCR) and cytokine receptor pathways.

    b. Metabolism. Metabolized in the liver by CYP3A and to a minor extent by CYP2D6; eliminated mainly in feces

  3. Toxicity

    a. Dose limiting. Myelosuppression

    b. Common. Hypertension (6% to 17%), atrial fibrillation and atrial flutter (6% to 9%), thrombocytopenia, diarrhea, neutropenia, anemia, fatigue, musculoskeletal pain, peripheral edema, upper respiratory tract infection, nausea, bruising, dyspnea, constipation, rash, abdominal pain, vomiting, and decreased appetite

    c. Occasional. Tumor lysis syndrome. Bleeding events (intracranial hemorrhage [including subdural hematoma], GI bleeding, hematuria, and postprocedural hemorrhage) have occurred in up to 6% of patients.

    d. Rare. Other malignancies (range, 5% to 16%) including nonskin carcinomas (range, 1% to 4%)

CDK (cyclin-dependent kinase) 4/6 inhibitors

O. **Palbociclib** (Ibrance)

1. **Indications.** ER-positive, HER2-negative advanced breast cancer as initial endocrine-based therapy for their metastatic disease in combination with letrozole.
2. **Pharmacology**
   a. **Mechanisms.** It is an inhibitor of CDK 4 and 6. Cyclin D1 and CDK4/6 are downstream of signaling pathways, which lead to cellular proliferation.
   b. **Metabolism.** Metabolized in the liver by CYP3A and sulfotransferase (SULT) enzyme SULT2A1; eliminated mainly in feces, 17% in urine
3. **Toxicity**
   a. **Dose limiting.** Neutropenia
   b. **Common.** Neutropenia, leukopenia, fatigue, anemia, upper respiratory infection, nausea, stomatitis, alopecia, diarrhea, thrombocytopenia, decreased appetite, vomiting, asthenia, peripheral neuropathy, and epistaxis
   c. **Occasional.** Diarrhea. Pulmonary embolism has been reported at a higher rate.

EGFR (Epidermal growth factor receptor) inhibitors

P. **Afatinib** (Gilotrif)

1. **Indications.** The first-line treatment in metastatic NSCLC that has epidermal growth factor receptor (EGFR) exon 19 deletions or exon 21 (L858R) substitution mutations
2. **Pharmacology**
   a. **Mechanisms.** It binds to the kinase domains of EGFR (ErbB1), HER2 (ErbB2), and HER4 (ErbB4) and irreversibly inhibits tyrosine kinase autophosphorylation, resulting in downregulation of ErbB signaling. It has also activity against secondary mutations in EGFR such as T790M.
   b. **Metabolism.** Covalent adducts to proteins are the major circulating metabolites of afatinib and enzymatic metabolism of afatinib is minimal. Excreted mainly in feces (85%)
3. **Toxicity**
   a. **Dose limiting.** Diarrhea
   b. **Common.** Diarrhea, rash/dermatitis acneiform, stomatitis, paronychia, dry skin, decreased appetite, pruritus
   c. **Occasional.** Keratitis, elevation of LFTs, dehydration, epistaxis, pyrexia
   d. **Rare.** Interstitial lung disease (1.5%); severe bullous, blistering, and exfoliating lesions (0.15%); symptomatic left ventricular dysfunction

Q. **Erlotinib** (Tarceva)

1. **Indications.** Locally advanced or metastatic NSCLC that has not progressed after four cycles of platinum-based first-line chemotherapy. Locally advanced or metastatic NSCLC after failure of at least one prior chemotherapy regimen. First-line treatment in pancreatic cancer, in combination with gemcitabine. Erlotinib is not recommended in patients with NSCLC with *KRAS* mutations (or EGFR gene amplification) as they are not likely to benefit from erlotinib treatment. EGFR mutations, specifically exon 19 deletions and exon 21 mutations (L858R), are associated with better response to erlotinib in patients with NSCLC.
2. **Pharmacology**
   a. **Mechanisms.** A selective small molecule inhibitor of the epidermal growth factor receptor (EGFR) TK that results in inhibition of proliferation, growth metastasis, and angiogenesis

   b. **Metabolism.** Metabolized in the liver primarily by the CYP3A4 microsomal enzyme and, to a lesser extent, by CYP1A2. More than 90% of the drug metabolites are excreted in the bile.

3. **Toxicity**
   a. **Dose limiting.** Diarrhea (55%) and rash (75%)
   b. **Common.** Pustular, acneiform rash (oral or gel forms of clindamycin, 2% erythromycin topical gel b.i.d., or minocycline, 100 mg b.i.d. for 5 days, may help); mild dyspnea, cough
   c. **Occasional.** Interstitial lung disease (<1% of patients), keratoconjunctivitis
   d. **Rare.** Interstitial lung disease, microangiopathic hemolytic anemia when combined with gemcitabine

R. **Gefitinib** (Iressa)
   1. **Indications.** The first-line treatment in metastatic NSCLC that has epidermal growth factor receptor (EGFR) exon 19 deletions or exon 21 (L858R) substitution mutations
   2. **Pharmacology**
      a. **Mechanisms.** It reversibly inhibits the kinase activity of wild-type and certain activating mutations of EGFR. The affinity of gefitinib for EGFR exon 19 deletion or exon 21 point mutation L858R mutations is higher than its affinity for the wild-type EGFR.
      b. **Metabolism.** Metabolized in the liver by CYP3A and excreted mainly in feces (86%)
   3. **Toxicity**
      a. **Dose limiting.** Diarrhea, rash
      b. **Common.** Skin reactions (47%) and diarrhea (29%)
      c. **Occasional.** Keratitis, elevation of LFTs, hemorrhagic cystitis, nausea, asthenia, pyrexia, dry mouth, dehydration
      d. **Rare.** Interstitial lung disease (1.3%), GI perforation (0.1%), severe bullous, and exfoliating lesions

S. **Osimertinib** (Tagrisso)
   1. **Indications.** Epidermal growth factor receptor (EGFR) T790M mutation–positive NSCLC
   2. **Pharmacology**
      a. **Mechanisms.** It is a kinase inhibitor of the epidermal growth factor receptor (EGFR), which binds irreversibly to certain mutant forms of EGFR (T790M, L858R, and exon 19 deletion) at approximately 9-fold lower concentrations than wild type.
      b. **Metabolism.** Metabolized in the liver by oxidation (predominantly CYP3A) and dealkylation and excreted mainly in feces (68%)
   3. **Toxicity**
      a. **Dose limiting.** Diarrhea, cardiomyopathy
      b. **Common.** Diarrhea (42%), rash (41%), dry skin, and nail toxicity
      c. **Occasional.** QTc prolongation, neutropenia, fatigue, cough, headache, hyponatremia, hypomagnesemia
      d. **Rare.** Interstitial lung disease (3.3%), cardiomyopathy (1.4%)

HDAC (histone deacetylase) inhibitors:

T. **Belinostat** (Beleodaq)
   1. **Indications.** Relapsed or refractory peripheral T-cell lymphoma
   2. **Pharmacology**
      a. **Mechanisms.** An HDAC inhibitor. HDACs catalyze the removal of acetyl groups from the lysine residues of histones and some nonhistone proteins.

  b. Metabolism. Metabolized in the liver by UGT1A1, to a lesser degree by CYP2A6, CYP2C9, and CYP3A4; excreted mainly in urine
  3. Toxicity
   a. Dose limiting. Thrombocytopenia, neutropenia
   b. Common. Nausea, lymphopenia, fatigue, pyrexia, dyspnea, rash, anemia, and vomiting
   c. Occasional. Hepatotoxicity, tumor lysis syndrome, cough, peripheral edema, pruritus, chills, phlebitis, headache
   d. Rare. Serious and fatal infections

U. Panobinostat (Farydak)
  1. Indications. Multiple myeloma in combination with bortezomib and dexamethasone
  2. Pharmacology
   a. Mechanisms. An HDAC inhibitor. HDACs catalyze the removal of acetyl groups from the lysine residues of histones and some nonhistone proteins.
   b. Metabolism. Metabolized in the liver by CYP3A; excreted mainly in feces
  3. Toxicity
   a. Dose limiting. Thrombocytopenia, neutropenia
   b. Common. Diarrhea, fatigue, nausea, peripheral edema, decreased appetite, pyrexia, vomiting, hypophosphatemia, hypokalemia, hyponatremia, increased creatinine, thrombocytopenia, lymphopenia, leukopenia, neutropenia, and anemia
   c. Occasional. Hepatotoxicity, infections, hypothyroidism, hyperglycemia, dehydration, rash, joint swelling, fatigue
   d. Rare. Fatal and serious cases of GI and pulmonary hemorrhage, cardiac ischemic events

V. Romidepsin (Istodax)
  1. Indications. Cutaneous T-cell lymphoma (CTCL), peripheral T-cell lymphoma (PTCL)
  2. Pharmacology
   a. Mechanisms. An HDAC inhibitor. HDACs catalyze the removal of acetyl groups from the lysine residues of histones and some nonhistone proteins.
   b. Metabolism. Metabolized in the liver by CYP3A4
  3. Toxicity
   a. Dose limiting. Thrombocytopenia, leukopenia (neutropenia and lymphopenia), and anemia
   b. Common. Infections, nausea, fatigue, vomiting, anorexia, anemia, and ECG T-wave change
   c. Occasional. Supraventricular arrhythmia, central line infection, hypotension, hyperuricemia, edema (5%), ventricular arrhythmia, nausea, dehydration, pyrexia, aspartate aminotransferase increased, sepsis, hypophosphatemia and dyspnea (4%), tumor lysis syndrome
   d. Rare. Reactivation of DNA viruses (Epstein-Barr and hepatitis B), pneumonitis

W. Vorinostat (Zolinza)
  1. Indications. Cutaneous T-cell lymphoma (CTCL)
  2. Pharmacology
   a. Mechanisms. It inhibits the enzymatic activity of histone deacetylases HDAC1, HDAC2, and HDAC3 (Class I) and HDAC6 (Class II).

HDACs catalyze the removal of acetyl groups from the lysine residues of histones and some nonhistone proteins.

  b. **Metabolism.** Metabolized by glucuronidation and hydrolysis followed by β-oxidation; eliminated predominantly through metabolism with <1% of the dose recovered as unchanged drug in urine

3. **Toxicity**
   a. **Dose limiting.** Thrombocytopenia, anemia
   b. **Common.** Diarrhea, fatigue, nausea, thrombocytopenia, anorexia, dysgeusia
   c. **Occasional.** Vomiting, hyperglycemia, GI bleeding, muscle spasms, alopecia, dry mouth, increased creatinine level, dizziness, peripheral edema
   d. **Rare.** Pulmonary embolism and deep vein thrombosis

HER2 (human epidermal growth factor receptor 2) inhibitors
X. **Lapatinib** (Tykerb)
  1. **Indications.** In combination with capecitabine for the treatment of patients with advanced or metastatic breast cancers that overexpress HER2 and who have received prior therapy, including an anthracycline, a taxane, and trastuzumab. Also, in combination with letrozole for the treatment of postmenopausal women with hormone receptor–positive metastatic breast cancer that overexpresses the HER2 receptor for whom hormonal therapy is indicated
  2. **Pharmacology**
     a. **Mechanisms.** Lapatinib is a 4-anilinoquinazoline kinase inhibitor of the intracellular TK domains of both EGFR (ErbB1) and of HER2 (ErbB2). *In vitro* studies showed an additive effect with 5-FU, the active metabolite of capecitabine.
     b. **Metabolism.** Lapatinib undergoes extensive metabolism, primarily by CYP3A4, CYP3A5, and P-glycoprotein. There is negligible renal excretion.
  3. **Toxicity** of lapatinib plus capecitabine
     a. **Dose limiting.** Diarrhea, serious adverse events
     b. **Common.** Diarrhea (65%), nausea, vomiting; fatigue, palmar–plantar erythrodysesthesia (50%, due to capecitabine), rash; elevated LFTs (40%); hematosuppression (20%); prolonged QT interval
     c. **Occasional.** Decreased left ventricular ejection fraction (LVEF, 2%)
     d. **Rare.** Pulmonary toxicity, hepatotoxicity (including fatalities)

JAK (Janus-associated kinase) inhibitors
Y. **Ruxolitinib** (Jakafi)
  1. **Indications.** Intermediate or high-risk myelofibrosis, including primary myelofibrosis, post–polycythemia vera myelofibrosis and post–essential thrombocythemia myelofibrosis
  2. **Pharmacology**
     a. **Mechanisms.** It inhibits JAK1 and JAK2. JAK signaling involves recruitment of STATs (signal transducers and activators of transcription) to cytokine receptors and activation and subsequent localization of STATs to the nucleus leading to modulation of gene expression.
     b. **Metabolism.** Metabolized in the liver by CYP3A and excreted mainly in urine (74%), and partially in feces
  3. **Toxicity**
     a. **Dose limiting.** Thrombocytopenia (reversible, managed by reducing the dose or temporarily withholding the drug)

   b. Common. Thrombocytopenia, anemia, neutropenia, bruising, dizziness, and headache

   c. Occasional. Weight gain, flatulence, herpes zoster reactivation, urinary tract infections

   d. Rare. Liver enzyme elevation, cholesterol elevation

mTOR (mammalian target of rapamycin) inhibitors

Z. **Everolimus** (Afinitor)

1. **Indications.** Hormone receptor–positive, HER2-negative breast cancer in combination with exemestane, neuroendocrine tumors of pancreatic origin (PNET), neuroendocrine tumors (NET) of GI or lung origin, advanced renal cell carcinoma, renal angiomyolipoma, and tuberous sclerosis complex

2. **Pharmacology**

   a. Mechanisms. Inhibitor of mTOR, a serine–threonine kinase, downstream of the P13K/AKT pathway. Everolimus binds to an intracellular protein resulting in a complex that inhibits mTOR kinase activity and downstream effectors of mTOR involved in protein synthesis. Additionally, the drug reduces expression of hypoxia-inducible factors (HIF-1) and of VEGF.

   b. Metabolism. Extensively metabolized in the liver by CYP3A4. Metabolites are excreted in the feces.

3. **Toxicity**

   a. Dose limiting. Immunosuppression resulting in bacterial or fungal infections

   b. Common. Stomatitis, GI disturbance; fatigue; hematosuppression; hyperglycemia, hyperlipidemia, hypophosphatemia, transaminase elevation; fever; peripheral edema; nephrotoxicity; cough, dyspnea, anemia, thrombocytopenia, leukopenia.

   c. Occasional. Epistaxis, interstitial pneumonia, nail disorders, hand–foot syndrome; hypertension, headache, tremor

   d. Rare. Angioedema, renal failure

AA. **Temsirolimus** (Torisel)

1. **Indications.** Advanced renal cell carcinoma

2. **Pharmacology**

   a. Mechanisms. Inhibitor of mTOR that controls cell division, resulting in growth arrest in the G_1 phase of the cell cycle and reduced levels of hypoxia-inducible factors (HIF-1 and HIF-2) and of VEGF

   b. Metabolism. Extensively metabolized via the CYP 3A4 hepatic microsomal pathway into metabolites, including sirolimus (the principle active metabolite). Elimination is primarily through the feces.

3. **Toxicity**

   a. Dose limiting. Hypersensitivity reactions or end organ damage (see below)

   b. Common. Myelosuppression, anorexia; dysgeusia; mucositis, diarrhea, constipation; rash, asthenia, edema; delayed wound healing; hyperglycemia, hyperlipidemia (may require cholesterol-lowering agents), hypokalemia, hypophosphatemia, elevated serum creatinine, abnormal LFTs

   c. Occasional. Interstitial lung disease, headache, lacrimation, arthralgia/myalgias, chest pain, intracerebral hemorrhage (with brain metastasis or anticoagulant therapy)

   d. Rare. Fatal interstitial lung disease, bowel perforation, or acute renal failure

PARP (poly (ADP-ribose) polymerase) inhibitors

BB. **Olaparib** (Lynparza)

1. **Indications.** Patients with deleterious or suspected deleterious germline BRCA-mutated advanced ovarian cancer who have been treated with three or more prior lines of chemotherapy

2. **Pharmacology**
   a. **Mechanisms.** It inhibits PARP1, PARP2, and PARP3. PARP enzymes are involved in normal cellular homeostasis, such as DNA transcription, cell cycle regulation, and DNA repair.
   b. **Metabolism.** Metabolized in the liver by CYP3A4 and excreted in urine (44%) and in feces (42%)

3. **Toxicity**
   a. **Dose limiting.** Anemia
   b. **Common.** Anemia, nausea, fatigue (including asthenia), vomiting, diarrhea, dysgeusia, dyspepsia, headache, decreased appetite, nasopharyngitis/pharyngitis/URI, cough, arthralgia/musculoskeletal pain, myalgia, back pain, dermatitis/rash, abdominal pain/discomfort, increase in creatinine, mean corpuscular volume elevation, anemia, lymphopenia, neutropenia, thrombocytopenia
   c. **Occasional.** Stomatitis, peripheral neuropathy, pyrexia, hypomagnesemia, hyperglycemia, anxiety, depression, insomnia, dysuria, urinary incontinence, vulvovaginal disorder, dry skin/ eczema, pruritis, hypertension, venous thrombosis (including pulmonary embolism), and hot flush
   d. **Rare.** Pneumonitis, MDS/AML

PI3Kδ (phosphatidylinositol 3-kinase) inhibitors

CC. **Idelalisib** (Zydelig)

1. **Indications.** Relapsed CLL, in combination with rituximab, relapsed follicular B-cell NHL (FL), relapsed small lymphocytic lymphoma (SLL)

2. **Pharmacology**
   a. **Mechanisms.** It inhibits PI3Kδ, inhibits several cell signaling pathways, including B-cell receptor (BCR) signaling and the CXCR4 and CXCR5 signaling, which are involved in trafficking and homing of B cells to the lymph nodes and bone marrow.
   b. **Metabolism.** Metabolized in the liver by aldehyde oxidase and CYP3A and excreted in urine (49%) and in feces (44%)

3. **Toxicity**
   a. **Dose limiting.** Hepatotoxicity (fatal and/or serious hepatotoxicity occurred in 14% of patients), diarrhea (severe diarrhea or colitis occurred in 14%)
   b. **Common.** Diarrhea, pyrexia, fatigue, nausea, cough, pneumonia, abdominal pain, chills, rash, neutropenia, hypertriglyceridemia, hyperglycemia, ALT elevations, and AST elevations
   c. **Occasional.** Peripheral edema, upper respiratory infections, headache, insomnia
   d. **Rare.** Pneumonitis, intestinal perforation

Proteasome inhibitors

DD. **Bortezomib** (Velcade)

1. **Indication.** Multiple myeloma, mantle cell lymphoma

2. **Pharmacology.**
   a. **Mechanisms.** Reversible inhibitor of the chymotrypsin-like activity of the 26S proteasome, which is a large protein complex that degrades ubiquitinated proteins, which are involved in regulating the intracellular

concentration of specific proteins. Disruption of this pathway affects multiple signaling pathways within the cell, leading to cell death. Down-regulates the NK-κB pathway, leading to inhibition of cell growth

    b. Metabolism. Metabolized via hepatic P450 3A4 (CYPEA4) enzymes. Elimination is not well characterized.

  3. Toxicity

    a. Dose limiting. Peripheral neuropathy (predominantly sensory), hematosuppression (especially dose-related thrombocytopenia with nadir at day 11)

    b. Common. Fatigue, fever (up to 40%), headache, GI disturbance (anorexia, nausea, vomiting, diarrhea, constipation), arthralgia, neuralgia, vomiting, lymphopenia, neutropenia

    c. Occasional. Hypotension (10%); motor neuropathy, blurred vision, myalgia; congestive heart failure; toxic epidermal necrolysis

    d. Rare. Interstitial pneumonia and acute respiratory distress syndrome, reversible posterior leukoencephalopathy syndrome, acute hepatic failure

EE. Carfilzomib (Kyprolis)

  1. Indication. Multiple myeloma

  2. Pharmacology.

    a. Mechanisms. A tetrapeptide epoxyketone proteasome inhibitor that irreversibly binds to the N-terminal threonine-containing active sites of the 20S proteasome, the proteolytic core particle within the 26S proteasome

    b. Metabolism. Metabolized in the liver by peptidase cleavage and epoxide hydrolysis; it is largely cleared extrahepatically, 25% excretion in the urine.

  3. Toxicity

    a. Dose limiting. Thrombocytopenia

    b. Common. Anemia, fatigue, thrombocytopenia, nausea, pyrexia, dyspnea, diarrhea, headache, cough, edema peripheral, infusion reactions

    c. Occasional. Insomnia, muscle spasm, cough, upper respiratory tract infection, hypokalemia, heart failure, hypertension, hypotension, venous thrombosis (thromboprophylaxis is recommended)

    d. Rare. Acute renal failure, tumor lysis syndrome, pulmonary toxicity, pulmonary hypertension, reversible posterior leukoencephalopathy syndrome, acute hepatic failure, thrombotic microangiopathy

FF. Ixazomib (Ninlaro)

  1. Indication. Multiple myeloma

  2. Pharmacology

    a. Mechanisms. A reversible proteasome inhibitor. Ixazomib preferentially binds and inhibits the chymotrypsin-like activity of the beta 5 subunit of the 20S proteasome.

    b. Metabolism. Metabolized in the liver by multiple CYP enzymes and non-CYP proteins; it is mainly excreted in urine (62%) and feces (22%).

  3. Toxicity

    a. Dose limiting. Thrombocytopenia, peripheral neuropathy, diarrhea

    b. Common. Diarrhea, constipation, thrombocytopenia, neutropenia, peripheral neuropathy, rash, nausea, peripheral edema, vomiting, and back pain

    c. Occasional. Liver enzyme elevation, blurred vision, conjunctivitis

    d. Rare. Acute febrile neutrophilic dermatosis (Sweet syndrome), Stevens-Johnson syndrome, transverse myelitis, posterior reversible encephalopathy syndrome, tumor lysis syndrome, and thrombotic thrombocytopenic purpura

SMO (Smoothened)/Hedgehog pathway inhibitors

GG. **Sonidegib** (Odomzo)
1. **Indications.** Locally advanced basal cell carcinoma (BCC)
2. **Pharmacology**
   a. **Mechanisms.** It is an inhibitor of the Hedgehog pathway. Sonidegib binds to and inhibits Smoothened, a transmembrane protein involved in Hedgehog signal transduction.
   b. **Metabolism.** Metabolized in the liver by CYP3A and excreted in feces (70%) and in urine (30%)
3. **Toxicity**
   a. **Dose limiting.** Muscle spasm, dysgeusia
   b. **Common.** Muscle spasms, alopecia, dysgeusia, fatigue, nausea, musculoskeletal pain, diarrhea, decreased weight, decreased appetite, myalgia, abdominal pain, headache, pain, vomiting, pruritus, increased creatinine, CPK, lipase, amylase, LFTs, hyperglycemia
   c. **Occasional.** Anemia, lymphopenia
   d. **Rare.** It can cause embryo–fetal death or severe birth defects (verify the pregnancy status, use barrier contraception). Blood should not be donated for at least 20 months after the last dose.

HH. **Vismodegib** (Erivedge)
1. **Indications.** Metastatic or locally advanced basal cell carcinoma (BCC)
2. **Pharmacology**
   a. **Mechanisms.** It is an inhibitor of the Hedgehog pathway. Vismodegib binds to and inhibits Smoothened, a transmembrane protein involved in Hedgehog signal transduction.
   b. **Metabolism.** Metabolized in the liver by CYP2C9 and CYP3A4/5 and excreted mainly in feces (84%)
3. **Toxicity**
   a. **Dose limiting.** Muscle spasm, dysgeusia
   b. **Common.** Muscle spasms, alopecia, dysgeusia, weight loss, fatigue, nausea, diarrhea, decreased appetite, constipation, arthralgias, vomiting, and ageusia
   c. **Occasional.** Hyponatremia, azotemia, hypokalemia, amenorrhea
   d. **Rare.** It can cause embryo–fetal death or severe birth defects (verify the pregnancy status, use barrier contraception). Blood should not be donated for at least 7 months after the last dose.

VEGFR (Vascular Endothelial Growth Factor Receptor) inhibitors

II. **Axitinib** (Inlyta)
1. **Indications.** Advanced renal cell carcinoma after failure of one prior systemic therapy
2. **Pharmacology**
   a. **Mechanisms.** It inhibits VEGFR-1, VEGFR-2, and VEGFR-3.
   b. **Metabolism.** Metabolized in the liver mainly by CYP3A4/5 and excreted in feces (41%) and in urine (23%)
3. **Toxicity**
   a. **Dose limiting.** Hypertension (even hypertensive crisis has been observed)
   b. **Common.** Diarrhea, hypertension, fatigue, decreased appetite, nausea, dysphonia, palmar–plantar erythrodysesthesia (hand–foot) syndrome, weight decreased, vomiting, asthenia, and constipation
   c. **Occasional.** Hypothyroidism, liver enzyme elevation, proteinuria, dizziness, myalgia, abdominal pain, anemia, hemorrhoids, hematuria, tinnitus, increased lipase level

    d. Rare. Arterial and venous thrombotic events, bleeding, GI perforation and fistula formation, reversible posterior leukoencephalopathy syndrome

JJ. Cabozantinib (Cometriq, Cabometyx)

  1. Indications. Cabometyx: advanced renal cell carcinoma after failure of one prior systemic therapy. Cometriq: progressive, metastatic medullary thyroid cancer

  2. Pharmacology

    a. Mechanisms. It inhibits the tyrosine kinase activity of RET; MET; VEGFR-1, VEGFR-2, and VEGFR-3; KIT; TRKB; FLT-3; AXL; and TIE-2.

    b. Metabolism. Metabolized in the liver mainly by CYP3A4 and excreted in feces (54%) and in urine (27%)

  3. Toxicity

    a. Dose limiting. Thrombotic events (discontinue cabozantinib for myocardial infarction, cerebral infarction, or other serious arterial thromboembolic events), hypertension

    b. Common. Diarrhea, stomatitis, palmar–plantar erythrodysesthesia syndrome (PPES), decreased weight, decreased appetite, nausea, fatigue, oral pain, hair color changes, dysgeusia, hypertension, abdominal pain, constipation, increased AST, increased ALT, lymphopenia, increased alkaline phosphatase, hypocalcemia, neutropenia, thrombocytopenia, hypophosphatemia, and hyperbilirubinemia

    c. Occasional. Proteinuria, hypothyroidism, dehydration

    d. Rare. Wound dehiscence, osteonecrosis of the jaw, reversible posterior leukoencephalopathy syndrome

KK. Lenvatinib (Lenvima)

  1. Indications. Recurrent or metastatic, progressive, radioactive iodine-refractory differentiated thyroid cancer; renal cell carcinoma (in combination with everolimus)

  2. Pharmacology

    a. Mechanisms. It inhibits the kinase activities of VEGFR1 (FLT1); VEGFR2 (KDR); VEGFR3 (FLT4); fibroblast growth factor (FGF) receptors FGFR1, 2, 3, and 4; the PDGFR alpha (PDGFRα); KIT; and RET.

    b. Metabolism. Metabolized in the liver mainly by CYP3A and excreted in feces (64%) and in urine (25%)

  3. Toxicity

    a. Dose limiting. Hypertension, cardiac failure

    b. Common. Hypertension, fatigue, diarrhea, arthralgia/myalgia, decreased appetite, weight decreased, nausea, stomatitis, headache, vomiting, proteinuria, palmar–plantar erythrodysesthesia syndrome, abdominal pain, dysphonia

    c. Occasional. Hepatotoxicity, renal impairment, hypocalcemia, hypothyroidism, QTc prolongation

    d. Rare. Arterial thromboembolic events, GI perforation and fistula, hemorrhagic events, reversible posterior leukoencephalopathy syndrome

LL. Pazopanib (Votrient)

  1. Indications. Advanced renal cell carcinoma, advanced soft tissue sarcoma who have received prior chemotherapy

  2. Pharmacology

    a. Mechanisms. Pazopanib inhibits VEGFR-1, VEGFR-2, VEGFR-3, PDGFR-α and -β, fibroblast growth factor receptor (FGFR)-1 and -3, cytokine receptor (Kit), interleukin-2 receptor–inducible T-cell kinase

(Itk), leukocyte-specific protein tyrosine kinase (Lck), and transmembrane glycoprotein receptor tyrosine kinase (cFms).

b. **Metabolism.** The drug is extensively metabolized in the liver by CYP3A4 and eliminated primarily in the feces; <4% is eliminated in the urine.

3. **Toxicity**

a. **Dose limiting.** Hepatotoxicity, QT prolongation and torsades de pointes, GI perforation, hemorrhagic events, arterial thrombotic events

b. **Common.** Elevated serum transaminases (18%, particularly during the first 4 months of treatment); anorexia, nausea, vomiting, diarrhea; hypertension (40%); fatigue; hair color change; hematosuppression (about 33%), hypomagnesemia

c. **Occasional.** Alopecia, palmar–plantar dysesthesia, rash; dysgeusia, dyspepsia; QT prolongation and torsades de pointes (<2%), hemorrhagic events (13%), arterial thrombotic events, delayed wound healing, hypothyroidism, proteinuria

d. **Rare.** Arterial thromboembolic events, thrombotic microangiopathy, GI perforation and fistula, hemorrhagic events, interstitial lung disease, reversible posterior leukoencephalopathy syndrome

MM. **Regorafenib** (Stivarga)

1. **Indications.** Metastatic colorectal cancer (CRC) that has been previously treated with fluoropyrimidine-, oxaliplatin-, and irinotecan-based chemotherapy, an anti-VEGF therapy, and, if KRAS wild type, an anti-EGFR therapy; locally advanced, unresectable or metastatic GIST that has been previously treated with imatinib mesylate and sunitinib malate

2. **Pharmacology**

a. **Mechanisms.** It inhibits RET, VEGFR1, VEGFR2, VEGFR3, KIT, PDGFR-alpha, PDGFR-beta, FGFR1, FGFR2, TIE2, DDR2, TrkA, Eph2A, RAF-1, BRAF, BRAFV600E, SAPK2, PTK5, and Abl.

b. **Metabolism.** Metabolized in the liver by CYP3A4 and UGT1A9, and excreted in feces (71%) and in urine (19%)

3. **Toxicity**

a. **Dose limiting.** Hypertension, cardiac ischemia, and infarction

b. **Common.** Asthenia/fatigue, hand–foot skin reaction, diarrhea, decreased appetite/food intake, hypertension, mucositis, dysphonia, infection, pain (not otherwise specified), decreased weight, GI and abdominal pain, rash, fever, and nausea

c. **Occasional.** Hepatotoxicity, elevation of amylase, lipase, hypokalemia, hypophosphatemia, hyponatremia, leukopenia, thrombocytopenia, QTc prolongation

d. **Rare.** Wound healing problems, GI perforation and fistula, hemorrhagic events, reversible posterior leukoencephalopathy syndrome

NN. **Sorafenib** (Nexavar)

1. **Indications.** Metastatic renal cell carcinoma; unresectable hepatocellular carcinoma

2. **Pharmacology**

a. **Mechanisms.** It inhibits multiple intracellular (CRAF, BRAF, and mutant BRAF) and cell surface kinases (KIT, FLT-3, RET, VEGFR-1, VEGFR-2, VEGFR-3, and PDGFR-ß).

b. **Metabolism.** Metabolized by CYPA34 and hepatic UGT1A9 glucuronidation. Approximately 80% of the drug and its metabolites are excreted in the feces and 20% in the urine.

3. **Toxicity**
   a. **Dose limiting.** Skin reactions or unacceptable toxicities
   b. **Common.** Rash/desquamation, hand–foot skin reaction; hypertension; diarrhea, alopecia, anemia; fatigue
   c. **Occasional.** Granulocytopenia, thrombocytopenia; bleeding events, vomiting, myocardial ischemia, increased serum lipase or amylase; sensory neuropathy, headache; arthralgia/myalgia
   d. **Rare.** Hypothyroidism, pancreatitis

OO. **Sunitinib malate** (Sutent)
   1. **Indications.** Metastatic renal cell carcinoma; GIST after progression on imatinib; progressive pancreatic neuroendocrine tumors
   2. **Pharmacology**
      a. **Mechanisms.** It inhibits PDGFRs (PDGFRα and PDGFRβ); VEGFR1, VEGFR2, and VEGFR3; SCF receptor (KIT); Fms-like tyrosine kinase-3 (FLT3); colony-stimulating factor receptor type 1 (CSF-1R); and the glial cell line–derived neurotrophic factor receptor (RET).
      b. **Metabolism.** The drug and its active metabolite are metabolized primarily by the p450 enzyme CYP3A4. More than 80% of the drug is eliminated via feces.
   3. **Toxicity**
      a. **Dose limiting.** Hematosuppression, bleeding
      b. **Common.** Bleeding events (epistaxis and elsewhere); hypertension; anorexia, diarrhea, mucositis, nausea/vomiting; fatigue; altered taste; yellow skin discoloration (one-third of patients), rash
      c. **Occasional.** Peripheral neuropathy, anorexia, periorbital edema, lacrimation; prolonged QT interval on electrocardiogram, left ventricular dysfunction, deep vein thrombosis; hypothyroidism, adrenal insufficiency, hypoglycemia, hypocalcemia, hypophosphatemia, hyponatremia, hypernatremia, hypokalemia, hyperkalemia, elevated serum lipase or amylase levels; musculoskeletal pain, reversible hair depigmentation, alopecia; fever
      d. **Rare.** Adrenal insufficiency, severe hemorrhage, microangiopathic hemolytic anemia (with bevaciz+umab)

PP. **Vandetanib** (Caprelsa)
   1. **Indications.** Medullary thyroid cancer in patients with unresectable locally advanced or metastatic disease
   2. **Pharmacology**
      a. **Mechanisms.** It inhibits VEGFR.
      b. **Metabolism.** Metabolized in the liver by CYP3A4 and FMO1 and FMO3, and excreted in feces (44%) and in urine (25%)
   3. **Toxicity**
      a. **Dose limiting.** QTc prolongation (torsades de pointes and sudden death have occurred), hypertension
      b. **Common.** Diarrhea/colitis, rash, acneiform dermatitis, hypertension, nausea, headache, upper respiratory tract infections, decreased appetite, and abdominal pain
      c. **Occasional.** Hypothyroidism, asthenia, fatigue, pyrexia, elevated creatinine, dysgeusia
      d. **Rare.** Interstitial lung disease, ischemic cerebrovascular events, hemorrhage, heart failure, reversible posterior leukoencephalopathy syndrome

VII. MONOCLONAL ANTIBODIES

A. **Monoclonal antibodies** are proteins secreted by one clone of immune cells and each type has single specificity. They are currently used as a part of anticancer systemic therapy, but they are also extensively used in the diagnostic processes.

1. **Mechanisms**
   a. **Direct binding of antigens on cancer cells,** for example, CD20 on lymphoma cell (rituximab), Her2 on breast cancer cells (trastuzumab, pertuzumab), and EGFR on colon cancer cells (cetuximab, panitumumab)
   b. **Binding of soluble antigens** that affect tumor growth/survival, for example, bevacizumab binds to soluble VEGF or siltuximab binds to interleukin 6
   c. **Binding of antigens on immune cells** and enhancing anticancer immune responses, for example, CTLA4 (ipilimumab) or PD-1 (pembrolizumab, nivolumab)
   d. **Delivery of toxins into cancer cells,** for example, ado-trastuzumab emtansine that carries DM1 (a microtubule inhibitor) recognizes Her2 and allows for delivery of DM1 specifically to cells that are Her2+.
   e. **Bispecific antibodies.** These are antibodies of 2, and not 1, specificity. Bispecific T-cell engager (BiTE) is an example of the use of bispecific antibodies. Blinatumomab binds to CD19 on leukemic cells and CD3 on T cells and directs T cells into proximity of leukemic cells.

2. **Structure**
   a. **Chimeric antibodies** (e.g., rituximab, cetuximab) are antibodies made by fusing the antigen-binding region (variable domains of the heavy and light chains, VH, and VL) from one species like a mouse, with the human constant domain.
   b. **Humanized antibodies** (e.g., trastuzumab, pembrolizumab) in which only CDR-coding segments (responsible for the desired binding properties) originated from mice and are inserted into a fully human antibody backbone
   c. **Human antibodies** (e.g., nivolumab, panitumumab) are fully human proteins generated in transgenic mice in which the genes encoding antibodies have been replaced with human genes.

B. **Ado-trastuzumab emtansine** (Kadcyla)

1. **Indications.** HER2-positive, metastatic breast cancer that has previously been treated with trastuzumab and a taxane

2. **Pharmacology**
   a. **Mechanisms.** Ado-trastuzumab emtansine is a HER2-targeted antibody–drug conjugate. The antibody is the humanized anti-HER2 IgG1, trastuzumab. The small molecule cytotoxin, DM1, is a microtubule inhibitor. Upon binding to subdomain IV of the HER2 receptor, ado-trastuzumab emtansine undergoes receptor-mediated internalization and subsequent lysosomal degradation, resulting in intracellular release of DM1-containing cytotoxic catabolites.
   b. **Metabolism.** Metabolized primarily in the liver by CYP3A4/5. The elimination half-life ($t_{1/2}$) is approximately 4 days.

3. **Toxicity**
   a. **Dose limiting.** Hepatotoxicity and cardiac failure
   b. **Common.** Fatigue, nausea, musculoskeletal pain, hemorrhage, thrombocytopenia, headache, increased transaminases, constipation, and epistaxis
   c. **Occasional.** Pneumonitis, infusion reactions, bleeding, peripheral neuropathy, hypokalemia
   d. **Rare.** Liver failure and death have occurred.

C. **Alemtuzumab** (Campath)
1. **Indications.** T-cell prolymphocytic leukemia; relapsed or refractory B-cell CLL
2. **Pharmacology**
    a. **Mechanisms.** It binds to CD52, an antigen present on the surface of B and T lymphocytes, a majority of monocytes, macrophages, NK cells, and a subpopulation of granulocytes. The proposed mechanism of action is antibody-dependent cellular-mediated lysis following cell surface binding of alemtuzumab to the leukemic cells.
    b. **Metabolism.** The half-life is about 12 days with minimal clearance by the liver and kidneys. Steady-state levels are reached by the sixth week. CD4+ and CD8+ counts may take more than 1 year to return to normal.
3. **Toxicity**
    a. **Dose limiting.** Significant immunosuppression with increased incidence of opportunistic infections; myelosuppression
    b. **Common.** Infusion reaction usually occurs within the first week of therapy. Hypertension, rash, fever, rigors
    c. **Occasional.** Pancytopenia, supraventricular tachycardia; nausea, vomiting, diarrhea
    d. **Rare.** Anaphylaxis
D. **Atezolizumab** (Tecentriq)
1. **Indications.** Locally advanced or metastatic urothelial carcinoma and non-small cell lung cancer
2. **Pharmacology**
    a. **Mechanisms.** Atezolizumab is an Fc-engineered, humanized, monoclonal antibody that binds to PD-L1 and blocks interactions with the PD-1 and B7.1 receptors. PD-L1 may be expressed on tumor cells and/or tumor-infiltrating immune cells and can contribute to the inhibition of the antitumor immune response in the tumor microenvironment.
    b. **Metabolism.** The elimination half-life is approximately 27 days.
3. **Toxicity**
    a. **Dose limiting.** Immune-mediated adverse events such as pneumonitis, colitis, endocrinopathies, encephalitis, hepatitis, pancreatitis, myasthenia gravis
    b. **Common.** Fatigue, decreased appetite, nausea, urinary tract infection, pyrexia, and constipation
    c. **Occasional.** Meningitis, encephalitis, motor and sensory neuropathy, abdominal pain, venous thromboembolism, urinary tract obstruction
    d. **Rare.** Infusion reactions
E. **Bevacizumab** (Avastin)
1. **Indications.** Advanced colorectal cancer, nonsquamous NSCLC, glioblastoma, cervical cancer, ovarian cancer, fallopian tube cancer, primary peritoneal carcinoma
2. **Pharmacology.** Bevacizumab is a humanized monoclonal antibody from genetically engineered cells designed to block the action of vascular endothelial growth factor (VEGF). VEGF is a protein that is secreted from malignant and nonmalignant hypoxic cells and stimulates new blood vessel formation by binding to specific receptors. Metabolism of bevacizumab has not been characterized.
3. **Toxicity**
    a. **Dose limiting.** Thromboembolism (e.g., transient ischemic attack, stroke, angina pectoris, myocardial infarction), GI perforation, wound dehiscence
    b. **Common.** Hypertension (severe in 15%), proteinuria, bleeding (especially epistaxis or GI), infusion reactions, fatigue, abdominal pain, impaired wound healing, constipation, diarrhea

   c. **Occasional**. Leukopenia, thrombocytopenia, hypersensitivity, taste disorders, sensory neuropathy
   d. **Rare.** Bowel perforation, reversible posterior leukoencephalopathy syndrome (RPLS), nephrotic syndrome, hypertensive crisis
F. **Blinatumomab** (Blincyto)
   1. **Indications.** Philadelphia chromosome–negative relapsed or refractory B-cell precursor ALL
   2. **Pharmacology**
      a. **Mechanisms.** Blinatumomab is a bispecific CD19-directed CD3 T-cell engager that binds to CD19 expressed on the surface of cells of B-lineage origin and to CD3 expressed on the surface of T cells. It activates endogenous T cells by connecting CD3 in the T-cell receptor (TCR) complex with CD19 on benign and malignant B cells. Blinatumomab mediates the formation of a synapse between the T cell and the tumor cell, upregulation of cell adhesion molecules, production of cytolytic proteins, release of inflammatory cytokines, and proliferation of T cells, which result in redirected lysis of CD19+ cells.
      b. **Metabolism.** The mean half-life is 2 hours.
   3. **Toxicity**
      a. **Dose limiting.** Cytokine release syndrome (CRS), which may be life-threatening or fatal. Neurological toxicities have occurred in approximately 50% of patients (encephalopathy, convulsions, speech disorders, disturbances in consciousness, confusion and disorientation, and coordination and balance disorders). The majority of events resolved following interruption.
      b. **Common.** Pyrexia, headache, peripheral edema, febrile neutropenia, nausea, hypokalemia, tremor, rash, constipation
      c. **Occasional**. Increased alanine aminotransferase, increased aspartate aminotransferase, increased total bilirubin, anemia, thrombocytopenia, neutropenia, infections, electrolyte abnormalities
      d. **Rare.** Tumor lysis syndrome, leukoencephalopathy
G. **Brentuximab vedotin** (Adcetris)
   1. **Indications.** Refractory Hodgkin lymphoma and refractory systemic anaplastic large cell lymphoma
   2. **Pharmacology**
      a. **Mechanisms.** An antibody drug conjugate consisting of a CD30-specific chimeric IgG1 antibody, a microtubule-disrupting agent (monomethyl auristatin E, MMAE), and a protease cleavable dipeptide linker that covalently binds MMAE to the antibody. MMAE disrupts the cellular microtubule network and induces cell cycle arrest at the G2/M phase.
      b. **Metabolism.** Minimally metabolized, primarily in the liver via oxidation by CYP3A4/5. A terminal half-life of approximately 4 to 6 days
   3. **Toxicity**
      a. **Dose limiting.** Neutropenia, neuropathy
      b. **Common.** Hematosuppression; infusion reactions; fatigue, fever; peripheral sensory neuropathy, arthralgia/myalgia, headache, dizziness, insomnia, anxiety; anorexia, nausea, vomiting, diarrhea, constipation; upper respiratory tract infections; rash, pruritus.
      c. **Occasional.** Peripheral motor neuropathy, oropharyngeal pain; alopecia; chills, shortness of breath; supraventricular arrhythmia, edema; antibrentuximab antibody formation
      d. **Rare.** Anaphylaxis, progressive multifocal leukoencephalopathy, Stevens-Johnson syndrome, tumor lysis syndrome

H. Cetuximab (Erbitux)

1. **Indications.** EGFR-expressing metastatic colon cancer after failure of both irinotecan- and oxaliplatin-based regimens; squamous cell carcinoma of the head and neck. Metastatic colorectal cancer trials have not shown a benefit with EGFR inhibitor treatment in patients whose tumors have *KRAS* mutations (codons 12 or 13); use of cetuximab is not recommended in these patients. Similar findings and conclusions pertain to *BRAF* gene point mutation V600E and EGFR gene amplification.

2. **Pharmacology**

   a. **Mechanisms.** Monoclonal antibody that binds to the EGFR (HER1, ErbB-1), which is a transmembrane glycoprotein of the TK growth factor receptor family, and thus inhibits ligand-induced TK autophosphorylation, which affects multiple mechanisms of action (cell growth, apoptosis, production of vascular endothelial growth factor, production of matrix metalloproteinase). There is no evidence to indicate that the level of EGFR expression can predict for the drug's clinical activity.

   b. **Metabolism.** Metabolism of cetuximab has not been characterized. In steady state, the mean half-life of cetuximab in the serum is approximately 5 days.

3. **Toxicity**

   a. **Dose limiting.** Severe infusion reactions characterized by rapid onset of airway obstruction, hypotension, and/or cardiac arrest (particularly during the first infusion); mild or moderate reactions are managed by slowing the infusion rate in subsequent doses. Severe reactions require the immediate and permanent discontinuation of cetuximab therapy. An acneiform rash develops in 90% of patients (severe in 12%), usually within 2 weeks of starting therapy. Treatment of the rash involves topical and oral antibiotics, but not topical corticosteroids.

   b. **Common.** Asthenia/malaise; skin drying and fissuring; abdominal pain, diarrhea, nausea, vomiting; hypomagnesemia (with accompanying hypokalemia and hypocalcemia) during or following infusions; headache

   c. **Occasional.** Stomatitis, fever, mild anemia, depression

   d. **Rare.** Interstitial lung disease, severe infusion reactions (up to 3%)

I. Daratumumab (Darzalex)

1. **Indications.** Multiple myeloma treated with at least three prior lines of therapy

2. **Pharmacology**

   a. **Mechanisms.** Daratumumab is an IgG1k human monoclonal antibody (mAb) that binds to CD38 and inhibits the growth of CD38 expressing tumor cells by inducing apoptosis directly through Fc-mediated cross-linking as well as by immune-mediated tumor cell lysis through complement-dependent cytotoxicity (CDC), antibody-dependent cell-mediated cytotoxicity (ADCC), and antibody-dependent cellular phagocytosis (ADCP). Myeloid-derived suppressor cells (MDSCs) and a subset of regulatory T cells (CD38+Tregs) express CD38 and are susceptible to daratumumab-mediated cell lysis.

   b. **Metabolism.** The mean (SD) estimated terminal half-life associated with linear clearance was approximately 18 days.

3. **Toxicity**

   a. **Dose limiting.** Severe infusion reactions (bronchospasm, dyspnea, hypoxia, and hypertension). Premedicate with corticosteroids, antipyretics, and antihistamines.

  b. Common. Infusion reactions (46% with the first infusion, 5% with the second infusion), fatigue, nausea, back pain, pyrexia, cough, and upper respiratory tract infection

  c. Occasional. Nasal congestion, chills, dyspnea, arthralgia, pneumonia, diarrhea, constipation, headache, decreased appetite, anemia, thrombocytopenia, neutropenia

  d. Rare. Herpes zoster reactivation. Prophylaxis for virus reactivation is recommended.

J. Dinutuximab (Unituxin)

 1. Indications. High-risk neuroblastoma after at least a partial response to prior first-line multiagent, multimodality therapy

 2. Pharmacology

  a. Mechanisms. Dinutuximab binds to the glycolipid GD2. This glycolipid is expressed on neuroblastoma cells and on normal cells of neuroectodermal origin, including the central nervous system and peripheral nerves. Dinutuximab binds to cell surface GD2 and induces cell lysis of GD2-expressing cells through antibody-dependent cell-mediated cytotoxicity (ADCC) and complement-dependent cytotoxicity (CDC).

  b. Metabolism. The terminal half-life is 10 days.

 3. Toxicity

  a. Dose limiting. Severe infusion reactions. CLS and hypotension: Administer required prehydration and monitor patients closely during treatment.

  b. Common. Pain (severe neuropathic pain in the majority of patients; administer intravenous opioid prior to, during, and for 2 hours following completion of the infusion), pyrexia, infections, thrombocytopenia, lymphopenia, infusion reactions, hypotension, hyponatremia, increased alanine aminotransferase, anemia, vomiting, diarrhea, hypokalemia, CLS, neutropenia, urticaria, hypoalbuminemia, increased aspartate aminotransferase, and hypocalcemia

  c. Occasional. Bone marrow suppression, electrolyte abnormalities

  d. Rare. Neurological disorders of the eye, atypical hemolytic uremic syndrome

K. Elotuzumab (Empliciti)

 1. Indications. Multiple myeloma in combination with lenalidomide and dexamethasone

 2. Pharmacology. It can interfere with assays used to monitor M-protein.

  a. Mechanisms. Elotuzumab is a humanized IgG1 monoclonal antibody that specifically targets the SLAMF7 (Signaling Lymphocytic Activation Molecule Family member 7) protein. SLAMF7 is expressed on myeloma cells independent of cytogenetic abnormalities. SLAMF7 is also expressed on natural killer cells, plasma cells, and at lower levels on specific immune cell subsets of differentiated cells within the hematopoietic lineage. Elotuzumab directly activates natural killer cells through both the SLAMF7 pathway and Fc receptors. Elotuzumab also targets SLAMF7 on myeloma cells and facilitates the interaction with natural killer cells to mediate the killing of myeloma cells through antibody-dependent cellular cytotoxicity (ADCC).

  b. Metabolism. 97% is predicted to be eliminated in 82 days.

 3. Toxicity

  a. Dose limiting. Severe infusion reactions (premedication is required)

  b. Common. Fatigue, diarrhea, pyrexia, constipation, cough, peripheral neuropathy, nasopharyngitis, upper respiratory tract infection, decreased appetite, pneumonia

  c. Occasional. Hepatotoxicity

  d. Rare. Second primary malignancies

L. Ipilimumab (Yervoy)

 1. Indications. Unresectable or metastatic melanoma, adjuvant treatment for stage III melanoma

 2. Pharmacology. A recombinant human IgG1 immunoglobulin monoclonal antibody that binds to the cytotoxic T-lymphocyte–associated antigen 4 (CTLA-4). Blockade of CTLA-4 has been shown to augment T-cell activation and proliferation, including the activation and proliferation of tumor infiltrating T-effector cells. Inhibition of CTLA-4 signaling can also reduce T-regulatory cell function, which may contribute to a general increase in T-cell responsiveness, including the antitumor immune response.

 3. Toxicity

  a. Dose limiting. Severe and fatal immune-mediated adverse effects due to T-cell activation may occur and involve *any* organ. Reactions generally occur during treatment, although some reactions have occurred weeks to months after treatment discontinuation. Common severe effects include dermatitis, endocrine disorders, enterocolitis, hepatitis, and neuropathy. Corticosteroid treatment is recommended for immune-mediated reactions.

  b. Common. Fatigue; pruritus, rash; anorexia, nausea, vomiting, diarrhea, constipation, abdominal pain

  c. Occasional. Headache, fever, enterocolitis; anemia, eosinophilia; hepatotoxicity; nephritis; hypopituitarism, hypothyroidism, hyperthyroidism, hypophysitis, adrenal insufficiency (≤2% each); ophthalmic toxicity (episcleritis, iritis, uveitis)

  d. Rare. Postmarketing and/or case reports include but are not limited to acute respiratory distress syndrome, Guillain-Barré syndrome, motor or sensory neuropathy, leukocytoclastic vasculitis, myasthenia gravis, and myelofibrosis.

M. Necitumumab (Portrazza)

 1. Indications. First-line treatment of metastatic squamous NSCLC in combination with gemcitabine and cisplatin

 2. Pharmacology

  a. Mechanisms. A recombinant human IgG1 monoclonal antibody that binds to EGFR and blocks the binding of EGFR to its ligands

  b. Metabolism. The elimination half-life is approximately 14 days.

 3. Toxicity

  a. Dose limiting. Severe infusion reactions

  b. Common. Hypomagnesemia (83%), rash (44%), vomiting (29%), diarrhea (16%), and dermatitis acneiform (15%)

  c. Occasional. Venous and thromboembolic events, hemoptysis, paronychia, headache, conjunctivitis

  d. Rare. Cardiopulmonary arrest and/or sudden death occurred in 3% of patients. Monitor serum electrolytes, including serum magnesium, potassium, and calcium before each dose and for at least 8 weeks after the last dose. Offer aggressive replacement if needed.

N. Nivolumab (Opdivo)

 1. Indications. Unresectable or metastatic melanoma as a single agent or in combination with ipilimumab, metastatic NSCLC, advanced renal cell carcinoma, classical Hodgkin lymphoma

 2. Pharmacology

  a. Mechanisms. Nivolumab is a human IgG4 kappa monoclonal antibody that blocks the interaction between PD-1 and its ligands, PD-L1 and

PD-L2. Binding of the PD-1 ligands, PD-L1 and PD-L2, to the PD-1 receptor found on T cells, inhibits T-cell proliferation and cytokine production. Upregulation of PD-1 ligands occurs in some tumors and signaling through this pathway can contribute to inhibition of active T-cell immune surveillance of tumors.

   b. Metabolism. The elimination half-life is approximately 27 days.

3. **Toxicity**

   a. Dose limiting. Immune-mediated adverse events such as pneumonitis, colitis, endocrinopathies, encephalitis, hepatitis, nephritis. Combination of ipilimumab and nivolumab is associated with a similar spectrum of side effects, but they are of increased frequency and severity.

   b. Common. Fatigue, rash, musculoskeletal pain, pruritus, diarrhea, and nausea

   c. Occasional. Increased amylase, increased lipase, iridocyclitis, dizziness, peripheral and sensory neuropathy, exfoliative dermatitis, erythema multiforme, vitiligo, psoriasis, extremity pain, musculoskeletal pain, peripheral edema

   d. Rare. Infusion reactions

O. **Obinutuzumab** (Gazyva)

   1. **Indications.** CLL in combination with chlorambucil

   2. **Pharmacology**

      a. Mechanisms. A humanized anti-CD20 monoclonal antibody of the IgG1 subclass. Upon binding to CD20, obinutuzumab mediates B-cell lysis through engagement of immune effector cells, by directly activating intracellular death signaling pathways and/or activation of the complement cascade. The immune effector cell mechanisms include antibody-dependent cellular cytotoxicity and antibody-dependent cellular phagocytosis.

      b. Metabolism. The elimination half-life is approximately 28 days.

   3. **Toxicity**

      a. Dose limiting. Infusion reactions. Premedicate patients with glucocorticoid, acetaminophen, and antihistamine.

      b. Common. Neutropenia, thrombocytopenia, anemia, pyrexia, cough, and musculoskeletal disorder

      c. Occasional. Tumor lysis syndrome, hyperkalemia, hypokalemia, liver enzyme elevation, hypocalcemia

      d. Rare. Progressive multifocal leukoencephalopathy (PML), which can result in death; hepatitis B virus (HBV) reactivation, in some cases resulting in fulminant hepatitis, hepatic failure, and death

P. **Ofatumumab** (Arzerra)

   1. **Indications.** CLL refractory to fludarabine and alemtuzumab

   2. **Pharmacology.** A CD20-directed cytolytic monoclonal antibody generated via transgenic mouse and hybridoma technology

      a. Mechanisms. It is an IgG1κ human monoclonal antibody that binds specifically to both the small and large extracellular loops of the CD20 molecule, which is expressed in normal and CLL B cells. The Fab domain of ofatumumab binds to the CD20 molecule and the Fc domain mediates immune effector function s to result in B-cell lysis.

      b. Metabolism. The mean half-life is approximately 14 days after the first three doses.

   3. **Toxicity**

      a. Dose limiting. Prolonged severe neutropenia (40%) and thrombocytopenia

    b. Common. Infusion reactions occur in 40% of patients on the first infusion, 30% on the second infusion, and less frequently thereafter. Premedicate patients with glucocorticoid, acetaminophen, and antihistamine. Fever, cough, upper respiratory infections, dyspnea; nausea, diarrhea, rash

    c. Occasional. Bowel obstruction

    d. Rare. Progressive multifocal leukoencephalopathy (PML), which can result in death; hepatitis B virus (HBV) reactivation, in some cases resulting in fulminant hepatitis, hepatic failure, and death

Q. Panitumumab (Vectibix)

    1. Indications. Metastatic colorectal cancer that expresses EGFR and that has progressed with 5-FU-, oxaliplatin-, and irinotecan-containing regimens. Panitumumab is not effective for tumors that have *KRAS* or BRAF mutations.

    2. Pharmacology

        a. Mechanisms. Panitumumab is a recombinant human IgG2 kappa monoclonal antibody that binds specifically to EGFR on normal and tumor cells and competitively inhibits the binding of ligands for EGFR. The interaction of EGFR with its ligands activates a series of intracellular TKs.

        b. Metabolism. Panitumumab concentrations reach a steady state by the third infusion. Its half-life is about 1 week.

    3. Toxicity

        a. Dose limiting. Infusion reactions; severe dermatologic toxicity (potentially complicated by infection and septic death); pulmonary infiltrates

        b. Common. Skin toxicities (90% of patients, severe in 15%), paronychia, fatigue, abdominal pain; nausea, diarrhea, constipation; hypomagnesemia/hypocalcemia; ocular toxicity (conjunctivitis, irritation)

        c. Occasional. Mucositis

        d. Rare. Pulmonary fibrosis (<1%)

R. Pembrolizumab (Keytruda)

    1. Indications. Unresectable or metastatic melanoma, metastatic NSCLC that is positive for PDL1 expression and head and neck cancer

    2. Pharmacology

        a. Mechanisms. Pembrolizumab is a humanized IgG4 kappa monoclonal antibody that blocks the interaction between PD-1 and its ligands, PD-L1 and PD-L2. Binding of the PD-1 ligands, PD-L1 and PD-L2, to the PD-1 receptor found on T cells inhibits T-cell proliferation and cytokine production. Upregulation of PD-1 ligands occur in some tumors and signaling through this pathway can contribute to inhibition of active T-cell immune surveillance of tumors.

        b. Metabolism. The elimination half-life is approximately 27 days.

    3. Toxicity

        a. Dose limiting. Immune-mediated adverse events such as pneumonitis, colitis, endocrinopathies, hepatitis, nephritis

        b. Common. Fatigue, pruritus, rash, dyspnea, constipation, diarrhea, cough, nausea, and decreased appetite

        c. Occasional. Hypertriglyceridemia, hypercholesterolemia, increased liver enzymes

        d. Rare. Infusion reactions

S. Pertuzumab (Perjeta)

    1. Indications. HER2-positive metastatic breast cancer, in combination with trastuzumab and docetaxel. HER2-positive, locally advanced, inflammatory, or early-stage breast cancer, in combination with trastuzumab and docetaxel, as neoadjuvant therapy

2. Pharmacology

a. Mechanisms. Pertuzumab is a humanized monoclonal antibody that targets the extracellular dimerization domain (subdomain II) of HER2 and, thereby, blocks ligand-dependent heterodimerization of HER2 with other HER family members, including EGFR, HER3, and HER4. As a result, it inhibits ligand-initiated intracellular signaling through MAP kinase and phosphoinositide 3-kinase (PI3K). Inhibition of these signaling pathways can result in cell growth arrest and apoptosis. In addition, pertuzumab mediates antibody ADCC.

b. Metabolism. The elimination half-life is approximately 18 days.

3. Toxicity

a. Dose limiting. Left ventricular dysfunction (evaluate cardiac function prior to and during treatment)

b. Common. Diarrhea, alopecia, neutropenia, anemia, thrombocytopenia, nausea, fatigue, rash, and peripheral neuropathy

c. Occasional. Paronychia, pleural effusion, headache

d. Rare. Infusion reactions

T. Ramucirumab (Cyramza)

1. Indications. Advanced gastric or gastroesophageal junction adenocarcinoma, metastatic NSCLC, metastatic colorectal cancer

2. Pharmacology

a. Mechanisms. Ramucirumab is a recombinant human IgG1 monoclonal antibody that specifically binds to VEGFR2 and blocks binding of VEGFR ligands, VEGF-A, VEGF-C, VEGF-D, thereby inhibiting ligand-induced proliferation, and migration of human endothelial cells.

b. Metabolism. The elimination half-life is approximately 14 days.

3. Toxicity

a. Dose limiting. Hemorrhage and GI perforation

b. Common. Hypertension, diarrhea, fatigue, neutropenia, epistaxis, stomatitis, decreased appetite

c. Occasional. Arterial thrombotic events, impaired wound healing, proteinuria, increased lacrimation, peripheral edema

d. Rare. Infusion reactions, reversible posterior leukoencephalopathy syndrome

U. Rituximab (Rituxan, MabThera)

1. Indications. CD20-positive, B-cell NHL, CLL, rheumatoid arthritis, microscopic polyangiitis, granulomatosis with polyangiitis (Wegener granulomatosis)

2. Pharmacology

a. Mechanisms. Rituximab is a chimeric murine/human monoclonal IgG1 kappa antibody–directed against the CD20 antigen found on the surface of normal and malignant B lymphocytes. Upon binding to CD20, rituximab mediates B-cell lysis. Possible mechanisms of cell lysis include complement-dependent cytotoxicity (CDC) and antibody-dependent cell-mediated cytotoxicity (ADCC).

b. Metabolism. Rituximab has been detectable in the serum 3 to 6 months after completion of treatment. Administration results in a rapid and sustained depletion of circulating and tissue-based B cells. B-cell levels return to normal by 12 months after completion of treatment.

3. **Toxicity**
   a. **Dose limiting.** Hypersensitivity reactions, severe mucocutaneous reactions, serious cardiac arrhythmias
   b. **Common.** Infusion reaction occurs in 25%, particularly during the first infusion (decreasing in occurrence substantially on subsequent infusions).
   c. **Occasional.** Severe granulocytopenia or thrombocytopenia; arthralgia/myalgia, malaise, headache, diarrhea, dyspepsia, taste perversion, hypertension, hypotension, tachycardia, bradycardia, dyspnea, lacrimation, paresthesia, hypesthesia, agitation, insomnia; hyperglycemia, hypocalcemia, pain in chest, back, abdomen or tumor site, rash, night sweats, angioedema, tumor lysis syndrome, bowel obstruction
   d. **Rare.** Arrhythmias, angina; aplastic anemia, hemolytic anemia; mucocutaneous reactions (e.g., Stevens-Johnson syndrome); pneumonia; progressive multifocal leukoencephalopathy related to Jakob-Creutzfeldt virus infections up to 1 year after treatment, reactivation of hepatitis B virus infection

V. **Siltuximab** (Sylvant)
   1. **Indications.** Multicentric Castleman disease (MCD)
   2. **Pharmacology**
      a. **Mechanisms.** Siltuximab is a human-mouse chimeric monoclonal antibody that binds human interleukin-6 (IL-6) and prevents the binding of IL-6 to both soluble and membrane-bound IL-6 receptors. IL-6 has been shown to be involved in diverse normal physiologic processes such as induction of immunoglobulin secretion. Overproduction of IL-6 has been linked to systemic manifestations in patients with MCD.
      b. **Metabolism.** The mean terminal half-life for siltuximab is 21 days.
   3. **Toxicity**
      a. **Dose limiting.** Severe infections
      b. **Common.** Pruritus, increased weight, rash, hyperuricemia, and upper respiratory tract infection
      c. **Occasional.** Thrombocytopenia, dry skin, eczema, edema, hypertriglyceridemia, hypercholesterolemia, renal impairment, headache, hypotension
      d. **Rare.** GI perforation

W. **Trastuzumab** (Herceptin)
   1. **Indications.** Cancers of the breast (adjuvant or metastatic) and metastatic adenocarcinomas of the stomach or gastroesophageal junction (GEJ) that overexpress the HER2 protein
      a. **Adjuvant breast indication:** In combinations for ER/PR-negative or high-risk ER/PR-positive (tumor size > 2 cm, or age < 35 years, or tumor grade >1) breast cancers
      b. **Metastatic breast indication:** As a single agent or in combinations
      c. **Metastatic gastric/GEJ adenocarcinoma indication**: In combination with cisplatin and capecitabine or 5-FU for patients who have not received prior treatment for metastatic disease
   2. **Pharmacology.** The *HER2* (*HER2/neu, c-erb-B2*) protooncogene encodes a transmembrane receptor protein that is structurally related to EGFR. Trastuzumab is a recombinant DNA-derived humanized monoclonal antibody that selectively binds to the extracellular domain of HER2. The humanized IgG-κ antibody against HER2 is produced by a mammalian cell (Chinese hamster ovary) suspension culture. It inhibits the proliferation of tumor cells that overexpress HER2. The metabolism of trastuzumab is not well characterized.

3. **Toxicity.** During pregnancy, it can result in oligohydramnios and oligohydramnios sequence.
   a. **Dose-limiting.** Cardiomyopathy
   b. **Common.** Infusion reaction occurs in 40% during the first infusion (reactions can be serious).
   c. **Occasional.** Asthenia, headache, rash, nausea and vomiting, arthralgia, pain, fever
   d. **Rare.** Anemia, leukopenia; severe pulmonary toxicity, hypersensitivity reaction, nephritic syndrome (4 to 18 months after treatment)

VIII. MISCELLANEOUS AGENTS

A. **Aldesleukin** (Proleukin)
   1. **Indications.** Metastatic renal cell carcinoma and melanoma
   2. **Pharmacology**
      a. **Mechanisms.** It is a human recombinant interleukin-2 that enhances lymphocyte cytotoxicity and killer and natural killer cell activity and induces interferon gamma production.
      b. **Metabolism** is characterized by high plasma concentrations following a short intravenous infusion, rapid distribution into the extravascular space, and elimination from the body by metabolism in the kidneys with little or no bioactive protein excreted in the urine.
   3. **Toxicity.** The treatment with aldesleukin is associated with significant side effects, and therefore, it should be used only in experienced medical centers. Patients should be treated in the intensive care unit setting.
      a. **Dose limiting.** CLS begins immediately after aldesleukin treatment starts and is marked by increased capillary permeability to protein and fluids and reduced vascular tone. In most patients, this results in a concomitant drop in mean arterial blood pressure within 2 to 12 hours after the start of treatment. With continued therapy, clinically significant hypotension and hypoperfusion will occur. In addition, extravasation of protein and fluids into the extravascular space will lead to the formation of edema and creation of new effusions.
      b. **Common.** Chills, fever, malaise, asthenia, infections, hypotension, tachycardia, arrhythmias, increased creatinine, hyperbilirubinemia, elevation of liver enzymes, confusion, somnolence, diarrhea, nausea, vomiting, thrombocytopenia, anemia, dyspnea, cough, rash
      c. **Rare.** malignant hyperthermia; cardiac arrest; myocardial infarction; pulmonary emboli; stroke; intestinal perforation; liver or renal failure; severe depression leading to suicide; pulmonary edema; respiratory arrest; respiratory failure

B. **Anagrelide** (Agrylin)
   1. **Indications.** Thrombocytosis in myeloproliferative disorders
   2. **Pharmacology**
      a. **Mechanisms.** Anagrelide reduces the platelet count by uncertain mechanisms. It does not affect the leukocyte count and does not affect DNA synthesis.
      b. **Metabolism.** The drug is extensively metabolized by CYP1A2 and also inhibits this enzyme; <1% is excreted in the urine as unaltered drug.
   3. **Toxicity.** Adverse effects are treated symptomatically and usually abate with transient discontinuation of therapy. Cardiovascular complications that occur are usually related to underlying diseases.
      a. **Dose limiting.** Thrombocytopenia (platelet counts return to normal 4 days after discontinuing the drug).

   b. Common. Headache (45%), asthenia, palpitations, tachycardia, fluid retention, diarrhea, bloating, abdominal pain, asthenia, dizziness

   c. Occasional. Nausea, vomiting, other GI disturbances; dyspnea, chest pain, paresthesia, rash, pruritus, fever, malaise

C. Arsenic trioxide (Trisenox)

   1. Indications. Refractory or relapsed acute promyelocytic leukemia (APL) that is characterized by the presence of the *t*(15;17) translocation or PML/RAR-alpha gene expression

   2. Pharmacology

   a. Mechanisms. The mechanism of action is not understood.

   b. Metabolism. Involves reduction of pentavalent arsenic to trivalent arsenic by arsenate reductase and methylation of trivalent arsenic to monomethylarsonic acid and monomethylarsonic acid to dimethylarsonic acid by methyltransferases, which appear to be mostly in the liver. Trivalent arsenic is mostly methylated and excreted in urine.

   3. Toxicity. A litany of side effects is associated with this drug; refer to the package insert for details. The following are the most important:

   a. Dose limiting. QT interval prolongation can lead to *torsades de pointes* and complete heart block and occurs in 40% of patients.

   b. Common. Leukocytosis, GI disturbances, fatigue, fever, edema, cough, dyspnea, hypotension; rash, pruritus; headaches, insomnia, paresthesia dizziness; arthralgias, myalgias; hypokalemia, hyperkalemia, hypomagnesemia, hyperglycemia

   c. APL differentiation syndrome occurs in about 25% of patients and is characterized by fever, dyspnea, pulmonary infiltrates, pleural or pericardial effusions, and weight gain, with or without leukocytosis (this topic is further discussed in Chapter 26, Acute Leukemia). High-dose dexamethasone is administered when clinical signs develop.

D. Bexarotene (Targretin)

   1. Indication. Cutaneous T-cell lymphoma that is refractory to at least one prior systemic therapy

   2. Pharmacology

   a. Mechanisms. Selectively binds and activates retinoic X receptors (RXRs), which form heterodimers with various other receptors, including retinoic acid receptors (RARs), vitamin D receptors, and thyroid receptors. The activated receptors function as transcription factors, which then regulate the expression of various genes involved in controlling cell differentiation, growth, and proliferation.

   b. Metabolism. Extensively metabolized by the hepatic P450 microsomal system to both active and inactive metabolites. Primarily eliminated through the hepatobiliary system and in feces

   c. Toxicity

   (1) Photosensitivity, dry skin, rash, exfoliative dermatitis

   (2) Hypothyroidism (up to 50% of patients), hypoglycemia, hypertriglyceridemia, hypercholesterolemia

   (3) Ocular problems: retinal complications, cataracts, xerophthalmia, conjunctivitis, blepharitis, periorbital edema

   (4) Headache, asthenia

   (5) Mild, dose-related leukopenia

E. Denileukin diftitox (Ontak) is a recombinant fusion protein composed of amino acid sequences of human interleukin-2 (IL-2) and the enzymatic and translocation domains of diphtheria toxin. This protein binds specifically to the

CD25 component of the IL-2 receptor and is then internalized via endocytosis. Cellular protein synthesis is inhibited, and apoptosis occurs on release of diphtheria toxin into the cytosol.

1. **Indications.** Persistent or recurrent cutaneous T-cell lymphomas whose malignant cells express the CD25 component of the IL-2 receptor (must be confirmed on tumor biopsy)

2. **Toxicity**

   a. **Infusion reactions** are observed in 70% of patients within 24 hours and resolving within 48 hours of the last infusion of a course. Serious hypersensitivity reactions occur in about 8% of patients.

   b. **Common.** A CLS characterized by edema, hypotension, and/or hypoalbuminemia is usually a self-limited process but can be serious and even result in death (the onset may occur up to 2 weeks after infusion); asthenia, mild, transient flulike symptoms; rash, diarrhea (may be prolonged), abnormal LFTs; hypoalbuminemia (85% with nadir at 2 weeks)

   c. **Occasional.** Loss of visual acuity, usually with loss of color vision, has been reported and may be persistent; hyperthyroidism; nausea, vomiting, constipation; tachycardia, chest pain; paresthesia, confusion; arthralgia/myalgias; hematosuppression

F. **Interferon alpha-2b** (Intron A, Sylatron). Interferons exert their cellular activities by binding to specific membrane receptors on the cell surface. Once bound to the cell membrane, interferons initiate a complex sequence of intracellular events. These include the induction of certain enzymes, suppression of cell proliferation, immunomodulating activities such as enhancement of the phagocytic activity of macrophages and augmentation of the specific cytotoxicity of lymphocytes for target cells, and inhibition of virus replication in virus-infected cells.

Sylatron is a pegylated version of interferon that is characterized by a long half-life and it is administered weekly.

1. **Indications.** Hairy cell leukemia, melanoma, Kaposi sarcoma, follicular lymphoma

2. **Toxicity**

   a. **Dose limiting.** It can cause or aggravate fatal or life-threatening neuropsychiatric, autoimmune, ischemic, and infectious disorders.

   b. **Common.** "Flulike" symptoms, particularly fever, headache, chills, myalgia, and fatigue, neutropenia, anorexia, vomiting/nausea, elevation of liver enzymes, depression, diarrhea, alopecia, altered taste sensation, dizziness/vertigo, and anemia. More severe toxicities are observed generally at higher doses and may be difficult for patients to tolerate.

   c. **Occasional.** Severe depression with suicidal behaviors, ischemic and hemorrhagic cerebrovascular, hypotension, arrhythmia, tachycardia, decrease or loss of vision, retinopathy, hypothyroidism or hyperthyroidism, dyspnea, pulmonary infiltrates, pneumonia, bronchiolitis obliterans, interstitial pneumonitis, pulmonary hypertension, sarcoidosis, vasculitis, Raynaud phenomenon, rheumatoid arthritis, lupus erythematosus, and rhabdomyolysis

G. **Lenalidomide** (Revlimid)

1. **Indications.** Multiple myeloma; MDS with deletion 5q abnormality, myelofibrosis; mantle cell lymphoma

2. **Pharmacology**

   a. **Mechanisms.** Lenalidomide is a thalidomide analogue with immunomodulatory, antiangiogenic, and antineoplastic properties.

  b. Metabolism. The majority of the drug is excreted unchanged in the urine.

 3. Toxicity. Lenalidomide is an analogue of thalidomide, which is a known human teratogen that causes life-threatening human birth defects.

  a. Dose-limiting. Neutropenia and thrombocytopenia

  b. Common. Fatigue, diarrhea, anemia, nausea, cough, pyrexia, rash, dyspnea, pruritus, constipation, peripheral edema, and leukopenia

  c. Occasional. Deep vein thrombosis; myalgia/arthralgias, peripheral neuropathy, dizziness, headache, fever; hypokalemia, hypomagnesemia; hypertension, hypothyroidism, tumor flare reactions

  d. Rare. Serious and fatal cardiac adverse reactions, hepatotoxicity, angioedema

H. Lanreotide (Somatuline)

 1. Indications. Unresectable, well or moderately differentiated, locally advanced or metastatic gastroenteropancreatic neuroendocrine tumors

 2. Pharmacology

  a. Mechanisms. It is a synthetic octapeptide with a biological activity similar to naturally occurring somatostatin. It has a high affinity for human somatostatin receptors (SSTR) 2 and 5 and a reduced binding affinity for human SSTR1, SSTR3, and SSTR4. Lanreotide inhibits the basal secretion of motilin, gastric inhibitory peptide, and pancreatic polypeptide but has no significant effect on the secretion of secretin.

  b. Metabolism. The steady-state concentrations were reached after 4 to 5 injections.

 3. Toxicity

  a. Dose limiting. Diarrhea

  b. Common. Abdominal pain, musculoskeletal pain, vomiting, headache, injection site reaction, hyperglycemia, hypertension, cholelithiasis

  c. Occasional. Hypoglycemia, thyroid function abnormalities, flatulence

  d. Rare. Bradycardia

I. Pomalidomide (Pomalyst)

 1. Indications. Multiple myeloma that has been treated with at least two prior therapies including lenalidomide and a proteasome inhibitor

 2. Pharmacology

  a. Mechanisms. Pomalidomide is a thalidomide analogue with immunomodulatory, and antineoplastic properties. Pomalidomide inhibited the proliferation of lenalidomide-resistant multiple myeloma cell lines.

  b. Metabolism. It is primarily metabolized in the liver by CYP1A2 and CYP3A4 and excreted mainly in urine.

 3. Toxicity. Pomalidomide is an analogue of thalidomide, which is a known human teratogen that causes life-threatening human birth defects.

  a. Dose-limiting. Neutropenia, thrombocytopenia

  b. Common. Fatigue and asthenia, neutropenia, anemia, constipation, nausea, diarrhea, dyspnea, upper respiratory tract infections, back pain, and pyrexia

  c. Occasional. Tumor lysis syndrome, deep venous thrombosis, pulmonary embolism, myocardial infarction, stroke (thromboprophylaxis is recommended), dizziness, confusion, neuropathy, hyperkalemia, hyponatremia

  d. Rare. Angioedema, severe dermatologic reactions, hepatic failure

J. Sipuleucel-T (Provenge)

 1. Indications. Asymptomatic or minimally symptomatic metastatic castrate resistant (hormone-refractory) prostate cancer

2. **Pharmacology.** Sipuleucel-T consists of autologous peripheral blood mononuclear cells, including antigen presenting cells (APCs), that have been activated during a defined culture period with a recombinant human protein, PAP-GM-CSF, consisting of prostatic acid phosphatase (PAP, an antigen expressed in prostate cancer tissue), linked to granulocyte-macrophage colony-stimulating factor (GM-CSF, an immune cell activator). The patient's peripheral blood mononuclear cells are obtained via a standard leukapheresis procedure approximately 3 days prior to the infusion date. Sipuleucel-T is classified as an autologous cellular immunotherapy; it is designed to induce an immune response targeted against PAP.

3. **Toxicity.**
    a. **Dose limiting.** Acute infusion reactions
    b. **Common.** Chills, fatigue, fever, back pain, nausea, joint ache, and headache
    c. **Occasional.** Paresthesia, muscle ache, rash, sweating, tremor
    d. **Rare.** Cerebrovascular events, including hemorrhagic and ischemic strokes

K. **Talimogene laherparepvec** (Imlygic)
1. **Indications.** Unresectable cutaneous, subcutaneous, and nodal lesions in patients with melanoma recurrent after initial surgery
2. **Pharmacology.** Talimogene laherparepvec is a live, attenuated HSV-1 that has been genetically modified to express huGM-CSF; it can proliferate in tumor cells, but not in normal cells. It causes lysis of tumors, followed by release of tumor-derived antigens, which together with virally derived GM-CSF may promote an antitumor immune response.
3. **Toxicity.**
    a. **Dose limiting.** None. All patients who have easily injectable lesions can be treated.
    b. **Common.** Fatigue, chills, pyrexia, nausea, influenza-like illness, and injection site pain
    c. **Occasional.** Headache, dizziness, diarrhea
    d. **Rare.** It should not be administered to immunocompromised patients.

L. **Thalidomide** (Thalomid)
1. **Indications.** Myeloma; MDS
2. **Pharmacology**
    a. **Mechanisms.** Incompletely understood; inhibits TNF-α, down-modulates certain surface adhesion molecules, may exert an antiangiogenic effect
    b. **Metabolism.** Not well defined
3. **Toxicity.** Thalidomide's teratogenic effect is its most serious toxicity. All women of childbearing age should have a baseline β-human chorionic gonadotrophin before starting therapy with thalidomide. Women should practice two forms of birth control throughout treatment: one highly effective form (intrauterine device, hormonal contraception, partner's vasectomy) and one additional barrier method. Men taking the drug must use latex condoms for every sexual encounter with a woman of childbearing potential, because the drug may be in the semen.
    a. **Dose limiting.** Neurologic side effects (70% and dose related), including fatigue, sensory and motor neuropathy, sedation, dizziness, confusion, tremor, agitation, orthostatic hypotension, etc. Manifestations may resolve slowly or be irreversible.
    b. **Common.** Constipation, anorexia, skin rash (maculopapular or urticarial), venous thromboembolism, edema

      c. Occasional. Leukopenia, hypersensitivity, fever, hypotension, LFT abnormalities

      d. Rare. Stevens-Johnson syndrome

M. Tretinoin (all-trans-retinoic acid [ATRA], Vesanoid)

    1. Indication. Acute promyelocytic leukemia

    2. Pharmacology

      a. Mechanisms. On entry into cells, tretinoin binds to cellular retinoic acid–binding protein. This complex is transported to the nucleus, where it binds to retinoic acid receptors (RARs) and/or retinoic X receptors. This process induces differentiation of acute promyelocytic cells to normal myelocytes and induces apoptosis by mechanisms that have not been fully elucidated.

      b. Metabolism. Extensively metabolized by the hepatic P450 microsomal system. Excreted both in feces and urine

    3. Toxicity

      a. Vitamin A toxicity (nearly all patients): headache (which improves after the first week), fever, dryness of skin and mucous membranes, skin rash, mucositis, conjunctivitis, and fluid retention

      b. Retinoic acid syndrome (25% of patients): Fever, leukocytosis, dyspnea, diffuse pulmonary infiltrates, pleural and/or pericardial effusions, and weight gain. The syndrome usually occurs during the first month of therapy and can be dose limiting. Development of these manifestations mandates discontinuance of the drug and treatment with dexamethasone (10 mg IV q12h for 3 days or until the syndrome has completely resolved). Therapy can be resumed in most cases once the syndrome has completely resolved.

      c. Other common events. Fatigue and weakness, hyperlipidemia (60%), GI symptoms; bone pain, myalgia, chest discomfort, arrhythmias, flushing, abnormal LFTs (50%), ear discomfort (25%), visual disturbances

      d. Occasional. Alopecia, photosensitivity; cardiac ischemia or failure, myocarditis, pericarditis, hypertension, pulmonary hypertension; renal dysfunction; central nervous system toxicity in various forms including encephalopathy

      e. Rare. Venous or arterial thrombosis, vasculitis, genital ulceration

N. Ziv-aflibercept (Zaltrap)

    1. Indications. Metastatic colorectal cancer

    2. Pharmacology

      a. Mechanisms. It is a soluble receptor that binds to human VEGF-A, VEGF-B, and PLGF. By binding to these endogenous ligands, ziv-aflibercept can inhibit the binding and activation of their cognate receptors. This inhibition can result in decreased neovascularization and decreased vascular permeability.

      b. Metabolism. The elimination half-life was approximately 6 days.

    3. Toxicity.

      a. Dose limiting. Severe, sometimes fatal hemorrhage, GI perforation

      b. Common. Leukopenia, diarrhea, neutropenia, proteinuria, AST increased, stomatitis, fatigue, thrombocytopenia, ALT increased, hypertension, weight decreased, decreased appetite, epistaxis, abdominal pain, dysphonia, serum creatinine increased, and headache

      c. Occasional. Dehydration, proteinuria, thromboembolic events, nasopharyngitis

      d. Rare. Impaired wound healing, fistula formation

IX. HORMONAL AGENTS

A. Glucocorticoids

1. **Indications.** Broad variety of oncologic problems that include the following:

   a. Component of combination chemotherapy regimens for lymphoproliferative disorders and plasma cell dyscrasias

   b. Symptomatic lymphangitic lung carcinomatosis; bronchial obstruction by tumor

   c. Symptomatic brain metastases with or without cerebral edema; spinal cord compression

   d. Painful liver metastases

   e. Immune-mediated cytopenias

   f. Prevention of chemotherapy-induced vomiting

   g. Appetite stimulant and mood elevator in patients with terminal cancer

   h. Management of immune-related adverse events of therapy with checkpoint inhibitors

2. **Toxicity and side effects** (usually associated with long-term therapy)

   a. Peptic ulcer disease

   b. Sodium retention (edema, heart failure, hypertension)

   c. Potassium wasting (hypokalemia, alkalosis, muscle weakness)

   d. Glucose intolerance, accumulation of fat on trunk and face, weight gain

   e. Proximal myopathy

   f. Personality changes, including euphoria and psychosis

   g. Osteoporosis, aseptic hip necrosis

   h. Thinning and fragility of the skin

   i. Suppression of the pituitary–adrenal axis

   j. Susceptibility to infection

B. Adrenal inhibitors: Mitotane (Lysodren)

1. **Indications.** Adrenal carcinoma, ectopic Cushing syndrome

2. **Pharmacology**

   a. **Mechanism.** Causes adrenal cortical atrophy; the exact mechanism is unknown. Blocks adrenocorticosteroid synthesis in normal and malignant cells. Aldosterone synthesis is not affected.

   b. **Metabolism.** Degraded slowly in the liver and extensively distributed in fatty tissues. Its action is antagonized by spironolactone; the two drugs should not be administered together. Metabolites are excreted in the bile and urine.

3. **Toxicity**

   a. **Dose limiting.** Nausea and vomiting; adrenocortical insufficiency

   b. **Common.** Depression, lethargy, maculopapular rash

   c. **Occasional.** Orthostatic hypotension; diarrhea, abnormal LFTs; headache, irritability, confusion, tremors; diplopia, retinopathy, lens opacity; myalgia; hemorrhagic cystitis, fever

   d. **Rare.** Long-term (>2 years) use may lead to brain damage or functional impairment.

C. Androgens

1. **Indications.** Breast carcinoma, short-range anabolic effect, stimulation of erythropoiesis

2. **Toxicity and side effects** vary among preparations. Virilization, fluid retention, and hepatotoxicity (abnormal LFTs or cholestasis), which is usually reversible, are frequent with certain preparations. May cause hypercalcemia in immobilized patients.

3. **Administration.** Use with caution in patients with cardiac, hepatic, or renal disease.

   a. **Fluoxymesterone** (Halotestin and others): 10 to 40 mg/d in two to four divided doses (supplied as 2-, 5-, and 10-mg tablets)

   b. **Methyltestosterone** (Android and others): 50 to 200 mg/d in two or three divided doses (supplied as 10- and 25-mg tablets)

D. **Antiandrogens** (bicalutamide, flutamide, nilutamide, enzalutamide, abiraterone)

   1. **Indications.** Prostate cancer in combination with medical therapy or orchiectomy that reduces testicular but not adrenal androgen production

   2. **Pharmacology**

      a. Bicalutamide, flutamide, nilutamide: androgen receptor blockers, they bind to cytosol androgen receptors and competitively inhibit the uptake or binding of androgens in target tissues and do not prevent androgen receptor nuclear translocation.

      b. Enzalutamide: inhibits androgen binding to androgen receptors and inhibits androgen receptor nuclear translocation and interaction with DNA

      c. Abiraterone: inhibits 17 α-hydroxylase/C17,20 lyse and stops androgen synthesis in the testis, adrenal gland, prostate tissue

   3. **Toxicity**

      a. **Common.** Impotence, gynecomastia, and other manifestations of hypogonadism; diarrhea

      b. **Occasional.** Nausea and vomiting, myalgia, depression; mild hypertension or pulmonary disorder (bicalutamide, nilutamide)

      c. **Rare.** Hepatitis, including cholestatic jaundice (all three), hemolytic anemia or methemoglobinemia (flutamide), iron-deficiency anemia (bicalutamide), interstitial pneumonitis, or visual disturbances (nilutamide)

E. **Estrogens** [diethylstilbestrol (DES)]

   1. **Indication.** Breast carcinoma, prostate cancer

   2. **Pharmacology.** It acts as an estrogen at the level of the hypothalamus and downregulates hypothalamic luteinizing hormone (LH) production.

   3. **Toxicity.** Nausea, uterine bleeding; hypercalcemic "flare"; thromboembolic disorders; abnormal LFTs, cholestatic jaundice (rare); chloasma, optic neuritis, retinal thrombosis; rash, pruritus; fluid retention, hypertension, headache, dizziness, hypertriglyceridemia

F. **Antiestrogens** (tamoxifen, toremifene, fulvestrant)

   1. **Indication.** Breast carcinoma

   2. **Pharmacology.** Tamoxifen and toremifene are nonsteroidal agents that bind to estrogen receptors and may exert antiestrogenic, estrogenic, or both activities. Fulvestrant is an estrogen receptor antagonist without known agonist effects.

   3. **Toxicity**

      a. **Common.** Hot flashes, menstrual changes, vaginal discharge, uterine bleeding; lowered serum cholesterol (especially low-density cholesterol); thrombocytopenia (mild and transient)

      b. **Occasional.** Retinopathy or keratopathy (reversible), cataracts; leukopenia, anemia; nausea, vomiting; hair loss (mild), rash; "flare" in first month of therapy of patients with bone metastases; thrombophlebitis or thromboembolism, particularly in patients with cofactors for thrombosis (e.g., inheritance of factor V[Leiden])

  c. Rare. Abnormal LFTs; altered mental state; slightly increased occurrence of endometrial adenocarcinoma on prolonged use

  d. Toxicity of fulvestrant includes transient pain at injection site, GI symptoms, headache, back pain, and vasodilatation.

G. Aromatase inhibitors (anastrozole, letrozole, exemestane, aminoglutethimide)

 1. Indication. Breast cancer in postmenopausal women

 2. Pharmacology. These nonsteroidal inhibitors interfere with aromatase, the enzyme that converts androgens from the adrenals and peripheral tissues to estrogens. Anastrozole and letrozole are competitive inhibitors, whereas exemestane permanently binds to and irreversibly inactivates aromatase. None of these agents inhibit adrenal corticosteroid or aldosterone biosynthesis. All are significantly more potent inhibitors of aromatase than aminoglutethimide (Cytadren), which also inhibits corticosteroid or aldosterone biosynthesis, requires q.i.d. dosing with hydrocortisone, is more toxic than the newer alternatives, and is no longer recommended.

 3. Toxicity. Antiestrogen effects, peripheral edema, thromboembolism, osteopenia, vaginal bleeding

H. Gonadotropin-releasing hormone (GnRH) agonists (leuprolide, goserelin)

 1. Indications. Prostate and breast cancer

 2. Pharmacology. GnRH agonist analogs are potent inhibitors of gonadotropin secretion. Continuous administration decreases serum levels of luteinizing hormone (LH) and follicle-stimulating hormone (FSH) and results in castration levels of testosterone in men and of estradiol in women within 2 to 4 weeks of treatment.

 3. Toxicity and side effects. A small but statistically significant increased risk of diabetes mellitus and/or cardiovascular disease has been observed in men receiving GnRH agonist therapy.

  a. Common. Hot flushes, decreased libido; impotence and gynecomastia in men; amenorrhea and uterine bleeding in women; osteoporosis, depression

  b. Occasional. Hypercholesterolemia, local discomfort at site of injection

  c. Rare. GI upset, rash, hypertension, azotemia, headache, depression

I. Progestins

 1. Indications. Endometrial and breast carcinomas; or as an appetite stimulant in malignant cachexia; or for hot flashes in patients with breast carcinoma

 2. Toxicity and side effects

  a. Menstrual changes, uterine bleeding, hot flashes, gynecomastia, galactorrhea

  b. Fluid retention, thrombophlebitis, thromboembolism

  c. Nervousness, somnolence, depression, headache

 3. Drugs

  a. Medroxyprogesterone acetate

  b. Megestrol (Megace)

ACKNOWLEDGMENT

The author would like to acknowledge Dr. Dennis A. Casciato who significantly contributed to earlier versions of this chapter.

Cancer Immunotherapy

Siwen Hu-Lieskovan, Bartosz Chmielowski, and Antoni Ribas

I. TUMOR IMMUNOLOGY

A. **Cancer immunosurveillance.** Paul Ehrlich proposed the concept of cancer immune surveillance in 1957. He suggested that the emergence of malignant clones of cells is a frequent event, but in majority of people, this can be suppressed by the host's natural immunity. When this immunity is weakened either by old age or other conditions, cancer becomes prevalent. Burnet and Thomas added in 1971 that lymphocytes were responsible for this process. This concept has since been proven directly and indirectly in immune-deficient animal models and humans with immune-suppressed conditions.

B. **Cancer immunoediting** is a hypothesis introduced by Schreiber et al. in 2001, stating that the host immunity could have a dual role of an extrinsic tumor suppressor and a facilitator of tumor growth and progression. It was supported by a study using carcinogen-induced sarcomas generated from both wild-type and RAG2$^{-/-}$ mice (mice devoid of T, B, and NK cells) and subsequently implanted in wild-type or RAG2$^{-/-}$ hosts. The tumor cells generated from wild-type mice grew progressively when implanted in both wild-type and RAG2$^{-/-}$ hosts. The tumors generated from RAG2$^{-/-}$ mice also grew progressively in RAG2$^{-/-}$ hosts, but nearly half of the tumors implanted in the immune-competent wild-type mice were rejected, indicating that tumors arising from immune-competent hosts are less immunogenic than those from immune-deficient hosts.

The process of immunoediting consists of three phases:

1. **Elimination.** Tumors are recognized and destroyed by the immune system before becoming clinically evident.

2. **Equilibrium.** Tumor cells start to mutate/escape and at the same time the immune system try to adapt and control the tumor growth.

3. **Escape.** The constant selection of tumors of lower immunogenicity make the tumor cells evolve to the state that can no longer be recognized and controlled by the immune system, and the tumor becomes clinically evident.

C. **Mechanisms of antitumor responses**

1. **T cells and interferon gamma (IFNγ)**

a. **Thymus.** The thymus provides an inductive environment for development of T cells (thymus-derived cells) from hematopoietic progenitor cells, and the thymic stromal cells allow for the selection of a functional (through positive selection) and self-tolerant (through negative selection) T-cell repertoire. This process ensures that the host's own immune system does not recognize self-antigens.

The importance of the thymus was first realized in the 1960s when neonatal-thymectomized mice were used to study lymphocytic leukemia induced by the Gross leukemia virus, which has to be given at birth. Thymectomy at 1 month of age could prevent the development of the leukemia. This phenomenon was not seen in adult-thymectomized mice and indicates that the virus needs cells only present in the newborn thymus to multiply. Grafting of a foreign thymus could induce tolerance to skin graft of the same donor.

b. **T-cell activation.** T cells recognize antigen through a tightly regulated process. The **T-cell receptor** (TCR) only recognizes antigen presented by **major histocompatibility complex** (MHC) molecules on the surface of **antigen-presenting cells** (APC) or viral infected cells. T-cell activation requires two signals, recognition of antigen-derived peptide presentation on the MHC molecules and interaction of costimulatory molecules CD28 on the T cells to the ligands B7 on the APC. T cells with high affinity to self-antigens are deleted by negative selections in the thymus. Several **T-cell subsets** were identified, including CD4 helper T cells, CD8 cytotoxic T cells, natural killer T cells (NKT), and regulatory T cells (Tregs). Treg cells are immune-suppressive T cells in the periphery designed to tone down autoimmunity and promote self-tolerance.

c. **IFNγ.** Not only lymphocytes but also IFNγ are important in the process of immunosurveillance and protection of the host against tumor growth. IFNγ up-regulates MHC class I antigen-presenting machinery in the tumor cells, has antiproliferative and proapoptotic effects, inhibits angiogenesis, and can influence the host cells by polarizing CD4 cells into Th1 cells.

IFNγ-insensitive (IFNGR1$^{-/-}$ or STAT1$^{-/-}$), IFNγ$^{-/-}$, or RAG2$^{-/-}$ mice (lack T, B, and NKT cells) were found to have significantly higher rate of carcinogen-induced or spontaneous tumors than their wild-type counterparts. This was found to be a direct effect to the tumor cells because a highly immunogenic tumor cell line that rendered IFNγ insensitive by introducing a dominant negative IFNGR1 grew aggressively in immune-competent mice, while the wild-type cells were rejected by the murine immune system.

d. **Patients with congenital or acquired immune deficiency** have a higher risk of cancer development (tumors of the colon, lung, bladder, kidney, ureter, endocrine, pancreas, skin), and it is an indirect evidence of the importance of immunosurveillance in human. It is still unclear whether immune-suppression promotes de novo tumor growth or allows an existing tumor to outgrow. On the contrary, the presence of tumor-infiltrating lymphocytes (TILs) was found to be an independent prognostic factor for survival in several tumor types, including melanoma, ovarian cancer, colorectal cancer, esophageal squamous carcinoma, or adenocarcinoma.

2. **Innate immune response.** The innate immune system can discriminate cancer cells and normal cells and participate in the cancer immunosurveillance process. When tumor cells become malignant with uncontrolled growth, the constant tissue disruption and remodeling, as well as angiogenesis, could alert and activate the innate immune system. Proinflammatory cytokines and chemokines are released, and NK cells, NKT cells, γδ T cells, dendritic cells, and macrophages are recruited to the site, forming a positive feedback and production of IFNγ, which kills tumor cells through IFNγ-dependent or IFNγ-independent processes.

NK and NKT cells are components of the innate immune response and have been shown to be critical effectors of cancer immunosurveillance. Mice depleted of NK cells (anti-asialo-GM1 treatment), invariant NKT cells (Jα281$^{-/-}$), or both (NK1.1mAb treatment) were all more susceptible to carcinogen-induced tumor formation and developed higher incidence of tumors than the wild-type counterparts. Studies have shown that NK cell infiltration in the tumors is a positive prognostic factor in gastric cancer, squamous lung carcinoma, and colorectal cancers. MHC class I chain-related protein (MIC) has limited expression in normal gastrointestinal epithelium but are expressed constitutively in many human primary carcinomas. MIC is recognized by the activating receptor NKG2D on effector cells and subsequently triggers downstream signaling and tumor killing. On the other hand, NKG2D expression was found to be reduced by immune cells infiltrating the MIC + tumors, indicating a mechanism of tumor escape from immunosurveillance.

3. **Adaptive immune response**
   a. **Mechanism.** Tumor antigens are released and picked up by activated dendritic cells (DCs), which in turn migrate to the draining lymph nodes and activate tumor-specific naïve CD4+ Th1 cells and CD8+ cytotoxic T lymphocytes (CTLs) via MHC class I restriction. CD4+ cells facilitate the activation of tumor-specific CD8 CTLs, which kill tumor cells directly or indirectly through IFNγ.
   b. **Tumor-specific antigens.** Over the years with the advance of the techniques to detect immune responses *in vitro* and gene cloning, several classes of tumor antigens that can be recognized by T cells or antibodies have been identified, including differentiation antigens, mutational antigens, overexpressed antigens, viral antigens, and cancer–testis antigens. Of these, the cancer–testis antigen has gained much interest due to their limited expression in normal adult human tissues and wide range of expression in different tumors types, thus potential targets for immunotherapy.
   c. **Paraneoplastic neurologic disorders (PND)** provide evidence for the adaptive immune response toward tumor cells. In PND, the host's immune response toward tumor cross-reacts with normal cells, frequently from the nervous system. High titers of neuronal-reactive antibodies can be identified in these patients, and interestingly, the presence of these antibodies is associated with improved survival of the patients.

4. **Tumor microenvironment.** The tumor has a complex microenvironment comprised of not only tumor cells and debris but also immune cells, fibroblasts, cytokines and chemokines, stroma, etc. They interact with the tumor cells and influence their growth, survival, as well as metastatic and immunogenic potential. On the other hand, the tumor cells can manipulate the microenvironment they are residing in and can transform a hostile environment to be more permissive. Although TILs are frequently found in the tumors, they are often debilitated by the overwhelmingly suppressive immune microenvironment, including down-regulation of tumor-specific antigen or antigen-presenting machinery; recruitment of immune suppressive cells such as Tregs, tumor-associated macrophages (TAM), or myeloid-derived suppressor cells (MDSCs); and production of immunosuppressive cytokines such as IL-8, IL-10, TGFß, VEGF, as well as ligands such as programmed death-ligand 1 (PD-L1).

5. **Microbiota.** Microbes are implicated in many human malignancies, and the intimate relationship of the host's microbiota and carcinogenesis is well established but poorly understood. When mucosal barriers are breached, the

environmental insult and repair process trigger a chronic low-grade inflammatory state that can facilitate microbe's influence on tumor growth and metastasis. Many of these processes involve activation of NF-kB, a regulator of cancer-associated inflammation, and both innate and adaptive immune responses can occur. One example is the modulation of colon tumorigenesis by the gut microbiota independent of genetic considerations. An immune-deficient state induced by microbes can also increase the risk of cancers, such as in HIV-infected individuals. The question whether microbiota can influence a host's susceptibility to immunotherapy has gained much interest lately due to the exciting success of modern cancer immunotherapies. Recent data showing impaired response to CpG oligonucleotide treatment in antibiotics-treated mice seem to support this hypothesis.

II. IMMUNOTHERAPY

The earliest observations that certain bacterial infection could induce regression of cancers dates back to the 1700s, and in the 1890s, a New York surgeon Dr. William B. Coley recognized the power of the host's immune system to eradicate cancer and pioneered the Coley toxin, a mixture of the gram-positive Streptococcus and gram-negative Serratia, both heat inactivated, which reportedly can induce a 10% response rate by local injections in patients with advanced sarcoma. Subsequently, cytokines, vaccines, and adoptively transferred immune effector cells were developed throughout the last century in attempts to activate the patient's antitumor immunity with small but consistent success rates. It was only recently, with the advance of our understanding of immunobiology, that successful immunotherapies were developed and consistent benefits have been observed in multiple tumor histologies. There are objective tumor responses to immunotherapy in cancers that are not traditionally considered "immunotherapy sensitive," such as lung cancers, head and neck cancers, urothelial cancers, etc., and this list has been continuously expanding. In 2013, cancer immunotherapy was named "breakthrough of the year" by the magazine Science.

A. Innate Immune Modulators

1. **Interleukin-2 (IL-2)** was the first immunotherapy approved for treatment of human cancers. IL-2 is a T-cell growth factor that allows for expansion of T cells while maintaining their functional activity. IL-2 gene was cloned in 1983, and subsequently, recombinant IL-2 (**aldesleukin**) has been used in clinical practice, given in bolus doses every 8 hours until grade 3 to 4 toxicities occur. With this schedule, a low objective response rate (ORR) but durable disease regressions in the majority of the complete responders (CR) was observed in renal cell carcinoma (ORR 20%, CR 9%) and malignant melanoma (ORR 16%, CR 6%), which led to the approval of this approach by the Food and Drug Administration (FDA) in 1992 and 1998, respectively. High-dose IL-2 administration is associated with significant toxicities due to the underlying capillary leak syndrome that causes fluid extravasation into visceral organs and impairs their functions. These toxicities are reversible after the therapy is interrupted and treatment-related mortality is <1%.

B. Cancer Vaccines

Despite decades of attempts to develop tumor-specific therapeutic vaccines in the hope to activate the host's immune system against cancers that are non- or low immunogenic, the overall experience has not been fruitful. The fundamental problem lies in the suboptimal antigen vaccine design and the immune-suppressive tumor microenvironment that prohibits the effector function that is activated by the vaccine. Targeting neoantigens that are consequence of tumor-specific mutations represents a new promising personalized immunotherapy modality that has been made possible with the recent advance in next-generation sequencing and epitope prediction techniques.

1. **Bacillus Calmette-Guérin (BCG) vaccine** is a live attenuated strain of *Mycobacterium bovis*, and it is given intravesically as a part to adjunctive therapy for superficial bladder cancer (see Chapter 14).

2. **Sipuleucel-T** is a DC vaccine that is designed to enhance the T-cell response against prostatic acid phosphatase. Patient-derived DCs are expanded *in vitro* and loaded with tumor-specific antigen, before giving back to the patients. The trial in men with castration-resistant prostate cancer without visceral metastasis showed a small improvement in overall survival (26 vs. 22 months) when compared to placebo (see Chapter 14).

3. **GVAX** is a whole-cell vaccine that is composed of two irradiated prostate cancer cell lines that expresses granulocyte–macrophage colony-stimulating factor (GM-CSF) that promote the activation of T cells with low affinity for self-antigens expressed by tumors. Clinical testing has not shown survival benefit by randomized trials. Besides the common challenges associated with cancer vaccine, immunization with allogeneic cells against antigens from patient's own tumor could be misleading.

4. **Gp100 vaccine** is a peptide vaccine with a melanocyte differentiation antigen, glycoprotein 100 (gp100). When it was used in combination with high-dose IL-2 in patients with melanoma, it improved ORR and progression-free survival (PFS) when compared to high-dose IL-2 alone in a phase III clinical trial.

C. **Adoptive Cell Transfer (ACT) Therapy**

1. **Tumor-infiltrating lymphocytes (TILs).** The number of TILs favorably correlates with cancer patient survival. A new treatment approach pioneered by Steven Rosenberg and his colleagues in the 1980s was based in isolating **TILs** from the patient's surgical melanoma specimens, expanding them *in vitro* under stimulating culture conditions, and reinfusing with systemic cytokine (IL-2) back to the lympho-depleted patient. The reported response rate was 50% for melanoma, and most responses were durable. Of the 20% CR, 95% of them had more than 5 years of survival. This approach, however, requires large surgical samples, is restricted to limited academic centers with experience, and seems only applicable to melanoma, where larger number of antitumor T cells can be found in the tumors and is a rare event in other tumor types.

2. **T-cell receptor engineering.** The advance of the gene transfer technologies and T-cell engineering enabled a more versatile and feasible approach, adoptive transfer of the patients' own peripheral T cells that are genetically engineered to target cancer-specific antigens back to preconditioned lympho-depleted patients.

a. **Viral transduction of physiologic TCR.** A physiologic TCR usually is cloned from TILs specific for a cancer antigen, such as NY-ESO-1, a cancer–testis antigen that has very limited expression in normal adult tissue, but expressed by certain cancers. It contains variable α and ß chains that recognize tumor antigen presented in the context of MHC. Clinical success has been documented using autologous T cells transduced with NY-ESO-1 TCR to treat melanoma, sarcomas, and multiple myeloma. The advantage of the TCR approach is that the antigen target can be intracellular, but it is MHC restricted, therefore is only available to patients with the matched Human Leukocyte Antigen (HLA) subtype, and can be subject to treatment failure for tumors that have down-regulated their MHC surface expression.

   b. **Chimeric antigen receptor (CAR)** technology was initially developed by genetically engineering T cells with chimeric genes linking single-chain antibodies (scFv) targeting tumor cell surface antigens to intracellular signaling adaptors for TCR, the ζ chain of the CD3 complex (first generation), a T-cell–specific chain that has activating function of T cells. Subsequent modification of the design with the incorporation of the intracellular domains of costimulatory molecules such as CD28 (second generation) and 41BB agonist (third generation) has enabled the expansion of T cells while retaining function upon repeated antigen exposure. Engineered CAR T-cell therapy does not require MHC restriction as it recognizes a full surface protein not requiring MHC presentation. Therefore, this approach can be applied to patients regardless of their HLA typing or whether the tumor has altered self-antigens and can be engineered to enhance T-cell function. However, the repertoire of potential antigens is much more restricted.

   Recent clinical data using autologous T cells transduced with CD19 targeting CAR to treat CD19+ B-cell malignancy, including diffuse large B-cell lymphoma (DLBCL), chronic lymphocytic leukemia (CLL), and acute lymphoblastic leukemia (ALL), have shown impressive results. A remarkable 90% complete remission (CR) was reported in 30 relapsed or refractory ALL patients, and two-thirds of these patients remained in remission after 6 months.

   The biggest challenge facing the field of ACT is the identification of target tumor antigens that are not expressed by normal tissues, to maximize specificity and efficacy and minimize target toxicity. A commonly seen toxicity in ACT therapy is cytokine release syndrome, which is managed by steroids and IL-6 receptor antibody (tocilizumab) and can be life-threatening.

D. **Bispecific T-Cell Engager (BiTE).** BiTE is a new form of immunotherapy. BiTEs are bispecific monoclonal antibodies that are able to form a link between a T cell and a cancer cell and activate the T cell so it can exert its cytotoxic activity. **Blinatumomab** is a bispecific antibody that binds to CD19 antigen, expressed on normal and malignant B cells, and to CD3, a molecule on T cells. The drug allows to bring T cells in the proximity of cancer cells. Blinatumomab is approved for the treatment of B-cell precursor ALL (see Chapter 26).

E. **Checkpoint Inhibitors.** T-cell activation requires not only TCR recognition of antigen presented by the MHC molecule on the surface of APC but also interaction of costimulatory molecules CD28 and B7. Activated T cells will then be regulated by inhibitory checkpoints to avoid collateral damage and autoimmunity.

   1. **CTLA (cytotoxic T-lymphocyte associated protein)-4** is a receptor on activated T effector cells and Tregs, discovered by Pierre Goldstein in the 1980s. Seminal work done by James Allison and colleagues showed that CTLA-4 competes with CD28 for B7 ligands and transmits inhibitory signals to attenuate effector T-cell function in the initiation phase of T-cell activation, and CTLA-4–blocking antibodies could treat tumors in immune-competent animal models. Interestingly, immunosuppressive Treg cells express high levels of CTLA-4, which paradoxically enhances Treg cell activity. Deficiency of CTLA-4 in Treg cells in mice results in spontaneous autoimmune disease,

and loss of CTLA-4 also potentiates tumor immunity. Ipilimumab is a CTLA-4–blocking antibody and it is the first approved checkpoint inhibitor (2011). Clinical trials showed that the treatment with ipilimumab led to the improvement in the overall survival in patients with advanced melanoma (see Chapter 17). A recent long-term follow-up analysis showed a 15% durable response at 5 years. Ipilimumab was also approved by the FDA as an adjuvant therapy for locally advanced melanoma. Due to the immune activation at the early stage of T-cell activation, significant immune-related toxicity has been observed, including skin, bowel, liver, thyroid, pituitary glands, etc., that can be managed by systemic steroid therapy. Evaluation of anti-CTLA-4 treatment in other cancer types has been ongoing.

2. **Programmed death 1 (PD-1)** is another checkpoint in the effector phase of T-cell activation. PD-1 was cloned in 1992 by Tasuku Honjo, and its ligand PD-L1 was characterized by Lieping Chen and Gordon Freeman in 1999 and 2000. PD-1 is expressed by activated T cells, and expression of PD-L1 can be induced by many tumor cells on their surface in response to IFNγ to evade immune attack. Antibodies blocking the PD-1/L1 inhibitory axis can unleash activated tumor-reactive T cells to proliferate and attack tumor cells and has been shown in clinical trials to induce durable antitumor responses in increasing numbers of tumor histologies, including the tumor types that is not traditionally considered "immunotherapy sensitive," such as lung cancer, bladder cancer, head and neck cancers, Hodgkin disease, cancers with microsatellite instability, hepatocellular cancers, etc.

   Two anti-PD-1 antibodies, **pembrolizumab** and **nivolumab**, have been approved for treatment of advanced melanoma with around 30% to 40% of response rate and advanced NSCLC with 20% to 30% response rate. Nivolumab is also approved for treatment of patients with renal cell carcinoma and Hodgkin disease. **Atezolizumab**, an anti-PD-L1 antibody, is approved for the treatment of bladder cancer. Other anti-PD-1/PD-L1 antibodies are in various stage of clinical testing. The treatment can be associated with immune-related side effects, but possibly because PD-1/L1 checkpoint is at the last step of T-cell activation, with more restricted T-cell reactivity toward tumor cells, the frequency of side effects is much lower than in the case of ipilimumab.

3. **Combination of ipilimumab and nivolumab.** Due to the nonoverlapping mechanism of action of anti-CTLA-4 and anti-PD-1 antibodies, clinical testing of combination of these two classes of checkpoint inhibitors were conducted with improved clinical response (up to 60%) in melanoma at the expense of significantly increased toxicities. This combination of ipilimumab and nivolumab has been approved for patient with melanoma (see Chapter 17).

F. **Oncolytic Viruses**

Talimogene laherparepvec (T-VEC, formerly known as OncoVEXGM-CSF) is an oncolytic virus, first-in-class approved agent for treatment of cancer. T-VEC is a modified herpes simplex virus type 1 (HSV1) that is designed to selectively replicate in tumor tissue and to stimulate a systemic antitumor immune response. The HSV1 viral genes that are responsible for replication in normal cells have been deleted. In addition, the coding sequence for human GM-CSF was inserted to enhance the immune response to tumor antigens released during oncolysis. Intralesional administration of T-VEC results in oncolysis of cells and local release of progeny virus as well as of tumor cell antigens. This strategy results in the destruction of injected tumors as well as uninjected sites of disease (including micrometastases) via a systemic antitumor immune response. Success of T-VEC in the pivotal phase 3 trial (OPTiM) in melanoma indicated that this treatment could induce a systemic immune response against melanoma with favorable toxicity profile. The data on combination with checkpoint inhibitors suggest much higher complete and ORRs; the confirmatory trials are currently ongoing.

G. Other Immune Modulatory Agents

Agonists or antagonists targeting other immune modulatory targets have been studied and are in the clinical testing, including immune-stimulating antibodies toward 41BB/CD137, OX40, and GITR (glucocorticoid-induced TNFR family-related gene); CSF1R (colony-stimulating factor 1 receptor) inhibitors targeting the immunosuppressive TAM; intratumoral injection of toll-like receptor (TLR) agonists; inhibitors of indoleamine 2,3-dioxygenase (IDO), which is a critical immune-resistant mechanism in the tumor microenvironment; and inhibitors against other immune checkpoint modulators on the cell surface such as TIM3, LAG3, etc.

H. Immune-Related Response Criteria (irRC). The patterns of response to checkpoint inhibitors may differ from those seen in patients treated with traditional chemotherapy or molecularly targeted agents. The following patterns of response were noted:

1. **Conventional response** in baseline lesions with a decrease in the size of measurable disease. It is the identical pattern to the one seen with traditional chemotherapy.

2. **Prolonged stable disease** followed by a gradual decrease in size of measurable disease. This type of response may be seen with traditional chemotherapy and molecularly targeted therapy. In case of immunotherapy, the steady decline in tumor burden may continue although the treatment by itself was discontinued because of toxicity or because the course of the therapy was completed (e.g., ipilimumab is given for a total of 4 doses).

3. **Response after initial increase in total tumor volume.** The initial restaging scans show an increase in the tumor burden, but subsequent scans show improvement in the tumor volume.

4. **Reduction in total tumor burden after the appearance of new lesions.** Traditionally, the appearance of a new lesion is consistent with a lack of efficacy of chemotherapy. When immunotherapy is used, new lesions may appear, while the baseline lesions decrease or increase in size. Eventually, all lesions start decreasing in size.

5. **When to switch the therapy.** Clinicians must be aware of these different patterns of response so they do not discontinue immunotherapy prematurely. Usually, patients who are destined to achieve a response have a stable performance status and frequently experience an improvement in symptoms. If imaging studies show worsening of tumor burden and patient's condition deteriorates, it is extremely unlikely a delayed response would be seen. These patients should be offered alternative therapy. Atypical patterns of response to immunotherapy are much less common than traditional ones, and they are seen in about 1% of melanoma patients treated with ipilimumab and in about 5% of patients treated with anti-PD-1 antibodies.

I. Immune-Related Adverse Events (irAEs). The treatment with checkpoint inhibitors is associated with a unique spectrum of toxicities that are related to nonspecific T-cell activation and general immunologic enhancement. The side effects resemble autoimmune diseases, but standard immunologic tests used in rheumatology are mostly negative. In some patients, these side effects may be life threatening or fatal, especially when not recognized and treated early. Most commonly, they affect skin, gastrointestinal tract, liver, endocrine glands, and lungs, but they can occur in almost any organ.

1. **Dermatologic irAEs:**
   a. Vitiligo
   b. Rash—typically reticular, maculopapular, faintly erythematous
   c. Toxic epidermal necrolysis Stevens-Johnson syndrome—rare, but can be life threatening

2. **Gastrointestinal irAEs:**
   a. Diarrhea—about 30% patients are treated with ipilimumab, and 10% of patients experience severe diarrhea.
   b. Colitis—defined as diarrhea with abdominal pain, cramps, possibly fever, or imaging and/or endoscopic evidence of colonic inflammation. Colitis resembles Crohn disease. Colonic biopsies showed lymphocytic and neutrophilic infiltrates with cryptitis and, in some cases, crypt abscesses and granuloma.
   c. Bowel perforation—colitis, when untreated, may lead to bowel perforation.

3. **Endocrine irAEs:**
   a. Hypothyroidism—more common than hyperthyroidism; TSH should be monitored during therapy.
   b. Hyperthyroidism—usually self-limited; beta-blockers can be used to ameliorate symptoms; methimazole is prescribed when free T4 continues to rise.
   c. Adrenal insufficiency—characterized by low cortisol and elevated ACTH levels; symptoms/signs are often nonspecific such as fatigue and orthostatic hypotension; it may lead to dehydration, hypotension, and electrolyte disturbances.
   d. Hypophysitis with pituitary insufficiency—the symptoms/signs are frequently nonspecific such as headache, fatigue, decreased blood pressure, visual problems, muscle weakness, nausea, and constipation; MRI of the pituitary gland can show pituitary enlargement/edema; laboratory tests revealed decreased TSH, ACTH, LH, and FSH; sometimes, only one line is affected; thyroid and adrenal replacement is required.

4. **Hepatic irAEs:**
   a. Immune-related hepatitis—characterized by unexplained elevation of serum levels of hepatic alanine aminotransferase or aspartate aminotransferase enzymes; other causes of liver injury such as biliary obstruction and infection should be excluded; serum assays for ANAs, antismooth muscle antibodies, antiliver kidney microsomal antibody type 1, and antiliver cytosol type 1 are usually negative.
   b. Liver failure—very rare; may be fatal.

5. **Pulmonary irAEs:** Pneumonitis is uncommon in patients treated with CTLA-4–blocking antibodies, more common with PD-1/PD-L1–blocking antibodies; it presents with dry cough, progressive shortness of breath, and fine inspiratory crackles; if untreated, it may proceed to hypoxia and respiratory failure; imaging studies reveal ground-glass opacities and/or disseminated nodular infiltrates, predominantly in the lower lobes.

6. **Ophthalmologic irAEs:** Episcleritis, conjunctivitis, uveitis, and orbital inflammation

7. **Neurologic irAEs:** Neuropathy, Guillain-Barré syndrome, aseptic or lymphocytic meningitis or meningoencephalitis, posterior reversible encephalopathy syndrome, and transverse myelitis.

8. **Renal irAEs:** Uncommon, but more commonly seen in patients treated with PD-1/PD-L1–blocking antibodies; interstitial nephritis with inflammatory cortical renal enlargement or granulomatous nephritis and glomerular lupus-like nephropathy; some patients may require temporary hemodialysis.

9. **Pancreatic irAEs:** Cases of endocrine and exocrine insufficiency have been described. Exocrine pancreatic insufficiency should be considered in patients who present with chronic foul-smelling diarrhea and weight loss. Pancreatic enzymes replacement leads to a fast improvement in symptoms.

10. **Hematologic irAEs:** Very rare, red cell aplasia, autoimmune neutropenia or pancytopenia, and acquired hemophilia A.

11. **Musculoskeletal irAEs:** Polyarthritis or arthralgia has been reported in around 5% of patients with immune checkpoint blockade.

12. **Management of irAEs:** Steroids are the mainstay of the management of irAEs. There is a single institution retrospective study of 254 patients treated with ipilimumab with short follow-up showing no impact of immunosuppression on efficacy or patient survival, but there are no long-term prospective studies to prove the hypothesis.

    a. **Mild severity.** The therapy with a checkpoint inhibitor can be continued, and symptomatic treatment should be offered. The patient must be educated; the symptoms/signs may worsen.

    b. **Moderate severity.** The therapy with a checkpoint inhibitor should be withheld, and symptomatic treatment offered. If symptoms persist for 5 to 7 days, the treatment with methylprednisolone or oral equivalent should be started at the dose of 0.5 to 1 mg/kg/d. After symptoms improve, steroids are tapered over a period of 1 month or longer. Prophylactic antibiotics for opportunistic infections should be considered for patients treated with 20 mg of prednisone equivalent daily for at least 4 weeks. Pneumocystis prophylaxis with trimethoprim–sulfamethoxazole, atovaquone, or pentamidine is strongly recommended; the benefits of antiviral and antifungal prophylaxis are less clear.

    c. **Severe toxicity.** The therapy with a checkpoint inhibitor should be discontinued permanently. Methylprednisolone or oral equivalent should be started at the dose of 1 to 2 mg/kg/d. If the patient is very symptomatic, hospitalization and intravenous steroids are preferred. Prophylactic antibiotics for opportunistic infections should be considered. After symptoms improve, steroids are tapered over a period of 1 month or longer.

    d. **Persistent/recurrent toxicity.** If toxicity does not resolve on steroids, patients can be treated with a single-dose infliximab 5 mg/kg (it may be repeated in 2 weeks if symptoms improved, especially helpful in the management of gastrointestinal irAEs, and contraindicated in hepatic irAEs) or mycophenolate mofetil at the dose of 1 g twice a day (especially helpful in the management of hepatic irAEs).

J. **Future direction.** Despite these recent breakthroughs in developing checkpoint inhibitors to treat advanced melanoma and other cancers, a significant number of patients do not respond to PD-1/PD-L1 blockade, and a significant number of patients experience disease progression after an initial response. Emerging evidence has suggested that response to anti-PD-1/L1–based therapies relies on the patients' ability to mount a tumor-specific response, which is then turned off by PD-1/PD-L1 engagements. Failure of therapy is likely due to lack of sufficient immune activation against the cancer or overwhelming suppressive tumor microenvironment that is hard to overcome, and can be addressed by combination therapies strategies to increase T-cell activation and tumor infiltrations, as well as to improve tumor immune microenvironment. Critical questions remain as to how to choose patients for different combination options and how best to combine these immunotherapy modalities while avoiding toxicities. Careful study of patient-derived samples at baseline and while patient is on treatment and development of predictive biomarkers is key to answer these questions.

Suggested Readings

Chen DS, Mellman I. Oncology meets immunology: the cancer-immunity cycle. *Immunity* 2013;39:1.

Dunn GP, Old LJ, Schreiber RD. The three Es of cancer immunoediting. *Annu Rev Immunol* 2004;22:329.

Garrett WS. Cancer and the microbiota. *Science* 2015;348:80.

Miller JF, Sadelain M. The journey from discoveries in fundamental immunology to cancer immunotherapy. *Cancer Cell* 2015;27:439.

Ribas A. Adaptive immune resistance: how cancer protects from immune attack. *Cancer Discov* 2015;5:915.

Rosenberg SA. IL-2: the first effective immunotherapy for human cancer. *J Immunol* 2014;192:5451.

Shankaran V, Ikeda H, Bruce AT, et al. IFNgamma and lymphocytes prevent primary tumor development and shape tumour immunogenicity. *Nature* 2001;410:1107.

Sharma P, Allison JP. The future of immune checkpoint therapy. *Science* 2015;348:56.

Sharma P, Allison JP. Immune checkpoint targeting in cancer therapy: toward combination strategies with curative potential. *Cell* 2015;161:205.

Smyth MJ, Ngiow SF, Ribas A, et al. Combination cancer immunotherapies tailored to the tumour microenvironment. *Nat Rev Clin Oncol* 2016;13:143.

Tumeh PC, et al. PD-1 blockade induces responses by inhibiting adaptive immune resistance. *Nature* 2014;515:568.

6 Palliative Care in Oncology: Symptom Management and Goals of Care

David Wallenstein, Shireen N. Heidari, and Andrew Huy Cao Nguyen

PALLIATIVE CARE

Palliative care encompasses a wide variety of clinical disciplines and management skills and has many definitions. One aspect of palliative care is the strategic management of symptoms in the context of serious illness. A misconception is that palliative care is reserved for the end of life, when in fact it can be offered in conjunction with curative treatment, such as surgery or chemotherapy. Most oncologists perform palliative symptom assessments and interventions on a regular basis in clinic, as side effects are common with curative treatments. Additionally, understanding a patient's goals of care and expectations of each treatment option can dramatically inform the treatment plan. The goal of this chapter is to address some of the basic principles of palliative care assessments and challenges in addressing goals of care with seriously ill patients.

I. PATIENT ASSESSMENT

Studies have shown that implementing regular standardized symptom screenings during active treatment, with triggers for nursing and clinician intervention, may cost very little and have a measurable impact on symptom improvement and patient-reported quality of life. In addition, they also have a potential for reducing emergency department visits and hospital admissions. In essence, when symptoms are managed, patients are better able to tolerate their therapies.

A. **Assessing symptoms:** One often-used symptom management tool is the **Edmonton Symptom Assessment Scale (ESAS)**, which has patients rate 10 common symptoms on a scale of 1 to 10 (0 = no symptom → 10 = worst possible). These symptoms include pain, tiredness, nausea, depression, anxiety, drowsiness, appetite, well-being, shortness of breath, and others. These symptom assessments can then be tracked over time, with triggers for intervention and response to oncologic therapy monitored based on changes in symptom severity.

B. **Assessing performance:** It is also important to assess a patient's functional status both at the start and during the course of treatment. There are several tools that are used in both the oncology setting as well as by palliative providers. These include the Eastern Cooperative Oncology Group (**ECOG**) Performance Status and **Karnofsky** Performance Status (KPS) (Table 6-1).

II. PAIN

Pain is a common symptom in the management of cancer patients, affecting approximately 30% to 40% of those receiving therapy and almost 90% of those with advanced disease. **Inadequate pain control can adversely affect quality of life regardless of prognosis.**

TABLE 6-1	Measurements of Performance Status
ECOG Performance Status	**Karnofsky Performance Status**
0 = Fully active, able to carry on all predisease performance without restriction	100 = Normal, no complaints; no evidence of disease
	90 = Able to carry on normal activity; minor signs or symptoms of disease
1 = Restricted in physically strenuous activity but ambulatory and able to carry out work of a light or sedentary nature, for example, light house work, office work	80 = Normal activity with effort, some signs or symptoms of disease
	70 = Care for self but unable to carry on normal activity or to do active work
2 = Ambulatory and capable of all self-care but unable to carry out any work activities. Up and about more than 50% of waking hours	60 = Requires occasional assistance but is able to care for most of personal needs
	50 = Requires considerable assistance and frequent medical care
3 = Capable of only limited self-care, confined to bed or chair more than 50% of waking hours	40 = Disabled; requires special care and assistance
	30 = Severely disabled; hospitalization is indicated although death not imminent
4 = Completely disabled. Cannot carry on any self-care. Totally confined to bed or chair	20 = Very ill; hospitalization and active supportive care necessary
	10 = Moribund
5 = Dead	0 = Dead

Information from Karnofsky DA, Burchenal JH. The clinical evaluation of chemotherapeutic agents in cancer. In: MacLeod CM, ed. *Evaluation of Chemotherapeutic Agents.* Columbia University Press, 1949:196; information from Oken M, et al. Toxicity and response criteria of the Eastern Cooperative Oncology Group. *Am J Clin Oncol* 1982;5(6):649–655.

A. **Barriers to adequate pain control include:**
   1. Patient reluctance to report pain, fears about addiction, or side effects of medications
   2. Physician failure to screen for or appreciate severity of pain
   3. Undertreatment of pain
B. **Assessment of pain**
   1. Take a careful pain history including site of pain, onset, acute or chronic, constant or intermittent, provoking and alleviating factors, and associated symptoms.
   2. Quality of the pain. Can help to distinguish between nociceptive somatic, nociceptive visceral, and neuropathic pain, which can guide therapy decisions.
   3. Impact on activities of daily living.
   4. The pain interventions already tried and their level of effectiveness.
   5. Screen for history of alcohol or drug dependence. Note: the presence of active drug addiction is not a contraindication to the effective treatment of cancer pain with an opioid; however, specialist consultation with addiction medicine may be necessary.
   6. Evaluation for depression.
   7. Physical examination.
C. **Initiation of pain medication**
   1. What medication you choose and the route of administration will depend on the severity of the pain and the patient's current clinical status (ability to tolerate medication, organ dysfunction).
   2. One often-used tool is the WHO ladder, which advises a **stepwise progression** from nonopioids (NSAIDs, acetaminophen) and adjuvants for mild pain, to the addition of "weak" opioids (tramadol, hydrocodone, oxycodone–acetaminophen, codeine) to the adjuvants for moderate pain,

to "strong" opioids (morphine, oxycodone, hydromorphone, fentanyl, methadone) for severe pain nonresponsive to the previous steps. It is a useful tool for many patients, though starting at step 1 may not apply in cases of oncologic pain crisis in the inpatient setting.

3. There are three very important pharmacology concepts when dosing pain medications:
   a. **Time to Cmax** = amount of time it takes for medication to reach maximum levels in bloodstream.
   b. **Half-life** = amount of time it takes for half the medication to be eliminated from the body.
   c. **Steady state** = when the amount of drug entering the bloodstream is the same as the amount leaving (generally takes between 5 and 6 half-lives to reach steady state). This is an important concept when assessing the efficacy of a certain dose, and whether adjustments should occur, both for oral medications and infusions. Adjusting too frequently may result in overmedication.

   Example: in the case of morphine:
   - Half-life = 2 to 4 hours
   - Time to Cmax IV = 15 minutes, IM/SC = 30 min, PO = 1 hour
   - Steady state = 5 half-lives

4. If a patient has uncontrolled pain, it is reasonable to give breakthrough doses every Tmax (since you would see max effect at that time), so with IV morphine, every 15 minutes until pain is controlled.

5. **Start with short-acting opioids** when determining a patient's daily opioid requirement (no extended release or long-acting medications as first line).

6. Once the daily opioid requirement is determined, you can start long-acting formulations. Consider giving between 50% and 100% of the daily total in divided doses.

7. Then 10% and 20% of daily opioid requirement can be scheduled as a breakthrough dose.
   a. Example: if you started a patient with severe pain from metastatic disease on 15 mg of morphine orally q4h as needed, and he took a total of 75 mg over 24 hours, with excellent pain relief and minimal sedation, you could consider scheduling 30 mg of long-acting morphine twice daily and continue to use 15 mg of the short acting every 4 hours as a breakthrough dose.
   b. Conversely: if your patient was taking sublingual morphine 5 mg q4h p.r.n. for shortness of breath, and only needed 2 doses in 24 hours, he or she may not need scheduled doses.

8. **If patient is requiring more than 4 p.r.n. doses of short-acting breakthrough opioid a day,** he or she may need an adjustment to the dose of the long-acting medication.

D. **Commonly used pain medications** (with typical starting doses)
   1. Hydrocodone–acetaminophen (5 to 325 mg; 1 tabs q4h p.r.n. moderate to severe pain).
   2. Oxycodone–acetaminophen (5 to 325 mg; 1 tabs q4h p.r.n. moderate to severe pain).
   3. Morphine (starting dose varies based on severity of pain; consider 15 mg PO q4h p.r.n., 1 mg IV q3–4h p.r.n.).
   4. Oxycodone (5 mg q4h p.r.n.).
   5. Hydromorphone (2 to 4 mg PO q4h p.r.n., 0.5 mg IV q3–4h p.r.n.).
   6. Fentanyl (see section on transdermal fentanyl; not recommended as first line or in opioid-naive patients).

TABLE 6-2 Converting Between Different Opioid Medications

Oral/Rectal Dose (mg)	Analgesic	Parenteral Dose IV/SC/IM (mg)
150	Tramadol	–
150	Codeine	50
15	Hydrocodone	–
15	**Morphine**	5
10	Oxycodone	–
5	Oxymorphone	–
3	Hydromorphone	1
2	Levorphanol	1
–	Fentanyl[a]	0.050

[a]Additional notes on fentanyl transdermal patches below.
Adapted from Bodtke S, Ligon K. *Hospice and Palliative Medicine Handbook: A Clinical Guide.* San Diego, CA, 2016:192.

7. Methadone—less common as first line but can be helpful for severe and neuropathic pain as it has *N*-methyl-D-aspartate (NMDA) receptor antagonism in addition to affinity for opioid receptor. Consider involving pain or palliative care team for assistance as conversions are not straightforward.

E. **Converting between different medications** (Table 6-2): In general, when converting between different pain medications, providers will convert dosing to oral morphine equivalents. Oral morphine equivalents will also provide guidelines for the initiation of some more regulated long-acting medications.

  1. **Example 1**: if a patient was getting 2 mg IV morphine every 4 hours as needed, and got 3 doses, he would have received 6 mg IV morphine, or (since 5 IV morphine is equal to 15 oral morphine) 18 mg oral morphine equivalents.

  2. **Example 2**: if a patient is taking oxycodone 5-mg tablets at home, but is hospitalized for inability to tolerate oral intake, an equianalgesic table can help provide guidelines on starting doses for IV medications.

  3. **Adjusting for cross-tolerance**

    a. When converting between medications, it is important to remember that switching medications is exposing the patient to a new analgesic and that they may not need as much medication as they did previously. In general, **unless they had very poor pain control, the dose of the new medication should be reduced from the calculated direct conversion dose** (Table 6-3).

F. **The use of transdermal fentanyl**

  1. There are multiple possible conversions used for transdermal fentanyl. One of the most generous is that approximately 50 oral morphine equivalents per day are approximately equal to a 25 mcg/hr patch. This does not decrease for cross-tolerance, which is an important consideration. Conversions provided by the manufacturer typically urge for more conservative estimations (e.g., patients on between 60 and 134 oral morphine equivalents per day should be started on a 25 mcg/hr patch).

TABLE 6-3 Adjustments for Cross Tolerance

Pain Control Prior to Switch	Adjustment to Calculated Dose
Poor	No adjustment
Moderate	Reduce by 25%
Excellent	Reduce by 50%

Adapted from Bodtke S, Ligon K. *Hospice and Palliative Medicine Handbook: A Clinical Guide.* San Diego, CA, 2016:193.

    2. By FDA guidelines, patients need to be on at least 60 oral morphine equivalents a day for 1 week to be considered "opioid tolerant" and therefore appropriate for a fentanyl patch. The fentanyl patch is not designed for "opioid-naive" patients, and there are significant risks in doing so.

    3. Patches are typically not as effective in patients with severe cachexia, poor circulation, edema, or intermittent pain.

    4. Fevers or temperature changes (including local application of heat) will also lead to variable absorption of the medication and potentially increase dramatically the intended dose.

G. Patients with renal dysfunction

    1. Morphine is well known to have metabolites that can accumulate in renal dysfunction and cause side effects (including but not limited to myoclonus, seizures).

    2. Hydromorphone may not be an appropriate alternative to morphine in the setting of renal dysfunction, as it also is renally cleared.

    3. Consider methadone or fentanyl for patients who have significant kidney dysfunction.

H. Common side effects of opioid therapy

    1. GI: constipation, nausea, and vomiting

    2. CNS: sedation, confusion, and myoclonus

    3. Urinary retention

    4. Tolerance

I. Additional routes of administration for opioids

    1. Epidural and intrathecal anesthesia. Consider when other routes are ineffective or opioids cause excessive toxicity.

    2. Sublingual/buccal or rectal if oral route not available or not tolerated.

    3. Topical for painful ulcerative lesions or oral mucositis.

    4. Pumps: patient-controlled analgesia (PCA) can be useful for cancer patients. Consider involving pain management or palliative care team when initiating, particularly if the patient is in pain crisis. When you initiate a PCA, it is probably best to start with a conservative dose and increase the demand dose if there is inadequate relief. Begin with a 1- to 3-mg demand dose of morphine sulfate with a delay interval of 10 minutes ("lockout"); the patient can thus receive this dose up to six times an hour. The amount given over 4 hours is determined and may be converted (averaged) to an hourly (basal) dose. The new, every 10-minute *demand dose* becomes 50% of the hourly dose. For patients already on morphine or other pain medications, the same method is used except that the 24-hour dose is converted to an hourly (basal) dose and then a new demand dose can be formulated. Keep in mind that the patient may need adjustments as the underlying reasons for the patient's pain are treated during the course of the hospitalization, and both scheduled and as-needed doses should be evaluated regularly.

J. Opioid-induced hyperalgesia

    1. This is an important consideration in patients who have been taking opioid pain medications long term with increasing pain despite dose escalation, mechanism not well understood.

    2. The solution may be to decrease their opioid dose (may be helpful to consult palliative care or pain management for guidance).

K. Adjuvants

    1. Antidepressants

        a. Tricyclic antidepressants (**TCAs**): nortriptyline is most commonly used because of fewer side effects (25 mg qhs).

    b. Selective serotonin reuptake inhibitors (**SSRIs**): fluoxetine, sertraline, citalopram, and escitalopram.

    c. Serotonin–norepinephrine reuptake inhibitors (**SNRIs**): duloxetine and venlafaxine.

    d. **Atypicals**: mirtazapine—often used for its effect on appetite as well as mood, be advised that it is less helpful for both effects if the dose is raised beyond 15 mg (start at 7.5 mg nightly).

    e. Caution: avoid using more than one antidepressant at once without input from psychiatry or neurology.

2. Anticonvulsants: particularly helpful for neuropathic (burning) pain.

    a. **Gabapentin**: start with 300 mg at bedtime. Can increase every few days, max dose 3,600 mg/d (typically dosed t.i.d. or q.i.d.) unless CrCl < 60 (will need to adjust dose). If discontinuing, recommend taper to avoid side effects.

    b. **Pregabalin**: start with 75 twice daily, may increase to 150 mg b.i.d. in 1 week. Max dose 600 mg/d (but rarely get improved effect over 300 mg). Again, taper over at least 1 week if planning to discontinue.

    c. **Topiramate**: start with 25 mg nightly.

    d. **Lamotrigine**: start with 25 mg nightly.

3. Muscle relaxants

    a. **Baclofen**: start 5 mg t.i.d. for spasticity. Can also be used intrathecally.

    b. **Cyclobenzaprine**: start 5 mg PO t.i.d. p.r.n.

    c. **Tizanidine**: alpha adrenergic—2 mg PO nightly. Can also be used intrathecally.

    d. **Methocarbamol**: start 250 mg 4 times daily.

    e. Carisoprodol: DO NOT USE—high levels of dependence, abuse, and withdrawal.

4. Topical medications

    a. **Lidocaine**: cream or patch form for local anesthetic action. Up to 3 patches (5%) placed on area of discomfort for 12 hours.

    b. Additional combination creams of lidocaine and prilocaine are also available.

5. NSAIDs: caution with GI upset and bleeding risk. Avoid long-term daily use of nonselective COX inhibitors when possible.

    a. **Acetaminophen**: starting dose 650 four times daily, generally want to stay below 3,000 mg daily.

    b. **Ibuprofen** (nonselective) 200 to 800 mg up to 4× daily (max 2,400 daily).

    c. **Naproxen** (nonselective), typical dose 500 twice daily (max 1,500/d × 6 months).

    d. **Indomethacin** (nonselective) 25 mg two to three times daily (max 200 mg/d, or 150 mg of ER formulation/d).

    e. **Meloxicam** (selective COX-2 inhibitor): 7.5 mg one to two times daily (max 15 mg/d).

    f. **Celebrex** (selective COX-2 inhibitor): 100 to 200 mg one to two times daily.

    g. **Toradol** (available IM and IV): if planning to give single dose can give 15 mg, 30 mg, or 60 mg ×1 or if planning to give multiple doses, can be given in 30 mg q6h but not to exceed 120 mg/d for 5 days (15 mg q6h not to exceed 60 mg/d in elderly patients or patients with weight <50 kg, again not to exceed 5 days).

6. **Steroids**: often helpful for refractory bone pain, brain metastases, neuropathic pain, and pain associated with abdominal distention. Consider starting with dexamethasone 4 mg b.i.d. and scheduling doses in morning and afternoon (steroids in evening can cause agitation and difficulty sleeping).

L. **Other treatments**

1. **Ketamine** is an *N*-methyl-D-aspartate (NMDA) receptor antagonist that can be considered for refractory pain.

2. **Bisphosphonates** are useful to treat bone pain and fracture prevention from osteolytic lesions of multiple myeloma. They may also be helpful in controlling bone pain in up to 25% of patients with breast cancer or prostate cancer. Either pamidronate (90 mg IV over 3 hours) or zoledronic acid (4 mg IV over 15 minutes) can be used.

3. For targeted areas, consider involvement of interventional pain team, for example, a subcostal block for severe rib pain or celiac plexus block for abdominal visceral pain related to pancreatic cancer. Local radiation can also be considered.

M. **Important principles**

1. All patients on chronic opioid pharmacotherapy should also be started on prophylaxis for opioid-induced constipation (i.e., senna 2 tablets once or twice daily).

2. It is important to consider route of administration and organ dysfunction while selecting medications.

3. For a patient on chronic opioid pharmacotherapy with suboptimal pain control, consider rotation to another opioid.

4. In cases of refractory pain, psychosocial and spiritual causes need to be addressed.

5. An increase in cancer pain often indicates progression of disease.

6. Always attempt to identify the underlying cause of the pain as this will guide its treatment.

III. CONSTIPATION

Constipation is a common symptom among cancer patients. It is important to be aware of causes and institute preventive measures when possible.

A. **Causes**

1. Side effects of opioids and other medications (i.e., serotonin receptor antagonists, vincristine, thalidomide)

2. Decreased oral intake and immobility

3. Autonomic neuropathy

4. Metabolic imbalance such as hypercalcemia

5. Secondary to intra-abdominal malignancy (i.e., with bowel obstruction or spinal cord compression)

B. **Treatments**

1. It is important to rule out bowel obstruction prior to escalating bowel regimen. If a patient does have bowel obstruction, surgical versus nonsurgical management will depend on individual patient characteristics, comorbidities, and goals of care. Medications that can be helpful in the symptomatic management of bowel obstruction include steroids and octreotide.

2. Most inexpensive and effective are combinations of a stimulant (senna) and hyperosmolar agent (miralax), which can be titrated to effect.

3. **Stimulants**

a. **Senna**: 8.6 mg tabs or liquid. For patients on scheduled opioids, consider starting with 2 tabs nightly (not as needed). May increase to 2 tabs b.i.d.

and again to 4 tabs b.i.d. as needed. All patients on scheduled opioids should be on scheduled senna to counteract opioid-induced constipation.

   b. Bisacodyl: also comes in suppository form.
4. **Hyperosmolar agents**
   a. Miralax: 17 g daily p.r.n., can be scheduled daily and increased to b.i.d.
   b. Lactulose: start with 15 to 30 mL/d.
5. **Emollients** (i.e., docusate, mineral oil): particularly in patients with advanced cancer, a stool softener such as docusate is not likely to have much benefit without a motility agent.
6. **Enemas**
7. **Opioid antagonists**
   a. Methylnaltrexone: note that this should be reserved for patients in whom bowel regimen has already been optimized, is not a first-line agent, and is contraindicated in suspected bowel obstruction and **dose is based on weight** of the patient (subcutaneous: 8 mg if 38 kg to <62 kg, 12 mg if 62 kg to 114 kg, and 0.15 mg/kg if >114 kg).
   b. Naloxegol: also for opioid-induced constipation, not tested against other bowel regimens or in cancer patients. Try other things first. Dose is 25 mg daily (unless CrCl < 60, then 12.5 mg/d).
8. **Other medicines** used for chronic constipation such as linaclotide and lubiprostone have mainly been used for treatment of IBS and have not been well studied in cancer patients.

C. **Important principles**
   1. All patients on an opioid should be started prophylaxis for opioid-induced constipation (i.e., senna 2 tablets once or twice daily).
   2. Always consider the possibility of an evolving small bowel obstruction.
   3. Consider underlying constipation when evaluating urinary obstruction, nausea/vomiting, and mental status changes.

IV. NAUSEA/VOMITING

Nausea and vomiting are common symptoms in cancer patients and relate to multiple factors.

A. **Causes:** Nausea and vomiting are frequently the resultant side effects of treatments (chemotherapy, radiation, or other medications), but can be due to tumor effects (CNS metastases, GI obstruction) or to other causes such as metabolic abnormalities (hyponatremia, hypercalcemia), pain, infection, or constipation.

B. **Treatments:** Diverse receptor populations are involved in the transmission of sensation of nausea; for that reason, it is important to choose agents with varied mechanisms of action to target nausea comprehensively.
   1. **Serotonin (3HT3) antagonists**: start doses prior to initiation of emetogenic chemotherapy and continue afterward.
      a. Ondansetron: 8 mg PO/SC/IV q8h
      b. Granisetron: 1 mg PO/IV q12h
   2. **Dopamine antagonists** (D2)
      a. Haloperidol: 0.5 to 1 mg PO/SC/IV q6h p.r.n.
      b. Olanzapine: can start with 2.5 mg b.i.d. p.r.n. and will likely need to increase dose. Blocks both dopamine and serotonin.
      c. Metoclopramide: 10 to 20 mg PO/SC/IV q6h p.r.n. This agent acts both centrally as a dopamine antagonist and also acts by stimulating gastric and small bowel motility (preventing gastric stasis and dilation).
      d. Prochlorperazine: 10 to 20 mg PO q6h p.r.n. or 25 mg PR q12h p.r.n.

3. **Centrally acting**
   a. Lorazepam: 0.5 to 1 mg q6h p.r.n. Often helpful for anticipatory nausea.
   b. Dexamethasone: 2 to 4 mg PO/SC/IV daily, may need to increase. It can have a synergistic effect when used with other classes of agents.
   c. Tetrahydrocannabinol (THC/Marinol): start with 2.5 mg b.i.d.
4. **Acetylcholine antagonists**
   a. Scopolamine (transdermal)—place 1 patch q72h.
5. **Histamine Antagonists (H1)**
   a. Diphenhydramine: 25 mg PO/SC/IV q6h p.r.n.
   b. Hydroxyzine: 25 mg q6h p.r.n.
6. **Somatostatin analogues for cases of obstruction**
   a. Octreotide: start at 100 mcg SC/IV q8h; can increase dose if needed. Has a prokinetic effect with improvement for cases of intestinal obstruction who are not surgical candidates. It can also be beneficial in chronic nausea after transplantation.
C. **Important principles**
   1. When combining medications, use drugs from different classes or that have different mechanism of action.
   2. Start with serotonin antagonist, then add dopamine antagonist, and continue to add medications from different classes. Adding two medications from the same category is not as helpful.

V. DYSPNEA

There are many reasons for dyspnea in cancer patients (see Chapter 30). It is important to look for reversible causes.
A. **Causes**
   1. Lung pathology: pleural effusion, pneumothorax, bronchospasm, COPD, primary tumor or metastases, and radiation pneumonitis
   2. Infections: pneumonia and bronchitis
   3. CHF, fluid overload, and ascites
   4. Anxiety
   5. Aspiration and reflux
B. **Evaluation**
   1. Physical exam, with particular attention to the lung exam, measurement of respiratory rate, and use of accessory muscles
   2. Chest x-ray, CT scan, and echo as indicated. Blood gas and other laboratory evaluations
C. **Treatments** (will be based on cause)
   1. Optimize current cardiac and pulmonary medications.
   2. Low-dose opioids (morphine 2.5 to 5 mg orally q2h p.r.n. to start) can blunt the air hunger effect, particularly in COPD and advanced cancer.
   3. Anxiety medications may be helpful if there is underlying anxiety.
   4. Oxygen may be helpful.
   5. Bronchodilators as may be indicated.
   6. Thoracentesis, guided drainage for significant effusions.
   7. Repositioning and improving air circulation by fans may also be helpful for comfort.
   8. Whenever possible, try to treat underlying cause of dyspnea in addition to treating symptom.
D. **Terminal congestion or "death rattle"**
   1. This may not distress the patient, but can cause significant distress to providers and family.

   2. Decrease IV fluids as you are able.
   3. Attempt to reduce secretions: glycopyrrolate (0.4 mg IV/SQ/SL q4h p.r.n.) has less CNS effects (does not cross the blood–brain barrier). If sedation or CNS effects are less of a concern, can also use hyoscyamine (0.125 mg SL q2–4h p.r.n.), scopolamine (0.2 to 0.4 mg SQ p.r.n.), or atropine (0.4 mg SQ q4h p.r.n.). A scopolamine patch will take 12 hours to work; as such, it will not provide immediate effect. Mouth care and positioning may be helpful, but suctioning is more likely to cause discomfort and not relieve congestion.

VI. ANXIETY/DEPRESSION
   A. Both anxiety and depression can heighten a patient's experience of additional symptoms as well as affect their performance status.
   B. Can be related to uncertainty about disease trajectory or prognosis.
   C. Anxiety and depression are expected reactions to a diagnosis of cancer. Consider treating them with an SSRI or an SNRI, if they are chronic. Psychiatric consultation may be useful.
   D. Benzodiazepines can worsen agitation paradoxically. Make sure to identify cause of anxiety or agitation prior to medicating with benzodiazepines, particularly in older patients.
   E. Consider using some of these medications for patients with multiple symptoms (e.g., anxiety and nausea).

VII. DELIRIUM
   A. Look for underlying cause first.
      1. Infection
      2. Medication side effect
      3. Renal or hepatic dysfunction
      4. Electrolyte abnormality
      5. CNS disease
      6. Hypoxemia
   B. In the terminal patient, delirium can be a normal part of the dying process. In that case, it would be appropriate to use medications such as neuroleptics, antipsychotics, or benzodiazepines.
   C. Treatments
      1. Nonpharmacologic interventions (e.g., reassurance, softly lighted room, reorientation) are useful both in prevention and treatment of delirium.
      2. Benzodiazepines can paradoxically worsen agitation. Make sure to identify cause of anxiety or agitation prior to medicating with benzodiazepines, particularly in older patients.
      3. Exercise caution when using anticholinergics since these may precipitate and exacerbate delirium.

VIII. STOMATITIS
   Stomatitis (a painful inflammation of the inside of the mouth) can develop after treatment with many cytotoxic agents and during radiation therapy to the head or neck. The development of stomatitis may be reduced, by sucking on ice chips or popsicles during a short infusion of cytotoxic agents.
   A. Symptoms and signs: Stomatitis is usually first noted by the patient as pain or sensitivity to certain foods. Erythema and aphthous ulcers develop. In severe cases, extensive ulceration and sloughing of the oral mucosa may be seen. *Candida albicans* or herpesvirus infection can have a similar appearance and must be considered in all cases.

B. Treatments

1. Avoid foods that trigger the pain (citrus, spicy or hot food), and abstain from alcohol (including mouthwashes that contain alcohol which can exacerbate mucositis). Suck on popsicles and drink cold beverages for relief.
2. Frequently rinse the mouth with solutions of saline and/or baking soda.
3. Swish and spit certain commercial suspensions.
   a. Ulcerease: glycerin, sodium bicarbonate, and sodium borate
   b. Bioadherent oral gel (Gelclair)
4. Various formulations can be prepared containing combinations of diphenhydramine, viscous lidocaine, and Maalox or Mylanta, +/- sucralfate, +/- nystatin. Rinse with 15 mL 4 to 6 times/d.
5. Opioids may be useful.
6. Appropriate antimicrobial treatment for bacterial, candidal, or herpesvirus infections.
7. Palifermin, a recombinant human keratinocyte growth factor, has reduced the incidence of moderate to severe mucositis in some series.

DISCUSSIONS WITH PATIENTS AND FAMILY

I. DISCUSSING GOALS OF CARE

While communication between physicians and patients about treatment is a fundamental piece of cancer care, and of effective medical treatment of any sort, many physicians feel that they have inadequate training in how to initiate and to manage discussions regarding a patient's goals of care. There are several barriers to initiating these conversations, both from the patient and the physician perspectives. There are also a number of misconceptions about how to carry them out.

Many physicians, and patients, believe that discussions about goals of care are appropriate only at the end of life or in instances of acute, life-threatening illness when, in fact, postponing these dialogues to times of crises often makes them more difficult and less effective. Further, many physicians feel that clarifying a patient's goals of care occurs in one or two discrete discussions when, in reality, identifying a patient's goals of treatment is a dynamic process that takes place over a long period of time and is usually subject to revision as the clinical scenario unfolds. It is of immeasurable benefit for providers who have the longest standing relationships with the patient to participate in these dialogues.

A. A goals of care discussion at the beginning of treatment should address the following topics:

1. What is the patient's level of understanding of his/her disease?
2. What are the patient's hopes for treatment?
3. What are the patient's fears regarding their disease?
4. Are there any symptoms or treatment side effects that are unacceptable to the patient?
5. Are there things the patient is hoping to accomplish in the next few weeks/months?
6. What are things that bring the patient joy now?
7. Has the patient decided who they would like to be involved in decision making now, as well as in potential situations when they would be unable to speak for themselves?
8. Does the patient have a completed advance directive on file?
9. Has the patient completed a Physician Orders for Life-Sustaining Treatment (POLST) form?

10. Does the patient have a designated power of attorney?
11. How do they like to make decisions? Themselves? With family?
12. What is the follow-up plan?

Addressing these and other questions early helps the treating oncologist tailor the treatment plan more precisely to the individual patient's goals and needs, which may have a salutary effect on both patient adherence and functional status. It is also vital to begin to discuss, and to clarify, particular treatments, outcomes, and clinical scenarios that are unacceptable to the patient keeping in mind that these may change during the treatment course.

If the patient responds well to treatment, there may be no immediate need to revisit these conversations. But if the patient's cancer progresses during therapy or if the patient is admitted to the hospital with worsening symptoms and/or complications, it can be useful to build on these conversations. Finally, an effective goals of care discussion, in which the patient's wishes, hopes, fears, and preferences are clarified, is an exercise in trust building between patient and provider that can be built upon to facilitate further dialogue at a later time.

B. **Setting up the goals of care conversation.** When setting up a goals of care conversation, there are several useful tools that can be used to structure the conversation. One commonly used tool is the S-P-I-K-E-S protocol for giving news, which gives a framework for setting up what may be a difficult conversation.

S—Setting: Make sure there are chairs, that there is minimal noise, that the room is private, and that the appropriate people are present (Who did they want present?). Do not stand over the patient—make sure you can make eye contact on the same level. Silence your pager. Make sure there are tissues nearby.

P—Perception: What is their understanding of what's going on? Allow the patient/family a chance to explain what they think is happening. The patient should do most of the talking at this stage.

I—Invitation: A time to assess what they want to know; you might ask, "Are you the type of person who likes to know all the details or do you tend to focus on the big picture?"

K—Knowledge: When you share information regarding their current status, you should avoid medical jargon and explain things in terms they will understand. Remember to pause often, and to ask them to repeat things back to you. Also, if you are going to break bad news in this conversation, remember to give them warning, such as starting with: "I need to share something serious with you" or "it's not what we had hoped..." so that they have a chance to stop you if they're not ready to hear what you are trying to say right then.

E—Empathy: Listen. Allow for emotion. If you're able, name the emotion ("I can see that this is upsetting"), you may also choose to validate the emotion with a statement like "I wish the news were different." In service of empathic listening, it is important to allow periods of silence without attempting to resume the conversation. The patient may just have had his/her greatest fears confirmed and is trying to process the information. At this point in the conversation, if the patient appears severely distressed, it may be useful to offer to stop the discussion and return to it when the patient feels more able to participate. Finally, it is always important, even when speaking with patients who are medically sophisticated, to acknowledge that they have been just been presented with a large amount of information and will likely have further questions in the future, that you will do your best to answer.

S—Strategy and Summary: Now that you've gotten a sense of the patients mindset and shared information with them, it's important to make a plan for next steps and to summarize what has been discussed. Patients often feel both a loss of autonomy and a sense of helplessness when confronted with serious illness, and including them in the formulation of their treatment plans empowers them to be actively involved in their medical care.

It is important to also **update other providers involved in the patient's care** about the outcome of these discussions.

C. **Additional important strategies and issues include:**

1. Break discussion of the patient's illness and treatment plan into small, manageable bits of information.
2. Taking time to pause, reflect, and recap.
3. Refocus the conversation when necessary.
4. Brainstorming with the patient and their family:
5. Remember: It is extremely difficult for a patient to participate in a productive goals of care discussion, when pain and symptoms are uncontrolled. Unless absolutely necessary, pain and symptoms should be under acceptable control before embarking upon a discussion of the patient's goals.
6. Sometimes, with refractory pain, the psychosocial and spiritual issues need to be addressed.
7. Quality of life may have a different meaning to different people.
8. Take yourself out of the equation, and focus on what the patient wants.
9. Compromise and negotiation are key.

II. DISCUSSING STOPPING PALLIATIVE CHEMOTHERAPY

As with any intervention, when the burdens and the risks of chemotherapy outweigh the potential benefits, a careful re-evaluation of both the treatment and the patient's goals of care are appropriate. These discussions are often the most challenging for both patient and oncologist, and it is vital that they be done with empathy, clarity, tact, and, above all, with honesty.

When breaking any bad news, it is important to prepare the patient for a serious discussion by clearing as much time and physical space as is possible for uninterrupted dialogue with the patient and those who the patient wishes to be present. While the oncologist should be careful not to appear patronizing—since most providers lack the personal experience being cancer patients—it is often reassuring to the patient to convey that the therapy is a joint effort both of you have undertaken together; now, things are not proceeding as hoped and a discussion of next steps is necessary.

It's often useful to start the conversation with a statement like, "Well, the therapy hasn't gone as planned and we need to talk about what to do next." It is very important NOT to convey the message to the patient that the treatment's lack of efficacy is their fault. For this reason, it's best to avoid statements such as "Well, you've failed the last two protocols…." since what has actually taken place is that the treatment has failed the patient and not the other way around.

It's often helpful to reframe the decision to stop palliative chemotherapy in a proactive light since this can help address the patient's fear of abandonment by the oncologist. But at the same time, it's important to be as honest and as realistic as possible with the patient about prognosis and not try to give the patient comfort by providing either unrealistic hope or postponing a discussion of end-of-life issues, if appropriate. Too often, patients whose performance status will not permit them to receive further chemotherapy are told "…just take some time and get stronger and when you can walk into the office, then you can resume chemotherapy" when the reality that this will ever take place is little to none. Although said with the intention to comfort a desperate and terminally ill patient, statements such as this can prevent the patient's process of accepting the end of life and may cause them to focus on attaining the unattainable rather than attending to important personal tasks or attainable goals.

As the next phases of medical treatment are explained to the patient (e.g., a shift in focus to more comfort-focused interventions that enhance quality of life rather than attempt to cure the cancer) another "goals of care" discussion may need to take place, as previous goals of care are reviewed and renegotiated.

Finally, honesty about your future involvement with the patient now that chemotherapy is suspended is important in managing the patient's expectations. Often, the patient will want the oncologist to remain involved in his/her medical treatment, but if this is not possible in one's practice environment, it is imperative to let the patient know this and to make sure that they are connected to their primary care physician or a palliative care physician.

III. DISCUSSING HOSPICE CARE

Hospice care, which in the United States is a capitated and bundled group of services for patients with an estimated prognosis of 6 months or less, is often misunderstood by health care providers, patients, and their loved ones. Broadly defined, hospice care is intended for terminally ill patients whose goals include an emphasis on comfort, enhancing quality of life, and avoiding rehospitalization rather than on attempting to prolong life. It is helpful to think of hospice as a "philosophy of care" as opposed to location. Many patients mistakenly believe that in order to receive hospice services, they have to go to a facility, but the majority of patients on hospice receive services at home. The range of these services is also poorly understood.

A. What hospice can and can't provide:

1. Coordinated interdisciplinary services with visits from nurses, social workers, and chaplains can be provided. Generally, patients receive visits a few times a week.

2. Hospice can provide 24-hour phone support for families and ability to send staff to the home in cases of escalating symptom needs.

3. Medications and medical equipment, including a hospital bed and oxygen, can be provided.

4. Hospice does not provide routine caregiver support. For this reason, family provides the majority of caregiving needs for patients on home hospice.

5. Hospice care is provided in patient's home, in skilled nursing facilities, and, under certain circumstances, in inpatient settings.

6. Patients are certified as appropriate for hospice care for an initial period of 90 days and then recertified for one additional 90-day period. Patients are then recertified, if appropriate, for 60 days periods of hospice care.

7. Patients receiving hospice care can revoke hospice services or can be discharged for extended prognosis but can re-enroll if they meet the admission criteria.

8. Being on hospice does not preclude treatment of respiratory or bladder infections that may make patients more uncomfortable. They are generally treated with oral antibiotics.

IV. BESIDES HOSPICE, WHAT PALLIATIVE CARE SERVICES ARE AVAILABLE OUTSIDE THE HOSPITAL?

A. Palliative Care Outpatient Clinic

Can follow longitudinally along with oncologists for additional symptom management and goals of care discussions for ambulatory patients

B. Home Palliative Care

1. For patients who have difficulty getting outside the home but wish to continue therapies and are not opposed to possible hospitalizations for acute exacerbations.

2. Similar to home health services, with intermittent visits (usually every few weeks) provided in the home by visiting nurses, sometimes also with social workers and physicians.

3. Emergencies will still require hospitalization. This is not 24-hour support.

V. WHAT IS THE BENEFIT OF PALLIATIVE CARE SPECIALISTS INVOLVEMENT IN MY PATIENT'S CARE?

A. The most immediate benefit may be symptom relief.

B. Studies show that early palliative care involvement can improve quality of life and patient satisfaction, as well as confer longer median survival for patients with metastatic cancer undergoing treatment.

C. Additional studies show that patients with in-hospital consultation by palliative care teams have cost savings 48 hours after consultation.

ACKNOWLEDGMENT

The authors would like to acknowledge Drs. Eric Prommer, Lisa Thompson, and Dennis Casciato, who significantly contributed to earlier versions of this chapter.

Suggested Readings

Palliative Care Fast Facts. Available online at www.mypcnow.org and as online application for mobile phones.

Basch E, Deal AM, Kris MG, et al. Symptom monitoring with patient-reported outcomes during routine cancer treatment: a randomized controlled trial. *J Clin Oncol* 2015;34 (6):557–565.

Bodtke S, Ligon K. *Hospice and Palliative Medicine Handbook: A Clinical Guide*. San Diego, CA, 2016:192–193.

Bruera E, Hui D, Dalal S, et al. Parenteral hydration in patients with advanced cancer: a multicenter, double blind, placebo-controlled randomized trial. *J Clin Oncol* 2013;31 (1):111.

Ekstrom MP, Bornefalk-Hermansson A, Abernethy AP, et al. Safety of benzodiazepines and opioids in very severe respiratory disease: national prospective study. *BMJ* 2014;348:g445.

Ernecoff NC, Curlin FA, Buddadhumaruk P, et al. Health Care Professionals' responses to religious or spiritual statements by Surrogate Decision Makers during goals-of-care discussions. *JAMA Intern Med* 2015;175 (10):1662.

Morrison RS, Penrod JD, Cassel JB, et al. Cost savings associated with US Hospital Palliative Care Consultation Programs. *Arch Intern Med* 2008;168 (16):1783–1790.

Steinhauser KE, Christakis NA, Clipp EC, et al. Factors considered important at the end of life by patients, family, physicians, and other care providers. *JAMA* 2000;284 (19):2476.

Tarumi Y, Wilson MP, Szafran O, et al. Randomized, double-blind, placebo-controlled trial of oral docusate in the management of constipation in hospice patients. *J Pain Symptom Manage* 2013;45 (1):2.

Temel JS, Greer JA, Muzikansky A, et al. Early palliative care for patients with metastatic non-small-cell lung cancer. *N Engl J Med* 2010;363:733.

Teno JM, Gozalo PL, Mitchell SL, et al. Does feeding tube insertion and its timing improve survival? *J Am Geriatr Soc* 2012;60 (10):1918.

Weeks JC, Catalano PJ, Cronin A, et al. Patients' expectations about effects of chemotherapy for advanced cancer. *N Engl J Med* 2012;367:1616.

Wright AA, Zhang B, Ray A, et al. Associations between end-of-life discussions, patient mental health, medical care near death, and caregiver bereavement adjustment. *JAMA* 2008;300 (14):1665.

Wright AA, Zhang B, Keating NL, et al. Associations between palliative chemotherapy and adult cancer patients' end of life care and place of death: prospective cohort study. *BMJ* 2014;348:g1219.

7 Cancer Survivorship

Mary E. Sehl, Amy A. Jacobson, and
Patricia A. Ganz

I. INTRODUCTION

Long-term survival from cancer is increasing, and the number of cancer survivors is growing, emphasizing the demand for greater attention to the specialized needs of disease-free cancer survivors. According to a recent report by the National Cancer Institute, the number of people living beyond a cancer diagnosis reached nearly 14.5 million in January 2014 and is expected to rise to almost 19 million by 2024. There are many challenges to delivering optimal health care to these individuals, including preexisting conditions that are exacerbated by cancer and its treatment and new chronic conditions that arise from the persistent effects of cancer treatment. Approximately 39.6% of men and women will be diagnosed with cancer at some point during their lifetimes based on 2010 to 2012 data, highlighting the need to increase awareness and emphasize how to best care for this growing population.

Because of the improvements in cancer therapies, the 5-year and extended disease-free survival rates for early-stage breast, colorectal, prostate, thyroid, and kidney cancer are over 90%. Likewise, early-stage melanoma, Hodgkin lymphoma, and cancers of the bladder, uterine corpus and cervix, and testes are associated with excellent survival outcomes. Because of the improvements in targeted therapies and immunotherapy strategies, the 5-year survival rates for advanced cancers are also rising. As a result, for most cancer survivors, death is more likely to occur from competing illnesses. However, cancer treatment modalities, including surgery, radiotherapy, chemotherapy, endocrine therapy, and immunotherapy, have been shown to be associated with late effects that may persist for up to 20 years after initial treatment, including cognitive effects, physical effects, psychosocial adjustments, and functional decline. The effects of cancer treatment can precipitate new chronic conditions and exacerbate coexisting medical conditions. Optimal cancer rehabilitation involves a multidisciplinary team of providers who can address the patient's physical, psychologic, vocational, and social functioning given the limits imposed by the chronic or late effects of cancer treatment and other coexisting conditions. Cancer survivors are also at increased risk of a secondary cancer developing, suggesting the need for close surveillance and screening. In this chapter, we will discuss the optimal care of the cancer survivor, including recognizing and addressing late effects of cancer treatment, developing a treatment summary and survivorship care plan, and a shared care model for comprehensive care for survivors.

II. DEFINITION OF A CANCER SURVIVOR

According to a broad definition developed in 1986 by the National Coalition for Cancer Survivorship (NCCS), any cancer patient or close family member of a cancer patient, from the time of diagnosis until death, may be considered a cancer survivor. More recently, the survivorship phase of care has been used to describe the period of time after the completion of initial treatment with curative intent, when the patient is being seen post treatment and in follow-up. This period of time is the focus of this chapter. Important issues that arise after curative intent treatment include managing persistent symptoms and preventing late effects of treatment, as well as health care maintenance and screening for other cancers.

III. LATE EFFECTS OF CANCER TREATMENT AND TARGETED INTERVENTIONS

   A. Late effects of treatment. Late effects arise following cancer treatment modalities, including chemotherapy, surgery, radiotherapy, endocrine therapy, and post stem cell transplant, and can persist for decades. These effects are widespread and occur in nearly every organ system. Table 7-1 summarizes the late effects by physiologic system and treatment modality. In addition to physiologic changes, cancer treatment can have a profound effect on general physical functioning, social well-being, and vocational and financial status.

   B. Interventions for prevention and recovery. There are many strategies that can be effective in addressing the late effects of cancer treatment. Diabetes, cardiovascular disease, congestive heart failure, bone loss, adverse body composition, and renal disease can be managed through rehabilitation interventions including medication, counseling, behavior change, and promotion of healthy diets, physical activity, and weight control. Fatigue, depression, anxiety, fear of recurrence, cognitive dysfunction, pain syndromes, peripheral neuropathy, sexual dysfunction, balance and gait problems, upper or lower extremity mobility issues, lymphedema, bladder and bowel problems, stoma care, problems with swallowing or dysphagia, and communication difficulty are amenable to rehabilitation interventions. Self-management skills and health promotion interventions provided in the context of comprehensive cancer rehabilitation also have the potential to decrease the risk of additional late effects including the cardiac, pulmonary, endocrine, or bone complications of cancer treatment and may even reduce the risk of second malignancies.

   Risk for therapy-related malignancy is related not only to the type, dose, and duration of therapy received but also in some cases to an underlying genetic predisposition. A careful family history should be taken on each patient and referral for genetic counseling and testing should be considered for high-risk patients.

   C. Late effects after immunotherapy. In the early era of immunotherapy and increased durable response rates in both solid tumors and leukemias, oncologists will need to be vigilant in monitoring for the as yet unknown long-term effects of immunotherapy. While little is known about the anticipated prevalence of autoimmune phenomena from newer immune therapies such as PD-1 inhibitors or cellular-based therapies such as CAR-T cells, there is experience in the setting of the long-term effects of immune activation after allogeneic stem cell therapy.

   D. Late effects after stem cell transplantation. Survivors of allogeneic hematopoietic stem cell transplant (HSCT) experience a variety of late effects, some of which are in common with those of other cancer survivors related to high doses of chemotherapy and radiation, as well as the unique long-term sequelae associated with acute and chronic graft versus host disease. With broadening indications for allogeneic stem cell transplant and improvement in survival, there may be up to half a million long-term survivors after allo-HSCT worldwide. Table 7-1 lists the late effects that are experienced by allogeneic stem cell recipients across physiologic systems. Notable complications include the effects of chronic steroids, including bone loss, avascular necrosis, diabetes,

TABLE 7-1	Late Effects of Cancer Therapy by Physiologic System and Treatment Modality				
System	**Chemotherapy**	**Radiotherapy**	**Surgery**	**Endocrine Therapy**	**HSCT**
Cardiovascular	Cardiomyopathy and congestive heart failure	Scarring, inflammation, pericardial effusion, and coronary artery disease		Venous thrombotic events	Restrictive or dilated cardiomyopathy, arrhythmia, autonomic neuropathy, endothelial damage, metabolic syndrome, and dyslipidemia
Pulmonary	Pulmonary fibrosis, inflammation, and interstitial pneumonitis	Pulmonary fibrosis and decreased lung function	Atelectasis		Obstructive changes, bronchiolitis obliterans, bronchiolitis obliterans–organizing pneumonia, and restrictive lung disease
Gastrointestinal	CASH, hepatic fibrosis, and cirrhosis	Malabsorption, biliary stricture, and liver failure	Intestinal obstruction, hernia, altered bowel function, nausea, and vomiting		
Genitourinary	Hemorrhagic cystitis	Bladder fibrosis and small bladder capacity	Incontinence	Vaginitis	
Renal	Decreased creatinine clearance and delayed-onset renal failure	Decreased creatinine clearance and hypertension			Nephropathy and nephrotic syndrome Hypertension, chronic kidney disease, nephropathy and nephrotic syndrome Iron overload
Hematologic	Myelodysplasia and acute leukemia	Myelodysplasia, cytopenias, and acute leukemia			
Musculoskeletal	Avascular necrosis	Osteonecrosis, fibrosis, atrophy, and deformity	Accelerated arthritis	Osteopenia	Avascular necrosis and bone loss
CNS	Problems with thinking, learning, and memory; structural brain changes; seizure; paralysis; and fatigue	Problems with thinking, learning, and memory; structural brain changes; hemorrhage; and fatigue	Impaired cognitive function, motor sensory function, vision, swallowing, language, bowel and bladder control, phantom pain (amputation), and fatigue	Mood changes, fatigue, generalized weakness, and hot flashes	Anxiety, depression, PTSD, and fatigue

TABLE 7-1	Late Effects of Cancer Therapy by Physiologic System and Treatment Modality (Continued)				
System	**Chemotherapy**	**Radiotherapy**	**Surgery**	**Endocrine Therapy**	**HSCT**
Peripheral nervous system	Peripheral neuropathy and hearing loss		Neuropathic pain		
Pituitary	Diabetes	Growth hormone deficiency and other hormone deficiencies			Diabetes mellitus
Thyroid		Hypothyroidism and thyroid nodules			Hypothyroidism
Gonadal	Infertility and early menopause	Infertility, ovarian failure, early menopause, and Leydig cell dysfunction	Retrograde ejaculation, sexual dysfunction, and testosterone deficiency		Hypogonadism, infertility, and decreased intimacy
Oral health	Tooth decay	Dry mouth, poor enamel, and dental carries			
Ophthalmologic	Cataracts	Cataracts, dry eyes, visual impairment, and retinopathy		Cataracts	Keratoconjunctivitis and cataracts
Skin	Rashes	Burn			
Lymphatic		Lymphedema	Lymphedema		
Immune	Impaired immune function and immunosuppression	Impaired immune function and immunosuppression	Impaired immunity and risk of sepsis (splenectomy)		
All tissues	Second cancer	Second cancer		Endometrial cancer	New solid tumors at twice the rate of the general population

dyslipidemia, muscle weakness, and restrictive pulmonary changes secondary to muscle weakness, as well as the endothelial damage and diffuse fibrosis of graft-versus-host disease (GVHD) causing cardiovascular disease, vision changes, and debilitation.

1. **New solid cancers.** Survivors of allogeneic stem cell transplant have an increased risk of developing new solid cancers at twice the rate in the general population with the risk increasing over time reaching 3-fold among patients followed for 15 years or more. Risk factors for solid tumors, including cancers of the breast, thyroid, brain, central nervous system, bone and connective tissue, and melanoma, include younger age at transplantation and the use of radiation in the conditioning regimen. Chronic GVHD and immunosuppressive therapy are associated with squamous cell cancers of the skin and mucosa. These elevated risks highlight the importance of adherence to cancer screening guidelines for skin, cervical, and colon cancer, with more systematic skin evaluations by health care providers and yearly gynecologic examinations, including Pap smears.

2. **Infections.** Patients on chronic immunosuppressive therapy are at risk of reactivation of varicella–zoster virus, hepatitis B and C, and cytomegalovirus. Prophylaxis with antiviral medications, antifungal medications, as well as antibiotics for *Pneumocystis jiroveci* and encapsulated organisms is indicated until immunosuppression is discontinued.

3. **Ocular manifestations.** Annual ophthalmologic evaluations are important given the frequency of keratoconjunctivitis and cataracts.

4. **Psychosocial aspects.** Finally, while the psychosocial aspects of quality of life following allogeneic stem cell transplant tend to improve during the years following transplantation, a large proportion of HSCT survivors experience fatigue (80% to 96%), posttraumatic stress disorder (45% have intrusive thoughts pretransplant compared with 7% to 8% posttransplant), anxiety and depression (26% to 36%), fluctuating social well-being, and concerns about intimacy and fertility. Despite these ongoing effects, the majority of survivors are able to return to work and resume school or household activities. It is important to recognize survivors with adjustment difficulties and incorporate factors that may aid in positive adjustment.

IV. GENETIC TESTING IN CANCER SURVIVORS

Second primary malignancies among cancer survivors account for 16% of all cancer incidences. While lifestyle, environment, hormone exposures, host factors, and their interactions may underlie the increased risk, the exact molecular mechanisms are not well understood. While second malignant neoplasms are one of the most serious effects of successful cancer treatment, genetic testing is often overlooked at the time of diagnosis. Because many treatments including chemotherapy and radiation are linked to secondary malignancies, and because individuals at high familial risk are at increased risk of developing treatment-related malignancies (e.g., through aberrations in DNA repair pathways), it is important to screen and provide counseling to patients regarding familial cancer syndromes and testing for inherited mutations conferring increased risk of cancer.

V. TREATMENT SUMMARY AND SURVIVORSHIP CARE PLAN

On the basis of reviews of Surveillance, Epidemiology, and End Results (SEER) Medicare claims data, it became apparent that a shared survivorship care plan is needed to ensure better preventive care for cancer survivors. The provision of treatment summaries and survivorship care plans is becoming a standard of care across the country. In addition to the standard follow-up in oncology practice that focuses on surveillance for cancer recurrence and management of the adverse effects of treatment, the survivorship care plan addresses the long-term effects of cancer and its treatment. The care plan also addresses the ongoing psychosocial burden of a cancer diagnosis. Survivorship care plans lead to improvements in perceived knowledge and quality of survivorship care.

A. **Models of care.** A clinical program designed to meet the special health needs of cancer survivors should be multidisciplinary in nature. This care is coordinated by the patient's physician or advanced practiced nurse, with availability of a mental health provider. Aspects of nutritional evaluation, psychological evaluation, social work assessment, and evaluation by physical therapy and occupational therapy should be available if necessary for referral. A very important component of the survivorship care plan is to facilitate the coordination of care with other physicians. Multiple models of integrated care have been implemented, including the academic cancer center model, the integrated community survivorship model, and survivorship care within a nationalized health care system, and these are being increasingly adopted and tested.

B. **Who provides survivorship care?** There has historically been some ambiguity about the responsibility for providing ongoing medical care for cancer survivors. According to a survey conducted by the ASCO Cancer Prevention Committee, when oncologists were asked the question, "To what extent do you provide ongoing medical care, including health maintenance, screening, and preventive services," 31% responded always, 48% sometimes, 15% rarely, and 5% not at all. The majority (74%) felt that it was the role of the oncology specialist to provide this type of continuing care to cancer survivors and 66% felt comfortable providing it. In a study examining attitudes of patients, oncologists, and primary care providers, patients expected their oncologists to be primarily responsible for cancer recurrence, while they expected both their oncologists and primary care providers to be involved in surveillance for cancer recurrence and other cancer screening, and they preferred their primary care physicians to be solely involved in general preventive care and treatment of other coexisting illnesses. Generally, primary care providers and oncologists agreed with their patients. Although primary care providers expected most of the responsibility for preventive care, oncologists expressed interest in shared care for prevention.

C. **Early interventions.** Under the shared care model, it will be important for both oncologists and primary care providers to take responsibility for incorporating interventions into routine care for cancer survivors. Many patients spontaneously initiate positive behaviors, and it will be important to encourage modification of behaviors and initiate preventive exercise programs for patients early in the course of their treatment.

D. **Elements of the treatment summary.** The treatment summary provides both disease and treatment history information, including tumor characteristics and staging and cancer treatments received. The survivorship care plan is a guide for outlining and coordinating follow-up care, including surveillance tests, recommended health behaviors and resources, and education about and monitoring of potential long-term effects of cancer treatment. Table 7-2 lists the contents of the treatment summary and survivorship care plan. Important elements of the individual treatment summary include:

1. **Diagnosis**
2. **Stage, grade, and receptor status**
3. **Surgery**
4. **Chemotherapy**
5. **Radiotherapy**

TABLE 7-2	Elements of the Treatment Summary and Survivorship Care Plan

Treatment Summary

Provider contact information
    Medical oncologist
    Radiation oncologist
    Surgical oncologist
    Primary internist
Surgical history
    Procedures and dates
    Complications
Pathology and stage
    Histopathology, TNM stage, and biologic marker data
Chemotherapy history
    Treatments and dates
    List all agents and number of cycles received
    Total dose (e.g., anthracycline)
    Growth factors received and blood transfusions
    Complications
Endocrine therapy toxicity
    Dates
    Side effects
Other therapies (e.g., biologically targeted therapies and immunotherapies)
    Dates
    Side effects
Radiation history
    Date started and date finished
    Fields radiated
    Total dose (Gy)

Survivorship Care Plan

Persistent medical conditions
List of current medications and allergies
Family history and social history
Current symptom review
Current psychosocial assessment
Recent screening and diagnostic tests
Recommendations
    Cancer management and surveillance
    Late effects monitoring
    Psychosocial concerns
    Symptom management
    Health promotion
    Prevention
        Bone health
        Weight management and physical activity
    ASCO guidelines for follow-up care for specific cancer

      6. Clinical trials information
      7. Targeted therapy
      8. Toxicity
   E. **Elements of the survivorship care plan.** Items of the survivorship care plan include:
      1. Toxicities and late effects
      2. Cancer surveillance
      3. Psychosocial effects
      4. Referrals and resources
      5. Prevention and health promotion
      6. Genetic testing recommendations

F. **Coordinating delivery of care.** There is a great deal of variation in clinical settings and organization of care during the initial phase of cancer treatment. While patients are often seen by several different cancer care providers, including surgical oncologists, medical oncologists, and radiation oncologists, the medical oncologist will need to develop strategies to incorporate survivorship care planning in the office practice. The treatment summary and survivorship care plan should first be delivered at the completion of surgery and adjuvant radiation and/or chemotherapy and updated at the end of a course of adjuvant endocrine therapy or after additional treatment decisions are made, such as genetic testing that necessitates preventive surgery and other interventions. The care plan should be summarized in a report for the patient to keep and should be placed in the chart so that it can be accessed by primary care providers and specialists involved in the care of the patient and so that all involved care providers can ensure that components of the survivorship care plan are complete and comprehensive care has been addressed.

G. **Guidelines and resources for survivors and providers.** The treatment summary and survivorship care plan can serve as both a communication vehicle and an educational resource for the cancer survivor. The American Society of Clinical Oncology (ASCO) promotes the use of written treatment plans and summary care plans and has developed templates to support effective communication of a survivor's health status and long-term care needs.

  1. **ASCO Resources**. ASCO provides guidelines resources for breast, colorectal, non–small cell lung, small cell lung, and prostate cancer, as well as diffuse large B-cell lymphoma (https://www.asco.org/practice-guidelines/quality-guidelines/guidelines/patient-and-survivor-care). There is also a survivorship toolbox available, as well as guidelines for various symptoms and fertility preservation and guidelines for screening, assessment, and management of fatigue and anxiety and depressive symptoms and prevention and management of chemotherapy-induced peripheral neuropathy.

  2. **ACS guidelines**. The American Cancer Society provides guidelines on survivorship care for breast cancer, prostate cancer, colorectal cancer, head and neck cancer, and nutrition and physical activity guidelines for survivors (http://www.cancer.org/healthy/informationforhealthcareprofessionals/acsguidelines/).

  3. **OncoLife Survivorship Care Plan.** This resource is a comprehensive care plan that is individualized based on responses to an online questionnaire and is a tool intended for health care providers in busy clinics or for patients to create and review with their providers. These and other resources are listed in Table 7-3. Patient empowerment is critical to ensuring successful implementation of the care plan.

  4. **Journey Forward.** This Web-based platform provides a variety of treatment and care plan resources for providers and patients, including a survivorship care plan builder with disease-specific templates and drop-down menus to facilitate completion. A recently developed Journey Forward app for iOS and android platforms allows patients to initiate a treatment summary and posttreatment plan to discuss with their oncology provider. It is part of an effective strategy to increase patient empowerment. There is also a survivorship resource library on the website (www.journeyforward.org).

VI. SPECIAL CONSIDERATIONS IN THE GERIATRIC POPULATION

In patients older than 65 years, the toxicity of cancer and its treatment is a heterogeneous process in a heterogeneous population. This heterogeneity is a result of the number and severity of coexisting illnesses, cognitive function,

TABLE 7-3	Important Web Links/Resources

Resources for Survivors

American Cancer Society Survivors Network: available at www.cancer.org, csn.cancer.org
CancerCare: available at www.cancercare.org
IOM report "From Cancer Patient to Cancer Survivor: Lost in Transition": available at
www.iom.edu/CMS/28312/4931/30869.aspx
Susan G. Komen for the Cure: available at www.komen.org
Living Beyond Breast Cancer: available at www.lbbc.org
NCI Office of Cancer Survivorship: available at http://cancercontrol.cancer.gov/ocs/
The Cancer Support Community at www.cancersupportcommunity.org
The National Coalition for Cancer Survivors: available at www.canceradvocacynow.org/
CancerNet: available at www.cancer.net
People Living with Cancer: available at www.cancer.net
Cancer Information and Support Network: available at www.cisncancer.org
National Marrow Donor Program: https://bethematchclinical.org/post-transplant-care/
long-term-care-guidelines

Resources for Health Care Providers

ASCO treatment summary and care plan templates for breast and colon cancer: available at
www.asco.org/treatmentsummary
Haylock PJ, Mitchell SA, Cox T, et al. The cancer survivors's prescription for living. *Am J Nurs*
2007;107:58–70
Livestrong Care Plan from the OncoLink website: available at http://www.livestrongcareplan.org
Children's Oncology Group guidelines for pediatric cancer survivorship www.survivorship-
guidelines.org
ASCO guidelines for survivor care: available at https://www.asco.org/practice-guidelines/
quality-guidelines/guidelines/patient-and-survivor-care
American Cancer Society guidelines for survivor care available at http://www.cancer.org/
healthy/informationforhealthcareprofessionals/acsguidelines/
ASCO Survivorship Clinical Tools and Resources https://www.asco.org/practice-guidelines/
cancer-care-initiatives/prevention-survivorship/survivorship/survivorship-11
Journey Forward Patient and Provider Tools http://www.journeyforward.org/
National Marrow Donor Program: https://bethematchclinical.org/post-transplant-care/
long-term-care-guidelines

physical activity, performance status, and social connectedness. Age-associated physiologic changes occur across physiologic systems and put the older patient at increased risk for both acute toxicities and increased susceptibility to the late effects of cancer treatment modalities. These changes occur across physiologic systems and put patients at increased risk for the effects outlined in Table 7-1. They include decreased cardiac output, decreased maximum oxygen consumption, increased inflammatory cytokines, decreased FEV1, decreased total lung capacity, impaired peristalsis and absorption, delayed gastric emptying time, decreased liver blood flow, enlarged prostate, diminished bladder capacity, decreased creatinine clearance, anemia, decreased bone density, decreased muscle strength, increased reaction times, impaired circadian rhythm, decreased growth hormone, decreased thyroxine secretion, decreased testosterone, decreased salivary flow rate, epidermal atrophy, slower wound healing, and impaired cell-mediated immunity. Functional decline is an important late effect in cancer survivors and is a significant concern in the older cancer patient. Cancer survivors are twice as likely as persons without a history of cancer to report limitation in an activity of daily living. Functional decline that persists two years after a cancer diagnosis in early-stage breast cancer survivors predicts shorter 10-year survival. Disability is an important concern in the older patient, highlighting the need for functional assessment in older cancer survivors.

VII. SPECIAL CONSIDERATIONS IN SURVIVORS OF CHILDHOOD CANCERS

Almost 80% of children and adolescents who receive a diagnosis of cancer become long-term survivors, prompting the study of the long-term health consequences of treatments for childhood cancer demonstrating damage to organ systems that only becomes clinically evident many years after diagnosis. Among 10,397 survivors treated in the 1970s and 1980s and their siblings followed in the Childhood Cancer Survivor study, the cumulative incidence over 30 years following cancer diagnosis reaches 73.4% for diagnosis of a chronic health condition and 42.4% for severe, disabling, or life-threatening conditions or death due to a chronic condition. The conditions that were reported as severe, disabling, or life-threatening included major joint replacement (relative risk 54.0 when compared with siblings), congestive heart failure (relative risk 15.1), second malignant neoplasm (relative risk 14.8), cognitive dysfunction (relative risk 10.5), coronary artery disease (relative risk 10.4), cerebrovascular accident (relative risk 9.3), renal failure or dialysis (relative risk 8.9), hearing loss not corrected by aid (relative risk 6.3), legally blind or loss of an eye (relative risk 5.8), and ovarian failure (relative risk 3.5). The incidence of chronic conditions and serious outcomes was further shown to increase over time without approaching a plateau, raising concerns for the development of multiple coexisting debilitating conditions in this population and suggesting the need for close monitoring and interventions to promote healthy living in this population. Survivors of childhood cancers are also at risk for psychological distress and pain. While most survivors report satisfaction with their lives, certain groups of childhood cancer survivors, including those with a chronic medical condition, female sex, and lower education and socioeconomic status, are at high risk for psychological distress, neurocognitive dysfunction, and poor health-related quality of life, suggesting the need for targeting interventions in these high-risk groups.

Adolescent and young adult cancer survivors have a higher relative risk of secondary malignant neoplasms (SMNs) compared with the general population and have a higher absolute risk of SMNs compared with younger or older cancer survivors. In those with a history of radiotherapy, the risk of breast cancer is 40.2% in individuals treated at ages 15 to 39, compared with 23.7% in those age ≤14 years and 35.1% in those age ≥40 years when treated. The risk of breast cancer is also a concern in those receiving systemic treatments other than radiotherapy. In those without radiotherapy, breast cancer risk is 30.5% in individuals treated at ages 15 to 39, compared with 11.9% in those ≤14 years and 26.6% in those ≥40 years when treated.

It is important to consider early interventions to prevent the late effects of cancer treatment in this population. Physical exercise training has been found to have positive effects on physical fitness, including body composition, flexibility, cardiorespiratory fitness, muscle strength, and health-related quality of life.

The Children's Oncology Group Long-Term Follow-Up Guidelines for Survivors of Childhood, Adolescent, and Young Adult Cancers are a resource for health care providers that provide screening recommendations and management of late effects and ongoing issues related to treatment of pediatric malignancies (Table 7-3). These guidelines are intended to increase awareness of late effects and enhance follow-up care provided to survivors of pediatric malignancies throughout their lifespan.

II Solid Tumors

8 Head and Neck Cancers

Steve P. Lee, Maie A. St. John, and Deborah J. Wong

I. GENERAL ASPECTS OF HEAD AND NECK CANCERS

Head and neck cancers include a heterogeneous group of malignant tumors arising in all structures cephalad to the clavicles, except for the brain, spinal cord, base of the skull, and usually the skin. A meaningful understanding of these malignant tumors requires anatomic separation into those cancers arising in the oral cavity, oropharynx, hypopharynx, nasopharynx, larynx, nasal fossa, paranasal sinuses, thyroid and salivary glands, and vermilion surfaces.

A. Epidemiology and etiology

1. **Incidence.** Cancers arising in the head and neck comprise the sixth leading cancer diagnosis and constitute about 3% of all newly diagnosed cancers in the United States. In 2015, over 61,000 people were diagnosed with head and neck cancer with approximately 13,000 deaths.

2. **Etiology.** Cigarette smoking and substantial alcohol intake are the major risk factors. *Field cancerization* is a concept based on the prolonged exposure of the oral and pharyngeal mucosa to carcinogens. Twenty percent of the survivors of one cancer of the head and neck develop another primary head and neck cancer, and such patients are at increased risk for lung and esophageal cancers. Human papilloma virus (HPV) is a recognized risk factor for a rising number of oropharyngeal cancers, and Epstein-Barr virus (EBV) is associated with nasopharyngeal cancers, more commonly in Southeast Asian populations.

B. Pathology

1. **Histology.** Nearly all cancers of the oral cavity and pharynx are squamous cell carcinomas of varying differentiation. Adenoid cystic and mucoepidermoid cancers arise from salivary glands. A range of histologically different cancers, such as papillary, follicular, giant cell, Hurthle cell, and anaplastic carcinomas, arise in the thyroid gland.

2. **Metastases.** Most primary cancers of the head and neck spread by invasion of adjacent tissues and metastases to regional lymph nodes (LNs). Metastases to distant sites are infrequent.

C. Diagnosis

1. **Common symptoms/signs**
   a. Painless mass
   b. Local ulceration with or without pain
   c. Referred pain to teeth or ear
   d. Dysphagia, mechanical or painful
   e. Alteration of speech such as difficulty pronouncing words (tongue) or change in character (larynx, nasopharynx)
   f. Persistent hoarseness (larynx)
   g. Unilateral tonsillar enlargement in an adult
   h. Persistent unilateral "sinusitis"
   i. Persistent unilateral nosebleed or obstruction

  j. Unilateral hearing loss often with serous otitis
  k. Cranial nerve palsies
 2. Biopsy and imaging. Primary cancers of the head and neck must be documented by biopsy. In addition to presenting as a mass at the primary site, head and neck cancer may present as a new, firm, usually nontender mass or masses, in the neck, either unilateral or bilateral. In adults, these should be considered metastatic (or primary in the thyroid) cancer involving the LN until proven otherwise. In addition to direct biopsy of the neck mass, search for a primary cancer is important. In some circumstances, when carcinoma has been identified in a cervical LN and there is no obvious primary tumor on physical or imaging exams, biopsies of Waldeyer's ring are appropriate. When an LN biopsy is HPV+, transoral robotic surgery (TORS) is recommended as a means of identifying the occult primary site in the tonsils or tongue base. This technique has allowed for the identification of the primary tumor in 75% to 90% of cases. Magnetic resonance imaging (MRI) and computed tomography (CT) from the base of the skull to the thoracic inlet are essential in establishing the local/regional extent of the tumor. Chest x-rays remain part of the evaluation, although intrathoracic metastases are infrequent.
 3. Endoscopy. Visualization of the oral cavity, nasal cavity, nasopharynx, oropharynx, hypopharynx, larynx, cervical esophagus, and proximal trachea is essential in establishing the presence and extent of tumor. These exams have been facilitated by the development of flexible, small caliber, bright-light endoscopes. Biopsies may be done at the time of endoscopy.
D. Staging. Staging can be done clinically or pathologically, based on information found at surgery. Clinical staging is important because many patients are managed by radiation therapy (RT). Clinical staging is based on physical examination and information from MRI and/or CT examinations. All primary cancers must be documented histologically. For detailed staging, refer to the current AJCC Cancer Staging atlas for TNM staging system.
E. Prognostic factors. The most important prognostic factors for patients with primary cancers of the head and neck are primary tumor site, size and extent, and regional/distant metastases. Histologic differentiation of epidermoid carcinomas is less important. A major risk factor is a previous head and neck cancer. Continued cigarette smoking and consumption of alcoholic beverages expose the mucosa to known carcinogens.
F. Prevention. The main preventatives for cancer of the head and neck are abstinence from the tobacco and alcohol. Avoidance or elimination of chronic irritants such as an irregular sharp tooth or ill-fitting dentures is desirable.
G. Management principles of head and neck cancers. Prior to commitment to a therapy program for a specific patient, there should be input from all members of the multidisciplinary oncology group who will be involved. Included are surgeons, radiation oncologists, medical oncologists, dentists, nurses, social workers, and rehabilitation personnel. Proper management includes posttreatment close, periodic examinations. Persistent or "recurrent" cancers usually can be recognized within 2 years of the completion of treatment. Figure 8-1 shows a simplified algorithm of the management of patients with localized or locoregional disease; it must be noted this algorithm encompasses most, but not all, clinical scenarios (Fig. 8-1).
 1. Surgery has long been a mainstay of the treatment of patients with cancers of the head and neck. Treatment of the primary tumor requires removal of the tumor and its locoregional extensions. Sometimes, involvement of vital

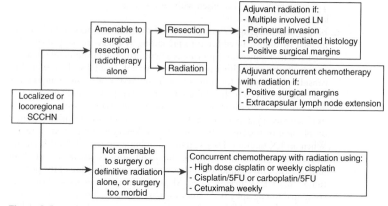

Figure 8-1 Management of patients with localized or locoregional SCCHN.

structures such as carotid artery encasement or base of the skull erosion makes such complete removal unlikely. In such situations, adjuvant RT and/or chemotherapy may facilitate or even negate the need for radical surgery. Recent advances have promoted adequate resection of some tumors involving the base of the skull.

    a. Preservation of functions, such as swallowing, voice or vision, and cosmesis, must be considered in any management plan. Tumor extension into bone, such as the mandible or maxilla, usually requires resection. Often, reconstruction can minimize the long-term morbidity. Speech therapy and swallow therapy when started prior to therapy or at the outset of therapy increase the likelihood that the patient's function will be preserved after therapy has concluded.

    b. Metastases to cervical LNs, particularly from the oral cavity, paranasal sinuses, hypopharynx, and thyroid, are best treated surgically, although postoperative irradiation frequently is indicated. Removal of cervical nodes containing metastatic cancer can be accomplished by *en bloc* resection (radical neck dissection) or a limited procedure, such as modified radical neck dissection or selective neck dissection.

2. RT, with or without concurrent chemotherapy, is often utilized for definitive treatment of head and neck cancer, particularly when patients are not operative candidates. In such cases, RT can control many cancers of the head and neck, usually with better consequent function and cosmesis than following radical resection. There are no anatomical barriers to RT, although there are specific tissue tolerance limitations. Basic radiobiologic principles must be observed in devising specific treatment approach (see Chapter 3). Speech therapy and swallow therapy when started prior to therapy or at the outset of therapy increase the likelihood that the patient's function will be preserved after therapy has concluded.

    a. Primary treatment. RT used as the initial and possibly only therapy. This is done mainly to either preserve organs and functions or substitute surgery for unresectable tumors.

    b. Adjuvant treatment. RT planned for use before or after surgery. The irradiated volume can be the preoperative or the postoperative tissue volume at risk, or it can be separate from the operative site such as the treatment of cervical nodes after surgical removal of the primary tumor.

c. **Volume treated.** RT should include all known tumor-bearing anatomic sites plus any sites of suspected tumor spread, such as the neck in a patient with aggressive oral tongue or pharyngeal cancers.

d. **RT doses.** In general, daily doses should be 180 to 200 cGy per fraction. For epidermoid carcinomas of the head and neck without surgery, the total doses are usually 6,500 to 7,500 cGy. When used as a postoperative adjuvant, the total doses can be lower (5,500 to 6,000 cGy), and when used preoperatively, even lower doses (4,500 to 5,000 cGy) are appropriate.

e. **Altered fractionation schemes.** Special fractionation regimens have been created to exploit certain radiobiologic advantages for treatment of head and neck cancers (see Chapter 3, Section III.E). They have been tested in numerous international phase III multicenter randomized trials, and the results have in general been favorable as compared to conventional fractionation practice, especially for locoregionally advanced disease.

f. **Hyperfractionation** delivers more fractions with smaller dose per fraction to a higher total dose than conventional fractionation, over the same length of overall treatment time. It aims to enhance tumor cell killing while maintaining the same level of late normal tissue damage.

g. **Accelerated fractionation** aims to overcome the therapy-induced *accelerated repopulation* of cancer cells and delivers a conventional amount of total dose while shortening the overall treatment time with more intensely fractionated patterns.

h. **Combined chemoradiotherapy.** Cytotoxic chemotherapy as well as biologic response modifiers have been shown to augment the therapeutic effect of RT. Most randomized trials have shown the benefit of concurrent chemo-RT (CCRT; see Section I.J.3), while induction or neoadjuvant chemotherapy before definitive RT continues to be evaluated.

i. **Precision-oriented RT.** Recent advances in computer technology have enabled the development of ultra-precision treatment techniques such as *stereotactic irradiation* and *intensity-modulated RT* (IMRT). *Particle therapy* with protons and heavy ions are also available in a few centers worldwide (see Chapter 3, Sections V.A and V.B).

H. **Management of the primary cancer**

1. **Most T1 and T2 primary cancers** can be controlled equally well by surgery or RT. The choice of treatment may be influenced by tumor site, accessibility, histologic grade, the patient's health status, vocation, or preference. Organ or functional preservation may be provided by RT for cancers of the oral and pharyngeal tongue, floor of the mouth, larynx, orbit, or tonsil. Surgery is preferable when tumor involves bone.

2. **Most T3 and T4 primary cancers** often require combinations of surgery and RT. If resection is not possible, high-dose RT may still be effective and adjuvant chemotherapy may be useful. Although preoperative irradiation may reduce the tumor size and theoretically facilitate the surgery, postoperative irradiation is nearly always preferable because the extent of tumor can be better determined and tissue healing is less impaired. The total radiation doses after complete resection of the primary and regional tumors may be reduced to 5,500 to 6,000 cGy. Indications for postoperative RT include:

a. Close or inadequate resection margins

b. Poorly differentiated cancers

    c. Involvement of lymphatics, including cervical nodes

    d. Perineural invasion

  3. When cancer reappears clinically at the initial site following a complete response to the primary treatment, this is considered local recurrence of cancer. If a tumor arises at a different site, especially if the histology is different, it is considered a new cancer. The retreatment of cancers may be difficult, with reduced effectiveness and increased morbidity, although surgery may "rescue" failures of RT, and irradiation may control surgical failures.

    a. Recurrence of a tumor usually indicates a biologically aggressive cancer and the prognosis is worse than that prior to initial treatment.

    b. If the local failure is at the margin of the treatment site, it may be a direct result of "geographical miss," and additional focal salvage treatment may still provide effective cure.

I. **Treatment of metastases to cervical LNs** is related to extent of the metastases (massive, fixed, bilateral), the location of the metastases, the histology, and the primary tumor site. The most frequent treatment is surgery either at the time of resection of the primary cancer or later.

  1. The types of neck dissection (ND) are:

    a. Classic radical ND removes *en bloc* all tissues from the clavicle to the mandible and from the anterior margin of the trapezius muscle to the midline strap muscles between the superficial layer of the deep cervical fascia (platysma) and the deep layer of the deep cervical fascia. Included are the sternocleidomastoid muscle, internal jugular vein, and accessory (11th) cranial nerve.

    b. A **modified radical ND** usually spares the accessory (11th) nerve and/or sternocleidomastoid muscle. This operation is usually used when the neck is "clinically negative," but at high risk for metastases or when the metastases to cervical nodes are minimal and when RT is to be used. A variant is the **supraomohyoid dissection** that removes nodes only from the upper neck.

    c. When a **partial or selective neck dissection** is done, only a limited number of LNs are removed. This might be a single, suspicious node.

  2. The risk of clinically undetected metastases varies with primary tumor site and size and the histology. For example, approximately 40% of patients with squamous cell carcinomas of the oral tongue will eventually develop cervical adenopathy. This risk is higher, and often bilateral, for patients with carcinomas of the pharyngeal tongue. In contrast, cervical metastases do not develop in patients with cancers limited to the true vocal cords because there are no lymphatics.

  3. Selection of treatment. When metastases to cervical LNs are present at the time of diagnosis, treatment of the neck is usually dictated by the treatment modality selected for the primary tumor. For squamous cell carcinomas primary in the oral cavity and paranasal sinuses, surgery may be preferable. When the cancers arise in the nasopharynx, RT is the choice because these tumors are radioresponsive, often are bilateral, and may not be resectable because of anatomic barriers. Other pharyngeal and laryngeal primary tumors would require both surgery and RT, but with cervical nodal metastases, primary RT with or without chemotherapy is preferable, often followed by planned neck dissection.

J. Role of chemotherapy in squamous cell carcinomas of the head and neck (SCCHN). Chemotherapy does not have a role in most early-stage (I and II) SCCHN. The greatest benefit derived from chemotherapy is in patients with locally advanced disease when chemotherapy is used either sequentially or concurrently with RT, with or without surgery. It has been shown in this setting to increase the possibility of larynx preservation and improve survival. Data supporting adjuvant chemotherapy alone is largely restricted to nasopharyngeal carcinoma. In the metastatic setting, it may be used as a palliative measure, and one regimen has also been shown to improve overall survival.

1. **Effective agents.** Many drugs have shown activity as single agents in the recurrent and metastatic setting, usually in the range of 10% to 20%. Specific examples from published phase II studies include methotrexate (RR 10% to 45%), cisplatin (RR 15% to 40%), bleomycin (RR 5% to 45%), 5-fluorouracil (5-FU; RR 0% to 33%), capecitabine (24%) paclitaxel (RR 30% to 40%), docetaxel (RR 30% to 40%), carboplatin (RR 10% to 30%), gemcitabine (13%), ifosfamide (RR 25%), cetuximab (RR 16%), and erlotinib (RR 4%).

2. **Induction chemotherapy** (before surgery or RT) has been evaluated extensively. Despite very high RR, studies have not clearly shown survival benefit with this approach. A meta-analysis has shown, however, a small but significant survival benefit when cisplatin and 5-FU are used in combination. A benefit of adding a taxane (usually docetaxel) to cisplatin/5-FU, given either before RT or CCRT, has been shown. The Dana Farber group (TAX 324) showed a significant improvement in 3-year overall survival from 48% to 62% when docetaxel was added to cisplatin/5-FU and then followed by carboplatin given concurrently with RT. What is not known is whether the addition of any induction chemotherapy will improve survival compared with the optimal CCRT and studies are ongoing to address this question. Use of induction chemotherapy is sometimes considered with bulky N3 disease or if there is a significant delay with initiation of RT. Side effects of multiagent chemotherapy with TPF include neutropenia and other cytopenias, mucositis, nausea and vomiting, and hearing loss. Given the potential toxicity of multiagent chemotherapy, induction chemotherapy should be additionally reserved for patients with good performance status and minimal comorbidities.

3. **Induction chemotherapy regimens for SCCHN** include:
   a. TPF, given in 21-day cycles
      Docetaxel (**T**axotere), 75 mg/m^2, IV on day 1
      Cis**p**latin, 75 mg/m^2, IV on day 1
      5-**F**U, 750 mg/m^2/d by continuous IV infusion over 24 hours on days 1 through 5
   b. TPF, also given in 21-day cycles
      Docetaxel, 75 mg/m^2, IV on day 1
      Cisplatin, 100 mg/m^2, IV on day 1
      5-FU, 1,000 mg/m^2/d by continuous IV infusion over 24 hours on days 1 through 4

4. **Concurrent chemoradiotherapy (CCRT)** is an established standard for definitive treatment of locally advanced squamous cell head and neck cancer. It has been shown to improve larynx preservation rates in intermediate, locally advanced laryngeal cancer by the Radiation Therapy Oncology Group (RTOG 91-11). A meta-analysis of CCRT used in patients with locally advanced SCCHN has shown a statistically significant improvement in overall survival (absolute improvement 8%) compared to RT alone. Survival benefits have been seen in randomized studies using various chemotherapy regimens, such as cisplatin alone, cisplatin with 5-FU, and carboplatin with 5-FU.

A study with cetuximab, a monoclonal antibody to the epidermal growth factor receptor, in combination with RT, has shown a significant survival benefit compared with RT alone (55% vs. 45% 3-year overall survival). Although CCRT using conventional cytotoxic agents will increase mucosal toxicity compared with RT alone, this increase in toxicity was not seen with cetuximab.

The combination of cisplatin, cetuximab, and RT was tested in a phase III cooperative group study (RTOG 05-22) of 895 patients, which showed that the addition of cetuximab did not improve either progression-free survival or overall survival. Thus, single-agent cisplatin or cetuximab remains the standard of care for combination with RT for locally advanced HNSCC. Definitive CCRT regimens for SCCHN include:

a. Given in 21-day cycles for three cycles with RT:
Cisplatin, 100 mg/m^2, IV on day 1

b. Given in 21-day cycles for 3 cycles with RT:
Carboplatin, 70 mg/m^2, IV on days 1 through 4
5-FU, 600 mg/m^2/d by continuous IV infusion over 24 hours on days 1 through 4

c. Cetuximab, 400 mg/m^2 IV loading dose given on the week before RT starts, then 250 mg/m^2 IV weekly for 7 weeks

d. Acceptable cisplatin alternative schedules for improved tolerability include 30 to 40 mg/m^2 weekly, or 20 mg/m^2 daily for 5 days on first and fifth weeks of RT.

e. If induction TPF is used, carboplatin or cetuximab given weekly with RT is acceptable. High-dose cisplatin is typically not utilized after induction TPF given toxicity concerns

In the postoperative/adjuvant setting, several studies have evaluated CCRT in "high-risk" patients. The two largest phase III randomized studies completed were the European Organization for Research of Cancer (EORTC 22931) and the RTOG (RTOG 95-01) studies. Both randomized patients to either high-dose cisplatin concomitant with RT or RT alone and showed significant improvement in disease-free survival with cisplatin added. However, only EORTC 22931 showed a significant improvement in overall survival (absolute 13% survival benefit at 5 years). Subset analyses of both studies have shown that *significant improvement in survival is seen only for patients with either extracapsular LN extension or positive surgical margins.* Therefore, addition of platinum-based chemotherapy with RT is considered standard adjuvant treatment in patients when these two adverse features are found at the time of surgery.

5. **Adjuvant chemotherapy** is not recommended as standard of care after RT, with the single exception of **nasopharyngeal carcinoma**. In the Intergroup Study 0099, patients with stage III/IV nasopharyngeal carcinoma were randomized to RT alone or concurrent cisplatin and RT followed by three cycles of adjuvant cisplatin and 5-FU. The 3-year overall survival was 47% and 78%, respectively ($P = 0.005$), establishing this regimen with CCRT followed by adjuvant chemotherapy as the standard of care.

a. **CCRT plus adjuvant regimen for nasopharyngeal carcinoma.** Cisplatin, 100 mg/m^2, IV on day 1 of 21-day cycles for three cycles concurrently with RT (alternatively, carboplatin AUC 6 may be substituted for cisplatin); followed by three 28-day cycles (after RT is completed) of cisplatin, 80 mg/m^2 IV on day 1 (or carboplatin AUC 5 if carboplatin used for combined portion), and 5-FU, 1,000 mg/m²/d by continuous IV infusion over 24 hours on days 1 through 4.

6. **Reirradiation.** The standard of care for patients with recurrent unresectable disease in a previously irradiated field is palliative chemotherapy, especially if reirradiation option does not exist. Several investigators have evaluated the use of reirradiation concurrently with chemotherapy with overall 2- to 5-year survival rates ranging from 15% to 25%. Despite these results, this approach remains experimental.

7. **Metastatic SCCHN** is generally treated with systemic therapy alone and is not curable. Multiple chemotherapy agents have shown activity in this setting. Although multiple combination regimens have shown superior improvement in responses compared with single agents, only one randomized study to date has demonstrated an improvement in overall survival. Examples of regimens with activity in the recurrent/metastatic setting are:

   a. **Single-agent chemotherapy.** In general, response rates of 10% to 20% have been seen with several chemotherapy regimens given as single agent. These include methotrexate 40 to 60 mg/m² IV weekly, taxanes (paclitaxel or docetaxel), cisplatin or carboplatin, ifosfamide, 5-flurouracil, and cetuximab.

   b. **Cisplatin/5-FU combination** has been an acceptable standard largely due to an improved response rate. However, when tested in a randomized phase 3 trial versus single-agent methotrexate, despite an improved response rate (32% vs. 10%), no statistically significant difference was seen in survival. Most practitioners reserve this regimen and other multiagent platinum-based chemotherapy regimens for younger, more fit patients who can tolerate cisplatin.

   c. **The roles of platinum/5-FU and cetuximab**

      (1) The EXTREME trial is the only multiagent regimen that has demonstrated improved overall survival. EXTREME compared cisplatin (100 mg/m² on day 1) or carboplatin (AUC 5 on day 1) plus 5-FU (1,000 mg/m²/d by continuous infusion on days 1 through 4), with and without cetuximab (400 mg/m² loading dose followed by 250 mg/m² weekly). This study showed a significant improvement in median survival with the addition of cetuximab from 7 to 10 months. However, compared to platinum plus 5-FU, addition of cetuximab resulted in increased rate of sepsis, hypomagnesemia, skin rash, and infusion reactions. Furthermore, since no crossover to cetuximab was allowed in the study, it is unclear whether sequential treatment with cetuximab after progression on platinum plus 5-FU would result in similar overall survival benefit.

      (2) A randomized phase III trial by the Eastern Cooperative Oncology Group compared cisplatin and placebo with cisplatin and cetuximab in 117 eligible patients. The median and progression-free survivals were 8 and 3 months in the control group versus 9 ($P = 0.21$) and 4 months ($P = 0.07$) in the experimental arm. Crossover was allowed in this study.

   d. **Platinum/taxane** combinations with cisplatin or carboplatin and paclitaxel or docetaxel are similarly reserved for patients with good performance status. In an ECOG phase III study, cisplatin with paclitaxel compared with cisplatin and 5-FU yielded similar objective response rates (26% vs. 27%), overall survival (8.1 months vs. 8.7 months), and 1-year response rates (32% vs. 41%).

   e. Immunotherapy. The immune checkpoint inhibitors, such as PD-1 or PD-L1 blocking, are likely to become a standard treatment for patients with platinum-refractory recurrent/metastatic squamous cell head and neck cancer. A phase III trial of nivolumab versus standard of care treatment of physician's choice in platinum-refractory disease showed an overall survival of 7.5 months for nivolumab versus 5.1 months for chemotherapy. Pembrolizumab has been approved by FDA for the treatment of patients with metastatic squamous head and neck carcinoma whose disease progressed on standard chemotherapy. The approval was granted based on a clinical trial showing a 16% response rate. Most of the responders (82%) had a durable control of the disease for 6–24 months.

K. Adverse effects of treatment. All treatments of cancer, even when properly administered by current standards, may have unintended adverse consequences.

1. Radical surgery

   a. Interference with swallowing
   b. Loss or change in quality and forcefulness of voice
   c. Aspiration
   d. Shoulder/upper limb weakness
   e. Localized cutaneous sensory change/loss
   f. Need for thyroid replacement
   g. Diplopia, visual loss
   h. Cosmetic changes

2. Radiation therapy

   a. Acute, self-limiting effects

      (1) Erythema of skin.
      (2) Conjunctivitis.
      (3) Mucositis in oral cavity, oropharynx, hypopharynx, nasopharynx, larynx, and nasal fossa.
      (4) Epilation, dose related, involving scalp, facial hair, eyelashes, and eyebrows. Returning hair may be more sparse and even of a different color and texture.
      (5) Edema. Laryngeal is the most serious.
      (6) Lhermitte syndrome is an infrequent problem manifested as an "electric shocklike" sensation, usually in the upper limbs precipitated by flexion of the neck. This syndrome is secondary to radiation-induced change, probably temporary demyelination. It is not a precursor of permanent myelopathy.
      (7) Alteration or absence of taste senses.
      (8) Xerostomia, which may be minimized by total radiation dose reduction through use of techniques such as IMRT (intensity-modulated radiation therapy). Medications, such as pilocarpine, have been tried without scientifically documented success.
      (9) Infection, the most frequent of which is candidiasis controllable by fluconazole.

   b. Long term/permanent

      (1) Xerostomia. Recovery from acute change may be minimal with long-term adverse consequences, including tooth decay, oral infections, problems swallowing, and associated weight loss. Xerostomia also may be associated with autoimmune disorders (Sjögren syndrome), diabetes, scleroderma, and many medications, including antidepressants, antihypertensives, and medication for allergies.
      (2) Altered taste: usually for salt or sweet.

(3) Cataract. Develops slowly (more frequent in diabetics).

(4) Osteoradionecrosis, usually of the mandible (worse with poor oral hygiene).

(5) Cervical myelopathy appears over several months and is permanent.

(6) Soft tissue change: atrophy, telangiectasia, and rarely ulceration.

(7) Second malignancies: reported in literature but rare.

(8) Epilation.

3. **Chemotherapy** as an adjunct can increase adverse side effects of RT.

4. **Toxicity of CCRT.** Moderately severe to severe toxicities, particularly those affecting swallowing and eating, are experienced by the majority of patients undergoing CCRT. The incidence of grade 3 to 4 mucositis is doubled with CCRT compared with RT alone. The use of gastrostomy tubes for feeding and hydration are usually necessary. About 10% of patients develop severe granulocytopenia.

   a. Xerostomia develops in 75% of patients and persists in 60% at 1 year after CCRT treatment. Persistent problems with sticky saliva, swallowing, chewing, or tasting develop in 25% to 35%.

   b. At 12 months following treatment, half of the patients are still able to eat only soft foods or liquids. Feeding tubes continue to be necessary after 2 years in 25% of patients treated with RT alone and in 50% of patients treated with CCRT.

   c. Because of toxicity, compliance with the treatment protocol is often compromised. About 40% of patients do not undergo the third planned course of high-dose cisplatin and 30% require delays in the RT schedule.

L. **Supportive care**

   1. **Acute mucositis.** Discomfort can be decreased by use of bland foods at room temperature, ice chips, topical analgesics/anesthetics, preparations such as Ulcerease or Gelclair, and pain medications.

   2. **Opportunistic infections,** most frequently candidiasis, can be controlled by specific medications.

   3. **Adequate nutrition** is very important. Frequent meals, diet supplements, and high calorie intake usually are adequate. Hyperalimentation is rarely used.

   4. **Dental care**

      a. All patients who plan to receive high-dose RT to the head and neck region, especially if major salivary glands are in the irradiated fields, should have dental consultation prior to the start of treatment.

      b. Fluoride gel treatment should be used before, during, and after RT. Continuation of treatment should be based on consultation with the involved dentist.

      c. Dentures should not be worn during treatment or until healing of the oral mucosa is complete (several months). Special dentures may be advisable.

      d. Prophylactic tooth extraction may need to be performed before RT, and 1 to 2 weeks of recovery time may be necessary before any irradiation begins.

      e. Special devices such as intraoral shielding or bite opener may need to be constructed by specialty dentist before the RT planning session.

      f. Chemotherapy can exacerbate significantly the dental sequelae of RT.

M. **Special clinical problems**

   1. **Local/regional regrowth** of the previously treated cancer needs to be distinguished from the side effects of treatment. Cancer usually increases in mass and firmness, and the overlying skin may become brawny, purple in color,

and fixed to adjacent tissue. There may be associated ulceration. Although radiation side effects may persist or temporarily increase, usually, there is tissue decrease with fibrosis and atrophy. Secondary radiation changes will be limited to the irradiated volume, whereas the regrowing cancer may extend outside the treatment volume. Biopsies of radiation-induced changes may be hazardous with the development of poorly or nonhealing ulceration and infection. Therefore, treatment, if potentially useful, usually can be instituted based on clinical appearance.

2. **Cosmetic defects** may be devastating to the patient. These usually are distortions such as secondary to VIIth nerve palsy, reduction in size of the oral cavity, loss of portions of the nose or ear, loss or alteration of orbital contents, permanent absence of dentures, and unsightly grafts. Often, reconstructive surgery is indicated. Psychological support is imperative. Interactions with support groups with similar problems may be useful.

3. **Massive facial edema** is an infrequent problem, fortunately. The underlying cause is extensive venous and/or lymphatic obstruction secondary to uncontrolled cancer. Management is symptomatic and usually unsatisfactory. This usually is an end-stage problem with death secondary to cerebral edema, hemorrhage, or inanition.

4. **Arterial rupture with rapid exsanguination** due to disruption of the carotid artery secondary to cancer or necrosis is a rare problem. Prevention is based on local tumor control, avoidance of progressive infection with necrosis, and proper technique of neck dissections.

5. **Upper airway obstruction** may be secondary to progressive cancer, edema, or a combination. The edema can be treated with high doses of prednisone (40 to 60 mg/d orally). Tracheostomy may bypass the obstruction and produce temporary relief. Associated infection should be vigorously treated. For patients who have tumor regrowth after irradiation, chemotherapy may provide tumor reduction.

6. **Obstructive dysphagia.** If this is secondary to progressive, previously treated cancer, there probably are accompanying adverse findings such as airway obstruction and pain. Management usually accomplishes very little.

7. **Infection** associated with progressive, necrotic cancer can be treated with broad spectrum antibiotics, although the effect usually is minimal and temporary.

N. **Specific head and neck cancer sites.** The relative occurrence, sex predominance, most common site, and histology of the constituents of head and neck cancers are compared in Table 8-1.

II. LIP

A. **Definition.** Cancers of the lip arise on the vermilion surfaces and mucosa. Cancers arising on the skin of the lower lip are considered separately as primary skin cancers.

B. **Pathology.** Nearly all lip cancers are squamous cell carcinomas, usually well differentiated.

C. **Natural history**

1. **Presentation.** Ninety-five percent of primary lip cancers arise on the lower vermilion surface. The gross appearances range from minimal erythematous change, through dry scaling to ulcerated masses, occasionally with destruction of underlying muscle and bone. The prognosis may be worse with a need for more aggressive treatment when the lateral commissure is involved by tumor.

2. **Risk factors.** Long-time exposure to sun or wind; chronic irritation.

TABLE 8-1 Features of Head and Neck Cancers by Site of Origin

Primary Tumor	Most Common Site	Relative Occurrence (%)	Cervical Lymph Node Metastases at Time of Presentation (%)
Lip[a]	Lower lip (90%)	15	5
Oral cavity[a]	Tongue (lateral border)	20	40
Oropharynx[a]	Tonsillar region	10	80 for tonsillar fossa and base of tongue 40 for other sites
Hypopharynx[a]	Pyriform sinus	5	80
Larynx[a]	True vocal cord	25	<5 for early glottic 35 for other sites
Nasopharynx[a]	Roof	3	80
Nasal cavity and sinuses	Maxillary antrum	4	15
Salivary glands	Parotid (80%)	15	25

[a]At least 97% are squamous cell carcinomas.

3. **Lymphatic drainage.** From the upper lip primarily to the submandibular LNs; from the lower lip to the submental, submandibular, and subdigastric nodes. The risk of metastases to regional LNs increases with less differentiated tumors, large size and extension of tumor to the lateral commissures. Five to ten percent of patients are likely to have spread to regional LNs at the time of diagnosis, and another 5% to 10% will develop adenopathy later.

D. **Differential diagnosis**
   1. Keratoacanthoma is an exophytic lesion that arises rapidly and usually resolves spontaneously within a few months. Small doses of RT accelerate this resolution, but usually are not advisable.
   2. Hyperkeratosis, often with irritation and/or infection.
   3. Leukoplakia.
   4. Chancre when syphilis was more frequent.

E. **TNM staging.** Refer to the current AJCC Cancer Staging atlas for TNM staging system.

F. **Management of the primary cancer.** Lip cancer, when detected early, can be cured equally well by limited surgery, RT, or surgery (Mohs method)
   1. **Vermilionectomy** (lip shave) can be used to treat leukoplakia, severe dysplasia, and limited carcinoma *in situ*.
   2. **T_{is} and T_1 carcinomas** (≤1.0 cm). RT (external beam, isotope surface application or implantation) or surgery (minimal resection with primary closure without reduction of oral stoma) is highly effective with good resulting cosmesis.
   3. **T_{1-4} carcinomas** (>1.0 cm). RT has some cosmetic and functional advantages over surgery if there is no destruction of underlying normal tissues. If bone is involved or there is substantial loss of normal tissue, surgery with reconstruction is preferable.
   4. **Commissure involvement.** RT has advantage over surgery.
   5. **Local tumor control rate.** Failure rates are related to tumor size and extent. For the primary cancer, the failure rate is <10% for T_1 lesions. Failure in the neck is <10% when the neck initially is N_0, but may increase to 45% when there is gross metastatic adenopathy.

G. **Treatment of regional LNs**

1. **Clinically negative neck.** Observation is preferable. RT may be used for primary cancers that are large or histologically poorly differentiated.

2. **Clinically involved nodes.** Surgery is preferable. When the primary cancer crosses the midline, both sides of the neck are at risk. The major adenopathy is best treated surgically. Subclinical tumor on the other side of the neck can be irradiated or treated with a limited neck dissection.

3. **Delayed neck dissections** can effectively treat metastatic adenopathy that appears clinically after previous treatment of the primary cancer.

H. **Treatment of locally "reappearing" cancer** can be effective. Surgery is preferable for the treatment of failures of RT and additional resections can be used for surgical failures.

III. ORAL CAVITY

A. **Definition.** Includes primary cancers of the oral tongue, floor of the mouth, buccal mucosa, retromolar trigone, gingiva, alveolar ridge, hard palate, and anterior tonsillar pillar.

B. **Pathology.** Nearly all primary cancers are squamous cell carcinomas. Less than 5% are adenocarcinomas (adenocystic, mucoepidermoid carcinomas arising from minor salivary glands).

C. **Natural history**

1. **Risk factors** include use of tobacco products, long-time ingestion of alcoholic beverages, poor oral hygiene, and prolonged focal irritation from teeth/dentures. Recently, there has been a rise in the incidence of oral tongue cancers in young (20 to 40 year old) Caucasian males and females who are never smokers and nondrinkers.

2. **Presentation**

a. Patients with **oral tongue cancers** may notice a local mucosal irritation or a mass that may become ulcerated, infected, and painful. A foul odor or taste may be associated with infection. Pain may be local or referred to the ear. Infiltration of muscle can give rise to problems transporting boluses or speaking.

b. Early **buccal mucosa cancers** may be asymptomatic or felt by the tongue. Ulceration can result in local pain. Obstruction of Stensen duct may be the basis of tender enlargement of the parotid gland. Pain referred to the ear follows tumor involvement of the lingual or dental nerves. Local tumor extension can cause trismus.

c. **Gingival cancers** may be noted as local mucosal changes often with accompanying leukoplakia. More extensive cancers cause loosening of teeth, interference with denture use, bleeding, or pain. Underlying bone may be invaded. Tumor may extend to involve adjacent anatomic structures such as floor of mouth, buccal mucosa, hard and soft palate, or maxillary sinus.

d. Cancers of the **retromolar trigone** may cause trismus by involving the pterygomandibular space, pterygoid, and buccinator muscles.

e. Cancers arising on the **hard palate** are likely to invade bone.

f. Cancers arising from the mucosa of the **floor of the mouth** may be seen as a localized mucosal change, often with leukoplakia, or felt as a mass by the patient. When localized with ulceration and tenderness, these lesions initially may be misdiagnosed as canker sores. With local extension, there may be a submandibular mass, obstruction of the submaxillary ducts with gland enlargement, and invasion of the oral tongue or mandible.

3. **Lymphatic metastases** most often involve subdigastric, upper jugular, and submandibular nodes. The frequency varies with site, extent, and differentiation of the primary cancer but may range up to 30% to 35% at the time of diagnosis with a later increase in untreated necks secondary to the growth of initial subclinical metastases. The risk of bilateral metastases increases as the primary tumor approaches or involves the anatomic midline.

4. **Metastases** below (caudad) the clavicles or above (cephalad) the base of the skull are infrequent, whether lymphatic or hematogenous.

D. **Diagnosis.** Establishment of a diagnosis of cancer arising in the oral cavity should be relatively straightforward because patients usually have distinctive symptoms and signs and the tumors can easily be visualized and palpated. A diagnosis must be established by biopsy. Imaging exams (CT, MRI) have become a major part of the appraisal of tumor extent, bone involvement, and LN metastases.

E. **TNM staging.** Refer to the current AJCC Cancer Staging atlas for TNM staging system.

F. **Management of the primary tumor**

1. **Oral tongue and floor of mouth carcinomas**

   a. **Small tumors (<1.0 cm).** Resection with primary closure; interstitial RT; or external beam RT using oral cone (rarely used).

   b. **T_1 or T_2 tumors.** Resection if minimal deformity or combination of external beam RT and interstitial RT. The choice can vary with patient preference, health status, occupational, or social or psychological factors.

   c. **Extensive tumors.** Resection followed by external beam RT. Surgery is preferable when the mandible is invaded by tumor and for verrucous carcinomas and unreliable patients.

2. **Gingival and hard palate carcinomas**

   a. **Small tumors:** resection

   b. **Extensive tumors:** resection and postoperative RT

   c. **Local control rate of T_1 tumors:** 60%

3. **Buccal mucosal carcinomas**

   a. **Small tumors (<1.0 cm):** resection and primary closure.

   b. **T_{1-3}:** RT or resection, probably with a graft.

   c. **Larger superficial cancers ($T_{1,2}$):** RT effective.

   d. **Extensive tumors (T_{3-4}) with invasion of muscle:** resection and postoperative RT.

   e. **Tumor extension to commissure:** RT should be considered.

4. **Retromolar trigone:** faucial pillar carcinomas

   a. **T1–T2 tumors:** RT or resection with or without RT

   b. **T3 superficial tumors:** RT

   c. **Large tumors, deep infiltration:** resection and postoperative RT (special problems exist with extension of tumor into the pharyngeal tongue or bone)

5. **Management of the neck.** When the primary cancer is controlled, death due to uncontrolled metastatic cancer in the neck should be uncommon. The risk of subclinical involvement of neck nodes is related to the T-stage and histologic differentiation. Although adenopathy usually can be treated successfully after observation of an N_0 neck, elective treatment may lessen the risk of uncontrolled tumor in the neck and development of distant metastases. *Some general guidelines are as follows:*

   a. **Clinically "negative" neck**

      (1) T_1, low-grade primary cancers: observation if the patient is reliable

(2) T_2 to T_4 and/or poorly differentiated primary cancers:
  (a) If the primary tumor is treated surgically, perform elective neck dissection.
  (b) If the primary cancer is irradiated, the neck should be concurrently irradiated.
  (c) If the primary cancer is managed by combined treatment methods, either treatment method may be used.

  b. **Clinical lymphadenopathy**
  (1) If the primary tumor is treated surgically, add ND.
  (2) If the primary tumor is treated with RT, irradiate the neck and follow with ND for residual adenopathy after adequate observation or if an initially enlarged node was large (i.e., > 3.0 cm).
  (3) When the tumor-involved nodes are "fixed," start with RT. If the adenopathy becomes resectable, perform ND after about 5,000 cGy. If not, give RT to full total dose.

IV. OROPHARYNX

A. **Definition.** Includes pharyngeal ("base of") tongue, tonsillar region (fossa and pillars although anterior pillar often included in oral cavity), soft palate, and pharyngeal walls between the pharyngoepiglottic fold and the nasopharynx.

B. **Pathology.** Ninety-five percent are squamous cell carcinomas, usually less histologically differentiated than those of the oral cavity. A few tumors may be adenocarcinomas arising in the minor salivary glands or primary lymphomas.

C. **Natural history**
  1. **Risk factors** include:
    a. Prolonged intake of alcoholic beverages, especially for primary carcinomas of the anterior tonsillar pillar and posterior pharyngeal wall.
    b. **HPV**: HPV infection, and in particular type 16 (HPV-16), is now recognized as a significant player in the onset of oropharyngeal SCC, with different epidemiologic, clinical, anatomical, radiologic, behavioral, biologic, and prognostic characteristics from HPV-negative SCC. Indeed, the only subsite in the head and neck with a demonstrated etiologic viral link is, at present, the oropharynx. HPV+ oropharyngeal carcinoma is on the rise. HPV is causal in 70% of OP SCCA. These tumors can be treated with primary RT, CRT, or TORS +/- adjuvant RT. Ongoing ECOG and RTOG trials are investigating the possibility of de-escalating adjuvant therapy in patients who are TORS candidates.
  2. **Clinical presentation**
    a. May be clinically "silent," especially those cancers arising in the pharyngeal tongue where the tumor may be submucosal, but indurated.
    b. Pharyngeal tongue and tonsillar carcinomas may appear clinically as cervical adenopathy.
    c. Symptoms include localized pain aggravated by swallowing, ipsilateral otalgia, difficulty swallowing secondary to pain, or decreased mobility of the tongue. The patient may feel a mass at the primary site or in the neck.
  3. **Lymphatic drainage.** The lymphatics of the pharyngeal tongue, tonsil, and pharyngeal wall are abundant. The lymphatics of the pharyngeal tongue drain into the deep cervical nodes, and involvement often is bilateral. The lymphatics of the tonsillar region and faucial arch drain into the subdigastric, upper and middle cervical, and parapharyngeal nodes. Metastases

usually are ipsilateral unless the primary tumor approaches the midline. Lymphatic drainage from the pharyngeal wall is to the retropharyngeal and level II to III cervical nodes.

D. Diagnosis. Cancers arising in the oropharynx can be visualized and palpated. The diagnosis must be documented by biopsy. Differential diagnoses on physical exam include tonsillar abscess, benign lymphoid hyperplasia, or benign ulceration with induration.

E. TNM staging. Refer to the current AJCC Cancer Staging atlas for TNM staging system.

Staging is for epithelial malignant tumors arising in the sites defined above. Nonepithelial tumors arising in lymphoid tissue, soft tissue, bone, and cartilage are not included. Clinical staging often is used because many of these cancers are managed by primary RT. Assessment for clinical staging is based on inspection, palpation, CT, and MRI examination. Pathologic staging adds information found at surgery.

F. Management of the primary tumor
  1. Pharyngeal tongue
    a. Small tumors: surgery if lateralized or RT
    b. Larger tumors: especially if approaching midline, RT
  2. Tonsillar region
    a. Small tumors: surgery or RT
    b. Extensive primary tumors: surgery plus postoperative RT
  3. Soft palate
    a. Small tumors: usually RT or surgery if minimal resulting dysfunction
    b. Large tumors: RT
  4. Pharyngeal wall
    a. Small tumors: RT can be effective with minimal morbidity
    b. Extensive tumors: RT and surgery if applicable

G. Management of the neck. Primary carcinomas arising in the pharyngeal tongue, soft palate, and pharyngeal wall are likely to metastasize to nodes in both sides of the neck. Limited primary cancers of the tonsillar region may metastasize only to ipsilateral nodes.

For primary carcinomas managed by RT, the neck should be part of the initial treatment plan. As the cervical adenopathy becomes larger or more nodes are involved, ND becomes part of the management. If the initial treatment of the primary site and the neck is surgery, postoperative RT is advisable when the primary tumor is extensive, the histology is poorly differentiated, the adenopathy is large (i.e., > 3.0 cm), or multiple nodes are involved or when tumor extends through the capsule of the node. CCRT may also be considered under these circumstances.

H. Treatment of "recurrence." Repeated thorough examinations at intervals of a few months are an important part of patient management. Most persistence or regrowth of tumor can be recognized within 2 years of treatment of the initial cancer. Salvage treatment by either surgery or RT or both may be successful. These patients are also at high risk to develop other cancers.

V. NASOPHARYNX

A. Definition. Carcinomas of nasopharynx arise in a small anatomic site bordered by the nasal fossae, the posterior wall continuous with the posterior wall of the oropharynx (anterior to the first and second cervical vertebrae), the body of the sphenoid and basilar part of the occipital bones, and the soft palate.

B. **Pathology.** World Health Organization (WHO) classification should be used. About 90% of malignant tumors are squamous cell carcinoma, whereas 5% are lymphomas and 5% are of other various subtypes. The squamous cell carcinomas are 20% keratinizing (WHO-I); 40% to 50% nonkeratinizing, differentiated (WHO-II); and 40% to 50% nonkeratinizing, undifferentiated (lymphoepitheliomas; WHO-III).

C. **Natural history**
   1. **Risk factors**
      a. Incidence higher in Asians, particularly those from southern China, Eskimos, and Icelanders. This risk prevails in first-generation immigrants to other parts of the world.
      b. Nonkeratinizing nasopharyngeal carcinomas are uniformly associated with EBV; patients usually have increased levels of immunoglobulin A antibody to the viral capsid antigen and early antigen. Monitoring EBV DNA in the serum of affected patients using real-time polymerase chain reaction technology appears to be useful tool for gauging responses to therapy.
      c. It may occur in pediatric age group.
      d. Affected often have increased titers of antibodies to EBV.
   2. **Presentation**
      a. Often initially noted as high posterior cervical adenopathy, which may be bilateral
      b. Epistaxis, nasal obstruction
      c. Change in voice
      d. Unilateral hearing loss or "fullness" in one ear, serous otitis
      e. Trismus
      f. Headache
      g. Proptosis
      h. Cranial nerve syndromes secondary to tumor invasion of base of the skull
         (1) **Retrosphenoidal syndrome** from involvement of cranial nerves II through VI manifests as unilateral ophthalmoplegia, ptosis, pain, trigeminal neuralgia, and unilateral weakness of muscles of mastication.
         (2) **Retroparotid syndrome** from compression of cranial nerves IX through XII and sympathetic nerves manifests as mechanical dysphagia, problems with taste, salivation, or respiration; weakness of the trapezius, sternocleidomastoid muscles, or tongue muscles; and Horner syndrome.
      i. Distant metastases more frequent with nasopharyngeal carcinoma than with any other head and neck cancer.
   3. **Lymphatic drainage.** The abundant lymphatics drain to the retropharyngeal and deep cervical LNs (internal jugular and spinal accessory nerve chains). Drainage is bilateral. Lymphadenopathy is present in 80% of patients at presentation with 50% being bilateral.
   4. **Prognostic factors**
      a. Tumor extent, particularly invasion of the base of the skull
      b. Size and level of cervical node metastases
      c. Age (prognosis is better with age under 40 to 50 years)
      d. Tumor type

D. **Diagnosis**
   1. Endoscopy to identify the primary cancer, which may be a minimal mucosal alteration or mass.

2. Palpation of the neck for adenopathy, which usually is high posterior cervical and often is bilateral.
3. CT or MRI to identify the extent of primary tumor and adenopathy and involvement of the base of the skull.
4. Cranial nerve examination.
5. Differential diagnoses include benign adenopathy of Waldeyer's ring, nasopharyngitis, and cervical adenopathy of other etiology.

E. **TNM staging.** Refer to the current AJCC Cancer Staging atlas for TNM staging system. In addition to T staging, nasopharyngeal cancer has unique N-staging categories distinct from other SCCHN. Other staging systems have been published from Asian investigators.

F. **Management of the primary tumor.** Surgery usually is not applicable because tumor-free margins cannot be obtained at the base of the skull. RT with high-energy x-rays, often combined with chemotherapy, is the treatment of choice. **Treatment sequelae** may be severe after RT with the necessary high total doses. These include local ulceration, occasionally with necrosis, retinopathy, fibrosis of soft tissues in the neck, and middle ear changes. These sequelae can be reduced with modern treatment planning.

G. **Management of regional LNs.** External beam RT is the choice because the adenopathy frequently is bilateral in the neck and often involves the retropharyngeal LNs. Control of regional adenopathy also is related to N stage but has not been well documented. Neck dissection may be useful for tumor that persists or regrows after primary irradiation.

H. **Chemotherapy for nasopharyngeal carcinoma.** About 60% of patients have stage III or IV disease and often develop distant metastases. Induction chemotherapy resulted in high response rates but no change in overall survival and is not recommended. CCRT involving cisplatin with or without 5-FU (see Section I.J.3) for three cycles is considered standard therapy in the Western world. CCRT appears to double the 5-year survival rate to 67%, but about half of the patients cannot complete planned therapy because of toxicity.

I. **Treatment of local recurrence.** Retreatment is more often successful for nasopharyngeal carcinoma than after failure of treatment of other head and neck cancers. Reirradiation of the primary tumor site still requires a high total dose and may be done with precision-oriented external beam treatment such as IMRT or brachytherapy. Limited post-RT failures in the neck may be controlled by surgery.

VI. HYPOPHARYNX

A. **Definition.** The "low pharynx" is between the level of the hyoid bone and the entry to the esophagus at the level of the lower border of the cricoid cartilage. It contains the piriform sinuses, aryepiglottic folds, postcricoid region, and lateral pharyngeal walls.

B. **Pathology.** More than 95% of malignant tumors are squamous cell carcinomas. Histologic differentiation varies with the anatomic site. For example, squamous cell carcinomas of the aryepiglottic fold are twice as likely to be well differentiated than are tumors arising in the piriform sinus.

C. **Natural history**
1. **Risk factors**
   a. Use of tobacco and alcoholic beverages
   b. Having had other cancers in the aerodigestive tract
   c. Women more likely to develop postcricoid carcinomas than men

2. Clinical presentation
   a. May be asymptomatic and notice mass in the neck
   b. Pain aggravated by swallowing
   c. Blood-streaked saliva
   d. Mechanical dysphagia
   e. Ear pain
   f. Voice change
   g. Aspiration with pneumonia
   h. Cervical adenopathy in more than 50% (in 25%, a mass in the neck will be the initial finding)

3. Lymphatic drainage
   a. Extensive lymphatics with frequent metastases to midcervical chain (jugulodigastric nodes may be first affected), posterior cervical triangle, and paratracheal LNs.
   b. Frequency of metastases to cervical nodes related to primary tumor site and extent:
      (1) Piriform sinus: 60%
      (2) Aryepiglottic fold: 55%
      (3) Pharyngeal wall: 75%

4. Prognostic factors
   a. Anatomic site and extent of primary tumor
   b. Cervical node metastases
   c. Distant metastases (20% at diagnosis)

D. Diagnosis. These cancers usually are locally advanced at diagnosis.
   1. History and physical exam to include palpation and direct and indirect laryngoscopy.
   2. CT and MRI are essential to determine extent of primary tumor and cervical node metastases.

E. TNM staging. Refer to the current AJCC Cancer Staging atlas for TNM staging system.

F. Management of the primary tumor
   1. Piriform sinus:
      a. T_1 and some T_2 tumors: RT might be preferable. Partial laryngopharyngectomy with neck dissection is effective but with greater morbidity.
      b. Advanced carcinoma extending into the apex or outside piriform sinus often with invasion of the larynx, thyroid cartilage, or soft tissues of the neck: total laryngopharyngectomy, radical ND, and postoperative RT. If resection not possible, RT for palliation.
   2. Aryepiglottis:
      a. T_{1-2} tumors: RT or supraglottic resection
      b. T_{3-4} tumors: surgery with laryngeal conservation if possible, followed by RT
      c. Local tumor control rate for T_{1-2} tumors: 90%
   3. Hypopharyngeal walls:
      a. RT or resection with unilateral neck dissection plus postoperative RT
   4. Management of local recurrence at the primary site: RT if patient only had surgery; further RT is not effective in previously irradiated patients.

G. Management of the neck
   1. No clinical adenopathy: RT to primary site and neck, with or without planned ND.
   2. Clinical cervical node metastases: RT plus planned ND.

3. **Management of recurrence in the neck:** ND if failure of RT, or RT if failure of ND. Unfortunately, the patient often has already had both ND and RT.

VII. LARYNX

A. **Definition.** Laryngeal cancer involves three anatomic sites:
  1. Glottis—paired true vocal cords
  2. Supraglottis—epiglottis, false vocal cords, ventricles, aryepiglottic folds (laryngeal surface), and arytenoids
  3. Subglottis—arbitrarily begins 5.0 mm below free margin of true vocal cord and extends to inferior border of cricoid cartilage

B. **Pathology.** More than 95% of malignant tumors arising from the epithelium are squamous cell carcinomas. The remainder is sarcomas, adenocarcinomas, or neuroendocrine tumors

C. **Natural history**
  1. **Risk factors**
     a. Use of tobacco
     b. Prior occurrence of other carcinomas of aerodigestive tract
  2. **Presentation**
     a. Vocal cord: persistent hoarseness
     b. Supraglottis: often no symptoms; sore throat; intolerance to hot or cold food; ear pain
     c. Subglottis: usually no symptoms until locally extensive
  3. **Lymphatic drainage**
     a. True vocal cords: none (the true vocal cords are devoid of lymphatics)
     b. Supraglottis: rich network draining to subdigastric and midinternal jugular nodes
     c. Subglottis: sparse network draining to inferior jugular nodes

D. **Diagnosis**
  1. Palpation of neck for cervical adenopathy and laryngeal crepitus
  2. Endoscopy
  3. CT and MRI to assess site and extent of primary tumor and cervical adenopathy

E. **TNM staging.** Refer to the current AJCC Cancer Staging atlas for TNM staging system

F. **Management of the primary tumor**
  1. **Principles.** After the initial objective of tumor control with preservation of the patient's life, preservation of voice and the swallowing reflex becomes of major importance. RT alone or limited surgery can accomplish these objective in many laryngeal cancers.
     a. **Partial laryngectomy** for selected situations may result in tumor control and preservation of a useful voice.
     b. **Salvage (total) laryngectomy** may be successful after failure of conservative treatment.
     c. **Locally extensive cancers**, especially with edema, usually require total laryngectomy often followed by RT.
     d. **Chemotherapy.** Induction chemotherapy followed by definitive RT achieves laryngeal preservation in a high percentage of patients with advanced cancer, but does not improve overall survival. CCRT (Section I.J.3) has been more successful for both laryngeal preservation and survival than induction chemotherapy, however, and is recommended

as the treatment of choice for locally extensive cancers. High total radiation doses with modern techniques such as IMRT, conformal planning, accelerated fractionation, and hyperfractionation may be comparably successful.

   e. Sequelae of treatment

      (1) RT. Edema, usually temporary, and chondritis, which is rare; infrequent persistent minimal voice change.

      (2) Partial laryngectomy. Some voice deterioration, interference with swallowing reflex.

      (3) Total laryngectomy. Loss of voice; over 50% of patients can develop effective esophageal speech.

2. True vocal cords including anterior or posterior commissures

   a. T_{is}. RT or "cord stripping."

   b. T_{1-2}. RT preferable; cordectomy and vertical hemilaryngectomy have more sequelae.

   c. T_3, **limited tumors** may respond to RT, surgical salvage can follow.

   d. T_3, **extensive tumors.** Surgery, usually followed by RT or CCRT.

   e. T_4. Total laryngectomy and postoperative RT or CCRT for larynx preservation.

   f. Persistent or recurrent cancer:

      (1) Surgery for RT failure

      (2) RT or more extensive surgery or both for failure of limited surgery

      (3) RT for failure after total laryngectomy

   g. Local tumor control rates:

      (1) T_1, 90% to 95% with RT and most failures can be salvaged surgically; voice preservation in 95%.

      (2) T_2, 75% to 80% with RT and most failures can be salvaged by surgery; voice preservation in 80% to 85%.

      (3) T_3, **favorable tumors** with minimal fixation of vocal cords: 60% by RT increased to 85% by salvage surgery.

      (4) T_3, **more extensive tumors.** 40% with RT, increased to 60% by salvage surgery; total laryngectomy—55% to 70%.

      (5) T_{4a}, **favorable with early invasion of thyroid cartilage.** 65% with RT; extensive with involvement of piriform sinus 20% with RT; laryngectomy—40% to 50%.

3. Supraglottic carcinoma

   a. T_{1-2}. RT or supraglottic laryngectomy.

   b. T_3. RT often controls exophytic tumors; and surgery can be reserved for salvage; for infiltrating tumors, surgery is preferable often with postoperative RT.

   c. T_4. Surgery followed by postoperative RT. In a group of medically inoperable patients, RT resulted in a 35% local tumor control.

   d. Treatment of recurrent cancer:

      (1) Surgery for RT failures

      (2) RT for surgery failures

      (3) Chemotherapy

4. Subglottic carcinoma

   a. Usually extensive when discovered; treat with surgery + RT

   b. Local tumor control <25%

G. Management of the neck

   1. Glottic carcinomas. When tumor limited to true vocal cords, there are no metastases to be treated.

2. **Extensive glottic tumors and supraglottic carcinomas.** The neck can initially be managed by the method used for treatment of the primary tumor. Persistent adenopathy after primary RT should be treated surgically. Surgical failures can be irradiated.

VIII. NASAL CAVITIES AND PARANASAL SINUSES

A. **Definition.** Knowledge of the complex anatomy is basic to understanding these tumors. The *nasal vestibule* is the entrance to the *nasal fossa*. It is bounded by the columella, nasal ala, and floor of the nasal cavity. The nasal fossa extends from the vestibule (limen nasi) to the choana posteriorly, communicating with the nasopharynx, paranasal sinuses, and lacrimal sac and conjunctiva. The boundaries of the *maxillary sinus* are the orbit, lateral wall of the nasal fossa, hard palate (the roots of the first two molar teeth may project into the floor), infratemporal fossa, and pterygopalatine fossa. The multiple *ethmoidal sinuses* are in the ethmoid bone between the nasal cavity and orbit. The left and right *frontal sinuses* in the frontal bone are separated by a septum. The dual *sphenoid sinuses* are surrounded by the pituitary fossa, cavernous sinuses, ethmoidal sinuses, nasopharynx, and nasal cavities.

B. **Pathology**
   1. **Nasal vestibule.** Nearly all are squamous cell carcinomas; a few are basal cell or adnexal carcinomas; <1% are melanomas.
   2. **Nasal cavity and paranasal sinuses.** Most are squamous cell carcinomas; 10% to 15% arise in minor salivary glands; 5% are lymphomas; other tumors include chondrosarcoma, osteosarcoma, Ewing tumor, and giant cell tumor of the bone.
   3. **Esthesioneuroblastomas** arise from neuroepithelium.
   4. **Inverting papilloma.**
   5. **Midline lethal granuloma** (including extranodal NK/T-cell lymphoma, nasal type).

C. **Natural history**
   1. **Risk factors.** Etiologies are unknown, but carcinoma is more frequent in workers exposed to nickel or wood dust and, historically, in patients exposed to radioactive thorium as an x-ray contrast agent.
   2. **Presentation:**
      a. **Nasal vestibule.** Small, crusted plaques, ulceration, bleeding.
      b. **Nasal fossa.** Unilateral discharge, bleeding, obstruction.
      c. **Maxillary sinus:** Findings may mimic inflammation, pain, upper dental problems, proptosis.
      d. **Ethmoid sinuses.** Anatomic distortion, pain, local extension.
      e. **Sphenoid sinus:** Ill-defined headache, neuropathy of cranial nerves III, IV, V, and VI
   3. **Lymphatic drainage:**
      a. **Nasal fossa, ethmoidal and frontal sinuses**—to submaxillary nodes; to nodes at base of skull when olfactory region involved
      b. **Maxillary sinus**—to ipsilateral subdigastric and submandibular nodes
      c. **Sphenoid sinus**—to jugulodigastric nodes
   4. **Prognostic factors:**
      a. Anatomic site, that is, cancers of nasal fossa, nearly always are cured, whereas cancers of the sphenoid sinus are rarely controlled.
      b. Tumor extent.
      c. Patient's general health (treatment usually is demanding).

D. **Diagnosis**
   1. Clinical symptoms and signs
   2. Direct visualization of nasal vestibule and fossa, palate, alveolar ridge, external orbit (proptosis)

    3. Endoscopy of nasopharynx for tumor extension

    4. Cranial nerve evaluation

    5. MRI and CT examinations of primary site and neck

    6. Differential diagnoses:

        a. Nasal polyps (inverting papillomas)

        b. Inflammatory disease

        c. Upper dental problems

        d. Destructive mucoceles

E. TNM staging. Refer to the current AJCC Cancer Staging atlas for TNM staging system.

F. Management of primary tumors

    1. Nasal vestibule

        a. Small tumors: RT if surgery will produce deformity; chemosurgery or laser surgery

        b. Large tumors: RT or surgery + RT (plastic surgery repair if possible)

        c. Persistence of tumor: surgery for RT failures; more extensive surgery or RT for surgery failures; chemosurgery, laser surgery

    2. Nasal fossa

        a. Small tumors: RT if surgery will produce deformity; surgery with or without RT if bone involved.

        b. Large tumors: combined surgery and RT; RT for lymphomas and melanomas.

        c. Esthesioneuroblastomas: probably combined surgery and RT; chemotherapy (i.e., cisplatin + etoposide) may be helpful.

    3. Maxillary sinus. Fenestration of the palate allows direct inspection and access for biopsy and drainage

        a. Small tumors: surgery alone except for infrequent highly radiation-responsive tumors such as lymphomas.

        b. Advanced tumors: surgery and postoperative RT; chemotherapy and radiotherapy may be used preoperatively in an attempt to make resection possible.

        c. Unresectable tumors: RT and chemotherapy.

        d. Local treatment failure: usually, all modalities have been used; trial of chemotherapy, cautery, or cryosurgery.

    4. Ethmoid sinus

        a. Limited lesions: surgery

        b. Most tumors: surgery and postoperative RT

    5. Sphenoid sinus. RT, possibly with chemotherapy (nearly always extensive when recognized)

    6. Local tumor control rates

        a. Nasal vestibule: most tumors are small and nearly 100% controlled.

        b. Nasal fossa: stage I, nearly 100%; control decreases with increasing extent.

        c. Esthesioneuroblastoma: 90% for Kadish stage A tumors.

        d. Ethmoid sinuses: about 60%.

        e. Maxillary sinus: 75% to 80%.

        f. Sphenoid sinuses: usually extensive when discovered with very infrequent local tumor control.

G. Management of the neck

    1. Nasal vestibule: small tumors; observation with ND if adenopathy develops

    2. Nasal fossa: observation and ND if adenopathy develops (for tumors smaller than 5 cm, <10% ever develop adenopathy)

3. **Esthesioneuroblastoma:** ND, usually as part of primary surgery
4. **Maxillary sinus:** ND, usually as part of primary surgery

H. **Treatment of local recurrence**
  1. **Small tumors** may be salvaged by surgery after RT failures or additional surgery after failure of initial surgery.
  2. **Extensive tumors** usually have received both surgery and RT and retreatment usually not feasible; palliative chemotherapy.

IX. SALIVARY GLANDS

A. **Definition**
  1. **Major salivary glands:** parotid, submandibular, sublingual
  2. **Minor salivary glands:** widespread in mucosa of upper aerodigestive tract

B. **Pathology.** A range of histologic tumor types arise from ductal and acinar cells of the epithelium. The most frequently involved site is the parotid gland with tumors being 10-fold more frequent than in the submaxillary or minor salivary glands. The histologic subtypes and approximate frequencies are:

Mucoepidermoid: 35%
Adenocarcinoma: 25%
Adenoid cystic: 25%
Acinic cell: 10%
Epidermoid: 5% to 10%
Other: 1% to 5%

C. **Natural history**
  1. **Risk factors**
    a. Previous exposure to ionizing radiations
    b. Skin cancer of the face
  2. **Clinical presentations**
    a. Mass, often painless, in salivary gland
    b. Neurologic changes with involvement of facial nerve
    c. Younger women older men
  3. **Lymphatic drainage**
    a. Parotid gland to preauricular, jugulodigastric, intraglandular nodes
    b. Submaxillary gland to submental, jugulodigastric, intraglandular nodes
  4. **Prognostic factors**
    a. Tumor type and grade
    b. Tumor site and extent
    c. Tumor involvement of surgical margins; attempts to spare facial nerve resulting in inadequate resection
    d. Regional node metastases

D. **Diagnosis.** Differentiate from inflammatory changes with tenderness of mass and warmth of overlying skin plus hematologic changes.
  1. Mass in salivary gland, usually painless, often fixed
  2. Paresis and/or numbness related to involvement of facial nerve
  3. Biopsy
  4. CT or MRI of primary site and neck

E. **TNM staging.** Refer to the current AJCC Cancer Staging atlas for TNM staging system.

F. **Management of primary tumor**
  1. **Surgery** is the treatment of choice, if the tumor is resectable. Minimal surgery for parotid tumors is superficial parotidectomy with preservation of the facial nerve. Unwelcome sequelae, if extensive surgery is performed, include facial nerve palsy and auriculotemporal syndrome with gustatory sweating.

2. **RT** has a secondary role as postoperative adjuvant therapy when the histology is poorly differentiated, when significant perineural invasion is seen, or the surgical margins are not tumor-free. RT is also used when the tumor has recurred. Primary irradiation for medically inoperable patients has had some success. Salivary gland tumors seem responsive to fast neutron teletherapy.

3. **Local tumor control rates**
   a. **Surgery alone**
      Stages I to II: 95% to 100%
      Stages III to IV: 40% to 50%
      Low grade: 90%
      High grade: 40%
   b. **Surgery plus RT**
      Stages I to II: 95% to 100%
      Stages III to IV: 75%
      Low grade: 90%
      High grade: 80%
   c. **RT for nonresectable disease**
      Using photons 25%
      Using fast neutrons 65%

G. **Management of the neck**
   1. **Small, low-grade tumors**—Surgery when adenopathy is present.
   2. **Extensive, poorly differentiated tumors**—Surgery plus postoperative RT.

X. METASTASES OF CANCER OF UNKNOWN PRIMARY (CUP) TO NECK LYMPH NODES

A. **Definition.** CUPs are metastatic solid tumors (hematopoietic malignancies and lymphomas are excluded) for which the site of origin is not identified despite thorough history, physical examination, chest radiograph, routine blood and urine studies, and thorough histologic evaluation.

B. **Pathology.** Metastases are located in the upper jugular chain in the majority of patients. The histologic type of metastasis to neck nodes varies in incidence according to anatomic location (Table 8-2); the probability for squamous carcinoma rises the higher the node is on the chain. Involved nodes are single in 75% of patients, multiple but ipsilateral in 15%, and bilateral in 10%. Multiplicity is often associated with adenocarcinoma or metastases from the nasopharynx or infraclavicular sites.

C. **Natural history.** CUPs account for 3% to 9% of head and neck cancers. The occurrence of CUP to cervical LNs is six times higher in men than in women. Patients are usually heavy smokers and heavy drinkers who have noted the mass for several months. Despite the absence of a detected

TABLE 8-2	Histology of Neck Node Metastases from Unknown Primary Site			
	Histopathology: Relative Frequencies (%)			
Lymph Nodes	Squamous Cell Carcinoma	Undifferentiated Carcinoma	Adenocarcinoma	Other[a]
Upper to middle cervical	60	25	10	5
Lower cervical	45	40	5	10
Supraclavicular	20	45	35	

[a]Malignant melanoma accounts for most cases with other histologies.

primary site, both long-term survival and cures are observed in a significant percentage of patients.

1. **Upper cervical nodes.** The primary site is the upper respiratory passages for most squamous tumors that present as CUP in the upper half of the neck. About 35% of these patients can potentially be cured. With CT or MRI scanning and skillful endoscopic evaluation, a primary site can be determined in at least 30% of cases.

   Carcinomas of the nasopharynx, hypopharynx, base of the tongue, and tonsil present with cervical node metastasis as the first manifestation of disease in 30% to 50% of cases. These sites or the larynx harbors the primary tumor 95% of the time when the primary site is ultimately found after initially manifesting as metastasis of CUP to cervical nodes.

2. **Lower cervical nodes.** About 65% of metastases to the low cervical nodes originate in sites below the clavicle, most commonly in the lung. Thus, this presentation is usually associated with a poor prognosis.

3. **Supraclavicular nodes.** Involvement of this group of LNs with malignancy nearly always indicates disease that is far advanced. The primary site is usually the lung, breast, or gastrointestinal tract. The expected survival time is <6 months.

4. **HPV+ unknown primary**. Carcinoma of unknown primary remains an uncommon presentation of head and neck squamous cell carcinoma. p16 testing of FNAB specimens helps the surgeon classify patients as low or high risk, and a positive p16 result mandates a rigorous inspection of the oropharynx. When examination under anesthesia with directed biopsies does not reveal the primary source, patients with a p16+ cancer should undergo lingual tonsillectomy in an effort to identify the primary site. When the primary site is identified on frozen section, the surgeon may proceed to a definitive negative margin resection. Patients with a known primary site benefit from more focused radiation fields, increased survival, and improved quality of life. Using this technique, primary cancers are identified up to 90% of the time.

5. **Prognostic factors.** Prognosis is predominantly affected by the N stage of neck disease, by the location in the neck (see above), by the histopathology, and by whether the primary site is ever found (the prognosis is much better if the primary tumor never becomes manifest).

D. **Diagnosis.** Excisional biopsy of cervical nodes should not be performed because it distorts surgical planes and may result in poor outcomes if it proved to be a squamous cell carcinoma originating in an occult site in the head and neck. Supraclavicular lymphadenopathy, on the other hand, rarely represents curable disease; these nodes may be excised directly for histologic examination. **The recommended sequence of evaluation of cases of potentially cancerous cervical nodes** is as follows:

1. **Initial evaluation.** Carefully inspect and palpate all accessible areas of the mouth and nose. Then evaluate the upper airways, especially the nasopharynx, with mirrors or Hopkin's laryngoscope.

2. **Imaging.** Obtain a CT or MRI scan of the neck and paranasal sinuses to search for a primary tumor. PET may detect more metastatic sites and provide a higher rate of positive biopsy results during panendoscopy for cervical LN CUP, but the clinical relevance of this information is marginal.

3. **Fine-needle aspiration** (FNA) is performed if these efforts fail to demonstrate any hint of a primary cancer. The results of cytologic evaluation direct further evaluation, as follows:

   a. **Squamous cell or undifferentiated carcinoma.** Perform panendoscopy and manage the patient for a primary head and neck cancer.

    b. Indeterminate or equivocal histology. Excise the node, and perform immunoperoxidase stains and other special studies on the tissue as necessary.

    c. Adenocarcinoma. Manage as for metastasis of CUP to viscera (see Chapter 21). The outlook is nearly hopeless unless originating in a major salivary gland (which is rare).

    d. Melanoma. Manage as discussed in Section V.A of Chapter 20.

    e. Lymphoma. Manage accordingly (see Chapter 22).

4. Panendoscopy (nasopharyngoscopy, laryngoscopy with tracheoscopy, bronchoscopy, and esophagoscopy) is performed under general anesthesia. All suspected lesions and random areas of apparently normal tissue at the base of tongue, pyriform sinus, and nasopharynx are subjected to biopsy in search of a primary source. Ipsilateral tonsillectomy has a better yield than tonsillar fossa biopsy and is often performed as well. If a primary tumor is found, treatment is planned with consideration of the primary site and neck metastasis.

5. Lingual tonsillectomy. Carcinoma of unknown primary remains an uncommon presentation of head and neck squamous cell carcinoma. p16 testing of FNAB specimens helps the surgeon classify patients as low or high risk, and a positive p16 result mandates a rigorous inspection of the oropharynx. When examination under anesthesia with directed biopsies does not reveal the primary source, patients with a p16+ cancer should undergo lingual tonsillectomy in an effort to identify the primary site. When the primary site is identified on frozen section, the surgeon may proceed to a definitive negative margin resection. Patients with a known primary site benefit from more focused radiation fields, increased survival, and improved quality of life. Using this technique, primary cancers are identified up to 90% of the time.

6. Biopsy of the suspect node should be done only when:

    a. Thorough physical examination fails to reveal a primary tumor.

    b. CT or MRI examination does not disclose a primary tumor.

    c. FNA cytology fails to reveal the diagnosis.

    d. Panendoscopy fails to reveal a primary site.

    e. Lymphoma is suspected (excluded in the definition of CUP).

E. Treatment alternatives. Treatment should follow the guidelines for locally advanced squamous cell carcinoma arising in the head and neck. Treatment must be comprehensive at the outset because salvage therapy has a low yield.

1. Comprehensive RT (encompassing the nasopharynx, oropharynx, hypopharynx, and both sides of the neck) achieves a high rate of local control in the neck. In theory, RT fields should encompass the undiscovered primary tumor. However, less extensive RT has been shown to be associated with the same good results and less morbidity.

2. Surgery. The use of surgical treatment alone should be discouraged in these patients because primary sites in the head and neck become manifest in approximately 40% of patients treated with ND alone. Furthermore, 20% to 50% of patients treated with surgery alone develop contralateral neck disease or subsequently manifest a primary tumor site. The incidences of subsequent manifestation of a primary site or development of contralateral neck disease are both much less after RT than after ND.

3. Chemotherapy. Randomized trials have demonstrated the superiority of cisplatin-based CCRT in patients with known primary site head and neck squamous cell carcinomas at high risk for local recurrence (see Section I.J.3).

The application of CCRT to CUP involving cervical LNs in appropriately selected patients appears to be a logical extension of those findings.

F. **Recommended treatment.** Many centers use RT for all cases and CCRT for patients at particularly high risk for local recurrence.

1. **Stages N1 and N2a involving upper or middle neck node.** Treat patients with RT alone. Alternatively, perform ND (particularly if the metastasis is <3 cm in diameter); if the specimen reveals other involved nodes (stage N2b) or extracapsular invasion, administer postoperative RT or CCRT.

2. **Stage N2b involving upper or middle neck nodes.** Use RT or CCRT followed by ND in 3 to 6 weeks.

3. **Stage N3** (massive or bilateral nodes). Use RT alone or CCRT in medically suitable patients.

4. **Squamous cell carcinoma of lower cervical or supraclavicular nodes or adenocarcinomas.** Administer RT alone (survival rates are poor no matter what is done; the goal of treatment is control of local disease).

G. **Results of treatment**

1. **Patients with upper cervical LN metastasis.** The 5-year survival rate for all patients is 30% if the primary tumor is eventually found and 60% if it is never found.

a. **Stage N1 or N2a.** The 5- and 10-year survival rates are both 70% to 80%. At 10 years after treatment, the risk of finding a primary site is about 30%, which is the same as the odds of developing a second cancer after successful treatment.

b. **Stage N2b.** The reported survival rates are variable.

c. **Stage N3.** The 5-year survival is about 20%.

2. **Patients with low cervical or supraclavicular LN metastasis.** The 5-year survival rate is 5% (median survival time is 7 months).

ACKNOWLEDGMENT

The authors would like to acknowledge Drs. Steven G. Wong, Robert G. Parker, and Dennis A. Casciato, who significantly contributed to earlier versions of this chapter.

Suggested Readings

Adelstein DJ, Li Y, Adams GL, et al. An intergroup phase III comparison of standard radiation therapy and two schedules of concurrent chemoradiotherapy in patients with unresectable squamous cell head and neck cancer. *J Clin Oncol* 2003;21:92.

Al-Sarraf M, Pajak TF, Byhardt RW, et al. Post-operative radiotherapy with concurrent cisplatin appears to improve locoregional control of advanced, resectable head and neck cancers: RTOG 88-24. *Int J Radiat Oncol Biol Phys* 1997;37:777.

Al-Sarraf M, LeBlanc M, Giri PG, et al. Chemoradiotherapy versus radiotherapy in patients with advanced nasopharyngeal cancer: phase III randomized intergroup study 0099. *J Clin Oncol* 1998;16:1310.

Ang KK, Zhang Q, Rosenthal DI, et al. Randomized phase III trial of concurrent accelerated radiation plus cisplatin with or without cetuximab for stage III to IV head and neck carcinoma: RTOG 0522. *J Clin Oncol* 2014;32:2940.

Balz V, Scheckenbach K, Götte K, et al. Is the p53 inactivation frequency in squamous cell carcinomas of the head and neck underestimated? Analysis of p53 exons 2-11 and human papillomavirus 16/18 E6 transcripts in 123 unselected tumor specimens. *Cancer Res* 2003;63:1188.

Bernier J, Bentzen SM. Altered fractionation and combined radio-chemotherapy approaches: pioneering new opportunities in head and neck oncology. *Eur J Cancer* 2003;39:560.

Bonner JA, Harari PM, Giralt J, et al. Radiotherapy plus cetuximab for squamous-cell carcinoma of the head and neck. *N Engl J Med* 2006;354:567.

Browman GP, Hodson DI, Mackenzie RJ, et al. Choosing a concomitant chemotherapy and radiotherapy regimen for squamous cell head and neck cancer: a systematic review of the published literature with subgroup analysis. *Head Neck* 2001;23:579.

Chan AT, Teo PM, Ngan RK, et al. Concurrent chemotherapy-radiotherapy compared with radio-therapy alone in locoregionally advanced nasopharyngeal carcinoma: progression-free survival analysis of a phase III randomized trial. *J Clin Oncol* 2002;20:1968.

Clark JR, Busse PM, Norris CM Jr, et al. Induction chemotherapy with cisplatin, fluorouracil, and high-dose leucovorin for squamous cell carcinoma of the head and neck: long term results. *J Clin Oncol* 1997;15:3100.

Cohen EE, Lingen MW, Vokes EE. The expanding role of systemic therapy in head and neck cancer. *J Clin Oncol* 2004;22:1743.

Forastiere AA, Metch B, Schuller DE, et al. Randomized comparison of cisplatin plus fluorouracil and carboplatin plus fluorouracil versus single-agent methotrexate in advanced squamous-cell carcinoma of the head and neck: a Southwest Oncology Group study. *J Clin Oncol* 1992;10:1245.

Forastiere AA, Goepfert H, Maor M, et al. Concurrent chemotherapy and radiotherapy for organ preservation in advanced laryngeal cancer. *N Engl J Med* 2003;349:2091.

Gibson MK, Li Y, Murphy B, et al. Randomized phase III evaluation of cisplatin plus fluorouracil versus cisplatin plus paclitaxel in advanced head and neck cancer (E1395): an intergroup trial of the Eastern Cooperative Oncology Group. *J Clin Oncol* 2005;23:3562.

Gillison ML, Blumenschein G, Fayette J, et al. Nivolumab (nivo) vs investigator's choice (IC) for recurrent or metastatic (R/M) head and neck squamous cell carcinoma (HNSCC): CheckMate-141. Proceedings of the 107th Annual Meeting of the American Association for Cancer Research; 2016 April 16–20; New Orleans, LA. Philadelphia, PA: AACR, 2016 (CT099).

Haas I, Hoffmann TK, Engers R, et al. Diagnostic strategies in cervical carcinoma of an unknown primary (CUP). *Eur Arch Otorhinolaryngol* 2002;259:325.

Lo YM, Chan AT, Chan LY, et al. Molecular prognostication of nasopharyngeal carcinoma by quantitative analysis of circulating Epstein-Barr virus DNA. *Cancer Res* 2000;60:6878.

Parker RG, Janjan NA, Selch MT, eds. Cancers of the head and neck. Chapter 13. In: *Radiation Oncology for Cure and Palliation*. Springer-Verlag, 2003:187–234.

Pignon JP, Bourhis J, Domenge C, et al. Chemotherapy added to locoregional treatment for head and neck squamous-cell carcinoma: three meta-analyses of updated individual data. MACH-NC Collaborative Group Meta-Analysis of Chemotherapy on Head and Neck Cancer. *Lancet* 2000;355:949.

Psyrri A, Cohen E. Oropharyngeal cancer: clinical implications of the HPV connection. *Ann Oncol* 2011;22:997.

Staar S, Rudat V, Stuetzer H, et al. Intensified hyperfractionated accelerated radiotherapy limits the additional benefit of simultaneous chemotherapy: results of a multicentric randomized German trial in advanced head-and-neck cancer. *Int J Radiat Oncol Biol Phys* 2001;50:1161.

9 Lung Cancer

Martin J. Edelman and David R. Gandara

I. EPIDEMIOLOGY AND ETIOLOGY

A. Incidence. Lung cancer is the most common visceral malignancy, accounting for roughly one-third of all cancer deaths, and it is the most common cause of cancer-related death in both men and women. Annually, there are approximately 225,000 new cases in the United States. Although rates for men are decreasing, there is a continued increase for women. Even more disturbing is a possible increase in incidence of non–small cell lung cancer (NSCLC) in patients who never smoked or had a minimal smoking history (i.e., <10 to 15 pack-years).

B. Etiology

1. **Smoking.** Cigarette smoking is the cause of 85% to 90% of lung cancer cases; the risk for lung cancer in smokers is 30 times greater than in non-smokers. Passive smoking probably increases the risk of lung cancer about twofold, but because a proportion of the risk associated with active inhalation is about 20-fold, the actual risk is small. Further, a recent report showed that the tumor molecular profile in never-smoking lung cancer patients with a high secondhand smoke exposure mimicked that of never smokers rather than smokers with lung cancer.

   a. The risk for lung cancer is related to cumulative dose of tobacco carcinogens, which for cigarettes is quantified in "pack-years." The incidence of death from lung cancer begins to diverge from the nonsmoking population at 10 pack-years.

   b. After cessation of smoking, the risk steadily declines, approaching, but not quite reaching, that of nonsmokers after 15 years of abstinence for patients who smoked for <20 years. With the decline in smoking in the United States, a large percentage of new diagnoses of lung cancer occur in former smokers.

   c. The risk of the major cell types of lung cancer is increased in smokers. Some adenocarcinomas, especially in women, are unrelated to smoking.

   d. Small cell lung cancer (SCLC) is almost always associated with smoking, though there are well-documented cases in never smokers. These should not be confused with extrapulmonary small cell carcinomas.

2. **Asbestos** is causally linked to malignant mesothelioma. Asbestos exposure also increases the risk for lung cancer, especially in smokers (three times greater risk than smoking alone).

3. **Radiation exposure** may increase the risk for SCLC in both smokers and nonsmokers. Radon has been associated with up to 6% of lung cancer cases.

4. **Other substances** associated with lung cancer include arsenic, nickel, chromium compounds, chloromethyl ether, and air pollutants.

5. **Lung cancer** is itself associated with an increased risk for a second lung cancer occurring both synchronously and metachronously. Other cancers of the upper aerodigestive tract (head and neck, esophagus) are associated with an increased risk for lung cancer because of the "field cancerization" effect of cigarette smoking.

181

6. **Other lung diseases.** Lung scars and chronic obstructive pulmonary disease are associated with an increased risk for lung cancer, typically associated with a history of cigarette smoking.

7. **Never and minimal smokers and lung cancer.** A substantial portion of the lung cancer population has no obvious toxic exposure. Approximately 10% to 15% of patients in the United States with NSCLC are never smokers. However, in some East Asian countries, over 30% are never smokers. Many of these cases are associated with mutations of the epidermal growth factor receptor (EGFR). Other oncogenic driver mutations, such as ALK translocations, have also been reported in the never-smoker population. Patients with EGFR or ALK mutations have a markedly different prognosis from other patients with lung cancer. There is an expanding list of additional "driver" mutations, occurring in NSCLC (primarily in nonsquamous subtypes) with no, scant, or distant use of tobacco products.

II. PATHOLOGY AND NATURAL HISTORY

Small specimens from fine needle aspiration (FNA), through bronchoscopy or transthoracic CT-guided biopsy, can make specific histologic classification of lung cancer difficult and may preclude molecular testing. A needle core biopsy or paraffin fixation of FNA material is preferable as these allow for better histologic analysis as well as immunohistochemistry and molecular analysis for the presence of targetable mutations.

A. **Small cell lung cancer** (SCLC; 15% of all lung cancers)

1. **Location.** More often central or hilar (95%) than peripheral (5%)

2. **Clinical course.** Patients with SCLC often have widespread disease at the time of diagnosis. Rapid clinical deterioration in patients with chest masses often indicates SCLC.

   a. **Hematogenous metastases** commonly involve the brain, bone marrow, or liver. Pleural effusions are common.

   b. **Relapse** after radiation therapy (RT) or chemotherapy occurs in the sites initially affected as well as in previously uninvolved sites.

3. **Associated paraneoplastic syndromes** include the syndrome of inappropriate antidiuretic hormone (SIADH; most common), hypercoagulable state (common), ectopic adrenocorticotropic hormone (ACTH) syndrome (uncommon), and Eaton-Lambert (myasthenic) syndrome (rarely seen with any other tumor). Hypercalcemia occurs rarely in SCLC, even in the presence of extensive bony metastases.

B. **Non–small cell lung cancer** (NSCLC; 85% of all lung cancers)

1. **Squamous cell carcinoma** (20% to 25% of NSCLC)

   a. **Location.** Previously, adenocarcinomas were thought to occur in a predominantly peripheral location, whereas squamous cell cancers occurred centrally. Studies indicate a changing radiographic presentation, with the two cell types now having similar patterns of location.

   b. **Clinical course.** Compared with other kinds of lung cancers, squamous cell lung cancers are most likely to remain localized early in the disease and to recur locally after either surgery or RT.

   c. **Associated paraneoplastic syndromes.** Hypercalcemia resulting from ectopic production of parathyroid hormone–related peptide (PTH-RP) is the more frequent syndrome. Hypertrophic osteoarthropathy (occasional), paraneoplastic neutrophilia (sometimes associated with hypercalcemia), prominent joint symptoms (occasional), or hypercoagulability is also seen.

2. **Adenocarcinoma** (50% to 60% of NSCLC). Adenocarcinoma is the most common cell type occurring in nonsmokers, especially young women. Most cases, however, are smoking associated.

   a. **Location.** These tumors present as peripheral nodules more commonly than squamous cell carcinoma.

   b. **Clinical course.** More than half of patients with adenocarcinoma, apparently localized as a peripheral nodule, have regional nodal metastases. Adenocarcinomas and large cell carcinomas have similar natural histories and spread widely outside the thorax by hematogenous dissemination, commonly involving the bones, liver, and brain.

   c. **Associated paraneoplastic syndromes** include hypertrophic osteoarthropathy, hypercoagulable state, hypercalcemia due to PTH-RP or cytokines, and gynecomastia (large cell).

3. **Large cell and "not otherwise specified" lung cancer.** The remainder of NSCLC consists of large cell and other histologies. Large cell NSCLC with neuroendocrine features is increasingly diagnosed on the basis of immunohistochemical features of neuroendocrine differentiation (e.g., chromogranin, neuron-specific enolase).

C. **Uncommon tumors of the lung and pleura**

   1. **Bronchial carcinoids** may present with local symptoms from airway obstruction, ectopic ACTH production, or carcinoid syndrome (see Chapter 16).

   2. **Cystic adenoid carcinomas** ("cylindromas") are locally invasive cancers. Locoregional recurrence is most common, but they may also metastasize to other areas of the lung and to distant sites (see Chapter 20, Section V).

   3. **Carcinosarcomas** are large lesions that have a tendency to remain localized and are more often resectable than other lung malignancies.

   4. **Mesotheliomas** are caused by exposure to asbestos and occur primarily in the pleura, peritoneum, or tunica vaginalis or albuginea of the testis. A history of asbestos exposure of any duration at any time is *prima facie* evidence that it caused the mesothelioma.

      a. **Histopathology.** Mesotheliomas consist of several histologic variants: sarcomatous, epithelioid, and others that have the histologic appearance of adenocarcinoma. The latter type can be distinguished from other adenocarcinomas by the absence of mucin staining and the loss of hyaluronic acid staining after digestion by hyaluronidase.

      b. **Clinical course.** The diffuse (usual) form of mesothelioma spreads rapidly over the pleura and encases the lung. It may develop multifocally and invade the lung parenchyma. Distant metastases are not common and usually occur late in the course. If there is a sarcomatous pattern, liver, brain, and bone may be involved.

III. DIAGNOSIS AND FURTHER EVALUATION

The primary effort should be directed at establishing a histologic diagnosis because this will determine the need for, and type of, additional tests as well as therapeutic options.

If NSCLC is diagnosed, the subsequent staging evaluation is directed to determine which modalities of therapy (surgery, radiotherapy, or chemotherapy) should be employed. In the past, surgery has been the mainstay of therapy for NSCLC and remains the primary mode in early-stage (I and II) disease. Therefore, the initial evaluation determines whether the tumor is potentially **resectable** (the tumor can be surgically removed with clear margins) and **operable** (the patient is physiologically capable of withstanding such a procedure).

The fundamental question must also be asked: What are the long-term results for surgical resection of any given stage of NSCLC? If surgery is not warranted, then the next question is whether the patient is a potential candidate for nonsurgical management with curative intent (i.e., chemoradiotherapy).

If SCLC is diagnosed, the evaluation is directed at determining whether the patient has limited- or extensive-stage disease because stage dictates prognosis and the appropriate therapeutic approach. Generally, the therapeutic approach to SCLC involves chemotherapy with or without radiotherapy. Only occasionally does surgery play a role in this disease.

A. **Symptoms and signs**

1. **Symptoms.** The majority of patients present with symptomatic disease. Symptoms may be referable to the primary disease in the chest (new or changing cough, hoarseness, hemoptysis, chest pain, dyspnea, pneumonia), metastatic disease (new nodal masses, bone pain, pathologic fracture, headache, seizure), or paraneoplastic manifestations (anorexia, weight loss, nausea due to hypercalcemia, etc.). Patients may also be completely asymptomatic and present as a consequence of an incidental finding on a radiographic study obtained for another reason.

   a. Patients with cancers located in the lung apices or superior sulcus (Pancoast tumor) may have paresthesias and weakness of the arm and hand as well as Horner syndrome (ptosis, miosis, and anhidrosis) caused by involvement of the cervical sympathetic nerves.

   b. Evidence of metastatic disease includes bone pain; neurologic changes; jaundice, bowel, and abdominal symptoms with a rapidly enlarging liver; subcutaneous masses; and regional lymphadenopathy.

2. **Physical findings.** In addition to local findings in the chest and lungs, physical examination should be directed at determining whether there is metastatic disease.

B. **Laboratory studies**

1. **Radiographs**

   a. **Chest radiograph.**

   b. **Computed tomography (CT) scan of the chest and abdomen** through the level of the adrenal glands. CT of the chest for the staging of lung cancer is clearly superior to chest radiographs and has been reported to have an overall accuracy of 70%. Mediastinal lymph nodes are generally considered abnormal when larger than 1.5 cm in diameter and normal when smaller than 1.0 cm. CT scanning provides information about the extent of invasion of the primary tumor, the presence of pleural effusion, and lymph node status.

      (1) **Adrenal masses.** Unsuspected adrenal metastases are common in NSCLC and alter management if the patient otherwise appears to have early-stage disease. It is sometimes possible to distinguish between metastatic disease and adrenal adenomas based on the density characteristics on CT or MRI. If the diagnosis is unclear and the adrenal is the only site of suspected metastases, biopsy is indicated.

      (2) **Other single areas that are suspect** for, but not diagnostic of, malignancy (i.e., liver, brain) warrant a similar approach (see also Section VII.B).

C. **Obtaining pathologic proof of lung cancer.**

1. **Sputum cytology** has been largely replaced by the flexible fiberoptic bronchoscope. Even in the best series, repeated sputum cytology is positive in only 60% to 80% of centrally located NSCLC and 15% to 20% of peripheral NSCLC.

2. **Flexible fiberoptic bronchoscopy** if symptomatic or radiologic evidence indicates a central and accessible cancer or nodal disease. Most cancers can be directly visualized. Additional tumors are evident only as extrinsic bronchial narrowing, which may be diagnosed through the bronchoscope by transbronchial biopsy. Bronchoscopy is unnecessary if histologic or cytologic diagnosis of metastatic lung cancer has already been made. **Endoscopic bronchial ultrasound (EBUS)** and GPS-guided bronchoscopy significantly improves the ability of bronchoscopy to sample mediastinal lymph nodes and evaluate more distal lesions, in many cases replacing more invasive procedures such as mediastinoscopy.

3. **Suspicious cutaneous nodules** may undergo biopsy to establish a histologic diagnosis and for staging.

4. **Lymph nodes.** Enlarged, hard, peripheral lymph nodes represent another potential site for biopsy.

D. **Subsequent evaluation.** After the histologic diagnosis of lung cancer, the evaluation should focus on determining whether disease is confined to the chest and may therefore be treated with curative intent (limited-stage SCLC and stages I to III NSCLC) or whether the patient has distant disease.

1. **Positron emission tomography** (PET). Although PET scanning has demonstrated superiority to CT scanning and is complementary to mediastinoscopy in the evaluation of mediastinal nodes, it is most useful in excluding distant occult metastases. PET may also be useful in restaging after a preoperative therapy (i.e., chemotherapy or chemoradiotherapy) or in follow-up. PET–CT scanners are now in common use and further improve the ability to accurately stage patients.

2. **Spinal MRI** for patients who have suspected epidural metastases in the spinal canal or suspected lung cancer with back pain or brachial plexopathy.

3. **Brain CT or MRI** should be obtained as part of routine staging for patients with SCLC, which is associated with a 10% incidence of neurologically asymptomatic brain metastases. These studies are not recommended for staging most patients with small stage I NSCLC in the absence of clinical signs. All patients with more advanced NSCLC and all who are symptomatic should undergo a brain scan.

4. **Mediastinoscopy** is useful in the following circumstances:

   a. For *routine* preoperative staging of NSCLC (radiologic assessment alone of the mediastinum is inadequate).

   b. In patients with mediastinal masses, negative sputum cytology, and negative bronchoscopy.

   c. To evaluate mediastinal lymphadenopathy. Hyperplastic nodes related to postobstructive infection are common. Mediastinoscopy may permit the patient to be considered for curative resection if enlarged nodes on CT scan are demonstrated to be pathologically negative.

   d. Restaging after preoperative chemotherapy or chemoradiotherapy in patients with stage III NSCLC based on pathologic documentation of N2 positive lymph nodes.

5. **Percutaneous and transbronchial needle biopsy** are frequently used to diagnose lung cancer. Some argue that if NSCLC is found by these techniques and medical resectability is assumed, mediastinoscopy or thoracotomy inevitably follows in the absence of evidence of metastatic disease, and therefore, the procedure is unnecessary. Furthermore, if cancer is suspected and the needle biopsy reveals a granuloma, the cancer may have been missed. If the diagnosis is SCLC, however, thoracotomy may be avoided.

Additionally, medically inoperable patients with negative bronchoscopy still require a tissue diagnosis.

6. **Bone scans** have largely been supplanted by PET. However, the bone scan offers complementary information regarding bone disease to PET and is substantially less expensive. There may be value for obtaining a bone scan in a patient with known metastatic disease in whom new bone involvement is suspected.

E. **Evaluation of the solitary pulmonary nodule** requires a diagnostic strategy that maximizes the chance of detecting cancer and minimizes the chance of performing a needless thoracotomy if the nodule is benign. *The diagnostic approach must be individualized.* Facts that should be considered include the following:

1. **Characteristics that define a solitary pulmonary nodule** are as follows:
   a. *A peripheral lung mass* measuring <6 cm in diameter.
   b. The nodule is asymptomatic.
   c. Physical examination is normal.
   d. CBC and LFTs are normal.

2. **Calcification** of the nodules has little bearing on the diagnostic approach. Calcified nodules are more likely to be malignant unless the pattern is circular, crescentic, or completely and densely calcified.

3. **Risk that a solitary pulmonary nodule is malignant.**
   a. **According to age**
      (1) Younger than 35 years of age: <2%
      (2) 35 to 45 years of age: 15%
      (3) Older than 45 years of age: 30% to 50%
   b. **According to tumor volume doubling time** (DT).
      (1) DT of 30 days or less: <1%
      (2) DT of 30 to 400 days: 30% to 50%
      (3) DT of >400 days: <1%
   c. **According to smoking history.** The risk of a solitary nodule being cancerous in a smoker compared with a nonsmoker is not known. The incidence is generally higher for smokers in the older age group.

4. **Needle biopsies** of solitary nodules are falsely negative in 15% of cases. In a patient with a high likelihood of cancer (e.g., a smoker who is older than 40 years of age), who is also a good surgical candidate, proceeding directly to thoracotomy without a tissue diagnosis is reasonable.

5. **FDG–PET scanning** has demonstrated considerable value in the diagnostic evaluation of the solitary pulmonary nodules, with sensitivity and specificity exceeding all other diagnostic modalities short of thoracotomy. However, if there is a high probability of malignancy, functional imaging is not necessary as a diagnostic procedure (though it may be needed for staging). A nodule with a high likelihood of malignancy should be biopsied or resected.

IV. STAGING SYSTEM AND PROGNOSTIC FACTORS

A. **Staging system:** Refer to the AJCC Cancer Staging Manual. Though there are four stages of disease, it is conceptually useful to think of disease as localized (stage Ia, b, IIa, b), characterized by tumors that do not involve major structures and lymph nodes (if present) that are peribronchial or hilar; locally advanced (IIIa, b), characterized by tumors that involve major structures and/or involvement of ipsilateral or contralateral mediastinal or supraclavicular lymph nodes); or advanced (stage IV) disease, characterized by distant metastases (including pleural or pericardial effusions).

B. **Performance status** (PS) has direct bearing on patient survival and should be accounted for in studies evaluating treatment modalities for lung cancer. Criteria for assessment of functional PS are described on the inside of the back cover. Patients who feel well and have few symptoms of disease (PS of 0 to 1) survive longer than ill patients (PS of 2 or more) and are more likely to tolerate chemotherapy, independent of other prognostic factors. In general, patients with NSCLC not characterized by driver mutations are not considered suitable for chemotherapy if PS is ≥3. It is important to note that patients with severe symptomatology (i.e., PS 3 and 4) may have rapid benefit from molecularly targeted agents.

C. **Weight loss.** Involuntary weight loss of 5% or more is an independent and negative prognostic factor.

D. **Tumor histology.** Survival is not greatly influenced by cell type if PS and extent of disease are taken into account. Patients with SCLC, however, have debility and extensive disease more often than those with the other cell types.

E. **Molecular prognostic factors.** Suppressor oncogene alterations are common in NSCLC and are associated with a poor prognosis; mutated *p53* (17p) oncogene occurs in half of patients with NSCLC and in almost all patients with SCLC. The *k-ras* oncogene is the most frequently mutated gene in NSCLC (primarily adenocarcinoma). Since the mid-2000s, an increasing number of "driver mutations" have been identified that can be specifically targeted.

1. **EGFR mutations** appear to be associated with a better overall prognosis as well as to be predictive for benefit from anti-EGFR therapies, notably the tyrosine kinase inhibitors (TKIs) afatinib, erlotinib, gefitinib, and osimertinib. Numerous abnormalities that predict benefit to the EGFR TKIs ("sensitizing mutations") have been described between exons 18 and 21 of the gene. The most common are deletions in exon 19 and missense mutations in exon 21. Other mutations, most notably on exon 20 (e.g., T790M), predict for resistance to EGFR TKIs, except osimertinib that has been approved for treatment of patients with tumors harboring acquired T790M mutations.

2. **ALK fusion genes.** Patients with this abnormality are demographically similar to those with EGFR mutations (never/scant smokers, adenocarcinoma), with the exception of ethnicity. Crizotinib is highly active in this setting and approved for NSCLC with ALK translocation as defined by a fluorescence *in situ* hybridization (FISH) assay; however, immunohistochemistry or RT-PCR may define additional ALK-positive patients who benefit from crizotinib. Patients, whose disease progresses on crizotinib, may benefit from alectinib or ceritinib.

3. **ROS translocations.** Patients almost always have nonsquamous disease and are most frequently never, scant, or distant smokers. Crizotinib has been approved for treatment in this setting.

4. **Other mutations** include B-Raf, Trk, RET, and others.

V. PREVENTION AND EARLY DETECTION

A. **Prevention** is the best way to reduce the death rate from lung cancer. More than 90% of patients with lung cancer would not have developed the disease if they had not smoked. Every smoking patient should be advised of the enormous risks. Trials of vitamin A analog supplementation and beta-carotene have failed to demonstrate benefit. Epidemiologically, aspirin use in individuals who have quit smoking has been associated with reduced risk of developing lung cancer.

B. **Early detection** of lung cancer by screening high-risk populations with chest radiographs and sputum cytology has not been clearly demonstrated to improve survival rates. New antibody tests and fluorescent bronchoscopy are also under study.

The National Lung Screening Trial (NLST) accrued over 50,000 subjects considered to be at high risk for lung cancer on the basis of age and smoking history. This study compared 3 years of screening with CT versus CXR. The results, reported in late 2010, showed that spiral CT scans were associated with a 20% reduction in risk of death from lung cancer as well as reduction in all-cause mortality. However, false-positives occurred due to the prevalence of lung abnormalities in patients at risk for lung cancer. Because the value of a screening test is dependent on the prevalence of a disease in a population, the determination that smokers with minimal degrees of obstructive disease are at substantially higher risk for lung cancer may improve the sensitivity and specificity of screening tests.

VI. MANAGEMENT

A. **NSCLC.** See Figure 9-1. Surgery remains the mainstay of management in stage I and II disease. Stage III disease (characterized by mediastinal nodal disease or involvement of major structures) is frequently resectable but almost invariably relapses, resulting in the patient's death within 5 years (90% to 95%) when managed by surgery alone. Therefore, multimodality therapy is increasingly employed in this large subset (about 40,000 patients per year). Patients with only a single mediastinal nodal "station" positive for disease or with incidentally discovered stage III disease (i.e., patients who undergo surgery for stage I or II disease and who are found to have microscopic mediastinal nodal disease) fare substantially better than other stage III patients.

After histologic proof of NSCLC is obtained, resectability is determined by the extent of the tumor and operability according to the overall medical condition of the patient. About half of patients with NSCLC are potentially operable. About half of tumors in operable patients are resectable (25% of all patients), and about half of patients with resectable tumors survive 5 years (12% of all patients or 25% of operable patients).

1. **Determinants of resectability. Signs of unresectable NSCLC** are as follows:
    a. Distant metastases, including metastases to the opposite lung. If solitary adrenal, hepatic, or other masses are detected by scans, these areas should be evaluated by biopsy because there is a significant incidence of benign masses that masquerade as tumor (see also Section VII.B).
    b. Persistent pleural effusion with malignant cells. Cytologic examination of 50 to 100 mL of fluid is positive for malignant cells in about 65% of patients. Repeat thoracentesis may provide the diagnosis in most of the remaining patients. In the event of negative cytology and in the absence of other contraindications to surgery, thoracoscopy should be undertaken at the time of surgery. Pleural involvement with malignant cells would preclude surgery. Transudative and parapneumonic effusions that clear do not contraindicate surgery. Most exudative effusions in the absence of pneumonia are malignant, regardless of cytologic findings.
    c. Superior vena cava obstruction.
    d. Involvement of the following structures:
        (1) Supraclavicular or neck lymph nodes (proved histologically)
        (2) Contralateral mediastinal lymph nodes (proved histologically)
        (3) Recurrent laryngeal nerve
        (4) Tracheal wall
        (5) Mainstem bronchus <2 cm from the carina (resectable by sleeve resection technique)
2. **Determinants of operability**
    a. **Age and mental illness** *per se* are not factors in deciding operability. Elderly patients, arbitrarily defined as individuals >70 years of age,

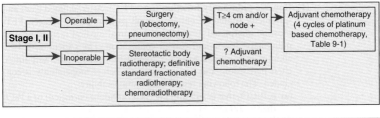

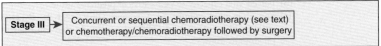

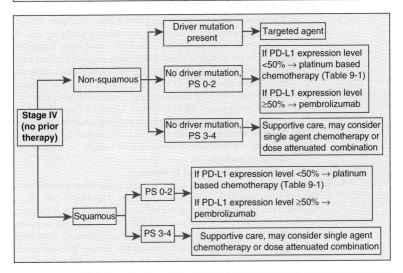

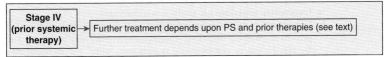

Figure 9-1 Algorithm of the Management of NSCLC.

experience the same degree of benefit from therapy as younger patients provided that they have adequate nutritional and PS.

b. Cardiac status. The presence of uncontrolled cardiac failure, uncontrolled arrhythmia, or a recent myocardial infarction (within 6 months) makes the patient inoperable.

c. Pulmonary status. The patient's ability to tolerate resection of part or all of a lung must be determined. The presence of pulmonary hypertension or inadequate pulmonary reserve makes the patient inoperable. *It is critical that any patient for whom surgery is contemplated stop smoking for at least several weeks before the operation.*

(1) **Routine pulmonary function tests** (PFTs). Arterial blood gases and spirometry should be obtained in all patients before surgery. PFTs must be interpreted in the light of optimal medical management of pulmonary disease and patient cooperation. The patient with PFT abnormalities should receive a trial of bronchodilators, antibiotics, chest percussion, and postural drainage before inoperability is concluded. The following results suggest inoperability:

(a) A $PaCO_2$ that is >45 mm Hg (that cannot be corrected) or a PaO_2 that is <60 mm Hg.

(b) Forced vital capacity (FVC) <40% of predicted value.

(c) Forced expired volume at 1 second (FEV_1) ≤1 L. Patients with an FEV_1 of >2 L or >60% of predicted value can tolerate pneumonectomy.

(2) **Special PFTs**

(a) **The quantitative perfusion lung scan** is done when patients with impaired pulmonary function are suspected of not being able to tolerate excision of lung tissue. The FEV_1 is measured before the scan. The percentage of blood flow to each lung is calculated from the results of the scan. The percentage of flow in the noncancerous lung is multiplied by the FEV_1, giving a measure of the anticipated postoperative FEV_1. Pneumonectomy is contraindicated if the calculated postoperative FEV_1 is 700 mL because the patient is likely to develop refractory cor pulmonale and respiratory insufficiency.

(b) **Exercise testing.** If maximal oxygen consumption is >20 mL/kg, perioperative morbidity is low; if it is <10 mL/kg, morbidity and mortality are high.

B. **NSCLC: Management of stage I and II disease**

1. **Surgery.** Surgical resection of the primary tumor is the treatment of choice for patients who can tolerate surgery and who have stage I or II NSCLC.

Definition of nodal involvement during surgical resection is mandatory to determine prognosis and to evaluate the results of treatment; the anatomic boundaries of 13 nodal stations have been described. Although considered technically resectable, most patients with stage IIIa disease (predominantly N2 disease) do poorly (see Section VI.C). An exception is the patient with malignant involvement of a single mediastinal nodal station.

a. **Incomplete resections** are rarely, if ever, indicated.

b. **Lobectomy** is the procedure of choice in patients whose lung function permits it. Sublobar resections (e.g., segmentectomy) may be appropriate for elderly and/or compromised populations, where the increased risk of local failure is balanced by the decreased physiologic impact of the procedure.

c. **Bilobectomy, sleeve lobectomy, or pneumonectomy** with or without lymph node dissection are used in other clinical presentations.

d. **Video-assisted thoracoscopic surgery** (VATS) is associated with results comparable to open procedures.

e. **Surgical mortality.** A multicenter study of contemporary operative mortality due to lung surgery documented the following death rates within 30 days of operation: pneumonectomy, 7.7%; lobectomy, 3.3%; and segmentectomy or wedge resection, 1.4%. Advanced age, weight loss, coexisting disease, reduced FEV_1, and more extensive resection are significant risk factors. Hospitals with higher surgical volumes tend to have lower surgical mortality.

2. **Pancoast tumor.** Historically, RT has been employed as the preliminary treatment for Pancoast tumors (T3 N0 M0, stage IIb) before surgical resection of the primary tumor and involved chest wall. Mature results from a national intergroup trial using preoperative chemotherapy and RT (chemoradiotherapy) in the treatment of this disease entity, however, demonstrated a median survival of 37 months and 5-year survival of 42%, far exceeding the historical approach of radiation followed by surgery. Given the relative rarity of this entity, the use of preoperative chemoradiotherapy can now be considered the standard of care.

3. **Adjuvant chemotherapy.** The majority of patients undergoing complete resections for NSCLC relapse and die within 3 years of resection. Platinum-based adjuvant chemotherapy has now been unequivocally established. The International Adjuvant Lung Trial (IALT) detected a 4% to 5% absolute benefit in long-term survival for patients treated with adjuvant platinum-based chemotherapy. Although this trial was characterized by heterogeneous chemotherapy regimens and premature closure, it was the largest trial ever performed studying this question. The results of this trial have now been confirmed by the North American Intergroup trial (JBR-10) and another European trial (ANITA). The latter two studies employed cisplatin/vinorelbine as the adjuvant regimen and demonstrated an approximately 10% absolute reduction in mortality. This level of benefit is comparable to the degree of benefit seen in breast and colon adjuvant studies. Routine use of adjuvant therapy with a cisplatin-based, two-drug regimen is now recommended for patients with resected stage IIa, IIb, and IIIa disease (Table 9-1).

The role of adjuvant chemotherapy in patients with resected stage Ib is controversial. Only one trial has specifically addressed this issue, and although it demonstrated improved disease-free survival, overall survival was not significantly improved. Retrospective analysis indicates that patients with tumors ≥4 cm may enjoy a benefit comparable to that of stage II and III patients, but this is not established. Adjuvant therapy should be discussed on an individual basis with patients with stage Ib disease characterized by tumors ≥4 cm. Preoperative chemotherapy in localized NSCLC is an alternative approach.

The role of "targeted agents" has been addressed with the anti–vascular endothelial growth factor (VEGF) antibody bevacizumab and with the EGFR TKI erlotinib. Randomized trials combining these agents with standard regimens did not demonstrate any advantage over standard therapy. Current studies are addressing this issue in patients with EGFR mutations or ALK translocations. Other studies are addressing the role of immunotherapy in the adjuvant setting.

TABLE 9-1	Second- and Subsequent-Line Chemotherapy Regimens for Advanced Non–Small Cell Lung Cancer		
Regimen	**Dose (mg/m²)**	**Days Given**	**Cycle Length (Days)**
Docetaxel	75	1	21
Docetaxel	75	1	
Ramucirumab	10 mg/kg	1	21
Pemetrexed	500	1	21

4. **Adjuvant RT** does not improve long-term survival in node negative or in N1 disease, but it is likely of benefit in patients with resected N2 disease.
5. **Resectable but inoperable.**
   a. **Definitive RT** should be the primary treatment for medically inoperable but resectable patients. The overall survival rate at 5 years is about 20%, depending on the size of the primary tumor and associated comorbidities. The sterilization rate for small tumors ranges from 25% to 50%.
   b. **Stereotactic body radiotherapy (SBRT)** has been recently demonstrated to provide a degree of local control comparable to surgical resection for small (<3 cm) tumors.
   c. **Chemoradiotherapy** may also be considered for these patients, particularly those with N1 disease, for whom the outcome is very poor with RT alone.

C. **NSCLC: Management of stages IIIa and IIIb**
   1. **Combined-modality therapy.** Multiple randomized clinical trials indicate a survival advantage with the use of chemoradiotherapy (vs. radiation alone) in this setting (with or without surgery); long-term survival of 20% to 30% of patients entered on study has been reported.
      a. Conceptually, there are two major approaches: "systemic full-dose chemotherapy" with concurrent radiotherapy and "radiosensitizing" chemotherapy concurrent with radiation and followed by consolidative chemotherapy. For the former approach, the most mature data utilize cisplatin/etoposide and concurrent radiation to 61 Gy. For the latter, the most commonly utilized approach combines weekly low doses of carboplatin (AUC 2) and paclitaxel (45 to 50 mg/m^2) concurrent with 61 Gy followed by full doses of carboplatin/paclitaxel. Unfortunately, there has not been and is unlikely to be a randomized trial comparing the regimens. Two recent analyses have demonstrated that the outcomes are similar in terms of median and overall survival with less toxicity for the low-dose carboplatin/paclitaxel regimen. Going forward, the approaches are best thought of as complementary in that for some new agents, it might be best to combine concurrently with the existing approach, which would favor the low-dose treatments while others may be best utilized sequentially as a single agent and would favor the "full-dose" approach.
      b. Most chemoradiotherapy trials entered patients with good PS, minimal weight loss, and little comorbid illness. The use of chemoradiotherapy is also appropriate, however, in many poor-risk patients, defined by weight loss and other medical problems.
      c. An emerging problem in stage III disease patients treated with combined-modality therapy is the occurrence of CNS metastases, which may be the sole site of relapse in 10% to 20% of patients. Despite a high risk of relapse in the brain, prophylactic cranial radiation is not recommended.
   2. **Preoperative "neoadjuvant" chemotherapy** (with or without RT) for patients with locally advanced disease may downstage the malignancy and make it resectable. Adjuvant surgical resection after chemoradiotherapy was compared with chemoradiotherapy alone in stage IIIa (N2). This study demonstrated that an increase in early mortality in the surgical group, primarily in patients undergoing pneumonectomy, offsets a possible long-term advantage from surgery. There was an unusually high rate of pneumonectomy on the trial. At this time, the role of surgical resection after chemoradiotherapy

remains to be established and should not be done outside of centers with substantial expertise in this approach.

3. **Technical aspects of RT** are important, both as a single modality and in combination with chemotherapy. Issues of dose, schedule, and fields are crucial. A randomized trial failed to demonstrate an advantage for twice-a-day fractions when combined with chemotherapy over standard chemoradiotherapy. Additionally, the use of three-dimensional conformal techniques may reduce or prevent toxicity to normal lung within the radiation field and allow dose escalation.

4. **Concurrent versus sequential treatment.** Several randomized controlled trials have demonstrated the superiority of concurrent chemoradiotherapy over sequential therapy.

5. **Specific management recommendations** should be individualized. In the absence of a clinical trial, patients with documented N2 or N3 disease should receive concurrent chemoradiotherapy. Patients with T4 N0 disease may be considered for induction chemotherapy with or without RT followed by surgery.

6. **Radiographic responses.** In all cases, patients treated with multimodality therapy may have variable radiographic responses. Except for those who demonstrate progressive disease (and consequently have a dire prognosis), there is no correlation between degree of radiographic response (complete response, partial response, or stable disease) and outcome. It is unclear that PET scanning improves the ability to assess these patients noninvasively.

D. **NSCLC: Management of stage IV disease**

1. **Overview.** Treatment of advanced NSCLC is in considerable flux. As recently as 2005, treatment could be easily divided into first-line, second-line, and subsequent therapies with no regard for histology or molecular variables. The emergence of histology, rapid molecular analysis and molecularly targeted agents, and, most recently, immunotherapy has greatly altered the landscape.

2. **Fully ambulatory patients** have increased survival, and symptoms are often palliated by the use of platinum-containing (cisplatin or carboplatin) chemotherapy. Regimens developed in the 1990s (carboplatin plus paclitaxel, cisplatin plus vinorelbine, cisplatin plus gemcitabine, cisplatin plus pemetrexed) have resulted in median survivals of 9 to 10 months and 1-year survival rates of 30% to 40% in large multicenter randomized trials. Economic analysis has demonstrated that it is more cost-effective to treat patients with chemotherapy because of the reduced need for hospitalization, RT, and other interventions.

Pemetrexed-platinum regimens, while highly active, have been *restricted to nonsquamous cell histologies* of NSCLC due to the results of a prospective randomized phase III trial and retrospective review of other pemetrexed studies in NSCLC. These results may relate to thymidylate synthase (TS), which is a molecular target of pemetrexed and generally higher in squamous cell cancers of the lung. In phase III trials of advanced NSCLC, cisplatin/pemetrexed demonstrated superiority over cisplatin/gemcitabine in nonsquamous histology cancers, while the gemcitabine regimen was more favorable in squamous histology cancers. In second-line therapy, pemetrexed was superior to docetaxel in nonsquamous histologies, as discussed below.

Bevacizumab, an antibody to the VEGF, has been demonstrated to result in superior survival in selected patients with advanced NSCLC. Bevacizumab is *contraindicated in squamous carcinoma* due to toxicity. Studies with bevacizumab have also excluded patients with bleeding disorders, significant cardiovascular or thrombotic disease, CNS metastases, or cavitary lesions. The approved dose is 15 mg/kg every 21 days. A European trial has reported that bevacizumab, in addition to cisplatin/gemcitabine, improved progression-free survival but not overall survival. The treatment with ramucirumab, an antibody to VEGF2, when combined with docetaxel in the second line, led to a modest improvement in overall survival (10.5 vs. 9.1 months).

A recent trial of an anti-EGFR antibody, necitumumab, in combination with first-line chemotherapy in advanced squamous cell carcinoma, demonstrated improved overall survival over chemotherapy alone. However, the relatively small degree of benefit and lack of a validated biomarker should be considered in determining which patients should receive this new therapy.

The major recent change in the treatment of NSCLC is the role of checkpoint immunotherapy, as described in detail below. Additionally, three agents are approved for use after progression with first-line chemotherapy. Pembrolizumab has obtained approval as first line therapy for patients with tumors demonstrating PD-L1 expression of >50% (approximately one third of patients).

3. **Patients who are less than fully ambulatory** (PS of ≥2) have poor outcomes, but they still do benefit from treatment with carboplatin-based two-drug therapy. However, management must be individualized, and options are ultimately dependent on the presence of comorbid disease and the patient's wishes.

   Patients with cancers containing activating mutations in the EGFR or ALK translocations (and others such as Ret, ROS, B-Raf, etc.) may have substantial, rapid, and sustained benefit from the specific targeted agent with almost any PS. Though this group represents only 10% to 15% of patients in the United States, it is critical that they be identified as rapidly as possible. Randomized trials in patients with EGFR-activating mutations or ALK translocations have demonstrated that the appropriate TKI (e.g., erlotinib with EGFR mutation) is superior to chemotherapy in terms of progression-free survival, though not overall survival. The current consensus is that a patient who has an identified activating mutation should receive the appropriate TKI as first-line therapy, though it is appropriate to hold these agents in reserve if a patient has begun on chemotherapy and is having an excellent response.

4. **Patients who have progressed after initial chemotherapy** may be treated with immunotherapy (anti–PD-1 agents) (Table 9-2) or chemotherapy. Two anti–PD-1 agents (nivolumab and pembrolizumab) and one anti-PD-L1 agent (atezolizumab) have been demonstrated to improve overall survival and response rate when compared to docetaxel. These drugs in general are well tolerated. However, it should be noted that they may produce severe and occasionally fatal immune-related adverse events (see Chapter 5). Considerable effort has been devoted to the evaluation of PD-L1 by immunohistochemistry as a predictive marker for the use of anti–PD-1

TABLE 9-2	Immunotherapy for NSCLC		
Anti–PD-1	**Dose**	**Schedule**	**Comments**
Nivolumab	240 mg	q14d	
Pembrolizumab	200 mg	q21d	For PD-L1–positive patients
Atezolizumab	1200 mg	q21d	

therapeutics. There are a number of tests employing different antibodies and different criteria for positivity under development. For pembrolizumab, PD-L1 positivity is a companion diagnostic required for the use of the agent.

Treatment with docetaxel (75 mg/m² IV over 1 hour q21d) can be considered in second-line therapy for those who may be unlikely to benefit from immunotherapy (known to have low PD-L1 expression) or as a third-line treatment after progression on a second-line immunotherapy. Pemetrexed (500 mg/m² q21d) was demonstrated to have similar efficacy to docetaxel (retrospectively for nonsquamous histology) with a favorable toxicity profile in a randomized phase III trial.

It is important to recognize that most of the benefit for second-line therapy with docetaxel or pemetrexed occurs in patients who had at least some benefit from initial chemotherapy. Individuals who progress rapidly on initial chemotherapy are unlikely to experience benefit from subsequent chemotherapy (in the absence of sensitizing mutations).

5. **Gefitinib, erlotinib, and afatinib** (Table 9-3). Recent evidence indicates that these agents are likely the preferred choice for first-line treatment in patients with EGFR mutations (deletions in exon 19 and missense in exon 21; see above), which occur in 10% to 15% of NSCLC patients in the United States. These patients tend to be those who are minimal (<15 pack-years), never, or distant smokers (quit > 20 years earlier). Some patients with reportedly wild-type EGFR may benefit, likely as a result of the presence of undetected rare mutations.

The use of an EGFR TKIs as first-line therapy based upon clinical factors (e.g., nonsmokers, female, Asian ancestry) without evidence of EGFR mutation is discouraged because in a randomized trial, patients with wild-type EGFR who received initial treatment with EGFR TKI experienced inferior progression-free survival compared with those treated with platinum-based chemotherapy. For patients in whom EGFR mutation is uncertain, initial use of platinum-based chemotherapy is preferred with a switch to an EGFR TKI when a sensitizing mutation is confirmed.

a. **The major toxicities** of this therapy are skin rash, diarrhea, and, rarely, interstitial pneumonitis. Interstitial pneumonitis is predominantly seen in Asians and may be fatal; the incidence is 1%. Cessation of drug, steroid

TABLE 9-3	**Molecularly Targeted Agents**		
Molecular Abnormality	**Agent(s)**	**Dose (mg) (All Agents Orally Administered)**	**Schedule**
EGFR-activating muta-tions (del19, L858r)	Gefitinib	250	Daily
	Erlotinib	150	Daily
	Afatinib	40	Daily
EGFR T790M	Osimertinib	80	Daily
ALK translocations	Crizotinib	250	b.i.d.
ALK translocations (second line, intolerant of crizotinib)	Alectinib	600	b.i.d.
	Ceritinib	750	Daily
ROS translocations	Crizotinib	250	Daily
B-Raf (V600E)	Vemurafenib[a]	960	b.i.d.
	Dabrafenib[a]	150	b.i.d.
Ret mutations	Vandetanib[a]	300	Daily

[a]Not FDA approved for this indication.

therapy, and hospitalization (as appropriate) should be undertaken in the patient with worsening dyspnea and radiographic changes consistent with interstitial pneumonitis. It is frequently difficult to distinguish pneumonitis from disease progression.

   b. Skin rash is a very common toxicity, and its occurrence may correlate with tumor response.

   (1) For mild rash (grade 1), use topical hydrocortisone 1% or 2.5% cream and/or clindamycin 1% gel b.i.d. to affected areas. Make sure to apply the topicals at least 1 hour apart. Continue the EGFR inhibitor at current dose, and monitor for change in severity. If after 2 weeks the reactions do not improve, then proceed to treatment for moderate rash.

   (2) For moderate rash (grades 2 or 3), use hydrocortisone 2.5% cream and/or clindamycin 1% gel or pimecrolimus 1% cream *plus* doxycycline 100 mg PO b.i.d. or minocycline 100 mg b.i.d. Continue the EGFR inhibitor at the current dose, and monitor for change in severity. If there is no improvement in 2 weeks and symptoms worsen, then treat as above with the addition of a methylprednisolone dose pack. If reaction continues to worsen, then dose interruption or discontinuation may be necessary.

   (3) For the patients who report pruritic, dry, erythematous eyes when the onset could be attributed to treatment with EGFR inhibitors, use prednisolone sodium phosphate ophthalmic (0.125%), 1 to 2 drops to the affected eyes b.i.d. to q.i.d. If condition increases in severity, it is recommended that the patient follow up with an ophthalmologist.

   c. Diarrhea should be managed with loperamide or diphenoxylate/atropine. If toxicities persist despite adequate management (i.e., >grade I), dose interruption followed by reductions is indicated.

6. **Osimertinib** is a third-generation TKI that targets a mutation (T790M), which results in resistance to other EGFR TKIs in 50% of patients. The drug should not be used unless this secondary mutation is identified (i.e., after rebiopsy or possibly the use of circulating DNA).

7. **Crizotinib** is effective in patients with ALK fusion genes and can result in rapid and sustained benefit in 65% of patients. **Ceritinib** and **alectinib** are actually more specific for the ALK translocations than crizotinib and may ultimately supplant that drug in the first-line setting.

8. **Duration of therapy.** The maximum benefit from any specific chemotherapy regimen is achieved in six cycles. Fewer cycles may be adequate. Two studies have demonstrated equivalent response and survival when three or four cycles of a platinum-based regimen were compared with more cycles of the same regimen.

   Maintenance treatment (i.e., continued treatment with either one of the same agents utilized for first-line treatment or with a different agent) is an area of considerable controversy. Two agents, pemetrexed and erlotinib, are FDA approved for this indication. Much, if not all, of the benefit may be a consequence of early initiation of appropriate second-line therapy. An alternative strategy to maintenance therapy is close follow-up with frequent staging and early institution of second-line treatment at the first indication of progressive disease.

9. **The choice of which platinum-based chemotherapy** regimen to use as first-line therapy can be based on several considerations. As noted

above, histology plays an increasing role in the decision as well as the presence or absence of EGFR, ALK, or other activating mutations. In addition to efficacy, the considerations include convenience of administration, cost, and toxicity profiles. Cisplatin-based regimens are less expensive and in one randomized trial demonstrated a survival advantage compared with a carboplatin-based treatment. However, these cisplatin regimens are less convenient and cause more nausea, vomiting, renal toxicity, and ototoxicity. Taxane-based regimens universally result in alopecia and may have significant cumulative neurotoxicity. Gemcitabine-platinum regimens are more myelotoxic but usually do not cause alopecia. Bevacizumab has been safely combined with carboplatin/paclitaxel and cisplatin/gemcitabine in large phase III studies. This issue can be summarized as a choice of regimens but no regimen of choice with the exception of cisplatin/pemetrexed for nonsquamous histologies. Table 9-4 provides details of the most commonly utilized regimens for advanced NSCLC.

10. **The evolving landscape of therapy in lung cancer.** There has been an explosion in knowledge of the biology of lung cancer and in particular in the number and types of therapeutics available. Immunotherapy is now validated as an approach, with unquestionable benefit as single agents in advanced disease. Current trials are exploring the use of immunotherapy as initial treatment of NSCLC, as well as SCLC. The use of next-generation sequencing approaches as well as the increasing ease of obtaining biopsies after progression of disease or obtaining circulating DNA has improved the understanding of mechanisms of disease resistance that occurs with TKIs and has resulted in the development and approval of drugs to overcome resistance. Single arm studies designed with the understanding of the mutational

TABLE 9-4	First-Line Chemotherapy Regimens for Advanced Non–Small Cell Lung Cancer		
Regimen	**Dose (mg/m²)**[a]	**Days Given**	**Cycle Length (Days)**
Cisplatin	100	1	28
Vinorelbine	25	1, 8, 15	
Carboplatin	AUC = 6	1	21
Paclitaxel	225 (over 3 hr)	1	
Carboplatin	AUC = 5.5	1	21
Gemcitabine	1,000	1, 8	
Cisplatin	75	1	21
Gemcitabine	1,250	1, 8	
Necitumumab	800 mg (flat dose)	1	
Cisplatin	75	1	21
Docetaxel	75	1	
Carboplatin	AUC = 6	1	21
Paclitaxel	200	1	
Bevacizumab[b]	15 mg/kg	1	
Cisplatin	75	1	21
Pemetrexed[b]	500	1	
Carboplatin	AUC = 6	1	21
Pemetrexed[b]	500	1	

[a]AUC, area under the curve.
[b]Restricted to nonsquamous histology.

profile have accurately reflected the activity of molecularly targeted therapies and have been the basis for regulatory approval.

E. **Small cell lung carcinoma: Management**

1. **Limited stage (I, II, III)** is confined to one hemithorax, including contralateral supraclavicular adenopathy. Less than 5% of patients with SCLC have stage I or II disease. About one-third, however, has disease that is clinically confined to the hemithorax and draining regional nodes at presentation (stages IIIa and IIIb).

   a. **Combined-modality therapy.** The available data indicate that these patients should receive concurrent chemotherapy and thoracic RT. Sequential chemotherapy followed by RT results in inferior long-term survival and should be discouraged. At this time, the most accepted chemotherapy regimen is cisplatin and etoposide (Table 9-5). RT given twice daily (hyperfractionated) has been demonstrated to be superior to once-daily therapy (4,500 cGy). If given concurrently as induction, combined-modality therapy yields a median survival of 23 months and a 5-year survival rate of 25%.

   b. **Prophylactic cranial irradiation** (PCI) decreases the rate of brain metastases. The use of PCI is controversial because the occurrence of synchronous metastases has made it difficult to demonstrate a survival advantage. The best evidence is that the use of PCI results in about a 5% improvement in survival in patients who responded to the initial chemotherapy.

2. **Extensive stage (ESCLC).** Some effective chemotherapy regimens for ESCLC are shown in Table 9-5. Fully ambulatory patients with ESCLC have good responses to cisplatin and etoposide (PE regimen) or the combination of cyclophosphamide, doxorubicin, and vincristine. Only 15% to 20% of such patients achieve complete response. The median survival of fully ambulatory patients is about 1 year, and the 2-year survival rate is 20%. Survival for 5 years, however, is unusual.

   a. A randomized trial from Japan comparing cisplatin/irinotecan with PE demonstrated superior survival for cisplatin/irinotecan. However, a similar study from the United States failed to demonstrate an advantage for either regimen. Either PE or cisplatin/irinotecan can be considered an

TABLE 9-5	Regimens for Small Cell Lung Cancer		
Regimen	**Dose (mg/m^2)**	**Days Given**	**Cycle Length (Days)**
Cisplatin	60	1	21
Etoposide	120	1, 2, 3	
Chest RT	1.5 Gy (45 Gy total)	Twice daily	For 5 wk
PCI	2.5 Gy (25 Gy total)	Daily	For 3 wk (after completion of other therapy)[a]
Cisplatin	100	1	21
Etoposide	100	1, 2, 3	
Cisplatin	60	1	28
Irinotecan	60	1, 8, 15	
Topotecan (IV)	1.5	1, 2, 3, 4, 5	21
Topotecan (oral)	2.3	1, 2, 3, 4, 5	21

[a]PCI (prophylactic cranial irradiation) is indicated in patients with limited disease who have obtained a good partial response or a complete response after the completion of other therapy. Chest RT and PCI are administered Monday to Friday.

acceptable regimen for the treatment of ESCLC. In elderly or compromised patients, carboplatin is frequently substituted for cisplatin.

b. Topotecan has demonstrated activity as second-line therapy for SCLC. Other agents (paclitaxel, gemcitabine, vinorelbine, and docetaxel) also have activity in ESCLC.

c. Patients with SCLC who are less than fully ambulatory may still be appropriate candidates for chemotherapy. Patients who respond may have significant improvement in PS.

d. PCI has been demonstrated to reduce the risk of CNS metastases and improve event-free and overall survival in patients with ESCLC who have had any degree of response (including stable disease) to initial chemotherapy. However, this trial did not require radiographic assessment of the brain prior to treatment and may simply represent the benefits of therapy for asymptomatic CNS disease after initial systemic therapy.

VII. SPECIAL CLINICAL PROBLEMS

A. Positive sputum cytology with a negative chest radiograph (TX N0 M0) and no other evidence of disease is an occasional problem, usually occurring in screening programs. Patients should be examined by CT scan of the chest and fiberoptic bronchoscopy with selective washings.

1. When these measures fail to identify a lesion, patients must be informed that the likelihood that they have a cancer too small to be detected is significant. Such patients should be followed with monthly chest radiographs and should be strongly advised to stop smoking.

2. The cytologic discovery of an unequivocal small cell cancer in the absence of other findings should be confirmed by repeat sampling and solicitation of a second pathologist's opinion at another institution. After the diagnosis is confirmed, patients should be treated as described previously.

B. Solitary brain metastasis. Patients with NSCLC who present with a single site of metastatic disease, most commonly in the brain, can be treated with curative intent. There are two situations in which this occurs: patients who have received definitive therapy and relapse with a single CNS metastasis (and no other disease) and those who at initial presentation have chest disease and the CNS as the sole site of metastasis.

For the relapsed patient, resection of the CNS metastasis may lead to long-term survival. For patients with synchronous disease, resection of the primary chest tumor and resection or the use of radiosurgery for the CNS disease are appropriate. If the patient has otherwise locally advanced disease (stage IIIa or IIIb), one could consider resection of the CNS disease followed by chemoradiotherapy with or without surgery for the chest disease in selected patients.

C. Oligoprogression. There have probably always been a small fraction of patients who initially present with advanced disease who achieve an excellent response and then progress in one or two areas that are amenable to local therapy. However, this phenomenon has become more common in the past few years, particularly in the context of "targeted therapies" such as the EGFR and ALK TKIs. These patients can frequently be managed by employing a local modality to eradicate the area of progression (e.g., surgery, stereotactic radiotherapy) and continuation of the systemic treatment.

VIII. FOLLOW-UP

A. After primary therapy with curative intent (**i.e., surgery or definitive radiotherapy/chemoradiotherapy**). Although most cases of SCLC and NSCLC recur, there is little evidence that frequent laboratory or radiologic studies detect disease before the development of symptoms or that early detection improves outcome. We recommend history and physical examination every 2 to 3 months and chest CT twice yearly for the first few years after resection. The follow-up visit is an excellent opportunity to reinforce the importance of smoking cessation in individuals who continue to abuse tobacco.

B. Radiologic abnormalities. Patients who undergo chemoradiotherapy frequently demonstrate scarring and infiltrates on radiologic studies, which may evolve with time. These abnormalities are frequently misinterpreted as progressive disease. PET–CT is of limited utility in the follow-up of patients treated with chemoradiotherapy. While higher standard uptake values in imaged areas are associated with worse outcomes, no specific cutoff has been identified.

C. Patients undergoing therapy for metastatic disease should have periodic reassessments of the known sites of disease. Progression of disease (>20% increase in the sum of unidimensional measurements of indicator lesions or the appearance of new disease) or deteriorating PS is a reason to stop therapy and consider second- or third-line treatment. Occasional patients progress in only one or two areas after an excellent response elsewhere and should be managed as described above under "oligoprogression." The benefits of second and subsequent lines of therapy are primarily confined to patients who maintain reasonable PS (ECOG ≤ 2). These patients should be offered additional treatment after appropriate discussion. For more compromised patients, the use of chemotherapy is frequently associated with toxicity and relatively little benefit. An exception is those patients with mutations that predict for benefit from molecularly targeted agents.

Suggested Readings

Aberle DR, DeMello S, Berg CD, et al. Results of the two incidence screenings in the National Lung Screening Trial. *N Engl J Med* 2013;369(10):920.

Albain KS, Crowley JJ, LeBlanc M, et al. Determinants of improved outcome in small-cell lung cancer: an analysis of the 2,580-patient Southwest Oncology Group Data Base. *J Clin Oncol* 1990;8:1563.

Albain KS, Swann RS, Rusch VW, et al. Radiotherapy plus chemotherapy with or without surgical resection for stage III non-small-cell lung cancer: a phase III randomised controlled trial. *Lancet* 2009;374(9687):379.

Auperin A, Arriagada R, Pignon JP, et al. Prophylactic cranial irradiation for patients with small cell lung cancer in complete remission. *N Engl J Med* 1999;341:476.

Borghaei H, Paz-Ares L, Horn L, et al. Nivolumab versus docetaxel in advanced nonsquamous non–small-cell lung cancer. *N Engl J Med* 2015;373:1627–1639.

Bradley JD, Paulus R, Komaki R, et al. Standard-dose versus high-dose conformal radiotherapy with concurrent and consolidation carboplatin plus paclitaxel with or without cetuximab for patients with stage IIIA or IIIB non-small-cell lung cancer (RTOG 0617): a randomised, two-by-two factorial phase 3 study. *Lancet Oncol* 2015;16(2):187.

Ciuleanu T, Brodowicz T, Zielinski C, et al. Maintenance pemetrexed plus best supportive care versus placebo plus best supportive care for non-small-cell lung cancer: a randomised, double-blind, phase 3 study. *Lancet* 2009;374(9699):1432.

Fossella FV, DeVore R, Kerr RN, et al. Randomized phase III trial of docetaxel versus vinorelbine or ifosfamide in patients with advanced non-small cell lung cancer previously treated with platinum containing regimens. *J Clin Oncol* 2000;18:2354.

Garon EB, Ciuleanu TE, Arrieta O. Ramucirumab plus docetaxel versus placebo plus docetaxel for second-line treatment of stage IV non-small-cell lung cancer after disease progression on platinum-based therapy (REVEL): a multicentre, double-blind, randomised phase 3 trial. *Lancet* 2014;384:665.

Gould MK, Donington J, Lynch WR, et al. Evaluation of individuals with pulmonary nodules: when is it lung cancer? Diagnosis and management of lung cancer, 3rd ed: American College of Chest Physicians evidence-based clinical practice guidelines. *Chest* 2013;143(5 Suppl):e93S.

Groome PA, Bolejack, V, Crowley JJ et al. The IASLC Lung Cancer Staging Project: validation of the proposals for revision of the T, N, and M descriptors and consequent stage groupings in the forthcoming (seventh) edition of the TNM classification of malignant tumours. *J Thorac Oncol* 2007;2:694.

Herbst RS, Baas P, Kim D-W, et al. Pembrolizumab versus docetaxel for previously treated, PD-L1-positive, advanced non–small-cell lung cancer (KEYNOTE-010): a randomised controlled trial. *Lancet* 2016;6736(15):1281.

Kelly K, Bunn PA Jr. Is it time to reevaluate our approach to the treatment of brain metastases in patients with non–small cell Lung Cancer? *Lung Cancer* 1998;20:85.

Kelly K, Crowley J, Bunn PA Jr. Randomized phase III trial of paclitaxel plus carboplatin versus vinorelbine plus cisplatin in the treatment of patients with advanced non–small-cell lung cancer: a Southwest Oncology Group trial. *J Clin Oncol* 2001;19:3210.

Kwak EL, Bang Y-J, Camidge DR, et al. Anaplastic lymphoma kinase inhibition in non–small-cell lung cancer. *N Engl J Med* 2010;363:1693.

Machtay M, Duan F, Siegel BA, et al. Prediction of survival by [18F]fluorodeoxyglucose positron emission tomography in patients with locally advanced non-small-cell lung cancer undergoing definitive chemoradiation therapy: results of the ACRIN 6668/RTOG 0235 trial. *J Clin Oncol* 2013;31(30):3823.

Maemondo M, Inoue A, Kobayashi K, et al. Gefitinib or chemotherapy for non–small-cell lung cancer with mutated EGFR. *N Engl J Med* 2010;362:2380.

Noda K, Nishiwaki Y, Kawahara M, et al. Irinotecan plus cisplatin compared with etoposide plus cisplatin for extensive small cell lung cancer. *N Engl J Med* 2002;346:85.

Paez JG, Janne PA, Lee JC, et al. EGFR mutations in lung cancer: correlation with clinical response to gefitinib therapy. *Science* 2004;304:1497.

Paul S, Mirza F, Port JL, et al. Survival of patients with clinical stage IIIA non-small cell lung cancer after induction therapy: age, mediastinal downstaging, and extent of pulmonary resection as independent predictors. *J Thorac Cardiovasc Surg* 2011;141(1):48.

Reck M, Rodríguez-Abreu D, Robinson AG, et al. Pembrolizumab versus chemotherapy for PD-L1-positive non-small-cell lung cancer. *N Engl J Med.* Published online, 2016 Oct 8.

Sandler A, Gray R, Perry MC, et al. Paclitaxel-carboplatin alone or with bevacizumab for non–small-cell lung cancer. *N Engl J Med* 2006;355:2542.

Santana-Davila R, Devisetty K, Szabo A, et al. Cisplatin and etoposide versus carboplatin and paclitaxel with concurrent radiotherapy for stage III non–small-cell lung cancer: an analysis of Veterans Health Administration data. *J Clin Oncol* 2015;33:567.

Scagliotti G, Brodowicz T, Shepherd FA, et al. Treatment-by-histology interaction analyses in three phase III trials show superiority of pemetrexed in nonsquamous non-small cell lung cancer. *J Thorac Oncol* 2011;6(1):64.

Schiller JH, Harrington D, Belani CP, et al. Comparison of four chemotherapy regimens for advanced non–small cell lung cancer. *N Engl J Med* 2002;346:92.

Slotman B, Faivre-Finn C, Kramer G, et al. EORTC Radiation Oncology Group and Lung Cancer Group. Prophylactic cranial irradiation in extensive small-cell lung cancer. *N Engl J Med.* 2007;357(7):664.

Soda M, Choi YL, Enomoto M, et al. Identification of the transforming EML4-ALK fusion gene in non-small-cell lung cancer. *Nature* 2007;448(7153):561.

Thatcher N, Hirsch FR, Luft AV. Necitumumab plus gemcitabine and cisplatin versus gemcitabine and cisplatin alone as first-line therapy in patients with stage IV squamous non-small-cell lung cancer (SQUIRE): an open-label, randomised, controlled phase 3 trial. *Lancet Oncol* 2015;16(7):763.

Turrisi AT, Turisi AT III, Kim K, et al. Twice-daily compared with once-daily thoracic radiotherapy in limited small-cell lung cancer treated concurrently with cisplatin and etoposide. *N Engl J Med* 1999;340:265.

Von Pawel J, Schiller JH, Shepherd FA, et al. Topotecan versus cyclophosphamide, doxorubicin, and vincristine for the treatment of recurrent small-cell lung cancer. *J Clin Oncol* 1999;17:658.

Walsh GL, O'Connor M, Willis KM, et al. Is follow-up of lung cancer patients after resection medically indicated and cost-effective? *Ann Thorac Surg* 1995;60:1563.

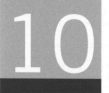

10 Gastrointestinal Tract Cancers

Pashtoon Murtaza Kasi and Axel Grothey

Cancers of the gastrointestinal (GI) tract account for about a fifth of all new visceral cancers and a quarter of cancer-related deaths in the United States. The noted improvements in survival for patients with metastatic GI cancers over the years are not the result of one particular drug or finding. It has been secondary to incremental benefits seen with the introductions of medical treatment options in the form of conventional chemotherapies and biologic agents. This is especially true for patients with metastatic colorectal cancer.

ESOPHAGEAL CANCER

I. EPIDEMIOLOGY AND ETIOLOGY

A. Epidemiology

1. Squamous cell esophageal cancer is the foremost malignancy in the Bantu of Africa. Some countries including South Africa, Japan, China, and the Caspian region of Iran also have relatively high incidence rates.
2. The incidence of adenocarcinoma of the esophagus (distal esophagus and gastroesophageal junction) is rapidly rising both in Western countries and in some parts of Asia due to lifestyle factors. Survival, however, from advanced esophageal cancer is still poor.

B. Etiology

1. **Carcinogens**
   a. Long-term use of tobacco and alcohol.
   b. *Human papillomavirus (HPV)* infection is associated with squamous cell carcinoma of the esophagus. *Helicobacter pylori* and adenocarcinomas of the esophagus have an inverse association.
   c. Other dietary carcinogens relevant to the development of squamous cell esophageal cancers include elevated nitrates in the drinking water and soup kettles that concentrate nitrate and food containing fungi: *Geotrichum candidum* (pickles, air-dried corn), *Fusarium* sp., and *Aspergillus* sp. (corn).

2. **Predisposing factors for squamous cell esophageal cancer**
   a. Howel-Evans syndrome or tylosis (hyperkeratosis of the palms and soles) is a rare genetic disease that is transmitted as a mendelian-dominant trait (nearly 40% develop esophageal cancer).
   b. Lye stricture (up to 30%).
   c. Esophageal achalasia (30%).
   d. Esophageal web (20%).
   e. Plummer-Vinson syndrome (iron deficiency anemia, dysphagia from an esophageal web, and glossitis, 10%).
   f. Short esophagus (5%).
   g. Peptic esophagitis (1%).

    h. Other conditions associated with squamous cell esophageal cancer
      (1) Patients with head and neck cancer ("field cancer effect")
      (2) Celiac disease
      (3) Chronic esophagitis without Barrett esophagus
      (4) Chronic thermal injury to the esophagus because of drinking boiling hot tea or coffee (Russia, China, and Middle East)

  3. Predisposing factors for adenocarcinoma of the esophagus
    a. Barrett esophagus is metaplastic replacement of squamous with intestinalized columnar epithelium. Adenocarcinomas associated with Barrett esophagus is on the rise worldwide, particularly in white men. In the United States, the incidence of adenocarcinoma of the esophagus has increased six- to sevenfold since 1970. Patients with Barrett esophagus have a 30- to 125-fold increased risk for esophageal adenocarcinoma compared with the average US population.
    b. Obesity.
    c. Reflux esophagitis.
    d. Advanced age.

II. PATHOLOGY AND NATURAL HISTORY

  A. Histology. While squamous cell tumors once constituted the majority of esophageal cancers, particularly in the upper and middle esophagus, adenocarcinomas are now the predominant form of esophageal cancer. Adenocarcinoma may arise from esophageal continuation of the gastric mucosa (Barrett esophagus) or may represent extension of a gastric adenocarcinoma.

  B. Location of cancer in the esophagus
    1. Cervical: 10%
    2. Upper thoracic: 40%
    3. Lower thoracic: 50%

  C. Clinical course. Esophageal cancer is highly lethal; >80% of affected patients die from the disease. About 75% present initially with advanced disease or distant metastasis. Death is usually caused by local disease that results in malnutrition or aspiration pneumonia.

III. DIAGNOSIS

  A. Symptoms and signs. Solid food followed by liquid food dysphagia is the most common complaint. Symptoms unfortunately only become apparent when the disease is advanced. Physical findings other than cachexia and palpable supraclavicular lymph nodes are rare.

  B. Diagnostic studies
    1. Preliminary studies include physical examination, CBC, LFT, chest radiograph, esophagoscopy, and barium esophagogram. Brushings can be obtained, and lesions can undergo biopsy using endoscopy.
    2. CT scan staging predicts invasion or metastases with an accuracy rate of >90% for the aorta, tracheobronchial tree, pericardium, liver, and adrenal glands; 85% for abdominal nodes; and 50% for paraesophageal nodes.
    3. Endoscopic ultrasound (EUS) is more accurate than CT in assessing tumor depth and allows for lymph node sampling.
    4. Positron emission tomography (PET) is a useful diagnostic tool and has a greater sensitivity for the detection of nodal metastases when compared with CT. It has now become part of diagnostic workup of patients with esophageal cancers.

5. **Laparoscopy** allows assessment of subdiaphragmatic, peritoneal, liver, and lymph node metastases. In patients who are getting chemotherapy and radiation, either preoperatively or in lieu of surgery, placement of a jejunostomy tube (and not gastrostomy tube if an esophagectomy with stomach pull-up is planned) for enteral alimentation during laparoscopy is clinically useful. Thoracoscopy can allow patients who are noted to have intrathoracic dissemination to be spared radical resections.

IV. STAGING SYSTEM AND PROGNOSTIC FACTORS

Refer to the current AJCC Cancer Staging atlas for TNM staging system. Stage groupings are different for squamous cell carcinomas and adenocarcinomas of the esophagus with regard to both TNM classification and histologic grades. Patients with earlier disease stage, particularly N0 and M0, have a better prognosis.

Prognosis of patients with esophageal cancer is poor. The 5-year survival rate ranges from approximately 35% with localized disease to <10% for distant disease.

V. SCREENING AND EARLY DETECTION

In high-risk populations, such as in portions of Asia, mass screening using balloon-assisted brushings or endoscopy has been used. Early detection by these methods is of uncertain benefit. In the United States, screening for esophageal cancer is not effective in the general population. However, patients who are higher risk, such as those with lye-induced strictures or Barrett esophagus, should undergo periodic screening via upper endoscopy as per guidelines.

VI. MANAGEMENT

A variety of options exist for the treatment of esophageal cancer depending on its stage.

A. **Resection of primary tumor.** Endoscopic mucosal resection (EMR) is a viable option for cancers confined to the mucosa. Results of surgical resection in cancer of the esophagus are poor. The operative mortality rate is about 5% to 10%. In the United States, the 5-year survival rate in patients undergoing R0 (complete) tumor resection is <20%. Aggressive surgery, however, may be justified, particularly for some patients with lesions in the lower half of the esophagus. For advanced and node-positive disease, a multimodality approach employing chemotherapy with radiation in the preoperative setting (trimodality therapy) is favored. Monitoring and maintaining nutritional status during therapy are important. Patients should be able to sustain an oral intake of at least 1,500 kcal/d; otherwise, a feeding tube should be considered.

B. **Palliating an obstructed esophagus** is an important issue and can be accomplished by several procedures and permits enteral nutrition. The most commonly employed approaches include:

1. **Esophageal stenting.** Multiple devices are available for esophageal intubation. About 15% of patients with malignant esophageal obstruction are candidates for tube placement and has a high success rate.

   a. **Advantages** of tube placement are improved ability to swallow saliva, pleasure of oral alimentation, relief from pulmonary aspiration related to esophagopulmonary fistula, independence from physician or hospital for constant care, and ability to spend time with family and friends in relative comfort.

   b. Contraindications to placement of endoprosthesis are carcinoma <2 cm below the upper sphincter, limited life expectancy (<6 weeks), and uncooperativeness.
   c. Complications include perforation, dislocation, tumor overgrowth, reflux symptoms with stricturing, pressure necrosis, foreign body impaction with obstruction, bleeding, and failure of intubation. The complication rate (early and late) is 10% to 25%. Restenting may be an option for some.
2. **External beam irradiation** or endoluminal brachytherapy can result in tumor regression with palliation in some cases. Up to 70% to 80% of patients with dysphagia may note improved swallowing after external beam irradiation. Endoluminal brachytherapy can be useful in previously irradiated patients with local tumor regrowth causing dysphagia.
3. **Feeding gastrostomy** is not advisable because it does not palliate dysphagia, which forces patients with complete or nearly complete esophageal obstruction to expectorate saliva and secretions, does not increase life expectancy, and has its own morbidity and mortality.

C. **Single-modality treatment**
1. **Radiotherapy (RT) alone** to a dose of 6,000 cGy resulted in 1-, 2-, 3-, and 5-year survival rates of 33%, 12%, 8%, and 7%, respectively, of patients treated on the radiation arm of a randomized trial in which responding patients were permitted to proceed to resection at physician discretion.
2. **Surgery alone.** The surgical procedures employed in esophagectomy depend on the location and preference of the surgeon and include principally transhiatal esophagectomy or the Ivor-Lewis procedure, which requires both thoracotomy and laparotomy. In the 25% to 30% of patients in whom complete resection is possible, 5-year survival rates are 15% to 20%.
3. **Chemotherapy alone** is seldom an effective palliative modality of the primary tumor in patients with esophageal cancer. When chemotherapy is employed, it should be coupled with mechanical or radiotherapeutic approaches for palliation of dysphagia. As in gastric cancer, discussed later, multiagent chemotherapy-induced responses tend to be short lived.

D. **Combined-modality therapy**
1. **Primary combined therapy without surgery.** "Definitive chemoradiation" (without surgery) is an option leading to long-term survival in some patients deemed as nonsurgical candidates. This approach is more attractive for esophageal cancers with squamous histology that are more sensitive to radiation therapy than adenocarcinomas and are more likely to be proximal tumors, which make surgical resection more challenging.
   a. Historically, the following regimen was most commonly used and is given during the first and fourth weeks of RT:
      Cisplatin, 75 mg/m^2 IV on day 1 of the cycle, and 5-fluorouracil (5-FU), 1,000 mg/m^2/d by continuous IV infusion for 4 days. Several other multiagent regimens have resulted in higher response rates (RRs) but have increased toxicity without a clear overall survival benefit.
      Today, a combination of weekly carboplatin (AUC2) and paclitaxel (50 mg/m^2) during radiation therapy has largely replaced the prior cisplatin-based approach with pathologic CR rates in squamous cell cancers and adenocarcinomas of 49% and 23%, respectively.
   b. In a prospective randomized trial of patients with squamous cell or adenocarcinoma of the thoracic esophagus, combined-modality treatment (5-FU plus cisplatin plus 5,000 cGy) resulted in improved median survival (9 vs. 12.5 months) when compared with RT alone

(6,400 cGy). The 2-year survival rate for patients randomized to combined chemotherapy and radiation was 38%, compared with 10% for those randomized to radiation alone. The patients receiving the combined-modality treatment experienced decreased local and distant recurrences but significantly more toxicity, much of which was serious or life threatening. Only half of these patients received all of the planned cycles of chemotherapy. Currently, this approach should be reserved for patients unable to undergo surgery and for selected patients with squamous cell cancers.

2. **Preoperative or postoperative RT alone** may reduce the local recurrence rate but has no apparent effect on median survival.

3. **Perioperative chemotherapy alone.** In general, neither preoperative (as reported in six randomized trials) nor postoperative chemotherapy alone has improved outcomes in patients with esophageal cancers. RR to multiagent neoadjuvant chemotherapy can be as high as 40% to 50%, and up to 25% of treated patients may have apparent pathologic complete remissions. Preoperative chemotherapy using cisplatin and 5-FU, however, did not improve overall survival when compared with surgery alone in a randomized trial of 440 patients with squamous esophageal cancer. The only exception is GEJ adenocarcinomas that were noted to derive benefit from perioperative chemotherapy employing epirubicin, cisplatin, and 5-FU (ECF).

4. **Triple-modality therapy.** The combination of preoperative chemotherapy and RT has led to an increase in the 3-year survival rates and prolonged median disease-free survival (DFS) in several randomized studies compared with surgery alone. While older trials have shown mixed results in regard to overall survival, more recent trials with predominantly adenocarcinoma patients have shown significant benefit to the use of neoadjuvant chemoradiotherapy followed by surgery compared to surgery alone. Current options for chemotherapy included (1) carboplatin and paclitaxel, (2) 5-FU and oxaliplatin, and (3) 5-FU and cisplatin. Based on outcomes and level of toxicity, carboplatin and paclitaxel appear to be the best option. Patients with complete pathologic response at surgery have about a 50% likelihood of long-term survival. The utility of biologics (anti–HER2-based therapy) in the preoperative setting is currently being explored in clinical trials.

E. **Advanced disease** (Fig. 10-1). The responses using single chemotherapeutic agents (15% to 20%) are usually partial and of brief duration (2 to 5 months). Combination chemotherapy, usually including cisplatin with 5-FU, a taxane, or both, is associated with reported RRs ranging from 15% to 80%, a median duration of response of 7 to 10 months, and many times with substantial toxicity. Higher RRs, however, do not necessarily translate into significant benefit for these patients, and the outcome remains poor. In most situations, the use of a doublet, rather than a triplet, chemotherapy combination will provide meaningful responses with acceptable levels of toxicity. For doublets, choices include FOLFOX, XELOX, and carboplatin and paclitaxel.

F. **Molecular markers and targeted therapies.** The most important predictive biomarker to consider in patients with metastatic esophageal adenocarcinomas is HER2. About 25% of adenocarcinomas have overexpression of this, allowing trastuzumab to be added to the chemotherapy. The so-called ToGA (trastuzumab for gastric cancer) trial, which included gastric and gastroesophageal junction (GEJ) tumors, showed improved overall survival of the addition of trastuzumab to platinum-based chemotherapy compared to chemotherapy alone in the metastatic setting (13.8 months vs. 11.1 months) in HER2-positive cancers. Guidelines have been revised on numerous occasions, and the current

	Classification Based on Molecular Testing and Performance Status			
Line of therapy	**Excellent Performance Status[a] and HER2-neu−**	**Excellent Performance Status and HER2-neu+**		**Poor Performance Status and/or Advanced age**
1	CT triplet[a] (EOX vs. ECF)	Fluoropyrimidine + cisplatin + trastuzumab[b]	CT triplet (EOX vs. ECF)	CT doublet vs. BSC
2	Ramucirumab ± paclitaxel	Ramucirumab ± paclitaxel	Fluoropyrimidine + cisplatin + trastuzumab	Ramucirumab ± paclitaxel vs. BSC
3	Doublet CT (FOLFOX vs. FOLFIRI)	Doublet CT (FOLFOX vs. FOLFIRI) + trastuzumab	Ramucirumab ± paclitaxel	
4	BSC	BSC		

[a] Usually excellent performance status refers to patients with an Eastern Cooperative Oncology Group (ECOG) of 0–1 and poor performance status as ECOG > 1. **Doublet CT are in General preferred over triplet CT regiments.**

[b] Trastuzumab should be added to the CT doublet in patients with tumors positive for HER2-neu expression based on standardized IHC and FISH criteria. Preferred doublet is fluoropyrimidine based with the addition of cisplatin every 3 weeks but can be potentially added to other CT combinations. Addition to anthracycline based regimens is avoided due to risk for cardiac toxicity.

Abbreviations: BSC, best supportive care; CT, chemotherapy, EOX: epirubicin, oxaliplatin, and capecitabine (Xeloda); ECF, epirubicin, cisplatin, and fluorouracil.

Figure 10-1 Treatment algorithm for the practical medical management of **metastatic gastric and gastroesophageal junction adenocarcinomas** based on molecular testing.

consensus is to follow the criteria laid out for patients with breast cancer utilizing immunohistochemistry (IHC) and fluorescence *in situ* hybridization (FISH) analyses. Baseline and periodic assessment of cardiac ejection fraction is an important consideration for patients receiving trastuzumab. Additionally, the anti–vascular endothelial growth factor receptor 2 (anti-*VEGFR2*) antibody, ramucirumab, has been approved for advanced gastroesophageal cancers after failure of first-line chemotherapy. Ramucirumab has a black box warning for increasing risk of hemorrhage and should be permanently discontinued in patients who experience severe bleeding. Proteinuria and hypertension need to be monitored as with all anti–VEGF-based therapies.

GASTRIC CANCER

I. EPIDEMIOLOGY AND ETIOLOGY

    A. Incidence. Currently, one-third of all gastric cancers arise in the proximal stomach, predominantly the cardia and gastroesophageal junction. The average age of onset is 55 years. Overall, the prevalence and death rates of distal gastric cancers have significantly decreased, while an increase in cardia and gastroesophageal tumors has been observed in the United States due to lifestyle changes. Factors conceivably responsible for the overall decline include reduction in toxic methods of food preservation (such as smoking and pickling), a decline in salt consumption, greater use of refrigeration, and increased consumption of fruits and vegetables.

Mortality from gastric cancer is highest in Costa Rica and East Asia (Hong Kong, Japan, and Singapore) and lowest in the United States. The incidence remains high in Japan and is intermediate in Japanese immigrants to the United States; first-generation Japanese Americans have an incidence comparable with other Americans.

B. Etiology. Two gastric cancer entities can be distinguished by their risk factors and histology. *Diffuse gastric cancer* is associated with hereditary factors and a proximal location and does not appear to occur in the setting of intestinal metaplasia or dysplasia. *Intestinal-type gastric cancer* is more distal, occurs in younger patients, is more frequently endemic, and is associated with inflammatory changes and with *H. pylori* infection.

1. **Diet.** Gastric cancer has been linked to the ingestion of red meats, cabbage, spices, fish, salt-preserved or smoked foods; a high-carbohydrate diet; and low consumption of fat, protein, and vitamins A, C, and E. Selenium dietary intake may be inversely proportional to the risk of gastric cancer but not to that of colorectal cancer.

2. ***H. pylori* infection** is associated with an increased risk for gastric adenocarcinoma and may be a cofactor in the pathogenesis of noncardiac gastric cancer. The *H. pylori* organism was identified in the malignant and nearby inflammatory tissue of 89% of patients with intestinal-type cancer, whereas it was present in 32% of tissues taken from patients with diffuse-type cancers. Eradicating *H. pylori* through antibiotics to prevent atrophic gastritis and intestinal-type gastric cancer is being studied in various populations. Treatment of asymptomatic individuals is debatable. Currently, therapy is reserved for patients with gastric ulcers or symptomatic GERD.

3. **Heredity and race.** African, Asian, and Hispanic Americans have a higher risk for gastric cancer than whites. The hereditary diffuse gastric cancer (HDGC) is often characterized by germline mutation of the E-cadherin gene (CDH-1); penetrance of which is in the autosomal-dominant fashion. Prophylactic total gastrectomy between ages 20 to 30 years is recommended in germline carriers of the mutation since given the high risk of development of gastric cancer.

4. **Pernicious anemia, achlorhydria, and atrophic gastritis.** Pernicious anemia carries an increased relative risk for gastric cancer that is said to be 3 to 18 times that of the general population, based on retrospective studies. Although some controversy surrounds this finding, follow-up endoscopy is generally suggested for patients known to have pernicious anemia.

5. **Previous gastric resection.** Gastric stump adenocarcinomas, which occur with a latency period of 15 to 20 years, are more common in patients after surgical treatment for benign peptic ulcer disease, particularly in those who have hypochlorhydria and reflux of alkaline bile. These cancers are associated with dysplasia of gastric mucosa, elevated gastrin levels, and a poor prognosis.

6. **Mucosal dysplasia** is graded from I to III, with grade III showing marked loss in cell differentiation and increased mitosis. The finding of high-grade dysplasia by experienced pathologists in two separate sets of endoscopic

biopsies is considered to be a marker for future gastric cancer. Intestinal metaplasia, replacement of gastric glandular epithelium with intestinal mucosa, is associated with intestinal-type gastric cancer. The risk for cancer appears to be proportional to the extent of metaplastic mucosa.

7. **Gastric polyps.** As many as half of adenomatous polyps show carcinomatous changes in some series. Hyperplastic polyps (>75% of all gastric polyps) do not appear to have malignant potential. Patients with familial adenomatous polyposis (FAP) have a higher incidence of gastric cancer. Patients with adenomatous polyps or FAP should have endoscopic surveillance.

8. **Chronic gastritis.** In chronic atrophic gastritis of the corpus or antrum, *H. pylori* infection and environmental and autoimmune (as in pernicious anemia) causes are thought to be associated with an increased risk for gastric cancer. In Ménétrier disease (hypertrophic gastritis), an increase in the incidence of gastric cancer is also observed.

9. **Other risk factors.** Gastric cancer is more common in men older than 50 years of age and in people with blood group A. Gastric cancer is consistently seen more commonly among those of lower socioeconomic class across the world.

II. PATHOLOGY AND NATURAL HISTORY

A. **Histology and classification.** About 95% of gastric cancers are adenocarcinomas; 5% are leiomyosarcomas, lymphomas, carcinoids, squamous cancers, or other rare types.

1. **Useful characteristics of gastric cancer**

   a. **Histologic classification (Lauren).** Diffuse (scattered solitary or small clusters of small cells in the submucosa), intestinal (polarized columnar large cells with inflammatory infiltrates localized in areas of atrophic gastritis or intestinal metaplasia), and mixed types. This classification has proved to be the most useful for adenocarcinomas because the two major types (diffuse and intestinal) represent groups of patients with differing ages, sex ratios, survival rates, epidemiology, and apparent origin. Studies have shown that diffuse histology affects younger patients, with slight predominance among women. Diffuse histology occurred in 50% of all cases and in 55% of unresectable cases. Intestinal-type predominates in high-risk regions of the world and among older people and affects more men than women.

   b. **Clinical classification (gross anatomy).** Superficial (superficial spreading), focal (polypoid, fungate, or ulcerative), and infiltrative (linitis plastica) types.

   c. **Japanese Endoscopic Society (JES) classification.** Type I (polypoid or mass-like), type II (flat, minimally elevated, or depressed), and type III (cancer associated with true ulcer).

2. **Location of cancers**

   a. Distal location: 40%

   b. Proximal: 35%

   c. Body: 25%

B. **Clinical course.** About 20% of gastric cancer patients are long-term survivors in the United States. Gastric carcinoma spreads by the lymphatic system and blood vessels, by direct extension, and by seeding of peritoneal surfaces. The ulcerative and polypoid types spread through the gastric wall and involve the serosa and draining lymph nodes. The scirrhous type spreads through the submucosa and muscularis, encasing the stomach, and in some instances spreads to the entire bowel. The physical examination is often normal.

Widespread metastatic disease may affect any organ, especially the liver (40%), lung (may be lymphangitic, 40%), peritoneum (10%), supraclavicular lymph nodes (Virchow node), left axillary lymph nodes (Irish node), and umbilicus (Sister Mary Joseph nodule). Sclerotic bone metastases, carcinomatous meningitis, and metastasis to the ovary in women (Krukenberg tumor) or rectal shelf in men (Blumer shelf) may also occur.

C. **Associated paraneoplastic syndromes**

1. Acanthosis nigricans (55% of cases that occur in malignancy are associated with gastric carcinoma)
2. Polymyositis, dermatomyositis
3. Circinate erythemas, pemphigoid
4. Dementia, cerebellar ataxia
5. Idiopathic venous thrombosis
6. Ectopic Cushing syndrome or carcinoid syndrome (rare)
7. Leser-Trélat sign (sudden eruption of multiple seborrheic keratoses)

III. DIAGNOSIS

A. **Symptoms and signs.** Similar to esophageal cancers, gastric cancer commonly presents in advance stages before symptoms or clinical signs develop. Symptoms of advanced disease include anorexia, early satiety, distaste for meat, weakness, and dysphagia. Abdominal pain is present in about 60% of patients, weight loss in 50%, nausea and vomiting in 40%, anemia in 40%, and a palpable abdominal mass in 30%. The abdominal pain is similar to ulcer pain, is gnawing in nature, and may respond initially to antacid treatment but remains unremitting. Hematemesis or melena occurs in 25% and, when present, is seen more often with gastric sarcomas.

B. **Diagnostic studies**

1. **Preliminary studies** include CBC, LFT, esophagogastroduodenoscopy (EGD) or upper GI barium studies, and chest radiographs.

2. **CT of the abdomen and pelvis** is useful for assessing the extent of disease. At laparotomy, however, half of patients are found to have more extensive disease than predicted by CT. Laparoscopy can identify patients with regionally advanced or peritoneal disseminated disease who are not candidates for immediate potentially curative surgical intervention.

3. **EUS** is up to six times more accurate in staging the primary gastric tumors than CT, but differentiation between benign and malignant changes in the wall is often difficult. EUS is useful in imaging the cardia, which may be difficult to evaluate by CT. This also allows for lymph node sampling.

4. **Endoscopy.** The combination of flexible upper GI endoscopy with biopsy of visible lesions, exfoliative cytology, and brush biopsy is able to detect >95% of gastric cancers. Biopsy of a stomach lesion alone is accurate in only 80% of cases. Positive gastric cytology with no endoscopic or radiographic abnormalities indicates superficial spreading gastric cancer.

5. **PET.** PET has more limited value in the diagnostic workup of patients compared to its use in esophageal cancer. It may help to identify malignant adenopathy not seen by CT. Its use in patients with gastroesophageal junction cancers appears to be more comparable to esophageal cancer.

C. **Differential diagnosis and gastric polyps.** The differential diagnosis of gastric cancer includes peptic gastric polyps, ulcer, leiomyoma, leiomyoblastoma, glomus tumor, malignant lymphoma (and pseudolymphoma), granulocytic sarcoma, carcinoid tumors, lipoma, fibrous histiocytoma, and metastatic carcinoma. Gastric polyps rarely undergo malignant transformation (3% after 7 years), but many contain independent carcinoma.

1. **Inflammatory gastric polyps** are not true neoplasms. They are usually located in the pyloric antrum and are associated with hypochlorhydria but not with carcinoma.
2. **Hyperplastic gastric polyps** (Ménétrier polyadenome polypeux) are the most common polyps (75%). Randomly distributed throughout the stomach, these polyps are usually small and multiple. Coexisting carcinoma is present in 8% of cases.
3. **Adenomatous polyps** are usually located in the antrum of the stomach and are frequently single and large. Coexisting carcinoma is present in 40% to 60% of patients.
4. **Villous adenomas** rarely occur in the stomach but are more often malignant.
5. **Polyposis syndromes**
   a. **Familial gastric polyposis** presents with multiple gastric polyps but no skin or bone tumors. The gastric wall is usually invaded with atypical carcinoma.
   b. **FAP** is associated with gastric involvement in more than half of patients. The gastric polyps are adenomatous, hyperplastic, or of the fundic gland hyperplasia type. Gastric carcinoma and carcinoid tumor may occur.

IV. STAGING AND PROGNOSTIC FACTORS

A. **Staging system.** Refer to the current AJCC Cancer Staging atlas for TNM staging system. The current TNM system does not take into account the location of the tumor within the stomach, the histologic type (Lauren classification), the pattern of growth (linitis plastica), or whether all disease could be resected (and if so, the type of resection).

B. **Prognostic factors.**
1. **Stage.** Multivariate analysis indicates that stage, invasion, and lymph node involvement are the most significant prognostic factors. The most important prognostic determinant appears to be the number of positive lymph nodes. Interestingly, patients with one to three lymph nodes involved with metastasis have as good a prognosis as those without nodal involvement.
2. **Clinical classification.** Survival is better with superficial than with focal cancer and worst with infiltrative types of cancer.
3. **JES classification.** Survival is better with type II (flat) than with type III (associated with ulcer) tumors and is worst with type I (polypoid) tumors.
4. **Grade.** Tumors with high histologic grade have a poor prognosis.
5. **Nature and extent of resection.** Survival is better with curative resection (a resection with uninvolved margins, or R0 resection) versus palliative resection, distal gastrectomy versus proximal gastrectomy, and subtotal gastrectomy versus total gastrectomy.

V. SCREENING AND EARLY DETECTION

Early detection of gastric cancers is clearly improved with relentless investigation of persistent upper GI symptoms. In Japan, mobile screening stations equipped with video gastrocameras have resulted in early detection of gastric cancer. Gastric cancer, which was detected in 0.3% of those screened, was associated with a 95% 5-year survival rate (50% of the patients had involvement of mucosa and submucosa only). Despite such screening programs, gastric cancer remains the most common cause of cancer death in Japan. Screening of populations with routine risk factors for gastric cancer is not recommended, however, in the United States.

VI. MANAGEMENT

A. Surgery

1. **Curative resection.** Subtotal gastrectomy with adequate margins of grossly uninvolved stomach (3 to 4 cm) and regional lymph node dissection is the treatment of choice and is generally considered the only potentially curative approach for patients with gastric cancer. Total gastrectomy is not superior to subtotal gastrectomy for achieving cures and should be used only when indicated by the local extent of the disease. A D2 lymph node dissection (removal of perigastric and celiac nodes) is considered standard of care. More extensive lymphatic dissection, known as D3 resections (e.g., of retroperitoneal lymph nodes), omentectomy, and splenectomy, are of uncertain benefit and do not appear to be advisable outside its use in Japan and specialized centers.

2. **Palliative resections** are performed to rid patients of infected, bleeding, obstructed, necrotic, or ulcerated polypoid gastric lesions. For these purposes, a limited gastric resection may suffice. Palliative resections succeed in ameliorating symptoms about half the time.

3. **Vitamin B_{12} deficiency** develops in all patients who undergo total gastrectomy within 6 years and in 20% of patients who undergo subtotal gastrectomy within 10 years unless parenteral B_{12} injections are administered.

B. Chemotherapy

1. **Neoadjuvant, adjuvant, or perioperative chemotherapy**
   a. **Neoadjuvant chemotherapy.** Patients with potentially resectable disease treated in phase II studies with preoperative chemotherapy, RT, or both have shown a high RR, and some have had pathologically negative resection specimens. There have not been any randomized trials published to help discern whether response translates into resectability, time to progression, or survival advantage over no neoadjuvant therapy.

   b. **Adjuvant chemotherapy with or without radiation.** Individual trials have shown mixed results in regard to the benefit of adjuvant chemotherapy over surgery alone. However, a recent meta-analysis showed that the use of adjuvant therapy with 5-FU–based regimens does reduce the risk of death related to gastric cancer compared to surgery alone. A combination of capecitabine plus oxaliplatin after gastrectomy with D2 lymph node dissection can be considered one standard of care in the adjuvant setting. Postoperative chemoradiation therapy (45 Gy) as a "sandwich" between 5-FU–based chemotherapies has shown to be superior to surgery alone; however, in this study, only a minority of patients underwent adequate lymph node resection, and the treatment effect was most pronounced in the reduction of the risk of local and not distant recurrence.

   c. **Perioperative chemotherapy.** In the Medical Research Council Adjuvant Gastric Infusional Chemotherapy (MAGIC) randomized phase III trial of perioperative ECF chemotherapy (epirubicin, cisplatin, and infusional 5-FU), with three cycles of preoperative and three cycles of postoperative therapy, a significant improvement was seen in overall survival compared with surgery alone. While this trial enrolled primarily patients with stomach cancer, similar benefit appeared to extend to those with adenocarcinoma of the gastroesophageal junction or lower esophagus. Cycles are given every 3 weeks as follows:

   Epirubicin 50 mg/m^2 IV on day 1
   Cisplatin 60 mg/m^2 IV on day 1
   5-FU 225 mg/m^2/d by continuous IV infusion on days 1 to 21

In a separate randomized phase III trial, perioperative chemotherapy with 5-FU and cisplatin provided similar results. In this trial, approximately two-thirds of patients had gastroesophageal junction cancers. In clinical practice, continuous infusion 5-FU is commonly replaced by capecitabine.

2. **Combined-modality therapy.** Several clinical trials for potentially resectable gastric cancer have assessed sequential chemotherapy and radiation. A previously completed intergroup trial (Intergroup 0116) involving nearly 600 patients undergoing potentially curative resection randomized patients to either observation alone or combined-modality therapy. Patients randomized to adjuvant therapy received one cycle of 5-FU and leucovorin followed by a combination of bolus 5-FU and RT. After the RT was completed, two additional cycles of 5-FU and leucovorin were given. Significant 3-year relapse-free and overall survivals were seen in the patients randomized to adjuvant therapy. The benefit of this approach appeared to be in a reduction of locoregional failures. Less benefit was seen with treatment in reducing distant failures.

3. **Chemotherapy for advanced disease** (Fig. 10-1). Single agents produce low RRs. Combination regimens produce higher RRs but are more toxic and more costly. Cisplatin has been increasingly used in new combinations that also yield higher RRs, but the incidence of important toxic events exceeds 10%. The reported RRs are about 20% for 5-FU alone and 10% to 50% for combination chemotherapy; the median survival times range from 5 to 11 months.

After nearly two decades of using combination chemotherapy, there is no regimen considered standard in the setting of advanced disease. It is of note that the value of anthracyclines in the management of advanced gastric cancer has recently been questioned and fluoropyrimidine–platinum combinations have emerged as standard of care.

   a. **ECF.** The chemotherapy regimen of epirubicin, cisplatin, and continuous infusion 5-FU (ECF) was shown to have superior activity over 5-FU, doxorubicin, and methotrexate (FAMtx) in a phase III trial. Dosages for ECF are shown in Section VI.B.1.c.

   b. **EOX.** A variation of ECF, EOX (epirubicin, oxaliplatin, and capecitabine) showed an improvement in overall survival and less toxicity compared with ECF. The dosage schedule for EOX is as follows; cycles are repeated every 3 weeks:

   Epirubicin, 50 mg/m^2 IV on day 1
   Oxaliplatin, 130 mg/m^2 IV on day 1
   Capecitabine, 625 mg/m^2/dose twice daily days 1 to 21

   c. **DCF.** The use of docetaxel has also been of benefit. As assessed in a trial comparing docetaxel, cisplatin (DCF), and 5-FU versus cisplatin and 5-FU (CF), the combination of DCF provided improved overall survival. However, both DCF and modified DCF may result in significant toxicity. Nearly 30% of patients receiving modified DCF were hospitalized. DCF is given in 3-week cycles as follows:

   (1) **DCF**
   Docetaxel 75 mg/m^2 IV on day 1
   Cisplatin 75 mg/m^2 IV on day 1
   5-FU 750 mg/m^2/d by continuous IV infusion on days 1 to 5

(2) **Modified DCF** using the following has shown comparable outcomes:
Docetaxel 40 mg/m² IV on day 1
Cisplatin 40 mg/m² IV on day 1
5-FU 400 mg/m²/d by continuous IV infusion on days 1 to 5

d. FOLFOX/XELOX. While triplets have generally shown the highest RRs and overall survivals, the toxicity of these combinations can make them difficult to administer. Doublet chemotherapy regimens, FOLFOX or XELOX, may provide similar outcomes with less toxicity. Doublet chemotherapies are now preferred over triplet regimens.

e. Carboplatin/paclitaxel. This combination also has meaningful activity with manageable toxicity.

f. Molecular markers and targeted therapies. As noted for earlier in esophageal cancers, in patients with gastric or gastroesophageal junction tumors overexpressing *HER2*, trastuzumab added to chemotherapy significantly enhances outcomes, including overall survival. Additionally, anti-VEGFR2 antibody ramucirumab has also been approved after failure of first-line chemotherapies (see details on this in the section for esophageal cancers and Figure 10-1).

C. RT

1. **Localized disease.** RT alone has not proved useful for treating gastric cancer. RT (4,000 cGy in 4 weeks) in combination with 5-FU (15 mg/kg IV on the first 3 days of RT), however, appears to improve survival over RT alone in patients with localized but unresectable cancers. Intraoperative radiation therapy (IORT) allows high doses of radiation to the tumor bed or residual disease while permitting the exclusion of mobile radiosensitive normal tissues from the area irradiated. Trials are limited to single institutional experiences; therefore, generalizing from such trials is difficult. Selected patients may benefit from IORT, particularly when combined with supplemental external beam radiation and chemotherapy. Long-term survival has been reported in some patients treated in this fashion for residual disease after surgery.

2. **Advanced disease.** Gastric adenocarcinoma is relatively radioresistant and requires high doses of radiation with attendant toxic effects to surrounding organs. RT may be useful for palliating pain, vomiting due to obstruction, gastric hemorrhage, and metastases to bone and brain.

COLORECTAL CANCER

I. EPIDEMIOLOGY AND ETIOLOGY

A. Incidence. Colorectal cancer is the second most common cause of cancer mortality after lung cancer in the United States and ranks third in frequency among primary sites of cancer in both men and women (after lung, breast, and prostate cancer). Nearly one million cases are diagnosed annually worldwide, accounting for 9% to 10% of human cancers. Peak incidence rates are observed in Europe, the United States, Australia, and New Zealand. A 10-fold variability is noted from highest to lowest regional incidence rates. Both the incidence and the mortality rates have declined in the United States since they peaked in 1985, a phenomenon thought to be a consequence of increased screening for and removal of premalignant polyps as well as potentially a more widespread use of aspirin and other nonsteroidal antirheumatic agents. Studies of migrant populations have discerned that the incidence of colorectal cancer reflects country of residence and not the country of origin. This suggests that overall environmental influences outweigh genetic trends for populations in which the experiences of those people with inherited special risk are pooled with those of lesser risk. Rural dwellers have a lower incidence of colorectal cancer than do urbanites.

The lifetime estimated risk for developing colorectal cancer in United States is about 5%, with 3% of colorectal cancers occurring in patients younger than 40 years of age. The median age of diagnosis is around 70 years. Based on Surveillance, Epidemiology, and End Results (SEER) statistics, it is estimated that, in the United States in 2016, there will be 134,490 new cases of colorectal cancer with an estimated 49,190 dying from the disease.

B. **Etiology.** Multiple forces drive the transformation of healthy colorectal mucosa to cancer. Inheritance and environmental factors, such as maintaining a low body mass index and exercising regularly, correlate with lower incidence rates, but the extent of the interdependence of these two factors as causative variables remains unknown.

1. **Polyps.** The main importance of polyps is the well-recognized potential of a subset to evolve into colorectal cancer. The evolution to cancer is a multistage process that proceeds through mucosal cell hyperplasia, adenoma formation, and growth and dysplasia to malignant transformation and invasive cancer. Oncogene activation, tumor suppressor gene inactivation, deficient DNA mismatch repair enzymes, and chromosomal deletion may lead to adenoma formation, growth with increasing dysplasia, and invasive carcinoma. The series of molecular alterations in the "adenoma–carcinoma sequence" have been well described.

   a. **Types of polyps.** Histologically, polyps are classified as neoplastic or nonneoplastic. Nonneoplastic polyps have no malignant potential and include hyperplastic polyps, mucous retention polyps, hamartomas (juvenile polyps), lymphoid aggregates, and inflammatory polyps. Neoplastic polyps (or adenomatous polyps) have malignant potential and are classified according to the World Health Organization system as tubular (microscopically characterized by networks of complex branching glands), tubulovillous (mixed histology), or villous (microscopically characterized by relatively short, straight glandular structures) adenomas, depending on the presence and volume of villous tissue. Polyps larger than 1 cm in diameter, those with high-grade dysplasia, and those with predominantly villous histology are associated with higher risk for colorectal cancer and are termed "*screen-relevant neoplasias.*" Colonoscopic polypectomy and subsequent surveillance can reduce the incidence of colon cancer by 90%, compared with that observed in unscreened controls.

   b. **Frequency of polyp types.** About 70% of polyps removed at colonoscopy are adenomatous, 75% to 85% of which are tubular (no or minimal villous tissue), 10% to 25% are tubulovillous (<75% villous tissue), and fewer than 5% are villous (>75% villous tissue). The incidence of synchronous adenomas in patients with one known adenoma is 40% to 50%.

   c. **Dysplasia** may be classified as low and high grade. About 6% of adenomatous polyps exhibit high-grade dysplasia and 5% contain invasive carcinoma at the time of diagnosis.

   d. **The malignant potential of adenomas correlates** with increasing size, the presence and the degree of dysplasia in a villous component, and the patient's age. Small colorectal polyps (smaller than 1 cm) are not associated with increased occurrence of colorectal cancer; the incidence of cancer, however, is increased 2.5- to 4-fold if the polyp is larger than 1 cm and 5- to 7-fold in patients who have multiple polyps. The study of the natural history of untreated polyps larger than 1 cm showed that the risk for progression to cancer is 2.5% at 5 years, 8% at 10 years, and 24% at 20 years. The time to malignant progression depends on the severity of dysplasia, averaging 3.5 years for severe dysplasia and 11.5 years for mild atypia.

e. Management of polyps. Because of the adenoma–cancer relationship and the evidence that resecting adenomas prevents cancer, newly detected polyps should be excised, and additional polyps should be sought through colonoscopy. The accuracy of colonoscopic examinations (94%) exceeds that of barium enema (67%), which is seldom used as a screening tool anymore. Additionally, with colonoscopy, therapeutic polypectomy can be accomplished during the diagnostic examination. CT colonography (virtual colonoscopy) is increasingly sensitive and specific, with refinements in software and radiologist expertise leading to sufficient improvements in the technique such that many centers offer this as a screening option, although a regular bowel preparation is required, and if relevant polyps are found, a colonoscopy will have to be performed. Fecal DNA assays that target genetic abnormalities specific to the malignant transformation of mucosal cells are now commercially available and are continuously being refined to improve their performance.

f. Intestinal polyposis syndromes. Table 10-1 summarizes familial polyposis syndromes and their histology distribution, malignant potential, and management.

2. Diet. Populations with high intake of fat, higher caloric intakes, and low intake of fiber (fruits, vegetables, and grains) characterized as a westernized diet tend to have increased risk for colorectal cancer in most but not all studies. Higher calcium intake, calcium supplementation, vitamin D supplementation, and regular aspirin use are associated with a lower risk for colorectal polyps and cancer in some studies. Fewer tumors that overexpress COX-2 occur in individuals who regularly use aspirin, which is known to reduce the incidence of both polyps and cancers. Increased intake of vitamins A, C, and E and β-carotene does not appear to decrease the risk for polyp formation.

3. Inflammatory bowel disease

a. Ulcerative colitis is a clear risk factor for colon cancer. About 1% of colorectal cancer patients have a history of chronic ulcerative colitis. The risk for the development of cancer in these patients varies inversely with the age of onset of the colitis and directly with the extent of colonic involvement and duration of active disease. The cumulative risk is 2% at 10 years, 8% at 20 years, and 18% at 30 years. Individuals with colon cancers associated with ulcerative colitis have a similar prognosis to sporadic cases.

The recommended approach to the increased risk for colorectal cancer in ulcerative colitis has been annual or semiannual colonoscopy to determine the need for total proctocolectomy in patients with extensive colitis of >8 years' duration. This strategy is based on the assumption that dysplastic lesions can be detected before invasive cancer has developed. An analysis of prospective studies concluded that immediate colectomy is essential for all patients diagnosed with a dysplasia-associated mass or lesion. Most important, due to inherent problems with sampling and

TABLE 10-1 Polyp Syndromes and Colorectal Cancer

Disease	Histology	Distribution of Polyps	Malignant Potential	Associated Manifestations	Age for First FOB Test (yr)	Age for First Colonoscopy (yr)	Surgery
Discrete polyps and CC	Few AP	Colon	High	None	≥45	≥45	Same as for general population
Hereditary discrete common polyps and CC	AP	Proximal colon	High	Lynch I[a]	30–35	35	Same as for general population
HNPCC	AP → Ac	Proximal colon	High	Lynch II[a]	None (ES)	20	Subtotal colectomy[d]
Familial CC	AP	Proximal colon; may be distal	High	None	30–35	35	Same as for general population
FAP and Turcot syndrome	Scattered AP → Ac	Colon	High	Central nervous system tumors	None (ES)	Teens	Prophylactic subtotal colectomy[d]
FAP and Oldfield syndrome	Scattered AP → Ac	Colon	High	Skin tumors	None (ES)	Teens	Prophylactic subtotal colectomy[d]
FAP and Gardner syndrome	Scattered AP → Ac	Usually colon; also stomach and SB	High	See Footnote[b]	None (ES)	Teens	Prophylactic subtotal colectomy[d,e]
Peutz-Jeghers syndrome	Hamartomas	Stomach, SB, colon, and ovary	Low	Buccal and cutaneous pigmentation	≥45	≥45	None
Generalized GI juvenile polyposis	JP	Stomach, SB, and colon	Low	None	None	≥45	None
Juvenile polyposis coli of infancy	JP	Stomach, SB, and colon	None	Protein-losing enteropathy	None	No special indications	None
Cronkhite-Canada syndrome	JP	Stomach, SB, and colon	None	Protein-losing enteropathy[c]	None	No special indications	None

[a]**Lynch syndrome I:** autosomal-dominant inheritance with susceptibility to early onset of colorectal cancer proximal to the splenic flexure in the absence of diffuse polyps; **Lynch syndrome II:** contains most of the features of Lynch I with excess incidence of carcinomas of the endometrium, ovary, kidney, ureter, bladder, bile duct, and small bowel and of lymphoma. (Lynch HT. The surgeon and colorectal cancer genetics. *Arch Surg* 1990;125:699.)

[b]Epidermoid cysts, fibromas, desmoids, dental and osseous abnormalities, intraperitoneal and retroperitoneal fibrosis, ampullary carcinoma, and tumors in other glandular structures. Follow with ophthalmoscopy for associated congenital hypertrophy of the retinal pigment epithelium.

[c]Hyperpigmentation, alopecia, and nail dystrophy.

[d]Prophylactic colectomy should be considered if 5 to 10 adenomatous polyps are present or if polyps recur.

[e]Or, total colectomy with pouch reconstruction. Nonsteroidal anti-inflammatory drugs decrease the number and size of polyps.

FOB, fecal occult blood; CC, colorectal cancer; AP, adenomatous polyps; HNPCC, hereditary nonpolyposis colorectal cancer ("cancer family syndrome"); SB, small bowel; JP, juvenile (retention) polyps.

interobserver agreement, the analysis demonstrated that the diagnosis of dysplasia does not preclude the presence of invasive cancer.

   b. Crohn disease. Patients with colorectal Crohn disease are at 1.5 to 2 times increased risk for colorectal cancer. The risk is less than that of those with ulcerative colitis.

4. **Genetic factors**
   a. Family history may signify either a genetic abnormality or shared environmental factors, or a combination of these factors. About 15% of all colorectal cancers occur in patients with a history of colorectal cancer in first-degree relatives. Individuals with a first-degree relative who has had colorectal cancer are more than twice as likely to develop colon cancer as those individuals with no family history.

   b. Gene changes. Specific inherited (adenomatous polyposis coli [*APC*] gene) and acquired genetic abnormalities (*RAS* gene point mutation; *c-MYC* gene amplification; allele deletion at specific sites of chromosomes 5, 8, 17, and 18) appear to be capable of mediating steps in the progression from normal to malignant colonic mucosa. About half of all carcinomas and large adenomas have associated point mutations, most often in the *K-RAS* gene. Such mutations are rarely present in adenomas smaller than 1 cm. Allelic deletions of 17p– are demonstrated in three-fourths of all colorectal carcinomas, and deletions of 5q– are demonstrated in more than one-third of colonic carcinoma and large adenomas.

   Two major syndromes and several variants of these syndromes of inherited predisposition to colorectal cancer have been characterized. The two syndromes, which predispose to colorectal cancer by different mechanisms, are FAP and hereditary nonpolyposis colorectal cancer (Lynch syndrome or HNPCC).

   (1) FAP. The genes responsible for FAP, *APC* genes, are located in the 5q21 chromosome region. Inheritance of defective *APC* tumor suppressor gene leads to a virtually 100% likelihood of developing colon cancer by 55 years of age, leading to the recommendation of a total proctocolectomy for affected individuals during their 20s or 30s. Screening for polyps should begin during early teenage years. The FAP syndrome can be associated with the development of gastric and ampullary polyps, desmoid tumors, osteomas, abnormal dentition, and abnormal retinal pigmentation. Variants of FAP include Gardner and Turcot syndromes.

   (2) HNPCC. The autosomal-dominant pattern of HNPCC includes Lynch syndromes I and II, both of which are associated with an increased incidence of predominantly right-sided colon cancer. This genetic abnormality in the DNA mismatch repair enzymes leads to defective excision of abnormal repeating sequences of DNA known as *microsatellites* (microsatellite instability [MSI]). Retention of these sequences leads to expression of a mutator phenotype characterized by frequent DNA replication errors (also called the *RER*+ phenotype), which predispose affected people to a multitude of primary malignancies, including cancers of the endometrium, ovary, bladder, ureter, stomach, and biliary tract.

   (a) Specific mutated genes on chromosomes 2 and 3, known as *hMSH2*, *hMLH1*, *hPMS1*, and *hPMS2*, have been linked to HNPCC. Patients with the RER+ phenotype may not have a germline abnormality and may instead have acquired abnormal methylation of DNA as the source of the absence of expression of the genes previously noted. Abnormal methylation, which silences the promoter region of mismatch repair genes preventing protein synthesis, is more common in older patients and women. Germline testing to determine if the RER+ phenotype is inherited or acquired is necessary as a part of genetic counseling when an individual is found to have a mismatch repair defect. Immunohistochemical stains can be used to determine if a tumor is devoid of the expression of mismatch repair enzymes, and then patients with absent gene expression should undergo germline testing to enable appropriate counseling of family members. Standardized algorithms now exist to screen for mismatch repair deficiencies in the tumor specimens, prompting a formal genetic consultation and germline testing of the patient and family if needed.

(b) Patients with HNPCC have a tendency to develop colon cancer at an early age, and screening should begin by 20 years of age or 5 years earlier than the age at diagnosis of the earliest affected family member for relatives of HNPCC patients. The median age of HNPCC patients with colon cancer at diagnosis was 44 years versus 68 years for control patients in one study.

(c) The prognosis for HNPCC patients is better than for those patients with sporadic colon cancer; the death rate from colon cancer for HNPCC patients is two-thirds that for sporadic cases over 10 years. One study suggests that patients with HNPCC may derive less benefit from adjuvant chemotherapy based on fluorouracil combinations than patients without this abnormality. The finding of immunotherapy being of immense benefit in patients with mismatch repair deficient (MMR-deficient) or microsatellite instability-high (MSI-high) tumors is leading to a paradigm shift as to how patients with advanced tumors would be treated in the near future. In a landmark study presented in 2015, immunotherapy with PD-1 blockade (pembrolizumab) showed substantial benefit in MMR-deficient tumors. Patients with this condition should be highly considered for immune checkpoint clinical trials. The benefit is thought to be due to a higher number of somatic mutations present in the tumors that are MMR deficient and that in turn result in potentially higher number of neoantigens making immunotherapy an effective option as compared to MMR-proficient (or MSI-stable) tumors.

(d) It is important to note that apart from the genetic deficiency in mismatch repair enzyme expression, about 15% of colon cancers exhibit the same biologic phenotype as HNPCC-derived tumors via the methylation of the promoter regions of DNA mismatch repair enzyme genes.

c. **Tumor location.** Proximal tumors have a higher likelihood to exhibit the defective DNA mismatch repair phenotype and MSI. Distal tumors show evidence of greater chromosomal instability and may develop through the same mechanisms that underlie familial polyposis-associated colorectal cancer. MSI was also noted to be higher in females and in tumors lacking the *KRAS* and/or *BRAF* mutations.

5. **Smoking.** Men and women smoking during the previous 20 years have three times the relative risk for small adenomas (<1 cm) but not for larger ones. Smoking for >20 years was associated with 2.5 times the relative risk for

larger adenomas. It has been estimated that 5,000 to 7,000 colorectal cancer deaths in the United States can be attributed to cigarette use.

6. **Other factors.** Personal or family history of cancer in other anatomic sites (such as breast, endometrium, and ovary) is associated with increased risk for colorectal cancer. Exposure to asbestos (e.g., in brake mechanics) increases the incidence of colorectal cancer to 1.5 to 2 times that of the average population.

II. PATHOLOGY AND NATURAL HISTORY

A. **Histology.** Ninety-eight percent of colorectal cancers above the anal verge are adenocarcinomas. Cancers of the anal canal are most often squamous cell or basaloid carcinomas. Carcinoid tumors cluster around the rectum and cecum and spare the rest of the colon and are distinguished from undifferentiated small cell neuroendocrine tumors of the colon by their tendency to be both well differentiated and indolent in their behavior.

B. **Location.** Two-thirds of colorectal cancers occur in the left colon and one-third in the right colon, although women more often develop right-sided tumors. About 20% of colorectal cancers develop in the rectum.

C. **Clinical presentation.** The common clinical complaints of patients with colorectal cancer relate to the size and location of the tumor. Right-sided colonic lesions are often asymptomatic, but when symptoms are manifested, these tumors most often result in dull and ill-defined abdominal pain, bleeding, and symptomatic anemia (causing weakness, fatigue, and weight loss), rather than in colonic obstruction. Left-sided lesions lead commonly to changes in bowel habits, bleeding, gas pain, decrease in stool caliber, constipation, increased use of laxatives, and colonic obstruction. Sometimes, distant metastases, in particular liver metastases, can cause the initial clinical symptoms and present with associated liver dysfunction.

D. **Clinical course.** Metastases to the regional lymph nodes are found in 40% to 70% of cases at the time of resection. Venous or lymphatic invasion is found in up to 60% of cases. Metastases occur most frequently in the liver, peritoneal cavity, and lung, followed by the adrenals, ovaries, and bone. Metastases to the brain, while rare, are noted more commonly as survival with distant disease is extended by better treatments. Rectal cancers are three times more likely to recur locally than are proximal colonic tumors, in part because the anatomic confines of the rectum preclude wide resection margins and in part because the rectum lacks an outer serosal layer through most of its course. Because of the venous and lymphatic drainage of the rectum into the inferior vena cava (as opposed to the venous drainage of the colon into the portal vein and variable lymphatic drainage), rectal cancers have a higher incidence of lung metastasis compared with colon cancers that more frequently recur first in the liver.

III. DIAGNOSIS

A. **Diagnostic studies.** After the clinical diagnosis of colorectal cancer is made, several diagnostic and evaluative steps should be taken.

1. **Biopsy confirmation** of malignancy via colonoscopy or via CT-guided fine-needle aspiration is important. US-guided biopsy of the liver metastases can also be diagnostic.

2. **General evaluation** includes a complete physical examination with digital rectal examination, CBC, LFT, and chest imaging.

3. **Carcinoembryonic antigen (CEA) screening** is recommended by the American Society of Clinical Oncology (ASCO) as a means of identifying early recurrence despite the lack of elevation in 40% of individuals with metastatic disease. A preoperative CEA can be useful as a prognostic factor

and in determining if the primary tumor is associated with CEA elevation. Preoperative CEA elevation implies that CEA may aid in early identification of metastases because metastatic tumor cells are more likely to result in CEA elevation in this circumstance.

4. **CT or MRI** with contrast of the chest, abdomen, and pelvis may identify small lung, liver, or intraperitoneal metastases.

5. **Endoscopy (or CT colonography)** is indicated to assess the entire colonic mucosa because about 3% of patients have synchronous colorectal cancers and a larger percentage have additional premalignant polyps. In patients where the initial full colonoscopy was not possible due to a distal obstruction, deserve a full evaluation after recovery from initial surgical resection.

6. **EUS** significantly improves the preoperative assessment of the depth of invasion of large bowel tumors, especially rectal tumors. The accuracy rate is 95% for EUS, 70% for CT, and 60% for digital rectal examination. In rectal cancer, the combination of EUS to assess tumor extent and digital rectal examination to determine mobility should enable precise planning of surgical treatment and definition of those patients who may benefit from preoperative chemoradiation (T3, T4, and N+). Transrectal biopsy of perirectal lymph nodes can often be accomplished under EUS direction. MRI with concomitant administration of rectal contrast is comparable to EUS in its sensitivity for staging the primary tumor and might be superior to EUS in the identification of perirectal lymph node metastases. Choice of MRI versus EUS is often a multidisciplinary decision between medical/radiation oncology and colorectal surgery.

7. **PET scanning** is of increasing utility to help distinguish if anatomic lesions of unclear origin are malignant or benign. Such scans are also useful to determine if localized or metastatic disease is potentially resectable. Its utility is increasingly being recognized for the small proportion of patients with oligometastatic disease that may be deemed potential candidates for resections of hepatic or pulmonary metastases.

B. **Biologic markers**

1. **CEA** is a cell surface glycoprotein that is shed into the blood and is the best known serologic marker for monitoring colorectal cancer disease status and for detecting early recurrence and liver metastases. CEA is too insensitive and nonspecific to be useful for screening of colorectal cancer. Elevation of serum CEA levels, however, does correlate with a number of parameters. Higher CEA levels are associated with histologic grade 1 or grade 2 tumors, more advanced stages of the disease, and the presence of visceral metastases. Although serum CEA concentration is an independent prognostic factor, its putative value lies in serial monitoring after surgical resection.

2. **Other markers.** Currently, light microscopic features and stage remain the most reliable prognostic measures. Other prognostic variables from a tumor mutational and circulating tumor cells' standpoint are still research tools only and have not made it to clinical practice.

IV. STAGING AND PROGNOSTIC FACTORS

A. **Staging system.** Refer to the current AJCC Cancer Staging atlas for TNM staging system.

B. **Prognostic factors**

1. **Stage** is the most important prognostic factor.

2. **Histologic grade** significantly influences survival regardless of stage. Patients with well-differentiated carcinomas (grades 1 and 2) have a better 5-year survival than those with poorly differentiated carcinomas (grades 3 and 4).

3. **The anatomic location of the tumor** appears to be an independent prognostic factor. For equal stages, patients with rectal lesions have a worse prognosis than those with colon lesions, and transverse and descending colon lesions result in poorer outcomes than ascending or rectosigmoid lesions.

4. **Clinical presentation.** Patients who present with bowel obstruction or perforation have a worse prognosis than patients who present with neither of these problems.

5. **Chromosome 18.** The prognosis of patients with an allelic loss of chromosome 18q is significantly worse than that of patients with no allelic loss.

6. **Other tumor characteristics.** Investigators have examined a number of tumor characteristics as judged by immunohistochemical or polymerase chain reaction–based assays for use either as factors for predicting prognosis or as characteristics that could potentially predict the likelihood of an individual patient's response to a specific regimen. These evaluations include levels in the tumor of thymidylate synthetase, dihydropyrimidine dehydrogenase (DPD), CDX2 expression, proliferation markers (Ki-67 or MIB-1), and tumor suppressor deletions (such as 18q deletions), among others. Molecular signature assays as prognostic markers have been developed and are commercially available for patients with stage II colon cancer, although their relevance for clinical practice is still unclear. Presence of MSI is an important adjunct in considering adjuvant chemotherapy for stage II colorectal cancers (see discussion on adjuvant chemotherapy).

V. SCREENING AND PREVENTION

A. **Screening.** The National Cancer Institute, the American College of Surgeons, the American College of Physicians, and the American Cancer Society (ACS) recommend a number of potential screening tests as alternatives for asymptomatic patients who are 50 years of age and older. One option is to have a sigmoidoscopic examination every 3 to 5 years. An annual digital rectal and three-sample fecal occult blood (FOB) test examination are recommended by the ACS, American College of Gastroenterology, and NCI for people 50 years of age and older. Screening colonoscopy has also been recommended for average-risk individuals every 10 years. Screening colonoscopy for high-risk patients with a family history of colorectal cancer in first-degree relatives but no clear evidence of FAP or HNPCC should begin at 40 years of age.

1. Three large randomized trials in which >250,000 patients were tested for FOB or followed according to the usual patterns of care have been reported. In the largest trial and the only one conducted in the United States, annual testing of a rehydrated fecal smear was associated with a 33.4% decrease in risk for death from colorectal cancer in 46,551 adults older than 50 years of age. Better markers for colorectal cancer are being sought because of the high false-positive and false-negative rates associated with FOB.

2. There has been burgeoning interest in the isolation of specific DNA sequences such as those in the *APC* or *p53* genes, and long segments of DNA that can be obtained from colonocytes shed into the stool and assayed using techniques for amplifying the amount of DNA present. These markers appear to be sensitive and specific for screening for malignancy in the aerodigestive tract. One of these multiple marker noninvasive stool DNA (sDNA) colorectal cancer screening tests, referred to as Cologuard, in a prospective study of more than 90 sites in United States and Canada showed excellent sensitivity and specificity. This led to this being one of the first tests being approved by the Food and Drug Administration (FDA) and Centers for Medicare & Medicaid Services (CMS) at the same time. It is noninvasive,

cost-effective, and orderable for individuals above the age of 50 who are deemed average risk for colorectal cancer.

B. Prevention

1. **Periodic sigmoidoscopy or colonoscopy** identifies and removes precancerous lesions (polyps) and reduces the incidence of colorectal cancer in patients who undergo colonoscopic polypectomy. However, no prospective randomized clinical trials have yet demonstrated that sigmoidoscopy is effective in the prevention of colorectal cancer death, although trials to test this strategy are in progress. The presence of even small rectosigmoid polyps is associated with polyps beyond the reach of the sigmoidoscope, and their presence should lead to full colonoscopy.

2. **Diets** that are high in fiber and low in fat or that contain calcium supplements, or both, may deter polyp progression to cancer.

3. **Nonsteroidal anti-inflammatory drugs (NSAIDs).** In a randomized, double-blind, placebo-controlled study of patients with familial polyposis, sulindac at a dose of 150 mg b.i.d. significantly decreased the mean number and mean diameter of polyps as compared with those in patients given placebo. The size and number of the polyps, however, increased 3 months after the treatment was stopped but remained significantly lower than at baseline. Data further suggest that aspirin reduces the formation, number, and size of colorectal polyps and reduces the incidence of colorectal cancer, whether familial or nonfamilial. These protective effects appear to require continuous exposure to at least 325 mg of aspirin per day for years. Selective COX-2 inhibitors have also been shown to be preventive for colon cancer but have been associated with an increased risk of cardiac events such that these are not routinely recommended outside of clinical trials

VI. MANAGEMENT

A. Surgery is the only universally accepted potentially curative treatment for colorectal cancer. Curative surgery should excise the tumor with wide margins and maximize regional lymphadenectomy such that at least 12 lymph nodes are available for pathologic evaluation. For lesions above the rectum, resection of the tumor with a minimum 5-cm margin of grossly negative colon is considered adequate, although the ligation of vascular trunks required to perform an adequate lymphadenectomy may necessitate larger bowel resections. Laparoscopic colectomy approaches have been developed and appear to be equally effective staging and therapeutic approaches to open colectomy, with modest decreases in hospital stay and pain medication use and improved cosmetic results. Subtotal colectomy and ileoproctostomy may be advisable for patients with potentially curable colon cancer and with adenomas scattered in the colon or for patients with a personal history of prior colorectal cancer or a family history of colorectal cancer in first-degree relatives.

1. **Arterial supply.** Excision of a tumor in the right colon should include the right branch of the middle colic artery as well as the entire ileocolic and right colic artery. Excision of a tumor at the hepatic or splenic flexure should include the entire distribution of the middle colic artery.

2. **Avoidance of permanent colostomy** in middle and low rectal cancers has been encouraged by the emergence of new surgical stapling techniques as well as the use of preoperative chemotherapy and radiation to shrink tumors prior to resection.

3. **Rectal tumors** may be treatable by primary resection and more distal anastomosis, usually without even a temporary (anastomosis-protective)

colostomy, if the lower edge is above 5 cm from the anal verge. Treatment options for rectal tumors include the following:

a. Middle and upper rectum (6 to 15 cm). Anterior resection of the rectum.

b. Lower rectum (0 to 5 cm). Coloanal anastomosis, with or without a pouch, transanal excision, transsphincteric and parasacral approaches, diathermy, primary radiation therapy, or abdominoperineal resection (APR).

c. Total mesorectal excision (TME). The mesorectum is defined as the lymphatic, vascular, fatty, and neural tissues that are circumferentially adherent to the rectum from the level of the sacral promontory to the levator ani muscles. Data from Europe suggest that local recurrence rates may be decreased with *en bloc* sharp dissection of the entire mesorectum at the time of tumor extirpation, and this procedure has now become standard.

4. Obstructing tumors in the right colon are usually managed by primary resection and primary anastomosis. Obstructing tumors in the left colon may be managed with initial decompression (proximal colostomy) or stent insertion followed by resection of the tumor and deferred closure of the colostomy. Recent trends, however, favor extending resection and primary anastomosis to include obstructing tumors in the transverse, descending, and even sigmoid colon.

5. Perforated colon cancer requires initial excision of the primary tumor and a proximal colostomy, followed later by reanastomosis and closure of the colostomy.

B. Adjuvant chemotherapy for stage III colon cancer (lymph node involvement) with 5-FU plus levamisole (mainly of historical interest) or 5-FU plus leucovorin (FU/L) reduced the incidence of recurrence by 41% ($p < 0.001$) in a number of large prospective randomized trials. The MOSAIC study in Europe randomized 2,200 patients (40% stage II, 60% stage III) to receive 5-FU infusion and leucovorin without or with oxaliplatin (FOLFOX). The primary end point of this trial was 3-year overall DFS rather than the more conventional end point of 5-year overall survival. There was a 73% 3-year DFS for the standard 5-FU/leucovorin arm and a 78% 3-year DFS for the FOLFOX regimen, with a 7.5% statistically significant advantage for stage III disease. More recent data have shown a 2.6% benefit in 6-year overall survival for FOLFOX over the two-drug regimen in all patients with a 4.4% difference for stage III disease. The National Surgical Adjuvant Breast Project (NSABP) C-07 study showed a similar outcome for DFS, but a higher rate of diarrhea for the specific regimen that employed a bolus-based 5-FU plus oxaliplatin regimen called *FLOX*.

The superiority of an oxaliplatin–fluoropyrimidine regimen to fluoropyrimidine alone was confirmed in a phase III trial comparing bolus 5-FU/LV to a combination of capecitabine plus oxaliplatin (XELOX) with increased DFS, comparable to the results found with FOLFOX and FLOX.

Three randomized trials have failed to show an advantage to irinotecan-containing regimens in the adjuvant setting. The use of irinotecan alone or in combinations is not recommended in the adjuvant setting.

Similarly, two large randomized phase III trials (NSABP C-08 and AVANT) have failed to show a benefit in terms of DFS and OS for the addition of bevacizumab to FOLFOX as adjuvant therapy in stage II and III colon cancer.

In addition, the cetuximab added to FOLFOX as tested in the phase III inter-group trial N0147 also did not improve outcomes as adjuvant therapy in stage III colon cancer, not even in patients with KRAS wild-type cancers.

As a consequence, the standard treatment for stage III colon cancer is now an oxaliplatin-containing regimen, most commonly FOLFOX or XELOX, unless there are contraindications to its use such as preexisting sensory neuropathy. In that case, FU/LV or capecitabine is recommended. In a large study known as the X-ACT trial, capecitabine, an oral 5-FU prodrug, was compared with bolus FU/LV, and outcomes were essentially equivalent. Adjuvant chemotherapy is begun 3 to 5 weeks after surgery.

1. **FU/LV regimens.** Two bolus 5-FU regimens commonly employed in the United States are as follows:
   a. **Dosage, Mayo Clinic regimen.** Leucovorin, 20 mg/m^2 by 30-minute IV infusion, followed by 5-FU, 425 mg/m^2 by rapid IV injection, daily for 5 consecutive days for two 4-week cycles and then every 5 weeks thereafter
   b. **Dosage, Roswell Park Memorial Institute (RPMI) regimen.** Leucovorin, 500 mg/m^2 by 30-minute IV infusion, followed by 5-FU, 500 mg/m^2 by rapid IV injection, weekly for 6 of every 8 weeks
   c. **The side effects of the Mayo and RPMI regimens and capecitabine** are different. Toxicity of grade III or more is based on the NCI common toxicity criteria. The principal difference in toxicity between the two regimens relates to rates of severe stomatitis and diarrhea. The Mayo regimen is associated with more grade III neutropenia and stomatitis, the RPMI regimen with a higher rate of grade III diarrhea. Nausea and vomiting are generally not severe. Dermatologic side effects are generally limited to erythema and desquamation of sun-damaged skin.

      Capecitabine is able to be administered orally and is associated with less GI toxicity and neutropenia than bolus FU regimens. However, it does cause hand–foot syndrome in which the skin of the palms and soles can become tender, erythematous, and if the drug is continued, exfoliation of the overlying skin may follow.
   d. **Dihydropyrimidine (DPD)** is the rate-limiting enzyme in the breakdown of 5-FU. Less than 1% of the US population has a deficiency of DPD. Such patients have severe toxicity and often die after exposure to standard doses because of profound and prolonged neutropenia and mucositis. Cerebellar toxicity occurs relatively commonly in DPD-deficient patients. An assay for DPD levels is commercially available and can be selectively ordered if DPD deficiency is suspected based on history or clinical parameters. Uridine triacetate is now available as an antidote to 5-FU or capecitabine toxicity.
2. **FOLFOX and XELOX** are the preferred regimens.
   a. **Dosage, mFOLFOX6.** Leucovorin, 400 mg/m^2, is given preceding a bolus of 5-FU of 400 mg/m^2. A 46-hour infusion of 2,400 mg/m^2 is then administered via infusion pump. Oxaliplatin is given at a dose of 85 mg/m^2 on day 1. The cycle is repeated every 2 weeks for a planned duration of 12 cycles (24 weeks). Modified FOLFOX6 has widely replaced the FOLFOX4 regimen used in the pivotal MOSAIC study. Other FOLFOX regimens explore variations on the oxaliplatin dose and have eliminated the 5-FU bolus like in FOLFOX7.
   b. **Dosage, XELOX.** Capecitabine 1,000 mg/m^2 b.i.d. PO days 1 to 14, oxaliplatin 130 mg/m^2 IV on day 1 of a 3-week cycle. Planned duration is eight cycles. Commonly, capecitabine has to be reduced to 850 mg/m^2 b.i.d. due

to hand–foot syndrome and diarrhea. Similar dose adjustments are recommended in individuals with decreased renal function and advanced age.

   c. Dosage, FLOX. Leucovorin 500 mg/m^2 is given preceding a bolus of 5-FU of 500 mg/m^2 weekly for 6 weeks in three 8-week cycles. Oxaliplatin, 85 mg/m^2, is given on weeks 1, 3, and 5 of each 8-week cycle. No pumps or prolonged infusions are used. Grade 3/4 diarrhea occurs in 40% of patients. This regimen is sometimes employed in individuals developing the rare 5-FU–induced coronary vasospasm that occurs with protracted fluoropyrimidine exposure.

   d. The side effects of FOLFOX. This regimen is commonly associated with grade 3 to 4 neutropenia (41% in the MOSAIC trial) but seldom causes neutropenic fever (1.8%). GI tract toxicity is less problematic than in the bolus-based 5-FU regimens, with 2.7% having stomatitis, 5.9% vomiting, and 10.8% diarrhea. Alopecia is relatively rare at 5%. Chronic sensory neuropathy, which is often aggravated by cold exposure and can limit the amount of oxaliplatin that can be administered over time, afflicted 12.3% of patients, but most patients with grade 3 neuropathy had recovered 1 year after the agent was stopped.

   e. The side effects of XELOX. Hand–foot syndrome, diarrhea, and sensory neuropathy as described above for FOLFOX are common. Myelosuppression is less common than with FOLFOX4.

C. Adjuvant chemotherapy for stage II colon cancer (no lymph node involvement) is controversial. Investigators from the NSABP advocate for adjuvant therapy in this setting because it has produced a small but consistent benefit in patients with stage II disease in serial NSABP trials. Conversely, a meta-analysis of five trials involving about 1,000 patients showed a statistically insignificant difference in 5-year survival rates of 82% versus 80%, treated versus untreated, respectively, for patients with stage II disease. The QUASAR group did show a 3% survival advantage at 5 years for FU/L over observation in a trial that enrolled >3,200 patients. There was no survival advantage for the 40% of stage II patients enrolled in the MOSAIC trial. The ASCO recommends against the routine use of chemotherapy in stage II colon cancer.

    Intense efforts have focused on differentiating stage II patients with higher risk for recurrence from those with lower risk through examination of molecular markers such as tumor ploidy (number of chromosomes), p53 status, levels of thymidylate synthesis, presence or absence of individual chromosomal mutations, and other parameters. Although none of these is accepted as a standard prognostic determinant, in one trial, patients with aneuploid tumors had a 5-year survival rate of 54%, compared with patients with diploid tumors who had a 74% 5-year survival rate.

    Several attempts have been made to characterize a population of stage II patients at high risk for tumor recurrence and metastases. The best validated high-risk factors are T4 tumor stage and the retrieval of <12 lymph nodes in the resected specimen. In contrast, obstruction, perforation, lymphovascular invasion, and undifferentiated histology have been found to be of lesser value in multivariate analysis. High-risk stage II colon cancers are commonly treated with oxaliplatin-containing regimens as adjuvant therapy. Patients with tumor expressing the defective mismatch repair phenotype (MMR-deficient or high microsatellite instability [MSI-high]) are at low risk of recurrence and should not be subjected to any adjuvant chemotherapy unless high-risk factors are present. For the group of patients with intermediate risk of recurrence, commercial molecular signature sets are available (Oncotype DX Colon and ColoPrint) that can help to refine the prognosis, although the utility of these tests in clinical practice has yet to be established.

D. Neoadjuvant therapy for rectal cancer. Because of the anatomic confines of the pelvic bones and sacrum, surgeons often cannot achieve wide, tumor-free margins during the resection of rectal cancer. Almost half of recurrences in rectal cancer are in the pelvis. This observation led a German group to compare preoperative chemotherapy with 5-FU and radiation to postoperative therapy in order to determine if the preoperative strategy could improve outcomes and reduce the number of APRs that result in a permanent colostomy. The trial randomized >800 patients and the outcomes favored preoperative therapy, which showed a lower local recurrence rate, less anastomotic stenosis, and fewer APRs. Patients who have a complete pathologic response to preoperative therapy have a favorable long-term prognosis. In general, postoperative adjuvant therapy with FOLFOX or FU/L based on preoperative staging is indicated for patients with known or suspected positive nodes. This trial has led to a widespread shift in practice to embrace preoperative chemotherapy plus RT.

   1. Variations in the use of RT alone or combined with chemotherapy and in surgical technique have been investigated in attempts to improve local control rates. Numerous randomized controlled studies of both preoperative and postoperative RT alone have demonstrated no improvement in survival; at best, there has been a small decrease in the rate of local recurrence. In the United States, radiation is generally given over 6 weeks to a dose approaching 50 Gy, and surgery is performed 4 to 6 weeks later. In some countries in Europe, it is common to give 25 Gy in five fractions (5 × 5 Gy) without chemotherapy and proceed promptly to surgery. These two approaches seem to demonstrate similar short-term results in terms of local recurrence rates.

   To minimize the risk of local recurrence, TME has become the standard of care. A Dutch trial showed that TME is associated with a lower local recurrence rate than conventional rectal resection but have also noted that rectal stump devascularization results in a higher rate of postoperative anastomotic site leakage. RT after TME reduces the rate of local recurrence at 2 years from the time of surgery, suggesting that RT is still a valuable tool in reducing local recurrence even after the more extensive *en bloc* resection done with TME.

   2. The current standard therapy for stage III rectal cancer, and sometimes for stage II disease, is preoperative chemotherapy using 5-FU and RT, followed by surgery, and then followed by adjuvant chemotherapy, which is modeled after experiences in colon cancer. Furthermore, some of the chemotherapy (FOLFOX) is also being moved to the neoadjuvant setting after patients have completed the chemoradiation portion of therapy. This appears to increase pathologic complete RRs. Whether or not this approach leads to increased overall survival still remains to be seen.

E. Postoperative follow-up. About 85% of all recurrences that are destined to occur in colorectal cancer are evident within 3 years after surgical resection, and nearly all recurrences are noted within 5 years. High preoperative CEA levels usually revert to normal within 6 weeks after complete resection.

   1. Clinical evaluation. After curative surgical resection, patients with stage II and III colon or rectal cancers are commonly seen more frequently during the first 2 postoperative years and less frequently thereafter. After 5 years, follow-up is mainly targeted at detection of new primary tumors. The primary goal of follow-up is to detect metastatic disease early. Some patients with colorectal cancer develop a single or a few metastatic sites (known as *oligometastases*) in the liver, in the lungs, or at the anastomotic site from which the primary bowel cancer was removed that can be resected with curative intent.

2. **Chest CT scanning has largely replaced chest radiographs** for detecting recurrence. They are advocated annually or semiannually.

3. **Colonoscopy.** Patients who presented with obstructing colon lesions that preclude preoperative imaging of the colon should have colonoscopy 3 to 6 months after surgery to ensure the absence of a concurrent neoplastic lesion in the remaining colon. The purpose of endoscopy done thereafter is to detect a metachronous tumor, suture line recurrence, or colorectal adenoma. In the absence of obstruction, colonoscopy is performed annually for 1 to 3 years after surgery and, if negative, at 5-year intervals thereafter.

4. **Rising CEA levels** call for further studies to identify the site of recurrence and are most often helpful in identifying hepatic recurrences. An elevated CEA calls for further testing using CT of the abdomen, pelvis, and chest as well as other studies as dictated by symptoms. If pelvic recurrence of a rectal cancer is suspected, MRI may be more helpful than CT. The use of hepatic imaging by CT, ultrasound, or MRI at regular intervals is now advocated by ASCO. PET scans may also be of value in identifying early signs of recurrent disease and for quantifying the number of metastatic deposits of disease visible at the time of recurrence.

F. **Management of isolated recurrence.** Early detection and surgical resection of isolated intrahepatic or pulmonary recurrence may be curative or result in improved survival. Those patients most likely to do well have a single lesion in a single site and a disease-free interval of 3 or more years between the primary diagnosis and evidence of metastatic disease. Resection of an isolated hepatic metastasis that involves one lobe of the liver may result in a 60% 5-year survival rate. Resection of an isolated pulmonary metastasis may result in 5- and 10-year survival rates of 40% and 20%, respectively. Even patients with multiple lesions can be resected and cured, although cure rates decrease with more widespread, albeit resectable, disease. In selected patients, multiple resections may be performed even for disease in the lung and liver with favorable outcomes. As more effective chemotherapy (FOLFOXIRI) and biologic therapy (anti-VEGF and anti-EGFR antibodies) are developed, the possibility of "converting" patients who were initially unresectable into resection candidates is more and more common ("conversion therapy"). Restaging with an eye toward resection when possible should be done on a frequent basis in patients who may be resection candidates.

G. **Management of advanced colorectal cancer: local measures**

1. **Surgery.** About 85% of patients diagnosed with colorectal cancer can undergo surgical resection. Patients with incurable cancer may benefit from palliative resection to prevent obstruction, perforation, bleeding, and invasion of adjacent structures. However, in the absence of symptoms, surgery can often be avoided when metastatic disease is present. It is common with newer CT scans to note the primary tumor on the scan and to observe shrinkage with chemotherapy treatment. The use of colonic stents and laser ablation of intraluminal tumors can often obviate the need for surgery even in symptomatic cases.

2. **RT** may be used as the primary and only treatment modality for small, mobile rectal tumors or in combination with chemotherapy after resection of rectal tumors. RT in palliative doses relieves pain, obstruction, bleeding, and tenesmus in about 80% of cases. In selected cases with locally advanced

disease, the use of IORT may provide an advantage. However, no randomized trials of external beam versus IORT or IORT plus external beam therapy have been reported.

3. **Hepatic arterial infusion** takes advantage of the dual nature of hepatic blood supply. Metastases in the liver derive their blood supply predominantly from the hepatic artery, whereas hepatocytes derive blood principally from the hepatic vein. The installation of floxuridine (FUDR) into the hepatic artery has been advocated and appears to improve the RR over 5-FU administered systemically. Problems with this approach include variable anatomy, which makes placement of a single catheter impossible; catheter migration; biliary sclerosis; and gastric ulceration. Progression of extrahepatic disease is a common pattern of failure with this modality. Randomized trials of systemic versus intrahepatic therapy have shown modest advantages to this approach, but the practical difficulties of managing these lines and ever-improving systemic therapies have kept this approach from widespread usage.

H. **Management of advanced colorectal cancer: chemotherapy** (Fig. 10-2). The most commonly used chemotherapeutic agents are 5-FU (alone or in combination with leucovorin, FU/L), capecitabine (the oral 5-FU prodrug), irinotecan, and oxaliplatin.

	Classification Based on Molecular Testing			
Line of therapy	*Any RAS* mutant ↓	*All-RAS* wild type		*BRAF* mutant ↓
1	CT doublet + anti-*VEGF*	CT doublet + anti-*EGFR*	CT doublet + anti-*VEGF*	FOLFOXIRI ± bevacizumab
	*Consider de-escalating (e.g., omit oxaliplatin) with maintenance chemotherapy after 4–6 cycles of upfront therapy if no progression; typically a fluoropyrimidine (capecitabine) with bevacizumab.			
2	CT doublet + anti-*VEGF*	CT doublet + anti-*VEGF*	CT doublet + anti-*VEGF*	Regorafenib
3	Regorafenib	Regorafenib	CT doublet + anti-*EGFR*	TAS-102
4	TAS-102	TAS-102	Regorafenib	BSC
5	BSC	BSC	TAS-102	
6			BSC	

Abbreviations: anti-VEGF, bevacizumab or aflibercept; anti-EGFR, cetuximab or panitumumab; BSC, best supportive care; CT, chemotherapy; EGFR, epithelial growth factor receptor; VEGF, vascular endothelial growth factor; TAS-102, trifluridine and tipiracil hydrochloride.

Figure 10-2 Treatment algorithm for the practical medical management of **metastatic colorectal cancer** (mCRC) based on clinically relevant molecular testing.

1. **Biochemical modulation of 5-FU with leucovorin.** The combination of 5-FU and leucovorin increases the activity as well as the toxicity of 5-FU, results in significant improvement in regression rate, and, according to some studies, culminates in improved survival. The partial RR is about 25%. The dose-limiting toxicities are diarrhea, mucositis, and myelosuppression. Regimens being used with essentially the same RR involve:

   a. 5-FU plus low-dose or high-dose leucovorin given weekly
   b. 5-FU plus low-dose or high-dose leucovorin given for 5 days every 4 to 5 weeks
   c. 5-FU plus leucovorin by infusion over 24 to 48 hours or for longer intervals

2. **Continuous IV infusion of 5-FU** changes the toxicity profile from hematologic to predominantly mucositis and dermatologic (hand–foot syndrome) when compared with bolus administration. Multiple randomized trials, however, have shown that continuous infusion of 5-FU using an ambulatory infusion pump, as compared with rapid injection, results in marginally improved survival, prolonging life on average for <1 month. Because of its favorable toxicity profile, the use of short-term infusion as the backbone of the FOLFOX and FOLFIRI regimens, and improvements in infusion pumps, has become common practice to treat advanced colorectal cancer.

3. **Therapy with irinotecan** has been shown to improve survival and quality of life in patients with advanced colorectal cancer. In patients with recurrent disease refractory to at least one 5-FU regimen, the survival at 1 year of patients treated with supportive care alone or with 5-FU was about 15%, compared with 36% when patients were treated with irinotecan. In the United States, a commonly used regimen for irinotecan is 125 mg/m^2 weekly for 4 of every 6 weeks or 2 of every 3 weeks. Irinotecan can also be administered as 350 mg/m^2 every 3 weeks.

   About 10% of the population in the United States has an inherited polymorphism of the *UGT1A1* gene that results in diminished activity of the enzyme that detoxifies irinotecan. Such patients have a higher risk of neutropenia, especially with the every-3-week higher dose regimen. A test for this abnormality is now commercially available, and testing is recommended in the package insert. These patients may require up to 50% dose upfront dose reductions and may require additional growth factor support for the significant and prolonged duration of neutropenia. In second-line therapy, there are no clear data supporting better outcomes from combinations of irinotecan with FU/L over single-agent irinotecan if a patient has had prior 5-FU exposure.

4. **Oxaliplatin** is a diaminocyclohexane-containing platinum agent that has been approved in combination with 5-FU and leucovorin for patients with metastatic colorectal cancer in the first- and second-line settings, as well as the adjuvant setting. It is generally administered in combination with 5-FU and leucovorin using one of a number of regimens called *FOLFOX1 to FOLFOX7* as data suggest greater efficacy in combination.

5. **First-line chemotherapy.** A number of randomized studies have compared three-drug regimens to FU/L as first-line therapy.

   a. Combination regimens being compared include
      (1) **IFL:** Irinotecan, 125 mg/m^2, with 5-FU, 500 mg/m^2, and leucovorin, 20 mg/m^2.
      (2) **FOLFIRI:** Irinotecan, 180 mg/m^2, followed by folinic acid (leucovorin), 200 mg/m^2, and then 5-FU, 2.4 g/m^2 infused over 24 hours.

Recent data have shown that the FOLFIRI regimen has advantages in both activity and toxicity over bolus 5-FU or capecitabine-based combinations.

(3) **FOLFOX4:** Folinic acid (leucovorin), 5-FU (given with a loading dose and 22-hour infusion repeated on consecutive days), and oxaliplatin (dosing schedule is defined in Section VI.B.2).

(4) **FOLFOX6:** Folinic acid (leucovorin), 5-FU (given with a loading dose and 46-hour infusion), and oxaliplatin.

(5) **FUFOX:** 5-FU given in high dose as a 24-hour infusion, folinic acid (leucovorin), and oxaliplatin.

(6) **IROX:** Irinotecan plus oxaliplatin.

b. **Results of some of these landmark randomized studies using chemotherapies** can be summarized as follows:

(1) Both the IFL and FOLFIRI regimens have been shown in randomized trials to offer an advantage to patients in median overall survival (OS), median time to tumor progression (TTP), and RR over FU/LV regimens.

(2) Several studies have compared oxaliplatin plus FU/LV to FU/LV alone. Both the FOLFOX and FUFOX regimens have been shown in randomized trials to offer a statistically significant advantage to patients with respect to TTP and RR but showed no statistically significant difference in OS over FU/LV regimens.

(3) Studies have compared regimens in which FU/LV is coupled to either irinotecan or oxaliplatin. In one large trial, 795 patients were randomly assigned to IFL versus FOLFOX versus IROX. The FOLFOX regimen was superior to both IFL and IROX with respect to overall MS, MTP, and RR. Toxicity also favored the FOLFOX regimen as patients had fewer episodes of severe diarrhea, febrile neutropenia, vomiting, and dehydration.

(4) A comparison of FOLFOX followed by FOLFIRI versus the reverse sequence has shown no significant differences in outcomes with respect to OS (21 months), RR in first-line therapy (55%), or TTP (8 months for first-line and 3 to 4 months for second-line therapy) based on the two sequences. Toxicity patterns were similar between the two regimens.

6. **Biologics and novel agents for colorectal cancer:**
Treatment of patients with colorectal cancer with biologics with or without the chemotherapy backbone has significantly improved outcomes and quality of life of these patients. These include antivascular endothelial growth factor (VEGF) antibodies (bevacizumab, ziv-aflibercept, and ramucirumab), antiepidermal growth factor receptor (EGFR) antibodies (panitumumab, cetuximab), regorafenib (an oral multikinase inhibitor), and trifluridine–tipiracil (a novel combination oral nucleoside antitumor agent).

a. **Anti-VEGF antibodies (bevacizumab, ziv-aflibercept, and ramucirumab)** are monoclonal antibodies that target the vascular endothelial growth factor system. Bevacizumab plus IFL was compared with IFL alone in a randomized trial involving 815 patients. The results for IFL alone were very similar to those reported in other phase III studies. The patients receiving IFL plus bevacizumab in this study achieved a better RR and MS compared with those receiving IFL alone. Toxicity was increased only modestly by the addition of bevacizumab, which led to hypertension and rare episodes of bowel perforation. Additional trials of bevacizumab with FOLFIRI and FOLFOX and capecitabine chemotherapy combinations have shown improvements in activity of lesser magnitude than that observed in IFL and bevacizumab study with similar toxicity profiles to the base regimens. Ziv-aflibercept is a VEGF receptor decoy fusion protein that has shown similar outcomes as compared to bevacizumab. Patients, however, were noted to have a higher incidence of toxicities, and therapy is relatively more expensive. Ramucirumab, an anti-VEGF2 antibody, is approved for colorectal cancer in combination with FOLFIRI in the second-line setting.

b. **Anti-EGFR antibodies (cetuximab and panitumumab)** are two monoclonal antibodies that target the EGFR and have been approved for use in advanced, refractory colorectal cancer. Multiple clinical trials have convincingly established that mutations in KRAS render these two antibodies ineffective in colorectal cancer. Consequently, cetuximab and panitumumab should only be used in KRAS wild-type colorectal cancer. Both have single-agent activity resulting in RRs of 10% to 15% in third-line therapy in KRAS wild-type cancers. Furthermore, tumor testing needs to include other activating RAS mutations in exons 2, 3, and 4 of KRAS and NRAS, since these patients also fail to benefit and may actually have a detriment from anti–EGFR-based therapies. Most of institutions now have tumor panel testing for BRAF, KRAS, HRAS, and NRAS for colorectal cancer.

In second-line treatment, the combination of either antibody with irinotecan is more active than irinotecan alone. Combinations of both agents with FOLFOX and FOLFIRI in first- and second-line therapy increase the efficacy of therapy with increases in RR and PFS in KRAS wild-type cancer in most, but not all, phase III trials. When compared with FOLFIRI alone, the combination of FOLFIRI + cetuximab increased overall survival in an unplanned subgroup analysis in KRAS wild-type colorectal cancer.

Cetuximab and panitumumab should *not* be combined with bevacizumab since two independent phase III trials demonstrated inferior outcomes when both antibody classes were combined in addition to chemotherapy in the first-line setting.

Cetuximab is a chimeric monoclonal antibody, and panitumumab is fully humanized. Both agents commonly cause an acne-like skin rash and paronychia in some patients, and development of this rash seems to correlate with benefit from the agents. Anaphylactic reactions are more common with cetuximab than with panitumumab.

c. **Regorafenib** is an oral multikinase inhibitor approved as an oral agent for treatment of refractory metastatic colorectal cancer. Regorafenib demonstrated improvement in overall survival and received FDA approval in 2012.

d. **Trifluridine and tipiracil hydrochloride** are oral combination nucleoside antitumor agents that also showed improvement in overall survival for patients with refractory metastatic colon cancer.

7. **FOLFOXIRI ± bevacizumab.** A study comparing a 5-FU plus irinotecan regimen to all three chemotherapy agents given together has shown an advantage for the FOLFOXIRI regimen, including a median survival for patients enrolled in the multidrug arm of 23 months and a high rate of liver resections among patients initially judged to be unresectable. The addition of bevacizumab to this regimen has also been studied and is another option

to be considered in the "conversion therapy" of potentially unresectable colorectal cancer lesions to resectable ones. This is also a regimen to consider in patients with *BRAF* mutations, which particularly have an aggressive tumor biology and a poor overall survival despite aggressive management.

8. **Serial sequential single agents versus combined chemotherapy.** Two trials done in Europe, the FOCUS study and the CAIRO study, have compared serial single agents with combinations. While trends favored combination therapies, neither study showed a significant advantage for combinations over serial single agents. However, median survivals were 15 to 17 months in all arms of both studies, which does not compare to the nearly 2-year median survivals seen with combinations. In addition, exposure to all three chemotherapy agents over the entire course of treatment for advanced disease is associated with better outcomes than less intensive therapy.

9. **Maintenance chemotherapy.** With more chemotherapy options being available for patients with metastatic colorectal cancer and realizing the potential long-term neurotoxic effects of upfront "induction" oxaliplatin-containing regimens, there has been a paradigm shift in management with the evolution of maintenance chemotherapy regimens. These regimens typically include a biologic with or without a chemotherapy backbone and are generally less toxic than the upfront induction chemotherapy regimens. The classic maintenance chemotherapy regimen arose from the so-called CAIRO-3 study employing capecitabine with bevacizumab after initial therapy in the form of capecitabine and oxaliplatin combination chemotherapy alongside bevacizumab for six cycles (CAPOX-B). Subsequently, bevacizumab in combination with erlotinib was also recently explored and showed overall survival advantage. The latter, however, cannot yet be regarded as a standard maintenance chemotherapy approach (Fig. 10-2).

10. **Immune checkpoint inhibitors.** The role of immunotherapy with PD-1–blocking antibodies for colorectal and other GI malignancies is being characterized further and appears to show significant benefit in tumors deemed MMR deficient or MSI-high as noted earlier. These tumors, however, constitute <5% of tumors in the metastatic setting. MSI testing, however, is recommended, and clinical trial participation is strongly encouraged.

11. **Other therapies and markers.** Anti–HER2-based therapies are also being explored given the finding that up to 4% of tumors in the refractory setting may have HER2 overamplification. This may be another option moving forward for our patients with metastatic colorectal cancer.

12. **Chemotherapy in the setting of liver dysfunction.** With the liver being a common site of metastases, it is not uncommon to encounter patients with varying degrees of liver dysfunction secondary to the colorectal cancer. Utilizing doublet chemotherapy with FOLFOX with or without a biologic is a standard approach recommended in these patients deemed not refractory to systemic therapy.

13. **Summary of chemotherapy recommendations for patients with advanced disease.** It appears that combination therapy with either irinotecan or oxaliplatin coupled to FU/LV is better than serial single-agent treatment with respect to overall survival. There are no clear data to favor FOLFOX, FOLFIRI, or FOLFOXIRI as the best first-line therapy. However, the protracted infusion of 5-FU seems to be better tolerated than bolus 5-FU, and use of the IFL regimen is not generally recommended. The toxicity profiles of the two regimens do differ, with FOLFOX causing more neutropenia and neuropathy and FOLFIRI more GI toxicity and alopecia; the side effect

profiles should be considered when choosing therapy on a patient-by-patient basis. Capecitabine can be substituted for 5-FU infusion in combination with oxaliplatin with similar outcomes. The overlapping GI toxicity of capecitabine and irinotecan limits the combination of these two drugs.

Most oncologists tend to begin patients on FOLFOX or FOLFIRI plus bevacizumab as first-line therapy in the United States. In patients deemed all-RAS wild type, comparative trials of chemotherapy with anti-VEGF versus chemotherapy with anti–EGFR-based therapies have essentially shown no significant overall difference. The choice of a particular biologic to be added to chemotherapy can be chosen based on patient-related factors and physician preference. If FOLFOX is used as chemotherapy backbone, oxaliplatin should be discontinued as soon as (or even before) neurotoxicity emerges. Considerations could be given to switching to "maintenance chemotherapy" approaches as noted earlier. Treatment can then be continued with 5-FU/LV (or capecitabine) plus bevacizumab until progression. Depending on the RAS/RAF status, a switch could be made to anti–EGFR-based therapies or continuing bevacizumab beyond progression with a different chemotherapy backbone.

In select patients, who require anatomical tumor shrinkage as prerequisite for resection of liver metastases, FOLFOXIRI with or without bevacizumab or a combination of doublet chemotherapy with anti-EGFR agents (in all-RAS wild-type cancers) can be considered.

Recent pooled analyses have suggested that patients older than 70 years and those with a performance status of 2 can tolerate and benefit from combination therapy similar to younger and asymptomatic patients.

ANAL CARCINOMA

I. EPIDEMIOLOGY AND ETIOLOGY

A. **Incidence.** Anal cancers constitute 1% to 2% of large bowel cancers, and approximately 8,000 new cases are diagnosed annually in the United States. Anal canal cancer most commonly develops in patients 50 to 60 years of age and is more frequent in women than in men (female-to-male ratio, 2:1). Cancer of the anal margin is more frequent in men. Therapy with upfront definitive chemoradiation for patients with advanced disease is still considered curative. Surveillance following this is important since surgery for relapsed cases is still with the intent to cure.

B. **Etiology.** In most patients with anal cancers, HPV appears to play a causal role.
   1. **Infectious agents.** HPV, particularly types 16 and 18, is a prime suspect as a causative agent for anal cancer. More than 70% of tumor tissues show HPV DNA by polymerase chain reaction techniques. An HPV-produced protein, E6, inactivates the tumor suppressor gene *p53*. The presence of genital warts increases the relative risk by a factor of 30.

   Although human immunodeficiency virus (HIV) has been suggested as a causative agent, anal tumors are extremely rare in IV drug abusers. The relative risk for homosexuals with acquired immunodeficiency syndrome (AIDS) is 84 and for heterosexuals with AIDS is 38. Other associated infections include herpes simplex virus type 2, *Chlamydia trachomatis* infection in women, and gonorrhea in men.

   2. **Diseases associated with anal cancer** include AIDS, prior irradiation, anal fistulas, fissures, chronic local inflammation, hemorrhoids, Crohn disease, lymphogranuloma venereum, condylomata acuminata, carcinoma of the cervix, and carcinoma of the vulva. The relative risk for anal cancer

development after a diagnosis of AIDS is 63. Sexual activity, particularly anal intercourse with multiple partners, is associated with an increased risk for anal canal cancer.

3. Immune suppression. Kidney transplant recipients have a 100-fold increase in anogenital tumors.

4. Cigarette smoking is associated with an eightfold increase in the risk for anal cancer.

5. Anal receptive intercourse in men but not in women is strongly associated with anal cancer at a risk ratio of 33. Studies have shown that the incidence of anal cancer (squamous and transitional cell carcinomas) is six times greater in single men than in married men. Single women are not at an increased risk.

II. PATHOLOGY AND NATURAL HISTORY

A. Anatomy. The anal canal is a tubular structure 3 to 4 cm in length. The junction between the anal canal and perineal skin is known as the anal verge (Hilton line). The pectinate (or dentate) line is located at the center of the anal canal.

The lining of the anal canal is composed of columnar epithelium in its upper portion and keratinized and nonkeratinized squamous epithelium in its lower portion. Intermediate epithelium (also known as transitional or cloacogenic epithelium, which resembles bladder epithelium) lines a middle zone (0.5 to 1 cm in length) that corresponds to the pectinate line. Anal tumors appear to originate near the mucocutaneous junction and grow either upward into the rectum and surrounding tissue or downward into the perineal tissue.

B. Lymphatics. Some of the upper lymphatics of the anus communicate with those of the rectal ampulla that lead to the sacral, upper mesocolic, and para-aortic lymph nodes. The lower lymphatics communicate with those of the perineum that lead to the superficial inguinal lymph nodes. Of patients undergoing abdominal perineal (AP) resection, 25% to 35% manifest pelvic lymph node metastases.

C. Histology. Squamous cell carcinoma accounts for 63% of cases; transitional cell (cloacogenic) carcinoma, 23%; and mucinous adenocarcinoma, 7% (often with multiple fistulous tracts). Basal cell carcinoma (2%) is curable either by local excision or by irradiation. Paget disease (2%) is a malignant neoplasm of the intraepidermal portion of the apocrine glands. Malignant melanoma (2%) usually begins at the pectinate line and progresses as single or multiple polypoid masses; the prognosis is poor and depends on tumor size and depth of invasion. Other forms include small cell carcinoma (rare but extremely aggressive), verrucous carcinoma (a polypoid neoplasm closely related to giant condyloma acuminata), Bowen disease, embryonal rhabdomyosarcoma (infants and children), and malignant lymphoma (in patients with AIDS).

III. DIAGNOSIS

A. Symptoms. Bleeding occurs in 50% of patients, pain in 40%, sensation of a mass in 25%, and pruritus in 15%. About 25% of patients do not have symptoms.

B. Physical examination should include digital anorectal examination, anoscopy, proctoscopy, EUS if available, and palpation of inguinal lymph nodes. Anorectal examination may have to be performed under sedation or general anesthesia in patients with severe pain and anal spasm.

C. Biopsy. An incisional biopsy is necessary and preferable to confirm the diagnosis. Excisional biopsy should be avoided. Suspicious inguinal lymph nodes should undergo biopsy to differentiate inflammatory from metastatic disease. Needle aspiration of these nodes may establish the diagnosis; if aspiration is negative, surgical biopsy should be performed.

D. **Staging evaluation** should include physical examination, chest radiograph, and LFT. Pelvic CT and EUS of the anal canal may be useful. MRI and PET/CT scans are increasingly being utilized to document the extent of disease. HIV testing is appropriate when warranted by individual patient risk factors.

IV. STAGING AND PROGNOSTIC FACTORS

A. **Staging system.** Refer to the current AJCC Cancer Staging atlas for TNM staging system. Anal margin tumors are staged as for skin cancer.

B. **Prognostic factors**

1. **TNM stage.** Patients with Tis have a propensity to progress to higher T stages and to have widespread superficial spread of disease, particularly among those that are HIV positive. Patients with T1 cancer (lesions smaller than 2 cm in diameter) have a significantly better prognosis than those with larger lesions. Five-year survival rates are >80% for patients with T1 and T2 cancers and <20% for those with T3 and T4 cancers. The survival is poor even with aggressive therapy for lesions larger than 6 to 10 cm in diameter. In a multivariate analysis, T stage was the only significant independent prognostic factor for anal cancers. Metastasis to lymph nodes also results in a poor outcome. Anal canal cancers tend to remain regionally localized, with distant metastases noted in <10% of cases.

2. **Other factors**

a. **Histology.** The histologic type (i.e., cloacogenic vs. epidermoid) has not been found to be prognostically relevant. Keratinizing carcinoma is associated with a better outcome than nonkeratinizing cancers. Patients with mucoepidermoid carcinoma and small cell anaplastic carcinoma have a worse prognosis.

b. **Symptoms.** Patients without symptoms do better than those with symptoms. Symptoms are usually directly related to the size of the tumor.

c. **Tumor grade.** Patients with low-grade tumors have a better 5-year survival rate than patients with high-grade tumors (75% vs. 25%, respectively).

V. PREVENTION AND EARLY DETECTION

A. **Early detection** depends on the patient's and physician's awareness of the disease, the presence of risk factors, and the histologic examination of all surgical specimens, even those removed from minor anorectal surgery. Yearly anoscopy may be indicated in high-risk patients. Anal examination should be performed routinely in patients with cervical and vulvar cancer.

B. **HPV vaccine.** Encouraging results from utilizing the HPV vaccination in high-risk groups have led to the use of quadrivalent and the 9-valent HPV vaccines being recommended in both males and females to prevent anal cancer and its precursor lesion. Ideally, these should be given before individuals become sexually active and exposed to HPV (aged 11 or 12 years). These measures will likely help reduce the burden of anal cancers in the long run.

VI. MANAGEMENT

Small tumors of the anal verge or the anal canal (<2 cm) can be cured in 80% of cases by simple excision with 1-cm margins, and cure by repeat local excision may be possible after local recurrence. An approach derived from Mohs surgery in which involved tissue is shaved and examined by a pathologist at the bedside until negative margins have been obtained is commonly done for Tis lesions. Combined chemotherapy and RT are the primary therapeutic modalities for more advanced anal verge or anal canal carcinoma. AP resection is now used as salvage treatment for chemoradiation-resistant disease (i.e., patients who fail to respond or who relapse after a complete response) and for patients who have fecal incontinence at presentation. Considering the rarity of anal canal cancer, randomized trials have led to considerable advances, shifting the standard of therapy from surgery, in which colostomy was routinely necessary as a first approach, to combined-modality chemoradiotherapy, leaving surgery as a last resort.

A. **Combined chemoradiation therapy** is the primary treatment of choice for anal carcinoma. This combination resulted in higher rates of both local control and survival (82%) and preserved anal function when compared with surgery. The administration of high-dose RT reduced the incidence of persistent carcinoma and eliminated the need for surgical lymphadenectomy. The radiation dose, the number of chemotherapy cycles required to improve the local control rate, and the role (if any) of invasive restaging after completion of therapy remain controversial.

1. **Primary therapy.** External beam RT appears to be superior to interstitial implants. RT doses of >5,000 cGy do not appear to be necessary. Using mitomycin C plus 5-FU with RT is superior to using 5-FU alone with RT at 4 years of median follow-up with respect to colostomy-free survival (71% vs. 59%), locoregional control (82% vs. 64%), and DFS (73% vs. 51%). The combination of these two drugs when administered concurrently with RT is superior to RT alone. RT regimens vary among institutions; 5-FU is given by continuous IV infusion in each case. Two useful regimens are as follows:

   a. **Radiation Therapy Oncology Group (RTOG)**
      Mitomycin C: 10 mg/m^2 IV bolus (day 2)
      5-FU: 1,000 mg/m^2/24 hours by continuous IV infusion (days 2 to 4 and days 28 to 32)
      RT: 170 cGy/d between days 1 and 28
      Total RT dose: 4,500 to 5,000 cGy

   b. **National Tumor Institute (Milan)**
      Mitomycin C: 15 mg/m^2 IV bolus (day 1)
      5-FU: 750 mg/m^2/24 hours by continuous IV infusion (days 1 to 5)
      RT: 180 cGy/d for 4 weeks with a 2-week rest
      Total RT dose: 5,400 cGy (in patients with locally advanced disease, the boost dose is increased but the total dose does not exceed 6,000 cGy)

2. **Follow-up therapy.** Additional 6-week cycles of chemotherapy with mitomycin C and 5-FU are given depending on tumor control or treatment toxicity. Patients are examined with imaging (PET/CT scans vs. MRIs) alongside digital examination and anoscopy at 3-month intervals for the first year and at 6-month intervals thereafter. AP resection is performed for biopsy-proven carcinoma during the follow-up period. Second-line chemotherapy with 5-FU plus cisplatin and AP resection are potentially curative salvage approaches after relapse. Myelosuppression can be significant from the mitomycin and 5-FU. Thrombotic thrombocytopenic purpura is an important side effect to be kept in mind in patients receiving mitomycin. This has been reported in the range of 4% to 15% in some studies.

B. **Surgery alone.** Wide, full-thickness excision is sufficient treatment for discrete, superficial, anal margin tumors and results in an 80% 5-year survival rate unless the tumor is large and deep. AP resection of the anorectum as the exclusive treatment for anal canal tumors and large anal margin tumors results in only a 55% 5-year survival rate.

C. **Follow-up** of patients with anal cancer every 3 months with digital rectal examination, anoscopy or proctoscopy, and biopsy of suspicious lesions is especially important during the first 3 years after initial treatment because salvage therapy may be curative.

PANCREATIC CANCER

I. EPIDEMIOLOGY AND ETIOLOGY

A. **Incidence.** In the United States, the incidence of pancreatic cancer has remained stable for several decades. There will be approximately 53,070 new cases diagnosed in 2016 in the United States and close to 41,000 deaths from pancreatic cancer, making it the third leading cause of US cancer deaths. The disease has a male-to-female ratio of 1:1 with a median age of 70 years at the time of diagnosis. Survival is extremely poor with approximately 5% of individuals surviving at the 5-years mark. Review of institutional databases reveals that even in individuals that receive an upfront surgical resection, the 10-year survival is <10% despite all the advances made in treatment over the years.

B. **Etiology and risk factors.** The cause of pancreatic adenocarcinoma remains unknown, but several factors show a modest association with its occurrence.

1. **Cigarette smoking** is a consistently noted risk factor for pancreatic cancer, with a relative risk of at least 1.5. The risk increases with increasing duration and amount of cigarette smoking. The risk is ascribed to tobacco-specific nitrosamines.

2. **Diet.** A high intake of fat, meat, or both is associated with increased risk, whereas the intake of fresh fruits and vegetables appears to have a protective effect.

3. **Partial gastrectomy** appears to correlate with a 2 to 5 times higher than expected incidence of pancreatic cancer 15 to 20 years later. The increased formation of N-nitroso compounds by bacteria that produce nitrate reductase and proliferate in the hypoacidic stomach has been proposed to account for the increased occurrence of gastric and pancreatic cancer after partial gastrectomy.

4. **Cholecystokinin** is the primary hormone that causes growth of exocrine pancreatic cells; others include epidermal growth factor and insulin-like growth factors. Pancreatic cancer has been induced experimentally by long-term duodenogastric reflux, which is associated with increased cholecystokinin levels. Some clinical evidence suggests that cholecystectomy, which also increases the circulating cholecystokinin, may increase the risk for pancreatic cancer.

5. **Diabetes mellitus** may be an early manifestation of pancreatic cancer or a predisposing factor. It is found in 13% of patients with pancreatic cancer and in only 2% of controls. Diabetes mellitus that occurs in patients with pancreatic cancer may be characterized by marked insulin resistance, which moderates after tumor resection. Islet amyloid polypeptide, a hormonal factor secreted by pancreatic B cells, reduces insulin sensitivity *in vivo* and glycogen synthesis *in vitro* and may be present in elevated concentrations in patients with pancreatic cancer who have diabetes.

6. **Chronic and hereditary pancreatitis** is associated with pancreatic cancer. Chronic pancreatitis is associated with a 15-fold increase in the risk for pancreatic cancer.

7. **Toxic substances.** Occupational exposure to 2-naphthylamine, benzidine, and gasoline derivatives is associated with a fivefold increased risk for pancreatic cancer. Prolonged exposure to DDT and two DDT derivatives (ethylan and DDD) is associated with a fourfold to sevenfold increased risk for pancreatic cancer.

8. **Socioeconomic status.** Pancreatic cancer occurs in a slightly higher frequency in populations of lower socioeconomic status.

9. **Coffee.** Analysis of 30 epidemiologic studies showed that only one case–control study and none of the prospective studies confirmed a statistically significant association between coffee consumption and pancreatic cancer.

10. **Idiopathic deep vein thrombosis** is statistically correlated with the subsequent development of mucinous carcinomas (including pancreatic cancer), especially among patients in whom venous thrombosis recurs during follow-up.

11. **Dermatomyositis and polymyositis** are paraneoplastic syndromes associated with pancreatic cancer and other cancers.

12. **Tonsillectomy** has been shown to be a protective factor against the development of pancreatic cancer, an observation that has been described for other cancers as well.

13. **Familial pancreatic cancer.** It is estimated that approximately 5% of pancreatic cancers are linked to inherited predisposition to the disease. Germline mutations have been identified in a few known cancer genes, such as the breast cancer susceptibility genes (especially *BRCA2*), that significantly increase the risk of developing pancreatic cancer especially earlier in life. There is, however, no clear consensus on screening in individuals identified with these germline mutations. Furthermore, individuals identified with these molecular alterations do not always have a family history. Genetic consultation and screening should be considered especially in younger patients and in those with a history of breast, ovarian, or early prostate cancers in the family.

II. PATHOLOGY

A. **Primary malignant tumors** of the pancreas involve either the exocrine parenchyma or the endocrine islet cells. Nonepithelial tumors (sarcomas and lymphomas) are rare. Ductal adenocarcinoma makes up 75% to 90% of malignant pancreatic neoplasms: 57% occur in the head of the pancreas, 9% in the body, 8% in the tail, 6% in overlapping sites, and 20% in unknown anatomic subsites. Uncommon but reasonably distinctive variants of pancreatic cancer include adenosquamous, oncocytic, clear cell, giant cell, signet ring, mucinous, and anaplastic carcinoma. Anaplastic carcinomas often involve the body and tail rather than the head of pancreas. Reported cases of pure epidermoid carcinoma (a variant of adenosquamous carcinoma) probably are associated with hypercalcemia. Cystadenocarcinomas have an indolent course and may remain localized for many years. Ampullary cancer (which carries a significantly better prognosis), duodenal cancer, and distal bile duct cancer may be difficult to distinguish from pancreatic adenocarcinoma.

B. **Metastatic tumors.** Autopsy studies show that for every primary tumor of the pancreas, four metastatic tumors are found. The most common tumors of origin are the breast, lung, cutaneous melanoma, and non-Hodgkin lymphoma.

C. **Genetic abnormalities.** Mutant *c-K-RAS* genes have been found in approximately 95% of all specimens of human pancreatic carcinoma and their metastases. Mutations in other DNA mismatch repair proteins and tumor suppressor genes including *BRCA1/2, PALB2, and ATM* genes are increasingly being recognized and constitute approximately 15% to 20% of the cases.

III. DIAGNOSIS

A. **Symptoms.** Most patients with pancreatic cancer have symptoms at the time of diagnosis. Predominant initial symptoms include abdominal pain (80%);

anorexia (65%); weight loss (60%); early satiety (60%); xerostomia and sleep problems (55%); jaundice (50%); easy fatigability (45%); weakness, nausea, or constipation (40%); depression (40%); dyspepsia (35%); vomiting (30%); hoarseness (25%); taste change, bloating, or belching (25%); dyspnea, dizziness, or edema (20%); cough, diarrhea because of fat malabsorption, hiccup, or itching (15%); and dysphagia (5%).

B. **Clinical findings.** At presentation, patients with pancreatic cancer have cachexia (44%), serum albumin concentration of <3.5 g/dL (35%), palpable abdominal mass (35%), ascites (25%), or supraclavicular lymphadenopathy (5%). Metastases are present to at least one major organ in 65% of patients, to the liver in 45%, to the lungs in 30%, and to the bones in 3%. Carcinomas of the distal pancreas do not produce jaundice until they metastasize and may remain painless until the disease is advanced. Occasionally, acute pancreatitis is the first manifestation of pancreatic cancer.

C. **Paraneoplastic syndromes.** Panniculitis–arthritis–eosinophilia syndrome that occurs with pancreatic cancer appears to be caused by the release of lipase from the tumor. Dermatomyositis, polymyositis, recurrent Trousseau syndrome or idiopathic deep vein thrombosis, and Cushing syndrome have been reported to be associated with cancer of the pancreas.

D. **Diagnostic studies**
   1. **Ultrasonography.** Abdominal ultrasound is technically adequate in 60% to 90% of patients and is noninvasive, safe, and inexpensive. Ultrasound can detect pancreatic masses as small as 2 cm, dilation of the pancreatic and bile ducts, hepatic metastases, and extrapancreatic spread. Intraoperative ultrasound facilitates surgical biopsy and may detect unsuspected liver metastases in 50% of patients.
   2. **CT** is less operator dependent than ultrasound and is not limited by air-containing abdominal organs, as is ultrasound. CT is favored over ultrasound because of its superior ability to demonstrate retroperitoneal invasion and lymphadenopathy. A pancreatic tumor must be at least 2 cm in diameter to become visible. *Dynamic CT* with continuous infusion of IV contrast (pancreas protocol) is the best test for assessing the size of the tumor and its extension. At least 20% of pancreatic tumors believed to be resectable may not be detectable by CT.
   3. **MRI** has no demonstrated advantage over CT in the diagnosis and staging of pancreatic cancer.
   4. **Endoscopic retrograde cholangiopancreaticography (ERCP)** is the mainstay in the differential diagnosis of the tumors of the pancreatobiliary junction, 85% of which originate in the pancreas (about 5% each in the distal common bile duct, ampulla, and duodenum). Ampullary and duodenal carcinomas can usually be visualized and biopsy performed with ERCP. The pancreatogram typically shows the pancreatic duct to be encased or obstructed by carcinoma in 97% of cases.

      It may be difficult to distinguish between pancreatic cancer and chronic pancreatitis because both diseases share clinical and radiologic characteristics. Pancreatic duct stricture usually does not exceed 5 mm in chronic pancreatitis; strictures longer than 10 mm (especially if irregular) indicate pancreatic cancer. Cytologic examination of cells in samples of pancreatic juice obtained during ERCP with secretin stimulation has been reported to be highly specific for the diagnosis of carcinoma and 85% sensitive. Brush biopsy of the pancreatic stricture (when possible) increases the diagnostic yield.

5. **EUS.** Prospective studies showed that EUS is more accurate than standard ultrasound, CT, and ERCP for diagnosis, staging, and predicting resectability of pancreatic tumors. EUS detected 100% of malignant lesions <3 cm, whereas angiography, CT, and ultrasound were of limited value for these small lesions. EUS can detect tumors smaller than 2 cm; ERCP cannot. The additional information obtained from EUS has been reported to result in a major change in the clinical management in one-third of patients and to aid in the clinical decision in three-fourths of patients.

The current limitations of EUS include a short optimal focal range of only 4 cm, inability to differentiate focal chronic pancreatitis from carcinoma reliably, and inability to differentiate chronic lymphadenitis from metastatic lymph node involvement. The ability to biopsy lymph nodes using EUS does allow assessment of lymph nodes for malignancy in some cases.

6. **Percutaneous fine needle aspiration cytology** is safe and reliable, with a reported sensitivity of 55% to 95% and no false-positive results for the diagnosis of pancreatic cancer. This procedure should be performed for histologic confirmation on all patients with unresectable or metastatic disease unless a palliative surgical procedure is planned. Needle aspiration cytology distinguishes adenocarcinoma from islet cell tumors, lymphomas, and cystic neoplasms of the pancreas, permitting therapy to be tailored to the specific diagnosis in each case.

The drawbacks to percutaneous aspiration biopsy include potential tumor seeding along the needle tract, potential to enhance intraperitoneal spread, and negative biopsy results that do not exclude the diagnosis of malignancy. Furthermore, the diagnosis of early and smaller tumors is most likely to be missed by this technique.

7. **Angiography** is excellent for assessing major vascular involvement but is not useful in determining the size and location of tumor (pancreatic cancer is hypovascular). In most cases, spiral CT scanning with proper administration of IV contrast allows resectability to be judged preoperatively.

8. **Laparoscopy** can demonstrate extrapancreatic involvement in 40% of patients without demonstrable lesions on CT.

9. **Tumor markers.** No available serum marker is sufficiently sensitive or specific to be considered reliable for screening of pancreatic cancer. CA 19-9 is widely used for the diagnosis and follow-up of patients with pancreatic cancer but is not specific for pancreatic cancer. Some studies have shown the actual levels of the CA-19-9 to be predictive of advanced disease at the time of diagnosis and the actual falls of the marker with therapy to be predictive of survival as well in a select proportion of patients. There is a lot of individual variations in this biomarker, and there are patients with advanced disease who have undetectable CA-19-9 levels ("nonproducers").

IV. STAGING AND PROGNOSTIC FACTORS

A. **Staging system.** Refer to the current AJCC Cancer Staging atlas for TNM staging system. The most important distinction to be made in patients with pancreatic cancer is metastatic versus nonmetastatic and, within the latter, resectable versus nonresectable.

B. **Preoperative evaluation.** Identifying patients with unresectable pancreatic tumor or with metastasis or vessel involvement would spare many patients a major operation. Operative mortality and morbidity for pancreatic surgery remain high, except in specialized centers. Modern diagnostic methods have reduced unnecessary laparotomies from 30% to 5% and have increased the resectability rate on patients judged to be potentially resectable on the basis of preoperative imaging from 5% to 20%. Accuracy in determining resectability before exploration has become even more important because of the availability of effective decompression of biliary obstruction endoscopically for palliation of obstructive jaundice without the need for laparotomy.

CT, angiography, and laparoscopy assess different aspects of resectability and are complementary. In general, if one of these studies indicates vascular invasion or local or regional spread, the resectability rate is about 5%, whereas if all are negative, the resectability rate is 78%. Gross nodal involvement is usually associated with other signs of unresectability and may be identified by CT or EUS.

C. Prognostic factors. Fewer than 20% of patients with adenocarcinoma of the pancreas survive the first year, and only 5% are alive 5 years after the diagnosis.

  1. Resectable disease. The 5-year survival rate of patients whose tumors were resected is poor; the reported range is 3% to 25%. The 5-year survival is 30% for patients with small tumors (≤ 2 cm in diameter), 35% for patients with no residual tumor or for patients in whom the tumor did not require dissection from major vessels, and 55% for patients without lymph node metastasis.

  2. Nonresectable or metastatic disease. The median survival of patients with such disease previously was 2 to 6 months. Performance status and the presence of four symptoms (dyspnea, anorexia, weight loss, and xerostomia) appear to influence survival; patients with the higher performance status and the least number of these symptoms lived the longest. With advent of more effective chemotherapy regimens, median survival in clinical trials has increased to close to 9 months with doublet chemotherapy regimens (gemcitabine/nab-paclitaxel) and approximately 11 months with a triplet chemotherapy regimen (FOLFIRINOX).

V. MANAGEMENT

A. Surgery. Only 5% to 20% of patients with pancreatic cancer have resectable tumors at the time of presentation.

  1. Surgical procedures

    a. Pancreaticoduodenal resection (Whipple procedure or a modification) is the standard operation. This implies that only cancer involving the head of the pancreas is resectable.

    b. A pylorus-preserving variation of Whipple procedure is a commonly used operation in the United States, in part because it has resulted in a significant reduction of postgastrectomy syndrome with no decrease in survival.

    c. An extended Whipple procedure, with a more extensive lymph node dissection, is used commonly in Japan but has not been widely accepted in the United States because of higher morbidity and lack of data from randomized trials to suggest that the procedure results in better survival.

    d. Regional pancreatectomy confers no survival advantage over conventional Whipple procedure.

    e. Total pancreatectomy produces exocrine insufficiency and brittle diabetes mellitus and should be performed only when necessary to achieve clear surgical margins.

  2. Surgical mortality and morbidity. The perioperative mortality rate from pancreatic resection is <5% when the operation is performed by expert surgeons. Nationally, however, the surgical mortality rate is about 18%. The major complication rate is 20% to 35% and includes sepsis, abscess formation, hemorrhage, and pancreatic and biliary fistulae.

3. **Relief of obstructive jaundice by surgical biliary bypass** (cholecystojejunostomy or choledochojejunostomy) is effective, but the average survival time is 5 months, and the postoperative mortality rate in large collected series is 20%. Jaundice can be relieved endoscopically by the placement of stents with a success rate of up to 85%, a procedure-related mortality rate of 1% to 2%, and significant reduction in the length of hospitalization and recovery compared with palliative surgery. Randomized trials showed no difference in survival between endoscopic stent placement and surgical bypass, but patients treated with stents had more frequent readmissions for stent obstruction, recurrent jaundice, and cholangitis.

B. **Adjuvant therapy** appears to be a reasonable approach to the patient who has undergone curative resection.

1. **Chemotherapy.** Prior trials assessing the potential benefit of adjuvant chemotherapy have shown mixed results. However, in a phase III trial, 368 patients were randomized to either observation alone or six cycles of gemcitabine following gross complete resection. Significant improvement was noted in DFS, but only a trend toward benefit in overall survival.

2. **Combined-modality therapy.** There is one prospective randomized study of only 43 patients (completed by the Gastrointestinal Study Group in the 1980s) that showed that adjuvant RT and 5-FU after a curative Whipple procedure improved survival. In that study, the median survival was 20 months for patients treated, and 3 of 21 patients survived 5 years or more. For patients not treated, the median survival was 11 months, and only 1 of 22 patients survived 5 years. The 5-year survival rate was 40% for patients with no lymph node involvement and <5% for patients with lymph node metastasis.

An RTOG trial randomized patients to either gemcitabine or infusional 5-FU after surgery. Both groups also received radiation. The results of this trial showed a nonsignificant improvement in survival for patients receiving gemcitabine, primarily in those with cancer arising from the head of the pancreas. The trial did not demonstrate the true benefit of adjuvant RT. Standard practices vary, and currently, combined-modality therapy employing chemoradiation is generally considered for patients with margin-positive and/or node-positive disease; however, its true benefit and utility are controversial.

C. **Therapy for locally advanced disease**

The recent years have seen a lot of therapy move from the adjuvant to the neoadjuvant setting. With the advent of more effective chemotherapy regimens, similar to colorectal cancers, a "conversion therapy" is now favored for patients deemed unresectable or borderline resectable initially. Since there is definite overall survival benefit to systemic chemotherapy, most of these approaches depending on institution and surgeons' preference would employ upfront chemotherapy in the form of FOLFIRINOX for approximately 4 cycles (2 months of treatment) or gemcitabine with nab-paclitaxel for approximately 2 cycles (2 months of treatment). This is followed by a reevaluation to assess tolerability and response to treatment followed by considerations toward more chemotherapy versus doing chemoradiation with later plans for surgical resection if possible. The overall survival benefit of chemoradiation is not entirely clear. This approach, however, does allow for better local control and longer time off of systemic therapy.

1. **External beam RT combined with 5-FU** (15 mg/kg IV on the first 3 and last 3 days of RT) significantly improves survival as compared with RT alone (10 vs. 5.5 months, respectively) in an older trial. Consideration should be

given to the use of continuous infusion 5-FU, capecitabine, or gemcitabine during irradiation, although there are no randomized trials to suggest incremental benefit of these options over bolus 5-FU in pancreatic cancer. The main benefit is in decreased toxicity.

2. **Intraoperative electron beam RT** delivered to a surgically exposed tumor from which radiosensitive bowel has been excluded by insertion of a field-limiting cone increased the median survival compared with historical controls in selected patients to 13 months, with excellent local control (5% of patients have lived 3 to 8 years). Intraoperative RT relieves pain in 50% to 90% of patients.

D. **Chemotherapy for metastatic disease** (Fig. 10-3).

1. **5-FU.** 5-FU has a RR of 0% to 20% in pancreatic cancer. Given its low RR and poor impact on overall survival, 5-FU used alone is not an option for most patients.

2. **Gemcitabine.** Weekly gemcitabine at a dose of 1,000 mg/m^2 for 3 of every 4 weeks has been shown to have activity and to provide palliative benefit exceeding that of 5-FU in a randomized trial of 126 patients with advanced disease. The median survival times were 5.6 versus 4.4 months ($p = 0.002$)

Line of therapy	Classification Based on Performance Status ± Age			
	Excellent Performance Status and Young Age	Excellent Performance Status and Advanced Age[a]	Poor Performance Status Young Age[a]	Poor Performance Status and/or Advanced age
1	FOLFIRINOX	Gemcitabine + nab-paclitaxel	Gemcitabine + nab-paclitaxel	Gemcitabine or Fluoropyrimidine-based CT
2	Gemcitabine + nab-paclitaxel	Irinotecan Nanoliposomal Injection (ILI) + 5 FU/LV	Irinotecan Nanoliposomal Injection (ILI) + 5 FU/LV	BSC
3	Irinotecan Nanoliposomal Injection (ILI) + 5 FU/LV[b]	BSC	BSC	
4	BSC			

[a] Usually excellent performance status refers to patients with an Eastern Cooperative Oncology Group (ECOG) of 0–1 and poor performance status as ECOG > 1. Age typically considered as advanced would be age > 70 years. The cutoff and definitions of both of these variables, however, are somewhat arbitrary. Aggressive chemotherapy maybe appropriate for somebody with advanced age who is in otherwise excellent health.

[b] Patients who have already received irinotecan chemotherapy with FOLFIRINOX may not derive as much benefit from the Irinotecan Nanoliposomal Injection.

Abbreviations: BSC, best supportive care; CT, chemotherapy; 5-FU/LV, 5-fluorouracil and leucovorin.

Figure 10-3 Treatment algorithm for the practical medical management of **metastatic pancreatic cancer**–based performance status ± age.

for gemcitabine versus 5-FU, respectively. A potentially promising alternative schedule for the administration of gemcitabine using fixed-dose rate infusion compared with the standard 30-minute infusion did not show benefit in a phase III trial. The administration of multiagent chemotherapy has generally not resulted in better outcomes than single-agent therapy. Several phase III trials comparing gemcitabine alone with gemcitabine and either oxaliplatin, bevacizumab, or cetuximab have all failed to show benefit. However, a statistically significant improvement was seen in overall survival (6.2 vs. 5.9 months) when erlotinib was added to gemcitabine. Since this benefit is not clinically meaningful, erlotinib is usually not used in this setting. The approval of erlotinib in this setting shows the dire need for active agents for patients with advanced pancreatic cancer.

3. **FOLFIRINOX.** In a randomized phase III trial, the combination of 5-FU, irinotecan, and oxaliplatin provided significantly better outcomes compared to gemcitabine. Overall survival improved from approximately 7 months with gemcitabine to 11 months with FOLFIRINOX. In good performance status patients, FOLFIRINOX should be considered as an option.

   Oxaliplatin 85 mg/m^2 over 2 hours, day 1

   Leucovorin 400 mg/m^2 over 2 hours, day 1

   Irinotecan 180 mg/m^2 as 90 min infusion, day 1

   5-FU 400 mg/m^2 bolus, day 1 (bolus 5-FU is commonly omitted in clinical practice)

   5-FU 2,400 mg/m^2 as a 46-hour infusion, days 1 to 2

4. **Gemcitabine with nab-paclitaxel.** In a randomized trial, the combination of gemcitabine with nab-paclitaxel provided significantly better overall survival as compared to gemcitabine alone (8.5 months vs. 6.7 months). This is one of the most frequently employed first-line chemotherapy regimens in patients with advanced pancreatic cancer.

5. **Irinotecan liposome injection (ILI) with 5-FU/LV.** More recently, 5-fluorouracil with leucovorin (5-FU/LV) in combination with MM-398 (nal-Iri, a nanoliposomal encapsulation of irinotecan) was approved for pancreatic cancer because the combination achieved a median OS of 6.1 months. This combination is approved for patients with advanced pancreatic cancer that are deemed gemcitabine refractory (Fig. 10-3).

E. **Neuroablation for pain control.** The relentless, boring, posterior abdominal and back pain caused when the celiac nerve plexus becomes invaded by pancreatic cancer can be extremely distressing and frequently requires the use of large doses of narcotics, particularly sustained-release morphine. Chemical splanchnicectomy (celiac axis nerve block) should be performed at the time of operation in nonresectable cases. Either 6% phenol or 50% alcohol (25 mL is injected on each side of the celiac axis) is used. This procedure results in relief of pancreatic cancer-related pain in >80% of patients. Percutaneous chemical neurolysis of the celiac ganglion, which may be attempted in patients who did not have an intraoperative splanchnicectomy or were not explored, is reported to be equally effective. Transient postural hypotension may occur. Celiac plexus block may be repeated if initially unsuccessful or if pain recurs.

F. **Other supportive measures.** Appetite suppression, decreased caloric intake, and malabsorption can all lead to cancer cachexia in patients with pancreatic cancer. Megestrol acetate suspension in doses up to 800 mg/d can be an effective appetite stimulant for treatment of anorexia. Calorie supplements are also potentially valuable. Fat malabsorption resulting from loss of the exocrine function of the pancreas responds to pancreatic enzyme replacement. Ascites can be managed with diuretics when possible and paracentesis when necessary. Removal of protein-rich ascitic fluid, however, can become an additional contributor to the negative protein balance in these already malnourished patients.

LIVER CANCER

I. EPIDEMIOLOGY AND ETIOLOGY

A. **Incidence.** Liver cancer is among the most common neoplasms and causes of cancer death in the world, occurring most commonly in Africa and Asia. Up to one million deaths due to hepatocellular carcinoma (HCC) occur each year worldwide. In the United States, 17,000 new cases of cancer of the liver and biliary passages develop annually. Incidence throughout the world varies dramatically, with 115 cases per 100,000 people noted in China and Thailand, compared with 1 to 2 cases per 100,000 in Britain. In countries with high incidence rates, there are often subpopulations also with high incidence rates living nearby lower risk subpopulations. For example, the incidence rates in black South Africans and Alaska Natives far exceed those of nearby white populations. HCC is four to nine times more common in men than in women.

B. **Conditions predisposing to HCC**

1. **Hepatitis B virus (HBV).** High titers of hepatitis B surface antigen (HBsAg) and core antibody (HBcAb) are frequently found in patients with HCC. HBsAg was found in the serum of 50% to 60% of patients with HCC and in 5% to 10% of the general population. In the United States, HCC is increased by 140-fold in HBsAg carriers. Anti-HBcAb was found in 90% of black South African and 75% of Japanese patients with HCC, as compared with 35% and 30% of matched controls, respectively. When HCC develops, the patient usually has had chronic HBV infection for three to four decades. The risk factors for the development of HCC in HBsAg carriers are the presence of cirrhosis, family history of HCC, increasing age, male sex, Asian or African race, cofactors (such as alcohol, aflatoxin, and perhaps smoking), and the duration of the carrier state. In Asia, HBV is transmitted vertically from mother to infant in the first few months of life; in Africa, HBV is transmitted horizontally.

2. **Cirrhosis.** HCC often develops in a cirrhotic liver. Autopsy studies showed that 60% to 90% of HBsAg-positive subjects have associated cirrhosis and 20% to 40% of patients with cirrhosis have HCC. Studies show that in Taiwan, the annual estimated incidence of HCC is 0.005% in HBsAg-negative patients, 0.25% in HBsAg-positive patients, and 2.5% in HBsAg-positive patients with liver cirrhosis (500 times higher than in HBsAg-negative patients). In France, the development of HCC in the presence of alcoholic cirrhosis was nearly always associated with HBV infection, and alcoholism was thought to hasten the development of HCC. In Italy, the prevalence of HCC in patients with cirrhosis was nearly 7%, with a yearly crude incidence of 3%; hepatitis C virus (HCV) chronic infection was the cause of cirrhosis in 45% of these patients. A clear association between alcohol-induced cirrhosis and HCC exists; associations between alcohol and HCC in the absence of cirrhosis are less clear.

3. **HCV infection** is a risk factor for the development of HCC. Apparently, HCV induces cirrhosis and to a lesser extent increases the risks for HCC in patients with cirrhosis. HCV infection acts independently of HBV infection, alcohol abuse, age, and gender. The ratios for HCC risk factors in patients with chronic liver disease, adjusted for age, sex, and other factors, are as follows:

a. Risk ratio six- to sevenfold: age, 60 to 69 years; HBsAg positive

b. Risk ratio fourfold: high-titer anti-HBcAb, anti-HCV positivity

c. Risk ratio twofold: presence of liver cirrhosis, currently smoking

4. **Aflatoxins** are produced by the ubiquitous fungi *Aspergillus flavus* or *Aspergillus parasiticus*, which commonly colonize peanuts, corn, and cassava in all except extremely cold climates. Aflatoxin B1 has been proved to be a potent hepatocarcinogen in experimental animals, and the amount of exposure is correlated with increased HCC risk in humans. For example, the daily intake of aflatoxin in Mozambique is four times greater than in Kenya, and the incidence of HCC is eight times greater.

5. **Mutations of tumor suppressor gene *p53*** have been reported in half of patients with HCC. These mutations, specifically of 249^{ser} *p53*, are correlated both with geographic areas where the ingestion of aflatoxin is common and with the prevalence of HBV infection.

6. **Sex hormones.** The risk for liver cell adenomas and HCC is increased in women who have used oral contraceptives for 8 or more years. Although liver cell adenomas regress with discontinuation of oral contraceptives in most cases, adenomas must be considered premalignant. Close and prolonged follow-up is necessary for women with adenomas who continue to use oral contraceptives. HCC has also been observed in people with a history of anabolic steroid use.

7. **Cigarette smoking, alcohol intake, diabetes, and insulin intake.** A study performed in Los Angeles showed that in non-Asian populations that have a low risk for HCC, cigarette smoking, heavy alcohol consumption, and diabetes mellitus, especially with insulin administration, appear to be significant risk factors for HCC.

8. **Nonalcoholic steatohepatitis (NASH).** It is becoming an increasingly important risk factor, accounting for approximately 10% of all risk factors for HCC. It is associated with fatty infiltration in the liver and is most commonly seen in obese patients.

9. **Other factors.** A relatively small number of HCCs develop in patients with various other diseases. The most common of these are a_1-antitrypsin deficiency, tyrosinemia, and hemochromatosis. Phlebotomy therapy can deplete hepatic iron and induce regression of hepatic fibrosis but does not prevent the development of HCC in hemochromatosis. Clonorchiasis, vinyl chloride exposure, and administration of thorium dioxide (an x-ray contrast agent used between 1930 and 1955) or methotrexate are also associated with the development of HCC.

II. PATHOLOGY AND NATURAL HISTORY

A. Pathology

1. **Liver cell adenoma** has low malignant potential. True adenomas of the liver are rare and occur mostly in women taking oral contraceptives. Most adenomas are solitary; occasionally, multiple (10 or more) tumors develop in a condition known as *liver cell adenomatosis*. These tumors are smooth, encapsulated masses and do not contain Kupffer cells. Patients usually have symptoms; hemoperitoneum occurs in 25% of cases.

2. **Focal nodular hyperplasia** (FNH) has no malignant potential. FNH occurs with a female-to-male ratio of 2:1. The relationship of oral contraceptives to FNH is not as clear as for hepatic adenoma; only half of patients with FNH take oral contraceptives. FNH tumors are nodular,

are not encapsulated, but do contain Kupffer cells. Patients usually do not have symptoms; hemoperitoneum rarely occurs.

3. **HCC** may present grossly as a single mass, as multiple nodules, or as diffuse liver involvement; these are referred to as *massive*, *nodular*, and *diffuse* forms. The growth pattern microscopically is trabecular, solid, or tubular, and the stroma, in contrast to bile duct carcinoma, is scanty. A rare sclerosing or fibrosing form has been associated with hypercalcemia. Fibrolamellar carcinoma, another variant, occurs predominantly in young patients without cirrhosis, has a favorable prognosis, and is not associated with elevation of serum α-fetoprotein (FP) levels. In the United States, almost half of HCCs in patients younger than 35 years of age are fibrolamellar, and more than half of them are resectable.

B. **Natural history.** Most patients die from hepatic failure and not from distant metastases. The disease is contained within the liver in only 20% of cases. HCC invades the portal vein in 35% of cases, hepatic vein in 15%, contiguous abdominal organs in 15%, and vena cava and right atrium in 5%. HCC metastasizes to the lung in 35% of cases, abdominal lymph nodes in 20%, thoracic or cervical lymph nodes in 5%, vertebrae in 5%, and kidney or adrenal gland in 5%.

C. **Associated paraneoplastic syndromes** include fever, erythrocytosis, hypercholesterolemia, gynecomastia, hypercalcemia, hypoglycemia, and virilization (precocious puberty).

III. DIAGNOSIS

A. **Symptoms and signs.** Pain in the right subcostal area or on top of the shoulder from phrenic irritation is common (95%). Severe symptoms of fatigue (31%), anorexia (27%), weight loss (35%), and unexplained fever (30% to 40%) are not uncommon. Many patients have vague abdominal pain, fever, and anorexia for up to 2 years before the diagnosis of carcinoma is made. Hemorrhage into the peritoneal cavity is often seen in patients with HCC and may be fatal. Ascites or the presence of an upper abdominal mass noticeable by the patient is an ominous prognostic sign. Any sudden deterioration in a patient with known liver disease or with positive HbsAg or hepatitis C serology should raise the suspicion of HCC. Physical findings include hepatomegaly (90%), splenomegaly (65%), ascites (52%), fever (38%), jaundice (41%), hepatic bruit (28%), and cachexia (15%).

B. **Diagnostic studies**

1. **LFTs** may be normal or elevated and are affected by liver cirrhosis. Elevated serum bilirubin and lactate dehydrogenase values and lowered serum albumin are associated with poor survival. Serum γ-glutamyl transferase (GGT) isoenzyme II (of 11 isoenzymes) was positive in 90% of patients with HCC. GGT-II was negative in most patients with acute and chronic viral hepatitis or extrahepatic tumors, in pregnant women, and in healthy controls. GGT-II was found to be valuable for the detection of small or subclinical HCC.

2. **Biopsy of liver nodules.** Some authors believe that percutaneous liver biopsy carries a high risk and has little or no role in the workup of liver tumors, whereas others believe that it can be performed without any significant risk. Nevertheless, liver biopsy is needed to establish the diagnosis and may be obtained either at operation or percutaneously.

3. **Serum tumor markers.** Serum AFP is often elevated in patients with HCC but can also be elevated in patients with benign chronic liver disease. In patients with liver cirrhosis and no HCC, serum AFP may be normal or elevated, with values ranging from 30 to 460 ng/mL (median, 30 to 70 ng/mL). In patients with HCC, the serum α-FP concentrations may range from 30 to 7,000 ng/mL (median, 275 ng/mL). Measurement of AFP fractions L3, P4, and P5 (different sugar chain structures) may allow the differentiation of HCC from cirrhosis in some cases. It may also be predictive for the development of HCC during follow-up of patients with cirrhosis. Serum ferritin levels are also frequently elevated in patients with HCC.

4. **Radiologic studies**
   a. **Ultrasound.** HCC is usually well circumscribed, hyperechogenic, and associated with diffuse distortion of the normal hepatic parenchyma. Metastatic deposits are usually hyperechogenic but may be hypoechogenic.
   b. **CT.** HCC typically appears as an area of low attenuation on CT. Lesions may occasionally be isodense with normal hepatic parenchyma, however. Metastatic tumors with low attenuation (close to the density of water) include mucin-producing tumors of the ovary, pancreas, colon, and stomach and tumors with necrotic centers, such as sarcomas. Mucin-producing metastases may have nearly normal attenuation values because of diffuse microscopic calcifications within the tumor.
   c. **MRI** has been reported to be superior to CT scanning and ultrasound for the detection of liver tumors.
   d. **Selective hepatic, celiac, and superior mesenteric angiography** can confirm portal vein involvement, define the arterial supply, and identify vascular lesions that are as small as 3 mm in diameter. Intra-arterial epinephrine injection can differentiate normal hepatic arteries from tumor vessels, which do not constrict because of the absence of smooth muscles in their walls.

IV. STAGING AND PROGNOSTIC FACTORS

A. **Staging.** The initial step is to establish whether the HCC is resectable. Indications of unresectability may be determined by exploratory laparotomy, by laparoscopy, or by CT, MRI, or angiography. Unresectable disease includes bilobar or four-segment hepatic parenchymal involvement, portal vein thrombus, and vena caval involvement with tumor or tumor thrombus. Metastatic disease includes involvement of regional lymph nodes, which is proved by biopsy at surgery. Liver failure or portal hypertension alone does not contraindicate surgery. Refer to the current AJCC Cancer Staging atlas for TNM staging system. While a variety of staging systems exist, the Barcelona Clinic Liver Cancer (BCLC) staging system has commonly been used to help direct therapeutic options. The BCLC staging system, the Child-Pugh and Okuda classification systems for underlying liver disease, and other clinical characteristics of the HCC help guide clinical decision making about treatment options such as resection, transplantation, ablation, embolization, or systemic therapy.

B. **Prognostic factors.** The number of liver lesions and the presence of vascular involvement are the most significant prognostic determinants in patients with disease limited to the liver. Neither the presence nor the degree of α-FP elevation has any prognostic importance. The prognostic factors that relate to survival in patients with resectable HCC are as follows:
   1. **Number, size, and location of liver lesions.** The 5-year survival rate for patients with a solitary tumor is 45%, and it is 15% to 25% for those with

multiple liver lesions. The 5-year survival rate is 40% to 45% for patients with small tumors (2 to 5 cm) and 10% for patients with tumors larger than 5 cm. Patients without cirrhosis with tumors located in the left lobe of the liver or in the right inferior segments (anteriorly or posteriorly) have the best prognosis.

2. **Vein involvement.** All patients with gross tumor thrombi involving the portal vein or the hepatic vein die within 3 years, whereas the 5-year survival rate for patients with no vascular involvement of any kind is 30%.

3. **Extent and type of resection.** The 5-year survival rate for patients undergoing curative resection is 55%, compared with 5% for those undergoing noncurative resections. The 5-year survival rate is 85% for hepatic lobectomy, 50% for subsegmentectomy, and 20% for wedge enucleation. In patients with resected HCC, the liver is the site of disease recurrence in 90% of cases.

4. **Hepatic reserve.** Determining underlying liver function is important in providing a prognosis as well as determining the ability of patients to tolerate therapy. The widely used Child-Pugh classification of severity of liver disease provides a simple clinical scoring system to estimate liver function and is commonly employed in HCC staging systems.

V. PREVENTION AND EARLY DETECTION

A. **Prevention.** Avoidance of the risk factors for HCC is difficult in those parts of the world where socioeconomic conditions are poor and where HBV infection is endemic. The widespread use of HBV vaccine may affect the incidence of HCC, but with a considerable lag time.

1. Almost four billion people (75% of the world population) live in areas of intermediate or higher prevalence of HBV. Infections with HBV and HCV can be treated with interferons, although prevention of initial infection is preferable. Protection against HBV, if attempted, is best done in infancy. In the United States, vaccination with recombinant HBsAg is recommended for health workers in contact with blood, for people residing for >6 months in areas that are highly endemic for HBV, and for all others at risk.

2. Steps should be taken to reduce the high levels of aflatoxin food contaminations that occur in many areas of Asia and southern Africa, as has been done in the Western world.

B. **Early detection.** Reports describing attempts for early detection of HCC in patients with liver cirrhosis have higher incidence of HCC (3% per year) in individuals with persistently high AFP levels than those with fluctuating levels. This screening program did not appreciably increase the rate of detection of potentially curable liver tumors, however. In another study from Japan, higher percentages of AFP L3, P4, and P5 fractions allowed the differentiation of HCC in some cases.

VI. MANAGEMENT

A. **Liver anatomy.** The liver is anatomically divided into four lobes: a larger right lobe, which is separated from a smaller left lobe by the attachment of the falciform ligament, and two small lobes (the quadrate lobe on the anterior inferior aspect and the caudate lobe). Practical surgical anatomy divides the liver into nearly equal halves, and each half is divided into two segments. The right half is divided into anterior (ventrocranial) and posterior (dorsocaudal) segments. The left half is divided into medial and lateral segments by a visible left sagittal accessory fissure. Each of the four segments is subdivided into superior and inferior subsegments. The French literature labels the eight liver subsegments with Roman numerals.

B. **Localized and resectable HCC.** Only 10% of HCCs are resectable with solitary or unilobar hepatic lesions at the time of diagnosis. The survival in resectable lesions depends on the prognostic factors as discussed earlier. In the United States, the median survival after surgical resection is about 22 months for patients with cirrhotic livers and 32 months for patients with normal livers (range, 2 months to 15 years). The perioperative morbidity is minimal and is slightly higher in the cirrhotic group. Morbidity includes subphrenic abscess, subhepatic abscess, pneumothorax, and wound infection. Total hepatectomy with orthotopic liver transplantation may be of benefit in patients with unresectable nonmetastatic fibrolamellar HCC, intrahepatic bile duct cancers, or hemangiosarcoma.

C. **Localized and nonresectable disease**
  1. **Preoperative multimodality treatment followed by surgery.** There are no current preoperative approaches that have been shown to be of benefit.
  2. **Transcatheter arterial chemoembolization (TACE)** of unresectable HCC using a mixture of Gelfoam powder, Lipiodol, and contrast media with chemotherapeutic drugs has been used with some success. TACE may also be used preoperatively to reduce intraoperative bleeding or as a palliative measure in patients with far advanced HCC. Recent trials with TACE suggest that there may be a survival advantage with its use.
  3. **Transcatheter arterial radioembolization (TARE)** is a newer modality that uses tumor ablation by transarterial injection of Y90 radioactive microspheres following the principles of transarterial chemoembolization. TARE has not been as rigorously studied as TACE. Early uncontrolled studies suggest that there is a risk of progressive long-term liver decompensation in patients with more advanced liver disease at the time of treatment initiation.
  4. **Other treatments.** Percutaneous intralesional installation of absolute ethanol under ultrasound guidance has resulted in a reported 5-year survival rate of nearly 80% in highly selected patients, particularly those with small tumors who are not surgical candidates. The use of radiofrequency ablation has become a common alternative to ethanol ablation. Radiofrequency ablation is performed by applying a high-frequency electrical current through a treatment probe that is inserted into the HCC. Cryosurgery has been reported to have similar efficacy in highly selected patients.

D. **Nonresectable and metastatic disease**
  1. **Targeted and antiangiogenic therapy** has shown early evidence of promise. In a randomized phase III trial comparing sorafenib with best supportive care, a significant increase in overall survival of approximately 2.5 months was seen with the use of sorafenib in patients with Child-Pugh A liver disease. Tolerability of the drug, however, can be an issue and does affect quality of life of these individuals. Therapy with sorafenib has to be weighed against the side effects associated with this drug.
  2. **Systemic chemotherapy** has a RR of 10% or less and does not affect median survival (3 to 6 months). Doxorubicin as a single agent or in combination with other drugs has been used. Doublet chemotherapy with FOLFOX has reported responses in isolated case reports. Other than in highly selected circumstances, the use of chemotherapy is generally not recommended.

GALLBLADDER CANCER

I. EPIDEMIOLOGY AND ETIOLOGY

A. **Incidence.** Primary gallbladder carcinoma (GBC) is the most common malignant tumor of the biliary tract and the fifth most common cancer of the digestive tract. It would be an estimated 39,230 new cases of GBC in 2016 in the United States. GBCs were found in 1% to 2% of operations on the biliary tract.

B. Risk factors. The cause of GBC remains unknown. Reported risk factors include the following:

1. **Sex.** The female-to-male ratio is 3:1 to 4:1. Acalculous carcinoma is also more common in women.

2. **Race.** The incidence of GBC is doubled in southwestern American Indians, who also have a twofold to threefold greater incidence of cholelithiasis. The incidence of GBC is also high in Peru and Ecuador among populations with Native American genealogy.

3. **Older age.** The mean age for the occurrence of GBC is 65 years; the disease is rare before 40 years of age.

4. **Chronic cholecystitis and cholelithiasis** are associated with the development of GBC in 50% and 75% of cases, respectively. Latency periods are lengthy; 1% of patients known to have gallstones for >20 years develop GBC. Those with larger stones are more prone to GBC than those with stones smaller than 1 cm. The incidence of GBC is decreasing among populations in the world where cholecystectomy is becoming more common. Calcification of the wall of the gallbladder (porcelain gallbladder) increases the risk for GBC by 10% to 60%. Cholecystitis associated with liver flukes and in chronic typhoid carriers is linked to the increased incidence of GBC.

5. **Benign neoplasms.** Both inflammatory and cholesterol polyps are associated with appreciable risk. Papillary and nonpapillary adenomas of the gallbladder may contain carcinoma *in situ*. Malignant transformation is rare, however.

6. **Ulcerative colitis** increases the risk for extrahepatic biliary cancer by a factor of 5 to 10; 15% of these cancers occur in the gallbladder.

7. **Carcinogens.** Rubber industry employees have a higher incidence and earlier onset of GBC.

II. PATHOLOGY AND NATURAL HISTORY

A. Pathology. Most GBCs are adenocarcinomas (80%) showing varying degrees of differentiation. The mucus secreted by this cancer is typically of the sialomucin type, in contrast to the sulfomucin type secreted by the normal or inflamed mucus-secreting glands. Other types of GBC include adenoacanthoma, adenosquamous carcinomas, and undifferentiated (anaplastic, pleomorphic, sarcomatoid) carcinomas. Some adenocarcinomas have choriocarcinoma-like elements, and others have morphology equivalent to small cell carcinoma.

B. Natural history. GBC has a propensity to involve the liver, stomach, and duodenum by direct extension. The common sites of metastasis are the liver (60%), adjacent organs (55%), regional lymph nodes (35%), peritoneum (25%), and distant visceral organs (30%).

C. Clinical presentation. GBC may present as one of the following clinical syndromes:

1. **Acute cholecystitis** (15% of patients). These patients appear to have less advanced carcinoma, a higher rate of resectability, and longer survival.

2. **Chronic cholecystitis** (45%).

3. **Symptoms suggestive of malignant disease** (e.g., jaundice, weight loss, generalized weakness, anorexia, or persistent right upper quadrant pain; 35%).

4. **Benign nonbiliary manifestations** (e.g., GI bleeding or obstruction; 5%).

III. DIAGNOSIS

A. **Symptoms.** The lack of specific symptoms prevents detection of GBC at an early stage. Consequently, the diagnosis is usually made unexpectedly at the time of surgery because the clinical signs commonly mimic benign gallbladder disease. Pain is present in 79% of patients; jaundice, anorexia, or nausea and vomiting in 45% to 55%; weight loss or fatigue in 30%; and pruritus or abdominal mass in 15%.

B. **Physical examination.** Certain combinations of symptoms and signs may suggest the diagnosis, such as an elderly woman with a history of chronic biliary symptoms that have changed in frequency or severity. A right upper quadrant mass or hepatomegaly and constitutional symptoms suggest GBC.

C. **Laboratory examination.** Elevated serum alkaline phosphatase is present in 65% of patients, anemia in 55%, elevated bilirubin in 40%, leukocytosis in 40%, and leukemoid reaction in 1% of patients with GBC. The association of elevated alkaline phosphatase without elevated bilirubin is consistent with GBC; about 40% of these patients have resectable lesions.

D. **Radiologic examination**

1. **Abdominal ultrasound** is abnormal in about 98% of patients. Cholelithiasis, thickened gallbladder wall, a mass in the gallbladder, or a combination of these constitutes the most common finding. Ultrasound is diagnostic of GBC in only 20% of cases, however.

2. **CT of the abdomen** may be diagnostic in half of patients.

3. **MRI** can differentiate gallbladder tumors from adjacent liver. Use of magnetic resonance cholangiography can help determine whether biliary tract encasement is present, and vascular enhancement techniques often permit preoperative diagnosis of portal vein involvement.

4. **Percutaneous transhepatic cholangiography (PTHC)** is abnormal in 80% of cases and diagnostic in 40%.

5. **ERCP** is abnormal in about 75% of cases and yields a tissue diagnosis in 25%.

6. **Laparoscopic exploration** may allow assessment of the peritoneal surfaces, liver, and tissues adjacent to the gallbladder to determine potential resectability.

IV. STAGING AND PROGNOSTIC FACTORS

A. **Staging.** Refer to the current AJCC Cancer Staging atlas for TNM staging system.

B. **Prognostic factors.** The overall median survival of patients with GBC is 6 months. After surgical resection, only 27% are alive at 1 year, 19% at 3 years, and 13% at 5 years. Disease stage is the most significant prognostic factor. The 5-year survival rate after surgical resection is 65% to 100% for stage I, 30% for stage II treated with simple cholecystectomy, <15% for stage III, and 0% for stage IV disease. Poorly differentiated (higher grade) tumors and the presence of jaundice are associated with poorer survival. Ploidy patterns do not correlate with survival.

C. **Molecular markers.** It is very interesting to note that molecular profiling of gallbladder cancers, intrahepatic cholangiocarcinomas, and extrahepatic cholangiocarcinomas has shown that these tumors that are anatomically so close to each other and resemble closely on pathology are very distinct based on the mutations and alterations present in these tumors. Commonly noted alterations included *BRAF, IDH1/2, ERBB2, BAP1, ARID1A, and PBRM1* among others. This is opening trial options for patients especially in patients with advanced disease with limited treatment options. These tumors may also benefit from immunotherapy if deemed MSI-high as noted in patients with colorectal cancers.

V. PREVENTION

Cholecystectomy has been recommended to prevent GBC. For every 100 gall-bladders removed, there is one patient with GBC. However, the overall mortality rate of cholecystectomy is also about 1% (including patients with diabetes and gangrenous gallbladder as well as patients with cholangitis or gallstone pancreatitis).

VI. MANAGEMENT

Despite the improvement of diagnostic capabilities, better perioperative care, and a more aggressive surgical approach, GBC remains a fatal illness in most patients.

A. Cholecystectomy. The best chance for long-term survival is the serendipitous discovery of an early cancer at the time of cholecystectomy. Simple cholecystectomy is curative for T1a tumors. Repeat resection with "extended cholecystectomy" (*en bloc* resection of the gallbladder bed, segments IVB and V of the liver, and regional lymph nodes) after the discovery of a GBC during cholecystectomy is recommended for stage T1b or stage II disease and is associated with a 5-year survival of 70% to 80%. Radical surgery for more advanced disease has not resulted in better survival.

B. RT appears to have no added benefit in the adjuvant setting, although the only reports of such therapy have been small retrospective series. Intraoperative RT has been reported to be of benefit in several small series of highly selected patients. RT may be useful as a primary treatment (without surgical resection) using either external beam RT alone or external beam RT plus ^{192}Ir implants. RT may relieve pain in a small number of patients.

C. Chemotherapy. The data on adjuvant systemic chemotherapy are anecdotal. 5-FU–based combinations are most commonly used, but the RRs are poor. Phase II trials have shown potential benefit to the use of gemcitabine.

For patients with metastatic disease, the combination of gemcitabine and cisplatin should be considered, based on the results of a randomized phase III trial as discussed in the next section. Alternative options include gemcitabine and oxaliplatin or gemcitabine and capecitabine.

BILIARY TRACT (INTRAHEPATIC AND EXTRAHEPATIC) CANCER

I. EPIDEMIOLOGY AND ETIOLOGY

A. Epidemiology. Biliary tract carcinomas (BTCs, cholangiocarcinomas) are rare and occur with equal frequency in men and women at the average age of 60 years. In American Indians, Israelis, and Japanese, the incidence of BTC is higher. However, cancer of the intrahepatic bile ducts appears to be increasing in incidence in both the United States and elsewhere. This increase is likely partly a result of more accurate diagnosis causing a shift from a classification of "unknown primary" to cholangiocarcinoma. Despite this possible shift, there appears to be a meaningful increase in the incidence of cholangiocarcinoma. The reasons for the observed increase have not been identified.

Extrahepatic bile duct cancers accounts for less than one-third of BTCs. When BTC is combined with GBC, GBC accounts for two-thirds of all BTCs. Half of patients with BTC have undergone cholecystectomy for cholelithiasis.

B. **Etiology and risk factors.** An increased incidence of BTC has been reported in patients with Crohn disease, choledocholithiasis, cystic fibrosis, chronic long-term ulcerative colitis, primary sclerosing cholangitis, and *Clonorchis sinensis* infestation. The incidence is also reportedly increased in patients with congenital anomalies of the intrahepatic and extrahepatic bile ducts (e.g., cysts, congenital dilation of the bile ducts, choledochal cyst, Caroli disease [congenital cystic dilation of multiple sections of the biliary tree], congenital hepatic fibrosis, polycystic disease, abnormal pancreaticocholedochal junction). Conditions that cause chronic bile duct stasis and infection are linked to increased risk for BTC. A history of exposure to the outmoded contrast agent thorotrast has also been associated with BTC.

II. PATHOLOGY

A. **Histology**

1. **Malignant tumors** of the bile ducts are adenocarcinoma in 95% of cases. Microscopically, BTCs generally extend to 1 to 4 cm beyond the gross margin of the tumor. Multiple foci of carcinoma *in situ* may be noted. Malignant tumors of intrahepatic bile ducts are less common than HCC and have no relation to cirrhosis. Mixed hepatic tumors with elements of both HCC and cholangiocarcinoma do occur; most of these cases are actually HCC with focal ductal differentiation.

   Other malignant tumors that involve the bile ducts include anaplastic and squamous carcinomas, cystadenocarcinomas, primary malignant melanoma, leiomyosarcoma, carcinosarcoma, and metastatic tumors (particularly breast cancer, myelomas, and lymphomas).

2. **Biliary tract adenomas** are solitary in 80% of cases and may grossly resemble metastatic carcinoma. Most are <1 cm in diameter and are located under the capsule.

3. **Biliary tract cystadenoma and cystadenocarcinoma.** Benign and malignant cystic tumors of biliary origin arise in the liver more frequently than in the extrahepatic biliary system.

4. **Biliary tract carcinoma** (cholangiocarcinoma; see Extrahepatic Bile Duct Cancer, later). Malignant tumors of intrahepatic bile ducts are less common than HCC and have no relation to cirrhosis. Mixed hepatic tumors with elements of both HCC and cholangiocarcinoma do occur; most of these cases are actually HCC with focal ductal differentiation.

B. **Location.** BTCs are divided anatomically into those that arise from the intrahepatic upper third of the biliary tract, including the hilum (50% to 70% of all tumors); the middle third (10% to 25%); the lower third (10% to 20%); and the cystic duct (<1%). Tumors found near the junction of the right and left hepatic duct (Klatskin tumors) are usually small and may be inconspicuous at laparotomy. Adenocarcinomas located in the right and left hepatic ducts or common hepatic duct are frequently scirrhous, constricting, diffusely infiltrating, or nodular and may mimic sclerosing cholangitis or stricture. Adenocarcinomas of the common bile duct or cystic duct are more often fungating and may have a better prognosis. Carcinoma of the cystic duct is rare, and distention of the gallbladder occurs before jaundice becomes apparent.

III. DIAGNOSIS

A. **Symptoms.** Jaundice is present in the majority of patients. Abdominal pain, weight loss, fever, malaise, or hepatomegaly occurs in half of cases, but generally in patients with advanced BTC. Patients with proximal tumors in the upper third of the biliary tract usually have symptoms for twice as long as those with tumors in the lower third.

B. Laboratory studies

1. **Serum chemistries.** Serum bilirubin levels >7.5 mg/dL are found in 60% of cases, alkaline phosphatase greater than twice normal in 80%, and increased transaminase level and prothrombin time in 25%.
2. **Tumor marker.** Serum CA 19-9 is elevated in 90% of patients.
3. **Radiologic examination.**
   a. **Abdominal ultrasound** shows dilation of the common bile duct or intrahepatic biliary ducts.
   b. **CT or MRI** may reveal a mass and suggest the site or origin of carcinoma.
   c. **PTHC** is the most specific test for proximal bile duct lesions.
   d. **ERCP** is the best diagnostic test for distal bile duct tumors.
   e. **Angiography and portovenography** can be useful in select cases in determining the extent of the disease for the preoperative evaluation of resectability.

IV. STAGING AND PROGNOSTIC FACTORS

A. **Staging.** Refer to the current AJCC Cancer Staging atlas for TNM staging system. All patients should be initially staged so that those with unresectable tumors are not subjected to needless surgery. If PTHC shows that the tumor extends into the parenchyma of both the right and left lobes of the liver, the tumor is unresectable and no surgery is performed. If angiography shows encasement of the main portal vein or hepatic artery, the tumor is also unresectable. If, however, the tumor extends into only one lobe, or if there is involvement of one branch of the portal vein or hepatic artery, surgical exploration is considered with the possibility of adding hepatic lobectomy to the hepatic duct resection.

B. **Prognostic factors.** The poor prognostic variables with statistical significance are mass lesion, cachexia, poor performance status, serum bilirubin 9 mg/dL or greater, multicentric disease, hilar or proximal sites, high tumor grade, sclerotic histology, liver invasion, lymph node involvement, and advanced stage.

C. **Molecular markers.** See section on Gallbladder Cancer.

V. MANAGEMENT

A. **Surgical resection** is the only treatment that may result in long-term survival. In specialized medical centers, about 45% of patients who undergo exploratory surgery also undergo complete resection with no gross tumor left behind, 10% undergo incomplete resection, and 45% have tumors that are not resectable. Tumors in the middle and distal ducts have a higher resectability rate than tumors in the proximal ducts, which have a maximal resectability rate of 20%. The median survival of patients with intrahepatic tumors following resection is 18 to 30 months, while that for patients with extrahepatic tumors is 12 to 24 months. The 5-year survival rate is about 10% to 45%. The 30-day operative mortality rate may be as high as 25%. The high postoperative complication rate includes wound infection, cholangitis, liver abscess, subphrenic abscess, pancreatitis, and biliary fistulas.

B. **Adjuvant therapy** has been advocated to reduce the high incidence of local recurrence (up to 100%), but it does not appear to improve survival after curative resection. The role of adjuvant RT remains unclear. Cholangiocarcinoma is radiosensitive, but bile duct tolerance to radiation is limited. The complications of RT include biliary and duodenal stenosis. The results of small series of selected patients treated with 5-FU combined with RT have led some authors to advocate this as an adjuvant to surgery or in cases with locally advanced and unresectable disease.

C. **Biliary tract bypass**
1. **Surgical biliary tract bypass** is carried out predominantly in those patients whose tumors are found to be unresectable at operation. Biliary-enteric anastomosis is usually performed using a Roux-en-Y jejunal loop. The operative mortality rate ranges from 0% to 30%, and the median survival varies from 11 to 16 months. The theoretical advantage of operative drainage is the decreased potential for recurrent cholangitis.
2. **Surgical stenting.** T-tube or U-tube catheters can be passed through the obstruction. A T-tube is hard to replace when it becomes clogged. The advantage of a U-tube is that both of its ends are externalized separately, easing replacement when the tube becomes obstructed. The 30-day mortality rate for operative stenting varies from 10% to 20%.
3. **Endoscopic stenting** has two advantages: a decreased morbidity and no creation of external fistulization. This method is more successful with distal bile duct tumors and is associated with a 30-day mortality rate of 10% to 20%.
4. **Percutaneous stenting** to provide drainage, either as an externalized stent or as an endoprosthesis, is associated with a 30-day mortality rate of 15% to 35%.

D. **Other methods of treatment**
1. **Liver transplantation** is generally not considered appropriate because of the high incidence of local recurrence. With orthotopic liver transplantation used alone, long-term survival is only 20% of highly selected patients with disease limited to the liver. The use of pretransplant chemotherapy and radiation has increased 5-year survival to 70% to 80%, making transplant a more meaningful option in selected patients.
2. **RT** appears to have some effect on the tumor size and may relieve jaundice in patients without biliary stenting. RT may be used (usually with biliary stenting) either as primary treatment or as adjuvant therapy. Conventional external beam RT has the advantage of giving a moderately high dose of radiation (5,000 to 6,000 cGy) to a relatively large volume of tissue and is more effective in treating bulky tumor masses. Implantation with ^{192}Ir seeds (effective radius of 1 cm from the seeds) delivers high-dose RT to localized residual disease after surgical resection or may provide palliation to patients with bile ducts obstructed by tumor. The typical dose with ^{192}Ir seeds is 2,000 cGy.
3. **Chemotherapy** is of potential benefit. 5-FU has a RR of 15%. Gemcitabine has been shown to have meaningful activity with an approximately 20% to 40% RR and improved overall survival of 8 to 14 months. Building on this observation, a variety of trials have looked at gemcitabine combined with other chemotherapy drugs including oxaliplatin, capecitabine, or low-dose cisplatin. In a phase III trial, the addition of low-dose cisplatin to gemcitabine compared to gemcitabine alone improved the RR from approximately 15% to 25% and significantly improved both progression-free and overall survival. The combination was well tolerated compared to gemcitabine alone. Based on this finding, the use of a gemcitabine–cisplatin doublet does appear to be warranted in patients with biliary tract or gallbladder cancer.

CANCER OF THE AMPULLA OF VATER

I. PATHOLOGY

Carcinoma of the ampulla of Vater is a papillary neoplasm arising in the last part of the common bile duct where it passes through the duodenum. Distinction between true ampullary tumor and periampullary tumors originating in the duodenal mucosa or pancreatic ducts is important because the periampullary cancers have a poor prognosis compared with ampullary cancers. The differentiation may be made by examination of the mucins they produce. Ampullary cancer produces sialomucins, whereas periampullary cancers produce sulfated mucins.

II. STAGING SYSTEM AND PROGNOSTIC FACTORS

The TNM staging system is used to stage ampullary cancer. The prognosis of patients with ampullary carcinoma is better than that of patients with cancer arising in any other site in the biliary tree. Pancreatic invasion and lymph node metastasis are the two most important prognostic factors. The 5-year survival rate is in excess of 50% when no nodal metastasis and no invasion of the pancreas have occurred. Nodal metastasis occurs much more frequently in patients with tumors larger than 2.5 cm.

III. MANAGEMENT

Surgery is the only curative treatment modality for ampullary carcinoma. Pancreaticoduodenal resection (Whipple procedure or a modification) is the surgical procedure of choice. The 5-year survival rate ranges from 5% to 55% depending on lymph node involvement, invasion of the pancreas, and histologic differentiation. Ampullectomy (local ampullary excision) performed on poor-risk patients with apparently localized disease is associated with a 10% 5-year survival rate.

ACKNOWLEDGMENT

The authors would like to acknowledge Dr. Steven R. Alberts, who significantly contributed to earlier versions of this chapter.

Suggested Readings

Esophageal and Gastric Cancer

Ajani JA, Moiseyenko VM, Tjulandin S, et al. Clinical benefit with docetaxel plus fluorouracil and cisplatin compared with cisplatin and fluorouracil in a phase III trial of advanced gastric or gastroesophageal adenocarcinoma: the V-325 study group. *J Clin Oncol* 2007;25:3205.

Bang Y-J, Van Cutsem E, Feyereislova A, et al. Trastuzumab in combination with chemotherapy versus chemotherapy alone for treatment of HER2-positive advanced gastric or gastro-oesophageal junction cancer (ToGA): a phase 3, open-label, randomized controlled trial. *Lancet* 2010;376:687.

Cunningham D, Allum WH, Stenning SP, et al. Perioperative chemotherapy versus surgery alone for resectable gastroesophageal cancer. *N Engl J Med* 2006;355:11.

Cunningham D, Starling N, Rao S, et al. Capecitabine and oxaliplatin for advanced esophagogastric cancer. *N Engl J Med* 2008;358:36.

Fuchs CS, Tomasek J, Yong CJ, et al. Ramucirumab monotherapy for previously treated advanced gastric or gastro-oesophageal junction adenocarcinoma (REGARD): an international, randomised, multicentre, placebo-controlled, phase 3 trial. *Lancet* 2014;383:31–39.

Macdonald JS, Smalley SR, Benedetti J, et al. Chemoradiotherapy after surgery compared with surgery alone for adenocarcinoma of the stomach or gastroesophageal junction. *N Engl J Med* 2001;345:725.

Tepper J, Krasna MJ, Niedzwiecki D, et al. Phase III trial of trimodality therapy with cisplatin, fluorouracil, radiotherapy, and surgery compared with surgery alone for esophageal cancer: CALGB 9781. *J Clin Oncol* 2008;26:1086.

The GASTRIC Group. Benefit of adjuvant chemotherapy for resectable gastric cancer. *JAMA* 2010;303:1729.

Wilke H, Muro K, Van Cutsem E, et al. Ramucirumab plus paclitaxel versus placebo plus paclitaxel in patients with previously treated advanced gastric or gastro-oesophageal junction adenocarcinoma (RAINBOW): a double-blind, randomised phase 3 trial. *Lancet Oncol* 2014;15:1224.

Colorectal Cancer

André T, Boni C, Mounedji-Boudiaf L, et al. Oxaliplatin, fluorouracil, and leucovorin as adjuvant treatment for colon cancer. *N Engl J Med* 2004;350:2343.

Bennouna J, Sastre J, Arnold D, et al. Continuation of bevacizumab after first progression in metastatic colorectal cancer (ML18147): a randomised phase 3 trial. *Lancet Oncol* 2013;14:29.

Bertagnolli MM, Eagle CJ, Zauber AG, et al. Celecoxib for the prevention of sporadic colorectal adenomas. *N Engl J Med* 2006;355:873.

Cunningham D, Humblet Y, Siena S, et al. Cetuximab monotherapy and cetuximab plus irinotecan in irinotecan-refractory metastatic colorectal cancer. *N Engl J Med* 2004;351:337.

de Gramont A, Figer A, Seymour M, et al. Leucovorin and fluorouracil with or without oxaliplatin as first-line treatment in advanced colorectal cancer. *J Clin Oncol* 2000;18:2938.

Falcone A, Ricce S, Brunetti I, et al. Phase III trial of infusional fluorouracil, leucovorin, oxaliplatin, and irinotecan (FOLFOXIRI) compared with infusional fluorouracil, leucovorin, and irinotecan (FOLFIRI) as first-line treatment for metastatic colorectal cancer: the Gruppo Oncologico Nord Ovest. *J Clin Oncol* 2007;25:1670.

Goldberg RM, Fleming TR, Tangen CM, et al. Surgery for recurrent colon cancer: strategies for identifying resectable recurrence and success rates after resection. *Ann Intern Med* 1998;129:27.

Goldberg RM, Sargent DJ, Morton RF, et al. A randomized controlled trial of fluorouracil plus leucovorin, irinotecan and oxaliplatin combinations in patients with previously untreated colorectal cancer. *J Clin Oncol* 2004;22:23.

Grothey A, Van Cutsem E, Sobrero A, et al. Regorafenib monotherapy for previously treated metastatic colorectal cancer (CORRECT): an international, multicentre, randomised, placebo-controlled, phase 3 trial. *Lancet* 2013;381:303.

Heinemann V, von Weikersthal LF, Decker T, et al. FOLFIRI plus cetuximab versus FOLFIRI plus bevacizumab as first-line treatment for patients with metastatic colorectal cancer (FIRE-3): a randomised, open-label, phase 3 trial. *Lancet Oncol* 2014;15:1065.

Le DT, Uram JN, Wang H, et al. PD-1 blockade in tumors with mismatch-repair deficiency. *N Engl J Med* 2015;372:2509.

Loupakis F, Cremolini C, Masi G, et al. Initial therapy with FOLFOXIRI and bevacizumab for metastatic colorectal cancer. *N Engl J Med* 2014;371:1609.

Mayer RJ, Van Cutsem E, Falcone A, et al. Randomized trial of TAS-102 for refractory metastatic colorectal cancer. *N Engl J Med* 2015;372:1909.

Mandel JS, Bond JH, Church TR, et al. Reducing mortality from colorectal cancer by screening for fecal occult blood. Minnesota Colon Cancer Control Study. *N Engl J Med* 1993;328:1365.

Moertel CG. Chemotherapy for colorectal cancer. *N Engl J Med* 1994;330:1136.

Rothenberg ML, Oza AM, Bigelow RH, et al. Superiority of oxaliplatin and fluorouracil-leucovorin compared with either therapy alone in patients with progressive colorectal cancer after irinotecan and fluorouracil-leucovorin: interim results of a phase III trial. *J Clin Oncol* 2003;21:2059.

Rougier P, Van Cutsem E, Bajetta E, et al. Randomised trial of irinotecan versus fluorouracil by continuous infusion after fluorouracil failure in patients with metastatic colorectal cancer. *Lancet* 1998;352:1407.

Simkens LH, van Tinteren H, May A, et al. Maintenance treatment with capecitabine and bevacizumab in metastatic colorectal cancer (CAIRO3): a phase 3 randomised controlled trial of the Dutch Colorectal Cancer Group. *Lancet* 2015;385:1843.

Tabernero J, Yoshino T, Cohn AL, et al. Ramucirumab versus placebo in combination with second-line FOLFIRI in patients with metastatic colorectal carcinoma that progressed during or after first-line therapy with bevacizumab, oxaliplatin, and a fluoropyrimidine (RAISE): a randomised, double-blind, multicentre, phase 3 study. *Lancet Oncol* 2015;16:499.

Tournigand C, André T, Achille E, et al. FOLFIRI followed by FOLFOX 6 or the reverse sequence in advanced colorectal cancer: a randomized GERCOR study. *J Clin Oncol* 2004;22:229.

Twelves C, Wong A, Nowacki MP, et al. Capecitabine as adjuvant treatment for stage III colon cancer. *N Engl J Med* 2005;352:2696.

Van Cutsem E, Peeters M, Siena S, et al. Open-label phase III trial of panitumumab plus best supportive care compared with best supportive care alone in patients with chemotherapy-refractory metastatic colorectal cancer. *J Clin Oncol* 2007;25:1658.

Van Cutsem E, Tabernero J, Lakomy R, et al. Addition of aflibercept to fluorouracil, leucovorin, and irinotecan improves survival in a phase III randomized trial in patients with metastatic colorectal cancer previously treated with an oxaliplatin-based regimen. *J Clin Oncol* 2012;30:3499.

Anal Cancer

Ajani JA, Winter KA, Gunderson LL, et al. Fluorouracil, mitomycin, and radiotherapy vs fluorouracil, cisplatin, and radiotherapy for carcinoma of the anal canal: a randomized controlled trial. *JAMA* 2008;299:1914.

Flam M, John M, Pajak TF, et al. Role of mitomycin in combination with fluorouracil and radiotherapy, and salvage chemoradiation in the definitive nonsurgical treatment of epidermoid carcinoma of the anal canal: results of a phase III randomized intergroup study. *J Clin Oncol* 1996;14:2527.

UKCCR Anal Cancer Trial Working Party. Epidermoid anal cancer: results of the UKCCR randomised trial of radiotherapy alone versus radiotherapy, 5-fluorouracil, and mitomycin. *Lancet* 1996;348:1049.

Pancreatic Cancer

Burris HA III, Moore MJ, Andersen J, et al. Improvements in survival and clinical benefit with gemcitabine as first-line therapy for patients with advanced pancreas cancer: a randomized trial. *J Clin Oncol* 1997;15:2403.

Gastrointestinal Study Group. Further evidence of effective adjuvant combined radiation and chemotherapy following curative resection of pancreatic cancer. *Cancer* 1987;59:2006.

Moore MJ, Goldstein D, Hamm J, et al. Erlotinib plus gemcitabine compared with gemcitabine alone in patients with advanced pancreatic cancer: a phase III trial of the National Cancer Institute of Canada Clinical Trials Group. *J Clin Oncol* 2007;25:1960.

Neoptolemos JP, Stocken DD, Friess H, et al. A randomized trial of chemoradiotherapy and chemotherapy after resection of pancreatic cancer. *N Engl J Med* 2004;350:1200.

Oettle H, Post S, Neuhaus P, et al. Adjuvant chemotherapy with gemcitabine vs observation in patients undergoing curative-intent resection of pancreatic cancer: a randomized controlled trial. *JAMA* 2007;297:267.

Regine WF, Winter KA, Abrams RA, et al. Fluorouracil vs gemcitabine chemotherapy before and after fluorouracil-based chemoradiation following resection of pancreatic adenocarcinoma. *JAMA* 2008;299:1019.

Von Hoff DD, Ervin T, Arena FP, et al. Increased survival in pancreatic cancer with nab-paclitaxel plus gemcitabine. *N Engl J Med* 2013;369:1691.

Wang-Gillam A, Li CP, Bodoky G, Dean A, et al.; NAPOLI-1 Study Group. Nanoliposomal irinotecan with fluorouracil and folinic acid in metastatic pancreatic cancer after previous gemcitabine-based therapy (NAPOLI-1): a global, randomised, open-label, phase 3 trial. *Lancet* 2016;387:545.

Liver Cancer

Farazi PA, DePinho RA. Hepatocellular carcinoma pathogenesis: from genes to environment. *Nat Rev Cancer* 2006;6:674.

Llovet JM, Ricci S, Mazzaferro V, et al. Sorafenib in advanced hepatocellular carcinoma. *N Engl J Med* 2008;359:378.

Louvet JM, Bruix J. Systematic review of randomized trials for unresectable hepatocellular carcinoma: chemoembolization improves survival. *Hepatology* 2003;37:429.

Marrero JA, Pelletier S. Hepatocellular carcinoma. *Clin Liver Dis* 2006;10:339.

Cholangiocarcinoma and Gallbladder Cancer

Churi CR, Shroff R, Wang Y, et al. Mutation profiling in cholangiocarcinoma: prognostic and therapeutic implications. *PLoS One* 2014;9:e115383.

Duffy A, Capanu M, Abou-Alfa GK, et al. Gallbladder cancer (GBC): 10-year experience at Memorial Sloan-Kettering Cancer Centre. *J Surg Oncol* 2008;98:485.

Heimbach JK, Gores GJ, Nagomey DM, et al. Liver transplantation for perihilar cholangiocarcinoma after aggressive neoadjuvant therapy: a new paradigm for liver and biliary malignancies? *Surgery* 2006;140:331.

Hejna M, Pruckmayer M, Raderer M. The role of chemotherapy and radiation in the management of biliary cancer: a review of the literature. *Eur J Cancer* 1998;34:977.

Jarnagin WR, Shoup M. Surgical management of cholangiocarcinoma. *Semin Liver Dis* 2004;24:189.

Lillemoe KD. Tumors of the gallbladder, bile ducts, and ampulla. *Semin Gastrointest Dis* 2003;14:208.

Reid KM, Ramos-De la Medina A, Donohue JH. Diagnosis and surgical management of gallbladder cancer: a review. *J Gastrointest Surg* 2007;11:671.

Valle J, Wasan H, Palmer DH, et al. Cisplatin plus gemcitabine versus gemcitabine for biliary tract cancer. *N Engl J Med* 2010;362:1273.

11 Breast Cancer

Mark D. Pegram

I. EPIDEMIOLOGY AND ETIOLOGY

A. Incidence

1. The American Cancer Society (ACS) estimated that breast cancer was diagnosed in 231,840 women and 2,350 men in the United States during 2015. Another 60,290 women were diagnosed with *in situ* breast carcinoma. Breast cancer was estimated to be the cause of death in 40,730 women and 440 men during that year. Overall breast cancer death rates in the United States decreased 36% from 1989 to 2012. These reductions are most likely owing to increased early detection and improved efficacy of adjuvant (and neoadjuvant) therapies.

2. Although breast cancer is the most common neoplasm in women, accounting for 29% of all cancers diagnosed annually, overall it is the second leading cause of cancer death (following lung cancer). Breast cancer, however, is the leading cause of cancer death in women $\geq$ age 65.

B. Genetic predisposition.

Approximately 10% of breast cancer patients have tumors that can be attributed to inherited germline mutations in genes that control DNA repair, cell growth regulation, or cell cycle control.

1. **Germline genetic defects** associated with an increased risk of breast cancer include the following:

   a. ***BRCA-1.*** The *BRCA-1* gene is assigned to chromosome 17q21. The gene product is a 1,863 amino acid nuclear protein with pleiotropic activities, including sensing or signaling DNA damage, transcriptional regulation, transcription-coupled DNA repair, and ubiquitin ligase activity. Several hundred different mutations have been identified by DNA sequence analysis. Particular *BRCA-1* mutations are prevalent in specific populations (e.g., del 185 mutation among patients of Ashkenazi Jewish ancestry). Mutation of *BRCA-1* accounts for about 20% of all familial breast cancers.

      (1) *BRCA-1* mutations are inherited in an autosomal dominant fashion with variable penetrance and are associated with an increased risk of breast, ovarian, prostate, and possibly colorectal cancers. Women with *BRCA-1* or *2* mutations have a fivefold increase in colorectal cancer risk, suggesting that heightened colon cancer screening in such populations (i.e., age 40 to 50) is warranted.

      (2) Breast tumors harboring *BRCA-1* mutations frequently lack expression of both ER and PR and lack amplification of the *HER2* gene. These tumors very frequently also have somatic mutations in the *P53* tumor suppressor gene.

      (3) Molecular classification of *BRCA-1* mutant tumors by gene expression profiling frequently demonstrates a "basal" breast cancer phenotype (see Section II.B).

      (4) Patients with inherited mutation of *BRCA-1* can expect a 50% to 85% lifetime risk for breast cancer and a 15% to 45% risk for ovarian cancer.

b. **BRCA-2.** The *BRCA-2* gene is assigned to chromosome 13q12. The gene encodes a 3,418 amino acid protein involved in DNA repair. As with *BRCA-1*, many different mutations have been described in the *BRCA-2* gene in affected individuals.

Germline mutations in *BRCA-2* are associated with an increased risk of a unique spectrum of human neoplasms, including melanoma, breast cancer (in both men and women), ovarian cancer, and pancreatic cancer. Breast cancers associated with *BRCA-2* mutation are frequently ER positive and tend to occur at an older age than do those with *BRCA-1* mutation.

c. **Li–Fraumeni syndrome** is caused by germline mutations in the *P53* tumor suppressor gene found on chromosome 17p13. In addition to breast cancer, there is an increased risk of other tumor types (sarcomas, brain tumors, leukemia, and adrenal tumors). The lifetime risk of breast cancer associated with this syndrome is about 50%.

d. **The *PTEN* gene** is assigned to chromosome 10q22–23 and encodes a tumor suppressor (see Chapter 29, Section III.C). The risk of breast cancer is increased by approximately 50% in subjects with mutation of the gene.

e. **CHEK-2.** This cell cycle checkpoint kinase gene is an important component of the cellular DNA repair pathway. Mutation of the gene increases the risk of breast cancer in women by 2-fold and in men by 10-fold.

f. **RAD-51.** The 339 amino acid RAD51 protein interacts with PALB2 and BRCA2 and is essential for homologous recombination repair; a biallelic missense mutation can cause a Fanconi anemia–like phenotype. Six monoallelic pathogenic mutations in RAD51C that confer an increased risk for breast and ovarian cancer were found within 480 pedigrees with the occurrence of both breast and ovarian tumors.

g. **PALB2.** This gene encodes a 1,186 amino acid protein that binds RAD-51 and functions in double-strand DNA break repair by stabilizing intranuclear localization and accumulation of BRCA-2. Variants in the *PALB2* gene are associated with increased breast cancer risk by a similar magnitude to that of BRCA-2.

h. **Mutations in other genes** have been associated with an increased risk of breast cancer (e.g., *ATM, CDH1, MRE11A, NBN, RAD50, RECQL, RINT1,* and *STK11*—Puetz-Jeghers syndrome). In approximately half of subjects with an apparent familial association with breast cancer based on analysis of the pedigree, no specific gene mutation can be found.

2. **Genetic testing for *BRCA-1* and *BRCA-2*** is commercially available but should be interpreted in consultation with a genetic counselor. Factors that indicate an increased likelihood of having germline *BRCA* mutations include the following:

a. Multiple cases of early onset breast cancer

b. Ovarian cancer with a family history of breast or ovarian cancer

c. Breast and ovarian cancer in the same individual

d. Bilateral breast cancer

e. Male breast cancer

f. Ashkenazi Jewish ancestry

3. **Next-generation sequencing panels** are commercially available to simultaneously analyze multiple genes associated with increased risk for breast cancer.

4. **American Society of Clinical Oncology (ASCO) guidelines** recommend that cancer predisposition genetic testing should be offered when (1) there is a personal or family history suggestive of a genetic cancer susceptibility condition; (2) the test can be adequately interpreted; and (3) the test result will influence medical management. Once a proband has been identified as a carrier for a heritable cancer predisposition condition, it is important that patients and their family members be counseled regarding additional screening and prevention strategies and be alerted to the risk of other primary neoplasms.

5. **Prophylactic surgery.** Prophylactic bilateral mastectomy reduces the risk of breast cancer among *BRCA* mutation carriers by more than 90%. Prophylactic bilateral salpingo-oophorectomy reduces the risk of ovarian cancer (although not primary peritoneal carcinoma) by 90% and also reduces the risk of breast cancer by approximately 65% in premenopausal women with *BRCA* abnormalities.

6. **Insurance issues.** The U.S. Health Insurance Portability and Accountability Act (HIPAA) of 1996 states that genetic information may not be treated as a preexisting medical condition for the purposes of denying insurance coverage or basing the cost of insurance. In addition to federal policy, many states have additional laws to prevent discrimination owing to genetic information. Consequently, most insurance companies will pay for genetic testing and any subsequent treatment that is indicated.

C. **Etiologic factors**

1. **Endogenous estrogen exposure.** The following factors affecting endogenous estrogen exposure have been associated with an increased risk of breast cancer in epidemiologic studies.

   a. Nulliparity.

   b. Late first full-term pregnancy (women who completed their first full-term pregnancy after age 30 are two to five times more likely to develop breast cancer compared with those who had had term pregnancies <18 years of age).

   c. Early menarche (<12 years of age).

   d. Late menopause (>55 years of age).

   e. Lactation may reduce the risk of breast cancer.

2. **Hormone replacement therapy (HRT) following menopause.** A preponderance of the evidence from previous historical cohort studies suggested that the risk of breast cancer was increased modestly by long-term estrogen use alone and that women on estrogen plus progestin were more likely to have tumors with more favorable biologic characteristics (hormone receptor–positive disease) and lower tumor stage. **The Women's Health Initiative (WHI) study** demonstrated a 24% increase in the risk of breast cancer among the women with an intact uterus randomized to receive conjugated equine estrogen (CEE, 0.625 mg/d) plus medroxyprogesterone acetate (MPA, 2.5 mg/d) ($P = 0.003$). Moreover, tumors detected in the CEE + MPA group had a larger mean tumor size (1.7 vs. 1.5 cm, $P = 0.038$) and were more likely to have lymph node metastasis (25.9% vs. 15.8%, $P = 0.033$). The study further demonstrated that the risk of both ER/PR-positive as well as ER/PR-negative disease was increased similarly. With longer follow-up (median = 11 years), breast cancer mortality also appears to be increased with combined use of estrogen plus progestin. Finally, the use of CEE + MPA was found to decrease the risk of colorectal cancer, although the colorectal cancers that were diagnosed were of more advanced stage.

The increased risk of invasive breast cancer was not seen in the women with prior hysterectomy who were randomized to receive CEE alone. The use of CEE alone increased the risk of stroke, decreased the risk of hip fracture, and did not affect the risk of coronary heart disease. These data led to a revised view of postmenopausal HRT because use of CEE + MPA potentially leads to delay in diagnosis of two of the three most common cancers in postmenopausal women:

    a. HRT with CEE + MPA should be used at the lowest possible dose and shortest duration sufficient to control vasomotor or vaginal symptoms.

    b. Women with prior hysterectomy treated with CEE for a short term have no significant increase in breast cancer risk, although the risk of stroke is increased.

        Subsequent to publication of findings from the WHI study, there was a sharp decline in the number of new prescriptions for HRT in the United States from 22.8 million in the first quarter of 2001 to 15.2 in the first quarter of 2003. Coincident with this practice was a sharp (7%) decrease in the breast cancer incidence, especially among older women with hormone receptor–positive disease, suggesting a possible link between decreased incidence and decreased exogenous estrogen and progestin exposure in the form of HRT.

3. Age. The incidence of breast cancer increases steadily with age. Approximately 75% of all cases are diagnosed in postmenopausal women.

4. Benign breast disease. Most forms of benign breast disease, such as fibrocystic disease, are not associated with increased risk. Hyperplasia with atypia, papillomas, sclerosing adenosis, and lobular carcinoma *in situ* (LCIS) have been reported to be associated with an increased risk. **Hyperplasia with atypia** is felt to be a proliferative disease that is associated with an 8% risk of developing invasive breast cancer in patients with a negative family history and a 20% risk in patients with a positive family history of breast cancer.

5. Physical activity. Most cohort studies suggest an inverse association between physical activity and breast cancer risk, regardless of the age at which the physical activity occurred.

6. Ionizing radiation. Exposure to radiation increases the risk of breast cancer. Medical radiation therapy (RT) to the chest, for example, to a mantle field for Hodgkin lymphoma, can increase subsequent risk of breast cancer. Exposure to fallout from nuclear weapons also appears to increase risk. Recent epidemiologic data following the Chernobyl nuclear power plant disaster suggest higher incidence of breast cancer in the years following the disaster. Breast cancers following radiation exposure typically have long latency, often a decade or more, following the exposure.

7. Ethanol. Studies have shown a positive linear relationship between incremental alcoholic beverage intake and increasing breast cancer risk.

II. PATHOLOGY, MOLECULAR CLASSIFICATION, AND NATURAL HISTORY

Breast cancer is a highly heterogeneous disease. Although classic histopathologic classification of breast cancer remains important, molecular characterization of the disease is rapidly emerging as a vital tool for understanding clinical prognosis, as well as for predicting response to systemic therapies.

    A. Classic histopathologic classification. Based on cellular morphology, breast tumors can be broadly categorized as tumors composed of cells of ductal origin (ductal adenocarcinomas) or of lobular origin (lobular carcinomas).

1. **Ductal adenocarcinoma** (70% to 80%) is the most common invasive histology. The clinical prognosis is highly variable, ranging from indolent to rapidly progressive. Prognosis may be estimated by evaluation of cellular morphologic characteristics and molecular markers, such as expression of ER, PR, Ki67 (a marker of cell proliferation, see Section V.B.5), and *HER2*.

2. **Lobular carcinoma** (10% to 15%). Invasive lobular carcinoma is capable of metastasis and has a stage-adjusted prognosis similar to infiltrating ductal carcinoma. Invasive lobular carcinomas may be especially difficult to diagnose because of their unique single-cell radial pattern of tissue invasion (so-called *Indian-filing* on light microscopy), rendering them frequently nonpalpable or mammographically silent. Invasive lobular carcinomas are somewhat more likely to be bilateral compared with infiltrating ductal carcinomas. Metastases from lobular breast carcinomas have a predilection for the gastrointestinal tract, peritoneal surfaces, gynecologic organs, and retroperitoneum. Loss of E-cadherin expression is common in lobular carcinoma.

   To be distinguished from invasive lobular carcinoma, LCIS is a benign lesion *associated* with an increase risk of developing subsequent invasive disease, either ductal or lobular. LCIS may be treated with close clinical follow-up and mammographic screening. Tamoxifen may be considered to reduce future risk of developing cancer.

3. **Special breast cancer subtypes with a favorable prognosis** include papillary, tubular, mucinous, and pure medullary carcinomas.

4. **Inflammatory breast cancer** (approximately 1%) is a particularly aggressive subtype that can be recognized microscopically based on presence of dermolymphatic invasion. Clinically, this is often associated with cutaneous erythema of the breast (which can mimic mastitis) and cutaneous edema ("peau d'orange").

5. **Paget disease of the breast**, which is characterized by unilateral eczematous change of the nipple, is frequently seen in association with underlying ductal carcinoma *in situ* (DCIS).

6. **Cystosarcoma phyllodes** constitute <1% of all breast neoplasms. About 90% of phyllodes tumors are benign and about 10% are malignant. Although these tumors rarely metastasize, they can recur locally. Surgical resection with ample margins is necessary to optimize local control.

7. **Rare tumors** include squamous cell carcinoma, lymphoma, and sarcoma.

B. **Molecular classification of breast malignancy.** Molecular classification of breast cancer can be based on single gene assays, such as ER, PR, *HER2* gene copy number, proliferation index, and Ki67; or on multigene expression platforms, which can measure dozens to even thousands of gene transcripts simultaneously. Example include the Oncotype DX assay (see Section VIII.A.2.b), the Prosigna Breast Cancer Prognostic Gene Signature Assay (formerly called the PAM50 test), and Mammaprint (see Section VIII.A.2.c).

   Gene expression profiling using DNA microarrays has defined intrinsic molecular subtypes of breast cancer associated with the cell-of-origin distinction. Based on these observations, breast cancer has been divided into at least five subgroups with distinct biologic features and clinical outcomes.

1. **Luminal A.** The luminal tumors express cytokeratins 8 and 18, have the highest levels of ER expression, tend to be low grade, will most likely respond to endocrine therapy, and have a favorable prognosis. They tend to be less responsive to chemotherapy.

2. **Luminal B.** Tumor cells are also of luminal epithelial origin, but with a gene expression pattern distinct from luminal A. Luminal B tumors are associated

with higher proliferation rates, and prognosis is somewhat worse than that of luminal A.

3. **Normal-like breast tumors.** These tumors have a gene expression profile reminiscent of nonmalignant "normal" breast epithelium. Prognosis is similar to the luminal B group.

4. *HER2*-**enriched.** These tumors often have amplification of the *HER2* gene on chromosome 17q and frequently exhibit coamplification and overexpression of other genes adjacent to *HER2*. *HER2*-positive cases have significantly decreased expression of ER and PR and have up-regulation of vascular endothelium growth factor (VEGF). Historically, the clinical prognosis of such tumors was poor. With the advent of trastuzumab therapy; however, the clinical outcome for patients with *HER2*-positive tumors has markedly improved.

5. **Basal-like.** These ER- or PR-negative and *HER2*-negative tumors (so-called *triple-negative*) are characterized by markers of basal or myoepithelial cells. They tend to be high grade and express cytokeratins 5/6 and 17 as well as vimentin, p63, CD10, smooth muscle actin, and epidermal growth factor receptor (EGFR). It is likely that the basal group is still somewhat heterogeneous; for example, patients with *BRCA-1* mutant tumors also fall within this molecular subtype. Overall, patients with basal breast cancers have a poor prognosis, although they likely benefit to some extent from chemotherapy.

6. **A new breast cancer intrinsic subtype**, known as Claudin-low, has been identified in human tumors. Clinically, the majority of Claudin-low tumors are poor prognosis ER-negative (ER–), PR-negative (PR–), and HER2-negative (HER2–) (i.e., triple-negative) invasive ductal carcinomas with a high frequency of metaplastic and medullary differentiation. Preliminary data shows that they have a response rate to standard neoadjuvant chemotherapy that is intermediate between basal-like and luminal tumors.

C. **Location and mode of spread.** The most common anatomic presentation of breast cancer is in the upper outer quadrant. Breast cancers spread by contiguity, lymphatic channels, and blood-borne metastases. The most common organs involved with symptomatic metastases are regional lymph nodes, skin, bone, liver, lung, and brain. Internal mammary nodes have evidence of tumor in 25% of patients with inner quadrant lesions and 15% with outer quadrant lesions. Internal mammary node metastases rarely occur in the absence of axillary node involvement.

D. **Clinical course.** The clinical course of breast cancer is highly heterogeneous, but generally, there are trends based on stage. Early breast cancer is curable, but has a chance of distant metastases occurring following long periods of dormancy (even 10 to 20 years) after treatment. Locally advanced cancer has an increased risk of latent distant metastasis. In some women, the course is quite rapid. Metastatic breast cancer (MBC) (except in rare cases of "exceptional responders") is not curable but typically has a course of stable or responsive disease on therapy, sometimes for many months (or years), and then progression in a stepwise fashion.

III. SCREENING AND EARLY DETECTION

A. **Mammography** detects about 85% of breast cancers. A distinction should be made between diagnostic mammography and screening mammography. A screening mammogram is an x-ray study of the breast used to detect breast changes in women who have no signs or symptoms of breast cancer. A diagnostic mammogram is an x-ray study of the breast that is used to check for breast cancer after a lump or other sign or symptom of breast cancer has been found. Although 15% of breast cancers cannot be visualized with mammography, 45% of breast cancers can be seen on mammography before they are palpable. **A normal mammographic result must not dissuade the physician from obtaining a biopsy of a suspicious mass.** Digital mammography has replaced film mammography.

1. **The American College of Radiology BI-RADS System** for reporting mammographic findings is as follows:

   Category 1: Negative

   Category 2: Benign finding

   Category 3: Probably benign finding. Short interval follow-up is suggested. The findings have a very high probability of being benign, but the radiologist would prefer to establish stability.

   Category 4: Suspicious abnormality: biopsy should be considered. These are lesions that do not have characteristic findings of breast cancer, but have a definite probability of being malignant.

   Category 5: Highly suggestive of malignancy.

2. **Meta-analysis** of eight randomized mammogram screening trials has shown a 24% reduction in the mortality rate of breast cancer. Mortality reductions have been observed in trials of women aged 40 to 69 years with mammography performed at intervals of 12 and 24 months.

3. **The ACS recommends** women ages 40 to 44 should have the choice to start annual breast cancer screening with mammograms if they wish to do so. The risks of screening as well as the potential benefits should be considered. Women age 45 to 54 should get mammograms every year. Women age 55 and older should switch to mammograms every 2 years, or have the choice to continue yearly screening. Screening should continue as long as a woman is in good health and is expected to live 10 more years or longer.

B. **Breast physical examinations.** The lack of data showing a reduction in risk of death from breast cancer owing to clinical breast examination (CBE) or breast self-examination (BSE) notwithstanding, both are reasonable to include in clinical practice.

   1. CBE is recommended for women at average risk of breast cancer beginning in their 20s. CBE should be part of a periodic health examination and should occur at least every 3 years. Women aged 40 years and older should receive CBE, preferably annually, and, ideally, before, or in conjunction with, the annual screening mammogram.

   2. Women should be told about the limitations of BSE. Women who choose to do BSE should receive instruction and have their technique reviewed on the occasion of a periodic health examination.

C. **High-risk patients.** The ACS reported that women at increased risk for breast cancer might benefit from additional screening strategies beyond those offered to women at average risk. These interventions may include initiation of screening at a younger age, shorter screening intervals, or the addition of other radiologic investigations in addition to mammography, including magnetic resonance imaging (MRI) or ultrasound.

   1. **ACS guidelines recommend MRI screening** in addition to mammograms for women who have at least one of the following conditions:

      a. A *BRCA1* or *BRCA2* mutation

      b. A first-degree relative (parent, sibling, child) with a *BRCA1* or *BRCA2* mutation, even if they have yet to be tested themselves

   c. A lifetime risk of breast cancer that has been scored at 20% to 25% or greater based on one of several accepted risk assessment tools that evaluate family history and other factors
   d. A history of radiation to the chest between the ages of 10 and 30 years
   e. Germline p53 mutation (Li–Fraumeni syndrome), or hamartoma syndromes associated with *PTEN* mutation (Cowden syndrome or Bannayan–Riley–Ruvalcaba syndrome), or one of these syndromes based on a history in a first-degree relative

2. **The ACS guideline indicates that sufficient evidence still does not exist to recommend for or against MRI screening** in women who have
   a. A 15% to 20% lifetime risk of breast cancer, based on one of several accepted risk assessment tools that evaluate family history and other factors
   b. LCIS or atypical lobular hyperplasia (ALH)
   c. Atypical ductal hyperplasia (ADH)
   d. Very dense breasts or unevenly dense breasts (when viewed on a mammogram)
   e. Already had breast cancer, including DCIS

3. **Contralateral breast cancer.** MRI scans can be a useful adjunct for finding contralateral breast tumors in women with newly diagnosed disease.

IV. DIAGNOSIS

A. Physical findings and differential diagnosis

1. **Breast lumps** are detectable in many patients with breast cancer and constitute the most common sign on history and physical examination. The typical malignant breast mass tends to be solitary, unilateral, solid, hard, irregular, and nontender.

2. **Spontaneous nipple discharge** through a mammary duct is the second most common sign of breast cancer. Nipple discharge develops in about 3% of women and 20% of men with breast cancer, but is a manifestation of benign disease in 90% of patients. Discharge in patients >50 years of age is more likely to represent cancer rather than benign conditions. Milky or purulent discharges are associated with a negligible chance of being cancer.

3. **Other presenting manifestations** include skin changes, axillary lymphadenopathy, or signs of locally advanced or disseminated disease. A painful breast is a common symptom, but it is usually a result of something other than the cancer. Paget carcinoma appears as unilateral eczema of the nipple. Inflammatory carcinoma appears as skin erythema, edema, and underlying induration in the absence of infection.

B. Evaluation of a breast mass

1. **Breast lump or mass in women <30 years of age.** Ultrasound is the preferred diagnostic modality for young women with a breast mass. If the mass is solid and suspicious, then mammography followed by tissue diagnosis is recommended. If the mass is thought to be benign ultrasonographically, then the option of tissue diagnosis versus observation with frequent physical and ultrasonographic surveillance is appropriate. If the breast mass appears to be a simple cyst on ultrasound, no intervention is required. If it appears to be a complex cyst, then aspiration is appropriate. If the mass disappears with aspiration and the aspirate is not bloody, then routine screening can again begin.

2. **Breast lump or mass in women >30 years of age.** Diagnostic mammography should be performed. If the mammographic features are indeterminate,

then ultrasonography should be performed. If the mammogram or ultrasound shows a suspicious lesion, tissue sampling is required.

  3. Breast biopsy. When a tissue diagnosis is required, then a choice must be made among the differing techniques.

    a. Fine needle aspiration (FNA) cytology may be performed if both technical and cytopathologic expertise are available. The sensitivity in diagnosing malignancy has been reported to be 90% to 95%, with 98% specificity. It is, however, impossible to distinguish invasive from *in situ* carcinoma.

    b. Ultrasound or stereotactic core biopsy. These techniques are the standard for mammographic changes without accompanying mass; wire- or needle-guided lumpectomies can follow the procedure. In addition, the core biopsy allows sufficient tissue to be removed to appropriately characterize the histology of the specimen. ER, PR, and *HER2* testing may be performed if an invasive malignancy is diagnosed.

    c. Excisional biopsy is a technique for diagnosis of a breast mass if stereotactic or ultrasound-guided core biopsy is unavailable. If excisional biopsy is performed, an adequate amount of normal tissue should be removed around the suspicious lesion in the event that a malignancy is found. This tactic allows for complete excision with clear margins and full histologic evaluation.

C. Pretreatment staging procedures for invasive breast cancer.

  1. Complete blood count, liver function tests, alkaline phosphatase and serum calcium

  2. Chest radiograph, diagnostic bilateral mammography

  3. A CT scan of the chest, abdomen and pelvis and a bone scan can be considered for patients with: clinically positive axillary nodes, large tumors (e.g., ≥ 5 cm), aggressive biology or clinical signs, symptoms or laboratory values suggesting the presence of metastases.

  4. Bone marrow aspiration if there is unexplained cytopenia or a leukoerythroblastic blood smear.

  5. The role of positron emission tomography (PET), with or without computed tomography, in the initial staging of breast cancer is being evaluated. In general, PET can accurately detect sites of distant disease with a sensitivity of 80% to 97% and specificity of 75% to 94%.

V. STAGING AND PROGNOSIS

A. Staging system. Refer to the current AJCC Cancer Staging atlas for TNM staging system.

B. Prognostic factors

  1. Tumor grade is an important prognostic variable; the higher the grade, the more guarded the prognosis. The Nottingham combined histologic grade (Elston–Ellis modification of the Bloom–Scarff–Richardson grading system) is recommended by the AJCC staging system. A tumor is graded by assessing three morphologic features (tubule formation, nuclear pleomorphism, and count of mitoses). A value of 1 (favorable) to 3 (unfavorable) is assigned to each feature. A combined score of 3 to 5 points is designated grade 1, 6 to 7 points is grade 2, and 8 to 9 points is grade 3.

  2. Pathologic stage has a clear impact on expected survival.

    a. Tumor size. The risk of recurrence increases linearly with tumor size for patients with fewer than four lymph nodes involved with metastases; thereafter, the prognostic weight of lymph node metastases generally supersedes tumor size. The effect of tumor size on prognosis is reflected by the following SEER 5-year survival data (adapted from Carter C, Allen C, Henson D. Relation of tumor size, lymph node status, and survival in 24,740 breast cancer cases. *Cancer* 1989;63:181).

Five-year survival rate according to the number of axillary lymph nodes with metastases		
Tumor size	No nodal metastasis	1–3 Nodes
≤5 mm	99%	95%
6–10 mm	98%	94%
11–20 mm	96%	87%

The 20-year breast cancer–specific, disease-free survival (DFS) for node-negative patients treated with mastectomy alone is about 92% for pT1a–b tumors and 75% to 80% for pT1c tumors. Tumor grade affects these probabilities.

b. Lymph node involvement is the greatest prognostic indicator for breast cancer recurrence.

c. Distant metastases. Many patients with stage IV disease survive 2 to 4 years, or even longer, depending on sites of metastases, their rate of progression, and response to therapy. Prolonged survival can be achieved, particularly in patients with hormone receptor–positive disease with bone-only metastasis.

3. Hormone receptor status. Patients with tumors that are negative for both ER and PR (measured by biochemical methods) have a slightly worse prognosis than do those patients who have cancers with either ER or PR being positive. It is felt that ER and PR as measured by current immunohistochemical (IHC) techniques represent very strong predictive factors for response to hormone therapy rather than being strong prognostic factors for survival.

Unfortunately, as many as 20% of current IHC determinations of ER and PR worldwide may be inaccurate (false negative or false positive), mostly because of variation in preanalytic variables, thresholds for positivity, and interpretation criteria. ER and PR assays are considered to be positive if there are at least 1% positive tumor nuclei in the sample in the presence of expected reactivity of internal (normal epithelial elements) and external controls.

4. *HER2* overexpression. All normal cells, including breast epithelial cells, carry two copies of the human epidermal growth factor receptor-2 gene (*HER2* or *HER2/neu;* also known as the *c-erbB2* gene). In about 20% of breast cancers, multiple copies of the gene are found owing to gene amplification. *HER2* gene amplification results in increased expression of the gene product, a 185-kDa transmembrane receptor tyrosine kinase. Pathologic overexpression of p185^{HER2} leads to constitutive activation of the *HER2* kinase, resulting in increased proliferation, survival, and metastasis of tumor cells.

a. Tumors that overexpress *HER2* tend to metastasize earlier and to have a worse prognosis. HER2-positive breast cancers have a propensity for metastasis to the brain. Tumors that exhibit amplification of the *HER2* gene by fluorescence *in situ* hybridization (FISH) are among the most likely to benefit from systemic therapy with trastuzumab.

b. **Common methods of identifying *HER2 alteration*** are IHC and FISH. *HER2* status should be determined for all invasive breast cancers. Laboratories performing the test must show 95% concordance with another validated test for positive and negative assay results. The recommended algorithm for defining results for both *HER2* protein expression and gene amplification is as follows:

(1) A positive *HER2* result is IHC 3+ based on circumferential membrane staining that is complete, intense.

(a) In situ hybridization (ISH) positive based on the following:

(i) Single-probe average *HER2* copy number ≥ 6.0 signals/cell

(ii) Dual-probe *HER2*/chromosome 17 centromere probe (CEP17) ratio ≥ 2.0 with an average *HER2* copy number ≥ 4.0 signals per cell

(iii) Dual-probe *HER2*/CEP17 ratio ≥ 2.0 with an average *HER2* copy number < 4.0 signals/cell

(iv) Dual-probe *HER2*/CEP17 ratio < 2.0 with an average *HER2* copy number ≥ 6.0 signals/cell.

(2) A negative result is an IHC staining of 0 or 1+, a FISH result of <4.0 *HER2* gene copies per nucleus, or a FISH ratio of <2.

(3) Equivocal results (e.g., IHC = 2+ or ISH *HER2* copy number between 4 and 6 per cell nucleus) require additional action for final determination. Also, be mindful that deletion of CEP17 may yield a *HER2*/CEP 17 ratio ≥ 2.0, but does NOT constitute *HER2* gene amplification (and are rarely *HER2* = 3+ on IHC).

5. **Other biomarkers**

a. **Ki-67 protein** is strictly associated with cell proliferation. The fraction of Ki-67–positive tumor cells (the Ki-67 labeling index) has been correlated with the clinical course. At present, an enormous variation in analytical practice markedly limits the value of Ki67.

b. **DNA flow cytometry** can be performed on tumor biopsy material following fluorescent staining with propidum iodide. From this analysis, total DNA content (and thus DNA ploidy) and the percentage of cells undergoing S-phase can be measured.

c. **Mutation of the *p53* tumor suppressor gene** frequently (but not always) leads to aberrant accumulation of dysfunctional p53 protein in the nucleus. Nuclear accumulation of p53 protein can be visualized using IHC staining and has been used as a surrogate marker for *p53* gene mutation. Overexpression of normal p53 protein can sometimes be seen in breast cancer cells, even in the absence of *p53* gene mutation. Conversely, some tumors harbor *p53* mutations that result in protein truncation, which cannot be accurately measured by IHC. Therefore, p53 IHC staining is not an accurate measure of p53 mutational statues and has limited (if any) clinical utility.

VI. MANAGEMENT OF NONINVASIVE BREAST CANCER

A. **Ductal carcinoma in situ (DCIS),** although noninvasive, is clearly a malignant disease and recurs in up to 1/3 of cases within 10 to 15 years if treated with excisional biopsy alone. The recurrence, if it occurs, is invasive carcinoma in as many as 50% of cases. When axillary node dissection has been performed, metastases have been found in <3% of DCIS cases. When mastectomy has been performed, the disease is often found to be *multicentric* (additional CIS lesions >2 cm away from the main lesion).

1. **Local treatment.**

   a. For women with multicentric DCIS, mastectomy, with or without reconstruction, should be performed. For women with unicentric disease, total mastectomy (without lymph node dissection) or lumpectomy with adequate negative margins are both acceptable options. Mastectomy cures at least 98% of patients with DCIS.
   b. The NSABP B-17 trial randomized 818 women with DCIS treated by lumpectomy to no further therapy or breast RT (see Fisher et al., 1999a). The trial demonstrated a reduction in ipsilateral recurrence (invasive plus noninvasive) from 27% to 12% with the use of RT at 8 years of follow-up. Half of the ipsilateral breast tumor recurrences were invasive for those who did not receive radiation. RT reduced the incidence of all noninvasive tumors from 13% to 8% ($P = 0.007$) and of all invasive tumors from 13% to 3%.
   c. The European Cooperative Group Study randomized 1,010 women to receive either 5,000 cGy of RT or observation following surgery (see Julien JP et al. in *Suggested Readings*). The relapse rate was 16% without RT and 9% with RT.
   d. A select group of women with DCIS might be considered for excision without radiation. These include women with low-grade DCIS with negative surgical margins by at least 1.0 cm in all directions.
2. **Adjuvant systemic therapy for DCIS.** The data from the NSABP B-24 trial support the use of adjuvant tamoxifen (20 mg/d for 5 years) for treatment of ER-positive DCIS (see Fisher et al., 1999b). The treatment resulted in 6% and 5% absolute risk reduction in ipsilateral and contralateral recurrence, respectively. Tamoxifen offers no benefit to women with ER-negative DCIS. The use of adjuvant tamoxifen for ER-positive DCIS must be carefully weighed against the known toxicities of the drug because there was no survival benefit.
B. **Lobular carcinoma *in situ* is also called *lobular neoplasia*.** LCIS is considered to be a nonmalignant disease. This tumor tends to be multicentric and is commonly bilateral (approximately 30%). The presence of LCIS is a marker for increased risk of subsequent invasive breast cancer. About 20% of patients with lobular CIS develop invasive breast cancer over 15 years.
   1. Surgery is not routinely recommended for LCIS. Annual diagnostic mammography is recommended to follow women with LCIS.
   2. Patients should be counseled regarding the potential benefit of tamoxifen for risk reduction in this circumstance (a 56% relative risk reduction in developing invasive breast cancer after 5 years of tamoxifen).
   3. In the prospective, double-blind, randomized NSABP STAR P-2 clinical trial, tamoxifen reduced the risk of invasive and noninvasive breast cancer by roughly 50% compared with a roughly 38% reduction in risk with raloxifene. Study participants who took raloxifene had fewer serious side effects than did study participants who took tamoxifen, both initially and after longer-term follow-up.

VII. MANAGEMENT OF EARLY INVASIVE BREAST CANCER: SURGERY AND RT

Management of the primary tumor does not substantially alter the risk of metastases. Variation in local therapies (radical, modified radical, or simple mastectomies, with or without RT) does not alter survival results.

Regional lymph nodes are harbingers of systemic disease and not barriers to tumor spread. Lymph nodes are removed because of the strong prognostic information gained by learning of their involvement. Removal of axillary nodes at surgery does not affect the frequency of breast recurrence, the development of distant metastases, or survival rates.

A. Surgical management

1. **Breast conservation therapy** involves the total gross removal of tumor by limited surgery (lumpectomy, segmental mastectomy) followed by RT to eradicate any residual tumor left in the remaining breast tissue. A *sentinel node* procedure, with or without an axillary nodal dissection, should be done for staging purposes.

   a. **Contraindications for breast conservation therapy**
      (1) Prior radiation to the breast or chest wall resulting in excessive exposure of radiation to the chest wall
      (2) Radiation to be delivered during pregnancy
      (3) Multicentric breast cancer (except in highly selected cases, or on a clinical trial)
      (4) Diffuse malignant-appearing microcalcifications on mammography

   b. **Relative contraindications for breast conservation therapy**
      (1) Multifocality requiring two separate incisions
      (2) Active connective tissue disease involving the skin, such as scleroderma or lupus erythematosus (which may preclude ability to give RT)
      (3) Tumors larger than 5 cm or a sizable tumor in a smaller breast where the subsequent cosmetic outcome is unacceptable

2. **Modified radical mastectomy** is the standard surgical procedure for patients who choose surgery as their only local treatment (e.g., to avoid radiation) or for those patients for whom breast conservation therapy is contraindicated. This procedure includes complete removal of the breast as well as axillary lymph node resection. A number of randomized trials have shown survival equivalence for women undergoing modified radical mastectomy versus breast-conserving surgery plus postlumpectomy radiation. The cosmetic deformity that results can be managed by reconstruction or the use of a prosthesis.

3. **Sentinel lymph nodes (SLN).** Most centers have replaced axillary lymph node dissection with the *SLN technique*, which allows a more limited removal of lymph nodes for staging purposes and results in a lower rate of complications (particularly lymphedema). Women with clinically negative axillae are candidates for SLN resection.

   a. **Completion axillary dissection** was traditionally offered to most patients with SLN metastases >0.2 mm in diameter. In 2011, the randomized phase III trial of ALND versus no ALND in women with invasive breast cancer smaller than 5 cm, no palpable adenopathy, and 1 to 2 SLNs containing metastases showed a 5-year overall survival (OS) of 92% in both groups, suggesting that the use of SLN dissection alone compared with ALND did not result in inferior survival. All patients underwent lumpectomy and tangential whole-breast irradiation. These findings are considered to be practice-changing.

   b. **The routine use of cytokeratin IHC for detection of SLN micrometastases should be discouraged.** Recently reported results of the ACOSOG Z0010 trial confirmed previous reports that the presence of IHC-detected nodal micrometastases (H&E negative) does not provide useful prognostic information.

4. **Breast reconstruction**

   a. **Indications for breast reconstruction** include the availability of adequate skin and soft tissue for a reasonable cosmetic result and realistic expectations on the part of the patient.
   b. **Contraindications to breast reconstruction** include inflammatory carcinoma, the presence of extensive radiation damage to the skin from prior treatment, unrealistic expectations on the part of the patient, and the presence of comorbid diseases that render surgery dangerous. Metastatic disease with an expected long natural history (i.e., years) is not necessarily an absolute contraindication to breast reconstruction.
B. **RT after breast conserving surgery (BCS).** Whole breast irradiation is considered standard of care after BCS in stage I and II breast cancer. The 2005 Early Breast Cancer Trialists' Collaborative Group meta-analysis of the randomized trials showed that the addition of radiation after BCS reduces the risk of local recurrence by 70% at 5 years with a 5% reduction in the 15-year breast cancer mortality (see *Clarke et al.*, 2005).
   1. **Whole breast RT fractionation**
      a. **Conventional fractionation**. The whole breast is usually treated to a dose of 45 to 50 Gy, in 1.8 to 2 Gy per fraction, over a period of 5 weeks.
      b. **Hypofractionation (shorter treatment length)**: Whole breast is treated to 42.5 Gy in 16 fractions over 3 weeks. Randomized trials have demonstrated that hypofractionated RT to the whole breast provides similar local control and toxicity compared with conventional fractionation (see *Whelan et al.*, 2010). For the use of hypofractionation, patients should
         (1) Be at least 50 years old with small or medium-sized breasts
         (2) Have tumor not larger than 5 cm without lymph node involvement
         (3) Not require chemotherapy
   2. **Use of boost of RT after whole breast RT.** The benefit of the boost is higher in patients who are 40 years of age or younger. The boost dose ranges from 10 to 16 Gy, in 2 Gy fractions, usually using electron beam therapy.
   3. **Accelerated partial breast irradiation (APBI).** Only part of the breast (lumpectomy cavity with margins) receives radiation with APBI. RT is usually delivered over 4 to 5 days. The rationale of APBI is that most of local recurrences after BCS occur close or at the lumpectomy site. APBI is still considered investigational and should be offered only for highly selected patients with low risk of recurrence.
   4. **Nodal RT after BCS and axillary surgery (SNL biopsy or ALND)**
      a. Regional nodal irradiation is not necessary in patients with pathologic node-negative disease.
      b. In the past, there was no consensus on regional nodal RT in patients with node-positive disease after BCS. The NCI Canada recently published analysis of the MA-20 trial (see *Whelan et al.*, 2015) which randomized patients who underwent BCS and axillary dissection to whole breast RT with or without regional nodal irradiation (internal mammary, supraclavicular and high axillary nodes). The stages evaluated were T1-2, N1 and high-risk N0 (T3N0 or T2N0 with <10 nodes removed). The tumors also had to manifest one of the following: ER-negative, grade 3, or the presence of lymphovascular invasion. At the 10-year follow-up, there was no significant between-group difference in survival. The rates of DFS were 82.0% in the nodal-irradiation group and 77.0% in the control group (hazard ratio [HR] 0.76, 95%

CI 0.61 to 0.94, $P = 0.01$). Patients in the nodal-irradiation group had higher rates of grade 2 or greater acute pneumonitis (1.2% vs. 0.2%, $P = 0.01$) and lymphedema (8.4% vs. 4.5%, $P = 0.001$).

C. Postmastectomy irradiation (PMRT) for patients with locally advanced breast cancer (LABC)

1. **Sites of locoregional recurrence (LRR).** At the time of LRR, the chest wall is the most common site, representing about two-thirds of the treatment failures. The second most common site of failure is the supraclavicular/infraclavicular region (43%), followed by axillary recurrences (12%) (see *Strom et al.*, 2005).

2. **Rationale for PMRT in patients with LABC.** In high-risk premenopausal breast cancer patients, treated with modified radical mastectomy and adjuvant chemotherapy the addition of radiation reduced the locoregional failure by 20% with a 10% gain in survival.

3. **ASCO guidelines for indications of PMRT:**
   a. Patients with T3N1, or stage III tumors
   b. Patients with ≥4 positive axillary nodes
   c. Positive or close (<1 mm) surgical margins (a NCCN guideline)

4. **Controversial issues with PMRT:**
   a. Patients with 1 to 3 positive axillary nodes
   b. In patients who had at least eight or more axillary nodes removed, the use of PMRT resulted in reduction of the 15-year LRR from 47% to 4% in patients with 1 to 3 positive nodes. There was also a 15-year survival benefit after PMRT in the 1 to 3 positive nodes (57% vs. 48%; see *Overgaard et al.*, 1997).
   c. Consider PMRT for patients with 1 to 3 positive axillary nodes if
      (1) The patient's age is ≤35 years
      (2) There is involvement of >20% of the axillary nodes, or gross extracapsular extension, or <10 nodes removed
      (3) The tumor is grade 3 or demonstrates the presence of lymphovascular invasion

5. **PMRT field design:**
   a. Chest wall irradiation is always given if PMRT is recommended.
   b. Supraclavicular and infraclavicular nodal irradiation is recommended for patients with ≥4 positive axillary nodes.
   c. Internal mammary nodal irradiation is controversial; consider treating if these lymph nodes are clinically or pathologically involved.
   d. Axillary nodal irradiation is not routinely used.

D. Radiotherapy or surgery of the axilla after a positive sentinel node in breast cancer. Patients with T1-2 primary breast cancer and no palpable lymphadenopathy were randomly assigned to receive either axillary lymph node dissection or axillary radiotherapy in case of a positive sentinel node (Donker *et al.*, 2014). Axillary recurrence occurred in four of 744 patients in the axillary lymph node dissection group and seven of 681 in the axillary radiotherapy group. The planned non-inferiority test was underpowered because of the low number of events. Lymphedema in the ipsilateral arm was noted significantly more often after axillary lymph node dissection than after axillary radiotherapy at 1 year, 3 years, and 5 years. Thus, axillary radiotherapy results in significantly less morbidity.

VIII. MANAGEMENT OF EARLY INVASIVE BREAST CANCER: ADJUVANT CHEMOTHERAPY

A. Principles. Application of about 6 months of polychemotherapy reduces the annual breast cancer death rate by about 38% for women <50 years of age,

TABLE 11-1 Approximate Reduction of Mortality at 10 Years with Adjuvant Chemotherapy for Breast Cancers

ER-negative and PR-negative patients treated with doxorubicin-based regimens

Reduction in mortality with adjuvant chemotherapy[a]

Stage	Age 35 yr		Age 60 yr	
	Grade 1	Grade 2/3	Grade 1	Grade 2/3
I (T1c N0)	3	6	2	4
IIA	6	12	4	8
IIB	9	15	6	10
IIIA	14	20	10	113
IIIC	18	21	12	14

ER-positive or PR-positive patients treated with doxorubicin-based regimens with or without hormonal therapy

Reduction in mortality with adjuvant chemotherapy[a]

Stage	Age 35 yr				Age 60 yr			
	Grade 1		Grade 2/3		Grade 1		Grade 2/3	
Stage	H	C-H	H	C-H	H	C-H	H	C-H
I (T1c N0)	1	2	4	8	1	1	4	6
IIA	3	5	8	15	3	4	7	11
IIB	6	16	12	25	4	6	10	13
IIIA	9	18	14	30	7	12	13	22
IIIC	12	26	14	35	11	14	13	20

[a]"Mortality" is the number of deaths caused by breast cancer among 100 patients. "Reduction" is the fewer number of deaths caused by breast cancer among 100 patients. Data do not account for *HER2* positivity or treatment with trastuzumab.
C-H, chemotherapy followed by hormonal therapy for 5 yr; H, hormonal therapy alone.
Adapted from *Adjuvant Online* and Woodward WA, Strom EA, Tucker SL, et al. Changes in the 2003 American Joint Committee on Cancer Staging for breast cancer dramatically affect stage-specific survival. *J Clin Oncol* 2003;21:3244.

and by about 20% for those aged 50 to 69. Table 11-1 shows the approximate reductions for mortality at 10 years by chemotherapy for patients who are 35 or 60 years of age and whose tumors are either negative or positive for hormone receptor activity. The algorithm for the adjuvant management is depicted in Figure 11-1.

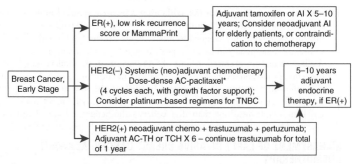

*See section VIII for other chemotherapy regimens used in the adjuvant setting

Figure 11-1 Algorithm for the (neo)adjuvant management of early-stage breast cancer.

1. **Candidates for adjuvant systemic therapy.** Women at sufficiently high risk to warrant adjuvant chemotherapy include nearly all women with positive axillary lymph nodes and many with high-risk, node-negative disease as well. Historically, node-negative patients with sufficiently high risk to be considered as candidates for adjuvant chemotherapy tend to be those with tumors that (1) are hormone receptor negative, high grade, or poorly differentiated; (2) overexpress *HER2*; (3) have markers of increased proliferation (e.g., mitotic index, high Ki-67, or elevated S-phase fraction); (4) have evidence of angiolymphatic invasion; (5) have a high-risk recurrence score (RS) based on the Oncotype DX assay; or (6) have high-risk disease based on MammaPrint analysis. The relative benefit of chemotherapy depends on many factors, including the woman's age at diagnosis, presence of comorbidities, and her hormone receptor status.

2. **Patient selection for adjuvant chemotherapy.** For early breast cancer but with poor prognostic markers, treatment discussion should include an explanation of both relative and absolute expected risk reduction. Moreover, patients with favorable prognostic features may be spared the toxicities of chemotherapy and treated appropriately with adjuvant endocrine therapy alone.

   a. ***Adjuvant! Online.*** Patient selection for appropriate systemic adjuvant therapy has been revolutionized by computerized decision-making tools such as *Adjuvant! Online* (www.adjuvantonline.com). Breast cancer outcome estimates made by *Adjuvant! Online* are for patients who have (1) unilateral, unicentric, invasive adenocarcinoma of the breast, (2) undergone definitive primary breast surgery and axillary node staging, and (3) no evidence of metastatic or known residual disease.

   In this online algorithm, professionals enter age, comorbidities, ER status, tumor grade, tumor size, and the number of positive lymph nodes. Then that person selects for type of adjuvant endocrine therapy (i.e., tamoxifen, aromatase inhibition) and adjuvant chemotherapy regimen (first, second or third generation). A report is then generated estimating 10-year recurrence risk or 10-year mortality (a) with no systemic adjuvant therapy, (b) with adjuvant endocrine therapy alone, (c) with adjuvant chemotherapy alone, or (d) both endocrine and chemotherapy. Graphic printouts of the results are available for counseling patients on both the risks and the benefits of adjuvant chemotherapy.

   Potential shortcomings of *Adjuvant!Online* include the relative lack of clinical data for patients who have very small lymph node–negative tumors or who are elderly, and the absence of important known risk factors such as *HER2* (although a new version will include data on *HER2* and adjuvant trastuzumab). An important update to *Adjuvant!Online* will include a genomic version that does include Oncotype DX RSs. Another shortcoming is that Adjuvant!Online has been offline for many months due to funding shortages.

   b. **Oncotype DX assay** quantifies the *likelihood* of breast cancer recurrence in women with newly diagnosed, early-stage, lymph node–negative, ER-positive breast cancer. The assay is performed using formalin-fixed, paraffin-embedded tumor tissue. This multiplex PCR assay measures messenger RNA (mRNA) transcripts of a panel of 16 breast cancer-associated genes that correlate with distant metastases and 5 control genes. The calculation of the RS then combines the gene expression data into a single result (0 to 100).

      (1) The Oncotype DX gene panel has a prognostic value in women treated with tamoxifen: they can be classified according to RSs into high risk (RS $\geq$ 31), intermediate risk (RS = 18 and <31), or low risk (RS < 18) based on 10-year distant DFS.

(2) In addition to prognostic information, the Oncotype DX assay may indicate the probability of response to adjuvant therapies. Patients with low or intermediate risk have a significant benefit from the use of adjuvant tamoxifen, whereas the high-risk group do not. Patients in the high-risk RS strata significantly benefit from adjuvant chemotherapy, whereas the intermediate and low-risk groups did not achieve statistical significance.

(3) Oncotype DX has also been evaluated in a pilot retrospective study in patients with lymph node–positive, ER-positive disease. Similar to observations in lymph node–negative disease, the pilot study indicated little (if any) benefit from anthracycline-based (but not containing a taxane) adjuvant chemotherapy for patients with low-risk RS, whereas patients with high-risk RS had a significant impact from adjuvant therapy. Prospective confirmation of these findings using modern adjuvant chemotherapy regimens is necessary for this observation to be practice changing.

c. **MammaPrint** analyzes a DNA microarray consisting of 70 genes regulating cell cycle, invasion, metastasis, and angiogenesis. By performing DNA microarray analysis on primary breast tumors of patients, a gene expression signature that was strongly prognostic for development of distant metastasis in lymph node–negative patients was identified. A potential advantage of the MammaPrint assay is its inclusion of both ER-negative and ER-positive early-stage patients.

The EORTC 10041/BIG 3-04 MINDACT study enrolled 6,693 patients who had undergone successful determination of their genomic risk G (with MammaPrint) and clinical risk C (modified version Adjuvant! Online). At 5 years, distant metastasis free survival (DMFS) was 94.7% for patients who were C- high/G- low and randomized to use G and received no chemotherapy (CT). When using the G assay MammaPrint® among the C-high patients, there was a 46% reduction in CT prescription, providing level 1A evidence for the clinical

---

TABLE 11-2   Selected Adjuvant Chemotherapy Options for Breast Cancer

Preferred Non–Trastuzumab-containing Regimens	Other Non–Trastuzumab-containing Regimens
DAC	FAC or CAF; FEC or CEF
AC → P weekly	FEC → P weekly
AC	EC
DC	AC → D every 3 wk
	FEC → D
	CMF
Dose dense: AC × 4 cycles → P × 4 cycles (regimen every 2 wk with filgrastim support)	Dose dense: A → P → C (regimen every 2 wk with filgrastim support)
Preferred Trastuzumab-containing Regimens	**Other Trastuzumab-containing Regimens**
H+ D-Carbo	D + H → FEC
AC → P + concurrent H	AC → D + concurrent H
	Chemotherapy followed by H sequentially

→, followed by; A, Adriamycin (doxorubicin); C, cyclophosphamide; Carbo, carboplatin; D, docetaxel (Taxotere); E, epirubicin; F, 5-fluorouracil; H, Herceptin (trastuzumab); P, paclitaxel (Taxol).
Regimen dosages are shown in Table 11-3.
Adapted from the National Comprehensive Cancer Network (NCCN) Guidelines, version 2.2011. All listed regimens are category 1 (based upon high-level evidence with uniform NCCN consensus that the treatment is appropriate).

| TABLE 11-3 | Adjuvant Chemotherapy Regimens for Breast Cancer[a] | | |

Regimen (Frequency and Numbers of Cycles)	Anthracycline or Antimetabolite	Taxane	Alkylator
AC (q 3 wk × 4)	Adr 60 (d 1)		Cyc 600 (d 1)
DC (q 3 wk × 4)		Doc 75 (d1)	Cyc 600 (d1)
DAC (q 3 wk × 6)[b]	Adr 50 (d 1)	Doc 75 (d 1)	Cyc 500 (d 1)
AC → P (AC q 3 wk × 4, then P)	Adr 60 (d 1)	Pac 80 (wkly × 12)	Cyc 600 (d 1)
AC → D (AC q 3 wk × 4, then D)	Adr 60 (d 1)	Doc 100 (q 3 wk × 4)	Cyc 600 (d 1)
FAC (q 3 wk × 6)	Adr 50 (d 1) 5-FU 500 (d 1 & 8)		Cyc 500 (d 1)
CAF (q 4 wk × 6)	Adr 30 (d 1 & 8)		Cyc 100 PO (days 1 to 14)
	5-FU 600 (d 1 & 8)		
EC (q 3 wk × 8)	Epi 100 (d 1)		Cyc 830 (d 1)
FEC (q 3 wk × 6)	Epi 50 (d 1 & 8) or 100 (d 1) 5-FU 500 (d 1)		Cyc 500 (d 1)
FEC → P (FEC q 3 wk × 4, then P)	Epi 90 (d 1) 5-FU 600 (d 1)	After 3 wk of no treatment: Pac 100 (wkly × 12)	Cyc 600 (d1)
FEC → D (FEC q 3 wk × 3, then D)	Epi 100 (d 1) 5-FU 500 (d 1)	Doc 100 (q 3 wk × 3)	Cyc 500 (d1)
Classic CMF (q 4 wk × 6)	Mtx 40 (d 1 & 8) 5-FU 600 (d 1 & 8)		Cyc 100 PO (days 1 to 14)
Dose dense: AC → P[b] (AC q 2 wk × 4, then P)	Adr 60 (d 1)	Pac 175 (q 2 wk × 4)	Cyc 600 (d 1)
Dose dense: A → P → C[b]	Adr 60 (q 2 wk × 4)	Pac 175 (q 2 wk × 4)	Cyc 600 (q 2 wk × 4)

Trastuzumab-containing regimens: see Section VIII.D.4.

[a]Drug doses are in mg/m[2] body surface area (days on which drugs are given in each cycle and frequency of cycles are in parentheses); all drugs are given intravenously except PO where indicated.

[b]Filgrastim or pegfilgrastim is given during each 2- or 3-week cycle.

Adr, Adriamycin (doxorubicin); Cyc, cyclophosphamide; Doc, docetaxel; Epi, epirubicin; 5-FU, 5-fluorouracil; Mtx, methotrexate; Pac, paclitaxel; wks/wkly, weeks/weekly.

utility of MammaPrint for assessing the lack of a clinically relevant chemotherapy benefit in the clinically high-risk (C-high) population.

B. Chemotherapy regimens. Commonly used regimens are shown in Table 11-2. Drug dosing and schedules for these options are shown in Table 11-3.

C. Role of taxanes in the adjuvant setting

1. Multiple clinical trials strongly suggest an additional benefit to adding a taxane to an anthracycline-based chemotherapy regimen for women with lymph node-positive breast cancer. Examples include

    a. Cancer and Acute Leukemia Group B (CALGB 9344) showed a 17% reduction in risk of recurrence and an 18% reduction in risk of death with the addition of paclitaxel given every 3 weeks for four cycles after four cycles of Adriamycin–cyclophosphamide (AC).

    b. NSABP B-28 showed a 17% reduction in risk of recurrence at a median of 65 months by adding paclitaxel sequentially to AC in a manner similar to the CALGB 9344.

   c. Breast Cancer International Research Group (BCIRG 001) showed that docetaxel/AC (DAC) delivered every 3 weeks for six cycles resulted in a 28% improvement in DFS compared with six cycles of CA-fluorouracil (CAF). In addition, a 30% improvement in OS was noted during this same time period.

   d. Four cycles of DC (docetaxel/cyclophosphamide) has been compared to four cycles of AC in patients with early breast cancer (about half of whom were lymph node negative). The difference in DFS between DC and AC was significant (81% DC vs. 75% AC; HR = 0.74, *P* = 0.033) as was OS (87% DC vs. 82% AC; HR = 0.69, *P* = 0.032).

   e. In a non-inferiority study designed to interrogate a role for adjuvant anthracycline-based chemotherapy, 4,156 patients were enrolled. The trial was stopped at the first interim analysis as the non-inferiority boundary was not met: TC was not as effective as anthracycline/taxane regimens. The hazard ration was 1.23 (*P* = 0.04 for superiority) favoring the use of anthracyclines. The benefit was greatest in patients with hormone-receptor negative disease and multiple lymph node involvement.

2. Because all ER-positive breast cancers respond less well to chemotherapy compared with ER-negative tumors, the additional benefit of adding a taxane for ER-positive patients is not as pronounced compared with ER-negative patients.

3. What these studies do not tell us is which is the best regimen and which taxane or taxane dosing schedule is superior. In an attempt to address this shortcoming, the Eastern Cooperative Oncology Group (ECOG) conducted a randomized, prospective clinical trial (E1199) designed to compare taxanes (docetaxel vs. paclitaxel) and taxane-dosing schedules (weekly vs. every 3 weeks) head to head. In this 2 × 2 factorial study design, patients received four cycles of AC every 3 weeks followed by (1) paclitaxel every 3 weeks for four cycles, (2) docetaxel every 3 weeks for four cycles, (3) paclitaxel weekly for 12 weeks, or (4) docetaxel weekly for 12 weeks.

   a. The primary comparisons failed to demonstrate any significant advantage of one taxane over another, or the weekly schedule over every-3-week schedule.

   b. In planned secondary comparisons, both the weekly paclitaxel arm and the every-3-week docetaxel arm were significantly superior to the every-3-week paclitaxel arm.

D. Adjuvant trastuzumab. Trastuzumab is a humanized, monoclonal antibody with specificity for the extracellular domain of the human *EGFR*-2 (*HER2*; *HER2/neu*).

1. Randomized trials. The adjuvant trastuzumab trials are remarkably consistent, with most analyses indeed reporting an OS benefit with trastuzumab treatment.

   a. In NSABP B-31, patients with *HER2*-positive, node-positive breast cancer were randomly assigned to AC for four cycles every 3 weeks followed by paclitaxel given every 3 weeks for four cycles or the same regimen with 52 weeks of trastuzumab commencing with the paclitaxel. In the North Central Cancer Treatment Group (NCCTG) N9831 intergroup trial, patients who were *HER2*-positive with early-stage cancer were similarly randomized except that paclitaxel was given by a low-dose weekly schedule for 12 weeks; a third arm testing sequential chemotherapy followed by trastuzumab was added.

      Because of their similarities, the B-31 and NCCTG N9831 trials with 3,351 patients together were analyzed jointly. With a median follow-up of 2 years, trastuzumab resulted in a 52% reduction in the risk of recurrence ($P < 0.001$) and a 33% reduction in the risk of death ($P = 0.015$).

b. A third trial (HERA) involving 5,081 patients tested trastuzumab for 1 versus 2 years (compared with no further treatment) following all local therapy and a menu of standard chemotherapy regimens. Two years of adjuvant trastuzumab is not more effective than is 1 year of treatment for patients with HER2-positive early breast cancer.

c. The BCIRG 006 study randomized 3,222 women with *HER2*-amplified, node-positive or high-risk node-negative breast cancer to AC followed by docetaxel, AC followed by docetaxel plus trastuzumab (DH) for 1 year, or carboplatin plus docetaxel plus trastuzumab. At a median follow-up of 10.3 years, a persistent significant DFS benefit is seen in both trastuzumab-containing arms compared to AC-T with only 10 DFS events separating the two trastuzumab-based regimens: AC-TH (HR = 0.70, $P < 0.001$) and TCH (HR = 0.76, $P < 0.001$). At this final analysis, the DFS HRs for AC-TH and TCH are closer than those observed in any prior protocol-directed study analyses (at 5 years follow-up the HRs were 0.64 and 0.75 for AC-TH and TCH respectively, and are not significantly different in an unplanned *post hoc* analysis). Also, an OS benefit was observed in both AC-TH (HR = 0.64, $P < 0.001$) and TCH (HR = 0.76, $P = 0.0081$). Importantly, TCH has significantly lower symptomatic congestive heart failure (CHF) events by five-fold compared to AC-TH; 21 (2.0%) for AC-TH versus 4 (0.4%) for TCH; $P = 0.0005$ (the AC-T control arm had 8 [0.8%] symptomatic CHF events). The incidence of patients with a relative LVEF decline >10% is doubled in the AC-TH compared to TCH regimens (206 vs. 97, $P < 0.0001$). Dosages and schedules for these regimens are shown in Table 11-3.

2. **Cardiac adverse events from adjuvant trastuzumab.** In the adjuvant trastuzumab trials, the rates of grade III/IV CHF or cardiac-related death for patients receiving treatment regimens containing trastuzumab ranged from 0% to 4.1%. The risk of cardiac dysfunction appears to be related to age, baseline left ventricular ejection fraction (LVEF), prior anthracycline treatment, and use of concomitant antihypertensive medications.

Candidates for treatment with trastuzumab should undergo thorough baseline cardiac assessment, including history and physical examination and assessment of LVEF by echocardiogram or radionuclide scan. Monitoring may not identify all patients who will develop cardiac dysfunction. Caution should be exercised in treating patients with pre-existing cardiac dysfunction. Discontinuation of trastuzumab treatment should be strongly considered in patients who develop a clinically significant decrease in LVEF.

3. *HER2* **status, topoisomerase II, and the role of anthracyclines.** Numerous large retrospective studies have linked *HER2* status with response to anthracyclines. Transfection and overexpression of *HER2* in breast cancer cell lines does not, however, increase sensitivity to doxorubicin *in vitro*. This observation suggests that some factor other than *HER2* confers drug sensitivity to anthracyclines.

The topoisomerase IIα gene is in close physical proximity to the *HER2* gene on the long arm of chromosome 17, and in 35% of patients with *HER2* gene amplification, the topoisomerase II gene is coamplified. The current hypothesis is that amplification of topoisomerase II confers sensitivity to anthracyclines, and not *HER2* gene amplification *per se*. Of note, topoisomerase II gene amplification is seen rarely (if ever) in the absence of *HER2* gene amplification. Thus, it is arguable whether or not anthracyclines are of any benefit in *HER2*-negative early-stage breast cancers.

The U.S. Oncology Network is currently testing docetaxel plus cyclophosphamide for six cycles, versus the DAC regimen for six cycles in *HER2*-negative early-stage patients. Whether or not to utilize anthracycline-containing adjuvant regimens in *HER2*-positive disease remains controversial (BCIRG 006 results notwithstanding). Published data indicate anthracyclines may be dispensable in lymph node–negative, *HER2*-positive early breast cancer.

4. **Trastuzumab combinations for adjuvant chemotherapy** (cardiac monitoring is done at baseline, 3, 6, and 9 months)
   a. **Docetaxel/carboplatin** (H + D-Carbo; TCH)
      Docetaxel, 75 mg/m² IV on day 1
      Carboplatin, area under the curve (AUC) 6 IV on day 1; cycled every 21 days for six cycles
      Trastuzumab, 4 mg/kg on week 1; followed by 2 mg/kg for 17 weeks; followed by 6 mg/kg every 3 weeks to complete 1 year of therapy.
   b. **Doxorubicin/cyclophosphamide/paclitaxel** (AC → P)
      Doxorubicin, 60 mg/m² IV on day 1 and
      Cyclophosphamide, 600 mg/m² IV on day 1; cycled every 21 days for four cycles
      Followed by paclitaxel, 175 mg/m² IV over 3 hours on day 1; cycled every 21 days for four cycles
      Trastuzumab, 4 mg/kg with first dose of paclitaxel; followed by 2 mg/kg weekly or 6 mg/kg every 3 weeks (after completion of paclitaxel) to complete 1 year of therapy
   c. **Doxorubicin/cyclophosphamide/docetaxel** (AC → P). Same as Section D.4.b except that docetaxel (100 mg/m² IV) is substituted for paclitaxel at the same schedule

E. **Dose-dense therapy.** Delivering identical doses of chemotherapy on a more frequent basis is described as *dose-dense* therapy. One large clinical trial (CALGB 9741) showed a 26% improvement in DFS and a 31% improvement in OS for women with lymph node–positive breast cancer receiving chemotherapy on an every-2-week basis with growth factors when compared with the same regimen delivered every 3 weeks without growth factor support. AC (every 2 weeks for four cycles) was followed by paclitaxel (every 2 weeks for four cycles).

F. **Adjuvant chemotherapy is not indicated in the following circumstances:**
   1. In women with a good prognosis without such treatment, including those with the following conditions:
      a. Noninvasive CIS of any size in women of any age
      b. Very small primary tumors (<0.5 cm; T1a) and negative axillary lymph nodes, irrespective of the status of hormone receptors
      c. Lymph node–negative, ER-positive cases with low-risk RS based on Oncotype DX
      d. Comorbid medical conditions that make survival beyond 5 years unlikely or that make the potential adverse effects of therapy unacceptable
   2. Controversy exists regarding the use of adjuvant systemic chemotherapy for women whose tumors are 0.6 to 1.0 cm with negative hormone receptors or with a grade interpreted as moderately or poorly differentiated.

G. **Radiation and chemotherapy.** For women who are prescribed both chemotherapy and RT, the modalities are usually used sequentially with chemotherapy delivered first. RT may be used concurrently with cyclophosphamide, methotrexate, 5-fluorouracil (CMF) chemotherapy (at times requiring dose modification of methotrexate), but not with other published regimens.

H. Adjuvant endocrine therapy

1. **Selective ER modifiers.** Tamoxifen has been considered the standard of care for all women with an invasive breast cancer that expresses either ER or PR. The benefit of tamoxifen is seen regardless of the patient's age, the number of involved lymph nodes, and whether or not chemotherapy is used. Historically, trials have demonstrated that patients did the best when taking 20 mg of tamoxifen daily for 5 years. However, in the ATLAS trial, among women with ER-positive disease, allocation to continue tamoxifen reduced the risk of breast cancer recurrence (617 recurrences in 3,428 women allocated to continue vs. 711 in 3,418 controls, $P = 0.002$), reduced breast cancer mortality (331 deaths vs. 397 deaths, $P = 0.01$), and reduced overall mortality (639 deaths vs. 722 deaths, $P = 0.01$). Similarly, in the aTTom trial, 6,953 patients were randomized to 5 vs. 10 years of tamoxifen. There were 580 versus 672 recurrences (RR = 0.85, $P = 0.003$) for the long vs. short duration tamoxifen, respectively (albeit in this case, without survival benefit). The risk of thromboembolic complications and endometrial cancer were higher with 10-years of tamoxifen.

2. **Aromatase inhibitors** (AIs) block the peripheral conversion of the adrenal androgens (androstenedione and testosterone) into estradiol and estrone in postmenopausal women. AIs should not be considered in those women who have any ovarian function because blockage of peripheral aromatization will not block the ovarian production of estrogen and progesterone.

   a. **The ATAC trial** randomized 9,366 postmenopausal women with early invasive breast cancer to one of three arms: anastrozole 1 mg daily for 5 years, tamoxifen 20 mg daily for 5 years, and the combination of both drugs daily for 5 years (see ATAC Trialists' Group, 2002). The outcome of those women taking the combination of anastrozole and tamoxifen was the same as that of the women taking tamoxifen alone. At a median follow-up of 48 months, however, findings were an 18% improvement in DFS and a 22% improvement in time to recurrence for those patients with ER-positive tumors who were randomized to anastrozole compared with tamoxifen. In addition, an additional 44% reduction was noted in new contralateral breast tumors for women receiving 5 years of anastrozole.

   b. **The BIG 1-98 trial** is a randomized, phase 3, double-blind study of tamoxifen versus letrozole in 6,182 postmenopausal women with steroid receptor–positive early breast cancer (see BIG 1-98 Collaborative Group, Mouridsen et al., 2009). Two years of treatment with one agent was followed by 3 years of the other agent. With a median follow-up of 71 months, DFS was not significantly improved with either of the sequential treatments compared to letrozole alone. Moreover, in the 4,922 patients randomized to tamoxifen or letrozole monotherapy, with a median follow-up of 76 months, DFS was superior in the letrozole arm (HR = 0.88, $P < 0.05$) with a nonsignificant trend toward improved OS (HR = 0.87, $P = 0.08$).

   Taken together, results from the ATAC and BIG 1-98 trials support the use of adjuvant AIs for postmenopausal women with hormone receptor–positive invasive early breast cancer.

   c. **The MA-17 trial** randomized 5,187 postmenopausal women with ER-positive and ER-negative invasive breast cancer who had received from 4.5 to 5.5 years of tamoxifen in the adjuvant setting (see Muss et al., 2008). These women were randomized to 5 years of further therapy with either placebo or letrozole. At 30-months median follow-up, letrozole significantly improved DFS in all patients and OS in node-positive patients. Additionally, letrozole decreased the incidence of contralateral breast cancer by 46%. Thus, for postmenopausal women, the addition of letrozole after 5 years of tamoxifen may be considered.

   d. Additionally, a double-blind, randomized trial to test whether, after 2 to 3 years of tamoxifen therapy, switching to exemestane was more effective than was continuing tamoxifen therapy for the remainder of the 5 years of treatment has been conducted. Exemestane therapy after 2 to 3 years of tamoxifen therapy significantly improved DFS and reduced the occurrence of contralateral breast cancer as compared with the standard 5 years of tamoxifen treatment.

   e. In summary, aromatase inhibition is superior to tamoxifen in postmenopausal ER-positive patients whether used first line in place of tamoxifen, following 2 to 3 years of tamoxifen, or following 5 years of tamoxifen. The optimal duration of AI therapy remains unknown.

   3. Ovarian ablation. Ovarian ablation via surgical oophorectomy or suppression with agonists of luteinizing hormone–releasing hormone (LHRH) is effective therapy for premenopausal ER-positive early-stage breast cancer. Available data suggest similar benefit from surgical ovarian ablation as there is with the use of CMF chemotherapy in such patients. In the SOFT and TEXT randomized trials, DFS at 5 years was 91.1% in the exemestane-ovarian suppression group and 87.3% in the tamoxifen-ovarian suppression group (HR for disease recurrence, second invasive cancer, or death, 0.72; $P < 0.001$). OS did not differ significantly between the two groups. Benefit from OFS is most striking in women under age 35.

   4. Combination chemohormonal therapy. When chemotherapy and tamoxifen are both used in the adjuvant setting, they are usually used sequentially, rather than in combination, because of a detrimental outcome when comparing concurrent versus sequential chemohormonal therapy. Whether this observation will also hold true for AIs is unknown.

I. **Preoperative (neoadjuvant) chemotherapy**

   1. The use of preoperative cytoreductive chemotherapy for those who desire breast conservation therapy may be considered. No published survival advantage exists to the delivery of the chemotherapy preoperatively compared with its postoperative use. The algorithm for the neoadjuvant management is depicted in Figure 11-1.

   2. For patients with inoperable locally advanced disease at presentation, the initial use of preoperative chemotherapy with an anthracycline and a taxane is standard treatment. Following neoadjuvant therapy, measures aimed at local control usually consist of total mastectomy with axillary lymph node dissection, with or without delayed breast reconstruction, or lumpectomy and axillary dissection. Both local treatment measures are considered to have sufficient risk of local recurrence to warrant the use of chest wall (or breast) and supraclavicular node irradiation. Involved internal mammary lymph nodes should also be irradiated. Tamoxifen (or an AI if postmenopausal) should be added for those with hormone receptor–positive tumors.

   3. In selected ER-positive patients, neoadjuvant endocrine therapy may be used; for example in elderly or frail patients, or patients with a contraindication to neoadjuvant chemotherapy.

   4. For *HER2*-positive patients, neoadjuvant chemotherapy regimens incorporating trastuzumab have been shown to have impressive pathologic complete response rates. Recently, incorporation of pertuzumab, along with trastuzumab plus chemotherapy has won accelerated approval by the U.S. FDA, based in part upon data from the NeoSphere trial (and a supporting cardiac safety trial). In this open-label, randomized phase II trial, patients given pertuzumab and trastuzumab plus docetaxel had a significantly improved pathologic complete response rate (49 of 107 patients; 45.8%) compared with those given trastuzumab plus docetaxel (31 of 107; 29.0%, $P = 0.0141$).

J. **Adjuvant bisphosphonates and adjuvant denosumab.** The Early Breast Cancer Trialists' Cooperative Group received data on 18,766 women (18,206 [97%] in trials of 2 to 5 years of bisphosphonate) with median follow-up 5.6 woman-years, 3,453 first recurrences, and 2,106 subsequent deaths. They observed a significant reduction in bone recurrence (RR 0.83, $2P = 0.004$), and among 11,767 postmenopausal women it produced highly significant reductions in recurrence (RR 0.86, $2P = 0.002$), distant recurrence (0.82, $2P = 0.0003$), bone recurrence (0.72; $2P = 0.0002$), and breast cancer mortality (0.82, $2P = 0.002$). Bone fractures were also reduced (RR 0.85, $2P = 0.02$).

In the prospective, double-blind, placebo-controlled, phase 3 ABCSG-18 trial, postmenopausal patients with early hormone receptor–positive breast cancer receiving treatment with AIs were randomly assigned in a 1:1 ratio to receive either denosumab 60 mg or placebo administered subcutaneously every 6 months in 58 trial centers in Austria and Sweden. Study results showed that after a median follow-up of 4 years, patients assigned denosumab had an 18% reduced risk of their disease recurring compared with those assigned placebo (HR = 0.816, $P = 0.051$). Denosumab also reduced the risk of clinical fractures in ABCSG-18.

K. **Adjuvant therapy for patients who do not achieve a pathologic complete response to neoadjuvant chemotherapy.** The phase III CREATE-X trial investigated whether the drug capecitabine, given for up to eight cycles, could improve DFS among 455 HER2-negative patients who had residual disease after neoadjuvant chemotherapy. At 5 years, DFS rates were 74.1% in the capecitabine arm vs. 67.7% in the control arm (HR = 0.70, $P = 0.00524$), and OS rates were 89.2% and 83.9% (HR = 0.40, $P < 0.01$), respectively.

L. **Adjuvant chemotherapy following isolated local-regional relapse (ILRR).** The CALOR trial was an open-label, randomized trial that accrued patients with histologically proven and completely excised ILRR after unilateral breast cancer who had undergone a mastectomy or lumpectomy with clear surgical margins. Eligible patients were centrally randomized (1:1) to chemotherapy (type selected by the investigator; multidrug for at least four courses recommended) or no chemotherapy. Five-year DFS was 69% with chemotherapy versus 57% without chemotherapy (HR = 0.59, $P = 0.046$). Adjuvant chemotherapy was significantly more effective for women with estrogen receptor–negative ILRR (p-interaction = 0.046).

IX. MANAGEMENT: DISSEMINATED DISEASE (STAGE IV)

Except in rare cases, stage IV breast cancer is considered incurable. Thus, the focus of treatment for advanced disease should be on palliation of disease-related symptoms. The algorithm for the management of metastatic disease is depicted in Figure 11-2.

A. **Hormone receptor–positive MBC.** For women who have non–life-threatening, ER-positive or PR-positive MBC, hormone therapy is recommended. Chemotherapy is reserved for hormone-resistant disease, or patients with symptomatic or life-threatening metastases.

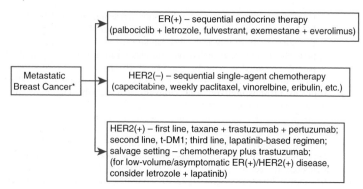

*Patients with bone metastasis also receive monthly denosumab or a bisphosphonate

Figure 11-2 Algorithm for the management of MBC.

1. **For postmenopausal women,** palbociclib has recently been introduced in the first line ER+ setting. Palbociclib is an oral, small-molecule inhibitor of cyclin-dependent kinases (CDKs) 4 and 6. In the PALOMA-1 (TRIO-18) randomized phase II study, 165 postmenopausal women with advanced estrogen receptor–positive and HER2-negative breast cancer who had not received any systemic treatment for their advanced disease were randomized to receive palbociclib plus letrozole versus letrozole alone. Median progression-free survival was 10.2 months for the letrozole group and 20.2 months for the palbociclib plus letrozole group (HR = 0.488, one-sided $P = 0.0004$). In another multi-center, double-blind, randomized phase 3 study (PALOMA 3), 521 women aged 18 years or older with hormone receptor–positive, HER2-negative MBC that had progressed on previous endocrine therapy were randomized (2:1) to fulvestrant plus palbociclib versus fulvestrant plus placebo. Median progression-free survival was 9.5 months in the fulvestrant plus palbociclib group and 4.6 months in the fulvestrant plus placebo group (HR = 0.46, 95% CI 0.36 to 0.59, $P < 0.0001$). For ER+ patients who progress following palbociclib plus letrozole in the first line metastatic setting, single agent fulvestrant (500 mg IM, monthly) is a common next choice.

   BOLERO-2 is a phase 3, double-blind, randomized, international trial comparing everolimus (10 mg/d) plus exemestane (25 mg/d) versus placebo plus exemestane in postmenopausal women with hormone receptor–positive advanced breast cancer with recurrence/progression during or after non-steroidal AIs. Final study results with median 18-month follow-up show that median PFS remained significantly longer with everolimus plus exemestane versus placebo plus exemestane [investigator review: 7.8 versus 3.2 months, respectively; HR = 0.45; log-rank $P < 0.0001$; central review: 11.0 versus 4.1 months, respectively; HR = 0.38; log-rank $P < 0.0001$] in the overall population and in all prospectively defined subgroups.

   Other endocrine agents can be used in a sequential manner:
   a. Tamoxifen (20 mg PO daily) or toremifene (60 mg PO daily)
   b. Fulvestrant 500 mg IM monthly
   c. Megestrol acetate 40 mg PO q.i.d.
   d. Fluoxymesterone 10 mg PO b.i.d. or t.i.d.

   e. Diethylstilbestrol 5 mg PO t.i.d.
   f. Estradiol 2mg PO t.i.d.
2. **For premenopausal women,** options include the following:
   a. Tamoxifen
   b. LHRH agonist or surgical or radiotherapeutic oophorectomy
   c. Megestrol acetate
   d. Fluoxymesterone
   e. Diethylstilbesterol
B. **Chemotherapy.** No gold standard chemotherapy regimen exists for MBC. Although somewhat more active than single agents, the combinations are associated with more treatment-related side effects. Consequently, sequential single agent chemotherapy (except in cases where rapid response is required) is most commonly used to manage advanced ER-negative (or hormone-refractory ER-positive) disease.
   1. *HER2*-negative, ER-negative MBC
      a. **Preferred single agents** include the anthracyclines (doxorubicin, epirubicin, or liposomal doxorubicin), the taxanes (paclitaxel, docetaxel, or albumin-bound paclitaxel), capecitabine, or vinorelbine. Effective treatment options for patients with MBC resistant to anthracyclines and taxanes are limited.
      b. **Other active agents** include gemcitabine, platinoids, vinblastine, irinotecan, mitomycin, ixabepilone, and eribulin. One study showed that ixabepilone plus capecitabine prolonged median progression-free survival (6 vs. 4 months), and increased objective response rate (35% vs. 14%, $P< 0.0001$) compared with capecitabine alone. In a phase 3 open label study of eribulin versus treatment of physician's choice (see Cortes et al., 2011) in patients with 2 to 5 previous lines of chemotherapy for advanced disease, OS was significantly improved in women ($N= 508$) assigned to eribulin compared with TPC ($N= 254$; HR $= 0.81$, $P= 0.041$).
      c. **Carboplatin in BRCA-mutant MBC.** In the Triple-Negative Trial (TNT), 376 patients were randomly assigned to receive carboplatin (AUC of 6 every 3 weeks) or docetaxel (100 mg/m^2 every 3 weeks) for six to eight cycles or until disease progression, with crossover possible on disease progression. Among the subset of 43 *BRCA*-mutant patients, a difference emerged between the regimens. The objective response rate was 68% with carboplatin and 33% with docetaxel, a 34.7% absolute difference (95% CI $= 6.3$% to 63.1%), which was statistically significant ($P= 0.03$). In contrast, for the 273 *BRCA*-negative patients, response rates were not significantly different at 28.1% and 36.6% (absolute difference = -8.5%, 95% CI $= -19.6$% to 2.6%), respectively ($P= 0.16$). There was a positive test for the interaction between the randomization arm and *BRCA1/2* status ($P= 0.01$).
      d. **Bevacizumab.** A randomized trial of weekly paclitaxel with or without bevacizumab as first-line treatment for patients with MBC has been conducted by ECOG (E2100). A significant improvement in progression-free survival was demonstrated, but no significant benefit seen in terms of OS. In another study, patients with metastatic disease previously treated with anthracyclines and taxanes were randomized to capecitabine alone versus capecitabine plus bevacizumab. The response rate was increased with bevacizumab, but no significant difference was found in time-to-progression or OS. Subsequent results

from other follow-on large, prospective, randomized phase III trials of multiple different chemotherapy backbones in the first of second line metastatic setting, with or without bevacizumab, have been far more modest as compared to the initial E2100 results. Consequently, FDA has removed the breast cancer label indication for bevacizumab in the United States.

2. **_HER2_-positive MBC**

a. **The _Clinical_ _Evaluation_ _Of_ _P_ertuzumab _And_ _Tra_stuzumab (CLEOPATRA) Trial.** In patients with MBC that is positive for HER2, progression-free survival was significantly improved after first-line therapy with pertuzumab, trastuzumab, and docetaxel, as compared with placebo, trastuzumab, and docetaxel. In the final pre-specified OS analysis, median OS was 56.5 months in the group receiving the pertuzumab combination, as compared with 40.8 months in the group receiving the placebo combination (HR favoring the pertuzumab group, 0.68; $P < 0.001$).

Data support the use of single-agent trastuzumab or the combination of trastuzumab with chemotherapy drugs. The anthracyclines are to be avoided, however, because of the risk of cardiotoxicity when trastuzumab is combined with these agents. Two randomized trials in women with MBC have shown a survival benefit for women who were placed immediately on trastuzumab therapy with concurrent chemotherapy.

b. **Antibody-drug conjugate ado-trastuzumab emtansine** (T-DM1) is an antibody-drug conjugate incorporating the HER2-targeted antitumor properties of trastuzumab with the cytotoxic activity of the microtubule-inhibitory agent derivative of maytansine 1 (DM1). In the phase 3, pivotal EMILIA study, 991 patients with HER2-positive advanced breast cancer who had previously been treated with trastuzumab and a taxane were randomized to T-DM1 or lapatinib plus capecitabine. Median progression-free survival as assessed by independent review was 9.6 months with T-DM1 versus 6.4 months with lapatinib plus capecitabine (HR for progression or death from any cause, 0.65; $P < 0.001$), and median OS at the second interim analysis crossed the stopping boundary for efficacy (30.9 months vs. 25.1 months; $P < 0.001$). T-DM1 should be considered as a new standard for patients with HER2-positive advanced breast cancer who have previously received trastuzumab and lapatinib.

c. **Lapatinib** is a small molecule, orally bioavailable tyrosine kinase inhibitor of _HER2_ and EGFR. It is active (in combination with capecitabine) in women with _HER2_-positive MBC that has progressed after trastuzumab-based therapy.

(1) In a randomized pivotal trial of lapatinib, patients with _HER2_-positive advanced or MBC that had progressed after treatment with regimens that included an anthracycline, a taxane, and trastuzumab were randomly assigned to receive either combination therapy (lapatinib at a dose of 1,250 mg/d continuously plus capecitabine at a dose of 2,000 mg/m^2 on days 1 through 14 of a 21-day cycle) or capecitabine alone. The median time to progression of 8 months in the combination-therapy group as compared with 4 months in the capecitabine alone arm. Notable toxicities of lapatinib include rash and diarrhea (similar to other EGFR kinase inhibitors) and only infrequent reports of cardiotoxicity.

(2) Cross-talk between human EGFRs and hormone receptor pathways may lead to endocrine resistance in breast cancer. In a placebo-controlled, randomized phase 3 study, combination of letrozole (2.5 mg PO daily) plus lapatinib (1,500 mg PO daily) significantly enhanced PFS and clinical benefit rates in patients with MBC that coexpresses hormone receptors and *HER2*.

(3) In one clinical study, patients with *HER2*-positive MBC who experienced progression on prior trastuzumab-containing regimens were randomly assigned to receive either lapatinib alone (1,500 mg PO daily) or lapatinib (1,000 mg PO daily) in combination with standard dose trastuzumab. The combination resulted in superior PFS and clinical benefit rate compared with single agent lapatinib. In an updated analysis, a significant trend in OS favoring the combination arm was also seen. This regimen offers a chemotherapy-free option with acceptable toxicities for selected patients with *HER2*-positive MBC.

C. Systemic agents for bone metastases (see also Chapter 34)

1. **Bisphosphonates** are recommended for women with breast cancer metastatic to bones. Both pamidronate (90 mg IV monthly) and zoledronate (4 mg IV monthly) are effective in reducing bone pain and pathologic fractures. Zoledronate may be superior to pamidronate for reducing (*1*) bone fractures, (*2*) spinal cord compression, (*3*) hypercalcemia of malignancy, and (*4*) the need for palliative RT in patients with metastatic disease.

2. **Denosumab**, a fully human monoclonal antibody against receptor activator of nuclear factor kappa B ligand (RANKL, 120 mg SQ) was superior to zoledronic acid in delaying time to the first skeletal-related event (HR = 0.82, $P = 0.01$). Rates of adverse events (including osteonecrosis of the jaw) were similar between the two groups.

D. Brain and orbital metastases. Patients who present with headache or nausea and vomiting and metastatic disease should alert the clinician to promptly investigate for brain metastases or meningeal carcinomatosis. Brain MRI, with and without gadolinium, is necessary to diagnose metastatic disease. Solitary lesions may be excised surgically or radiated with new modalities, such as cyberknife or gamma knife. Multiple lesions may be treated with stereotactic radiosurgery with or without whole brain radiation. In general, stereotactic radiosurgery alone for multiple metastasis is a consideration in patients with tumors less than approximately 4 cm, tumors without significant surrounding edema, a limited number of brain metastasis (four or less), and those with otherwise controlled extracranial systemic metastases with preserved performance status.

X. SPECIAL CLINICAL PROBLEMS

A. Postsurgical edema of the arm without pain was regularly associated with the traditional radical mastectomy but also occurs with less extensive surgery. The incidence is increased in patients who receive postoperative RT. The edema usually develops within 6 months after surgery, but may be delayed much longer. Therapy is not always helpful but includes elevation of the arm, arm compression sleeves, compression pump, lymphomassage, and physical therapy. Physical therapists or occupational therapists trained in lymphatic massage often benefit the patient.

B. Edema of the arm with pain or paresthesias occurring >1 month after surgery may reflect recurrent tumor. The cancer is often not clinically discernible because it resides high in the apex of the axilla or lung and involves the brachial plexus. Patients may complain of tingling or pain in the hands and progressive weakness and atrophy of the hand and arm muscles. If sufficient time passes, a tumor mass becomes palpable in the axilla or supraclavicular fossa, but the patient is usually left with a paralyzed hand unresponsive to therapy. These patients may receive RT to the axilla and supraclavicular fossa, if radiation has not previously been delivered to this region. The recurrence to the brachial plexus may not be easily seen on MRI or CT scanning. PET scanning may be useful in this circumstance. Occasionally, the pain of this nerve involvement is so severe that nerve blocks by a pain management specialist are necessary.

C. **Breast implants** can create a special challenge in both diagnosis and treatment of breast cancer. No relationship exists between breast implants and the development of breast cancer. Mammography techniques have been developed to assess the breast tissue in women with implants, and they appear to have the same sensitivity for picking up early breast cancers as in women without implants.

1. When an abnormality is seen on a mammogram in a woman with breast implants, special consideration is given to the type of biopsy techniques that must be used. Stereotactic techniques may be avoided to lessen the likelihood of puncturing the implant. Each case is taken on an individual basis depending on the proximity of the abnormality to the implant.

2. When a woman elects to have a mastectomy as part of her local breast cancer management and subsequently requires chest wall RT, placement of breast implants is sometimes avoided. A greater risk exists of scar tissue contracting around the implant with radiation, thus significantly reducing an optimal cosmetic benefit of breast reconstruction. If chest wall radiation is to be considered, many plastic surgeons would prefer to bring a flap of tissue from outside the radiation field to accomplish optimal reconstruction and cosmesis.

D. **Breast cancer during pregnancy.** In a California registry study, there were 1.3 breast cancers diagnosed per 10,000 live births. Breast cancer during pregnancy is most often associated with larger tumor size and with lymph node metastasis. Histologically, these tumors are often poorly differentiated, are more frequently ER negative and PR negative, and may be *HER2*-positive. Delay in diagnosis is typical because tumor masses can be masked by breast engorgement owing to lactation, and inflammatory changes may be mistaken for mastitis.

1. Mammography with shielding can be performed safely, although interpretation can be difficult because of increased breast density. Ultrasonography of the breast and regional lymph nodes is used to assess the extent of disease and also to guide biopsy.

2. Core needle biopsy is preferred for histologic diagnosis and biomarker analysis.

3. Staging assessment of the pregnant patient can be problematic. In addition to complete blood count and serum chemistries, including hepatic function testing, a chest radiograph (with shielding) is feasible. Additionally, in patients who have clinically node-positive or T3 breast lesions, an ultrasound of the liver and directed screening MRI of the thoracic and lumbar spine without contrast can be used. Documentation of metastases may alter the treatment plan and influence the patient's decision regarding maintenance of the pregnancy.

4. Assessment of the pregnancy should include a maternal fetal medicine consultation.

5. Indications for systemic chemotherapy do not differ for the pregnant patient with breast cancer, although chemotherapy is to be avoided during the first trimester of pregnancy because of the risk of fetal malformation. Fetal

malformation risks in the second and third trimester fall to approximately 1.3%, no different than those of unexposed fetuses.

a. The greatest treatment experience in pregnancy has been with anthracycline and alkylating agent chemotherapy. Limited data are found on the use of taxanes during pregnancy, although taxanes have less propensity to cross the placental barrier. One popular strategy is to complete cycles of anthracycline plus cyclophosphamide during second or third trimester, followed by a taxane postpartum.

b. Chemotherapy during pregnancy should be avoided following week 35 to avoid hematologic complications at the time of delivery. Ondansetron, lorazepam, and dexamethasone may be used for the antiemetic regimen.

c. There are several case reports of trastuzumab use during pregnancy. Oligohydramnios has been reported in such cases. Accordingly, trastuzumab should be delayed until the postpartum period.

d. Endocrine therapy and radiation therapy are contraindicated during pregnancy and should not be initiated until the postpartum period.

ACKNOWLEDGMENT

The author would like to acknowledge Drs. Cristiane Takita and Dennis A. Casciato, who significantly contributed to earlier versions of this chapter.

Suggested Readings

ATAC Trialists' Group. Anastrozole alone or in combination with tamoxifen versus tamoxifen alone for adjuvant treatment of postmenopausal women with early breast cancer: first results of the ATAC randomised trial. *Lancet* 2002;359:2131.

Bartelink H, et al. Impact of a higher radiation dose on local control and survival in breast-conserving therapy of early breast cancer: 10-year results of the randomized boost versus no boost EORTC 22881-10882 trial. *J Clin Oncol* 2007;25:3259.

Bear HD, et al. Sequential preoperative or postoperative docetaxel added to preoperative doxorubicin plus cyclophosphamide for operable breast cancer: National Surgical Adjuvant Breast and Bowel Protocol B-27. *J Clin Oncol* 2006;24:2019.

BIG 1-98 Collaborative Group; Mouridsen H, et al. Letrozole therapy alone or in sequence with tamoxifen in women with breast cancer. *N Engl J Med* 2009;361:766.

Carter C, Allen C, Henson D. Relation of tumor size, lymph node status, and survival in 24,740 breast cancer cases. *Cancer* 1989;63:181.

Citron ML, et al. Randomized trial of dose-dense versus conventionally scheduled and sequential versus concurrent combination chemotherapy as postoperative adjuvant treatment of node-positive primary breast cancer: first report of Intergroup Trial C9741/Cancer and Leukemia group B Trial 9741. *J Clin Oncol* 2003;21:1431.

Clarke M, et al. Effects of radiotherapy and of differences in the extent of surgery for early breast cancer on local recurrence and 15-year survival: an overview of the randomised trials. *Lancet* 2005;366(9503):2087.

Coombes RC, et al. A randomized trial of exemestane after two to three years of tamoxifen therapy in postmenopausal women with primary breast cancer. *N Engl J Med* 2004;350:1081.

Cortes J, et al. Eribulin monotherapy versus treatment of physician's choice in patients with metastatic breast cancer (EMBRACE): a phase 3 open-label randomised study. *Lancet* 2011;377(9769):914.

Davies C, et al. Long-term effects of continuing adjuvant tamoxifen to 10 years versus stopping at 5 years after diagnosis of oestrogen receptor-positive breast cancer: ATLAS, a randomised trial. *Lancet* 2013;381(9869):805–816.

Donker M, et al. Radiotherapy or surgery of the axilla after a positive sentinel node in breast cancer (EORTC 10981-22023 AMAROS): a randomised, multicentre, open-label, phase 3 non-inferiority trial. *Lancet Oncol* 2014;15(12):1303–1310.

Early Breast Cancer Trialists' Collaborative Group. Effects of chemotherapy and hormonal therapy for early breast cancer on recurrence and 15-year survival: an overview of the randomised trials. *Lancet* 2005;365:1687.

Early Breast Cancer Trialists' Collaborative Group (EBCTCG); Coleman R, Powles T, Paterson A, et al. Adjuvant bisphosphonate treatment in early breast cancer: meta-analyses of individual patient data from randomised trials. *Lancet* 2015;386(10001):1353–1361.

Fan C, et al. Concordance among gene expression-based predictors for breast cancer. *N Engl J Med* 2006;355:560.

Finn RS, et al. The cyclin-dependent kinase 4/6 inhibitor palbociclib in combination with letrozole versus letrozole alone as first-line treatment of oestrogen receptor-positive, HER2-negative, advanced breast cancer (PALOMA-1/TRIO-18): a randomised phase 2 study. *Lancet Oncol* 2015;16(1):25–35.

Fisher B, et al. Tamoxifen in treatment of intraductal breast cancer: National Surgical Adjuvant Breast and Bowel Project B-24 randomised controlled trial. *Lancet* 1999a;353:1993a.

Fisher ER, et al. Pathologic findings from the National Surgical Adjuvant Breast Project (NSABP) eight-year update of protocol B-17. Intraductal carcinoma. *Cancer* 1999b;86:429.

Geyer CE, et al. Lapatinib plus capecitabine for HER2-positive advanced breast cancer. *N Engl J Med* 2006;355:2733.

Gianni L, et al. Efficacy and safety of neoadjuvant pertuzumab and trastuzumab in women with locally advanced, inflammatory, or early HER2-positive breast cancer (NeoSphere): a randomised multicentre, open-label, phase 2 trial. *Lancet Oncol* 2012;13(1):25–32.

Giuliano AE, et al. Axillary dissection vs no axillary dissection in women with invasive breast cancer and sentinel node metastasis: a randomized clinical trial. *JAMA* 2011a;305:569.

Giuliano AE, et al. Association of occult metastases in sentinel lymph nodes and bone marrow with survival among women with early-stage invasive breast cancer. *JAMA* 2011b;306:385.

Gnant M, et al. The impact of adjuvant denosumab on disease-free survival: results from 3,425 postmenopausal patients of the ABCSG-18 trial. 2015 San Antonio Breast Cancer Symposium. Abstract S2-02.

Hillner BE, et al. American Society of Clinical Oncology 2003 update on the role of bisphosphonates and bone health issues in women with breast cancer. *J Clin Oncol* 2003;21:4042.

Julien JP, et al. Radiotherapy in breast-conserving treatment for ductal carcinoma in situ: first results of the EORTC randomised phase III trial 10853. EORTC Breast Cancer Cooperative Group and EORTC Radiotherapy Group. *Lancet* 2000;355:528.

Lee S-J, Toi M, Lee ES, et al. A phase III trial of adjuvant capecitabine in breast cancer patients with HER2-negative pathologic residual invasive disease after neoadjuvant chemotherapy (CREATE-X, JBCRG-04). 2015 San Antonio Breast Cancer Symposium. Abstract S1-07.

Lehman CD, et al.; ACRIN Trial 6667 Investigators Group. MRI evaluation of the contralateral breast in women with recently diagnosed breast cancer. *N Engl J Med* 2007;356:1295.

Mansel RE, et al. Randomized multicenter trial of sentinel node biopsy versus standard axillary treatment in operable breast cancer: the ALMANAC Trial. *J Natl Cancer Inst* 2006;98:599.

Morrow M, et al. Standard for the management of ductal carcinoma in situ of the breast (DCIS). *CA Cancer J Clin* 2002a;52:256.

Morrow M, et al. Standard for breast conservation therapy in the management of invasive breast cancer. *CA Cancer J Clin* 2002b;52:277.

Muss HB, et al. Efficacy, toxicity, and quality of life in older women with early-stage breast cancer treated with letrozole or placebo after 5 years of tamoxifen: NCIC CTG intergroup trial MA.17. *J Clin Oncol* 2008;26:1956.

NCCN Clinical Practice Guidelines in Oncology. *Breast Cancer Version.3.2015.* www.nccn.org

Olivotto IA, Bajdik CD, Ravdin PM, et al. Population-based validation of the prognostic model ADJUVANT! for early breast cancer. *J Clin Oncol* 2005;23:2716.

Overgaard M, et al. Postoperative radiotherapy in high-risk premenopausal women with breast cancer who receive adjuvant chemotherapy. Danish Breast Cancer Cooperative Group 82b Trial. *N Engl J Med* 1997;337:949.

Pagani O, et al. Adjuvant exemestane with ovarian suppression in premenopausal breast cancer. *N Engl J Med* 2014;371(2):107–118.

Paik S, et al. Gene expression and benefit of chemotherapy in women with node-negative, estrogen receptor-positive breast cancer. *J Clin Oncol* 2006;24:3726.

Piccart-Gebhart MJ, et al. Trastuzumab after adjuvant chemotherapy in HER2-positive breast cancer. *N Engl J Med* 2005;353:1659.

Recht A, et al. Postmastectomy radiotherapy: clinical practice guidelines of the American Society of Clinical Oncology. *J Clin Oncol* 2001;19:1539.

Romestaing P, et al. Role of a 10-Gy boost in the conservative treatment of early breast cancer: results of a randomized clinical trial in Lyon, *France. J Clin Oncol* 1997;15:963.

Romond EH, Perez EA, Bryant J, et al. Trastuzumab plus adjuvant chemotherapy for operable HER2-positive breast cancer. *N Engl J Med* 2005;353:1673.

Slamon DJ, et al. Use of chemotherapy plus a monoclonal antibody against HER2 for metastatic breast cancer that overexpresses HER2. *N Engl J Med* 2001;344:783.

Slamon DJ, et al. Ten year follow-up of BCIRG-006 comparing doxorubicin plus cyclophosphamide followed by docetaxel (AC → T) with doxorubicin plus cyclophosphamide followed by docetaxel and trastuzumab (AC → TH) with docetaxel, carboplatin and trastuzumab (TCH) in HER2+ early breast cancer. Proceedings of the San Antonio Breast Cancer Symposium, 2015. Abstract S5-04.

Smith BD, et al. Accelerated partial breast irradiation consensus statement from the American Society for Radiation Oncology (ASTRO). *Int J Radiat Oncol Biol Phys* 2009;74:987.

Smith BD, Bentzen SM, Correa CR, et al. Fractionation for whole breast irradiation: An American Society for Radiation Oncology (ASTRO) Evidence-Based Guideline. *Int J Radiat Oncol Biol Phys* 2010;81:59.

Sorlie T, et al. Gene expression patterns of breast carcinomas distinguish tumor subclasses with clinical implications. *Proc Natl Acad Sci USA* 2001;98:10869.

Strom EA, et al. Clinical investigation: regional nodal failure patterns in breast cancer patients treated with mastectomy without radiotherapy. *Int J Radiat Oncol Biol Phys* 2005;63:1508.

Swain SM, et al. Pertuzumab, trastuzumab, and docetaxel in HER2-positive metastatic breast cancer. *N Engl J Med* 2015;372(8):724–734.

Tan-Chiu E, et al. Assessment of cardiac dysfunction in a randomized trial comparing doxorubicin and cyclophosphamide followed by paclitaxel, with or without trastuzumab as adjuvant therapy in node-positive, human epidermal growth factor receptor 2-overexpressing breast cancer: NSABP B-31. *J Clin Oncol* 2005;23:7811.

Taylor ME, et al. ACR appropriateness criteria on postmastectomy radiotherapy expert panel on radiation oncology-breast. *Int J Radiat Oncol Biol Phys* 2009;73:997.

Tolaney SM, et al. Adjuvant paclitaxel and trastuzumab for node-negative, HER2-positive breast cancer. *N Engl J Med* 2015;372(2):134–141.

van de Vijver MJ, et al. A gene-expression signature as a predictor of survival in breast cancer. *N Engl J Med* 2002;347:1999.

Verma S, et al. Trastuzumab emtansine for HER2-positive advanced breast cancer. *N Engl J Med* 2012;367(19):1783–1791.

Warner E, et al. American Cancer Society Guidelines for Breast Screening with MRI as an Adjunct to Mammography. *CA Cancer J Clin* 2007;57:75.

Whelan TJ, et al. Long-term results of hypofractionated radiation therapy for breast cancer. *N Engl J Med* 2010;362:513.

Weiss RB, et al. Natural history of more than 20 years of node-positive primary breast carcinoma treated with cyclophosphamide, methotrexate, and fluorouracil-based adjuvant chemotherapy: a study by the Cancer and Leukemia Group B. *J Clin Oncol* 2003;21:1825.

Whelan TJ, et al. Regional nodal irradiation in early-stage breast cancer. *N Engl J Med* 2015; 373:307–316.

Wooster R, Weber BL. Genomic medicine: breast and ovarian cancer. *N Engl J Med* 2003;348:2339.

Yardley DA, et al. Everolimus plus exemestane in postmenopausal patients with HR(+) breast cancer: BOLERO-2 final progression-free survival analysis. *Adv Ther* 2013;30(10):870–884.

12 Gynecologic Cancers

Margaret I. Liang and Sanaz Memarzadeh

GENERAL ASPECTS

I. EPIDEMIOLOGY

Malignancies of the genital tract constitute about 20% of visceral cancers in women. The incidence and mortality rates according to primary site are shown in Table 12-1.

II. DIAGNOSTIC STUDIES

A. **Staging evaluation** is necessary regardless of the site of the primary lesion after cancer of the female genital tract is proven histologically. Potentially valuable studies include the following:

1. Pelvic and rectal examinations (to determine whether the adnexa, vagina, or pelvic wall is involved)
2. CBC, serum electrolytes, creatinine, and LFTs
3. Chest radiograph: plain chest x-ray, or CT as indicated (to look for pulmonary metastases)
4. Abdominal–pelvic ultrasonography, CT or positron emission tomography (PET) with CT scans, or MRI (including evaluation of the ureters)
5. Sigmoidoscopy with biopsy of abnormal areas is optional (to look for mucosal involvement or mass lesions; especially in cervical cancer)
6. Cystoscopy with biopsy of abnormal areas is optional (to look for mucosal involvement or mass lesions; especially in cervical cancer)
7. Cytologic evaluation of ascites or pleural effusions

III. LOCALLY ADVANCED CANCER IN THE PELVIS

A. **Pathogenesis.** Massive pelvic metastases may develop in the course of gynecologic, urologic, or rectal carcinomas and some sarcomas. Locally advanced cancers in the pelvis can produce progressive pelvic and perineal pain, ureteral obstruction with uremia, and lymphatic and venous obstruction with pedal and genital edema. Invasion of the nearby rectum or bladder can lead to erosion with bleeding, sloughing of tumor into the urine or stool, and potentially bladder outlet or bowel obstruction.

B. **Management**

1. **Drug therapy** such as chemotherapy or targeted agents may be used in the neoadjuvant, adjuvant, or recurrent setting depending on the primary site.
2. **Radiation therapy** (RT) relieves symptoms and is useful when the tumor does not respond to chemotherapy.
3. **Surgery.** A bowel resection, colostomy, or suprapubic cystotomy may relieve bowel or urethral obstruction. Ureteral bypass can be accomplished by placement of ureteral stent catheters or by nephrostomy.

TABLE 12-1	Annual Rates for Cancers of the Female Genital Tract in the United States		
Primary Site	New Cases	Percentage (%)	Deaths from Cancer
Cervix	12,900	14	4,100
Uterine corpus	54,870	53	10,170
Ovary	21,290	25	14,180
Vulva	5,150	5	1,080
Vagina	4,070	3	910
Total	**92,280**	**100**	**30,440**

Siegel R, et al. Cancer Statistics, 2015. *CA Cancer J Clin* 2015;65:6, with permission from Wiley.

IV. ADVERSE EFFECTS OF RADIATION TO THE PELVIS

A. **Radiation cystitis**

   1. **Acute transient cystitis** may occur during RT to the pelvis. Urinary tract analgesics and antispasmodics may be helpful for pain.

   2. **Late radiation cystitis.** The bladder becomes contracted, fibrotic, and subject to mucosal ulcerations and infections. Urinary frequency and episodes of pyelonephritis or cystitis (often hemorrhagic) are the clinical findings. Hyperbaric oxygen therapy may help control severe hematuria. If symptomatic management is not successful, cystectomy may be required.

B. **Radiation vulvitis** of a moist and desquamative type usually begins at about 2,500 cGy and may require delay of treatment for 1 to 2 weeks in up to half of patients.

C. **Fistula formation.** Tumor extension and history of prior radiation increase the risk of fistula formation. Diverting procedures (i.e., nephrostomy, colostomy) may be required.

CANCER OF THE UTERINE CERVIX

I. EPIDEMIOLOGY AND ETIOLOGY

A. **Incidence** (Table 12-1). The mortality rate of cervical cancer has declined by 50% since the 1950s, largely as a result of early detection and treatment.

B. **Relationship to sexual history.** The common denominator for increased risk for cervical cancer is early age at first sexual intercourse. The incidence is also higher in patients with an early first pregnancy, multiple sexual partners, and sexually transmitted diseases, especially human papillomavirus (HPV) infection.

C. **Relationship to HPV.** A large body of evidence supports the relationship among HPV, cervical intraepithelial neoplasia (CIN; dysplasia), and invasive carcinoma. DNA transcripts of HPV have been identified by Southern blot analysis in >60% of cervical carcinomas. Types 16, 18, 31, and 33 are more likely to be associated with malignant transformation. HPV 16 and 18 are the causative agents for 70% of all cervical malignancies.

D. **Relationship to smoking.** There is evidence that a personal history of smoking significantly increases the risk for cervical cancer.

II. PATHOLOGY AND NATURAL HISTORY

A. **Histology.** About 80% of cervical carcinomas are squamous cancers and 20% are adenocarcinomas. The disease is believed to start at the squamocolumnar junction. A continuum from CIN to invasive squamous cell carcinoma is apparent. The average age of women with CIN is 15 years younger than that of women with invasive carcinoma.

B. **Metastases.** After invasive cancer is established, the tumor spreads primarily by local extension into other pelvic structures and sequentially along lymph node chains. Uncommonly, patients with locally advanced tumors may have evidence of hematologic route of metastatic spread, most often to the lung, liver, or bone.

III. PREVENTION AND EARLY DETECTION OF CERVICAL CANCER

A. **Vaccination.** Bivalent (HPV 16/18), quadrivalent (HPV 6/11/16/18), and most recently nonavalent (HPV 16/18/31/33/45/52/58/6/11) vaccines have shown efficacy by demonstrating protection against CIN, persistent HPV, and external genital warts. The vaccines are well tolerated, and they are recommended for females and males from ages 9 to 26. The HPV vaccine does not eliminate the need for cervical cytology screening and can be given regardless of history of prior dysplasia or HPV infection.

B. **Screening with Pap testing**
Most patients with cervical cancer do not have symptoms, and cases are detected by routine Pap test screening.

1. **Frequency.** Early detection has greatly reduced the morbidity and mortality of cervical cancer. The American Cancer Society's recommendations for Pap testing are as follows:

   a. Women should have yearly Pap smears starting at age 21, regardless of age at first sexual intercourse. Exceptions include patients with a history of cervical cancer and diethylstilbestrol (DES) exposure or who are immunocompromised.

   b. Women between ages 21 to 29 with normal risk for cervical cancer should be screened with cytology alone every 3 years.

   c. Women 30 and older with normal risk for cervical cancer should be screened with cytology every 3 years or cytology with HPV cotesting every 5 years.

   d. Women who have had their cervix removed at the time of hysterectomy for benign indications confirmed on final pathology do not need to have Pap tests.

   e. In patients who are ≥65 years of age, screening may be stopped in the presence of three consecutively normal and satisfactory Pap smears or two consecutive negative HPV tests. Exceptions include a history of CIN II or worse within the last 20 years.

2. **Technique.** There are many problems that contribute to the low sensitivity of Pap tests. Some of these include sample adequacy, slide preparation, and slide interpretation and receding of the squamocolumnar junction with age.

   a. **Conventional Pap smears.** When performing the conventional Pap smear, the cytobrush used together with an extended tip spatula is the most effective combination for cell collection. The specimens are smeared on clean glass slides and fixed immediately.

   b. **Liquid-based Pap smears.** This technique involves thin-layer, liquid-based systems. The cervical sample is taken and suspended in an alcohol-based preservative solution. This specimen can be used for detection of HPV.

3. **Pap smears are graded** using the 2001 Bethesda system as follows:
   Negative for Intraepithelial Lesion or Malignancy
   Epithelial Cell Abnormalities
       Squamous Cell
           Atypical squamous cells (ASC)
           Atypical squamous cells of undetermined significance (ASC-US)
           Atypical squamous cells—cannot exclude HSIL (ASC-H)
           Low-grade squamous intraepithelial lesion (LSIL)

Encompassing: mild dysplasia/cervical intraepithelial neoplasia type 1 (CIN 1)

High-grade squamous intraepithelial lesion (HSIL)

Encompassing: moderate and severe dysplasia, carcinoma *in situ* (CIS)/CIN II and CIN III

With features suspicious for invasion

Squamous cell carcinoma

Glandular Cell

Atypical

Endocervical cells (not otherwise specified, NOS)

Endometrial cells (NOS)

Glandular cells (NOS)

Endocervical cells, favor neoplastic

Glandular cells, favor neoplastic

Endocervical adenocarcinoma *in situ*

Adenocarcinoma

Endocervical

Endometrial

Extrauterine

NOS

Other Malignant Neoplasms

IV. DIAGNOSIS

A. **Symptoms and signs**

1. **Symptoms** of early-stage invasive cervical cancer include vaginal discharge, bleeding, and particularly postcoital spotting. More advanced stages often present with a malodorous vaginal discharge, weight loss, or obstructive uropathy.

2. **Signs.** Findings on pelvic examination include the appearance of obvious masses on the cervix; gray, discolored areas; and bleeding or evidence of cervicitis. If a tumor is present, the extent should be noted; involvement of the vagina or parametria (pelvic sidewall) is an important prognostic factor.

B. **Biopsy.** Biopsy specimens should be taken of all visibly abnormal areas, regardless of the findings on the Pap smear. Diagnostic conization may be required if the biopsy shows microinvasive carcinoma, if endocervical curettage (ECC) shows high-grade dysplasia, or if adenocarcinoma *in situ* is suspected from cytology.

C. **Patients with an abnormal Pap smear and no visible lesion** generally undergo colposcopy and directed biopsies, which can detect 90% of dysplastic lesions.

D. **Endocervical curettage (ECC)** is required when the Pap smear shows a high-grade lesion but colposcopy does not reveal a lesion; when the entire squamo-columnar junction cannot be visualized; when atypical endocervical cells are present on the Pap smear; or when women previously treated for CIN develop new high-grade findings on cytology. If the ECC reveals a HSIL, patients should undergo cervical conization with a knife or a loop electrosurgical excision procedure (LEEP).

V. STAGING SYSTEM AND PROGNOSTIC FACTORS

A. **The staging system** is clinical rather than surgical: refer to the AJCC Cancer Staging Manual.

B. **Prognostic factors** in each stage include size of primary tumor, presence of lymph node metastasis, tumor grade, and histologic cell type.

VI. MANAGEMENT

A. **Dysplasia/cervical intraepithelial neoplasia (CIN) I–III.** Treatment modalities include superficial ablative therapies, LEEP, cone biopsy, and hysterectomy (Fig. 12-1).

1. CIN I lesions may be observed if the patient has good follow-up because of the high rate of spontaneous regression of these lesions. In young patients, especially adolescents, CIN II may be followed expectantly.

2. Patients with high-grade (CIN II and III) squamous lesions are suitable for ablative or resection therapies, provided the entire transformation zone is visible on colposcopy, the histology of the biopsies is consistent with the Pap smear, the ECC is negative, and there is no suspicion of occult invasion.

3. For high-grade lesions, we recommend LEEP, which involves the use of wire loop electrodes with radiofrequency alternating current to excise the transformation zone under local anesthesia.

4. Cone biopsy with a scalpel is preferred for lesions that cannot be assessed colposcopically or when adenocarcinoma *in situ* is suspected.

5. If the patient has other gynecologic indications for hysterectomy, a vaginal or an extrafascial (type I) abdominal hysterectomy may be performed.

B. **Stage I invasive cervical cancer:** The management of patients with early carcinoma of the cervix is summarized in Table 12-2.

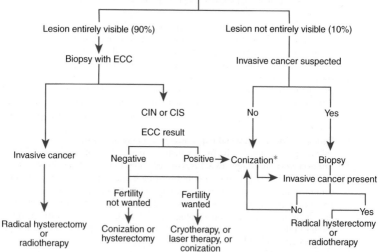

Figure 12-1 Management of patients with positive Pap smear cytology and early carcinoma of the uterine cervix. CIN, cervical intraepithelial neoplasia; CIS, carcinoma *in situ*; ECC, endocervical curettage. *If invasion is not found on conization, patients are followed with Pap smears, biopsies, or repeat conization, depending on the patient and patient's age. From Casciato DA. *Manual of Clinical Oncology.* 7th ed. Philadelphia, PA: Lippincott Williams & Wilkins, 2012.

TABLE 12-2	**Treatment of Stage I Cervical Carcinoma**

Stage	**Typical Treatment Options**
IA1 with ≤3-mm invasion but without LVSI	Therapeutic cone or type I hysterectomy
IA1 with ≤3-mm invasion with LVSI	Type I or II hysterectomy with bilateral pelvic lymphadenectomy
IA2 with >3- to 5-mm invasion (the risk for nodal metastases is 5%–10%)	Type II hysterectomy and bilateral pelvic lymphadenectomy or RT for inoperable patients
IB (the risk for nodal metastases is 15%–25%) and IIA	Type II or III hysterectomy with bilateral pelvic lymphadenectomy with para-aortic lymph node evaluation or RT for inoperable patients. In patients with intermediate-risk features (i.e., Sedlis criteria: tumor size, depth of stromal invasion, LVSI), postoperative RT should be given. In patients with high-risk features (i.e., Peters criteria: parametrial involvement, positive margins, or positive lymph node metastasis), postoperative RT with CCT with cisplatin as a radiation sensitizer should be given

C. **Concurrent chemotherapy (CCT) with RT** reduces recurrence by 30% to 50% and improves 3-year survival rates by 10% to 15% over adjuvant treatment with RT alone.

1. **CCT is indicated** in the following circumstances:

   a. **As adjuvant therapy for** high-risk stages I to IIA (i.e., parametrial involvement, positive margins, or positive lymph node metastasis)

   b. **As primary therapy for** stages IIB, III, and IVA

2. **Regimens.** Single agent cisplatin (40 mg/m² weekly for 6 weeks) or in combination with 5-fluorouracil (5-FU) has been effective. Cisplatin may be replaced by carboplatin or gemcitabine in patients with renal dysfunction.

D. **Stage II disease.** Stage IIA disease is treated in the same manner as stage IB disease.

E. **Stage IIB and III disease.** When the parametrium (IIB), the distal vagina (IIIA), or the pelvic sidewall (IIIB) is involved, clear surgical margins are not possible to achieve, and patients should be treated with maximum-dose (8,500 cGy) RT delivered both externally and by brachytherapy. CCT with cisplatin as radiation sensitizers improves survival rates when compared with RT alone (see Section VI.C).

F. **Recurrent and stage IV disease**

1. **Lower vaginal recurrence** can occasionally be cured by RT or exenteration.

2. **Pelvic exenteration.** A pelvic exenteration may also be considered for central pelvic recurrent disease after primary RT when spread is confined to the vagina, bladder, or rectum. Exenteration carries a high morbidity rate (up to 50%). Metastatic cancer outside the pelvis and poor medical condition of the patient are contraindications to exenteration. Ureteral obstruction, leg edema, and sciatic pain usually suggest sidewall disease. Surgery should be abandoned if there is more extensive cancer at the time of laparotomy than was clinically suspected.

3. **RT** alone or with chemotherapeutic sensitizers can occasionally cure stage IVA disease. External-beam RT is combined with intracavitary or interstitial radiation to a total dose of about 8,500 cGy. If disease persists after chemoradiation, pelvic exenteration can be performed.

4. **Chemotherapy** for metastatic disease is not curative. A number of chemotherapeutic drugs (i.e., cisplatin, carboplatin, paclitaxel, topotecan) produce

short-term responses in 10% to 30% of patients. The addition of angiogenesis inhibitors (i.e., bevacizumab) to doublet chemotherapy was associated with a higher response (48% vs. 36%), and overall survival was extended by 3.7 months in a randomized, controlled trial.

VII. SPECIAL CLINICAL PROBLEMS

A. **Incidental finding of cancer at hysterectomy.** Cancer found in hysterectomy specimens removed for other reasons carries a poor prognosis unless treated with additional surgery or postoperative RT soon after surgery.

B. **Uncertainty of recurrent cancer.** Recurrent cancer is usually manifested by pelvic pain, particularly in the sciatic nerve distribution; vaginal bleeding; malodorous discharge; or leg edema. Recurrence must be demonstrated by biopsy specimen because these symptoms and even physical findings can be similar to those associated with radiation changes. If no tumor is found using noninvasive measures, a surgeon experienced in pelvic cancer should perform diagnostic laparoscopy or exploratory laparotomy.

C. **Postirradiation dysplasia.** Abnormal Pap smears on follow-up examinations may represent postirradiation dysplastic changes or a new primary cancer. Suspected areas should undergo biopsy. If the biopsy findings show cancer, surgical removal may be necessary.

CANCER OF THE UTERINE BODY

I. EPIDEMIOLOGY AND ETIOLOGY

A. **Incidence** (Table 12-1). Endometrial cancer is the most common malignancy of the female genital tract in the United States. The peak incidence is in the sixth and seventh decades of life; 80% of patients are postmenopausal. Most premenopausal women with endometrial carcinoma have the Stein-Leventhal syndrome or polycystic ovarian syndrome. Fewer than 5% of all cases are diagnosed before age of 40 years, although younger age at diagnosis has become more prevalent with the obesity epidemic.

B. **Risk factors**

1. **Estrogen exposure** that is unopposed by progesterone increases the risk for endometrial carcinoma by four to eightfold. The use of tamoxifen is associated with a twofold increased risk for endometrial cancer.

2. **Medical conditions producing increased exposure to unopposed estrogens** and associated with increased risk of endometrial carcinoma include the following:
   a. Polycystic ovarian syndrome (anovulatory menstrual cycles with or without hirsutism and other endocrine abnormalities)
   b. Anovulatory menstrual cycles
   c. Obesity
   d. Granulosa cell tumor of the ovary, or any other estrogen-secreting tumor
   e. Advanced liver disease

3. **Other medical conditions** associated with increased risk for endometrial carcinoma
   a. Infertility, nulliparity, irregular menses
   b. Diabetes mellitus
   c. Hypertension
   d. History of multiple cancers in the family
   e. Personal history of breast or rectal cancer

4. **Hereditary factors** resulting from germline mutations in DNA mismatch repair (MMR) genes. Mutations in the MMR genes (*MSH2, MLH1, PMS2,*

or MSH6) can result in Lynch syndrome (hereditary nonpolyposis colorectal cancer or HNPCC). By age 70, up to 60% of these individuals may be diagnosed with endometrial cancer compared to 1.7% in the general population.

II. PATHOLOGY AND NATURAL HISTORY

A. **Histology.** About 95% of uterine cancers arise from the endometrium and the most common histologic subtype is endometrioid adenocarcinoma. Clear cell, papillary serous, and squamous cell carcinoma account for 10% of endometrial cancers.

B. **Role of estrogens.** Classically, unopposed estrogens cause a continuum of endometrial changes from simple hyperplasia to complex hyperplasia with atypia to invasive carcinoma. Progestin therapy is very effective in reversing endometrial hyperplasia without atypia, but less effective for endometrial hyperplasia with atypia. Pharmacologic options for reversing hyperplasia include continuous progestin therapy (i.e., oral progesterone) or placement of a progestin intrauterine device (IUD).

C. **Mode of spread.** Tumors are confined to the body of the uterus (stage I) in 75% of cases. Endometrial cancer most commonly spreads by direct extension. Deep myometrial invasion and involvement of the uterine cervix are associated with a high risk for pelvic lymph node metastases. It is rare to find positive para-aortic nodes in the absence of positive pelvic nodes. The presence of malignant cells in peritoneal washings suggests retrograde flow of exfoliated cells along the fallopian tubes. Hematogenous spread is an uncommon late finding in adenocarcinoma but occurs early in sarcoma. The lungs are the most frequent site of distant metastatic involvement.

III. DIAGNOSIS

A. **Symptoms and signs**
  1. **Abnormal vaginal bleeding** is the most common symptom (97%).
     a. **Premenopausal women** with prolonged menses, excessive menstrual bleeding, or intermenstrual bleeding must be evaluated for endometrial cancer, particularly if they have a history of irregular menses, diabetes mellitus, hypertension, obesity, or infertility.
     b. **All postmenopausal women with vaginal bleeding** >1 year after the last menstrual period are considered to have endometrial cancer unless proven otherwise.
  2. **Patients without symptoms** and with atypical endometrial cells on Pap smears should undergo endometrial sampling.
  3. **Women with AGC** (atypical glandular cells) on Pap smears who are >35 years, as well as younger women with AGC who have unexplained vaginal bleeding, must undergo an endometrial biopsy in addition to colposcopy.
  4. **Locally extensive tumors** may be palpable on pelvic examination.
  5. **Advanced disease** is the original manifestation of cancer in 5% of cases.

B. **Endocervical curettage and office endometrial biopsy** should be performed in all patients suspected of having endometrial carcinoma. Endometrial biopsy is associated with a 10% false-negative rate; thus, all patients with persistent symptoms and a negative biopsy must undergo dilation and curettage under anesthesia.

C. **Fractional curettage** is the diagnostic method of choice for endometrial cancer. The technique involves scraping the endocervical canal and then, in a set sequence, the walls of the uterus. If cancer is found by histologic evaluation, the fractional scrapings help to locate the tumor site.

D. **Pap smears** alone should not be used to exclude suspected endometrial cancer. Only half of patients with endometrial cancer have abnormal cells on Pap smear.

E. **Transvaginal ultrasound** with and without color flow imaging has been studied. Data suggest a strong association between thickness of the endometrial stripe and endometrial disease. The normal endometrium is usually <5-mm thick, but definitive diagnosis can only be obtained by tissue sampling.

IV. STAGING SYSTEM AND PROGNOSTIC FACTORS

A. **The staging system:** refer to the AJCC Cancer Staging Manual. Complete surgical staging for endometrial cancer involves total abdominal hysterectomy, bilateral salpingo-oophorectomy, pelvic and para-aortic lymphadenectomy, and sampling of any suspicious peritoneal implants.

B. **Prognostic factors**

1. **Histologic grade and myometrial invasion.** Increasing tumor grade and myometrial invasion have great prognostic value as they are associated with increasing risk for pelvic and para-aortic lymph node metastases, positive peritoneal cytology, adnexal metastases, local vault recurrence, and hematogenous spread.

2. **Tumor histology.** Histologic types ranked from best to worst prognosis are adenoacanthomas, adenocarcinomas, adenosquamous carcinomas, clear cell carcinomas, papillary serous carcinomas, and small cell carcinomas.

3. **Vascular space invasion.** Vascular space invasion is an independent prognostic factor for recurrence and death from endometrial carcinoma of all histologic types.

4. **Hormone receptor status.** The average estrogen receptor (ER) and progesterone receptor (PR) levels are, in general, inversely proportional to the histologic grade. However, ER and PR levels have also been shown to be independent prognostic indicators, with higher levels corresponding to longer survival.

5. **Nuclear grade** is a more accurate prognosticator than histologic grade.

6. **Tumor size.** The larger the tumor, the higher the risk for lymph node metastases.

7. **DNA ploidy.** Aneuploid tumors constitute a fairly small percentage (25%) of endometrial carcinomas as compared with ovarian and cervical cancers. Aneuploidy is, however, associated with increased risk for early recurrence and death.

V. PREVENTION AND EARLY DETECTION

A. **Prevention.** Unopposed exogenous estrogen administration should be avoided in postmenopausal women who have a uterus. Women who are anovulatory or who have endometrial hyperplasia should be treated with cyclic progestins.

B. **Early detection.** Patients in whom evaluation for endometrial carcinoma is necessary include postmenopausal women with vaginal bleeding or pyometra; premenopausal women with unexplained abnormal uterine bleeding, especially if they have risk factors (i.e., chronic anovulation, exogenous estrogen therapy, obesity, strong family history of cancers associated with Lynch syndrome).

VI. MANAGEMENT

A. **Early disease**

1. **Surgery.** Total abdominal hysterectomy with bilateral salpingo-oophorectomy (TAH/BSO), pelvic and para-aortic lymphadenectomy is the treatment for patients with early-stage endometrial cancer. Patients with an expanded (enlarged) cervix may be treated with a type II (modified radical) hysterectomy; those with microscopic involvement of the cervix may be treated with an extrafascial hysterectomy. Minimally invasive surgery via

standard laparoscopy or robotic-assisted surgery is an alternative and safe approach to open abdominal surgery in treating patients with endometrial cancer. Optimal tumor debulking is recommended for patients with metastatic extrauterine disease. Any enlarged pelvic or para-aortic lymph nodes are resected. Any peritoneal fluid should be sent for cytology.

a. **The role of lymphadenectomy.** During surgery, if the tumor measures <2 cm and superficial myoinvasion with grade 1 or 2 histology is noted, lymphadenectomy may potentially be deferred given the very low risk of lymph node spread. Suspicious lymph nodes should always be sampled.

b. **Patients with persistent complex atypical hyperplasia** after adequate progestin treatment are adequately treated with TAH/BSO in the absence of endometrial cancer. Up to 40% of these patients will have coexisting endometrial cancer.

c. **In young women who desire future fertility and who have well-differentiated (grade 1) lesions**, the use of high-dose progestin hormones can be curative. A durable complete response occurs in about 50% of patients. Oral pharmacologic options include progesterone 100 to 200 mg/d or megestrol acetate 80 to 320 mg/d in divided doses. An alternative well-tolerated option is placement of a Mirena IUD resulting in local release of progesterone in the uterine cavity. Therapy should be continued for up to 9 months with endometrial sampling every 3 months to assess response. If the disease completely resolves, the patient must undergo cyclic hormonal therapy to avoid anovulatory hyperplasia. Patients should be counseled that fertility sparing is not standard of care. Pelvic MRI should be obtained to rule out myometrial invasion prior to proceeding with fertility-sparing management. Hysterectomy is recommended in this group of patients after completion of childbearing.

2. **RT**

a. **RT alone** may be used only for patients at high risk for surgical mortality because of concomitant medical conditions, but the outcome is inferior to surgery.

b. **Postoperative RT.** To facilitate accurate risk stratification and selection for RT, surgical staging and the histopathologic findings in the uterine specimen and lymph nodes are essential. Based on the relative risk of recurrent disease, patients are categorized into three groups.

   (1) **Low-risk early-stage disease** is defined as well differentiated (i.e., grade 1 or 2 tumors) with no or superficial myometrial invasion and absence of LVSI or lymph node metastasis. These patients do not require any adjuvant treatment.

   (2) **Intermediate-risk early-stage disease** is considered based on age and the following three factors: grade 2 or 3 disease, deep myometrial invasion, and lymphovascular space invasion (LVSI). Adjuvant radiation is recommended if (a) patients are <50 years old with three of three risk factors present; (b) patients are 50 to 70 years old with two of three risk factors present; or (c) patients are age >70 years old with one of three risk factors present. Vaginal brachytherapy alone may be considered in certain patients as similar local control was noted with significantly less toxicity compared to pelvic radiation. If this group of patients has not undergone a thorough lymphadenectomy, external pelvic irradiation (about 5,000 cGy) should be considered.

(3) **High-risk early-stage disease** including patients with grade 3 disease associated with deep myometrial invasion or stage II disease may benefit from pelvic radiation, rather than brachytherapy alone.

3. **Chemotherapy** is sometimes used in patients with the highest risk of recurrence. (see Ovarian Cancer, Section VI.E.3 for regimen dosages).

4. **High-risk histology endometrial cancers, including serous, clear cell, and carcinosarcoma** (now considered an epithelial tumor rather than a sarcoma) have a significantly higher risk of recurrence, including systemic recurrence. Therefore, chemotherapy (carboplatin and paclitaxel as above) is considered for stage IA disease and recommended for all stage IB–IV. Carcinosarcoma may be treated with ifosfamide and paclitaxel or cisplatin and ifosfamide. Radiation may also be used in combination with chemotherapy.

B. **Advanced disease**

1. **Stage III or IV disease** is treated best with optimal cytoreduction. Surgery should be followed with systemic multiagent chemotherapy.

2. **Drug therapy.** Patients with widespread metastases or with previously irradiated, recurrent local disease can be treated with hormones or cytotoxic agents.

a. **Hormonal therapy.** Response to progestins occurs in 20% to 40% of patients. The average duration of response is 1 year, and expected survival in responding patients is twice that of nonresponders. A few patients survive in excess of 10 years. Hormone receptor studies are of some predictive value. The following drugs are most frequently used:

(1) Repository form of oral progesterone 100 to 200 mg/d or medroxyprogesterone acetate 1.0 g IM weekly for 6 weeks and monthly thereafter

(2) Megestrol acetate 40 mg PO four times daily

(3) Tamoxifen 20 mg PO twice daily for 3 weeks, alternating with megestrol acetate 80 mg PO twice daily or oral progesterone 100 to 200 mg daily for 3 weeks. This treatment cycle can be repeated as long as good response is noted.

b. **Chemotherapy** is the cornerstone of treatment for advanced stage III or IV disease and may be used in combination with pelvic radiation. While cisplatin and doxorubicin were historically used to treat endometrial cancers, carboplatin and paclitaxel have become widely accepted based on preliminary randomized data demonstrating noninferior outcomes and a markedly better toxicity profile (see Ovarian Cancer, Section VI.E.3 for regimen dosages).

VII. UTERINE SARCOMAS

A. Uterine sarcomas account for 3% of all uterine neoplasms and include from highest to lowest frequency: uterine leiomyosarcoma, endometrial stromal sarcoma (low-grade or high-grade), and undifferentiated uterine sarcoma.

B. **Uterine sarcomas differ from the subtypes of epithelial endometrial cancer:**

1. Endometrial biopsy is less sensitive for uterine sarcomas compared to epithelial endometrial cancers and diagnosis is often made after hysterectomy

2. Carcinosarcomas are staged using the same system as epithelial endometrial cancer. However, a different staging system is used for other types of uterine sarcomas (refer to the AJCC Cancer Staging Manual).

3. The initial treatment of choice is hysterectomy ± bilateral salpingo-oophorectomy. Morcellation should be avoided in cases of suspected sarcoma due to the risk of iatrogenic dissemination.

    4. Routine lymphadenectomy is controversial given the low risk of lymph node involvement.

  C. Leiomyosarcoma, high-grade endometrial stromal sarcoma, or undifferentiated uterine sarcoma carry a high risk of recurrence. The role of adjuvant therapy is poorly defined but typically includes chemotherapy ± radiation for surgically resected stage II–IV disease and can be considered after surgery for stage I disease. Doxorubicin (less toxic and equally efficacious) and combination of gemcitabine and docetaxel are most frequently used. There are no data showing that adjuvant chemotherapy prolongs survival. Metastatic disease is managed with chemotherapy (doxorubicin, ifosfamide, gemcitabine and docetaxel, pazopanib, dacarbazine, trabectedin).

  D. Low-grade endometrial stromal sarcoma can be observed after primary surgery or patients can be placed on hormone therapy (i.e., megestrol, medroxyprogesterone, aromatase inhibitors, GnRH analogs). These hormonal options can also be used in the recurrent setting or for unresectable disease given the hormonally responsive nature of these tumors.

VIII. SPECIAL CLINICAL PROBLEMS

  A. In premenopausal women with stage I endometrial cancer, ovarian preservation can be considered particularly in patients who are not carriers of Lynch syndrome (as these patients are at risk for synchronous tumors). If ovaries are preserved, surveillance and ultimately an oophorectomy should be considered after menopause. The decision should be individualized after thorough patient counseling. In patients who experience early surgical menopause, daily estrogen replacement therapy for younger patients with stage I disease may be considered to protect against osteoporosis and to improve quality of life. This treatment has not been associated with deleterious effects; however, it should be individualized for each patient, considering all their preexisting medical conditions.

VAGINAL CANCER

I. EPIDEMIOLOGY AND ETIOLOGY

  A. Incidence. Primary carcinoma of the vagina constitutes 1% to 2% of cancers of the female genital tract. Dysplastic changes of the vaginal mucosa are known as VAIN (vaginal intraepithelial neoplasia). The likelihood of vaginal carcinoma is increased in women with a history of cervical carcinoma. About 80% to 90% of cases of vaginal cancer are metastatic in origin (i.e., from the cervix or vulva) and are treated according to the primary lesion.

  B. HPV. HPV is associated with VAIN. The exact potential of VAIN to progress to frankly invasive carcinoma is unknown but appears to be in the range of 3% to 5%.

  C. Estrogens

    1. The 2 million daughters of women treated with DES during the first 18 weeks of gestation are at risk for developing vaginal clear cell adenocarcinomas. Use of DES was discontinued in the 1970s. As of April 2015, 775 cases of clear cell vaginal and cervical carcinomas have been reported by the Registry for Research on Hormonal Transplacental Carcinogenesis. DES exposure accounted for two-thirds of the reported cases.

    2. Vaginal adenosis is present in nearly 45% of women exposed to DES and 25% have structural abnormalities of the uterus, cervix, or vagina. Almost all women with vaginal clear cell carcinoma also have vaginal adenosis.

II. PATHOLOGY AND NATURAL HISTORY

A. Histology. About 85% of vaginal carcinomas are squamous cell carcinomas.

B. Location. Primary vaginal cancers most commonly arise on the posterior wall of the upper one-third of the vagina. If the cervix is involved, the disease is defined as cervical rather than vaginal cancer. If the vulva is involved, the disease is defined as vulvar cancer.

C. Mode of spread

1. Direct extension to adjacent soft tissues and bony structures, including paracolpos and parametria, bladder, urethra, rectum, and bony pelvis, usually occurs when the tumor is large.

2. Lymphatic dissemination occurs to pelvic and then para-aortic nodes from the upper vagina, whereas the posterior wall is drained by inferior gluteal, sacral, and deep pelvic nodes. The anterior wall drains into lymphatics of the lateral pelvic walls, and the distal one-third of the vagina drains into the inguinal and femoral nodes.

3. Hematogenous spread occurs late and is most often to lung, liver, bone, and supraclavicular lymph nodes.

III. DIAGNOSIS

A. Symptoms and signs. The most frequent presenting symptoms are vaginal discharge and bleeding. Vaginal adenosis is usually asymptomatic but may produce a chronic watery discharge.

B. Diagnostic studies

1. Diagnosis of vaginal carcinoma is often missed on initial examination, especially when the tumor is located in the distal two-thirds of the vagina, where the blades of the speculum may obscure the lesion. The speculum should always be rotated as it is withdrawn and the vaginal mucosa inspected carefully.

2. Vaginal Pap smears and biopsy of abnormal areas on pelvic examination are the mainstays of diagnosis.

IV. STAGING SYSTEM AND PROGNOSTIC FACTORS

A. Staging system: refer to the AJCC Cancer Staging Manual.

B. Prognostic factors. Generally, the greater the tumor size, the worse the prognosis. Cancers located in the upper vagina, however, have a better prognosis than those located in the lower vagina (upper posterior tumors can become large before invading the muscularis and changing the stage of disease).

V. PREVENTION AND EARLY DETECTION

A. Cytology and routine examination are the basis of screening the general population.

B. Females with a history of *in utero* **exposure to DES** should have a pelvic examination and Pap smear yearly from the time of menarche. All suspected areas should undergo biopsy, and careful palpation of all mucosal surfaces is extremely important.

VI. MANAGEMENT

A. Early disease

1. Surgery. The close proximity of bladder, urethra, and rectum often restricts the surgical margins that can be obtained without an exenterative procedure. In addition, attempts to maintain a functional vagina and the associated psychosocial issues play an important role in treatment planning. Vaginal reconstruction may be performed using split-thickness skin grafts from the thighs or with myocutaneous flaps, usually with gracilis muscle.

2. **RT** is an alternative treatment for patients with stage I disease; although, there are no controlled studies to prove that RT is as effective as surgery. Radiation is the treatment of choice for all higher stages, usually using combined external-beam and intravaginal RT. When the distal vagina is involved, the inguinal nodes are also treated.

3. **Chemotherapy.** Topical fluorouracil, applied twice daily, has been used for VAIN.

4. **Immune therapy** with 5% imiquimod cream—two to three times per week with close clinical observation and careful colposcopic exams to assess response is an alternative treatment for CIS.

5. **Laser therapy** is useful for stage 0.

B. **Advanced disease** is managed as for cancer of the cervix.

VULVAR CANCER

I. EPIDEMIOLOGY AND ETIOLOGY

A. **Incidence.** Carcinomas of the vulva constitute 3% to 4% of malignant lesions of the female genital tract. The disease is most common in women >50 years of age, with a mean age at diagnosis of 65 years.

B. **Etiology**

1. **HPV viruses** play a role in the development of vulvar cancer. High-risk subtypes of HPV (16, 18, 31, 33, and 45) have been isolated from invasive vulvar cancer.

2. **Vulvar intraepithelial neoplasia** (VIN) and CIN increase a woman's risk for carcinoma of the vulva. Vaccination with the HPV vaccine will provide protection against VIN, commonly a precursor lesion to invasive vulvar cancer.

3. **Medical comorbidities** associated with increased risk of vulvar cancer include obesity, hypertension, diabetes mellitus, arteriosclerosis, menopause at an early age, and nulliparity.

II. PATHOLOGY AND NATURAL HISTORY

A. **Histology.** Malignant tumors of the vulva are squamous cell carcinoma in >90% of cases and melanoma in 5% to 10%. Adenocarcinoma, sarcoma, basal cell carcinoma, and other tumors constitute the remainder.

B. **Location.** The sites of tumor in order of decreasing frequency are labia majora, labia minora, clitoris, and perineum.

C. **Natural history**

1. **Squamous cell carcinomas** in the vulva have not been shown to develop as a continuum from VIN to CIS to invasive carcinoma. Most studies report that only about 2% to 4% of VIN lesions become invasive cancer. These cancers tend to grow locally, spread to superficial and deep groin lymph nodes, and then spread to pelvic and distant nodes. Hematogenous spread usually occurs after lymph node involvement, and death usually results from cachexia or respiratory failure secondary to pulmonary metastases.

2. **Malignant melanoma** of the vulva accounts for 5% of all melanoma cases, despite the comparatively small surface area involved and the paucity of nevi at this site. Therefore, all pigmented vulvar lesions should be removed.

3. **Paget disease of the vulva** is a preinvasive lesion with thickened epithelium infiltrated with mucin-rich Paget cells, which are derived from the stratum germinativum of the epidermis. Approximately 10% to 12% of patients have invasive vulvar Paget disease, and 4% to 8% have an underlying adenocarcinoma. Underlying adenocarcinomas are usually clinically apparent. The natural course of this disease is characterized by local

recurrence over many years, and recurrences are almost always *in situ*. These patients are also predisposed to developing extragenital glandular cancers and need careful clinical evaluation (i.e., colonoscopy to rule out colorectal adenocarcinoma) and follow-up.

4. **Bartholin gland adenocarcinoma** is extremely rare and is usually seen in older women. Inflammation of this gland is uncommon in women >50 years of age and is virtually nonexistent in postmenopausal women; gland swelling in women in these age groups should arouse suspicion for the presence of cancer.

5. **Basal cell carcinomas and sarcomas** of the vulva have natural histories similar to that of primary tumors located elsewhere.

III. DIAGNOSIS

A. **Signs and symptoms**

1. Squamous cell carcinomas most often present with a vulvar lump or mass, often with a history of chronic vulvar pruritus. The tumors often ulcerate or become fungating. Bleeding, superinfection, and pain can develop with continued growth.

2. Paget disease has a characteristic lesion that is velvety red, with raised, irregular margins. Lesions are pruritic, with secondary excoriation and bleeding.

3. Basal cell carcinomas and melanomas are discussed in Chapter 17.

4. Lymph node enlargement may be palpable in the inguinal or femoral regions or in the pelvis.

B. **Indications for vulvar biopsy**

1. Patches of skin that appear red, dark brown, or white

2. Areas that are firm to palpation

3. Pruritic or bleeding lesions

4. Any nevus in the genital region

5. Enlargement or thickening in the region of Bartholin glands, particularly in patients >50 years of age

IV. STAGING SYSTEM AND PROGNOSTIC FACTORS FOR SQUAMOUS CELL CARCINOMA

A. **Staging system:** refer to the AJCC Cancer Staging Manual.

B. **Prognostic factors and survival.** Survival is determined by stage, structures invaded, and tumor location. The 5-year survival rate in patients with negative or one microscopically positive lymph node is 95%. In contrast, the 5-year survival rate for patients with two positive nodes is 80%, and that for patients with three or more positive nodes is 25%. Note that the risk for hematogenous spread with three or more positive nodes is 66%, in contrast to the risk with two or fewer nodes, which is only 4%.

V. PREVENTION AND EARLY DETECTION

The routine history and physical examination of all postmenopausal women should include specific questions regarding vulvar soreness and pruritus followed by careful inspection and palpation of the vulva and palpation for firm or fixed groin nodes. All suspicious lesions should undergo biopsy.

VI. MANAGEMENT

A. **Surgery is the treatment of choice for early-stage lesions.**

1. **Vulvar intraepithelial neoplasia.** Wide local excision is recommended for small lesions. Carbon dioxide laser of the warty variety is acceptable. Alternative treatments include topical administration of imiquimod or 5-FU. Before the use of either agent, the existence of invasive disease has to be ruled out.

2. **Paget disease.** As the Paget cells may invade the underlying dermis, this dermal layer should also be removed during surgical excision. Recurrent lesions may be treated with local excision in the absence of adenocarcinoma. If invasive adenocarcinoma is present, it should be treated in the same manner as an invasive squamous cell carcinoma of the vulva.

3. **Invasive carcinoma with ≤1-mm invasion.** Radical local excision is recommended. Lymphadenectomy is not required due to a <1% risk of lymphatic spread.

4. **Stage I disease with >1-mm invasion.** Radical local excision with ipsilateral groin lymphadenectomy for lateralized lesions and bilateral lymphadenectomy for centralized lesions within 2 cm of the midline in either direction.

5. **Stage II lesions** may be treated with bilateral groin lymphadenectomy and radical local excision (or modified radical vulvectomy) provided that at least 1 cm of clear margins in all directions can be achieved while preserving critical midline structures.

6. **Sentinel lymph node biopsy** can be performed to decrease surgical morbidity by injecting the vulvar lesion with a combination of blue dye and radiocolloid. Full lymphadenectomy is performed if a sentinel lymph node is not detected. Stage IB–II lesions are associated with a >8% risk of lymphatic metastases.

7. **Stage III or IV disease.** These lesions should be treated with RT and chemosensitization (with cisplatin or 5-FU). Selected cases can be treated with radical vulvectomy. Rare cases of persistent or recurrent disease can be salvaged with exenterative surgery.

B. **RT**

1. RT may be used to shrink stage III and IV tumors that involve the anus, rectum, rectovaginal septum, or proximal urethra preoperatively to improve resectability.

2. RT has been shown to improve survival and decrease groin recurrence when there is evidence of ≥3 micrometastases or macrometastasis (≥10 mm) in the groin nodes.

3. Postoperative RT to the vulva may be used to reduce local recurrence when tumors exceed 4 cm or there are positive surgical margins.

4. External-beam RT to 5,000 cGy with follow-up biopsy should be considered for small anterior tumors involving the clitoris, especially in young women, to prevent the psychosocial issues involved with surgery.

5. Patients who have medical conditions precluding surgery may be treated with RT alone.

C. **Chemotherapy**

1. 5-FU or cisplatin chemotherapy can be used as a radiation sensitizer.

2. Systemic treatment with agents active against cervical squamous cell carcinomas, such as cisplatin, carboplatin, paclitaxel, and topotecan, may be used for metastatic disease, but partial response rates are low (10% to 15%) and usually last only a few months.

OVARIAN CANCER

I. EPIDEMIOLOGY AND ETIOLOGY

A. **Incidence** (Table 12-1). About 21,290 American women are diagnosed with ovarian cancer, and 14,180 die due to this disease annually. It is the leading cause of death among all gynecologic cancers and the fifth most common female cancer in the United States, with a lifetime risk of 1 in 70. Despite the advances in surgical and chemotherapeutic management of this disease, the

5-year survival rate for women with stage III/IV epithelial ovarian cancer has remained as low as 15% to 40% over the past 30 years.

B. Predisposing factors are listed below

1. **Geographical.** The highest rates of ovarian cancer are recorded in industrialized countries.

2. **Genetic.** Germline mutations in DNA repair genes (i.e., *BRCA1, BRCA2, MLH1, MSH2, MSH6*, and *PMS2*) account for 10% to 15% of ovarian cancer cases. Identification of this group of women by genetic testing is essential as prophylactic risk reduction surgery with a bilateral salpingo-oophorectomy can decrease the risk of gynecologic cancers by 96%. All patients with epithelial ovarian cancer should be recommended genetic counseling and testing.

3. **Reproductive history** such as nulliparity with "incessant ovulation" is a risk factor. Endometriosis in now found to be an independent risk factor for ovarian cancer. The use of oral contraceptives reduces the risk of ovarian cancer, and postmenopausal estrogens may increase the risk.

4. **Environmental.** Intraperitoneal (IP) exposure to talc has been associated with a slight increase in the risk of ovarian cancer. Cigarette smoking may increase the risk of certain subtypes of ovarian cancer.

II. PATHOLOGY AND NATURAL HISTORY

A. Histology. The World Health Organization (WHO) classification of neoplasms of the ovary is shown in Table 12-3.

B. Histologic grade. The percentage of undifferentiated cells present in tissue determines the grade of the tumors.

Grade	Percentage of Undifferentiated Cells
G1	0–25
G2	25–50
G3	>50

C. Biologic behavior

1. **Borderline tumors,** also called "tumors of low malignant potential," tend to occur in premenopausal women and remain confined to the ovary for long periods of time. Metastatic implants may occur, and some may be progressive, leading to bowel obstruction and death. Borderline tumors have

TABLE 12-3	Histology of Ovarian Neoplasms

A. Epithelial Tumors (Approximate Frequency)	**B. Germ Cell Tumors**
Serous cystadenocarcinoma (75%–80%)	Dysgerminoma
Mucinous cystadenocarcinoma (10%)	Endodermal sinus tumor
Endometrioid carcinoma (10%)	Embryonal carcinoma
Clear cell (mesonephroma) (<1%)	Polyembryoma
Undifferentiated carcinoma (<1%)	Choriocarcinoma
Brenner tumor (<1%)	Teratoma
Mixed epithelial tumor	Mixed
Unclassified	
C. Sex Cord Stromal Tumors	**D. Other Tumors**
Sertoli–Leydig cell tumor	Lipid cell tumors
Granulosa–stromal cell tumor	Gonadoblastoma
Gynandroblastoma	Nonspecific soft tissue tumors
Androblastoma	Unclassified
Unclassified	

a <10% risk of recurrence, and the vast majority of these recurrences are borderline in nature and not invasive.

2. **Other histologic subtypes** behave similarly when grade and stage are considered. Even in suspected early stage disease, careful exploration frequently reveals subdiaphragmatic and omental implants. Organ invasion and distant metastases are less likely than is spread over serosal surfaces. The lethal potential of ovarian cancer is most frequently related to encasement of intra-abdominal organs, such as intestinal obstruction.

D. **Associated paraneoplastic syndromes**

1. Neurologic syndromes can occur. Peripheral neuropathies, organic dementia, amyotrophic lateral sclerosis–like syndrome, and cerebellar ataxia are the most frequent occurrences.

2. Peculiar antibodies that cause difficulties in cross-matching blood can be corrected with prednisone.

3. Cushing syndrome.

4. Hypercalcemia.

5. Thrombophlebitis.

III. DIAGNOSIS

A. **Symptoms and signs.** Early ovarian carcinoma is typically asymptomatic, thus making early diagnosis challenging. The majority of patients with advanced ovarian cancer present with vague symptoms of abdominal discomfort, such as bloating, constipation, gas, irregular menses if premenopausal, urinary frequency, or abnormal vaginal bleeding. Physical findings include ascites and abdominal masses. Any pelvic mass in a woman who is more than 1 year postmenopausal is suspicious for ovarian cancer.

B. **Tissue diagnosis.** Diagnosis requires tissue biopsy of ovarian or other suspected abdominal masses. When highly suspicious adnexal or pelvic masses are present in isolation, surgical removal of an intact ovary is recommended to avoid spillage of tumor and upstaging, which can result in the need for adjuvant chemotherapy.

1. **Masses that are smaller than 8 cm** in premenopausal women are most commonly benign cysts. Patients should undergo ultrasound to confirm the cystic nature of the mass and receive suppression with oral contraceptives for 2 months. Benign lesions should regress.

2. **Surgical evaluation** is necessary for masses with the following characteristics:
   a. Less than 8 cm in diameter and cystic but still present after 2 months of observation in premenopausal women
   b. Smaller than 8 cm in premenopausal women and solid or mural nodules present on ultrasound
   c. Larger than 8 cm in premenopausal women due to risk of torsion
   d. Present in any postmenopausal patient

C. **Serum tumor markers.** Potential biomarkers that can be used in workup of a patient with suspected epithelial ovarian cancer are CA-125, CEA, and CA 19-9. A very elevated CEA-to-CA-125 ratio should raise suspicion for possible gastrointestinal malignancy and may warrant colonoscopy prior to proceeding with surgery. If elevated initially, tumor markers may be useful to monitor the response to therapy in epithelial ovarian tumors. β-human chorionic gonadotropin (β-hCG), α-fetoprotein (α-FP), and lactate dehydrogenase (LDH) are useful tumor markers in germ cell malignancies. None of these markers is useful for screening purposes.

IV. STAGING SYSTEM AND PROGNOSTIC FACTORS

Staging for ovarian cancer is surgical.

A. Staging system: refer to the AJCC Cancer Staging Manual.

B. Prognostic factors. Stage, grade, and histology are prognostic. The extent to which the disease can be surgically debulked also affects prognosis.

V. PREVENTION AND EARLY DETECTION

The risk of developing ovarian cancer is 20% to 60% (average cumulative risk of approximately 45%) by age 70 for women with a mutation in *BRCA1* and 10% to 35% (average cumulative risk of approximately 15%) for women with *BRCA2* mutations. Mutations in the MMR genes responsible for the Lynch Type II syndrome portend a lifetime risk of 9% to 12% for ovarian cancer. Patients with a mutation associated with hereditary breast and ovarian cancer syndrome should consider prophylactic salpingo-oophorectomy by age 35 to 40 and when childbearing has been completed. Women should be advised that prophylactic salpingo-oophorectomy can decrease the risk of breast cancer up to 90%. The procedure, however, does not offer absolute protection from ovarian cancer because peritoneal carcinomas can occur in approximately 4% of women after bilateral salpingo-oophorectomy. Women should also be counseled regarding an approximately 5% to 12% risk of occult neoplasm identified at the time of risk-reducing salpingo-oophorectomy. The incorporation of closer pathologic sectioning of the fallopian tubes and ovaries after risk-reducing surgery has been shown to increase the detection of occult malignancy. The value and interval of CA-125 for screening and transvaginal ultrasound in these women have not been clearly established but are frequently utilized.

VI. MANAGEMENT OF EPITHELIAL OVARIAN, FALLOPIAN TUBE, AND PRIMARY PERITONEAL CANCERS

A. Surgical staging evaluation

1. The ovarian tumor should be removed intact, if possible, and sent for frozen section. If the tumor is confined to the pelvis, a thorough surgical staging procedure should be carried out.

2. Any free fluid, especially in the pelvic cul-de-sac, should be sent for cytologic evaluation. If no free fluid is found, peritoneal washings should be obtained with 50 to 100 mL normal saline.

3. Systematic exploration of all peritoneal surfaces and viscera is performed. Any suspicious areas or adhesions of peritoneal surfaces should undergo biopsy.

4. The omentum should be resected from the transverse colon (an infracolic omentectomy).

5. Peritoneal biopsies should be obtained of the vesical peritoneum, posterior cul-de-sac, bilateral pelvic sidewalls, bilateral paracolic gutters, and right diaphragm if obvious gross disease is not noted in the upper abdomen.

6. The retroperitoneal surfaces are then explored to evaluate the pelvic and para-aortic lymph nodes. Any enlarged lymph nodes should be resected and formal pelvic and para-aortic lymphadenectomy should be performed for comprehensive staging if obvious gross disease is not noted in the upper abdomen.

B. **Borderline tumors.** Treatment is surgical resection of the primary tumor. There is no evidence that subsequent chemotherapy or radiation improves survival. Even in most patients who have multifocal disease, adjuvant therapy probably has no role. Chemotherapy can be considered for patients with invasive implants.

C. **Stage IA and IB, grade 1**

1. **Premenopausal patients** in this category may, after staging laparotomy is completed, undergo unilateral oophorectomy to preserve fertility. Follow-up should include regular pelvic examinations and determinations of CA-125 levels. Generally, the other ovary and uterus are removed when childbearing is completed.

2. **Postmenopausal patients** and women in whom childbearing is not an issue should undergo TAH/BSO and staging.

D. **Stage IA and IB (grades 2 and 3) and stage IC are** treated with TAH/BSO and staging followed by chemotherapy. Carboplatin plus paclitaxel for three to six cycles is recommended for most patients (see Section VI.E.3 for regimen dosages). It may be preferable to give older patients a course of single-agent chemotherapy with carboplatin for four to six cycles.

E. **Stages II, III, and IV**

1. **Surgery** with exploration and removal of as much disease as possible should be carried out. Removal of the primary tumor and as much metastatic disease as possible is referred to as cytoreductive surgery or debulking. "Optimal debulking" is defined as having residual tumor diameters <1 cm in diameter. Ideally, no gross visible residual disease (or R0) is achieved. The volume of residual disease is a known prognostic factor.

2. **Neoadjuvant chemotherapy.** To reduce the potential morbidity of radical surgical procedures, the administration of neoadjuvant chemotherapy prior to interval cytoreductive surgery followed by additional chemotherapy has been recently investigated in two large randomized, controlled trials. Both trials demonstrate that administration of neoadjuvant chemotherapy is noninferior to primary debulking surgery as a treatment option in patients with bulky stage IIIC or IV ovarian cancer. Neoadjuvant chemotherapy may be particularly beneficial in patients with significant comorbidities (i.e., patients with acute venous thromboembolism, poor performance status, or severe malnutrition who may not be good surgical candidates at the time of diagnosis). Ongoing efforts are focused on defining strategies that can help select patients best suited for primary cytoreduction versus neoadjuvant chemotherapy. Scoring systems based on diagnostic laparoscopy and preoperative imaging are two such strategies being explored.

3. **Chemotherapy.** Platinum-based combination regimens have been the mainstay of treatment for advanced ovarian cancer. Combination of a platinum agent (carboplatin or cisplatin) with paclitaxel is the standard treatment for epithelial ovarian cancer. This regimen can be administered intravenously or intraperitoneally (in selected patients).

   a. **The intravenous regimen** is given to patients every 3 weeks for six cycles as follows:

   Paclitaxel 135 to 175 mg/m^2 over 3 hours (given before carboplatin or cisplatin)

   Carboplatin AUC 5 to 6 over 1 hour

   b. **The dose-dense intravenous regimen** can be considered based on evidence that this regimen may prolong progression-free and overall survival, particularly in patients who undergo suboptimal debulking.

Anemia is more common. This can also be given every 3 weeks for six cycles as follows:

Paclitaxel 80 mg/m^2 over 1 hour given weekly

Carboplatin AUC 6 over 1 hour every 3 weeks

c. The intraperitoneal (IP) regimen is an option in patients with stage III disease and microscopic residual disease after cytoreductive surgery. In this subset of patients, a significant improvement in progression-free and overall survival was noted compared with intravenous therapy. Due to increased side effects, such as abdominal pain, gastrointestinal discomfort, fatigue, hematologic toxicities, and neuropathy, many patients are not able to tolerate the full six courses of IP therapy. This regimen is administered in six cycles every 21 days as tolerated:

Day 1 IV Paclitaxel 135 mg/m^2 over 3 or 24 hours

Day 2 IP Cisplatin 75 to 100 mg/m^2

Day 8 IP Paclitaxel 60 mg/m^2

d. Relative toxicities. Carboplatin has fewer gastrointestinal, neurologic, and renal side effects than cisplatin but more hematologic toxicity. When paclitaxel is infused over 3 hours, it is associated with more neurologic toxicity and less hematologic toxicity than when it is infused over 24 hours.

e. Maintenance therapy in patients with advanced ovarian cancer who have achieved complete remission with standard induction chemotherapy is not the standard of care and does not improve outcomes.

f. Antiangiogenic agents. Using bevacizumab as adjuvant and maintenance therapy has been investigated without a survival benefit noted. Clinically, it is used in combination with chemotherapy or alone and often for platinum-resistant disease due to increased overall response rates and short improvements in progression-free survival. Hypertension and proteinuria are common toxicities. While the overall risk of gastrointestinal perforation is low (i.e., 1% to 3%), patients with bowel obstruction, fistula, or rectosigmoid disease involvement may be at heightened risk and were often excluded in randomized studies evaluating bevacizumab.

4. Serial CA-125 determinations should be followed. Rising CA-125 levels to a level >35 U/mL are associated with persistent or recurrent disease.

F. Second-line therapy

1. Cytotoxic drugs. If disease relapses more than 6 months (platinum-sensitive) after completion of primary therapy, a platinum doublet is often utilized. If disease progresses on first-line therapy (platinum-refractory) or less than 6 months after completion of primary therapy (platinum-resistant), other drugs are used.

a. Chemotherapeutic agents that may be helpful after failure of first-line therapy include liposomal doxorubicin, topotecan, gemcitabine, pemetrexed, etoposide. These agents are often used in combination with carboplatin in platinum-sensitive disease and as single agents in platinum-resistant disease. In most cases, single-agent therapy appears to be as effective as combinations. Response rates are about 15% to 25%.

b. Bevacizumab, a monoclonal antibody against vascular endothelial growth factor, has been used alone or in combination with cytotoxic agents in the treatment of recurrent epithelial ovarian cancer, particularly for platinum-resistant disease (see Ovarian Cancer, Section VI.E.3.f).

c. Hormonal treatment with tamoxifen has demonstrated 10% to 20% efficacy in this setting.

d. Poly-ADP ribose polymerase (PARP) inhibitors target DNA repair mechanisms. Tumor cells that are deficient in *BRCA1/2* are more sensitive to this therapy due to synthetic lethality. PARP inhibitors are administered orally and are well tolerated. Therapy with olaparib is FDA approved for patients with germline *BRCA1/2* mutations who have been treated with three or more prior lines of chemotherapy. An overall response rate of 34% was noted in a phase II trial with the most common adverse reactions including mild to moderate gastrointestinal symptoms, fatigue, and anemia.

2. Second-look laparotomy. A second-look operation is one performed to determine the response to therapy on a patient who has no clinical evidence of disease after a prescribed course of chemotherapy. Second-look laparotomy has not been shown to influence patient survival, although the information obtained at second look is highly prognostic. The operation should only be performed in a research setting, such as in patients receiving therapy in a setting where second-line therapies are undergoing clinical trial.

3. Secondary cytoreductive surgery may be beneficial for patients who have isolated residual disease at relapse, such as a persistent pelvic mass. This benefit depends on the ability to completely resect the residual disease. It is not beneficial for patients with disease that is unresponsive to chemotherapy or with a short disease-free interval.

4. Palliative surgery may be considered in patients who develop bowel obstruction and resistance to chemotherapy but have a reasonably good performance status; this is usually a difficult recommendation to make for all concerned. The goal is to allow the patient sufficient oral intake to maintain hydration or some nutrition at home. If successful, the procedure may allow 3 to 6 months of relief. Unfortunately, the complication and mortality rates from surgery are high, and the success rate is low. The patient and her family must clearly understand these limitations when decisions are made.

G. Patient surveillance is clinical because there are no reliable means of surveillance. CA-125 levels should be followed, but CT and ultrasound have proven too insensitive to detect early recurrent disease. Imaging may be used to follow measurable disease.

VII. GERM CELL TUMORS (see Table 12-3, Part B for subtypes)

A. General aspects of germ cell tumors

1. Epidemiology. Germ cell tumors make up 20% to 25% of all ovarian neoplasms, but only 3% of these tumors are malignant. These malignancies constitute <5% of all ovarian cancers in Western countries and up to 15% in Asian and African populations. Germ cell tumors constitute >70% of ovarian neoplasms in the first two decades of life, and in this age range, one-third are malignant. Malignant germ cell tumors have an excellent prognosis.

2. Signs and symptoms. These tumors grow rapidly and often present with subacute pelvic pain and pressure and menstrual irregularity. Acute symptoms related to torsion or adnexal ruptures can be confused with acute appendicitis. Adnexal masses >2 cm in premenarchal girls and in premenopausal women are suspicious; they usually require surgical investigation.

3. Diagnosis

a. Young patients should be tested for serum LDH, β-hCG, and α-FP titers along with other routine blood work.

   b. A chest radiograph is essential because germ cell tumors may metastasize to lungs or mediastinum.

B. **Dysgerminoma**

1. **Natural history.** Dysgerminomas are the most common germ cell malignancy and represent up to 10% of ovarian cancers in patients <20 years of age. Three-fourths of dysgerminomas occur between the ages of 10 and 30 years. About 5% are found in dysgenetic gonads. Three-fourths of cases are stage I, and 10% to 15% are bilateral. Unlike other ovarian malignancies, dysgerminomas often spread earlier through the lymphatics than to peritoneal surfaces. These tumors secrete LDH.

2. **Treatment** is primarily surgical; the minimal operation is unilateral oophorectomy with complete surgical staging. The chance of recurrence in the other ovary during the next 2 years is 5% to 10%, but these lesions are sensitive to chemotherapy. When fertility is an issue, the uterus and contralateral ovary should be preserved even in the presence of metastatic disease. If fertility is not an issue, TAH/BSO should be performed. If a Y chromosome is found by karyotyping, both ovaries should be removed, but the uterus may be left in place.

   a. Chemotherapy is the adjuvant treatment of choice for metastatic disease. A combination of bleomycin, etoposide, and cisplatin (BEP regimen) is most often used for 3 to 4 cycles. BEP dosages are as follows:

   Bleomycin 30 units per week
   Etoposide 100 mg/m²/d for 5 days every 3 weeks
   Cisplatin 20 mg/m²/d for 5 days every 3 weeks

   b. RT. If fertility is not an issue, metastatic disease may be treated with radiation because these tumors are extremely radiosensitive.

3. **Prognosis.** The 5-year survival rate for patients with stage IA disease is >95% when the disease is treated with unilateral oophorectomy alone. Recurrence is most likely in patients with lesions >10 to 15 cm in diameter, who are younger than 20 years of age, and who have an anaplastic histology. Patients with advanced disease that is treated with surgery followed by BEP chemotherapy have a 5-year survival rate of 85% to 90%.

C. **Immature teratoma**

1. **Natural history.** Pure immature teratomas account for <1% of all ovarian cancers but are the second most common germ cell malignancy. They constitute 10% to 20% of ovarian malignancies in patients younger than 20 years of age and account for 30% of ovarian cancer deaths in this group. Serum tumor markers (β-hCG, α-FP) are not found unless the tumor is of mixed type. The most common site of spread is the peritoneum; hematogenous spread is uncommon and occurs late.

2. **Treatment.** In premenopausal women in whom the lesion is confined to one ovary, a unilateral oophorectomy with surgical staging is warranted. In postmenopausal women, TAH/BSO is performed.

   a. For patients with stage IA, grade 1 tumors, no adjuvant therapy is required. For stage IA, grade 2 or 3, or stage II to IV disease, adjuvant chemotherapy with BEP should be used. Chemotherapy is also indicated for patients with ascites, regardless of grade.

   b. RT is reserved for patients with localized disease after chemotherapy.

   c. Second-look laparotomy is best reserved for patients at high risk for treatment failure (i.e., patients with macroscopic disease at the start of chemotherapy) because there are no reliable tumor markers for this disease.

3. **Prognosis.** The most important prognostic feature of immature teratomas is their histologic grade. The 5-year survival rate is 80% to 100%. Patients whose lesions cannot be completely resected before chemotherapy have a 5-year survival rate of only 50%, as compared with 94% for completely resected disease.

D. **Endodermal sinus tumors** (yolk sac carcinomas) are rare. The median age at diagnosis is 18 years. Pelvic or abdominal pain is the most common presenting symptom. Most of these lesions secrete α-FP, and serum levels are useful in monitoring response to treatment.

    1. **Treatment** consists of surgical staging, unilateral oophorectomy, and frozen section for diagnosis.

    2. **All patients** are given adjuvant or therapeutic chemotherapy. BEP appears to be most effective.

E. **Embryonal carcinoma** is an extremely rare tumor that occurs in young women and girls, with a median age of 14 years. These tumors may secrete estrogens, producing symptoms of precocious pseudopuberty or irregular bleeding. Two-thirds are confined to one ovary at presentation, and they frequently secrete α-FP and β-hCG, which are useful to follow response to therapy. Treatment is unilateral or bilateral oophorectomy followed by chemotherapy with BEP.

F. **Choriocarcinoma of the ovary** is extremely rare; most patients are younger than 20 years of age. β- hCG is often a useful tumor marker. Half of premenarchal patients present with isosexual precocity. The prognosis is usually poor, but complete responses have been reported with combination methotrexate, actinomycin D, and cyclophosphamide.

G. **Mixed germ cell tumors** most commonly have a dysgerminoma or endodermal sinus component. Secretion of α-FP or β-hCG depends on component parts. Lesions should be managed with unilateral oophorectomy and chemotherapy with BEP. A second-look laparotomy may be indicated when macroscopic disease is present at the start of chemotherapy to determine response to therapy in components that do not produce tumor markers.

VIII. **SEX CORD STROMAL TUMORS** (see Table 12-3, Part C for subtypes) account for 5% to 8% of all ovarian cancers. Most tumors are a combination of cell types derived from the sex cords and ovarian stroma or mesenchyme.

A. **Granulosa–stromal cell tumors** include granulosa cell tumors, thecomas, and fibromas. Thecomas and fibromas are rarely malignant and are then called fibrosarcomas. Granulosa cell tumors are low-grade, estrogen-secreting malignancies that are seen in women of all ages. Endometrial cancer occurs with granulosa cell tumors in 5% of cases, and 25% to 50% are associated with endometrial hyperplasia. Inhibin, which may be secreted by some granulosa cell tumors, may be a useful tumor marker. Surgery alone is usually sufficient therapy; RT and chemotherapy are reserved for women with recurrent or metastatic disease. Granulosa cell tumors have a 10-year survival rate of about 90%. DNA ploidy correlates with survival.

B. **Sertoli–Leydig tumors** have a peak incidence between the third and fourth decades. These rare lesions are usually low-grade malignancies. Most produce androgens, and virilization is seen in 70% to 85% of patients. Usual treatment is unilateral oophorectomy with evaluation of the contralateral ovary. TAH/BSO is appropriate for older patients. The utility of radiation or chemotherapy is yet to be proven.

IX. OTHER TUMORS (see Table 12-3, Part D for subtypes)

A. **Lipoid cell tumors** are extremely rare, with only slightly more than 100 cases reported. They are thought to arise from adrenal cortical rests near the ovary. Most are virilizing and are benign or low-grade malignancies. Treatment is surgical extirpation.

B. **Ovarian sarcomas** are also extremely rare, and most occur in postmenopausal women. They are aggressive lesions with no effective treatment. Most patients die within 2 years.

C. **Lymphoma** can involve the ovaries, usually bilaterally, especially with Burkitt lymphoma. A hematologist–oncologist should be consulted intraoperatively when lymphoma is found to determine the need for special studies; plans for cytoreductive surgery should be abandoned. Treatment is as for lymphomas elsewhere in the body.

X. SPECIAL CLINICAL PROBLEMS

A. **Pseudomyxoma peritonei** occurs in the setting of mucinous cystadenocarcinoma or "benign" mucinous adenomas. The peritoneum becomes filled with jelly-like material that compresses the bowel and produces painful abdominal distention. Chemotherapy may impede cellular production of the mucoid material but usually has little direct effect on the tumor. Periodic surgical debulking may be the only way to provide relief of abdominal symptoms. It is now believed that these lesions are typically associated with mucinous adenocarcinomas of the appendix.

B. **Fallopian tube cancers** account for 0.3% of all cancers of the female genital tract. Studies closely examining the fallopian tubes of patients who underwent risk-reducing salpingo-oophorectomy have identified a possible malignant precursor, referred to as serous tubal intraepithelial carcinoma (STIC). The fallopian tube is the site of origin for the vast majority of serous ovarian and primary peritoneal cancers. The classic triad of symptoms is a prominent watery vaginal discharge, pelvic pain, and pelvic mass; however, this triad is seen in <15% of patients. The histologic features, evaluation, and treatment are similar to those of epithelial ovarian cancer.

C. **Pregnancy with ovarian cancer** (see Chapter 27). Pregnancy is rarely complicated by the development of ovarian cancer. All pregnant patients have luteal cysts, which should be <5 to 6 cm in diameter. Masses that are larger or continue to enlarge over several weeks should be examined by laparoscopy at 16 weeks of gestation. Management of pregnant patients with ovarian cancer is the same as for nonpregnant patients who desire childbearing.

D. **Obstructive complications.** Intestinal obstruction is discussed in Chapter 31. Rectal or urinary tract obstruction or dyspareunia in patients with advanced pelvic cancers may respond to either systemic chemotherapy or local irradiation.

GESTATIONAL TROPHOBLASTIC NEOPLASIA

I. EPIDEMIOLOGY AND ETIOLOGY

Gestational choriocarcinoma accounts for <1% of malignancies in women. The etiology is unknown, but certain risk factors and the relationship with hydatidiform mole are well recognized.

A. **Hydatidiform mole** develops in about 1 in 1,500 to 2,000 pregnancies in North America and Europe. The incidence is 5 to 10 times greater in Asia, Latin America, and other countries.

B. **Other factors** that are associated with the occurrence of hydatidiform mole include the following:
1. Patients who have had a prior molar pregnancy
2. Extremes of reproductive age
3. Presence of twin pregnancy

II. PATHOLOGY AND NATURAL HISTORY

A. **Classification.** Molar pregnancies are classified as partial or complete based on morphology, histopathology, and karyotype. **Complete moles** have diploid karyotype, tend to have grape-like structures with diffuse hydropic villi, and can be accompanied with paraneoplastic sequelae. **Partial moles** have triploid karyotype, can resemble hydropic abortion with recognizable fetal tissue, and have focal trophoblastic hyperplasia.

B. **Malignant transformation.** Persistent gestational trophoblastic disease (GTD) is diagnosed when there is clinical, hormonal, pathologic, and/or radiologic evidence of gestational trophoblastic tissue. About 20% of patients with complete molar pregnancy will develop persistence; 15% will have localized uterine disease, whereas 4% have evidence of metastatic disease. In contrast, partial moles develop nonmetastatic persistence in 2% to 4% of cases. Choriocarcinoma results from the malignant transformation of the trophoblast and is characterized by the absence of villi. The clinical course determines whether the growth is benign or malignant. Occasionally, malignant growth may not become clinically evident until years after the last gestation.

C. **Dissemination.** Persistent GTD disseminates locally to the vagina and pelvic organs. Choriocarcinoma disseminates rapidly and widely through the bloodstream. The lungs are the most common site of metastases, followed by vaginal metastases. Hepatic and cerebral metastases are seen less commonly.

III. DIAGNOSIS

A. **Symptoms** of molar pregnancy or malignant trophoblastic disease include the following:
1. Vaginal bleeding during pregnancy (nearly all cases of molar pregnancy or malignant trophoblastic disease cause bleeding)
2. Hyperemesis gravidarum
3. Passage of grape-like villi from the uterus
4. Sweating, tachycardia, weight loss, and nervousness resulting from paraneoplastic hyperthyroidism (see Section VII.A)
5. Pulmonary symptoms as a consequence of lung metastases
6. Right upper quadrant pain or jaundice as a consequence of liver metastases
7. Any neurologic abnormality resulting from brain metastases
8. Abdominal (uterine) pain early in pregnancy

B. **Physical findings**
1. The uterus is usually, but not always, larger than expected for the duration of pregnancy.
2. Fetal heart tones are absent (the coexistence of a viable fetus and a partial hydatidiform mole is uncommon).
3. The patient develops signs of toxemia of pregnancy (hypertension, retinal sheen, sudden weight gain, proteinuria, or peripheral edema). If signs occur in the first or second trimester, a molar pregnancy is strongly suspected.

C. **Preliminary laboratory studies**
1. CBC, alkaline phosphatase level, LFTs.
2. β-hCG production is maximal in early pregnancy and decreases thereafter. Normal hCG values for pregnancy depend on the assay method used by the

laboratory. hCG is elevated in all patients with choriocarcinoma; the serum concentration directly reflects the tumor volume. The serum half-life of hCG is 18 to 24 hours.

D. Special diagnostic studies

1. Ultrasonography of the uterus and Doppler examination reveal no evidence of fetal parts or heartbeat in trophoblastic disease. If these examinations show no fetus, plain radiographs of the pelvic organs are obtained for confirmation.

2. A chest radiograph should be obtained in patients with molar pregnancy.

3. Radionuclide and CT scans are used to detect brain, liver, or other abdominal metastases. Scans and films of the abdomen and pelvis must be avoided until the absence of a fetus is proven.

4. Thyroid studies (serum thyroxine concentration and tri-iodothyronine–resin uptake) are obtained in patients with clinical evidence of hyperthyroidism.

IV. STAGING SYSTEMS AND PROGNOSTIC FACTORS

A. The staging system: refer to the AJCC Cancer Staging Manual.

B. The World Health Organization (WHO) scoring system for GTD is summarized in Table 12-4. *High-risk* patients are those with a score of ≥7 and *low-risk* patients are those with score of ≤6. In addition, another scoring system can be assigned by determining the risk of resistance to single-agent chemotherapy.

V. PREVENTION AND EARLY DETECTION

Early detection depends on careful attention to the signs and symptoms of trophoblastic disease in pregnant and postpartum patients, particularly in patients with a history of molar pregnancy.

VI. MANAGEMENT

All forms of gestational trophoblastic neoplasia, from hydatidiform mole to choriocarcinoma, are almost invariably lethal if not treated.

A. Early disease signifies a molar pregnancy without evidence of distant metastases by history, physical examination, LFTs, chest radiograph, or scans.

1. **Surgery.** Molar tissue is removed by suction curettage while oxytocin is being administered, and then by sharp curettage. Hysterectomy is recommended for women >40 years of age. Disappearance of hCG is achieved within

TABLE 12-4	The WHO Prognostic Scoring System for Gestational Trophoblastic Disease			
Parameter	**Score 0**	**Score 1**	**Score 2**	**Score 4**
Age (years)	≤39	>39		
Antecedent pregnancy	Mole	Abortion	Term	
Interval (months)	<4	4–6	7–12	>12
Pretreatment hCG (mIU/mL)	$<10^3$	$10^3–10^4$	$>10^4–10^5$	$>10^5$
Largest tumor, including uterine (cm)	<3	3–4	≥5	
Site of metastases	Lung, vagina	Spleen, kidney	Gut	Brain, liver
Number of metastases	0	1–4	5–8	>8
Prior chemotherapy drugs failed			1	≥2

WHO, World Health Organization.
Reprinted from Union for International Cancer Control. Gestational trophoblastic neoplasia. 2014 Review of Cancer Medicines on the WHO List of Essential Medicines. 2014:1–9. Accessed on March 6, 2016: http://www.who.int/selection_medicines/committees/expert/20/applications/GestationalTrophoblasticNeoplasia.pdf?ua=1.

8 weeks in 80% of patients treated by surgery; virtually all of these patients are cured. The patient is followed with weekly blood assays for hCG.

2. **RT** has no role in early disease.

3. **Chemotherapy.** After surgical treatment of a molar pregnancy with no suggestion of metastatic disease, weekly serum hCG titers are obtained. Chemotherapy is started for histologic diagnosis of choriocarcinoma, rising hCG titer (for 2 weeks), plateau of hCG titer (for 3 weeks), documentation of metastatic disease, or return of titers with no other explanation after achieving a zero titer. So long as titers continue to decrease, treatment is usually not started; in the past, treatment was started after a predetermined number of weeks.

   a. **Methotrexate** is the drug of choice in early gestational trophoblastic neoplasia. It can be administered in the following three ways:

   (1) Pulse methotrexate 40 mg/m^2 IM weekly

   (2) 5-day methotrexate 0.4 mg/m^2 IV or IM daily for 5 days; with response, retreat at same dose every 2 weeks

   (3) Methotrexate 100 mg/m^2 IV bolus in 250 mL of normal saline over 30 minutes, then 200 mg/m^2 IV in 500 mL normal saline over 12 hours; leucovorin is given 24 hours after starting methotrexate (15 mg PO or IM every 12 hours for 4 doses)

   b. **Actinomycin D** is used instead of methotrexate in patients with renal function impairment or when there is resistance to methotrexate. This drug can be administered every 2 weeks either as 12 μg/kg IV push daily for 5 days or as a pulse of 1.25 mg/m^2 IV.

B. **Advanced disease**

   1. **Surgery** is used to evacuate or excise the uterus for the same indications outlined in early disease (see Section VI.A.1).

   2. **RT,** in combination with chemotherapy, is clearly indicated for the primary management of patients with liver or brain metastases.

   3. **Chemotherapy** is the mainstay of management for metastatic trophoblastic disease. All patients undergo the restaging evaluation described in Section IV.

   a. **Low-risk patients** are treated with methotrexate or actinomycin D, as for early disease patients. Patients not responding to one of these agents are switched to the alternative drug.

   b. **High-risk patients** are treated with combination chemotherapy regimens, such as EMA-CO or EMA-CE (described subsequently). RT is given if the liver or brain is involved by metastases. Chemotherapy dosage schedules are as follows (cycle intervals should not be extended without good cause):

   (1) **EMA-CO** is given in 14-day cycles:
       Etoposide 100 mg/m^2 IV on days 1 and 2
       Methotrexate 100 mg/m^2 IV push, followed by 200 mg/m^2 by continuous IV infusion over 12 hours on day 1; leucovorin beginning 24 hours after the start of methotrexate, 15 mg PO or IM every 12 hours for four doses
       Actinomycin D 0.5 mg (*not* per m^2) IV push on days 1 and 2
       Cyclophosphamide 600 mg/m^2 IV on day 8
       Vincristine (Oncovin) 1.0 mg/m^2 IV on day 8 (maximum 2 mg)

   (2) **EMA-EP** is given in 14-day cycles:
       Cisplatin, 80 mg/kg over 12 hours on day 1

Etoposide 100 mg/m^2 IV on day 1 and day 8

Methotrexate 100 mg/m^2 IV push, followed by 200 mg/m^2 by continuous IV infusion over 12 hours on day 8; leucovorin 15 mg PO or IM every 12 hours for four doses beginning 24 hours after the start of methotrexate

Actinomycin D 0.5 mg (*not* per m^2) IV push on day 8

  c. Duration of treatment. Chemotherapy should be continued until hCG is no longer demonstrable in the serum for three consecutive weekly assays. If the hCG titer rises or plateaus between any two measurements, the chemotherapy regimen must be changed.

C. Patient follow-up
  1. The hCG level is the single most important tumor marker in trophoblastic neoplasia. For stage I, II, and III disease, weekly hCG levels are recommended until normal for 3 consecutive weeks. Then, hCG levels are monitored monthly until they are normal for 6 to 12 consecutive months. The duration is increased to 24 months for stage IV disease. Effective contraception during the entire interval of hormonal follow-up is essential.
  2. Other studies that demonstrated disease at the start of therapy should be repeated monthly until complete remission is documented.

VII. SPECIAL CLINICAL PROBLEMS

A. Thyrotoxicosis and even "thyroid storm" may result from the thyroid-stimulating hormone–like effect of high concentrations of hCG. Clinical evidence of hyperthyroidism in choriocarcinoma occurs in the presence of widespread metastases and is associated with a poor prognosis. Laboratory confirmation requires a serum thyroxine concentration and tri-iodothyronine–resin uptake levels compatible with hyperthyroidism. If the symptoms are mild, propylthiouracil or methimazole can be used. In severe cases, patients must be given propranolol and Lugol solution.

B. Development of choriocarcinoma can occur long after the last pregnancy or even hysterectomy. This development serves to emphasize that histologic diagnosis is necessary in metastatic cancer when the primary tumor is not evident. The diagnosis of choriocarcinoma can lead to lifesaving therapy as it is very responsive to treatment.

C. Subsequent pregnancies. Patients should be reassured that they can anticipate normal subsequent pregnancy outcomes. They are, however, at increased risk for repeat molar pregnancy. This risk is 1% after one molar pregnancy and 20% after two molar pregnancies.

ACKNOWLEDGMENT

The authors would like to acknowledge Dr. Jonathan S. Berek, who significantly contributed to earlier versions of this chapter.

Suggested Readings

Berek JS. *Berek & Novak's Gynecology.* 14th ed. Philadelphia, PA: Lippincott Williams & Wilkins, 2007.

Berek JS, Hacker NF, eds. *Practical Gynecologic Oncology.* 4th ed. Philadelphia, PA: Lippincott Williams & Wilkins, 2005.

Mutch DG, Prat J. 2014 FIGO staging for ovarian, fallopian tube and peritoneal cancer. *Gynecol Oncol* 2014;133:401–404.

Pecorelli S. Revised FIGO staging for carcinoma of the vulva, cervix, and endometrium. *Int J Gynaecol Obstet* 2009;105:103–104.

Cancer of the Uterine Cervix

Joura EA, et al. A 9-valent HPV vaccine against infection and intraepithelial neoplasia in women. *N Engl J Med* 2015;372:711.

Peters WA, et al. Concurrent chemotherapy and pelvic radiation therapy compared with pelvic radiation therapy alone as adjuvant therapy after radical surgery in high-risk early-stage cancer of the cervix. *J Clin Oncol* 2000;18:1606.

Rose PG, et al. Concurrent cisplatin-based radiotherapy and chemotherapy for locally advanced cervical cancer. *N Engl J Med* 1999;340:1144.

Sedlis A, et al. A randomized trial of pelvic radiation therapy versus no further therapy in selected patients with stage IB carcinoma of the cervix after radical hysterectomy and pelvic lymphadenectomy: a Gynecologic Oncology Group study. *Gynecol Oncol* 1999;73:177.

Tewari KS, et al. Improved survival with bevacizumab in advanced cervical cancer. *N Engl J Med* 2014;370:734.

Cancer of the Uterine Body

Cantrell LA, et al. Uterine carcinosarcoma: a review of the literature. *Gynecol Oncol* 2015;137:581.

Creasman WT, et al. Carcinoma of the corpus uteri. *Int J Gynaecol Obstet* 2003;83(suppl 1):79.

Hensley ML, et al. Fixed-dose rate gemcitabine plus docetaxel as first-line therapy for metastatic uterine leiomyosarcoma: a Gynecologic Oncology Group phase II trial. *Gynecol Oncol* 2008;109:329.

Keys HM, et al. A phase III trial of surgery with or without adjunctive external pelvic radiation therapy in intermediate risk endometrial adenocarcinoma: a Gynecologic Oncology Group Study. *Gynecol Oncol* 2004;92:744.

Randall ME, et al. Randomized phase III trial of whole-abdominal irradiation versus doxorubicin and cisplatin chemotherapy in advanced endometrial carcinoma: a Gynecologic Oncology Group study. *J Clin Oncol* 2006;24:36.

Vaginal Cancer

Iavazzo C, et al. Imiquimod for treatment of vulvar and vaginal intraepithelial neoplasia. *Int J Gynaecol Obstet* 2008;101:3.

Stock RG, et al. A 30-year experience in the management of primary carcinoma of the vagina: analysis of prognostic factors and treatment modalities. *Gynecol Oncol* 1995;56:45.

Vulvar Cancer

Berek JS, et al. Concurrent cisplatin and 5-fluorouracil chemotherapy and radiation therapy for advanced-stage squamous carcinoma of the vulva. *Gynecol Oncol* 1991;42:197.

Faul CM, et al. Adjuvant radiation for vulvar carcinoma. Improved local control. *Int J Radiat Oncol Biol Phys* 1997;38:381.

Rhodes CA, et al. The management of squamous cell vulvar cancer: a population-based retrospective study of 411 cases. *Brit J Obstet Gynaecol* 1998;105:200.

Ovarian Cancer

Armstrong DK, et al. Intraperitoneal cisplatin and paclitaxel in ovarian cancer. *N Engl J Med* 2006;354:34.

Coleman RL, et al. Latest research and clinical treatment of advanced-stage epithelial ovarian cancer. *Nat Rev Clin Oncol* 2013;10:211.

Homesley HD, et al. Bleomycin, etoposide, and cisplatin combination therapy of ovarian granulosa cell tumors and other stromal malignancies: a Gynecologic Oncology Group study. *Gynecol Oncol* 1999;72:131.

Katsumata N, et al. Dose-dense paclitaxel once a week in combination with carboplatin every 3 weeks for advanced ovarian cancer: a phase 3, open-label, randomized controlled trial. *Lancet* 2009;374:1331.

Ledermann J, et al. Olaparib maintenance therapy in platinum-sensitive relapsed ovarian cancer. *N Engl J Med* 2012;366:1382.

Memarzadeh S, et al. Advances in the management of epithelial ovarian cancer. *J Reprod Med* 2001;46:621.

Pujade-Lauraine E, et al. Bevacizumab combined with chemotherapy for platinum-resistant recurrent ovarian cancer: the AURELIA open-label randomized phase III trial. *J Clin Oncol* 2014;32:1302.

Vergote I, et al. Neoadjuvant chemotherapy or primary surgery in stage IIIC or IV ovarian cancer. *N Engl J Med* 2010;363:943.

Walker JL, et al. Society of Gynecologic Oncology recommendations for the prevention of ovarian cancer. *Cancer* 2015;121:2108.

Gestational Trophoblastic Neoplasia

Berkowitz RS, et al. Current management of gestational trophoblastic diseases. *Gynecol Oncol* 2009;112:654.

Lurain JR, et al. Gestational trophoblastic disease I: epidemiology, pathology, clinical presentation and diagnosis of gestational trophoblastic disease, and management of hydatidiform mole. *Am J Obstet Gynecol* 2010;203:531.

Lurain JR, et al. Gestational trophoblastic disease II: classification and management of gestational trophoblastic neoplasia. *Am J Obstet Gynecol* 2011;204:11.

13 Testicular Cancer

Lawrence H. Einhorn

I. EPIDEMIOLOGY AND ETIOLOGY

A. Epidemiology

1. **Incidence.** Testicular cancer constitutes only 1% of all cancers in men but is the most common malignancy that develops in men between the ages of 20 and 40 years. About 8,000 new cases are diagnosed annually in the United States.

2. **Racial predilection.** The incidence of testicular cancer in Blacks is one-sixth that in Whites. Asians also have a lower incidence than do Whites.

3. Bilateral cancer of the testis occurs in about 2% of cases.

B. Etiology

1. **Cryptorchidism.** Male patients with cryptorchidism are 10 to 40 times more likely to develop testicular carcinoma than are those with normally descended testes. The risk for developing cancer in a testis is 1 in 80 if retained in the inguinal canal and 1 in 20 if retained in the abdomen. Surgical placement of an undescended testis into the scrotum before 6 years of age reduces the risk for cancer. However, 25% of cancers in patients with cryptorchidism occur in the normal, descended testis.

2. **Testicular feminization syndromes** increase the risk for cancer in the retained gonad by 40-fold. Tumors in these patients are often bilateral.

3. **Other risk factors.** The magnitude of other suggested risk factors, such as a history of orchitis, testicular trauma, or irradiation, is not known.

II. PATHOLOGY AND NATURAL HISTORY

A. Histology.

1. Nearly all cancers of the testis in members of the younger age groups originate from germ cells (seminoma, embryonal cell, teratoma, and others). Other types, which account for <5% of cases, include rhabdomyosarcoma, lymphoma, and melanoma. Rarely, Sertoli cell tumors, Leydig cell tumors, or other mesodermal tumors develop.

2. In men >60 years of age, 75% of neoplasms are not germinal cancers. Lymphomas are the most common testicular tumors in this age group.

3. Metastatic cancer to the testis is rare and most often associated with small cell lung cancer, melanoma, or leukemia.

B. Histogenesis.
Each type of germinal cancer is thought to be a counterpart of normal embryonic development. Seminoma is the neoplastic counterpart of the spermatocyte. The tissues of the early cleavage stage are the most undifferentiated and pluripotential and give rise to both the embryo and the placenta; the malignant counterpart is embryonal cell carcinoma. Teratomas are the neoplastic counterparts of the developing embryo. Choriocarcinoma is actually a more highly undifferentiated cancer; its aggressive biologic behavior reflects the capacity of its normal counterpart (the placenta) to invade blood vessels.

The histologic similarity between germ cell cancer and normal embryology is illustrated by the following observations:

1. Pure choriocarcinomas usually metastasize only as choriocarcinomas, especially hematogenous. However, patients with pure choriocarcinoma in the orchiectomy specimen can have tumors in retroperitoneum composed of both choriocarcinoma and teratoma.

2. Seminomas usually metastasize as seminomas; those that do not are believed to represent mixed tumors undetected on the original histologic examination.

3. Metastases from embryonal carcinomas may be found to consist of teratoma or choriocarcinoma elements.

4. In metastases from mixed tumors, chemotherapy destroys the rapidly growing, drug-sensitive cell elements. The drug-resistant teratomatous elements persist after chemotherapy and require surgical resection.

C. **Natural history.** The natural history of testis cancer varies with the histologic subtype. Both blood-borne and lymphatic metastases occur. Lymphatic drainage usually occurs in an orderly progression. A right-sided primary will spread lymphatically to the interaortocaval nodes and a left-sided primary to para-aortic retroperitoneal nodes. Previous surgery, such as scrotal contamination with scrotal orchiectomy, disrupts normal lymphatic drainage patterns and can cause inguinal nodal metastases.

1. **Seminoma** (40% to 50% of testicular cancers) occurs in an older age group than do other germ cell neoplasms, most commonly after the age of 30 years. Sixty percent of patients with cryptorchidism who develop testicular cancer have seminoma. Seminomas tend to be large, show little hemorrhage or necrosis on gross inspection, and metastasize in an orderly, sequential manner along draining lymph node chains. About 25% of patients have lymphatic metastases, and 1% to 5% have visceral metastases at the time of diagnosis. Metastases to parenchymal organs (usually lung or bone) can occur late. Seminoma is the type of testicular cancer most likely to produce osseous metastases.

   a. **Spermatocytic seminoma** (4% of seminomas) occurs mostly after the age of 50 years and is the most common germ cell tumor after the age of 70 years. It is more often bilateral (6% compared with 2%) and appears to have a much lower incidence of both lymphatic and parenchymal metastases (even to draining lymph nodes) when compared with typical seminoma. These patients are usually cured with orchiectomy alone.

2. **Pure choriocarcinoma** (<0.5% of testicular cancers) metastasizes rapidly through the bloodstream to the lungs, liver, brain, and other visceral sites. They have very high serum human chorionic gonadotropin (hCG) levels with normal α-fetoprotein (AFP) levels.

3. **Yolk sac tumors** are common cancers in children and have a relatively nonaggressive clinical course. Yolk sac elements in testicular cancer found in adult patients, on the other hand, portend a worse prognosis compared with that of children. Pure yolk sac tumors have elevated AFP and normal hCG.

4. **Embryonal cell carcinoma** can be associated with elevated serum hCG, AFP, both, or neither tumor marker. When patients have clinical stage I testicular cancer with predominantly embryonal cell carcinoma, they are more likely to have occult microscopic disease in the retroperitoneum or elsewhere. Vascular invasion also predicts metastatic spread.

5. **Teratoma** appears pathologically inert as it is associated with cartilage, glandular, and glial tissue. Teratoma of and by itself usually does not have

the capacity to metastasize, but it is often associated with embryonal cell carcinoma, choriocarcinoma, yolk sac tumor, and seminoma in the testis and can metastasize as a template. In that situation, chemotherapy will often completely eliminate the nonteratomatous elements, but the teratoma will remain and require surgical resection for cure. When teratoma remains after chemotherapy, it can and will grow by local extension and can even cause death from teratoma alone. In addition, because teratoma is pluripotential tissue that can differentiate along endodermal, ectodermal, or mesodermal elements, it can undergo malignant transformation. The most common of these is mesodermal differentiation to sarcomatous elements associated with teratoma. Malignant transformation of teratoma does have the potential to metastasize. These elements can sometimes briefly respond to chemotherapy directed at the dominant cell type of malignant transformation.

6. **Rare testicular tumors**
    a. **Sertoli cell and Leydig cell tumors** are not germ cell tumors and are not associated with elevated serum hCG or AFP. They vary in malignant potential, but all can metastasize. Size, necrosis, and mitotic index predict the potential for spread and the need for retroperitoneal lymph node dissection. Leydig cell tumors rarely respond to chemotherapy. Sertoli cell tumors may benefit from platinum combination chemotherapy. These tumors are inhibin positive on immunohistochemical stain.
    b. **Rhabdomyosarcoma** of the testis occurs most often before 20 years of age. Its clinical behavior is similar to that of embryonal carcinoma; metastases to draining lymph nodes and lung are common at the time it first appears. They are usually paratesticular.

III. DIAGNOSIS

A. **Symptoms and signs.** Postorchiectomy, most patients will have an otherwise normal history and physical examination.

1. **Symptoms**
    a. **Mass and pain.** The most common symptom of testicular cancer is a painless enlargement, usually noticed during bathing or after a minor trauma. Painful enlargement of the testis occurs in 30% to 50% of patients and may be the result of bleeding or infarction in the tumor. Acute pain in a patient with a cryptorchid testis suggests the possibility of torsion of a testicular cancer.
    b. **Acute epididymitis.** Nearly 25% of patients with mixed teratoma and embryonal cell tumor present with findings indistinguishable from acute epididymitis. The testicular swelling from tumor may even decrease somewhat after antimicrobial therapy.
    c. **Gynecomastia** due to high levels of serum hCG is rarely a presenting sign.
    d. **Infertility** is the primary symptom in about 3% of patients.
    e. **Back pain** from retroperitoneal node metastases is a presenting feature in 10% of patients.
    f. **Other presenting symptoms.** Thoracic symptoms are rare even when extensive pulmonary metastases are present. When there is extensive replacement of pulmonary parenchyma, patients may develop hemoptysis, chest pain, or dyspnea.

2. **Physical findings**
    a. **Scrotum.** A testicular mass is nearly always present. The testis should be palpated using bimanual technique; the finding of irregularity,

induration, or nodularity is indication for further evaluation, including a testicular ultrasound to look for a hypoechogenic mass.

   b. Lymph nodes. Patients must be carefully examined for lymphadenopathy, particularly in the supraclavicular region. Scrotal contamination, such as following testicular biopsy, vasectomy, or herniorrhaphy, alters the normal lymphatic drainage; as a result, ipsilateral inguinal nodes may become involved. Large retroperitoneal masses may be palpable on abdominal examination.

   c. Breasts. Gynecomastia is associated with tumors that secrete high levels of hCG.

B. Differential diagnosis

   1. Hydroceles are usually benign, but about 10% of testicular cancers are associated with coexisting hydroceles. The finding of a hydrocele in a young man should increase suspicion for an associated neoplasm.

   a. Benign hydroceles extend along the spermatic cord, often cause groin swelling, and can give the penis a foreshortened appearance. Hydroceles can be transilluminated.

   b. If the fluid prevents adequate palpation of the testis, a testicular ultrasound should be performed.

   2. Epididymitis produces acute enlargement of the testis with severe pain, fever, dysuria, and pyuria. The same symptoms may be caused by an underlying testicular cancer.

   a. Persistent pain or swelling after treatment may result from a supervening testicular abscess or a coexisting tumor; testicular ultrasound is indicated.

   b. Recurrent epididymitis with a completely normal testis occasionally occurs. Surgical exploration should not be considered if physical examination between episodes is completely normal and there is no evidence of a tumor on testicular ultrasound. Recurrent epididymitis per se does not necessarily indicate cancer.

   3. Varicoceles are swollen veins in the pampiniform plexus of the spermatic cord. The scrotum feels like it contains a "bag of worms." The veins collapse when the patient is in Trendelenburg position.

   4. Spermatoceles are translucent masses that are located posterior and superior to the testis and feel cystic.

   5. Inguinal hernias generally are not a diagnostic problem.

   6. Other masses include gummatous and tuberculous orchitis, hematoma, and acute swelling from testicular torsion. None of these can be distinguished clinically from cancer, and all require exploratory surgery.

C. Tumor markers are the most crucial and sensitive indicators of testicular cancer. Serum hCG and AFP are the quintessential markers in oncology. One or both of these serum markers are present in more than 90% of patients with metastatic nonseminomatous germ cell cancer of the testis.

   1. hCG is markedly elevated with pure choriocarcinoma and also elevated in embryonal cell carcinoma and may be mildly elevated in patients with pure seminoma. The serum half-life of hCG is 18 to 24 hours. However, this refers to surgical resection for localized disease.

   a. hCG may also be found in patients with a variety of other tumors, including melanoma, large cell lung cancer, breast, ovary, or pancreatic cancer.

   b. Nonmalignant conditions associated with elevated hCG levels may occur with marijuana use or with testicular dysfunction due to cross-reactivity with luteinizing hormone. This may occasionally occur after chemotherapy. A repeat serum hCG level 2 weeks after the administration of 300 mg of depotestosterone intramuscularly will resolve this dilemma.

  c. In testicular cancer, a rising hCG after orchiectomy constitutes proof that the patient has residual cancer and requires further treatment. The absence of hCG, however, does not exclude the presence of active cancer, particularly in previously treated patients.

  2. AFP is produced by yolk sac elements and is most commonly associated with embryonal carcinomas and yolk sac tumors. Elevated levels of AFP are never found in patients with pure seminoma or pure choriocarcinoma. The blood half-life of AFP is 5 days, but may be much longer after successful chemotherapy.

  a. Elevated levels may also be explained by hepatocellular carcinoma, other cancers (occasionally), fetal hepatic production in pregnant women, infancy, and nonmalignant liver diseases (e.g., hepatitis, cirrhosis, necrosis).

  b. Rising levels of AFP after surgery or cytotoxic agent therapy for testicular cancer indicate the presence of residual disease and the need for further therapy.

D. Laboratory evaluation

  1. Routine preoperative studies

  a. Complete blood count, liver function tests, and renal function tests

  b. Chest radiograph, including posteroanterior (PA) and lateral projections

  c. Blood levels of hCG and AFP

  2. Routine postoperative studies are undertaken after the diagnosis of testicular cancer is proved. Studies performed in patients with all cell types include the following:

  a. Chest computed tomography (CT) scan can detect occult posterior mediastinal or pulmonary parenchymal metastases. This is not usually a necessary test if the PA and lateral chest x-rays are abnormal.

  b. Abdominal CT scans assist assessment of retroperitoneal adenopathy.

  c. Positron emission tomography (PET) scan is never indicated in the initial staging. It can be of assistance in deciding the necessity of postchemotherapy surgery, especially in patients with pure seminoma. A PET scan will not be "positive" when a residual mass is teratoma, and it will not detect microscopic disease.

IV. STAGING SYSTEM AND PROGNOSTIC FACTORS

A. Staging system and survival. The system presented is a pathologic staging system.

  1. Ninety-eight to hundred percent of patients presenting with stage I or early stage II will be cured, either with surgery alone or with subsequent cisplatin combination chemotherapy. Modern chemotherapy will cure 80% of patients with stage III disease.

  Stage

  I.   Confined to testis

  II. Metastases to retroperitoneal lymph nodes

  III. Supradiaphragmatic disease (mediastinal or supraclavicular nodes or hematogenous visceral metastases

B. Prognostic factors

  1. Elevated serum levels of AFP or hCG after orchiectomy is prima facie evidence that the patient has residual cancer. However, therapy should not be initiated until there is a rising AFP or hCG.

2. Serum LDH levels correlate fairly well with tumor burden, but should never be used as a sole indication for chemotherapy.

3. Nonseminomatous tumor patients receiving chemotherapy are categorized as having advanced (poor-risk) disease, with a 50% cure rate in the presence of the following:

   a. Very high markers (serum hCG > 50,000 IU/mL, AFP > 10,000 ng/mL) or LDH levels >10 times the upper limits of normal

   b. Nonpulmonary visceral metastases (such as liver, bone, or CNS)

   c. Primary mediastinal nonseminomatous germ cell tumors

4. Intermediate-risk disease comprises hCG 5,000 to 50,000 IU/mL, AFP 1,000 to 10,000 ng/mL, or seminoma with nonpulmonary visceral metastases; all other cases of metastatic disease defined as good risk.

5. Risk stratification made with hCG or AFP level at start of chemotherapy NOT preorchiectomy levels.

V. PREVENTION AND EARLY DETECTION

Cryptorchidism should be surgically corrected before puberty, usually before age 4 years, because the risk for malignancy is substantial. Prophylactic removal of undescended testes should be performed in postpubertal patients; the complication rate is minuscule, the testes are functionless, and prostheses are available to fill the empty scrotum.

The effectiveness of early detection by screening programs has not been tested. Most patients have symptoms or signs of a scrotal mass; few cases are detected by routine history and physical examination.

VI. MANAGEMENT

A. **Transinguinal orchiectomy** is performed to make the diagnosis for all testicular cancers in all stages and is the treatment for stage I disease. A transinguinal approach is essential; the blood supply of the spermatic cord is immediately controlled. Transscrotal orchiectomy has been proved to result in tumor seeding to the scrotum and inguinal nodes. Likewise, transscrotal needle biopsy of a suspected testicular mass is absolutely contraindicated.

B. **Management of seminomas: Stages I and II**

   1. **Surgery.** No further surgery is necessary after orchiectomy.

   2. **RT.** An abdominal CT is performed postoperatively in patients with seminoma. Most patients with clinical stage I seminoma should be managed with surveillance. Other options are RT or one dose of carboplatin. RT is preferred in patients with stage II seminoma with lymph nodes that are <3 cm in diameter.

   3. **Chemotherapy.** Patients with bulky stage II (>3-cm disease) or stage III disease are treated the same as those with nonseminomatous germ cell cancer, and the results are similar (see Section VI.D). Seminoma confers a favorable prognosis because none of these cases, even those with nonpulmonary visceral disease, is classified as poor-risk disease. Results with salvage chemotherapy are better for seminomatous than nonseminomatous patients.

   4. **Surveillance.** The cure rate with orchiectomy alone for clinical stage I seminoma is 80% to 85%. It is 95% if tumor is <4 cm and no rete testis involvement is present. Therefore, surveillance (vide infra) is the preferred option.

C. **Management of nonseminomatous germ cell cancer: Stages I and II**

   1. **Surgery.** Retroperitoneal lymph node dissection (RPLND) is the standard of practice at most centers in the United States for stage II disease when staging evaluation does not reveal distant metastases and when there is no lymph node with a maximal transverse diameter of 3 cm on abdominal CT

and postorchiectomy hCG and AFP are normal. Lymphadenectomy previously interrupted the sympathetic pathways and invariably resulted in sterility from failure of ejaculation, but not impotence. Modern nerve-sparing RPLNDs, however, now routinely preserve fertility and allow antegrade ejaculation. Options for stage I include surveillance, RPLND, or one course of BEP (see Section VI.D.2).

2. **Chemotherapy.** The agents used are discussed in Section VI.D. Indications for chemotherapy include the following:

   a. Rising serum levels of hCG or AFP after primary treatment or elevated levels of hCG or AFP with normal abdominal CT scan.

   b. The presence of bulky retroperitoneal disease (>3 cm in maximal transverse diameter of a node on abdominal CT) requires chemotherapy. If the abdominal CT scan becomes normal, retroperitoneal lymphadenectomy is not necessary. Postchemotherapy retroperitoneal lymph node dissection is usually performed for residual masses >1 cm for nonseminoma.

   c. A phase III study comparing one course of bleomycin and etoposide and cisplatin (BEP; see Section VI.D.1) with RPLND demonstrated superiority for chemotherapy for clinical stage I disease, with a relapse rate of only 1%.

3. **Surveillance is an appropriate strategy for compliant patients with clinical stage I disease** (normal markers, physical examination, and radiographic studies after orchiectomy). It is crucial that both the physician and the patient understand the necessity for close observation. Relapses are usually treated with chemotherapy. Surveillance is even appropriate in high-risk clinical stage I disease (embryonal predominant with vascular invasion).

   If surveillance is chosen, history and physical examinations and serum markers are obtained every 2 months during the 1st year. The same studies are obtained every 6 months during the 2nd year and annually during the 3rd, 4th, and 5th years after orchiectomy. Abdominal CT and PA and lateral chest x-ray are performed every 4 months during the 1st year and then every 6 months during the 2nd year and annually in years 3 to 5.

D. **Management of disseminated disease: Stage III**

1. **Standard chemotherapy** for good-risk patients is either BEP for three courses or EP for four courses. Patients with poor-risk (advanced) disease are treated with four courses of BEP.

2. **BEP** is administered every 3 weeks for three or four cycles. Dosages are as follows:
   Bleomycin: 30 U IV weekly on days 1, 8, and 15
   Etoposide: 100 mg/m^2 IV daily for 5 days
   Cisplatin: 20 mg/m^2 IV daily for 5 days

3. **Resection of residual disease.** After completion of chemotherapy, patients who do not achieve a complete remission are candidates for surgical resection of the residual localized disease in the chest or retroperitoneum. Radiologic findings cannot distinguish benign from malignant processes in these patients.

   a. The presence of elevated levels of tumor markers usually signifies the continued presence of carcinoma and the need for further chemotherapy. The absence of tumor markers signifies that the residual disease in the thorax or retroperitoneum can be necrosis, teratoma, or carcinoma.

   b. Surgical resection of residual disease defines the subsequent treatment strategy in all of these patients and is therapeutic in some.

    (1) If surgical resection of residual disease reveals fibrosis or teratoma, no further treatment is required. Follow-up CT scans are indicated after resection of teratoma, as microscopic teratoma may have been present outside the surgical field.

    (2) If surgical resection reveals carcinoma, usually two more cycles of EP therapy are given.

  4. Salvage chemotherapy. Patients who do not achieve a complete remission with BEP are still curable with salvage chemotherapy. Options include cisplatin plus ifosfamide plus either vinblastine or paclitaxel followed by high-dose chemotherapy with peripheral blood stem cell transplant or four courses of a cisplatin–ifosfamide combination triplet regimen. Occasionally patients may be cured with a nonplatinum salvage regimen such as paclitaxel plus gemcitabine, even after progression following high-dose chemotherapy.

VII. SPECIAL CLINICAL PROBLEMS

  A. Gynecomastia and elevated blood hCG levels are occasionally found in patients with clinically normal testes and no other evidence of cancer. A number of other cancers can also produce hCG. Patients should be evaluated with ultrasonography of the testes and CT of the abdomen and chest. Thereafter, it is best to follow such patients clinically until there is demonstrable cancer or rising hCG levels. Blind or random biopsies in this setting are not likely to reveal a diagnosis, can expose patients to unnecessary morbidity, and are contraindicated.

  B. Extragonadal germ cell neoplasms can occur in any anatomic site through which the normal germ cells migrate in the embryo. Such sites include the pineal gland, anterior mediastinum, and middle retroperitoneal areas. Tumor markers (hCG and AFP) should be measured. Chemotherapy with BEP should be used for nonseminomatous germ cell cancers. Results of treatment are less successful for primary mediastinal nonseminomatous germ cell tumors. Etoposide plus ifosfamide plus cisplatin (VIP) is preferred for such patients as it mitigates postoperative complications due to bleomycin.

  C. Solitary mediastinal or retroperitoneal masses with undifferentiated histology may represent germ cell cancer. Diagnosis by histopathology may be problematic. A reasonable approach would be to treat the patient for disseminated nonseminomatous germ cell cancer.

Suggested Readings

Albany C, Brames MJ, Fausel C, et al. Randomized phase III double blind placebo controlled crossover study evaluating the oral neurokinin-1 antagonist aprepitant in combination with a 5HT3 receptor antagonist and dexamethasone in patients with germ cell tumors receiving 5 day cisplatin combination chemotherapy regimens: a HOG study. *J Clin Oncol* 2012;30:3998.

Albany C, Einhorn LH. Pitfalls in management of germ cell tumor patients with slight "elevation" of AFP. *J Clin Oncol* 2014;32:2114.

Albers P, Siener R, Krege S, et al. Randomized phase III trial comparing RPLND with one course of BEP in the adjuvant treatment of clinical stage I nonseminomatous testicular germ cell tumors. *J Clin Oncol* 2008;26:2966.

Einhorn LH. Curing metastatic testicular cancer. *Proc Nat Acad Sci USA* 2002;99:4592.

Einhorn LH, Williams SD, Abonour R, et al. Prognostic variables and results with salvage chemotherapy with high dose carboplatin plus etoposide and peripheral blood stem cell transplant in patients with germ cell tumors. *NEJM* 2007;357:340.

Gilligan TD, Seidenfeld J, Basch EM, et al. American Society of Clinical Oncology clinical practice guidelines on uses of serum tumor markers in adult males with germ cell tumors. *J Clin Oncol* 2010;20:3388.

Hanna N, Einhorn LH. Testicular cancer: progress and updates. *NEJM* 2014;371:2005.

International Germ Cell Collaborative Group. International germ cell consensus classification: a prognostic factor-based staging system for metastatic germ cell cancers. *J Clin Oncol* 1997;15:594.

Kollmannsberger C, Tandstad T, Bedard PL, et al. Patterns of relapse in patients with clinical stage I testicular cancer managed with active surveillance. *J Clin Oncol* 2015;33:51–57.

Kondagunta GV, Bacik J, Donadio A, et al. Combination of paclitaxel, ifosfamide and cisplatin is an effective second-line therapy for patients with relapsed testicular germ cell tumors. *J Clin Oncol* 2005;23:6549.

Loehrer PJ, Gonin R, Nichols CR, et al. Vinblastine plus ifosfamide plus cisplatin as initial salvage therapy in recurrent germ cell tumors. *J Clin Oncol* 1998;16:2500.

Lorch A Kramar A, Einhorn L, et al. Conventional dose versus high dose chemotherapy as first salvage treatment in metastatic male germ cell tumors: Evidence from a large international database. *J Clin Oncol* 2011;29:2178.

Nichols C, Roth B, Albers P, et al. Active surveillance is the preferred approach to clinical stage I testicular cancer. *J Clin Oncol* 2013;28:3490.

14 Urinary Tract Cancer

Rekha A. Kumbla, Hyung L. Kim, and Robert A. Figlin

RENAL CANCER

I. EPIDEMIOLOGY AND ETIOLOGY

A. Incidence. Renal cell carcinoma (RCC) constitutes approximately 4% of all adult malignancies. The median age at diagnosis is 64. The worldwide incidence is increasing at an annual rate of about 2%, with approximately 61,000 new cases per year in the United States and 14,000 associated deaths. Men are affected twice as often as women. It is the seventh most common malignant condition among men and 12th leading among women. The incidence and mortality rates for blacks are higher than those for whites in the United States. In recent evaluation, a threefold higher incidence of RCC has been attributed to the earlier detection of these tumors, smaller size at diagnosis, and curative surgical resections.

B. Etiology. Approximately 70% of sporadic cases of clear cell RCC (the most common histologic variant) are associated with inactivating mutations of both copies of the *von Hippel–Lindau (VHL)* tumor suppressor gene. This results in overexpression of hypoxia-inducible factor-1 (HIF-1) and vascular endothelial growth factor (VEGF), leading to defective regulation of angiogenesis, which is of major importance in the pathophysiology of RCC.

  1. Factors that increase the risk for RCC include the following:
   a. Smoking
   b. Acquired cystic disease of the kidney
   c. Family history of renal cancer
   d. Hypertension
   e. Occupational exposure (cadmium, asbestos, petroleum by-products)
   f. Obesity
   g. Chronic use of analgesics (containing phenacetin and aspirin)

  2. Hereditary syndromes associated with RCCs include the following:
   a. Von Hippel–Lindau disease (associated with germline mutations of the *VHL* gene on chromosome 3; 35% to 45% of these patients have RCC, usually multiple and bilateral)
   b. Hereditary type 1 papillary RCC: associated with mutations in *MET* protooncogene
   c. Hereditary type 2 papillary RCC: associated with hereditary leiomyomatosis and fumarate hydratase mutations
   d. Birt-Hogg-Dube (BHD) syndrome associated with chromophobe and oncocytic kidney cancers

  3. Unproven factors that may increase the risk for RCC include polycystic kidney disease, diabetes mellitus, and chronic dialysis.

II. PATHOLOGY AND NATURAL HISTORY

A. **Renal cell carcinoma** makes up nearly all renal cancers in adults. They are typically round and have a pseudocapsule of condensed parenchyma and connective tissue. Bilateral tumors occur in 2% of sporadic cases, either synchronous or asynchronous.

   1. The most common histologic types include clear cell (75% to 85%), papillary (10% to 15%), chromophobe (5%), and unclassified RCC (<5%). Sarcomatoid tumors can arise from any cell subtype and are associated with a poor prognosis.

   2. These tumors originate from proximal tubular cells, invade local structures, and frequently extend into the renal vein. Metastasis occurs through the lymphatics and bloodstream. The most common sites of distant metastases are the lungs, liver, bones, and brain, but they may present with metastases to unusual sites, such as the fingertips, eyelids, and nose. A primary renal cancer may be diagnosed based on the characteristic histology of a metastatic deposit.

   3. The natural history of RCC is more unpredictable than that of most solid tumors. The primary tumor has variable growth patterns and may remain localized for many years. Metastatic foci may have long periods of indolent or apparently arrested growth and may be detected many years after removal of the primary tumor.

B. **Transitional cell carcinomas** are uncommon tumors that arise in the renal pelvis and often affect multiple sites of urothelial mucosa, including the renal pelvis, ureters, and urinary bladder, occasionally spreading over the posterior retroperitoneum in a sheet-like fashion, encasing vessels and producing urinary tract obstruction (see "Urinary Bladder Cancer," Section II). These tumors usually are low grade but are being discovered late in the course of the disease. Hematogenous dissemination occurs, particularly to lung and bone.

C. **Rare renal tumors**

   1. **Nephroblastomas** (Wilms tumors) appear as large, bulky masses in children but rarely occur in adults (see Chapter 19, "Wilms Tumor").

   2. **Lymphomas and sarcomas** arising in the kidney have clinical courses similar to their counterparts elsewhere in the abdomen.

   3. **Juxtaglomerular tumors** (reninomas) are rare causes of hypertension and are usually benign.

   4. **Chromophobe carcinomas** (4%) originate from intercalated cells of the collecting system, often associated with an up-regulation of the *KIT* oncogene and favorable prognosis.

   5. **Oncocytomas** (7%) are benign tumors originating from a subtype of collecting ducts.

   6. **Collecting duct RCC** (Bellini tumors, <1%) are aggressive cancers often in younger patients and originating from collecting ducts.

   7. **Medullary cancer** (<1%).

   8. **Translocation RCC** with a chromosomal translocation in TFE3 (microphthalmia transcription factor family) is found in pediatric populations but also younger adults associated with antecedent chemotherapy for malignancies, autoimmune disorders, or bone marrow transplant conditioning.

   9. **Benign renal adenomas.** The existence of benign renal adenoma is controversial because it is not possible to determine malignant or benign biologic behavior only by histology on any lesion <3 cm in diameter.

D. **Metastatic tumors.** The kidney is a frequent metastatic landing site for many malignancies, mainly cancers of the lung, ovary, colon, and breast.

E. Paraneoplastic syndromes commonly occur with renal adenocarcinomas.

1. **Erythrocytosis.** Renal adenocarcinomas are associated with erythrocytosis in 1% to 5% of patients and account for 15% to 20% of cases of inappropriate secretion of erythropoietin. Additionally, VHL inactivation is associated with impaired degradation of hypoxia-induced transcription factors and increased production of EPO, which is independent of oxygen levels in the tissue.

2. **Hypercalcemia,** which occurs in up to 15% of patients, is associated with overproduction of parathyroid hormone–like proteins. Hypercalcemia may also be associated with widespread lytic bony metastases.

3. **Fever** caused by tumor occurs in 10% to 20% of patients. It is often intermittent and associated with night sweats, anorexia, fatigue, and unintentional weight loss.

4. **Abnormal liver function (Stauffer syndrome)** occurs in 15% of patients. Leukopenia, fever, and areas of hepatic necrosis *without* liver metastases are noted. The resulting elevated serum levels of alkaline phosphatase and transaminase are reversed after nephrectomy. The dysfunction may be secondary to tumor-related production of cytokines.

5. **Hypertension** associated with renin production by the tumor occurs in up to 40% of patients and is alleviated by removal of the tumor.

6. **Hyperglobulinemia** can result in elevated erythrocyte sedimentation rate.

7. **Amyloidosis** occurs in 3% to 5% of patients secondary to an inflammatory response to amyloid (AA) fibrils.

8. **Thrombocytosis** is rare but associated with poor prognosis.

III. DIAGNOSIS

A. **Symptoms and signs.** Symptoms other than hematuria usually indicate large, advanced tumors. The classic triad of flank pain, a flank mass, and hematuria occurs in <10% of patients with RCC. The combined picture of anemia, hematuria, and fever is rare, but suggestive of renal cancer. The widespread use of diagnostic tests such as ultrasound, CT, and MRI has changed the typical presentation of RCC. More than three-fourths of all locally confined tumors are found serendipitously, and thus a substantial proportion of patients are symptom free at the time of diagnosis. Therefore, symptoms and signs (as listed below) become rare and currently are more characteristic in cases presenting with advanced disease.

1. **Symptoms**

   a. Gross hematuria is rare and generally only noted when tumor invades the collecting system.

   b. A steady, dull flank pain occurs in a few patients. Colicky pain may develop if blood clots are passed into the ureter.

   c. Weight loss may be a presenting feature in <15% of patients.

   d. Sudden onset of a left-sided or a right-sided varicocele is rare and usually suggests invasion into the renal vein or inferior vena cava, respectively.

   e. Lower extremity edema is the result of locally advanced disease, which causes venous or lymphatic obstruction.

   f. Fever, plethora, or symptoms of hypercalcemia or anemia may be presenting features.

   g. Symptoms related to metastases, including bone pain, fracture, and shortness of breath, may occasionally be a presenting symptom.

2. **Physical findings**

   a. A palpable flank mass is rarely present and usually only detected in thin adults.

b. Fever occurs in about 15% of patients.

c. Pallor from anemia may occur.

B. Diagnostic studies

1. **Urinalysis** may reveal proteinuria and hematuria. All patients with macroscopic or microscopic hematuria of any degree must have a thorough urologic evaluation.

2. **Routine studies**

   a. Complete blood count, liver function tests, and renal function studies.

   b. Hyperglobulinemia may be present in patients with RCC because acute-phase reactant proteins are elevated.

   c. Chest radiographs may reveal multiple, large, round (cannonball-like) metastatic deposits that are characteristic of metastatic genitourinary neoplasms.

3. **CT scanning of the kidneys** is the most cost-effective method for evaluating a suspected renal mass and should be the first study. CT does not detect minimal lymph node involvement.

4. **MRI** may be as accurate as CT. MRI images demonstrate extension of tumor into the renal vein and vena cava more reliably than CT when preparing for surgery.

5. **Ultrasonography** with duplex Doppler may assist in imaging tumor thrombus in the inferior vena cava and in defining its extension. It cannot be used for local staging because regional lymph node involvement cannot be imaged.

6. **Scans for staging** should be performed in the following situations:

   a. Bone scan, if there is bone pain or elevated serum alkaline phosphatase levels

   b. MRI of the brain, if there are signs of central nervous system abnormalities

7. **Percutaneous biopsy of a renal mass** has a controversial role and may be inaccurate in approximately 25% of the cases. It should be restricted to patients with medical conditions that make surgery unduly hazardous and patients with metastatic disease for which a tissue diagnosis is necessary.

C. Renal cysts are usually classified using CT based on the chance of harboring malignancy (Bosniak classification). The following approach is recommended to evaluate potential renal cysts:

1. If a renal cyst is suspected or demonstrated and the findings are not strongly suggestive of cancer, ultrasound is performed to determine whether the lesion is cystic or solid. If a simple cyst or a fatty tumor is demonstrated, no further follow-up is usually indicated. If a hyperechoic lesion is imaged, the patient should have follow-up studies.

2. Rarely, all imaging modalities are nondiagnostic, and surgical exploration is indicated.

3. Bosniak cyst types 3 and 4 are managed in the same fashion as renal cancers.

IV. STAGING SYSTEM AND PROGNOSTIC FACTORS

A. Staging system. Refer to the current AJCC Cancer Staging atlas for TNM staging system.

B. Prognostic factors

1. **Pathologic stage** is the most important prognostic indicator.

   a. Tumor size >10 cm is associated with poor prognosis compared to smaller lesions.

   b. Venous extension. Renal vein or vena caval involvement carries a poor prognosis; however, with proper surgical management, 25% to 50% of patients survive for 5 years.

2. **Histology.** Sarcomatoid and unclassified patterns of RCC have a poor prognosis.

   a. **Nuclear grade** correlates with survival across all tumor stages. A **four-tiered Fuhrman system** is most commonly used; it takes into consideration nuclear size, nuclear shape, and nucleolar appearance.

   b. **Nuclear ploidy** was proposed as a potential prognostic marker for survival. Nondiploid tumors are thought to harbor a less favorable prognosis.

3. **Disease-free interval.** The length of time between nephrectomy and the development of metastases affects the survival of patients with metastatic disease.

   a. Nearly all patients who have metastases at the time of surgery or who develop metastases or local recurrence within 1 year of surgery die within 2 years if untreated.

   b. Patients who develop metastases >2 years after nephrectomy have a 20% 5-year survival rate from the time metastases are recognized.

4. **Integrated prognostic systems.**

   a. Factors other than stage contribute to overall survival (OS). In patients with metastatic (stage IV) disease, using the Memorial Sloan Kettering Cancer Center (MSKCC) criteria first published in 1999, certain findings correlate with shorter survival times. Criteria: (1) high blood lactate dehydrogenase (LDH) level, (2) high blood calcium level, (3) anemia (low red blood cell count), (4) cancer spread to 2 or more distant sites, (5) less than a year from diagnosis to the need for systemic treatment (targeted therapy or chemotherapy), and (6) poor performance status. Patients with none of the above factors are considered to have a good prognosis; one or two factors are considered intermediate prognosis, and three or more of these factors are considered poor prognosis.

V. PREVENTION AND EARLY DETECTION

The incidence of renal cancer might be reduced if tobacco-smoking habits could be controlled. Early detection depends on prompt attention to hematuria and other symptoms suggestive of these cancers.

VI. MANAGEMENT

A. **Early disease**

1. **Surgery**

   a. **Radical nephrectomy** classically involves removal of all structures contained within Gerota fascia, including the kidney, adrenal gland, and superior ureter. Radical nephrectomy is generally used for large, locally advanced tumors. The adrenal gland can be safely spared when the tumor is in the lower pole or when a smaller tumor is clearly separate from the adrenal gland. A laparoscopic approach is generally preferred; however, an open approach may be necessary for tumors that involve adjacent structures such as the inferior vena cava.

   b. **Nephron-sparing surgery** (NSS, partial nephrectomy) is the treatment of choice when it is technically feasible. Maximal preservation of renal function is an important goal of surgery. Most tumors that are <4 cm in diameter are amenable to NSS. A minimally invasive approach using laparoscopy or robotics results in more rapid postoperative recovery when compared to an open approach. Although surgical resection is considered the standard of care, ablative procedures using cryotherapy or radiofrequency ablation can be considered for the smallest and most exophytic tumors.

   c. **Occlusion of the renal artery** using angiographic techniques has been advocated for locally advanced tumors associated with increased vasculature. Occlusion procedures may limit blood loss and make the operation technically easier. It may also provide palliation for symptomatic patients who are not candidates for surgery. However, renal artery occlusion will cause temporary pain, fever, and nausea.

d. **Contraindications to surgery** include high surgical risk because of unrelated medical diseases. Since the emergence of targeted therapies, the role of surgery ("adjunctive nephrectomy") in the presence of distant metastases is once again under investigation.

2. **Observation** is now recognized as an acceptable option for small renal tumors (e.g., tumor <4 cm) in patients who are poor surgical candidates or have a limited life expectancy. Many of these small tumors are benign; however, even if they are malignant, most small tumors are indolent and progress slowly.

3. **RT and chemotherapy** have no established role in the management of early renal cancers.

B. **Advanced disease**

1. **Surgery**

a. **Nephrectomy.** For patients treated with cytokine therapy, cytoreductive nephrectomy has been shown to extend survival. However, immunotherapy with IL-2 or interferon (INF) has been largely replaced by a growing number of targeted therapies. Therefore, ongoing clinical trials are revisiting the role of cytoreductive nephrectomy in patients treated with targeted therapies. Until these trials are completed, cytoreductive nephrectomy remains a well-accepted adjuvant to systemic therapy for patients with good performance status.

b. **Resection of metastases.** In select patients, metastatic lesions can be surgically resected for curative intent. Metastectomy is most likely to be curative in patients with a single metastatic lesion and in patients with a solitary recurrence identified more than 2 years after the definitive nephrectomy.

2. **RT** is used to palliate symptoms from metastases to the central nervous system and bone. Gamma knife radiotherapy is effective for control of brain metastasis.

3. **Pharmacotherapy (See Table 14-1)**

a. **Targeted Agents**

(1) **Vascular endothelial growth factor (VEGF)-directed therapies:**

(a) **Sunitinib** is one of the VEGF TKIs compared with interferon alpha (INFα) in the first-line setting of good to intermediate prognosis renal clear cell carcinomas. The treatment with sunitinib was notable for an improvement in objective response rate (ORR), progression-free survival (PFS), and OS. Initial trial dosing included sunitinib 50 mg orally daily for 4 weeks followed by 2 weeks off. Subsequent phase II trials have shown similar efficacy with 2 weeks on/1 week off with improvement on toxicity profile and less dosage adjustments.

(b) **Sorafenib** at the dose of 400 mg twice a day has been compared to placebo after cytokine failure and noted for improvement in PFS but with low ORR and no OS benefit.

(c) **Bevacizumab** at the dose of 10 mg/kg every 2 weeks in combination with INFα. The treatment resulted in the improvement on OS when compared to placebo; however, other newer effective therapies have made this approach less popular.

(d) **Pazopanib** at 800 mg daily orally has been compared to placebo and to sunitinib. The treatment led to improvement in PFS when compared to placebo, but no improvement in PFS and OS when

TABLE 14-1	Algorithm of Therapy in Renal Cell Carcinoma	
First-line treatment		
Risk group	**Standard**	**Options**
Good/intermediate	Sunitinib	High-dose IL-2
	Pazopanib	Bevacizumab + low-dose IFN alpha
Poor	Temsirolimus	Sunitinib
Second-line treatment		
Prior treatment	**Standard**	**Options**
TKI	Axitinib	Cabozantinib
	Everolimus	Sorafenib
		Nivolumab
Third-line treatment		
Prior treatment	**Standard**	**Options**
TKI (at least 2 lines)	Nivolumab	Levatanib + Everolimus
	Cabozantinib	Sorafenib

compared to sunitinib. However, the treatment with pazopanib resulted in fewer adverse events and improved quality of life.

- (e) **Axitinib** is administered at 5 mg orally twice daily and then increased stepwise to 7 mg followed by 10 mg twice daily as tolerated. The treatment resulted in an improved PFS when compared to sorafenib in the first- and second-line setting.
- (f) **Cabozantinib** at 60 mg orally daily has been compared to everolimus in the second-line setting after prior TKI therapy. Median PFS was significantly improved.

(2) **Inhibitors of the mammalian target of rapamycin (mTOR)**
- (a) **Everolimus** at the starting dose of 10 mg orally daily has been compared with sunitinib and showed worsened PFS. Also, when compared with nivolumab and cabozantanib, it was less effective. It is not recommended in the first-line setting.
- (b) **Temsirolimus** at the dose of 25 mg intravenously weekly improved median OS when compared with INFα in treatment-naïve patients with poor-risk disease. Uniquely, eligibility was not limited to those patients with clear cell RCC, and patients with treated brain metastases were allowed to enroll.

(3) **Side effects.** More extensive experience with VEGF-directed therapies and mTOR inhibitors have suggested class effects associated with these agents. VEGF-directed therapies appear to cause hypertension, proteinuria, hand–foot syndrome, impaired wound healing, and myelosuppression. In contrast, mTOR inhibitors have been associated with impaired metabolic profiles (i.e., hyperglycemia, hypertriglyceridemia, etc.), mucositis, and rash.

b. **Immunotherapy.** The role of immunotherapy for kidney cancer has increased once again with the exploration of monoclonal antibodies against the programmed cell death 1 protein PD-1. IL-2 still remains a therapeutic option in selected patients with favorable prognosis.

(1) **IL-2** administered alone in high-dose regimens produces a response rate of 15% to 20% in good-risk patients and durable remissions lasting for more than a decade in 10% of patients. Significant morbidity and 4% mortality associated with high-dose IL-2 make this therapy very difficult and applicable to only small minority of patients.

(2) **Nivolumab**, a human monoclonal antibody blocking programmed death 1 receptor (PD-1). PD-1 is expressed on T cells and interaction with its PD ligands (PD-L) expressed on immune cells and cancer cells blocks immune response. Nivolumab was compared to everolimus after one or two prior antiangiogenic therapies. The trial was stopped early because it showed a significant improvement in the OS (25 vs. 19.6 months for nivolumab versus everolimus, respectively). Nivolumab is dosed 3 mg/kg intravenously every 2 weeks until disease progression or unacceptable toxicity. Common toxicities with nivolumab are generally immune mediated and include colitis, diabetes mellitus, hypophysitis, pneumonitis, adrenal insufficiency and rash. (See Chapter 5)

(3) **IFN-α** as a single agent has modest antitumor activity in the setting of RCC, with a response rate of approximately 15%. With the emergence of effective targeted therapies, IFN-α is used rarely.

URINARY BLADDER CANCER

I. EPIDEMIOLOGY AND ETIOLOGY

A. Bladder cancers constitute 4.5% of all cancers in the United States and is the sixth most common cancer in the United States. The disease is 3 times more frequent in men than in women. The average age of onset is the sixth to seventh decade. The incidence doubles in men >75 years of age versus younger men. White males have almost twice the risk of bladder cancer than African American and Hispanic men.

B. **Risk factors and carcinogens**

1. **Occupational exposure** is associated with 20% of cases. Historically, aniline dye workers were afflicted 30 times more than the general population. Aromatic amines and related compounds are the most abundant bladder carcinogens. These are chemical intermediates of anilines, rather than the aniline dyes themselves. Leather, paint, and rubber industry workers also appear to have an increased risk for bladder cancer. Proven chemical carcinogens in these industries are 2-naphthylamine, benzidine, 4-aminobiphenyl, and 4-nitrobiphenyl.

2. *Schistosomum haematobium* infection of the bladder is associated with bladder cancer, particularly with squamous cell histology, in endemic regions of Africa and the Middle East.

3. **Smoking** increases the risk for bladder cancer fourfold in a dose-dependent fashion. Heavy smokers are more likely to have a high-grade tumor and muscle invasive disease compared to nonsmokers. Of men who die of bladder cancer, 85% have a history of smoking.

4. **Pelvic irradiation** for other cancers such as cervical, ovarian, prostate and testicular increases the risk for bladder cancer fourfold.

5. **Drugs.** Cyclophosphamide unequivocally increases the risk for bladder cancer. Other drugs that have been implicated in animal studies but not proved in humans are phenacetin, sodium saccharin, and sodium cyclamate.

II. PATHOLOGY AND NATURAL HISTORY

A. **Pathology**

1. **Histology.** Of bladder cancers, 90% are transitional cell carcinoma (TCC), and 8% are squamous cell types. Adenocarcinomas, sarcomas, lymphomas, and carcinoid tumors are rare.

2. **Sites of involvement.** The majority of TCCs are linked to carcinogen exposures such as smoking. Carcinogens in urine are believed to produce a field change in the urothelium that predisposes to formation of bladder cancer. Therefore, TCC can develop in any part of the urinary collecting system including the kidney and ureter; however, the bladder is the most common site for TCC because it functions to store urine and has the greatest contact time with urinary carcinogens.

3. **Types of bladder cancer**
   a. Single papillary cancers are the most common type (70%) and the least likely to show invasion.
   b. Diffuse papillary growths with minimal invasion
   c. Sessile cancers are often high grade and invasive.
   d. Carcinoma *in situ* (CIS; flat intraepithelial growth) appears either the same as normal mucosa or as a velvety red patch.

4. **The panurothelial abnormality or field defect.** Bladder cancer appears to be associated with premalignant changes throughout the urothelial mucosa. This concept is suggested by the following observations:
   a. Up to 80% of patients treated for superficial tumors develop recurrences at different sites in the bladder.
   b. Multiple primary sites are present in 25% of all patients with bladder cancer.
   c. Random biopsies of apparently normal areas of mucosa in patients with bladder cancer frequently show CIS.
   d. Depending on the reported series, patients with bladder CIS also have ureteral CIS (10% to 60%) and urethral CIS (30%).
   e. About 40% of patients presenting with carcinoma of the renal pelvis or ureter develop tumors elsewhere in the urinary tract, usually in the bladder.

B. **Natural history**
   1. **CIS of the bladder** is multifocal and can affect the entire urothelium. CIS is a high-grade malignancy. Up to 80% of patients with untreated CIS develop invasive bladder cancer within 10 years after diagnosis; the disease is lethal for most of these patients.
   2. **Low-grade superficial carcinomas** have a better prognosis than CIS. Although the recurrence rate is 80%, low-grade, superficial carcinomas do not metastasize. However, 10% of superficial carcinomas may progress to high-grade, invasive tumors with potential for metastasis. More than 80% of patients with both superficial cancers and CIS progress to invasive disease.
   3. **High-grade or invasive tumors** are associated with adjacent areas of CIS in 85% of cases. These tumors often invade into muscle and perivesical fat. Squamous cell cancers and adenocarcinomas are usually high grade and have an aggressive clinical behavior. Other uncommon and very aggressive histologic variants include sarcomatoid cancer, small cell carcinoma, and micropapillary tumors.
   4. **Mode of spread.** Bladder cancers spread both by lymphatic channels and by the bloodstream. High-grade lesions are more likely to metastasize. Of patients with distant metastases, 30% do not have involvement of the draining lymph nodes. Distant sites of metastases include bone, liver, lung, and, less commonly, skin and other organs. Uremia from ureteral compression by a large pelvic mass, inanition from advancing cancer, and liver failure are the usual causes of death.
   5. **Iatrogenic tumor implantation.** High-grade bladder cancer cells exfoliated by cystoscopy, brushing, transurethral biopsy, or resection were reported to

seed other areas of the bladder. Mucosal sites damaged by inflammation or instrumentation appear to be most receptive to such implants.

6. **Associated paraneoplastic syndromes:** systemic fibrinolysis, hypercalcemia, neuromuscular syndromes, leukemoid reaction.

III. DIAGNOSIS

A. Symptoms and signs

1. **Symptoms**
   a. Hematuria (gross or microscopic) occurs as a presenting feature in 90% of patients.
   b. Bladder irritability occurs in 25% of patients. Hesitancy, urgency, frequency, dysuria, and postvoiding pelvic discomfort may mimic prostatitis or cystitis. These symptoms occur in patients with CIS as well as in those with tumors that are large, extensive, or near the bladder neck.
   c. Pain in the pelvis or flank is associated with locally advanced disease.
   d. Edema of the lower extremities and genitalia develops from venous or lymphatic obstruction.

2. **Physical findings.** The patient is carefully examined for metastatic sites. It is mandatory that a bimanual examination is performed by the urologist through the rectum each time the patient is put under general anesthesia or having a cystoscopy done. The importance of the bimanual examination cannot be overemphasized. It supplies pertinent information concerning local extension of the disease not obtainable by current imaging modalities.

B. Diagnostic studies

1. **Routine studies**
   a. CBC, LFT, and renal function tests
   b. Urinalysis
   c. Chest radiograph

2. **Cystoscopy** is the cornerstone procedure for diagnosing bladder cancer. Biopsy is performed of abnormal areas. Random biopsies of normal areas are often performed to search for CIS. Cystoscopy is followed by bimanual pelvic examination under anesthesia in both men and women. Cystoscopy is indicated for patients with the following clinical features:
   a. Any gross or microscopic hematuria and a normal upper urinary tract imaging. Cystoscopy can be omitted in patients <35 years of age without risk factors for bladder cancer.
   b. Unexplained or chronic lower urinary tract symptoms.
   c. Urine cytology that is suspicious for cancer.
   d. A history of bladder cancer.

3. **Urography.** An intravenous pyelogram (IVP) is useful for imaging the upper urinary tract in patients with unexplained hematuria, or cystoscopic or cytologic evidence of tumor in an attempt to search for primary sites in the ureters or renal pelvis. It is advisable to perform an IVP before cystoscopy, because if a poorly visualized upper system or inconclusive filling defect is imaged, retrograde pyelography may be performed using a ureteral catheter inserted during the same cystoscopy session.

4. **CT urography (CTU).** CT scanning of the abdomen and pelvis typically includes three phases: a noncontrast phase, an early postcontrast phase, and the pyelographic phase. During the noncontrast phase, abnormal calcifications (i.e., urinary stones) can be identified. The early postcontrast phase obtained minutes after IV administration of contrast serves to discern renal lesions and to differentiate between abnormal lymph nodes and normal

anatomic structures. During the pyelographic phase, the contrast material is observed as it is excreted into the collecting system, allowing the identification of abnormal filling defects within the collecting system. Owing to its higher resolution and diagnostic accuracy, CTU has largely supplanted IVP as the imaging modality of choice for the upper urinary tract.

It is important to obtain a CTU in any patient with hematuria, a history of bladder cancer, or positive cytology. CTU is also useful for staging invasive bladder cancer or upper tract TCC to evaluate abnormally enlarged lymph nodes, visceral metastasis, or tumor infiltration into the perivesical fat. CT is not reliable for the detection of local invasion, however.

5. **Urine cytology** detects about 70% of bladder cancers that are subsequently diagnosed by cystoscopy. Cytologic evaluation should not be the primary diagnostic method for patients suspected of having bladder cancer as it has poor sensitivity. False positive results are rare; thus, any positive cytology should be worked up thoroughly for malignancy. Urine cytology is useful for the following purposes:
   a. Following patients with a history of bladder cancer
   b. Screening symptom-free patients who are exposed to environmental carcinogens
   c. Evaluating patients with chronic irritative bladder symptoms before cystoscopy is done

6. **Fluorescent *in situ* hybridization (FISH).** Because bladder cancers are associated with typical chromosomal aberrations, their detection in the urine is an accurate and noninvasive modality of TCC detection. The current commercially available FISH test uses four chromosomal probes to detect an abnormal number of chromosomal copies (CEP17, CEP3, and CEP7) and a single locus–specific indicator probe (9p21). FISH has a sensitivity of 81% and a specificity of 96%, far better than those of cytology. FISH has been reported to detect higher rates of CIS and high-grade tumors.

7. **Scans.** Bone scans should be performed in patients with bone pain or elevated serum alkaline phosphatase or transaminase levels.

IV. STAGING SYSTEM AND PROGNOSTIC FACTORS

A. **Staging system.** Refer to the current AJCC Cancer Staging atlas for TNM staging.

B. **Prognostic factors.** The most important clinical prognostic factors are tumor stage, tumor grade, and the presence of CIS. Untreated advanced stage patients have a 2-year survival rate <15% and a median survival of 16 months.

1. **Histology.** Squamous cancers and adenocarcinomas have poorer prognoses than TCC. Likewise, the other aggressive histologic subvariants confer a poor prognosis.

2. **Invasion** of muscle, lymphatics, or perivesical fat is associated with a poor prognosis. Invasive cancer is associated with a 50% mortality rate in the first 18 months after diagnosis. Delaying cystectomy >12 weeks following the diagnosis of muscle invasive disease (stage T2) may hamper patient survival.

3. **CIS** progresses to invasive carcinoma in 80% of patients within 10 years of diagnosis.

4. **Tumor grade**
   a. A close relationship exists between tumor grade and stage. Tumor grade alone affects survival in patients with superficial tumors. The 5-year survival rate is 85% with low-grade lesions and 30% with high-grade lesions. Virtually all high-grade superficial tumors become invasive if left untreated.

  b. Chromosome number correlates with tumor grade. Tetraploid and aneuploid cells, as opposed to diploid cells, are associated with invasive tumors.

  c. Several phenotypic properties that have been offered as markers for biologically more aggressive disease include enhanced expression of the Lewis x antigen; expression of defective p53, together with overexpression of the *Rb* gene and abnormal epidermal growth factor receptor; reduced expression of transforming growth factors b1, p27, and p15.

5. Size of the primary tumor does not correlate with the risk for dissemination. Large superficial lesions, however, are more likely to recur after therapy than are small lesions.

6. Multifocality is associated with an increased recurrence risk as compared with cases that have a solitary tumor.

V. PREVENTION AND EARLY DETECTION

A. Prevention. Protecting factory workers in certain industries from continuous exposure to bladder carcinogens (e.g., with protective clothing) may be beneficial. The benefit gained by reducing the intake of coffee or artificial sweetener has not been determined. All people should be discouraged from smoking. Folate-enriched diet has been associated with a decreased risk for bladder cancer.

B. Early detection depends on prompt evaluation of all patients with hematuria or chronic irritative bladder symptoms.

VI. MANAGEMENT

A. Early disease: overview

1. **Superficial low-grade tumors** not associated with CIS are managed by transurethral resection and, when indicated, intravesical chemotherapy. Although the recurrence rate is 80% with this management, the prognosis is good. Fulguration is effective treatment for small lesions.

2. **CIS** is usually multifocal, persistent, and recurrent. By definition, CIS is may evolve into invasive carcinoma. CIS is a superficial malignancy and cystoscopic resection or fulguration is effective treatment; however, CIS is usually flat and may not be visible by cystoscopy. Therefore, patients diagnosed with CIS should undergo additional treatment with intravesical bacillus Calmette-Guerin (BCG). Given the high risk of recurrence and progression, patients with CIS need to be followed closely with repeat cystoscopy every 3 months with routine cytology. CIS that recurs rapidly after BCG treatment should be managed with a cystectomy.

3. **Invasive tumors** that grow into the muscularis propria (>T2) are best treated by anterior pelvic exenteration in women and radical cystoprostatectomy in men. Pelvic lymph node dissection is performed to stage the nodes, and some advocate an extended node dissection to enhance the likelihood of a curative resection. Segmental resections of the bladder may be used in highly selected cases (see Section VI.B.2). Radiotherapy and chemotherapy may be appropriate in some cases (see Sections VI.C and VI.D).

B. Early disease: surgery

1. **Transurethral resection of bladder tumor (TURBT)** is the cornerstone for diagnosing and staging bladder cancer. Differentiating between superficial and muscle-invasive bladder is critical. One or more TURBT procedures and follow-up cystoscopy constitute sufficient treatment for most superficial tumors. Muscle invasive disease requires radical cystectomy; however, small solitary tumors that involve the bladder muscle may be treated with TURBT alone in patients who are poor candidates for radical surgery.

2. **Segmental resection** (partial cystectomy) is associated with a high risk for recurrence. Segmental resection can be considered for tumors with the following characteristics:
   a. Solitary
   b. Localized to the bladder dome
   c. CIS ruled out with multiple random biopsies
   d. Able to be removed with a 2-cm margin of healthy tissue
   e. Patients with adenocarcinomas are best suited for partial cystectomy since they are less likely to be due to a field change defect and therefore the tumors are less likely to be multifocal or recur.
3. **Intravesical instillations.** Because the bladder is a storage organ with no absorptive capacity, cytotoxic agents can be safely instilled into the bladder with virtually no systemic effects. Chemotherapy or immunotherapy has been used for the treatment and prevention of recurrence of superficial TCC. These agents have no role in the treatment of invasive bladder cancer. Chemotherapeutic agents include thiotepa, mitomycin C, valrubicin, and doxorubicin. Immunotherapy consists of BCG with or without IFN-α. Intravesical therapy should be administered for T1 disease, CIS, and for Ta disease that is multifocal or rapidly recurring.
   a. BCG is used only as prophylactic or adjuvant therapy. It is administered weekly for 6 weeks followed by maintenance administration of shorter courses. Maintenance BCG has been shown to augment the effects of a single 6-weekly course. BCG instillations are considered more effective in reducing the risks for recurrence and progression, as compared with chemotherapy. Therefore BCG is the treatment of choice for patients who have never received intravesical therapy. BCG is also curative for most patients with CIS. However, there is no proof that any intravesical therapy can alter long-term disease-specific survival.
   b. Mitomycin C is also given weekly at a dose of 40 mg each time. A single instillation of mitomycin C immediately following TURBT has been shown to dramatically decrease the risk of tumor recurrence, most likely owing to the prevention of cancer cell seeding. No proof exists that maintenance intravesical chemotherapy has any benefit.
   c. Both chemotherapy and BCG are frequently associated with local side effects, such as bladder irritability, and both can rarely induce systemic adverse reactions. Of particular importance, systemic infection with BCG affects 5% of the cases and may lead to significant morbidity.
4. **Radical cystectomy,** the standard treatment for invasive bladder cancer, includes excision of the bladder, perivesical fat, and attached peritoneum. Men undergo removal of the entire prostate and seminal vesicles; women undergo *en bloc* removal of the uterus, adnexa, and cuff of the vagina. Lymphadenectomy is controversial; it may improve survival and therefore, some surgeons advocate an extended node dissection that extends from the pelvis up to the inferior mesenteric artery. There is little doubt that lymphadenectomy provides useful staging information and a classic pelvic node dissection represents the minimal extent of the lymphadenectomy.
   a. **Urinary diversion procedures.** The ureters are diverted into either a loop of ileum that functions as a conduit to an abdominal stoma (ileal conduit) or a reservoir constructed from intestine. Generally, reservoirs are created by detubularizing and sewing a segment of small or large bowel into a new reservoir.

If a continent diversion is performed, the reservoir may be implanted orthotopically as a neobladder draining through the urethra using the native sphincter mechanism or attached to a catheterizable, continent stoma, which patients drain via intermittent self-catheterization. Alternative urinary drainage procedures, such as cutaneous implantation of the ureters and ureterosigmoidostomy, were largely abandoned because of a high rate of severe complications.

b. Indications for radical cystectomy
(1) Muscle invasive tumors
(2) CIS not responsive to intravesical therapy
(3) Superficial low-grade tumors that are diffuse, multiple, and frequently recurring and becoming difficult to control with recurrent TURBT and intravesical therapy
(4) High-grade tumors not responsive to intravesical therapy

c. Complications of cystectomy
(1) Mortality rate of 1% to 3%.
(2) Blood loss.
(3) Rectal injury, ureterocutaneous fistulas, wound dehiscence or infection; small bowel obstructions or fistulas. Small bowel fistulas are associated with a substantial mortality rate.
(4) Thrombophlebitis, pulmonary embolism, and other cardiocirculatory complications.
(5) Impotence in men; potency can be preserved in some men by sparing the corporal nerves.

d. Complications of urinary diversion
(1) Urinary tract infection.
(2) Obstruction owing to stenosis (fibrosis or tumor growth).
(3) Urinary calculi occasionally occur. Calcium stones are the most common.
(4) Acid–base imbalance: Hyperchloremic metabolic acidosis is the most common and results from the rapid reabsorption of ammonium followed by chloride from the urine by the intestine used for the urinary diversion. The type of diversion (reservoir vs. conduit) and the specific type of bowel segment used determine the type, extent, and gravity of the accompanied electrolyte impairment. The most severe metabolic derangements occur following diversions using sigmoid colon or jejunum.

C. Early disease: RT does not appear to alter the course of CIS favorably.
1. Indications for RT
a. RT is an alternative to surgery for highly motivated patients who desire to retain their bladder and potency using a bladder preservation protocol. These multiple modality treatment plans include aggressive TURBT, RT, and chemotherapy and are conducted in only a few dedicated institutions because such protocols mandate frequent follow-up visits and close coordination of multiple subspecialties. Following an attempt at bladder sparing, a salvage cystectomy is required in up to 20% of cases.
b. Preoperative RT is seldom used. RT does not appear to improve expected survival beyond that achieved by radical surgery alone, although local recurrence is reduced.
c. Postoperative radiation has no proved role in bladder cancer.

2. Complications of RT are discussed in Chapter 12, "General Aspects," (radiation cystitis) and Chapter 31, (radiation proctitis).

D. **Early disease: chemotherapy**

1. **Adjuvant therapy with systemic cytotoxic agents** for patients undergoing cystectomy has been associated with a delay in time to disease progression (8 to 12 months), but no conclusive evidence indicates improvement of survival. Several regimens have been used in this setting. M-VAC (methotrexate, vinblastine, doxorubicin, cisplatin) or GC (gemcitabine, cisplatin) are recommended. The treatment with neoadjuvant chemotherapy is a preferred approach.

2. **Neoadjuvant therapy** is an attempt to provide the earliest possible treatment of micrometastatic disease and to facilitate definitive local therapy. At present, the preferred neoadjuvant regimen is three cycles of M-VAC (see Section VI.E.3). Neoadjuvant therapy has been shown to improve survival. Other choices for chemotherapy include gemcitabine and cisplatin for patients with significant comorbidities who may not be able to tolerate M-VAC therapy. Retrospective analyses suggest similar pathologic complete responses. However, at present, the highest level of evidence supports the use of M-VAC as neoadjuvant therapy

E. **Advanced disease**

1. **Surgery.** An attempt to fulgurate large tumors that are bleeding uncontrollably or causing severe irritative symptoms is worthwhile.

2. **RT** ameliorates hemorrhage in about half of patients and provides substantial local pain relief in areas of bone involvement. Tumor masses that threaten extension through the skin, particularly in the perineum, should be irradiated early. Bacterial cystitis should be treated effectively before the use of RT, if possible.

3. **Chemotherapy.** Cisplatin-based combination chemotherapy regimens have produced sustained complete responses in up to 45% of patients and represent the best current therapy for advanced bladder cancer, although toxicity can be substantial. Using gemcitabine plus cisplatin (GC) appeared to have similar efficacy but reduced morbidity as compared to M-VAC in a randomized, phase III study.

 a. **M-VAC** is administered in 28-day cycles in the following dosages:

 (1) Methotrexate, 30 mg/m^2 IV on days 1, 15, and 22

 (2) Vinblastine, 3 mg/m^2 IV on days 2, 15, and 22

 (3) Doxorubicin (Adriamycin), 30 mg/m^2 IV on day 2

 (4) Cisplatin, 70 mg/m^2 IV on day 2

 b. **GC** is administered in 28-day cycles for up to six cycles in the following dosages:

 (1) Gemcitabine, 1,000 mg/m^2 IV on days 1, 8, 15, and

 (2) Cisplatin, 70 mg/m^2 IV on day 2

 There is no standard second-line therapy in metastatic or recurrent bladder cancer and clinical trials are recommended. Immunotherapy with checkpoint inhibitors (PD-1 and PD-L1) drugs is currently ongoing and may be promising in urothelial tract cancers based on initial phase one studies. If a patient is not a candidate for clinical trials, palliation may be considered with single agent therapy such a taxanes, pemetrexed, or gemcitabine.

F. **Patient follow-up**

1. Patients with severe urothelial dysplasia should have urine cytology repeated every 2 to 3 months and cystoscopy with random biopsies every 3 to 6 months.

2. Patients with superficial low-grade cancer treated with intravesical chemotherapy should have cystoscopy performed at 3-month intervals.

3. Patients who have undergone cystectomy should be evaluated every 3 months for the first 2 years, every 6 months for the next 3 years, and yearly thereafter. Urinalysis and urine cytology should be performed at 6-month intervals to search for the development of new primary cancers in the upper urinary tract. Hematuria or a positive cytology should be evaluated with IV urography.

4. For patients having an ileal conduit or continent diversion, urethral washing for cytology is advisable periodically to diagnose local recurrence in the urethra. For the same purpose, patients having orthotopic diversions should have follow-up cystoscopy.

VII. SPECIAL CLINICAL PROBLEMS

A. **Gross hematuria** can complicate the course of locally advanced bladder cancer treated with radiation. Transurethral fulguration may help control bleeding. In some retractable cases, the bladder may be treated with instillation of 4% formaldehyde into the bladder under general anesthesia; the agent is retained for 15 minutes. Prior to instillation of formaldehyde, a cystogram needs to be performed to rule out ureteral reflux since formaldehyde can scar and obstruct the ureter. Another option for severe, intractable hematuria is irrigation of the bladder with dilute alum. Alum should not be used in patients with renal insufficiency since alum that gets systemically absorbed is excreted by the kidney.

B. **Obstructive uropathy.** Uremia can develop in patients with any type of urinary diversion. Obstruction caused by benign conditions, such as stones or stenosis, must be excluded. The urine should be examined for malignant cells, crystals, and blood. If the ureteral orifice can be located, a retrograde pyelogram is performed. Otherwise, IVP or renal radionuclide scan may show obstruction.

Endoscopy may be used to dilate stenotic lesions with some success. Exploratory surgery should be considered to solve the problem in patients who otherwise are clinically free of cancer. Patients with advanced disease commonly benefit from diverting externally with percutaneous nephrostomies or internally with ureteral stents.

C. **Impotence.** Despite nerve-sparing technique, impotence complicates radical cystectomy in men. Oral agents, intraurethral preparations, intracavernosal injection, and penile prostheses are the available solutions that usually permit restoration of potency and, often, orgasm in these patients.

URETHRAL CANCER

I. EPIDEMIOLOGY AND ETIOLOGY

Urethral cancer is extremely rare. Women are affected four times as often as men. The differences in anatomy and etiology lead to differences in clinical presentation, diagnosis and treatment between women and men. The age of onset is usually >50 years. The etiology is not known, but urethral cancer may be associated with gonorrheal urethritis, HPV infection, urethral diverticulum strictures, or TCC in the bladder.

II. PATHOLOGY AND NATURAL HISTORY

A. **Histology.** Of cases, 80% are squamous cell carcinomas, usually arising from the stratified squamous epithelium of the posterior (proximal or bulbous) urethra (60%) or the anterior (distal or penile) urethra (30%). Fifteen percent are TCCs arising in the prostatic urethra. Adenocarcinomas possibly arise from Cowper glands.

B. **Diagnosis.** Patients have urinary hesitancy, dysuria, hematuria, palpable mass, urethral discharge, perineal pain, or enlarged inguinal nodes. Transurethral biopsy establishes the diagnosis. Additionally, patients may require cystoscopy and urethroscopy for complete staging and evaluation of etiology of urethral cancer. The biopsy and further locoregional imaging studies such as CT or MRI abdomen/pelvis contribute to TNM staging.

C. **Clinical course.** Urethral cancer is usually diagnosed late and involves inguinal nodes early on. Often patients are initially mistakenly treated for cystitis which delays diagnosis. It also spreads hematogenously to distant organs. Lesions of the anterior urethra are less likely to be associated with widespread metastases than are posterior lesions.

III. MANAGEMENT

Given the rare incidence of urethral cancer, most standard therapies are based on small series studies and basic oncologic principles. In both female and male patients, the extensiveness of therapy is determined by the stage, anatomic location of the tumor (anterior *vs.* posterior urethra), and need for local palliation. In women, treatment varies between total urethrectomy and more extensive surgery, which includes cystectomy (with total or partial resection of the vagina), urethrectomy, and pelvic lymph node dissection. For bulkier disease or proximal tumors, a multimodality approach with surgery, chemotherapy and radiation is favored.

In men who have anterior urethral cancer, transurethral resection of the tumor followed by wide local excision is usually sufficient. If the corpora are infiltrated with tumor, partial or total penectomy is usually required. For posterior urethral disease, the combination of radical cystoprostatectomy, total penectomy, and pelvic lymphadenectomy offers improved results. RT has a limited role in urethral cancer therapy for selected cases; it may be considered as neoadjuvant therapy to downstage locally advanced disease or to treat positive margins to reduce time to progression and likelihood of local recurrence. Additionally, definitive chemoradiation may be considered for patients who are not optimal candidates for surgery or for patients who have undergone neoadjuvant radiotherapy with good response.

PROSTATE CANCER

I. EPIDEMIOLOGY AND ETIOLOGY

A. **Incidence** of prostate cancer (CAP) has risen over the past 20 years. It is the second most common cancer in men worldwide. The current lifetime risk of prostate cancer for men in the United States is 1 in 6 based on 2012 estimates. The peak incidence was seen in 1992 (191/100,000) due to an increase in prostate-specific antigen (PSA) testing. The incidence declined from 1992 to 1995, and then leveled off but rates are still nearly twice as high as the pre-PSA era. The rise in incidence is basically explained by improved detection capability, mainly using PSA and transrectal ultrasound (TRUS) to direct prostate biopsies.

The risk for prostate cancer increases steeply with age. The annual incidence of new prostate cancers in white men in their 50s, 60s and 70s was 0.1%, 0.6% and 1%, respectively. Additionally, 1% incidence is reached at 67 and 72 years of age for black and white men, respectively. Prostate cancer rarely affects men before the age of 40 and the incidence declines after age 80 which may be due to less frequent screening. An age-adjusted death rate peak of 27/100,000 was reported in 1991 in the United States. Thereafter, death rates declined slowly, perhaps because of treatment efforts and novel therapies.

B. Etiology. The cause of prostate cancer is unknown. Several factors are associated with an increased risk.

1. **Demography.** The risk for developing prostate cancer is highest in Sweden, intermediate in the United States and Europe (and Japanese men who migrated to the United States), and lowest in Taiwan and Japan. Blacks are afflicted 30% more often than are whites and Hispanics, and they often present with higher PSA levels, higher Gleason scores, and more advanced stages.

2. **Positive familial history of prostate cancer** in the father or brother of a subject increases his risk sevenfold over the general population if the affected relative was diagnosed by 50 years of age. The relative risk declines to fourfold if the diagnosis of the first-degree relative was made after 70 years of age.

3. **BRCA1 or BRCA2 mutations** are associated with an increased risk of developing prostate cancer. BRCA2 mutations in families have been associated with a five fold increased risk of prostate cancer when compared with the general population. Additionally, it is associated with a higher Gleason score and poorer prognosis. BRCA1 mutations are associated with a younger age of diagnosis (age < 65) and have a twofold increased risk of prostate cancer. It is important to consider these mutations when counseling patients with a significant family history for breast and prostate cancer.

4. **Hormones.** Altered estrogen and androgen metabolite levels have been suggested as a causative mechanism leading to prostate cancer occurrence and have provided a rationale for clinical trials such as the Prostate Cancer Prevention Trial, which used finasteride to block the conversion of testosterone to its more active form dihydrotestosterone. Although finasteride prevented formation of new prostate cancers, its use was associated with more frequent diagnosis of high-grade cancers than in the control group.

5. **Other suggested risk factors,** which are not fully established, are increased intake of vitamin A, decreased intake of vitamin D, obesity, increased intake of animal fats (alpha-linolenic acid component), and occupational exposure to cadmium.

II. PATHOLOGY AND NATURAL HISTORY

A. Histology. Almost all prostate cancers are adenocarcinomas (95%). Transitional, small, and squamous cell carcinomas, lymphomas, and sarcomas are rare. The prostate may be the site of metastases from bladder, colon, or lung cancer or from melanomas, lymphomas, or other malignancies.

B. Location. Prostate cancer tends to be multifocal and frequently (70%) arises from the peripheral zone of the prostate (the surgical capsule). Both of these characteristics make removal by transurethral resection of the prostate (TURP) unfeasible for curative intent.

C. Mode of spread. The biology of adenocarcinomas of the prostate is strongly influenced by tumor grade. Low-grade tumors may remain localized for long periods of time. The disease locally invades along nerve sheaths and metastasizes through lymphatic chains. Lymphatic vessels produce cytokines that stimulate tumor cells promoting chemotactic diffusion of tumor cells into lymphatics. Additionally, the prostate tumors can secrete growth factors, creating new lymphatic vessels in a process known as lymphoangiogenesis. Distant metastases are often present when lymph nodes are involved; however, distant metastases can occur without evidence of nodal involvement.

   D. Metastatic sites. Bone is the most common site of prostate cancer metastases, almost always producing dense osteoblastic metastatic lesions. Occasionally, patients demonstrate uncharacteristic osteolytic lesions. Liver involvement also occurs, but metastases to the brain, lung, and other soft tissues are rare.

   E. Associated paraneoplastic syndromes: disseminated intravascular coagulation (DIC), thrombotic thrombocytopenic purpura (TTP), primary fibrinolysis, neuromuscular abnormalities. Paraneoplastic syndromes occur rarely and usually in patients with advanced disease.

III. DIAGNOSIS

A. Symptoms and signs

1. **Symptoms.** Currently, most patients with CAP are asymptomatic at diagnosis.

   a. Early prostatic cancer is usually asymptomatic and can be detected as a result of routine digital rectal examination (DRE). It is mainly discovered by serum PSA measurement or, rarely, during TURP for glandular hyperplasia. The presence of severe symptoms usually indicates advanced disease. Symptoms include hesitancy, urgency, nocturia, poor urine stream, dribbling, hematospermia, and terminal hematuria.

   b. The sudden onset and rapid progression of symptoms of urinary tract obstruction in men of the appropriate age are often caused by prostate cancer.

   c. Pain in the back, pelvis, or over multiple bony sites is the most common presenting complaint in patients with distant metastases.

   d. The sudden onset of neurologic deficiencies, such as paraplegia and incontinence resulting from extradural spinal metastases with cord compression, may be a presenting feature or may develop during the course of the disease.

2. **Physical examination**

   a. Check for asymmetrical induration or nodularity of the prostate, which often represents prostatic cancer. Frank nodules of prostatic cancer are typically stony hard and not tender.

   b. Examine lateral sulci and for palpable (abnormal) seminal vesicles.

   c. Evaluate inguinal nodes for metastatic disease.

   d. Evaluate for distant metastases by palpating the skeleton for tender foci and by performing an oriented neurologic examination looking for spinal cord compression.

B. Differential diagnosis of the enlarged prostate

1. **Acute prostatitis.** Bacterial infection causes dysuria, pain, and often fever. The prostate is tender and enlarged but not hard. Patients with acute bacterial prostatitis will have a positive urine culture.

2. **Chronic and granulomatous prostatitis** caused by bacterial, tuberculous (including following intravesical BCG instillation), fungal, or protozoan infection may produce a mass that cannot be clinically distinguished from cancer. Biopsy may be necessary to make the diagnosis.

3. **Nodular hyperplasia** (benign prostatic hypertrophy) is found in men >30 years of age and in 80% of men by 80 years of age. Urinary obstructive symptoms are common. Palpable nodules that are indistinguishable from cancer necessitate biopsy.

4. **Other possibilities.** Rarely, calculi, amyloidosis, benign adenomas, or infarction of a hyperplastic nodule can cause obstruction or a mass suggestive of cancer.

C. Diagnostic studies

1. **Routine studies.** Urinalysis, CBC, renal function tests, LFT, alkaline phosphatase, calcium, and chest radiographs

2. **PSA** is a serine protease that serves as a marker unique to the prostate. PSA is normally produced by the secretory cells that line the prostate glands (acini) and secreted into the lumen which eventually undergoes proteolysis generating a more inactive form of the PSA. In prostate cancer, there is a disruption of the basement membrane and normal lumen architecture allowing for more PSA to be leaked into the circulation. PSA screening increases the number of biopsies performed and the corresponding number of patients diagnosed. However, it is unable to differentiate between indolent and potentially lethal prostate cancer. Therefore, several major medical organizations have recommended against PSA-based prostate cancer screening. Patients undergoing PSA-based prostate cancer should understand the risks and potential benefits of early prostate cancer detection.

   a. **False-positive results.** About 15% of patients with nodular hyperplasia have elevated PSA levels. PSA values can also be increased with prostatic inflammation (prostatitis), ejaculation, perineal trauma, surgery, or endoscopy, but not with rectal examination. After a prostate biopsy, PSA is reported to be elevated for at least 6 to 8 weeks. Increased serum PSA concentration has been reported rarely in patients with cancers of the pancreas, parotid gland, and breast.

   b. **Free PSA** is the fraction of PSA that is not bound to the plasma antiproteases a_1-antichymotrypsin and a_2-macroglobulin. A *decreased ratio* of free PSA to total PSA is associated with increased probability of prostate cancer. For patients with elevated PSA and no abnormal findings on palpation of the prostate, conservative management with PSA monitoring is recommended after one negative biopsy if the free-to-total PSA ratio is >25%.

   c. **Age-specific PSA.** The normal range of PSA in patients without prostate cancer rises with age, mainly as a result of gland enlargement. See Table 14-2.

   d. **PSA density** indices are mathematic modifications of PSA. The transitional zone (TZ) is located centrally; it is one of the PSA-producing parts of the prostate and is usually increased in size when benign prostate hyperplasia occurs. The indices adjust serum PSA levels for the prostate gland volume (*PSA density* = PSA/gland volume) or for the TZ volume (PSA TZ = PSA/TZ volume). These indices were found to improve positive-predictive and negative-predictive values in patients with total PSA levels of 4 to 10 ng/mL. PSA TZ is also reported to assist in staging, screening, and sparing prostate biopsies in some patients.

   e. **Clinical utility of PSA.** PSA can detect primary or recurrent tumors of very low volume and is useful for both diagnosis and follow-up. Although PSA is not sufficiently sensitive to be the sole screening method

TABLE 14-2   Age-Specific Serum PSA

Age (yr)	Upper Limit of Normal (ng/mL)
40–50	2.5
50–60	3.5
60–70	4.5
70–80	6.5

for prostate cancer, it is useful when combined with DRE. About 25% of patients with biopsy-proven prostate cancer have serum PSA levels <4 ng/mL. When PSA is combined with TRUS-guided prostatic biopsies, cancer is detected in 20% of patients with PSA values between 4 and 10 ng/mL and in 60% of patients with values >10 ng/mL.

PSA values may show a progressive increase several years before metastatic disease becomes evident. Such a rise is an indication to look for local recurrence in previously treated patients using physical examination or TRUS. The search for metastatic disease in asymptomatic patients with PSA < 10 ng/mL is not routinely indicated.

3. **Biopsy techniques**
   a. **TRUS-guided true-cut biopsy** is the standard method to diagnose prostate cancer. A six to twelve-core biopsy under local anesthesia is taken by sampling the base, apex, and midgland on each side of the gland along two parallel lateral lines. Some cancers have a hypoechoic appearance on TRUS, although majority of cancers may be isoechoic. When the indication for TRUS-guided biopsy is a PSA > 4 ng/mL, the expected yield for diagnosing prostate cancer reaches 24%. When PSA is >4 ng/mL, the DRE is suspicious, and a hypoechoic lesion is imaged by TRUS, the yield rises to 45%.
   b. **TURP.** Prostate cancer may be found in approximately 5% of TURP performed for benign hyperplasia.
4. **Bone scans.** The probability of a positive scan is extremely low when the PSA is <10 ng/mL or symptoms are absent.
5. **CT scans and MRI** are used to assess tumor spread into lymph nodes or the pelvis. These studies are warranted in high-risk patients who have a tumor that is confluent with the pelvic side wall on DRE, a high Gleason score (see tumor grading in Section IV.B.1), or PSA > 20 ng/mL.

IV. STAGING AND PROGNOSTIC FACTORS
A. **Staging system.** Refer to the current AJCC Cancer Staging atlas for TNM staging.
B. **Prognostic factors**
   1. **Tumor grade** strongly affects prognosis. Higher tumor grades are more frequently associated with lymph node and distant metastases. The **Gleason scoring system** is most commonly used. This system is based on the glandular appearance/architecture and degree of differentiation at relatively low-power magnification. Two scores ranging from 1 to 5 points are given for a primary (predominant) site and a secondary (second most prevalent) site. These scores are summed to give a Gleason score between 2 and 10. In modern practice, prostate cancers are given a Gleason score ranging from 6 to 10, and higher scores are associated with worse prognosis.
   2. **Involvement of seminal vesicles** is associated with a poor prognosis, even in apparently early disease.
   3. **Extension of tumor beyond the prostate capsule** is associated with worse prognosis.
   4. **Perineural invasion** is generally a predictor of extraprostatic extension at the time of prostatectomy. It may be associated with higher grade disease, large tumor volume, and seminal vesicle invasion.
   5. High **PSA values** and elements of PSA kinetics, including rapid PSA rise (high PSA velocity) and short PSA doubling time, are associated with poor prognosis.

6. **Predictive Tools** such as OncotypeDx and Decipher are clinically useful for prognostication on a molecular level. OncotypeDx assay uses RT-PCR of 12 cancer genes to assess risk of identifying high risk disease on needle biopsy. Decipher assay is a genome classifier to assess risk of metastases after initial surgical treatment.

V. PREVENTION AND EARLY DETECTION

Screening for prostate cancer remains controversial. Early detection as a result of elevated PSA only (T1c disease) results, however, in the identification of more patients with organ-confined disease and perhaps contributes to a reduction in disease-specific mortality. American cancer society guidelines recommend that PSA screening and DRE begin at the age of 50 years. Screening at the age of 45 should be considered in African American men and in men with positive family history.

VI. MANAGEMENT

A. **Overview and philosophy.** The management of all stages of prostate cancer is controversial. This disease often has a long natural history; therefore, substantial numbers of patients survive 15 years or longer after the diagnosis (even without treatment). Furthermore, because the disease occurs in older men (who often have significant comorbid illnesses), many patients die from these conditions before they have symptoms or die from prostate cancer.

1. Expert options vary widely regarding the optimal use of surgery, RT, hormonal manipulation, and other measures for treating each stage of disease. Most clinicians agree, however, that treatment of early stage disease with either surgery or RT results in comparable survival.

2. All options should be explored when it comes to treatment selection for a specific patient. No prospective head-to-head data are available comparing radical retropubic prostatectomy (RRP) and RT. The long-term *survival* results of modern cryotherapy and modern brachytherapy have not been prospectively compared to gold standard therapies.

3. "Watchful waiting" implies that definitive local therapy is no longer under consideration as a management option. It is often the best option for patients with limited life expectancy.

4. *Active surveillance* also defers the application of definitive local therapy such as radical prostatectomy or radiation. However, a key difference from watchful waiting, is that the disease is actively monitored, and patients with signs of disease progression are treated with curative intent. It is generally used in younger men with low risk disease to defer treatment and their side effects. With active surveillance, PSAs can be monitored twice a year and tumor histology is re-evaluated with prostate biopsies every 1 to 3 years. Although the criteria for recommending active surveillance are evolving, there is a clear consensus that patients in the very low and low risk categories can safely undergo active surveillance. The latest version of the National Comprehensive Cancer Network guidelines recommends that some patients in the intermediate risk category can also undergo active surveillance.

These options should be carefully explained to the patient, exploring the advantages and disadvantages of each treatment modality. The treatment strategy should be tailored according to the patient's risk status, life expectancy and personal values.

B. **Surgery (stages T1 and T3)**

1. **Stage T1-T2.** Management options include watchful waiting, active surveillance, radical prostatectomy, and RT.

2. **Stage T3.** Clinical T3 disease without evidence of distant spread can be cured with surgery. To maximize the potential for cure, adjuvant radiation should be considered for patients with pathologically proven T3 disease, particularly if the surgical margin is positive.

3. **Radical prostatectomy.** In general, patients undergoing surgery should have a life expectancy >10 years. In the United States, the open RRP has been largely replaced by robotically assisted radical prostatectomy (RARP). The cancer control associated with RARP appears to be similar to RRP, and the decreased blood loss associated with RARP may translate into a more rapid recovery from surgery. At this time, it is unknown if the RARP is associated with greater likelihood of recovering erectile function and urinary control when compared to RRP. Other surgical options include a variety of ablative treatments such as cryotherapy, radiofrequency ablation, and high intensity focused ultrasound. However, in the United States, these options are considered experimental, particularly when used as primary therapy.

4. **Complications of radical prostatectomy and lymphadenectomy**

   a. **Radical prostatectomy** causes minor incontinence in 10% to 20% of patients. Severe incontinence is reported to occur in no more than 1% to 3%. Potency can be preserved by a skilled surgeon in up to 60% to 70% of younger patients who undergo nerve-sparing radical prostatectomy.

   b. **Staging lymphadenectomy** is performed during radical prostatectomy by sampling the pelvic nodes. Complications specifically due to the lymphadenectomy are rare and include lymphocele, pulmonary embolus, wound infection, and lymphedema.

   c. **Persistent or recurrent disease following radical extirpation of the prostate** is rare provided that patients were carefully selected for surgery. It may occur in 10% to 40% of patients after radical prostatectomy, depending on tumor stage, Gleason score, and pretreatment PSA. Patients who recur during follow-up can often be cured with salvage radiotherapy. Patients with high risk for disease recurrence may benefit from upfront adjuvant radiotherapy, which is administered to prevent a recurrence.

5. **Contraindications to radical prostatectomy and lymphadenectomy.** Generally speaking, radical prostatectomy is reserved for men who are likely to be cured and who have a life expectancy of at least 10 years.

C. **RT for early disease (stages T1 to T3)**

   1. **Indications.** RT is widely used in the treatment of patients with stages T1 and T2 disease. Adjuvant androgen deprivation therapy (ADT) for 6 months to 3 years has been shown to improve survival in this setting. The use of three-dimensional conformal technique and intensity-modulated RT (IMRT) allow improved results and with fewer side effects than standard RT. For patients with intermediate or high risk prostate cancers, doses up to 8100 cGy provide improved cancer control when compared to lower doses.

   For patients with locally advanced disease (stages T3 and T4), 2 to 3 years of adjuvant ADT has been shown to prolong survival in comparison with 6 months of ADT in a randomized clinical trial. Increasing the radiation dose is advisable in this selected group. This may be achieved by using conformal external-beam irradiation, proton therapy, or brachytherapy. Other indications for RT include the following:

   a. The patient's medical condition precludes surgery.

   b. Node involvement is found at staging lymphadenectomy (RRP is not performed).

   c. Residual malignant pelvic disease is found after prostate surgery (i.e., positive surgical margins and slowly rising PSA).

   d. Adjuvant RT should be considered for patients at high risk for recurrence following RRP. Several randomized studies show that patients with positive surgical margins, seminal vesicle invasion, or extracapsular extension benefit from adjuvant RT.

  2. Complications after approximately 7,000 cGy given in 7 to 8 weeks and their approximate incidence rates in treated patients are as follows:

   a. Impotence: 50% (may be less with IMRT or brachytherapy that can avoid structures such as corpus spongiosum, penile bulb)

   b. Radiation proctitis/enteritis with abdominal cramping, diarrhea, blood-streaked stools, and tenesmus: <5% (see Chapter 31)

   c. Dysuria, urinary urgency, and frequency secondary to cystitis or urethritis: <5%

   d. Perineal fistulas: <1%

   e. Rectal or anal strictures: <1%

   f. Fecal and urinary incontinence, bladder contracture: 1% to 2%

   g. Urethral stricture: 1% to 5%

   h. Persistent tumor or recurrent disease: 10% to 40%, depending on tumor stage, Gleason score, and pretreatment PSA

   i. Secondary malignancies such as bladder or rectal cancer

  3. Brachytherapy and cryotherapy are other therapies intended for cure. These modalities will be judged in the future when enough patients have been treated sufficiently long for ample follow-up data to become available.

   a. Brachytherapy involves implanting radioactive source (seeds) into the prostate to maximize delivery of radiation to the tumor while avoiding toxicity to nearby normal structures. Fewer number of treatments are needed compared with daily external beam RT. Brachytherapy alone can be used for low risk prostate cancer (≤T2a, Gleason score < 6, and PSA < 10). However, it is often used in conjunction with external beam therapy and hormonal deprivation therapy in patients with intermediate risk or high risk disease.

D. Advanced disease

  1. Surgery. TURP may be used to relieve bladder outlet obstruction due to cancer. Orchiectomy produces a rapid decline in testosterone level. It is an effective but irreversible procedure. Orchiectomy is advisable as primary treatment for advanced disease, particularly for patients who are noncompliant with androgen blockade or who require emergency blockade for spinal cord compression.

  2. RT is useful in treating the following problems commonly encountered in prostate cancer patients:

   a. Isolated, painful bony metastatic sites, despite endocrine therapy

   b. Pelvic pain syndromes and gross hematuria

   c. Metastases to retroperitoneal lymph nodes that produce back pain or scrotal and lower extremity edema

   d. Spinal cord compression from vertebral and extradural metastases is a common and rapidly progressive complication of prostate cancer. Cord compression is an emergency; MRI, administration of intravenous corticosteroids, and definitive therapy must be undertaken within a few hours after onset of symptoms (see Chapter 33).

  3. ADT is the mainstay of treatment for symptomatic advanced prostate cancer because testosterone is the main growth factor for prostate cancer cells. The timing of ADT is controversial because no conclusive evidence suggests that treatment of asymptomatic patients provides survival advantage. Prolonged androgen deprivation is associated with multiple side effects including hot flushes, gynecomastia, fatigue, loss of lean body mass, erectile dysfunction, osteoporosis, and increased risk of diabetes and cardiovascular disease. In patients with nodal metastasis, immediate ADT is associated with improved prostate cancer specific and OS when compared to delaying ADT until development of distal metastasis or symptomatic recurrence. The dosing of ADT has also been evaluated: continuous versus intermittent therapy. A large trial failed to demonstrate that intermittent ADT was noninferior to continuous ADT, and the increase in survival for continuous ADT when compared to intermittent ADT approached statistical significance.

Orchiectomy (see above), gonadotropin releasing hormone (GnRH) agonists, GNRH antagonist, and antiandrogens are used for ADT. Each produces symptomatic relief in 80% of patients. Improvement is often dramatic; many bedridden patients crippled with bone pain return to a more functional status.

a. **GnRH agonists,** such as leuprolide, goserelin, triptorelin, histrelin, appear to be as effective as orchiectomy. These synthetic analogs bind to the GnRH receptors on pituitary cells, leading to initial release of luteinizing hormone (LH) and follicle stimulating hormone (FSH). This signals testicular Leydig cells to produce testosterone. After 7 to 10 days of therapy, the GnRH receptors on the pituitary cells are down-regulated and there is a rapid decline in LH and FSH production resulting in castrate levels of testosterone (medical castration) within approximately 1 month of initiation therapy. Some depot forms of these drugs are given every 3 months (22.5 mg for leuprolide and 10.8 mg for goserelin). It is important to note that when initiating these drugs, a transient rise in LH usually causes a surge in testosterone which can enhance prostate cancer growth and cause a "flare" in bone pain, bladder obstruction or other symptoms. This is often avoided by using concurrent antiandrogen therapy. The cost of ongoing treatment with LHRH agonists is substantially greater than with orchiectomy.

b. **GnRH antagonists** such as degarelix suppress testosterone avoiding the "flare" phenomenon by binding to the GnRH receptors without initially stimulating release of LH or FSH. It is administered monthly (240 mg loading dose during the first month followed by 80 mg every 28 days).

c. **Antiandrogens combined with GnRH agonists** are believed by some investigators to be superior to LHRH agonists alone and to result in a small but significant survival benefit by "total androgen blockade." Flutamide (250 mg PO given t.i.d.), bicalutamide (50 mg PO daily), or other antiandrogens are given along with the LHRH agonist. The antiandrogens block the small amount of androgens produced by the adrenal gland.

d. **Other agents** that may be helpful include the following:
   (1) **Progestins,** such as megestrol acetate, 40 mg PO q.i.d.
   (2) **Other drugs that inhibit androgen synthesis,** such as ketoconazole (200 to 400 mg t.i.d.), have also been shown to be effective. These agents are often difficult to tolerate. However, ketoconazole has a rapid onset of action and is often used in the setting of cord compression, when rapid antitumor effects are needed. Corticosteroids are given simultaneously since these drugs block all steroid production by the adrenal gland.

(3) **Corticosteroids,** such as prednisone and dexamethasone, often provide symptomatic improvement and may be associated with reductions in PSA levels.

(4) **Zoledronic acid** (Zometa) is widely used for patients with bone metastases to reduce bone pain, time to first skeletal-related events (SRE), and incidence of fractures and other complications in castrate resistant patients. There is no benefit in castrate sensitive disease. Side effects to monitor include renal impairment, hypocalcemia, and osteonecrosis of the jaw.

(5) **Denosumab,** a monoclonal antibody that binds to RANK ligand, which is essential to osteoclast activation, has been compared to zoledronic acid in a pivotal phase III study in prostate cancer. These studies showed an approximate 18% reduction in SREs with denosumab therapy in castrate resistant prostate cancer (CRPC). Denosumab is administered as a monthly subcutaneous injection. It has a higher incidence of osteonecrosis of the jaw compared with zolendronic acid.

(6) **Strontium-89 infusion.** The beta emission of ^{89}Sr is used in selected hormone refractory patients to relieve skeletal pain. Responses last about 6 months. Hematologic toxicity is anticipated in the first 2 weeks after administration.

(7) **Radium-223.** This is an alpha particle indicated for treatment of symptomatic bone metastases without evidence of visceral metastases in CRPC. The treatment resulted in a significant improvement in OS (15 vs. 11 months).

(8) **α_5-Reductase inhibitors** (finasteride, dutasteride) are used for the treatment of benign prostatic hyperplasia. As a chemopreventive agent, finasteride decreases the overall incidence of prostate cancer, but patients on finasteride are more likely to be diagnosed with high-grade cancer when compared to the placebo group. Thus, the use of these agents in prevention is not routinely recommended.

4. **Other endocrine therapy.** In patients with CRPC, testicular androgens can produce autocrine/paracrine signaling that results in tumor progression. **Abiraterone** is an oral CYP17 lyase inhibitor (1,000 mg/d) that blocks the synthesis of testosterone in the tumor, testis and adrenal glands. The treatment with abiraterone significantly improved OS in patients with castration-resistant disease refractory to docetaxel and it improved PFS in chemotherapy naïve patients. Patients are concurrently treated with corticosteroids (prednisone 5 mg twice daily) given the risk of adrenal insufficiency. Side effects include hypokalemia, fluid retention, and hypertension.

   Enzalutamide, is an oral agent that blocks the androgen receptor, inhibiting nuclear translocation of the androgen receptor. The treatment with enzalutamide improved OS in both patients previously treated with docetaxel and chemotherapy naïve patients. Its benefit was small in patients who had been previously treated with abiraterone.

5. **Chemotherapy.** The first chemotherapy drug approved for the treatment of androgen-independent prostate cancer was **mitoxantrone** based on its palliative effects. Chemotherapy with **docetaxel**, given every 3 weeks, improved OS and provided superior palliation when compared with mitoxantrone in CRPC. Additionally, docetaxel with ADT improved OS when compared with ADT alone in castrate sensitive disease. In castrate sensitive disease, the treatment with docetaxel was notable for improvement in OS in men with high volume disease defined by visceral metastases and/or four or more bone

metastases. Adverse events with docetaxel included hepatic dysfunction and myelosuppression.

For patients refractory to docetaxel, the novel taxane **cabazitaxel** is another chemotherapeutic option. Treatment with cabazitaxel yielded a survival advantage when compared to mitoxantrone, albeit with an increased rate of neutropenic fevers (and associated deaths). Both agents were administered with prednisone (see Fig. 14-1).

6. **Vaccine therapy.** The autologous dendritic cell vaccine, **sipuleucel-T**, was compared to placebo in patients with asymptomatic or minimally symptomatic castration-resistant prostate cancer. Although no difference in time to progression was observed, treatment with sipuleucel-T yielded a survival advantage. The mechanism of action remains somewhat elusive, and the appropriate clinical utilization of the agent is unclear in the face of cost and introduction of other novel therapies. Treatment is not indicated in patients on corticosteroids or opioid therapy and in patients with significant liver metastases.

7. **Novel therapies.** In patients with germline DNA repair mutations (BRCA1/2, ATM, etc.), PARP inhibitors such as olaparib are being tested and appear promising. In a phase II trial TOPARP-A, all castrate resistant patients were treated with olaparib after failing docetaxel, abiraterone or enzalutamide. Patients with DNA repair mutations had better response compared with patients without mutations, suggesting this subset of patients may benefit from olaparib.

Immune checkpoint inhibition studies are also ongoing in advanced prostate cancer.

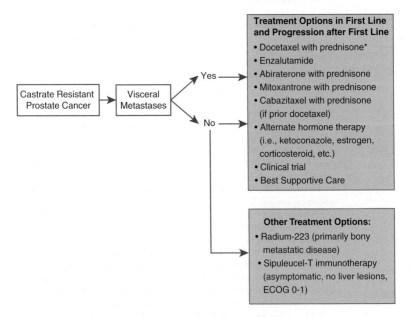

*Docetaxel may be used in castrate sensitive disease in patients with high volume disease (see text)

Figure 14-1 Algorithm for advanced prostate cancer treatments.

VII. SPECIAL CLINICAL PROBLEMS

A. **Cytopenias in prostate cancer** are usually part of the end-stage process caused by extensive tumor involvement of the bone marrow or by RT to major marrow-bearing sites.

B. **Obstructive uropathy and uremia** may be the fatal complication of prostate cancer. Ureteral obstruction can be palliated by placing a double-J ureteral stent or a percutaneous nephrostomy. Bladder outlet obstruction due to local extension of the prostate tumor into the urethra can be relieved with by TURP.

C. **Dense-bone sclerosis on radiograph** in an adult man of the appropriate age who has bone pain usually is diagnostic of prostate cancer. The radiologic appearance of Paget disease is distinguished by the fluffy, cotton-like appearance of lesions, by thickening of the bone cortex, and by the dense sclerosis of the pelvic brim (*brim sign*).

D. **Extraosseous extension** of prostate cancer is common. Extension of skull or vertebral lesions can produce neurologic deficits. Extension of rib lesions can produce subcutaneous or pleuropulmonary masses. Retroorbital and cavernous sinus masses can result in proptosis and visual loss. Extraosseous extension of bony lesions necessitates RT.

PENILE CANCER

I. EPIDEMIOLOGY AND ETIOLOGY

A. **Incidence.** Penile cancer constitutes about 0.5% of all cancers in men in the United States and Europe. The vast majority of cases occur in developing countries in Africa, Asia, and South America. The incidence is greatly increased in populations that do not uniformly practice circumcision. The average age of onset is about 60 years, peaking at about 80 years of age.

B. **Etiology.** The etiology of penile cancer is not known. Sexually transmitted diseases are not a causative factor. Circumcision appears to be preventative. The disease is almost nonexistent in Jewish men, who are all circumcised shortly after birth. In Africa and other countries where circumcision is not performed, penile cancer constitutes 20% of all cancers. Muslims have an intermediate risk for penile cancer. Muslim boys are circumcised at puberty.

II. PATHOLOGY AND NATURAL HISTORY

A. **Premalignant lesions**

1. **Carcinoma *in situ***
   a. **Erythroplasia of Queyrat** occurs on the glans or prepuce. It is an *in situ* squamous cell carcinoma. The lesions are flat, solitary, and reddened; or are velvety plaques and may progress to invasive cancer in 10% of patients. The development of ulceration may be a sign of progression.
   b. **Bowen disease** occurs on the penile shaft and appears as a small eczematoid, dull red plaque with associated crusting and oozing anywhere on the penis. Squamous CIS is demonstrated by histology.

2. **Leukoplakia.** Nonspecific plaques of leukoplakia on the glans are almost always associated with squamous carcinoma. Lesions of leukoplakia are often adjacent to squamous cell carcinoma lesions. Unlike leukoplakia lesions elsewhere, penile lesions are not white.

3. **Giant penile condyloma** (Buschke-Löwenstein tumor) grossly resembles a cauliflower-like squamous cell cancer and may have foci of cancer. Surgical excision is mandatory.

B. **Histology.** Squamous cell carcinoma, usually well differentiated, constitutes nearly all penile cancers. Rare penile cancers include melanoma, sarcoma, basal cell carcinoma, and metastatic tumor such as urethral carcinoma. Squamous carcinoma of the penis may demonstrate variable degrees of keratin formation.

C. **Clinical course.** If left untreated, penile cancers usually cause death within 2 years.

1. Squamous penile cancer usually starts on the glans or coronal sulcus. As the disease progresses, the corpora cavernosa are invaded. The urethra is usually spared until late in the disease course.

2. The rich lymphatic drainage of this region results in metastases to the inguinal nodes (only one-third of palpable nodes are involved with tumor by histology) followed by the pelvic nodes and then retroperitoneal nodes. Lymphatic metastases are not common if the tumor is confined to the glans or prepuce.

3. The tumor disseminates through the lymphatic system and the bloodstream to distant organs in up to 10% of patients, most often to the lungs and, less frequently, to bone and other sites.

D. **Paraneoplastic syndromes.** Hypercalcemia may develop with no evidence of bony metastasis (20% of patients).

III. DIAGNOSIS

Diagnosis is usually delayed substantially because of denial, personal neglect, shame, guilt, or lack of knowledge.

A. **Symptoms and signs**

1. The earliest lesion of penile carcinoma is described by patients as a nonhealing sore, often with an associated foul-smelling discharge. Phimosis may mask penile cancer until erosion through the prepuce occurs. Many patients have a long history of a painless mass. Urinary tract symptoms, such as pain and hematuria, are signs of locally advanced disease.

2. Physical examination usually reveals an exophytic mass. Infection of the tumor is usually present when the patient is examined for symptoms. In about 92% of patients, the tumor arises in the glans penis, prepuce, or both.

B. **Laboratory studies**

1. Routine blood tests, urinalysis, and chest radiographs are obtained.

2. Biopsy or imprint slides should be done for all patients with a penile mass or with any finding compatible with a precancerous lesion.

3. Liver and bone scans should be obtained only if abnormalities seen on physical examination or blood studies suggest liver or bone involvement.

4. MRI and ultrasound of the penis and pelvis are used in staging and surgical planning.

IV. STAGING SYSTEM AND PROGNOSTIC FACTORS

A. **Staging system.** Refer to the current AJCC Cancer Staging atlas for TNM staging.

B. **Prognostic factors.** Poor prognostic features include endophytic and high-grade lesions, invasion of the shaft, and involvement of draining lymph nodes, especially at the iliac level or higher. Of patients with clinical stage Tis, Ta, or T1 (Jackson stage I or II) tumors, 10% have inguinal node involvement proven by surgery.

V. PREVENTION AND EARLY DETECTION

Prevention of penile cancer can be accomplished by routine early circumcision of male babies. Circumcision should be performed in patients with phimosis and penile discharge, inflammation, or induration. Early detection of penile cancer requires regular inspection of the prepuce and glans at physical examination and biopsy of suspected lesions.

VI. MANAGEMENT

A. **Surgery** is the principal modality of therapy for penile cancer in the United States. Partial penectomy is sufficient therapy if there is a 2-cm tumor-free margin. Intraoperative frozen section should guide the extent of resection.

1. Total penectomy is necessary when you cannot leave at least 2 cm of penile stump, which will allow the urine stream to be directed.

2. In younger patients with tumor confined to the prepuce, circumcision may be used if close follow-up can be assured; however, the recurrence rate is high.

3. In most cases, palpable inguinal lymph nodes should be further evaluated with a biopsy. A biopsy is not necessary if lymph node sampling is already planned.

   a. Dynamic sentinel node biopsy involves intraoperative lymphatic mapping and sampling one or more nodes where the primary tumor is expected to spread.

   b. Inguinal lymph node dissection used to evaluate the most frequent site of metastasis. The typical boundaries include the inguinal ligament, the sartorius muscle, the fossa ovalis, and the adductor longus muscle.

4. Radical lymphadenectomy is routinely performed in patients with stage T3 tumors. The extensiveness of the lymph node dissection (deep *vs.* superficial inguinal *vs.* pelvic node dissection; unilateral *vs.* bilateral; full *vs.* limited) varies according to local and regional disease extension.

B. **RT.** The primary role of RT is to avoid penectomy, especially in younger patients. It may be administered via external beam or interstitial brachytherapy. This modality has been used for treating small primary stage I lesions (<3 cm in diameter); the results for RT alone (along with salvage surgery for failures) appear to be the same as those obtained when partial amputation is used as primary therapy. Complications of radiation are may include urethral edema/strictures, mucositis, infection, fistulas and even meatal stenosis.

C. **Chemotherapy.** Premalignant lesions may respond to topical therapy with fluorouracil or imiquimod cream or to laser therapy in selected cases. Penile cancer appears to be responsive to combination chemotherapy: vincristine, bleomycin, and methotrexate (VBM regimen) or cisplatin and 5-fluorouracil. Some authorities use these drugs as an adjunct to surgery or RT for stage T3 and T4 tumors. Response rates of advanced cancer to these drugs may be as high as 50%.

ACKNOWLEDGMENT

The authors would like to acknowledge Dr. Sumanta K. Pal, who significantly contributed to earlier versions of this chapter.

Suggested Readings

Renal Cancer

Bukowski R, et al. *Renal Cell Carcinoma. Molecular Targets and Clinical Applications.* 3rd ed. New York: Springer Press, 2015.

Choueiri T, et al. Cabozantinib versus everolimus in advanced renal cell carcinoma. *N Engl J Med* 2015;373:1814.

Hudes G, et al. Temsirolimus, interferon alfa, or both for advanced renal-cell carcinoma. *N Engl J Med* 2007;356:2271.

Motzer R, et al. Sunitinib versus interferon alfa in metastatic renal cell carcinoma. *N Engl J Med* 2007;356:115.

Motzer RJ, et al. Axitinib versus sorafenib as second-line treatment for advanced renal cell carcinoma: Overall survival analysis and updated results from a randomized phase 3 trial. *Lancet Oncol* 2013;14:552.

Motzer R, et al. Nivolumab versus everolimus in advanced renal cell carcinoma. *N Engl J Med* 2015;373:1803.

Rassweiler J, et al. Oncological safety of laparoscopic surgery for urological malignancy: experience with more than 1,000 operations. *J Urol* 2003;169:2072.

Sternberg CN, et al. Pazopanib in locally advanced or metastatic renal cell carcinoma: results of a randomized phase iii trial. *J Clin Oncol* 2010;28:1061.

Zisman A, et al. Risk group assessment and clinical outcome algorithm to predict the natural history of patients with surgically resected renal cell carcinoma. *J Clin Oncol* 2002;20:4559.

Urothelial Cancers

Borden LS, et al. Bladder cancer. *Curr Opin Oncol* 2003;15:227.

Grossman HB, et al. Neoadjuvant chemotherapy plus cystectomy compared with cystectomy alone for locally advanced bladder cancer. *N Engl J Med* 2003;349(9):859.

Raghavan D. Molecular targeting and pharmacogenomics in the management of advanced bladder cancer. *Cancer* 2003;97:2083.

Sternberg CN, et al. Chemotherapy for bladder cancer: treatment guidelines for neoadjuvant chemotherapy, bladder preservation, adjuvant chemotherapy, and metastatic cancer. *Urology* 2007;69 (1 suppl):62.

Von der Maase H, et al. Gemcitabine and cisplatin versus methotrexate, vinblastine, doxorubicin and cisplatin in advanced or metastatic bladder cancer: results of a large randomized, multinational, multicenter, phase III study. *J Clin Oncol* 2000;17:3068.

Prostate Cancer

Bill-Axelson A, et al. Radical prostatectomy versus watchful waiting in early prostate cancer. *N Engl J Med* 2005;352:1977.

de Bono JS, et al. Prednisone plus cabazitaxel or mitoxantrone for metastatic castration-resistant prostate cancer progressing after docetaxel treatment: a randomised open-label trial. *Lancet* 2010;376:1147.

de Bono JS, et al. Abiraterone and increased survival in metastatic prostate cancer. *N Engl J Med* 2011;364:1995.

Graefen M, et al. International validation of a preoperative nomogram for prostate cancer recurrence after radical prostatectomy. *J Clin Oncol* 2002;20:3206.

Hussain M, et al. Intermittent versus continuous androgen deprivation in prostate cancer. *N Engl J Med* 2013;368:1314.

Kantoff PW, et al. Sipuleucel-T immunotherapy for castration-resistant prostate cancer. *N Engl J Med* 2010;363:411.

Messing EM, et al. Immediate hormonal therapy compared with observation after radical prostatectomy and pelvic lymphadenectomy in men with node-positive prostate cancer. *N Engl J Med* 1999;341:1781.

Pisansky TM. External-beam radiotherapy for localized prostate cancer. *N Engl J Med* 2006;355:1583.

Sweeney CJ, et al. Chemohormonal therapy in metastatic hormone-sensitive prostate cancer. *N Engl J Med* 2015;373:737.

Tomasz MB, et al. Enzalutamide in metastatic prostate cancer before chemotherapy. *N Engl J Med* 2014;371:424.

15 Neurologic Tumors

Yoshie Umemura and Lisa M. DeAngelis

I. EPIDEMIOLOGY AND ETIOLOGY

A. **Incidence.** Malignant primary brain tumors represent 2% of all cancers and 2.5% of cancer deaths annually in the United States. The male-to-female ratio is 3:2 for all brain tumors. There is a bimodal incidence with a peak at 5 to 10 years of age and again at 50 to 55 years of age. Brain cancers are the most common solid tumors in children.

B. **Etiology**

1. **Environmental factors.** Exposure to ionizing radiation can induce the formation of meningiomas, nerve sheath tumors, sarcomas, and astrocytomas. Occupational exposure to vinyl chlorides may be a risk factor for astrocytomas; animal studies have shown that exposure to *N*-nitroso compounds, aromatic hydrocarbons, triazines, and hydrazines increases the risk for astrocytoma formation, but it is not clear whether these compounds play a role in human tumor formation.

2. **Hereditary neurocutaneous syndromes**

   a. **Neurofibromatosis I** is a dominantly inherited condition of multiple neurofibromas, café au lait spots, axillary freckling, and Lisch nodules of the iris that confers an increased risk for optic glioma, intracranial astrocytoma, neurofibrosarcoma, neural crest–derived tumors (glomus tumor, pheochromocytoma), embryonal tumors, leukemia, and Wilms tumor. The gene for this disorder, neurofibromin 1 (*NF1*), is on chromosome 17q11. The product of *NF1* is neurofibromin, which is a tumor suppressor gene.

   b. **Neurofibromatosis II** is a condition of multiple schwannomas, especially vestibular schwannomas, that is also associated with an increased risk for ependymoma and meningioma. The gene for this disorder, neurofibromin 2 (*NF2*) is located on chromosome 22q12, and its product, merlin, encodes a member of the ezrin–radixin–moesin (ERM) family of membrane and cytoskeletal linker proteins thought to be important for cell motility and adhesion.

   c. **Tuberous sclerosis** (Bourneville disease) is a dominantly transmitted disorder characterized by the development of hamartomas, including subependymal nodules and cerebral cortical tubers that have abnormal cortical architecture and can be associated with mental retardation, epilepsy, and behavioral disturbances such as autism. Hamartomatous lesions of other organ systems include facial angiofibromas, forehead plaques, shagreen patches, cardiac rhabdomyomas, and renal angiomyolipomas and cysts. This disorder is associated with the formation of subependymal giant cell astrocytomas. Two responsible tumor suppressor genes, TSC-1 (chromosome 9q34) encoding for hamartin and TSC-2 (chromosome 16p13) encoding for tuberin, have been identified.

   d. **Nevoid basal cell carcinoma syndrome** (Gorlin syndrome) is a dominantly inherited syndrome of multiple basal cell carcinomas that may be associated with medulloblastoma, meningioma, craniopharyngioma, and some systemic tumors (see Chapter 17).

    e. Neurocutaneous melanosis is a developmental rather than inherited condition of large, hairy, pigmented benign nevi of the skin associated with infiltration of the meninges by melanin-containing cells. Although the pigmented lesions of the skin remain benign, the pigmented cells in the meninges often undergo malignant transformation with neural invasion, resulting in primary central nervous system (CNS) melanoma.

3. Hereditary cancer syndromes

    a. von Hippel-Lindau disease is a dominantly transmitted disorder characterized by hemangioblastomas of the retina, cerebellum and, less commonly, spinal cord. Other associated tumors include renal carcinoma, pheochromocytoma, islet cell tumors, endolymphatic sac tumors, and benign renal, pancreatic, and epididymal cysts. The disorder is due to the loss of von Hippel-Lindau (*VHL*) tumor suppressor gene on chromosome 3p25-26. This loss results in the overexpression of vascular endothelial growth factor (VEGF) and erythropoietin, which are normally induced by hypoxia.

    b. Turcot syndrome is a rare autosomal dominant or recessive familial syndrome associated with colon cancer, glioblastoma, and medulloblastoma. It is due to a germ-line mutation of the adenomatous polyposis coli (*APC*) gene on chromosome 5q21, or germ-line mutations of genes governing the DNA replication mechanism including the mutL-homolog 1 (*hMLH-1*) or PMS1 homolog 2, mismatch repair system component (*hPMS-2*) genes, both of which encode proteins responsible for DNA mismatch repair.

    c. Li-Fraumeni syndrome is a clinical syndrome of familial breast cancer, sarcomas, leukemia, and primary brain tumors that is associated with germ-line p53 (chromosome 17) mutations.

4. Immune suppression. Transplant recipients and patients with acquired immunodeficiency syndrome (AIDS) have a markedly increased risk for primary CNS lymphoma (PCNSL).

II. DIAGNOSIS

A. Clinical presentation depends on the location of the tumor and its rate of growth. In general, slow-growing tumors cause little in the way of focal deficits because the brain tissue is slowly compressed and compensatory mechanisms appear to occur. Fast-growing tumors tend to be associated with considerable surrounding cerebral edema; the edema, in addition to the tumor mass, is more likely to cause focal deficits. Usually, the deficits caused by edema are reversible, whereas those caused by the tumor may not be reversible.

1. Headache occurs in about 50% of brain tumor patients. They are most likely to occur in younger patients with fast-growing tumors and are typically deep, dull, and not intense or throbbing. They are characteristically worse on arising in the morning and are exacerbated by straining or lifting. Lateralization of headache occasionally facilitates tumor localization.

2. Seizures are seen in 30% of all patients with brain tumor. Patients with low-grade gliomas are more likely to experience seizures at presentation (60% to 90%) compared to patients with glioblastoma (20% to 30%). The seizures may be generalized or partial (focal). Simple partial seizures commonly consist of transient sensory or motor phenomena of a single limb or side. Complex partial seizures, often of frontal or temporal lobe origin, consist of changes in the level of consciousness or awareness of surroundings, frequently in conjunction with abnormal olfactory or gustatory phenomena. Speech arrest may also occur. Generalized seizures result in loss of consciousness, bowel and bladder incontinence, and bilateral tonic–clonic movements.

3. **Increased intracranial pressure (ICP)** may result from a large mass or from obstructive hydrocephalus. Large supratentorial masses cause progressive obtundation and can lead to transtentorial herniation, which classically presents with an ipsilateral third cranial nerve palsy and contralateral hemiparesis. Hydrocephalus causes gait ataxia, nausea, vomiting, headache, and decreased alertness. If untreated, hydrocephalus can lead to central herniation, which is not heralded by a third nerve palsy. Papilledema is a sign of increased ICP, but it is rarely seen in current brain tumor patients because of the availability of modern neuroimaging, which facilitates early diagnosis. Unusual signs and symptoms of increased ICP include visual obscurations, dizziness, and false localizing signs, the most common of which is sixth cranial nerve dysfunction owing to stretching of the nerve from downward pressure caused by a large supratentorial mass.

4. **Supratentorial tumors** usually present with focal signs and symptoms, including hemiparesis (frontal lobe), aphasia (left frontal and posterior temporal lobes), hemineglect (parietal lobe), and hemianopsia (temporal, parietal, or occipital lobes). In 5% to 10% of patients with oligodendrogliomas or glioblastomas, intratumoral hemorrhage may lead to an acute presentation and sudden onset of lateralizing signs.

5. **Hypothalamic tumors** may be associated with disturbance of body temperature regulation, diabetes insipidus, hyperphagia, and, if the optic chiasm is involved, visual field deficit, typically a bitemporal hemianopsia.

6. **Brainstem tumors,** such as brainstem gliomas, present with multiple cranial nerve deficits, hemiparesis, and ataxia.

7. **Nerve sheath tumors,** such as vestibular schwannomas, result in deficits of the involved cranial or spinal nerve. As the tumor enlarges, surrounding neural structures may also be compressed, leading to further symptoms.

8. **Cerebellar tumors** are associated with dysmetria, ataxia, vertigo, nystagmus, headache, and vomiting.

9. **Spinal cord tumors** present with spastic paraparesis and sensory loss below the level of the tumor as well as disturbances of bowel and bladder function.

10. **Meningeal involvement** by primary CNS tumors is less common than with metastatic tumors (see Chapter 33) and is seen primarily with medulloblastoma, pineoblastoma, germ-cell tumor, PCNSL, and, to a lesser degree, ependymoma.

B. **Evaluation.** Imaging studies must be performed to evaluate patients suspected of having CNS mass lesions.

1. **Computed tomography (CT) and magnetic resonance imaging (MRI)** are the primary imaging modalities for evaluating presumed CNS tumors. MRI is preferable because of its greater sensitivity, especially for lesions in the brainstem, posterior fossa, medial temporal lobes, and spinal cord. Contrast studies should always be performed because many tumors show contrast enhancement.

2. **Lumbar puncture** is almost never a part of the initial evaluation of a suspected CNS tumor and, in fact, is often contraindicated in this setting.

3. **Angiography** may be useful in the preoperative evaluation of highly vascular tumors that require embolization to reduce the blood supply before surgical resection is performed.

4. **Systemic evaluation.** After a mass lesion is demonstrated on CT or MRI scan, its specific etiology must be determined. The differential diagnosis

includes a primary tumor of the nervous system, metastasis, stroke, and inflammatory or infectious process (e.g., multiple sclerosis, cerebral abscess). Radiographic features can help differentiate among these diagnoses; combined with the patient's history and physical examination, they can lead to a presumptive diagnosis with reasonable certainty in most patients.

A systemic evaluation is not necessary in the initial evaluation of a patient with a single lesion seen on MRI. Such patients should immediately undergo surgical resection and any subsequent testing based on the pathology. If a primary brain tumor is found, no systemic evaluation is necessary. If PCNSL is the leading differential diagnosis, a biopsy is preferred. If a metastasis is identified, a systemic workup can proceed accordingly.

5. **Surgery** is required for definitive diagnosis in most cases of suspected primary nervous system tumors and is usually a cornerstone of treatment as well. Exceptions include tumors not requiring surgical extirpation as a component of therapy and that can be diagnosed by characteristic imaging features (e.g., neurofibroma, optic nerve glioma, brainstem glioma).

III. GLIOMAS

A. **Pathology.** Gliomas are highly infiltrative tumors that are graded by their degree of anaplasia. Low-grade tumors are classified as astrocytoma or oligodendroglioma (WHO grade II) and those with more evidence of cytologic atypia and increased cellularity as anaplastic astrocytoma or anaplastic oligodendroglioma (WHO grade III), depending upon whether the histologic features of the cells most resemble astrocytes or oligodendrogliomas. Glioblastomas are gliomas with highly malignant features (GBM; WHO grade IV). The very low-grade pilocytic astrocytoma constitutes WHO grade I; it is seen almost exclusively in children.

B. **Molecular characteristics.** Recent molecular profiling has redefined these categories using the presence of an isocitrate dehydrogenase (*IDH*) mutation and the codeletion of chromosomes 1p and 19q to define prognostic subgroups (Table 15-1). Tumors that are *IDH* wild type and lack 1p19q codeletion tend to behave like GBMs (median survival 1.7 years) regardless of their histologic appearance. *IDH*-mutated tumors have a better prognosis (median survival 6.3 years), and those harboring both an *IDH* mutation and 1p19q codeletion have the best (median survival 8.0 years).

Glioblastoma remains a useful pathologic diagnosis and is characterized by vascular proliferation and necrosis in addition to cytologic atypia and increased cellularity. GBMs with sarcomatous features are gliosarcomas and behave in a fashion identical to GBMs. Methylation of the promotor of the O^6-methylguanine-DNA methyltransferase (*MGMT*) gene that encodes for a DNA repair enzyme confers a better prognosis and is predictive of response to alkylating agents, such as temozolomide (Table 15-1). Approximately 40% of all GBMs have amplification of the epidermal growth factor receptor (EGFR)

TABLE 15-1	Median Survivals of Gliomas Based on Molecular Subtypes	
	WHO Grade II/III	**WHO Grade IV**
IDH mutated: 1p19q codeleted (O)	8.0 yr	2.1 yr (regardless of 1q19p)
1p19q intact (A or O)	6.3 yr	
IDH wild type (A or O)	1.7 yr	1.1 yr
MGMT promotor methylated	NA	2.0 yr
MGMT promotor unmethylated	NA	1.1 yr

WHO, World Health Organization; O, oligodendroglioma; A, astrocytoma; NA, not applicable.

pathway, half of which harbor an activating mutation, EGFRvIII. Unexpected actionable mutations have been described in GBMs from isolated patients, but the frequency of this is uncertain.

The incidence of glioma increases with age, and as the patient's age increases, the glioma is more likely to be of higher grade. Astrocytomas are most commonly supratentorial but may occur in the cerebellum, brainstem, and spinal cord.

Immunohistochemical properties of neurologic malignancies are shown in Appendix B2.

C. **Radiology.** On CT or MRI scans, gliomas are usually solitary lesions primarily in the white matter. Grade II gliomas appear as a nonenhancing infiltrative mass best seen on T_2-weighted or fluid-attenuated inversion recovery (FLAIR) MRI sequences. High-grade gliomas (grades III and IV) usually enhance after administration of contrast material and are surrounded by focal edema; occasionally, anaplastic gliomas do not enhance on MRI. Oligodendrogliomas are most common in the frontal and temporal lobes, particularly in the insular cortex. Intratumoral calcifications and hemorrhage are more common in oligodendrogliomas, regardless of grade. GBMs often have central necrosis and may appear as ring-enhancing lesions. Uncommonly, cystic components may be associated with low- or high-grade astrocytomas.

D. **Treatment**
   1. **Dexamethasone** reduces the cerebral edema associated with malignant brain tumors by decreasing vascular permeability through its action on endothelial junctions. Treatment with steroids usually results in considerable clinical improvement. Dosing schedules vary, but the typical starting dose is 4 mg PO or IV twice a day. Doses should be reduced once definitive treatment has been undertaken.
   2. **Surgical resection** should be performed whenever technically feasible. Not only is surgery necessary for adequate tissue sampling for pathologic diagnosis, but it can also lead to neurologic improvement from reduction of mass effect. The degree of surgical resection has been shown to correlate with survival, especially for higher-grade lesions. The term gross total resection refers to removal of all or nearly all tumor visualized radiographically. Based on the infiltrative nature of all grades of astrocytoma, however, residual tumor always remains. Postoperative MRI scans should be performed within 3 to 4 days of surgery to determine the extent of surgical resection. If resection is not possible, biopsy should be performed for histologic diagnosis.
   3. **Radiation therapy** (RT) substantially improves survival, and a dose–response relationship has been documented for high-grade tumors. Low-grade astrocytomas are treated with 5,000 to 5,400 cGy and anaplastic astrocytomas and GBMs with 6,000 cGy of RT to the tumor and surrounding margins. RT may be deferred in some patients with low-grade astrocytomas who have seizures controlled by antiepileptic drugs and no other neurologic symptoms. Grade II gliomas in patients younger than 40 years and that have been completely resected may not require immediate postoperative therapy if they are *IDH* mutated. They can be followed with surveillance imaging, and a treatment decision can be made at progression. Radiation sensitizers are not beneficial in the treatment of astrocytomas.
   4. **Chemotherapy** with temozolomide has become the standard of care for patients with GBM. It is given concurrently during RT at 75 mg/m²/d continuously and for at least six cycles as adjuvant therapy at a dose of 150

to 200 mg/m^2 for 5 consecutive days every 4 weeks. Many continue the drug until progression or when 12 to 24 cycles have been completed. Treatment is usually well tolerated. Although efficacy has not been established for patients with anaplastic astrocytoma, many have adopted this regimen for all patients with malignant gliomas. Randomized controlled data on patients with anaplastic oligodendrogliomas that are 1p19q codeleted demonstrate that overall survival is better with RT and chemotherapy (median 14.7 years) than with RT alone (median 7.3 years). These studies used the combination of procarbazine, lomustine, and vincristine (PCV), but many clinicians prefer the GBM regimen with temozolomide because of lower toxicity; either may be considered.

5. **Other.** A recently developed device, tumor-treating fields (TTFields), was approved for treating supratentorial GBM. It delivers transcutaneous low-intensity intermediate-frequency alternating electrofields to disrupt spindle formation during cell division and aims to arrest mitosis. In newly diagnosed GBM, a statistically significant increase in progression-free survival by 3.1 months and overall survival by 4.9 months was achieved when used in combination with standard chemoradiation. The randomized controlled data in recurrent GBM did not show survival benefit. Given the modest benefit, high rate of skin irritation, weight of the battery pack potentially limiting patient mobility, the cosmetic consequences, and uncertain insurance coverage, most patients and physicians find TTFields unappealing.

6. **Treatment at recurrence.** Gliomas, including GBM, may respond to treatment at recurrence, and treatment strategies usually parallel those given at diagnosis. The antiangiogenic drug bevacizumab has become the standard at recurrence. It is usually combined with a chemotherapeutic drug such as a nitrosourea, carboplatin, or irinotecan. Optimally, patients should be offered participation in a clinical trial if available. Further irradiation, such as SRS combined with bevacizumab, may have a role in the treatment of these highly infiltrative neoplasms.

7. **Patient follow-up.** Patients with gliomas require lifelong follow-up. Low-grade astrocytomas can recur, often as higher-grade lesions, as long as 20 years after treatment. Tumor recurrence is usually at the primary site, but occasionally astrocytomas can become multifocal or recur at distal sites within the neuraxis. Metastasis to systemic tissues is exceedingly rare. Monitoring for tumor recurrence can be achieved best with serial neurologic examination and MRI scan. The rate of monitoring is individualized and depends on the grade of the tumor, the performance status of the patient, and the intention for further therapy.

E. **Survival.** Median survival with standard treatment is being redefined by molecular classification (Table 15-1).

IV. OTHER GLIAL NEOPLASMS

A. **Pilocytic astrocytoma (PA; formerly known as juvenile pilocytic astrocytoma)**
   1. **Pathology.** PAs (WHO grade I) differ in histology and clinical behavior from the astrocytomas. They are less invasive, more circumscribed, and much less likely to progress to a more anaplastic state. About 90% of PAs have activation of the BRAF pathway with over 70% carrying a *BRAF* fusion mutation and about 5% having a *BRAF* V600E mutation.
   2. **Clinical features.** PAs tends to occur in children and young adults and have a predilection for the cerebellum, hypothalamus, optic chiasm, and

thalamus. Radiographically, they are well-demarcated masses that enhance densely and homogeneously and may have cystic components.

3. **Treatment.** PAs are not infiltrative or histologically progressive and, therefore, can be cured by surgical excision. Subtotally resected tumors may be observed or rarely require immediate focal irradiation. Nonresectable tumors (e.g., optic gliomas) may also be followed or can be treated with RT (5,400 cGy, focal fields) or, in very young patients, with chemotherapy if symptoms dictate the need for immediate treatment. PAs respond to nitrosoureas, procarbazine, cyclophosphamide, vincristine, platinum compounds, and etoposide. A BRAF inhibitor, such as vemurafenib, can be used to treat PAs with *BRAF* V600E mutation; however, it should be avoided in patients with *BRAF* fusion mutation.

4. **Survival** depends on tumor location and extent of resection. The overall survival rate is over 90% at 10 years and 80% at 20 years.

B. **Ependymoma**

1. **Pathology.** Ependymomas arise from ependymal cells. Therefore, these tumors localize to the ventricular system and spinal canal, most often in the fourth ventricle and in the region of the cauda equina. They are more frequent in children but occur in adults as well. Most are histologically benign, but some, including the anaplastic ependymoma, ependymoblastoma, and myxopapillary ependymoma, can disseminate through the spinal fluid.

2. **Treatment.** Ependymomas can be cured by total resection, particularly the filum terminale myxopapillary ependymoma. Unfortunately, their location often prevents complete excision, and RT must often be administered postoperatively.

C. **Brainstem glioma**

1. **Pathology.** Brainstem gliomas are astrocytomas that arise in the brainstem, usually the pons, and are more common in children than adults. They can be any grade of astrocytoma, but their outcome is primarily determined by their location, so they are classified separately from the other astrocytomas. Patients present with multiple cranial nerve palsies and ataxia.

2. **Treatment.** Surgical resection is not possible because of the tumor location, and diagnosis is usually based on the typical radiographic and clinical findings. Treatment consists of focal RT, usually to 6,000 cGy. Chemotherapy is largely ineffective for brainstem gliomas. Median survival for patients with diffuse pontine gliomas is about <1 year.

V. PRIMARY CNS LYMPHOMA

Primary CNS lymphoma (PCNSL) is discussed in Chapter 22 and Chapter 37.

VI. MEDULLOBLASTOMA

A. **Pathology.** Medulloblastomas are embryonal tumors arising from primitive germinal cells in the cerebellum; they most commonly localize to the vermis and fourth ventricle. They are more common in childhood but occur in young adults as well (see also Chapter 19). Recent studies have described four molecular subgroups: wingless (*Wnt*), sonic hedgehog (*Shh*), group 3, and group 4. These subgroups differ in demographics, genetic profiles, and prognosis (Table 15-2). Group 4 is the most common (35%).

B. **Clinical features.** Medulloblastomas often cause obstructive hydrocephalus from compression of the fourth ventricle. Therefore, patients may present with signs of increased ICP (e.g., gait ataxia, headache, nausea, and vomiting) rather than with signs localizing to the site of their tumor.

TABLE 15-2	Medulloblastoma by Molecular Subgroups			
	Wnt	**Shh**	**Group 3**	**Group 4**
Frequency	10%	30%	25%	35%
Demographics	F = M	F = M	M > F	M > F
	Children > Adult	All ages, more in infants and adults	Children > Infants	All ages, mainly children
Genetics	Mutations in CTMMN1, APC	Mutations in PTCH1, SUFU, SMO	MYC amplification	CDK6 and MYCN amplification
Metastasis	Rare	Uncommon	Very frequent	Frequent
5 yr OS	94% (100% adults)	87%	32%	76%

F, female; M, male; OS, overall survival.

C. **Staging and treatment.** Patients require full staging of the neuraxis, including contrast-enhanced MRI of the head and full spine and cytologic examination of cerebrospinal fluid (CSF), because medulloblastoma disseminates in the CSF.

1. **Surgery.** The extent of surgical resection correlates with survival in patients with medulloblastoma, and gross total resection should be the goal. Patients with persistent hydrocephalus may require placement of a ventriculoperitoneal shunt.

2. **Radiation therapy,** consisting of craniospinal irradiation, is required for most patients, including those with negative staging studies. The standard dose ranges from 3,000 to 3,600 cGy to the whole brain and spine with an additional boost to the tumor for a total dose of 5,400 to 6,000 cGy. Recent data suggest that the craniospinal dose can be reduced to 2,400 cGy when adjuvant chemotherapy, which is now the standard of care, is used. RT is generally avoided in patients <3 years of age due to toxicity.

3. **Chemotherapy** allows for reduction of the dose of craniospinal irradiation and consequently a reduction in the long-term sequelae of treatment. Post-RT adjuvant chemotherapy is given to all patients ≥3 years of age. In patients <3 years of age, chemotherapy is usually given initially to delay or avoid RT. A standard adjuvant chemotherapy regimen usually consists of 8 cycles of lomustine, vincristine, and cisplatin given at 6-week intervals over approximately 1 year.

   Relapsed medulloblastoma may be treated with high-dose chemotherapy and autologous stem cell rescue. In addition, an inhibitor of the hedgehog pathway was shown to cause marked but transient tumor regression in a patient whose tumor had activation of the hedgehog pathway.

D. **Prognosis.** Patients with medulloblastomas who have had a gross total resection and show no evidence of tumor dissemination (standard risk) have a 5-year survival rate of 80% to 90%. In patients with disseminated tumor (high risk), the 5-year survival is 50% to 60%. The molecular subgroup Wnt is associated with the best prognosis with up to 100% 5-year survival in adults, and group 3 medulloblastomas have the worst prognosis with 32% 5-year survival.

VII. GERM-CELL TUMORS

A. **Pathology.** Germ-cell tumors arising in the nervous system are usually located in the pineal and suprasellar regions. They are of two basic types: germinomas and nongerminomatous germ-cell tumors. The former are highly sensitive to radiation and are analogous to systemic seminomas and dysgerminomas.

B. **Evaluation.** Because germ-cell tumors can readily disseminate in the neuraxis, all patients require complete staging, including contrast MRI of the brain and complete spine, CSF cytologic examination, and determination of serum and CSF alpha-fetoprotein and beta-human chorionic gonadotropin levels; CSF placental alkaline phosphatase may also be helpful.

C. **Treatment.** Surgical resection should be performed first with a goal of achieving a complete excision. If resection is not feasible, biopsy is necessary for histologic diagnosis. Resection constitutes complete therapy for the rare mature teratomas. Germinomas without evidence of neuraxis dissemination are treated with irradiation of the tumor and surrounding ventricular system; even those with positive markers can be treated with radiotherapy alone. Nongerminomatous germ-cell tumors and tumors with evidence of neuraxis dissemination are treated with craniospinal irradiation and chemotherapy. Regimens are similar to those used for systemic germ-cell tumors. The 5-year survival rate is over 90% for germinomas and may approach 75% for nongerminomas that are more resistant to therapy.

VIII. BENIGN NERVOUS SYSTEM TUMORS

A. **Meningiomas** are tumors arising from arachnoidal cells. Their incidence increases with age, and they are more common in women. Meningiomas may occur over the convexities, parasagittal along the falx, along the sphenoid wing, retroclival, or along the thoracic spine. Although most of these tumors are benign, some are histologically atypical or malignant. The tumors are recognized radiographically by their extra-axial location and their dense, homogeneous pattern of contrast enhancement. Patients with small asymptomatic meningiomas can be followed. Treatment is surgical resection, which is often curative. Recurrent tumors may be treated with RT or stereotactic radiosurgery. In addition to the classically known *NF2* mutations in meningiomas, additional unique mutations in *TRAF7*, *KLF4*, *AKT1*, and *SMO* have been identified; these mutations are potentially actionable but there are no data yet to confirm efficacy with targeted therapy.

B. **Craniopharyngiomas** are congenital, cystic suprasellar tumors thought to arise from epithelial remnants of Rathke pouch. They present with dysfunction of the optic chiasm or hypothalamic–pituitary axis as a result of tumor compression. The tumor may contain calcifications and an oily cellular debris that causes a severe chemical meningitis if a cyst ruptures into the spinal fluid. The tumor is histologically benign and can be cured by total resection. Unfortunately, this is often not possible, and RT may be required for tumor control.

C. **Pituitary adenoma.** Adenomas of the pituitary gland can be either secreting or nonsecreting tumors. Secretory tumors can cause acromegaly (growth hormone), infertility and galactorrhea (prolactin), or Cushing disease (adrenocorticotropic hormone, ACTH). These tumors are often microadenomas (<1 cm), but are usually visualized on MRI. Nonsecretory tumors are typically macroadenomas (>1 cm) and cause bitemporal hemianopsia because of optic chiasm compression, pituitary apoplexy resulting from hemorrhage into the tumor, or hypopituitarism. Treatment of either micro- or macroadenomas may consist of surgical resection, usually by the transsphenoidal route. However, secretory tumors may be treated pharmacologically: prolactinomas with cabergoline and growth hormone–secreting tumors with somatostatin or an analog such as octreotide. Recurrent tumors may require RT.

D. **Vestibular schwannoma (acoustic neuroma).** Vestibular schwannomas arise from the vestibular branch of the eighth cranial nerve. Initial symptoms are sensorineural hearing loss, tinnitus, and vertigo. Involvement of adjacent neural structures can cause facial weakness, facial numbness, dysphagia, and ataxia. On contrast-enhanced MRI scans, these tumors are seen as a homogeneous, densely enhancing mass that follows the eighth cranial nerve into the internal auditory canal; the diagnosis is usually clear on MRI. Management depends on the extent of hearing loss and whether bilateral tumors are present, but therapeutic options include surgical resection and stereotactic radiosurgery. Bilateral vestibular schwannomas constitute a diagnosis of neurofibromatosis II. Spinal schwannomas cause a radiculomyelopathy and can be cured by total resection. Rarely, these tumors can have sarcomatous degeneration.

IX. SPECIAL CLINICAL PROBLEMS

A. **Seizures.** Seizures occur in about 25% to 30% of all brain tumor patients. Once a patient has had a seizure, they are maintained on anticonvulsants. Anticonvulsants that induce hepatic enzymes (e.g., phenytoin, carbamazepine) can enhance chemotherapy metabolism, resulting in subtherapeutic serum levels. These drugs also tend to be associated with greater sedation and a worse toxicity profile. Therefore, newer agents are used more commonly. Prophylactic anticonvulsants are ineffective in the prevention of seizures in brain tumor patients who have not had a seizure. They should be avoided.

1. **Levetiracetam** is the first-line choice of antiepileptic agents in brain tumor patients because of its efficacy, favorable toxicity profile, lack of hepatic microsomal enzyme induction, and an option of IV administration. The starting dose is usually 500 mg bid and can be increased to 1,500 mg bid titrated to seizure control. Serum levels are available but do not correlate well with seizure control. Side effects include personality change, depression, and sedation.

2. **Lacosamide** is effective for focal seizures and is generally well tolerated. It has recently been used as an adjunctive agent to treat status epilepticus in patients with brain tumors, as it can be loaded intravenously to achieve a therapeutic serum level and has minimal interaction with other drugs. The starting dose is usually 50 mg bid and titrated up to 100 mg bid. When loading is indicated, 200 mg is given either orally or intravenously. Side effects include dizziness, headache, nausea, diplopia, fatigue, and sedation.

3. **Lamotrigine** is a highly effective antiepileptic for patients with brain tumors. It needs to be titrated slowly and can interact with valproic acid. The dose is usually 225 to 375 mg/d in two divided doses when used as an adjunct or monotherapy in patients not receiving valproate or other enzyme-inducing antiepileptics; it is only available in an oral preparation. Patients taking concurrent valproic acid usually require less and those taking concurrent enzyme-inducing antiepileptic agents may need more lamotrigine.

4. **Other anticonvulsants,** such as gabapentin, topiramate, vigabatrin, clobazam, and zonisamide, can be used at the discretion of the treating physician. Older agents such as carbamazepine, valproic acid, and phenytoin are usually reserved for patients with poorly controlled seizures.

B. **Hydrocephalus** can result from obstruction of CSF pathways, especially with intraventricular tumors or tumors in the upper brainstem. Patients with hydrocephalus present with headache, nausea, vomiting, gait ataxia, urinary incontinence, and progressive lethargy. Large ventricles above the level of obstruction can be diagnosed with a noncontrast CT scan. Communicating hydrocephalus may also develop in patients treated for a brain tumor; one sees progressive ventricular enlargement on serial neuroimaging. Patients who have received cranial RT are also at a higher risk for developing hydrocephalus. Treatment of both forms of hydrocephalus consists of placement of a ventriculoperitoneal shunt.

C. **Radiation necrosis** can result from RT and is common after high-dose and SRS. Clinically and radiographically, it is indistinguishable from tumor recurrence. PET or perfusion MRI may be useful in distinguishing tumor recurrence from radiation necrosis, but even these techniques cannot distinguish tumor progression from radiation necrosis reliably. Radiation necrosis can be treated with dexamethasone, but surgical debulking is often required to relieve mass effect and to provide a definite tissue diagnosis.

D. **Deep vein thrombosis (DVT)** occurs in about 20% of patients with high-grade gliomas and is optimally treated with anticoagulation. Studies have not shown that anticoagulation poses increased risk for intracranial hemorrhage into a brain tumor.

E. **Herniation** results from progressive mass effect in patients with large, edematous tumors. Herniation can be central in the case of midline tumors and hydrocephalus, uncal in the case of hemispheric lesions, or tonsillar in the case of posterior fossa tumors. Once recognized, herniation is an emergency that must be treated to decrease intracranial pressure. These interventions will reduce intracranial pressure, but they will only temporize until definitive treatment is initiated. The emergency methods include the following:

1. Elevation of the head of the bed
2. Hyperventilation to a P_{CO_2} of about 30 mm Hg
3. Creation of an osmotic gradient by administration of mannitol at 0.5 to 2 g/kg IV (usually 50 to 100 g in adults) or hypertonic saline, 300 mL 3% solution
4. Dexamethasone, up to 100 mg IV followed by 16 to 40 mg/24 hours depending on symptoms

Suggested Readings

Cairncross G, Wang M, Shaw E, et al. Phase III trial of chemoradiotherapy for anaplastic oligodendroglioma: long-term results of RTOG 9402. *J Clin Oncol* 2013;31:337.

Chinot OL, Wick W, Mason W, et al. Bevacizumab plus radiotherapy-temozolomide for newly diagnosed glioblastoma. *N Engl J Med* 2014;370:709.

Clark VE, Erson-Omay EZ, Serin A, et al. Genomic analysis of non-NF2 meningiomas reveals mutations in TRAF7, KLF4, AKT1, and SMO. *Science* 2013;339:1077.

Gajjar A, Bowers DC, Karajannis MA, et al. Pediatric brain tumors: innovative genomic information is transforming the diagnostic and clinical landscape. *J Clin Oncol* 2015;33:2986.

Gilbert MR, Dignam JJ, Armstrong TS, et al. A randomized trial of bevacizumab for newly diagnosed glioblastoma. *N Engl J Med* 2014;370:699.

Jordan JT, Gerstner ER, Batchelor TT, et al. Glioblastoma care in the elderly. *Cancer* 2016;122:189.

Preusser M, Lim M, Hafler DA, et al. Prospects of immune checkpoint modulators in the treatment of glioblastoma. *Nat Rev Neurol* 2015;11:504.

Shaw EG, Wang M, Coons SW, et al. Randomized trial of radiation therapy plus procarbazine, lomustine, and vincristine chemotherapy for supratentorial adult low-grade glioma: initial results of RTOG 9802. *J Clin Oncol* 2012;30:3065.

The Cancer Genome Atlas Research Network. Comprehensive, integrative genomic analysis of diffuse lower-grade gliomas. *N Engl J Med* 2015;372:2481.

Thomas AA, Brennan CW, DeAngelis LM, et al. Emerging therapies for glioblastoma. *JAMA Neurol* 2014;71:1437.

Thomas AA, Omuro A. Current role of anti-angiogenic strategies for glioblastoma. *Curr Treat Options Oncol* 2014;15:551.

Vecht CJ, Kerkhof M, Duran-Pena A. Seizure prognosis in brain tumors: new insights and evidence-based management. *Oncologist* 2014;19:751.

16 Endocrine Neoplasms

Carolyn Maxwell

I. GENERAL CONSIDERATIONS

Cancers of endocrine glands constitute about 3% of all malignancies. Most malignant neoplasms derived from endocrine organs are not associated with clinical endocrinopathies, although several do produce unique syndromes and biochemical markers.

A. Steroid hormones are usually produced by the adrenal cortex and gonads, whether that tissue is healthy or cancerous. Occasionally, human chorionic gonadotropin (hCG)-producing tumors of the placenta or other organs (e.g., lung) have the capacity to transform androgens into estrogens.

B. Peptide hormones and catecholamines

1. **Amine precursor uptake and decarboxylation (APUD) cells** are theoretically derived from embryonic neuroectoderm (melanocytes, thyroid C cells, adrenal medulla, paraspinal ganglia, argentaffin cells of the intestine). These cells produce hormone mediators such as serotonin, catecholamines, histamine, and kinins. Neoplasia of these tissues gives rise to carcinoid tumors, pheochromocytoma (PCC), and medullary thyroid cancer; these tumors may also produce peptide hormones (e.g., adrenocorticotropic hormone [ACTH] and vasoactive intestinal polypeptide [VIP]) in addition to their natural products. Other peptide-producing endocrine tissues (e.g., parathyroid, pancreatic islet) demonstrate some APUD characteristics, even though they may not be derived from neuroectoderm.

2. **Peptide hormones**, such as ACTH, hCG, and calcitonin, are produced by a wide variety of neoplastic tissues that may or may not synthesize detectable amounts of these hormones. Many of these peptides are synthesized as a *prehormone*. A segment of prehormone is enzymatically cleaved to form a storage molecule, a *prohormone*. The prohormone is further cleaved into the active hormone that is secreted into the blood.

3. **Gastrointestinal hormones**, such as insulin, glucagon, somatostatin, VIP, and gastrin, are normally produced by gut endocrine cells and the pancreatic islets. Neoplasms of these tissues commonly produce one or more of these hormones; gut hormones are also normally produced in the brain and may be products of a wide variety of other neoplasms.

C. Multiple endocrine neoplasias (MEN) are inherited, mendelian-dominant, endocrine tumor syndromes. Two categories of the syndrome are recognized.

1. **MEN1** (Wermer syndrome; menin tumor suppressor gene located at chromosome 11q13)

   a. Pituitary tumors (acromegaly, nonfunctioning adenoma, prolactinoma, or ACTH-producing adenoma)

   b. Pancreatic islet cell tumors, including gastrinoma, VIPoma, glucagonoma, and insulinoma

   c. Parathyroid adenomas

2. **MEN2.** Medullary carcinoma of the thyroid is present in all patients with this syndrome. Cushing syndrome may develop as a consequence of ectopic ACTH production by medullary carcinoma or PCC.

   a. **MEN2A** (Sipple syndrome; *ret* oncogene located at chromosome 10q11)

      (1) Medullary carcinoma of the thyroid

      (2) Pheochromocytoma (often bilateral)

      (3) Parathyroid hyperplasia or adenomas

   b. **MEN2B** (*ret* oncogene located at 10q11)

      (1) Medullary carcinoma of the thyroid.

      (2) Pheochromocytoma (bilateral).

      (3) Multiple mucosal ganglioneuromas (lips, tongue, eyelids).

      (4) Marfanoid body habitus, high-arched palate, pes cavus, diverticula, and sugar-loaf skull often accompany the endocrine abnormalities in MEN2B.

II. CARCINOID TUMORS

A. **Epidemiology.** Carcinoid cancers are rare, although the incidence is rising, probably due to increased rates of imaging and endoscopy.

B. **Pathology and natural history**

1. **Primary tumor.** Carcinoid tumors belong to the APUD system of tumors. The primary tumors are usually small. Previously, the majority of GI tract carcinoids were found in the small intestine. With the onset of routine screening colonoscopy, a greater number of rectal tumors are now being reported. They may also develop in the stomach, lung, ovary, and rarely other organs. Appendiceal carcinoids are common but are usually of no clinical significance.

2. **Classification.** Traditionally, carcinoid tumors have been classified according to their embryonic origin: foregut (gastric, bronchial), midgut (small intestine, appendix, cecum), and hindgut (distal colon, rectal, and genitourinary). This classification is generally useful in that it predicts the likelihood of the carcinoid syndrome, which is more common with tumors of midgut origin.

3. **Metastases** are common with all types of carcinoid tumors. They tend to develop primarily in the liver. Bone metastases, which are often osteoblastic, also occur. Carcinoid metastases are indolent or slowly progressive and evolve over many years. Carcinoid tumors tend to produce desmoplastic responses, which can result in mesenteric fibrosis and bowel obstruction ("parachute intestine").

4. **Tumor products.** Hormonally active tumors occur in 30% to 50% of patients and produce a variety of potentially lethal complications (*carcinoid syndrome*).

   a. **Small intestine carcinoids** never produce the carcinoid syndrome in the absence of liver metastases; the responsible hormonal mediators are degraded in their first pass through the liver.

   b. **Benign and malignant lung carcinoids** occur with about equal frequency; those that produce the carcinoid syndrome are malignant. Lung carcinoids can potentially produce hormonal effects without metastasizing; active tumor products may pass directly into the circulation without being filtered by the liver. Bronchial carcinoids that produce ACTH or growth hormone–releasing hormone (GH-RH) may be benign, and Cushing syndrome or acromegaly may be the only endocrine manifestation.

   c. **Symptomatic ovarian carcinoids** are rarely associated with liver metastases.

    d. Humoral mediators of the carcinoid syndrome are serotonin, histamine, kinins, prostaglandins, and other hormonally active tumor products.

      (1) The major source of serotonin is dietary tryptophan, which normally is mostly metabolized to nicotinic acid. In carcinoid syndrome, tryptophan metabolism is directed to the production of serotonin. Most patients with carcinoid syndrome develop chemical evidence of niacin deficiency, and some may develop clinically recognizable pellagra.

      (2) Other hormones and hormone metabolites that are found in some patients with carcinoid include calcitonin, gastrin, GH-RH, and ACTH. These substances may or may not produce clinical syndromes, but they should be searched for in patients with carcinoid and serum calcium abnormalities, peptic ulcer, acromegaly, or Cushing syndrome.

C. Diagnosis

  1. Symptoms: Endocrinologically inactive carcinoids. Most carcinoid tumors are endocrinologically inactive. Patients who have these tumors may have appendicitis, bowel obstruction, early satiety, or a painful, enlarged liver that results from metastases. Bronchial carcinoids may produce cough, hemoptysis, or frequent pulmonary infections.

  2. Symptoms: Endocrinologically active carcinoids

    a. Humoral mediators produce attacks of flushing, diarrhea, hypotension, light-headedness, and bronchospasm in various combinations. Attacks may be spontaneous or precipitated by emotional stress, alcohol ingestion, exercise, eating, or vigorous palpation of a liver that contains metastatic deposits.

    b. Heart failure commonly occurs in patients with long-standing carcinoid symptoms and appears to be related to serotonin excess. Ileal carcinoids with hepatic metastases produce tricuspid and/or pulmonic valve stenosis and insufficiency. A patent foramen ovale or bronchial carcinoids with venous drainage into the left atrium can occasionally produce mitral valve disease.

  3. Physical findings

    a. The characteristic flush differs somewhat according to the site of the primary tumor.

      (1) Ileal carcinoid. Purple flush involves the upper trunk and face and usually lasts <30 minutes.

      (2) Bronchial carcinoid. Deep, dusky purple flush over the entire body

      (3) Gastric carcinoid. Generalized urticaria-like, pruritic, and painful wheals, probably related to histamine production

    b. Chronic skin changes may result from repeated episodes of flushing, especially with bronchial carcinoids, which cause thickening of the facial features, telangiectasias, enlargement of the salivary glands, and leonine facies. A pellagrous skin rash characterized by photosensitivity, atrophy of the lingual mucosa, and thickened skin may develop.

    c. Right heart failure with evidence of tricuspid or pulmonic valve disease.

    d. Hepatomegaly.

    e. Cushing syndrome and, occasionally, acromegaly.

  4. Laboratory studies

    a. In all patients, routine blood tests, particularly liver function tests.

    b. In patients with symptoms, or tumors of midgut origin, measurement of 24-hour urine collection for 5-hydroxyindoleacetic acid (5-HIAA) is recommended. Measurement of plasma serotonin levels is not generally recommended due to low specificity.

    c. **Interpretation.** A urine level of 5-HIAA >9 mg per 24 hours in patients without malabsorption or >30 mg per 24 hours in patients with malabsorption is pathognomonic for carcinoid unless interfering foods or drugs have been ingested. The magnitude of 5-HIAA excretion in the urine roughly corresponds to the tumor volume; 5-HIAA excretion can also be used to monitor therapy.

    d. **Chromogranin A (CgA)** is a soluble protein found in secretory granules in a variety of neuroendocrine cell types. Plasma CgA is elevated in nearly all patients with carcinoid tumors but is nonspecific, as it is also elevated in patients with other neuroendocrine tumors. Serum CgA may also be elevated in patients receiving proton pump inhibitors. Due to this nonspecificity, CgA should not be used as a screening test for carcinoid tumor, but once the diagnosis is established by other means, it is a useful tumor marker in the monitoring of disease progression and response to therapy.

5. **Imaging**

    a. **Computed tomography (CT)** of the abdomen, or chest in the case of suspected bronchial carcinoid. Most tumors are hypervascular, and therefore, detection is enhanced with the use of intravenous contrast. The classic finding for midgut tumors is a mass with spoke-like projections radiating into the mesenteric fat. Calcifications are often present.

    b. **Magnetic resonance imaging (MRI)** may have better sensitivity in the detection of liver metastases.

    c. **Upper and lower endoscopy** may be helpful if unable to find the primary tumor with CT or MRI.

    d. **Somatostatin receptor scintigraphy (SRS)** using radiolabeled somatostatin to detect tumors that express high numbers of somatostatin receptors, as carcinoid tumors often do. It offers the advantages of whole body scanning (WBS), and provision of information as to the degree of receptor expression, which is useful if somatostatin-based therapy is to be considered.

6. A **histologic** diagnosis is essential for management. Biopsy the site that is associated with the least morbidity and that has been determined by noninvasive tests to be probably affected.

D. **Management.** These patients often survive for >10 years without antitumor treatment. Patients with endocrinologically active tumors are at especially high risk for complications from any procedure requiring anesthesia. Therapy should be focused on controlling the endocrine symptoms.

1. **Surgery** is the first-line treatment for patients with localized primary carcinoids or resectable metastatic tumors. The extent of and approach to surgery is dependent upon the size and location of the tumor. For example, appendiceal tumors <2 cm generally only require an appendectomy, whereas a right hemicolectomy may be considered for those >2 cm. For liver-predominant disease, surgical resection of metastatic disease, when possible, is recommended when potential for cure is present.

2. **Pharmacologic therapy** for tumor stability may be considered as a second-line treatment.

    a. **Somatostatin analogs** (octreotide, lanreotide) have some effect on delayed progression of tumor, in addition to their widely used effect of controlling symptoms of the carcinoid syndrome. Efficacy for tumor stability is best demonstrated in tumors with somatostatin receptor positivity arising from the small bowel. The use of radiolabeled somatostatin analogs to delay neuroendocrine tumor (NET) progression is currently being studied, but data are limited.

    b. Interferon is gathering evidence for utility in tumor size stabilization, as well as control of tumor secretion. It may be considered as a second-line agent, if somatostatin analog is ineffective. The potential benefit must be weighed against poor tolerability, with side effects including flu-like illness, depression, and autoimmune thyroid disease.

    c. Everolimus is an inhibitor of the mammalian target of rapamycin (mTOR), and treatment with it resulted in a significant improvement in progression-free survival when compared to placebo (11 vs. 4 months).

    d. Cytotoxic chemotherapy is not the first-line standard approach to treatment of carcinoid tumors but may be an option of last resort in progressive disease when other options have failed or are not feasible. There is no general agreement on when (or even if) chemotherapy should be started in patients with malignant carcinoid. Single-agent therapy with 5-fluorouracil (5-FU), streptozocin, cyclophosphamide, doxorubicin, dacarbazine, and temozolomide have been studied, as well as combination therapies, with variable results.

3. Hepatic artery occlusion via embolization, chemoembolization, or radio-embolization has been used to palliate endocrine symptoms or pain. Objective regression of manifestations occurs in 60% of patients for a median of 4 months. Side effects of arterial occlusion include fever, nausea, and liver function test abnormalities. No clear advantage of a single embolization modality has emerged.

4. Ablation of hepatic metastases may be of benefit for small tumors. This is done most often by radiofrequency, but cryoablation and microwave ablation techniques are also employed. This treatment is reserved for tumors <3 cm and can be used as an adjunct to surgery or in place of resection in nonsurgical candidates.

5. Radiation therapy (RT) is used to palliate liver or bone pain caused by far-advanced metastatic disease unresponsive to other treatments. However, carcinoid tumors are relatively radioresistant.

6. Pharmacologic management of carcinoid syndrome. It is probably not possible to control the symptoms of carcinoid syndrome completely with aggressive dietary tryptophan restriction and high-dose antiserotonin drugs alone.

    a. Somatostatin analogs such as octreotide and lanreotide reduce the production of 5-HIAA and ameliorate symptoms in about 90% of patients. They are the mainstay of treatment for nearly all symptoms of the carcinoid syndrome. The octreotide dosage is usually 100 to 600 mcg SC daily in two to four divided doses. More popular are long-acting depot forms of octreotide and lanreotide; octreotide LAR 20 to 30 mg IM or lanreotide 60 to 120 mg SC are given every 28 days. Side effects of both octreotide and lanreotide include abdominal cramping, cholelithiasis, and hyperglycemia.

    b. Hypotension, the most life-threatening complication of carcinoid syndrome, is mediated by kinins (and perhaps prostaglandins) and can be precipitated by catecholamines. β-Adrenergic drugs (e.g., dopamine, epinephrine) must be strictly avoided because they may aggravate hypotension. Pure α-adrenergic (methoxamine, norepinephrine) and vasoconstrictive (angiotensin) agents are preferred for treating hypotension in carcinoid syndrome.

    c. Flushing is mediated by kinins and histamine and may respond to several agents, including prochlorperazine, phenoxybenzamine, cyproheptadine, and methyldopa. Prednisone is useful in patients with bronchial carcinoids. The combined use of H_1- and H_2-receptor antagonists (e.g., diphenhydramine and cimetidine) has been effective in patients with carcinoid flush and documented hypersecretion of histamine. Monoamine oxidase inhibitors *are contraindicated* in carcinoid syndrome because they block serotonin catabolism and can aggravate symptoms.

  d. Bronchospasm is mediated by histamine and managed with aminophylline. Adrenergic agents, such as albuterol, do not appear to worsen bronchospasm and may also be used with caution, since they may cause hypotension.

  e. Diarrhea is mediated by serotonin and is often difficult to control. Treatment in refractory cases include

  (1) Loperamide or diphenoxylate and atropine

  (2) Tincture of opium and other opiates

  (3) Belladonna alkaloids and phenobarbital combination

  (4) Ondansetron

  f. Carcinoid crisis. Patients with carcinoid syndrome are at high risk for the development of severe flushing, bronchospasm, and hypotension (carcinoid crisis) during surgery. This is due to both effect of anesthesia as well as release of hormone from tumor manipulation. Stimulation of adrenergic hormone release and use of drugs that induce hypotension (morphine, succinylcholine, and curare) must be minimized.

  (1) Preoperative period. Patients with carcinoid syndrome, or with elevated urine 5-HIAA levels, should be given octreotide 100 mcg SC three times daily for 2 weeks prior to surgery to block the release of tumor products.

  (2) During and after surgery. Octreotide should be given intravenously at a rate of 50 to 200 mcg/h, starting before anesthesia. Increased doses should be given if flushing or hypotension occurs. Octreotide should be tapered gradually over 1 week postoperatively.

E. Special clinical problems associated with carcinoid syndrome

  1. Bowel obstruction may result from dense fibrosis of the mesentery. Surgical relief is often impossible. Patients may improve with simple nasogastric decompression and fluid replacement.

  2. Carcinoid heart disease manifests as right heart failure as a result of tricuspid and pulmonic valve lesions. These changes develop with far-advanced carcinoid syndrome, which has a poor prognosis independent of the heart lesions. Treatment of the tumor does not usually improve the valve lesions. Surgical valve repair is the only effective treatment for carcinoid heart disease and, despite a high surgical mortality rate, has been shown to result in overall better survival rates when compared to medical treatment of valve disease.

III. THYROID CANCER

A. Epidemiology and etiology

  1. Incidence. Thyroid cancer accounts for about 4% of visceral malignancies; there are approximately 63,000 new cases and 1,900 cancer deaths in the United States annually. The risk increases with age. Women are affected more than men in a ratio of 3:1. Increasing incidence of thyroid cancer over the past 10 to 15 years is likely attributable to the increased detection of small tumors via widespread availability of neck ultrasound.

  2. Radiation exposure. Radiation fallout and RT given to the neck region for both malignancy as well as benign conditions (such as acne in teenagers or enlarged tonsils or thymus glands in children) increase the risk for thyroid cancer, particularly the papillary type. There is a dose–response curve, with increased rates of thyroid cancer seen even with exposure to low radiation doses (100 mGy). This risk appears to diminish when radiation exposure occurs after the age of 20.

3. **Hereditary factors.** Medullary cancer of the thyroid may arise sporadically or as a dominantly inherited syndrome of MEN2 (see Section I.C.2). Thyroid tumors also occur frequently in Cowden multiple hamartoma syndrome, familial adenomatous polyposis, and Carney complex.

B. **Pathology and natural history.** The more aggressive histologic subtypes of thyroid cancer tend to affect older patients.

1. **Papillary cancers** (80% of thyroid cancers in adults) affect younger patients (peak incidence 30 to 50 years). Histologically, the tumor cells may be arranged in either papillary or follicular patterns; the diagnosis of papillary carcinoma is based on nuclear features, not on the presence or absence of follicles. Multifocal disease within the thyroid is common. Regional lymph nodes that drain the thyroid are involved in half of patients. 2% to 10% of patients have distant metastases at the time of diagnosis, usually to lungs and bone.

   a. **Noninvasive follicular thyroid neoplasm with papillary-like nuclear features (NIFTP)** is a recent reclassification of fully encapsulated tumors of the follicular variant of papillary thyroid cancer. The reclassification purposely omits the word carcinoma from the diagnosis, reflecting extensive evidence that these tumors are indolent and, once removed, have very low to zero risk of recurrence. Tumors classified as such do not need subsequent treatment with radioiodine nor radiographic or biochemical surveillance monitoring as is done for those classified as carcinoma.

2. **Follicular cancers** (10% of thyroid cancers) have a peak incidence at 40 to 60 years of age. They tend to invade blood vessels and to metastasize hematogenously to visceral sites, particularly bone. Lymph node metastases are relatively rare, especially compared with papillary cancers. Follicular carcinoma must be distinguished from adenoma by the presence of tumor extension through the capsule or by vascular invasion.

3. **Anaplastic cancers** (3% of thyroid cancers) occur most often in patients older than 60 years of age. Anaplastic thyroid cancers are aggressive cancers, which rapidly invade surrounding local tissues and metastasize to distant organs.

4. **Medullary thyroid cancer** (2% to 5% of thyroid cancers) is a neuroendocrine tumor of the C cells of the thyroid. About 25% of all tumors occur as part of the MEN2 syndrome. Medullary tumors secrete calcitonin and carcinoembryonic antigen (CEA). Metastases are mostly found in the neck and mediastinal lymph nodes and may calcify. Widespread visceral metastases occur late.

5. **Hürthle cell cancer** is a variant of follicular carcinoma and has a relatively aggressive metastatic course.

6. **Other tumors** found in the thyroid include lymphomas (1% to 2% of all thyroid cancers), a variety of soft tissue sarcomas, and metastatic cancers from kidney, colon and other primary sites.

C. **Diagnosis**

1. **Symptoms and signs**

   a. **Asymptomatic patients.** An increasing number of thyroid cancers are found incidentally, when thyroid nodules are noted during neck imaging for other reasons, or at the time of thyroidectomy done for other reasons.

   b. **Symptoms.** Some patients with thyroid cancer complain of an enlarging mass in the neck. Hoarseness may be the result of recurrent laryngeal nerve paralysis. Neck pain or dysphagia occasionally is a complaint.

   c. **Physical findings.** Thyroid cancer may be found on routine physical examination as a mass in the thyroid or in the midline up to the base of the tongue (thyroglossal duct remnant). The masses are often fixated to surrounding tissue. Thyroid masses <1 to 2 cm in diameter often are not palpable. Cervical lymph nodes are sometimes palpable. Anaplastic cancer is often manifested by obvious masses infiltrating the skin and soft tissues of the neck or by respiratory distress.

2. **Laboratory studies**
   a. **Routine studies.** Serum TSH should be measured in the initial evaluation of a thyroid nodule, to evaluate for a toxic nodule.
   b. **Radionuclide thyroid scan** (usually ^{123}I) should be obtained in nonpregnant patients with thyroid nodules who have a suppressed serum TSH, in order to document the existence of a "hot" nodule. If a nodule is found to be hyperfunctioning, the likelihood of the nodule harboring malignancy is quite low, and tissue sampling for cancer is not routinely recommended. Nonfunctional "cold" nodules are found in 90% of patients with palpable nodules, but only about 10% of cold nodules prove to be cancer. Routine isotope scanning of all thyroid nodules is therefore not indicated unless serum TSH is low.
   c. **Thyroid ultrasonography** is the gold standard imaging modality in determining the size and location of a nodule, diagnosing cystic lesions, detecting nonpalpable nodules or lymphadenopathy, and documenting the presence of features suggestive of malignancy (e.g., microcalcifications within the nodule, irregular borders, extrathyroidal extension). Purely cystic lesions, found in about 10% of patients with palpable nodules, are reported to be malignant in <1% of cases. Benign and malignant lesions cannot be confidently distinguished by ultrasonography if they contain mixed solid and cystic components or are entirely solid.
   d. **Serum calcitonin assay.** While it is not currently recommended for all patients, those with a family history of medullary thyroid cancer or other features of MEN2 should have serum calcitonin measured. This may also be pursued if there are cytologic features suggestive of medullary thyroid carcinoma. Patients with elevated serum calcitonin require neck exploration regardless of findings on physical examination or sonography.

3. **Thyroid gland biopsy**
   a. **Needle aspiration biopsy** is an invaluable tool for cytologic diagnosis of thyroid nodules and for preventing unnecessary thyroidectomies. Ultrasound-guided fine needle aspiration (FNA) has superior diagnostic value over palpation-guided and is now the standard of care. The overall accuracy of needle biopsy of the thyroid is >95%. For benign lesions, the false-negative rate is 5% to 10%. Only about 10% of nodules are cancerous.
   b. **Selection of nodules for biopsy** depends upon the size and sonographic features of individual nodules. Due to the high incidence of thyroid nodules and relatively low percentage that contain malignancy, biopsy of all nodules is neither recommended nor feasible. Criteria for pursuing cytologic evaluation of nodules have been set with the aim to avoid biopsying those nodules with low potential to cause clinically meaningful disease. There is mounting evidence that the presence of suspicious sonographic features is more predictive than size alone for detecting malignancy.
      (1) Nodules with a high suspicion pattern (solid, hypoechoic, irregular borders, microcalcifications, extrathyroidal extension) should be biopsied when >1 cm. A size cutoff of 1 cm may also be used for thyroid

nodules that demonstrate ^{18}F-fluorodeoxyglucose (FDG) uptake on positron emission scanning (PET), which increases the likelihood of malignancy.

(2) Nodules that lack these features should be biopsied when >1.5 to 2 cm.

(3) Nodules <1 cm should not routinely be biopsied, unless there is high suspicion for malignancy based on other clinical factors.

D. **Survival and prognostic factors**

1. **Papillary adenocarcinomas.** Only about 5% of patients die as a result of thyroid cancer. Even with distant metastases, patients often survive many years without therapy.

a. **Factors that adversely affect prognosis**, which both increase the recurrence rate and decrease the survival rate are as follows:

(1) Age > 45 years.

(2) Size of nodule >4 cm.

(3) Soft tissue invasion.

(4) Presence of extensive lymph node involvement (bilateral, or >3 cm metastatic node).

(5) Distant metastases.

(6) Residual tumor fails to take up ^{131}I.

(7) Subtotal thyroidectomy (compared with total or "near-total" thyroidectomy) for larger tumors.

(8) Probably, postoperative therapy with thyroid hormone alone (compared with thyroid hormone and ^{131}I) in patients with advanced tumors.

(9) There is mounting evidence that tumors with specific genetic mutations, particularly those of the *BRAF* and *TERT* genes, exhibit more aggressive disease courses. In some studies, these mutations have been linked to higher rates of both recurrence and cancer-specific mortality. Sufficient evidence of the prognostic value of these mutations does not yet exist to recommend routine testing.

2. **Follicular adenocarcinoma** without vascular invasion has essentially the same survival rate as papillary carcinoma for age-matched populations. With significant vascular invasion, the 10-year survival rate drops to 35%.

3. **Medullary carcinoma** without lymph node involvement is nearly always cured with surgery. With lymph node involvement, the 5-year survival rate decreases to 45%.

4. **Anaplastic carcinoma.** Nearly all patients die within 6 to 8 months. Aggressive therapy involving surgery, external RT, and chemotherapy may prolong survival in patients without distant metastases.

5. **Thyroid lymphoma.** Depending on the stage and histologic subtype, 5-year survival is 35% to 80%.

E. **Management of differentiated thyroid cancer (papillary and follicular)**; see Figure 16-1.

1. **Surgery** is the treatment of choice for all types of thyroid cancer. Total or near-total thyroidectomy is recommended for large (>4 cm) tumors or those with extrathyroidal extension or metastatic lymph nodes. For smaller tumors (1 to 4 cm) without evidence of spread beyond the thyroid, either total thyroidectomy or lobectomy may be considered. Lobectomy is the recommended operation for small, low-risk tumors (<1 cm) without clear indication for removal of the contralateral lobe, such as suspicious or large nodules in that lobe.

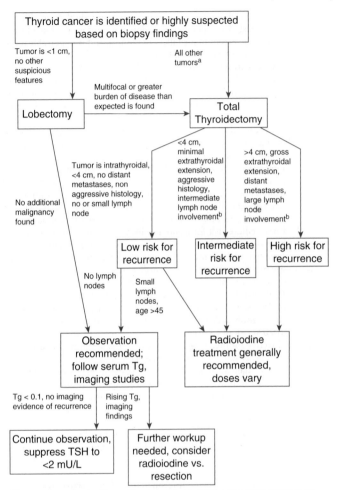

Figure 16-1 Papillary thyroid cancer initial management flow sheet.

[a]Tumors <4 cm without evidence of lymph node involvement, extrathyroidal extension, or suspicious nodules in the contralateral lobe may also be considered for lobectomy.

[b]Small lymph node involvement: ≤5 nodes with <0.2 cm focus of cancer; intermediate lymph node involvement: >5 nodes all of which are <3 cm; large lymph node involvement: any node >3 cm.

Recommendations based on the 2015 American Thyroid Association Guidelines (Haugen et al., *Thyroid* 2016;26(1):1).

    a. Lymph nodes that appear to be involved clinically or on sonography should be removed. A prophylactic central compartment dissection may be considered in advanced tumors without preoperative evidence of central nodal involvement or if there is known lateral node involvement. In the case of biopsy-proven central or lateral neck node metastases, therapeutic dissection is indicated. Routine radical or modified radical lateral neck dissection, however, does not improve the rate of survival or recurrence, except in medullary carcinoma, and is responsible for increasing the rate of major complications.

b. Complications. The major complications of thyroidectomy are hypoparathyroidism and vocal cord paralysis; death is rare. Combinations of these problems and other complications occur in 5% to 30% of patients subjected to total thyroidectomy; the incidence is doubled to tripled if neck dissection is added to the procedure.

2. **Risk stratification** to determine likelihood of disease recurrence is essential following surgery, as it informs the appropriate subsequent management and frequency of monitoring.

   a. Low risk for recurrence includes intrathyroidal tumors <4 cm, with no local or distant metastases (with the exception of low-volume cervical lymph node involvement), in which all macroscopic tumor has been resected, and the tumor does not have aggressive histologic subtype. Tumors in this category have a 1% to 10% risk of recurrence.

   b. Intermediate risk for recurrence includes tumors <4 cm with aggressive histology (tall cell, hobnail, columnar), vascular invasion, or minimal extrathyroidal extension. Presence of greater than five lymph nodes at a size of <3 cm are also at intermediate risk for recurrence. Tumors in this category have about a 15% to 30% risk of recurrence.

   c. High risk for recurrence includes tumors >4 cm, with gross extrathyroidal extension, known incomplete resection, distant metastases, or large lymph node burden (>3 cm). Tumors in this category have a 40% to 70% risk of recurrence.

3. **Radioactive iodine.** The true value of ^{131}I is not known and is difficult to determine because the isotope has been given to patients with thyroid cancer as part of standard practice for many years. In light of emerging evidence of minimal improvement of both disease-specific death as well as rates of recurrence with the use of ^{131}I in low-risk tumors, authorities have begun to recommend more constraint in the use of ^{131}I, with reservation of its use in those patients at highest risk for recurrence.

   a. Indications and dose recommendations for ^{131}I.

      (1) Tumors designated **low risk for recurrence** generally do not require ^{131}I therapy. If ^{131}I is to be given, lower ablative dose activity of 30 to 50 mCi is favored.

      (2) Tumors designated **intermediate risk for recurrence** have conflicting data as to whether ^{131}I therapy is beneficial. Those tumors that fall into the higher end of the spectrum with regard to aggressive potential, such as those with higher-volume lateral neck node involvement, or in patients >45 years of age are more favored for treatment. Dose activities in a range of 30 to 150 mCi are recommended.

      (3) In tumors designated **high risk for recurrence**, ^{131}I therapy is generally recommended. Clear benefit is seen in tumors >4 cm, those with gross extrathyroidal extension, and in the presence of distant metastases. In these patients, dose activities of 100 to 200 mCi is recommended, or alternatively, the use of dosimetry.

   b. Administration. ^{131}I may be given either when the patient demonstrates biochemical evidence of hypothyroidism or after treating the patient with recombinant human TSH. Both methods are based on the principle that

TSH stimulates ^{131}I uptake in both residual thyroid tissue and residual carcinoma and that it permits ablation of both.

  (1) Giving TSH. Recombinant human TSH (rh TSH, Thyrogen) stimulates ^{131}I uptake in thyroid remnants following thyroidectomy. 0.9 mg is injected intramuscularly, and then, a second dose is given 24 hours later. ^{131}I is then given 72 hours after the second rh TSH dose. Noninferiority to thyroid hormone withdrawal (see below) has been demonstrated in thyroid remnant ablation, and there is no evidence of difference in long-term outcomes as compared to the withdrawal method. Avoidance of prolonged hypothyroid symptoms and expedition of treatment make this an attractive option, and it is currently an acceptable alternative in patients at low and intermediate risk for recurrence.

  (2) Thyroid hormone withdrawal means allowing the patient to become hypothyroid following thyroidectomy. In some cases, patients are given triiodothyronine (T3) in a dose of 25 mcg PO twice daily for about 3 weeks to avoid prolonged hypothyroidism. T3 is then discontinued and serum TSH is measured 7 to 10 days later. If serum TSH exceeds 30 µU/mL, serum thyroglobulin (Tg) is measured and ^{131}I is given. This method is currently recommended for patients with distant metastases and with other features that place them at high risk for recurrence. It is also an acceptable option for patients with low and intermediate risk for recurrence.

  (3) Diet. To optimize ^{131}I uptake, patients must follow a low iodine diet for 7 to 10 days before and 2 to 3 days following ^{131}I administration.

4. **Thyroxine.** TSH suppression after thyroidectomy is essential because TSH stimulates the growth of most papillary and follicular tumors. Thyroxine is given in a dose sufficient to suppress serum TSH to low-normal or subnormal levels. Degree of appropriate TSH suppression is dependent upon the patient's risk for recurrence but must be balanced against risk of harm from excess thyroid hormone, such as in patients with concomitant tachyarrhythmia or low bone mass.

5. **Monitoring** for response to therapy and recurrence is achieved via biochemical testing and a variety of imaging modalities, most commonly neck ultrasonography. The interval at which monitoring should be performed, and what type of testing should be done is dictated both by the patient's initial risk for recurrence and their response to therapy.

  a. **Thyroglobulin.** Laboratory testing is centered around serum levels of Tg, which correlate with residual thyroid tissue (either normal or neoplastic) and can be used as a tumor marker after all normal thyroid remnants have been ablated. Serum Tg levels >1 to 2 ng/mL in patients receiving replacement thyroxine therapy indicate the presence of residual tumor. In a patient that has received ^{131}I ablation or therapy, the goal Tg is <0.2 ng/mL. In patients that have not undergone remnant ablation, a single Tg level is less specific for disease recurrence, as remaining nonresected thyroid tissue may physiologically produce Tg. It is useful, however, to follow Tg levels over time in these patients, as a steady increase is generally indicative of cancer recurrence. Within 6 to 12 months of initial surgery and radioiodine treatment, patients with an intermediate or high risk for recurrence should have an assessment of the serum Tg response to injected recombinant human TSH. Patients with residual tumor may demonstrate a Tg response even when the baseline serum Tg is <1 ng/mL. A stimulated Tg >2 ng/mL should prompt imaging workup to find recurrent disease. This testing is recommended at regular intervals for higher-risk patients. Low-risk patients with no biochemical or structural evidence of recurrence, and those with intermediate risk for recurrence with repeatedly low serum Tg upon stimulation, can be followed with measurement of unstimulated serum Tg levels. Measurement of stimulated Tg level is not routinely recommended in patients that have not undergone radioiodine ablation.

   b. **Neck ultrasonography** is done within 6 to 12 months of initial therapy, to evaluate for thyroid bed abnormalities and abnormal central and lateral neck lymphadenopathy. Biopsy of abnormal-appearing lymph nodes >8 to 10 mm is indicated. Subsequent routine neck ultrasound is performed on approximately a yearly basis, although this interval may be altered dependent upon risk for recurrence and response to therapy.

   c. **¹³¹I whole body scanning** (WBS) may be performed in conjunction with recombinant human TSH to seek focal areas of iodine uptake that correlate with metastatic disease. This testing is generally reserved for those with intermediate or high risk for recurrence, or when a stimulated Tg is elevated, suggesting disease recurrence. It is not generally useful in patients who have not had radioiodine ablation, as uptake in the thyroid remnant will be seen.

   d. **CT or MRI** of the neck and chest is useful in the detection of lymphadenopathy that is not well visualized with sonography, such as posterior cervical or mediastinal nodes.

   e. **¹⁸FDG-PET scanning** is recommended in patients with suspected recurrence in which ¹³¹I imaging does not reveal tumor. It is most useful in patients with high risk for recurrence or with poorly differentiated or aggressive histologic subtypes. Poorly differentiated tumors that lose the ability to concentrate iodine may uptake ¹⁸FDG and therefore be demonstrated on PET imaging.

6. **Relapsing disease** develops in about 12% of patients. Tumors that are not treatable by the combination of surgery, thyroxine therapy, and repeat doses of ¹³¹I respond poorly to external beam RT and systemic therapy. Tyrosine kinase inhibitors such as lenvatinib and sorafenib showed efficacy in metastatic disease. Vemurafenib or dabrafenib can be used in BRAF-mutated papillary thyroid cancer.

F. **Management of other forms of thyroid cancer**

   1. **Medullary**

      a. **Preoperative planning** with measurement of serum calcitonin and CEA is done as both may serve as a baseline tumor marker. Assessment for *RET* mutation is also recommended, with measurement of plasma metanephrines to preoperatively evaluate for PCC in those patients with known *RET* mutation or in whom *RET* status is unknown.

      b. **Surgery.** Total thyroidectomy is recommended in all cases of medullary thyroid carcinoma. Central and lateral neck dissections are done in the case of known metastatic nodal disease. Whether central and lateral neck dissection should be performed in patients without known nodal disease remains controversial.

      Postoperatively, thyroxine is indicated to replace thyroid function, but suppressing TSH does not serve to suppress tumor growth as in follicular-based cancers described above. Similarly, there is no role for radioiodine.

    c. Monitoring of calcitonin and CEA is done at regular intervals following surgery. The goal calcitonin is undetectable. Levels >150 pg/mL are strongly indicative of distant metastatic disease.

    d. Persistent disease is managed with a combination of surgical resection, external beam RT, local ablation, and, in some cases, observation, depending upon bulk of metastatic foci and tumor marker doubling time. Tyrosine kinase inhibitors (vandetanib, cabozantinib) have shown some efficacy in prolongation of disease-free survival.

  2. Anaplastic thyroid cancer has a mortality that approaches 100%. Treatment is therefore largely focused on palliation. Surgery is done for smaller intrathyroidal tumors, or those with resectable local disease, but most cases are detected after extrathyroidal invasion has occurred. External beam RT and chemotherapy are used both as primary and adjuvant therapy, and there is some evidence of benefit in the combination of these therapies. Special attention should be paid to end-of-life issues such as goals of care, airway securement, and nutrition.

G. Special clinical problems associated with thyroid cancer

  1. Hypoparathyroidism complicates total thyroidectomy in 10% to 30% of patients; it is rare after ^{131}I therapy. Hypoparathyroidism is transient in the majority of cases, and serum calcium levels normalize in 1 or 2 weeks.

    a. Acute therapy. Serum calcium levels and clinical evidence of hypocalcemia are checked daily following surgery for 1 to 2 days. If the serum calcium level is <8 mg/dL, oral calcium citrate (1 g four or five times daily) or calcium carbonate (2.5 g/d) is given; either preparation will provide about 1 g of elemental calcium per day. If the patient manifests tetany or the serum calcium is ≤6 mg/dL, intravenous calcium gluconate or lactate is given (1 g every 4 to 6 hours) and serum calcium levels are monitored more frequently.

    b. Chronic therapy. Patients with persistent hypocalcemia >1 to 2 weeks after thyroidectomy usually require chronic calcium supplements. Often, vitamin D therapy is necessary as well. Calcitriol is started at a dose of 0.25 mcg/d PO; calcium citrate or carbonate is continued. Serum calcium measurements are repeated weekly; if <8 mg/dL, the calcitriol is increased in 0.25-mcg increments weekly until the calcium level has normalized. Serum calcium should be maintained in the borderline low range (8.0 to 9.0 mg/dL) to avoid hypercalciuria.

  2. Permanent vocal dysfunction due to damage to the recurrent laryngeal or superior laryngeal nerves during thyroidectomy occurs in about 1% of patients. Transient voice symptoms occur in about 6%.

IV. PHEOCHROMOCYTOMA

A. Epidemiology and etiology. PCCs are rare tumors; they belong to the APUD system and produce symptoms by elaborating catecholamines. Extra-adrenal PCCs are called *paragangliomas*. Certain hereditary syndromes are associated with an increased risk for PCC or paraganglioma.

  1. Dominantly inherited MEN2 (see Section I.C)

  2. Dominantly transmitted PCC

  3. Neurofibromatosis type 1 (von Recklinghausen disease)

  4. von Hippel-Lindau disease

  5. Familial paraganglioma syndromes due to mutations in succinic dehydrogenase subunits B and D

As many as one-third of patients with an apparently sporadic PCC may, in fact, harbor a germ-line mutation in one of these genes. Screening for these mutations should be considered in all patients, and certainly performed in patients with bilateral, extra-adrenal, or malignant PCCs, patients with a family history of one of the syndromes, patients diagnosed with a PCC before the age of 20 years, or patients with other phenotypic features of one of the hereditary syndromes.

B. **Pathology and natural history**

1. **PCC originates** in the adrenal medulla (90% of patients) or in the paraganglia of the sympathetic nervous system. Bilateral PCC frequently occurs in inherited syndromes and in 10% of noninherited cases.

2. **Metastases** to bone, liver, and lung occur in 10% of cases of PCC, and about 20% of paragangliomas, despite a histologically benign appearance. Metastases frequently have an indolent growth pattern but are lethal because they often produce cardiovascular complications. Metastases are often detected at the time of diagnosis of the primary tumor but can appear up to 20 years later.

3. **Hyperglycemia** is common in patients with PCC. Patients also have an increased incidence of gallstones.

C. **Diagnosis**

1. **Symptoms and signs**

   a. **Symptoms.** The most common symptoms of PCC are episodes of various combinations of the following: headache, sweating, tachycardia, palpitations, pallor, nausea, and feeling of impending death. Episodes may be triggered by exercise, emotional upset, alcohol ingestion, physical examination in the area of the tumor, or micturition. Vague complaints of anxiety, tremulousness, fever, dyspnea, or angina are often mistaken for psychosomatic illness or thyrotoxicosis.

   b. **Hypertension** is present in 90% of patients. The hypertension is fixed (66% of patients) or paroxysmal (33%). Orthostatic hypotension occurs in 70% of patients.

   c. **Catecholamine cardiomyopathy.** Patients may have cardiovascular collapse after a vague history of arrhythmias and anxiety.

   d. **Patients with small tumors**, such as might be found when screening patients with a family history of a hereditary PCC syndrome or when evaluating patients with incidentally discovered adrenal masses, are often asymptomatic; the lack of symptoms does not exclude PCC.

2. **Selection of patients for study.** All patients with an incidentally discovered adrenal mass should be screened for PCC. The presence of PCC should be sought in patients with hypertension and any of the following:

   a. Age < 45 years.

   b. A family history of a hereditary PCC syndrome.

   c. Episodic attacks typical of the syndrome.

   d. Young patients without hypertension but with documented atrial arrhythmia, evidence of an unexplained hypermetabolic state, or cardiomyopathy should be screened for PCC and thyrotoxicosis.

3. **Chemical tests**

   a. **Catecholamine metabolites.** Measurement of plasma free metanephrines appears to be the most sensitive technique (98%) to detect PCC. Ideally, the sample should be drawn following an overnight fast and after the patient has been at rest, preferably supine, for 15 to 30 minutes. There is a 5% false-positive rate using this assay. Twenty-four–hour urine collections for measurement of fractionated metanephrines are nearly as sensitive and specific as plasma free metanephrines. Plasma catecholamine assays are also available but require meticulous technique in sample collection and handling and are susceptible to elevation from minimal stimulation. Elevated levels of catecholamines or their metabolites suggest the presence of PCC and mandate further studies.

(1) **Misleading elevations in catecholamine metabolites.** Many drugs affect either the metabolism or assay of catecholamines. In particular, phenothiazines, tricyclic antidepressants, drugs that are catecholamines (e.g., isoproterenol) or catecholamine releasers (e.g., ephedrine, amphetamines, methylxanthines), methyldopa, labetalol, phenoxybenzamine, acetaminophen, buspirone, monoamine oxidase inhibitors, sulfasalazine, and cocaine can falsely elevate both serum and urine catecholamines and their metabolites. If possible, these medications should be discontinued for up to 2 weeks before sampling. Additionally, physiologic stress from extreme illness and/or hospitalization raises catecholamines and should be taken into consideration when ordering and interpreting results collected from hospitalized patients.

(2) **Misleading low metanephrine values** may result from incomplete urine collections or from the use of α-methylparatyrosine, clonidine, reserpine, or guanethidine.

4. **Radiographic techniques** are used for localization of tumor in patients once clear biochemical evidence of PCC is established.

a. **CT** is preferred to MRI as the initial imaging modality. Chest, abdomen, and pelvis should be evaluated.

b. **MRI** is useful in patients with metastatic disease, particularly in the evaluation of head and neck paragangliomas.

c. **Isotope scanning** with ^{123}I-metaiodobenzylguanidine may be useful in demonstrating PCC, especially in extra-adrenal sites. Octreotide scanning appears to be less sensitive. Positron emission tomography scanning utilizing FDG or ^{18}F-fluoroDOPA has been reported to be particularly useful in cases of malignant PCC.

D. **Management**

1. **Pharmacologic control** of PCC is essential before invasive diagnostic tests or surgery is done.

a. Phenoxybenzamine, given in initial doses of 10 to 20 mg PO twice daily, is a pure α-adrenergic blocker that controls both episodic and fixed hypertension; doses are increased until blood pressure and episodes are well controlled. Other α-adrenergic blockers may also be used (e.g., doxazosin in doses up to 20 mg/d).

b. Propranolol, 10 to 40 mg PO given four times daily, is a β-adrenergic blocker that is useful for treating sweating, hypermetabolism, and arrhythmias. Propranolol should be used only after adequate α-adrenergic blockade is established to avoid worsening of hypertension.

c. Labetalol, a combined α- and β-adrenergic blocker, can also be used in doses of 200 to 600 mg given twice daily.

d. α-Methylparatyrosine (metyrosine) blocks catecholamine synthesis in doses of 2 to 4 g/d PO and may be added on to α-blockade. High cost and side effects of severe fatigue and extrapyramidal symptoms make this drug a less favorable option, but it can be used in high-risk patients.

e. Calcium channel blockers such as amlodipine (10 to 20 mg/d), nifedipine (30 to 90 mg/d), and verapamil (180 to 540 mg/d) may also be used.

2. Surgery

a. **Before surgery.** Long-acting α- and β-adrenergic blockers should be given for 7 to 14 days preoperatively and continued throughout surgery. Close attention should be paid to maintaining fluid and electrolyte balance. Preoperative volume expansion with high-sodium diet and fluid intake is recommended to prevent postoperative hypotension.

b. **During surgery.** The perioperative mortality rate due to catecholamine excess is up to 3%. Hypertensive episodes, which may occur while the tumor is being manipulated, are managed with nitroprusside infusion, rapid intravenous boluses of phentolamine, and nicardipine infusion. Hypotensive episodes, which occur after the tumor's blood supply has been isolated, should be treated with intravenous fluids.

c. **After surgery.** Hypertension may develop as a result of fluid overload during surgery and is treated with intravenous furosemide and fluid restriction until the blood pressure is controlled. Rebound hypoglycemia following removal of catecholamine excess is common, and plasma glucose levels should be monitored closely in the postoperative period, with dextrose infusion as needed. Monitoring for and treatment of adrenal insufficiency are indicated. All patients should have plasma free metanephrines or 24-hour urine metanephrines measured 2 to 4 weeks after surgery. Plasma or urine metanephrines should be repeated at yearly follow-up examinations indefinitely in all patients.

3. Metastatic disease

a. **RT is useful** for palliating locally symptomatic metastases.

b. The usefulness of chemotherapy for unresectable disease is not established, although the combination of cyclophosphamide, vincristine, and dacarbazine produces objective responses in many patients. Symptoms of catecholamine excess are managed pharmacologically (see Section IV.D.1).

c. Some patients may respond to therapeutic doses of ^{131}I-metaiodobenzylguanidine.

V. ADRENAL CORTICAL CARCINOMA

A. **Epidemiology.** Adrenal cancer is rare, with an incidence of 0.5 to 2.0 cases per million per year. It causes 0.2% of cancer deaths. The average age at diagnosis is 40 years, but the tumor occurs at all ages. About 60% of the patients are women. Adrenal cortical cancer may occur as a component of Li-Fraumeni syndrome, MEN1, Gardner syndrome, Lynch syndrome, and Beckwith-Wiedemann syndrome.

B. **Pathology and natural history.** Adrenal cancers are highly aggressive; they frequently metastasize to lungs, liver, and other organs and are large and bulky at the time of diagnosis. About two-thirds of these tumors produce functional corticosteroids, including cortisol, aldosterone, androgens, and estrogens.

C. **Diagnosis**

1. Symptoms and signs

a. **Hormonally inactive tumors** are discovered due to symptoms of abdominal mass effect in 30% of patients and as incidental tumors in 15% to 20% of patients with adrenal cancer.

  b. Hormonally active tumors present with the following:
   (1) Rapid virilization (hirsutism, clitoromegaly, oligomenorrhea, or amenorrhea) in women
   (2) Gynecomastia in men
   (3) Precocious puberty
   (4) Cushing syndrome with hypertension and glucose intolerance
2. Adrenal function tests. Patients with the above clinical symptoms, and/or a suspicious adrenal mass, should have basal serum cortisol, ACTH, dehydroepiandrosterone sulfate (DHEAS), 17-hydroxyprogesterone, androstenedione, testosterone, and estradiol measured. In addition, evaluation for excess cortisol production should be performed with the dexamethasone suppression test and the 24-hour urine collection for free cortisol.
  a. Dexamethasone suppression test. Following the administration of 1 mg of dexamethasone at 11:00 p.m., serum cortisol is measured before 9:00 a.m. the next morning; serum cortisol is usually suppressed to <1.8 mcg/dL in normal individuals without Cushing syndrome.
  b. Twenty-four–hour urine collection is obtained for urinary free cortisol (upper limit of normal is <50 mcg per 24 hours in most laboratories).
3. Imaging
  a. Abdominal CT is the standard modality to evaluate the adrenal glands. Imaging characteristics that make adrenal tumors more likely to be adrenal carcinoma include size >6 cm, heterogeneity, irregular borders, calcifications, necrosis, and hemorrhage. Malignant tumors tend to be dense, usually >10 to 13 Hounsfield units, and demonstrate <50% washout of contrast media.
  b. Abdominal MRI may enhance some features of adrenal tumors.
  c. Chest CT to search for metastases is recommended in all patients.
  d. FDG-PET scan may prove useful for staging and metastatic evaluation but is not routinely recommended.
4. Biopsy
  a. In patients with metastatic disease, biopsy is performed on the most readily accessible site (e.g., superficial lymph nodes or liver with evidence of metastases).
  b. If only intra-adrenal disease is evident, the adrenal tumor will either need to be biopsied, or, if this is not possible, surgery is necessary for proof of the diagnosis.
D. Management. The median survival for untreated patients is 3 months. Treated patients may survive much longer, depending on the extent of disease.
 1. Surgery should be utilized to resect as much tumor as possible. The contralateral adrenal gland should be inspected and removed if there is evidence of tumor.
 2. RT is used to palliate symptoms from local metastatic sites. Adjuvant tumor-bed RT has been reported to reduce tumor recurrence.
 3. Pharmacologic therapy
  a. Pharmacologic management of hypercortisolism is discussed in Chapter 28, Section VIII.A.3.
  b. Mitotane can improve endocrine symptoms and produce objective tumor regression. Important side effects include nausea, neurologic symptoms, and iatrogenic adrenal insufficiency, which requires replacement with both gluco- and mineralocorticoids.
  c. Cytotoxic chemotherapy. The combination of mitotane with etoposide, doxorubicin, and cisplatin has provided responses in 50% of patients.

VI. ISLET CELL TUMORS

A. **General aspects.** Islet cell tumors of the endocrine pancreas are uncommon. Peak age of presentation is 50 to 70 years. Many of these tumors are malignant and metastasize to the liver and regional lymph nodes. About 10% are associated with underlying genetic syndromes, the most common of which is MEN1.

1. **Diagnosis.** The diagnosis of islet cell tumor is usually suspected because of endocrine or biochemical abnormalities. Nonfunctional tumors may present with symptoms of mass effect and biliary obstruction. Signs and symptoms of islet cell tumors are described according to the specific type. After abnormal hormonal products are detected, the following studies may help to determine the tumor's location and extent:

   a. **CT or MRI** of the abdomen, to evaluate for isolated tumors of the pancreas or duodenum, as well as to identify liver metastases.

   b. **Endoscopic ultrasonography (EUS)** has emerged as a valuable tool in localizing small tumors in the head of the pancreas or duodenal wall. It offers the additional benefit of allowing for biopsy of observed tumors.

   c. **Somatostatin receptor scanning** using radioiodinated octreotide frequently demonstrates primary and metastatic islet cell tumors. More than 90% of pancreatic endocrine tumors possess somatostatin receptors. Detection of somatostatin receptors by this method correlates well with response to treatment with octreotide.

   d. **FDG-PET** does not visualize well-differentiated islet cell tumors well but may be useful in detecting poorly differentiated tumors.

   e. **Selective arterial secretagogue injection** is a useful technique in which the desired pancreatic hormone (e.g., gastrin, insulin) is measured in the hepatic vein immediately following selective injection of pancreatic hormone stimulants such as calcium or secretin into individual branches of the celiac artery axis; although technically difficult, it is highly effective in localizing the source of hormonal hypersecretion.

   f. Exploratory laparotomy is indicated if there is clinical or laboratory evidence of an islet cell tumor, even if preoperative localization is unrevealing.

2. **Management**

   a. **Surgery.** Intraoperative pancreatic ultrasonography and intraoperative duodenoscopy are used to localize tumors and guide resection. Laparoscopic pancreatic resection is gaining popularity. Cytoreductive surgery should be performed in all patients with malignant tumors when feasible. Palliative debulking surgery improves symptoms in over 90% of patients. In patients with liver metastases, partial hepatectomy, cryotherapy, and radiofrequency ablation have all been used for palliation, with some increase in both survival and quality of life.

   b. **Pharmacologic Therapy**

      (1) **Octreotide** and lanreotide are somatostatin analogs that inhibit hormone release from gastrinomas, insulinomas, VIPomas, glucagonomas, and GH-RHomas (tumors producing GH-RH) and often relieve the symptoms of the associated clinical syndrome. Both drugs may slow tumor progression in some patients. Sustained-release forms can be given as a monthly intramuscular or subcutaneous injection.

      (2) **Chemotherapy** is generally reserved for patients with documented progressive liver metastases or without control of symptoms by octreotide and other medical measures.

(a) **Streptozocin**-based therapies were the standard treatment for many years; however, the toxicity of this agent in addition to emerging evidence placing the efficacy of this drug in doubt has led to decreased popularity of this regimen.

(b) **Combination chemotherapy** with cisplatin plus etoposide is commonly used. Temozolomide, as monotherapy and in combination with capecitabine, may also be effective.

(c) **Molecularly targeted therapy**, specifically everolimus and sunitinib, is approved for well-differentiated pancreatic neuroendocrine tumors.

B. **Gastrinoma (Zollinger-Ellison syndrome).** About 60% of these tumors are malignant, 90% are multiple, and about 30% are associated with MEN syndromes; the majority are located in the duodenum, with smaller numbers in the pancreas. Duodenal gastrinomas have a 40% to 70% risk of spread to local lymph nodes, but a low (5%) risk of hepatic metastases, while pancreatic gastrinomas are more likely to spread to the liver. Prognosis is poorer in cases with hepatic metastases.

1. **Diagnosis**

   a. **Symptoms** include severe peptic ulcer disease (abdominal pain, heartburn), and severe diarrhea. Weight loss and gastrointestinal bleeding may also occur.

   b. **Laboratory studies**

      (1) **Upper gastrointestinal endoscopy** shows severe ulceration and hypertrophic gastric folds.

      (2) **Fasting serum gastrin level** (normal value is <100 pg/mL) is usually elevated to >1,000 pg/mL. This should be measured with confirmation of a gastric pH < 4 to rule out appropriately elevated gastrin due to achlorhydria. Other causes of increased gastrin levels (use of proton pump inhibitors, atrophic gastritis, vagotomy, retained antrum after Billroth II gastrojejunostomy, and G-cell hyperplasia) must be differentiated from gastrinoma.

      (3) **Stimulation studies.** If gastrinoma is suspected but serum gastrin levels are not elevated, gastrin stimulation with calcium or secretin may be attempted. Secretin is infused rapidly, 2 units/kg over 1 minute. Gastrin level is measured prior to infusion and at 5-minute intervals for the next 20 minutes. A rise of 120 pg/mL from basal is considered a positive test for gastrinoma. A similar infusion test using calcium may also be performed; however, it is more time consuming and carries a lower sensitivity and specificity.

2. **Management**

   a. Therapy with proton pump inhibitors controls symptoms in most patients. High initial doses are recommended, with gradual tapering to lowest effective maintenance dose.

   b. Total gastrectomy is rarely necessary because ulcer symptoms can be controlled with proton pump inhibitors. Curative tumor excision may be possible in patients with solitary tumors without hepatic metastases, and tumor debulking may improve quality of life in those with limited spread to the liver.

   c. Chemotherapy is used for metastatic disease (see Section VI.A.2.b.2).

C. **Insulinomas** are most likely to occur between the ages of 40 and 60 years. About 80% to 85% are benign, 90% are solitary, 90% are <2 cm, and 80% are hormonally functional. Insulinomas are sometimes found in association with gastrinomas. A family history of diabetes mellitus is present in 25% of patients.

Insulinomas occur with equal frequency in the head, body, and tail of the pancreas; about 3% develop outside the pancreas. Malignant tumors are more frequent in male patients. When malignant, they metastasize to the liver primarily.

1. **Diagnosis**
   a. **Symptoms.** Fasting hypoglycemia, often alleviated by meals, is usually the presenting feature of insulinoma. Symptoms are often episodic in nature due to intermittent tumor secretion. Symptoms include diaphoresis, nervousness, palpitations, hunger pangs, anxiety, asthenia, confusion, weakness, seizures, and coma. Many patients have personality or other psychiatric changes noticed by the family. Weight gain is occasionally reported. Weight loss and liver failure may develop with metastases to the liver.
   b. **Laboratory studies.** Classically, satisfying the criteria of Whipple triad has been the cornerstone in diagnosis of insulinoma: simultaneous measurements of fasting blood glucose, insulin, and C-peptide levels during hypoglycemia, with relief of symptoms upon correction of hypoglycemia.
      (1) **Fasting hypoglycemia.** A prolonged fast is initiated, up to 72 hours, in which blood glucose, insulin, C-peptide, and proinsulin measurements are obtained at regular intervals. Inappropriately elevated levels of plasma insulin (>6 mU/mL) or proinsulin (>20 pmol/L) and C-peptide (>0.6 ng/mL) in the presence of hypoglycemia (glucose < 55 mg/dL) usually is diagnostic of insulinoma or sulfonylurea ingestion. If symptoms of hypoglycemia develop at any time, blood glucose, insulin, and C-peptide levels should be measured; if the glucose concentration is <40 mg/dL, the test should be terminated by giving the patient food or a 50-mL intravenous bolus of 50% dextrose.
      (2) **Other insulin assays.** Proinsulin and C-peptide are absent from commercial insulin preparations; their measurement by radioimmunoassay determines the role of exogenous insulin administration in the causation of hypoglycemia. In fasting patients, proinsulin levels are normally <20% of total insulin; a higher percentage of proinsulin is suggestive of insulinoma.

2. **Management**
   a. **Surgery.** Surgical removal of the tumor is the treatment of choice for insulinoma.
   b. **RT** as an adjuvant to surgery has not been shown to be helpful.
   c. **Chemotherapy** may be used for advanced disease (see Section VI.A.2.b.2).
   d. **Treatment of hypoglycemia**
      (1) Diazoxide, up to 1,200 mg daily in divided doses, is effective in managing hypoglycemic symptoms. The drug can induce hyperglycemia, hyperosmolar coma, or ketoacidosis. Edema is a common side effect, often requiring the coadministration of a diuretic. Other complications of diazoxide therapy include cytopenias, lanugo hair growth, rashes, eosinophilia, and hyperuricemia.
      (2) Corticosteroids (prednisone, 40 mg/d, or hydrocortisone, 100 mg/d) may be given to patients who do not respond to diazoxide.
      (3) Subcutaneous injections of octreotide or lanreotide (or a monthly injection of a sustained-release preparation) inhibit insulin secretion and restore euglycemia in about half of insulinoma patients. By

suppressing glucagon and growth hormone secretion, somatostatin analogues will occasionally worsen hypoglycemia.

(4) Calcium channel blockers (e.g., verapamil, 80 mg t.i.d.) inhibit insulin secretion and have been successfully used to prevent hypoglycemic episodes.

(5) Everolimus has been used to improve hypoglycemia in patients with insulinoma.

(6) Continuous glucose monitoring devices alert patients to rapid changes in glucose concentration of interstitial fluid and can prompt the patient to correct hypoglycemia with oral glucose intake before neuroglycopenic symptoms occur.

D. **Glucagonomas** are usually malignant, and most have metastasized at the time of discovery. They are usually solitary, >3 cm at the time of diagnosis, and are more likely to arise in the distal pancreas.

These patients may present with weight loss, diarrhea, abdominal pain, depression or other personality changes, deep venous thrombosis, or necrolytic migratory erythema (a peculiar erythematous migratory skin rash that had waxed and waned over many years (often >6 years), especially involving perioral and perigenital regions, also the fingers, legs, and feet). They may have mild hyperglycemia, normocytic anemia, and elevated fasting blood glucagon levels, usually in the 500 to 1,000 pg/mL range (normal is <50 pg/mL). Because of high risk of thrombosis, prophylactic measures to prevent DVT during the perioperative period are mandatory.

E. **Pancreatic cholera syndrome** (VIPoma). These islet cell tumors secrete VIP (vasoactive intestinal peptide). The majority are solitary, >3 cm, and occur in the distal pancreas. About half have metastasized at the time of discovery.

1. **Diagnosis**

a. **Symptoms** include high-volume watery diarrhea, muscle weakness due to hypokalemia, flushing, psychosis, and hypotension.

b. **Laboratory studies**

(1) Serum chemistry studies may show hypokalemia, hypochlorhydria, hyperglycemia and hypercalcemia.

(2) Low stool osmotic gap (<50 mOsm/kg)

(3) Serum levels of VIP are elevated (normal is <60 pg/mL).

c. **Tumor location and extent.** See Section VI.A.1.

2. **Management**

a. **Fluid** and electrolyte repletion

b. **Surgery.** Removal of solitary tumors controls manifestations of the pancreatic cholera syndrome, including hypercalcemia. Debulking of extensive tumor may palliate the diarrhea.

c. **Chemotherapy** (see Section VI.A.2.b.ii) is useful for controlling symptoms in patients with metastatic tumor. Long-acting somatostatin analogs (octreotide or lanreotide) usually lower VIP levels and stop the diarrhea.

ACKNOWLEDGMENT

The author would like to acknowledge Dr. Harold E. Carlson, who significantly contributed to earlier versions of this chapter.

Suggested Readings

Carcinoid and Islet Cell Tumors

Basu B, Sirohi B, Corrie P. Systemic therapy for neuroendocrine tumours of gastroenteropancreatic origin. *Endocr Relat Cancer* 2010;17:R75.

Jensen RT, Delle Fave G. Promising advances in the treatment of malignant pancreatic endocrine tumors. *N Engl J Med* 2011;364:564.

Kulke MH. Clinical presentation and management of carcinoid tumors. *Hematol Oncol Clin North Am* 2007;21:433.

Luis SA, Pellikka PA. Carcinoid heart disease: diagnosis and management. *Best Pract Res Clin Endocrinol Metab* 2016;30(1):149.

Nakakura EK, Bergsland EK. Islet cell carcinoma: neuroendocrine tumors of the pancreas and periampullary region. *Hematol Oncol Clin North Am* 2007;21:457.

Okabayashi T, Shima Y, Sumiyoshi T et al. Diagnosis and management of insulinoma. *World J Gastroenterol* 2013;19(6):829.

Pavel M, Baudin E, Couvelard A, et al. ENETS consensus guidelines for the management of patients with liver and other distant metastases from neuroendocrine neoplasms of foregut, midgut, hindgut, and unknown primary. *Neuroendocrinology* 2012;95(2):157.

Pinchot SN, Holen K, Sippel RS, et al. Carcinoid tumors. *Oncologist* 2008;13:1255.

Poncet G, Faucheron J-L, Walter T. Recent trends in the treatment of well-differentiated endocrine carcinoma of the small bowel. *World J Gastroenterol* 2010;16:1696.

Zhou C, Zhang J, Zheng Y, et al. Pancreatic neuroendocrine tumors: a comprehensive review. *Int J Cancer* 2012;131:1013.

Thyroid Cancer

Haugen BR, Alexander EK, Bible KC, et al. 2015 American Thyroid Association guidelines for adult patients with thyroid nodules and differentiated thyroid cancer: the American Thyroid Association guidelines task force on thyroid nodules and differentiated thyroid cancer. *Thyroid* 2016;26(1):1.

Patel KN, Shaha AR. Poorly differentiated thyroid cancer. *Curr Opin Otolaryngol Head Neck Surg* 2014;22(2):121.

Sabet A, Kim M. Postoperative management of differentiated thyroid cancer. *Otolaryngol Clin North Am* 2010;43:329.

Thomas L, Lai SY, Dong W, et al. Sorafenib in metastatic thyroid cancer: a systematic review. *Oncologist* 2014;19(3):251.

Wells SA Jr, Asa SL, Dralle H, et al. Revised American Thyroid Association guidelines for the management of medullary thyroid carcinoma. *Thyroid* 2015;25:567.

Pheochromocytoma

Adjallé R, Plovin PF, Pacak K, et al. Treatment of malignant pheochromocytoma. *Horm Metab Res* 2009;41:687.

Lenders JWM, Quan-Yang D, Eisenhofer G, et al. Pheochromocytoma and paraganglioma: an endocrine society clinical practice guideline. *J Clin Endocrinol Metab* 2014;99(6):1915.

Mittendorf EA, Evans DB, Lee JE, et al. Pheochromocytoma: advances in genetics, diagnosis, localization and treatment. *Hematol Oncol Clin North Am* 2007;21:509.

Pacak K. Perioperative management of the pheochromocytoma patient. *J Clin Endocrinol Metab* 2007;92:4069.

Petri B-J, Van Eijck CHJ, de Herder WW, et al. Phaeochromocytomas and sympathetic paragangliomas. *Br J Surg* 2009;96:1381.

Adrenal Cortical Carcinoma

Baudin E. Adrenocortical carcinoma. *Endocrinol Metab Clin North Am* 2015;44:411.

Fassnacht M, Allolio B. What is the best approach to an apparently nonmetastatic adrenocortical carcinoma? *Clin Endocrinol (Oxf)* 2010;73:561.

Lacroix A. Approach to the patient with adrenocortical carcinoma. *J Clin Endocrinol Metab* 2010;95:4812.

Veytsman I, Nieman L, Fojo T. Management of endocrine manifestations and the use of mitotane as a chemotherapeutic agent for adrenocortical carcinoma. *J Clin Oncol* 2009;27:4619.

Young WF Jr. The incidentally discovered adrenal mass. *N Engl J Med* 2007;356:601.

Parathyroid Carcinoma

Adam MA, Untch BR, Olson JA. Parathyroid carcinoma: current understanding and new insights into gene expression and intraoperative parathyroid hormone kinetics. *Oncologist* 2010;15:61.

McClenaghan F, Qureshi YA. Parathyroid cancer. *Gland Surg* 2015;4(4):329.

Metastases to Endocrine Glands

Chung AY, Tran TB, Brumund KT, et al. Metastases to the thyroid: a review of the literature from the last decade. *Thyroid* 2012;22(3):258.

DeWaal YRP, Thomas CMG, Oei ALM, et al. Secondary ovarian malignancies. Frequency, origin and characteristics. *Int J Gynecol Cancer* 2009;19:1160.

Gittens PR, Solish AF, Trabulsi EJ. Surgical management of metastatic disease to the adrenal gland. *Semin Oncol* 2008;35:172.

Komninos J, Vlassopoulou V, Protopapa D, et al. Tumors metastatic to the pituitary gland: case report and literature review. *J Clin Endocrinol Metab* 2004;89:574.

17 Skin Cancers

Bartosz Chmielowski, Richard F. Wagner Jr, and Antoni Ribas

MALIGNANT MELANOMA

I. EPIDEMIOLOGY AND ETIOLOGY

A. Incidence. Malignant melanoma accounts for about 2% of all skin cancers, but it is responsible for 80% of deaths. The incidence of melanoma in the United States has been rising for the last 40 years. Before the age of 45, women have a higher risk than men, but after the age of 60, the risk for men is twice as high as for women. The estimated number of new cases in the United States in 2016 is 76,380, and 10,130 patients would die of melanoma.

The incidence of melanoma rose rapidly in the 1970s at about 6% per year; it continues to rise but at a lower rate of 2.7% per year from 2006 to 2010. White people have a 2.4% lifetime risk for the development of melanoma and African Americans 0.1%, but melanoma is diagnosed among all races.

B. Risk factors. The strongest risk factors for melanoma are a family history of melanoma, multiple benign or atypical nevi, and a previous melanoma. The list of additional risk factors includes immunosuppression, sun sensitivity, and exposure to ultraviolet (UV) radiation.

  1. Familial factors. Approximately 10% of melanomas are familial. The higher risk of melanoma in these families may be attributed to both shared susceptibility genes and shared environment.

  a. High-penetrance susceptibility genes. Two genes, *CDKN2A* and *CDK4*, are associated with high-penetrance susceptibility. Mutated *CDKN2A* is the most prevalent gene in families with melanoma. It is located on chromosome 9p21, and it encodes cyclin-dependent kinase inhibitor 2A (p16INK4a). *CDK4* encodes cyclin-dependent kinase 4, which is one of the binding partners of p16INK4a. Mutations in *CDK4* are found much less frequently than in *CDKN2A*. Other less common high-penetrance genes are *BAP1*, *TERT*, *XP* (various genes mutated in individuals with xeroderma pigmentosum).

  The higher the number of family members with melanoma, the higher the probability of carrying a high-penetrance gene. Mutated *CDKN2A* was found in 14% families with 2 cases of melanoma, in 67% families with 6 to 7 cases, and 100% families with 7 to 10 cases. Overall, between 20% (in Australia) and 57% (in Europe) of the cases of familial melanoma are associated with *CDKN2A*.

  b. Low-penetrance susceptibility genes. Epidemiologic studies suggest that low-penetrance susceptibility genes are found frequently among families with melanoma. The list includes *BRCA2*, *MC1R*, *MITF E318K*, shelterin complex genes (*POT1*, *ACD*, *TERF2IP*).

  c. Familial atypical multiple mole melanoma (FAMMM) syndrome, also known as the familial dysplastic nevus syndrome, was described in 1978 in families whose members suffered from melanoma and had multiple (usually >100) large moles of variable size and color (reddish brown to bright red) with pigmentary leakage. The median age of the development of melanoma in persons with this syndrome is 33 years, and 9% of affected people develop it before the age of 20. The syndrome is transmitted in autosomal dominant fashion, but there are sex differences in penetrance. Males develop melanoma less frequently and at an older age than women.

2. **Nevi.** Typical nevi are frequently precursors of melanoma, but more importantly, they are markers of increased risk. High common nevus counts (50 or more common nevi) account for 27% of melanoma cases, whereas individuals with few common nevi (0 to 10) account for only 4% of melanoma cases.

   Congenital nevi are benign neoplasms that are present at birth and composed of nevomelanocytes. The malignant potential of giant congenital nevi varies between different types. Pigmented giant nevi have especially high risk for malignant transformation. Nevus sebaceous is associated with the development of basal cell carcinoma. Verrucous epidermal nevi and woolly hair nevi do not have malignant potential.

3. **Previous melanoma.** The rate of a second primary cutaneous melanoma is 6% to 7%; the risk is higher among patients who initially presented with melanoma in situ than in those with invasive melanoma. The greatest risk is within the first 2 years, but it remains elevated for at least 20 years. Males, elderly patients, and individuals with the first melanoma on the face, the neck, and the trunk are at especially high risk. The incidence of a third primary melanoma from the time of second primary melanoma is 16% at 1 year and 31% at 5 years.

4. **Immunosuppression.** Among organ allograft recipients, melanoma constituted 5% of skin cancers and was significantly higher than in the general population (2.7%).

5. **Sun sensitivity.** Light-skinned and redheaded people frequently carry a polymorphism in the melanocortin receptor gene (MC1R) that results in a decreased melanin production after exposure to UV radiation and in an increased risk of melanoma.

6. **Exposure to sun and to UV radiation.** It is known that UV radiation causes genetic changes in the skin, impairs cutaneous immune function, increases the local production of growth factors, and induces the formation of DNA-damaging reactive oxygen species that affect keratinocytes and melanocytes. Epidemiologic studies revealed that intermittent sun exposure and frequent sunburns, especially during childhood, increase the risk of melanoma. Chronic low-grade sun exposure may be protective, although data also show that higher total exposure to the sun is associated with a higher risk of melanoma among non-Hispanic White individuals. In addition, exposure to UV light from recreational tanning salons is an important risk factor for melanoma.

7. **Occupational exposure.** Exposure to coal tar, pitch, creosote, arsenic compounds, or radium increases the risk of melanoma development.

8. **Other.** An increased rate of melanoma was seen in patients with Parkinson disease, prostate cancer, and endometriosis and patients treated with voriconazole, sildenafil, and tumor necrosis factor (TNF) inhibitors.

II. PREVENTION

Avoidance of exposure to the sun during the midday hours, wearing skin-protecting clothing, sunglasses, use of sunscreens with a sun protective factor (SPF) of 15 or higher, and avoidance of sunburns and tanning beds are recommended as a primary prevention. It is unclear if dietary vitamin D has any impact on development of melanoma. Patients with a family or personal history of melanoma should undergo at least one annual skin examination performed by a dermatologist as a secondary prevention.

III. PATHOLOGY AND NATURAL HISTORY

A. **Pathology.** Melanoma originates from melanocytes, the neural crest-derived cells that migrate into the epidermis during embryogenesis to reside in the basal layer of the epidermis. The overwhelming majority of melanomas originate in the skin, but some melanomas may arise from other primary sites. Potential extracutaneous sites include the choroidal layer of the eye and mucosal surfaces in the upper respiratory tract (most frequently, the nose and nasopharynx), gastrointestinal (GI) tract (most frequently, the anus), and genitourinary tract (most frequently, the vagina).

Several steps occur in the process of their malignant transformation. According to the Clark model, initially normal melanocytes proliferate and form a benign nevus. In the next phase, abnormal growth appears in the form of a dysplastic nevus. Melanoma may originate from a benign nevus, but it can also start from scattered melanocytes present in the normal skin. Next, in the radial growth phase, the cells acquire the ability to grow intraepidermally and have all the features of cancerous cells. Then, the lesion invades the dermis (vertical growth phase) and finally spreads to other organs and other areas of the skin (metastasis). Not all melanomas pass through each of these individual phases, however.

B. **Molecular events in the pathogenesis of melanoma.** Several molecular alterations have known pathogenic effects in the transformation of melanocytes and the evolution of melanoma.

1. **Alterations in signal transduction pathways.** Mutually exclusive somatic activating point mutations in *NRAS* (15% to 20% of melanomas) and *BRAF* (40% to 50% of melanomas), two members of the mitogen-activated protein kinase (MAPK) that provides proliferation signaling from surface receptors to the nucleus, are present in most melanomas of skin primary. More than 75 different mutations in the *BRAF* gene in melanoma have been described: V600E mutation 90% of cases, V600K 5% to 6%, V600R 1%, and V600D 0.1%; other *BRAF* mutations are less common. Mutations in *NF1* (neurofibromatosis 1) tumor suppressor gene leading to loss of its function are seen in 14% of melanomas and they also lead to activation of MAPK pathway. Paradoxically, *BRAF* mutation is also frequent in benign nevi, where its transforming effect may be counteracted by the phenomenon of oncogene-induced senescence.

   Somatic alterations in another signaling pathway important in cell growth, the phosphoinositide-3-OH kinase (PI3K) pathway, are also frequently found in melanoma, including loss of PTEN (phosphate and tensin homologue) and overexpression of Akt. About 20% to 40% of melanomas originating from mucosal membranes or from chronic sun damage skin and acral melanomas can harbor an activating mutation in KIT kinase. This mutation is not found in melanoma originating from the trunk.

   Finally, more than 80% of uveal melanomas have an activating mutation in GNAQ or GNA11, two small GTP-binding proteins that couple cell surface G-coupled receptors, and are involved in their signal transduction. BAP1 mutations are seen in 25% of uveal melanomas and its presence correlates with an increased risk for metastatic disease.

2. **Aberrant cell cycle control.** As described above, inherited mutations in the *CDKN2A* and *CDK4* genes are associated with high-penetrance susceptibility to melanoma. Somatic mutations in these and other cell cycle control genes seem a requisite for the development of melanoma and escape from oncogene-induced senescence.

3. **Other genetic events in melanoma pathogenesis.** *MITF* gene amplifications are noted in a small subset of melanomas, and this gene has a complex relationship with melanoma oncogenesis. Several genetic alterations common in melanoma reduce sensitivity to apoptosis, including overexpression of Bcl-2 (B-cell leukemia/lymphoma-2), silencing of APAF-1 (apoptotic peptidase activating factor-1), and activation of NF-κB (nuclear factor kappa B).

C. **Major clinical–histopathologic subtypes.** Traditionally, melanomas have been divided based on the histologic subtypes. Recently, it has become more important to sequence individual somatic mutations in key genes (i.e., *NRAS*, *BRAF*, *NF1*, *c-kit*, *GNAQ*, or *GNA11*) and use these findings to distinguish different melanoma subtypes. The progress in understanding the molecular biology of melanoma will soon lead to further subtyping of the disease.

1. **Superficial spreading melanoma** compromises about 70% of all melanomas. It is most common in middle age and develops most frequently on the upper back of both sexes and on the legs of women, but it can occur in any anatomic location. Only 25% of lesions are associated with a preexisting nevus. It spreads laterally (radial growth) for a period of time before it becomes invasive. The lesions appear as variably pigmented plaques or macules that have a bizarre shape with irregular borders. Progression correlates with the evolution of multiple shades of color from red (inflammation) through gray (regressed areas) to black (neoplastic melanocytes).

2. **Nodular melanoma** compromises about 15% to 20% of all melanomas. It is more common among older adults, and it occurs twice as frequently in male than in female patients. The lesion appears as a darkly pigmented dome-shaped or polypoid nodule that can ulcerate and bleed early. Occasionally, it can be amelanotic. These tumors grow rapidly and vertically from the onset.

3. **Lentigo maligna melanoma** (4% to 15% of melanomas) is most commonly seen in older individuals (in the sixth and seventh decade of life). It arises in sun-damaged areas of the skin, mainly on the face (90% cases). The lesion appears as a tan-brown macule, very often large in size (3 to 6 cm). The lesion grows slowly and the radial growth phase may last between 5 and 50 years before it starts growing vertically. Partial regression is not uncommon during evolution.

4. **Acral lentiginous melanoma** is the least common variant of radial growth phase melanomas. It compromises only 2% to 8% of melanomas in Whites, but 30% to 75% cases in Blacks, Hispanics, and Asians. It appears on the palms, soles, and terminal phalanges as a dark brown to black, unevenly pigmented patch.

5. **Rare types**
   a. **Nevoid melanoma** resembles benign nevi. It has verrucoid or dome-shaped appearance and can metastasize.
   b. **Desmoplastic melanomas** resemble a scar or fibroma and appear mainly on sun-exposed areas. Very often, they are amelanotic. They tend to recur locally or as isolated metastasis.

D. **Mode of spread.** Melanoma frequently first spreads through the lymphatic system forming satellite lesions and in-transit metastases and then it involves regional lymph nodes. *Satellite lesions* are skin or subcutaneous lesions within 2 cm of the primary tumor and represent intralymphatic extension of the tumor. *In-transit metastases* are defined as lesions that are >2 cm from the primary tumor, but not beyond the regional lymph node basin. Melanoma can also spread hematogenously, sometimes after the nodal spread or skipping the draining nodes, forming distant metastases in the skin, subcutaneous soft tissue, lungs, liver, brain, and other organs.

E. **Metastatic melanoma from an unknown primary site** accounts for approximately 2% to 6% of all melanoma cases. It is assumed that in most these cases, the primary cutaneous melanoma regressed spontaneously. Metastases most often develop as cutaneous or subcutaneous nodules or as lymph node metastases. The survival of patients with unknown primary melanoma is similar to that of patients with known primary tumors when corresponding stages are compared.

IV. DIAGNOSIS

A. **Symptoms**

1. **The ABCDE rule.** Warning signs of melanoma are as follows:
   a. **A**symmetry.
   b. Irregular **b**orders.
   c. **C**hanges in color; pigmentation is not uniform.
   d. **D**iameter >6 mm.
   e. **E**nlarging or evolving lesion.
      The **c**hanges in preexisting moles and appearance of a new mole with these features are highly suspicious for melanoma. More than 50% of the cases arise in apparently normal areas of the skin. Ulceration or bleeding usually represents deeper lesions.

2. **In-transit lesions and skin metastases** appear as skin or subcutaneous erythematous nodules between the primary tumor site and the regional nodal basin. The nodules do not have to be pigmented. As they grow, they can coalesce and ulcerate.

3. **Symptoms of the metastatic disease** are related to the involved site.

B. **Physical examination.** A complete skin examination of the whole body should be performed, including scalp, axillae, genital area, interdigital webs, and mouth. Skin lesions that follow the "ugly duckling rule" (i.e., look different from other skin lesions, even if they do not fully follow the ABCDE rule) should be biopsied. Melanoma in men occurs more frequently on the trunk or head and neck, and in women on the back and legs, but it can arise from any site on the skin surface. Although most primary lesions are usually pigmented, frequently skin metastases are not pigmented, and they may appear as red or subcutaneous nodules.

C. **Differential diagnosis.** Compound nevi, halo nevi, dermal nevi, basal cell carcinoma, seborrheic keratosis, angiomas, and dermatofibromas may have features that suggest melanoma. Biopsy specimens of these lesions should be obtained. Precision of the diagnosis can be increased by use of a dermatoscope, an instrument that magnifies pigmented lesions about 10 times. The dermatoscope is especially invaluable for examination of flat to slightly raised pigmented lesions.

D. **Biopsy.** Suspicious lesions should be biopsied and analyzed pathologically. A full-thickness excision with 1- to 3-mm margins should be performed if the tumor is highly suspected to be melanoma. Larger margins may interfere with planned sentinel lymph node biopsy (SNLB). Incisional biopsies (punch biopsy or tangential), where part of the pigmented lesion is sampled for pathologic diagnosis, may be used for very large lesions or lesions on the face, palmar surfaces of the hand, sole of the foot, ear, distal digits, genitalia, or under nails. Incisional biopsies may fail, however, to diagnose melanoma or result in a more favorable early staging impression owing to sampling error. If melanoma continues to be suspected or is diagnosed, the biopsy should be repeated or the lesion completely excised for pathologic reevaluation and staging. Incisional biopsies do not increase the chance for melanoma metastases.

V. PROGNOSTIC FACTORS

A. Prognostic factors
1. **Primary lesion.** Tumor thickness and ulceration are the most powerful predictors of survival.
   a. **Tumor thickness** as a prognostic factor was first described by Alexander Breslow and it is traditionally reported as Breslow thickness in millimeters. The AJCC staging system uses 1-, 2-, and 4-mm cutoffs, but tumor thickness is really a continuous prognostic variable.
   b. **Ulceration** (the absence of intact epithelium over the tumor determined by pathologic analysis) indicates aggressive biology of melanoma.
   c. **Mitotic rate.** Increased mitotic rate correlates with a decreased survival. It is the most important in staging melanomas with tumor thickness <1 mm.
   d. **Clark levels** specify the anatomic depth of invasion and are no longer utilized in the most recent staging system.
2. **Status of the regional lymph nodes.** The total number of nodal metastases is a significant predictor of outcome in patients with lymph node involvement. Moreover, patients in whom lymph node involvement was detected clinically have worse prognosis than those who required microscopic analysis. Satellite and in-transit lesions are considered an intralymphatic spread.
3. **Metastatic disease.** Patients who have nonvisceral metastases (skin, subcutaneous tissue, lymph nodes) carry a better prognosis than those who have visceral metastases. Elevated level of lactate dehydrogenase (LDH) is a poor prognostic factor.
4. **Survival.** The 5- and 10-year relative survival rates for people with melanoma are 91% and 89%, respectively. For localized melanoma (84% of cases), the 5-year survival rate is 98%; survival declines to 62% and 16% for regional and distant stage disease, respectively.

B. Staging workup
1. Breslow thickness, ulceration status, Clark level, mitotic rate, margin status, and the presence of satellite lesions should be reported by the pathologist. Reporting of location, regression, tumor-infiltrating lymphocytes, vertical growth phase, angiolymphatic invasion, neurotropism, and histologic subtype is encouraged.
2. Physicians should obtain a complete history and physical examination, including the entire skin and locoregional lymph nodes.
3. Patients with stage 0 or IA melanoma do not require further studies. For deeper primary melanomas (stages II and III), further tests may be performed (LFT, LDH, and baseline whole body imaging).
4. All patients with surgically incurable locally advanced melanoma (stage IIIb/IIIc) and metastatic melanoma (stage IV) should undergo complete blood work including LDH and whole body imaging. Specific brain imaging is required because approximately 20% of these cases will present with brain metastasis. Adequate brain imaging can be achieved with an MRI

(preferable, because it has higher sensitivity for metastasis) or a CT scan of the brain with IV contrast.

Imaging of the rest of the body can be obtained by CT of the chest, abdomen, and pelvis with both oral and IV contrast or a combined whole body [18]fluoro-deoxyglucose (FDG) positron emission tomography (PET) CT. PET scan may be especially helpful with the assessment of possible bone and bowel metastasis. If specific areas are involved that are not adequately imaged with CT scans (spinal, soft tissue, or bone metastasis), dedicated MRI may be required.

VI. MANAGEMENT

A. Surgery

1. **Management of the primary tumor**
   a. **Cutaneous melanoma.** The definitive surgical treatment for primary cutaneous melanoma is a wide excision. The usual recommended margin of the normal tissue depends on the depth of invasion of the primary tumor as follows:

Tumor Thickness (mm)	Recommended Surgical Margin (cm)
In situ	0.5–1
<1	1
1.01–2	1–2
2.01–4	2
>4	2

   Often, it is difficult to achieve a recommended excision margin in cases of melanoma located on the head or neck without skin grafting. Although some studies suggest that a narrower margin may result in better cosmetic results without influencing the overall survival, it is recommended that the tumor thickness—as opposed to cosmetic factors—guide the extent of the excisional surgery. Mohs micrographic surgery may contribute to favorable outcomes, especially on the head and neck where extensive subclinical spread is relatively common.

   b. **Melanoma of unusual sites**
      (1) **Subungual melanoma** is treated with partial digital amputation.
      (2) The wide excision of a **plantar melanoma** frequently requires a variety of flap reconstructive procedures, especially when the lesion is located on a weight-bearing surface.
      (3) **Mucosal melanoma** may arise from the epithelium lining the respiratory, GI, and genitourinary tracts. It often presents late with locally advanced or metastatic disease. If the disease is localized, it may require a major surgery (i.e., craniofacial resection for skull base tumors, radical vulvectomy for vulvar melanomas, or abdominal–perineal resection for anorectal melanomas).

2. **Management of regional lymph nodes**
   a. **Sentinel lymph node biopsy.** Lymph node mapping and biopsy of the first draining lymph node (the so-called *sentinel lymph node*) can adequately detect lymph node metastasis with decreased morbidity, and therefore, it is an important staging tool, but it has not been shown to improve disease-specific survival, it may improve survival in patients with intermediate-thickness (1.2- to 3.5-mm) melanoma. The SLN is identified by lymphoscintigraphy.

Patients who do not have clinically involved regional lymph nodes and whose primary tumor is thicker than >1 mm or thicker than 0.75 mm with high-risk features (ulceration, Clark level IV and V, histologic regression, or high mitotic rate) undergo SLNB. SLNB should be done before a wide excision of the primary site, which obfuscates mapping of the SLN location.

Only 1% to 2% of patients who have an uninvolved SLN have metastases to non-SLN. For patients with positive SLNB, the recommendation is to have elective lymph node dissection (ELND), although there are no randomized data supporting this approach available yet.

b. Enlarged regional lymph nodes together with other lymph nodes from the same lymph node basin are surgically removed (ELND). If inguinofemoral lymph nodes are clinically positive or three or more are involved microscopically or if Cloquet node is positive, elective iliac and obturator lymph node dissection should be considered. The procedure can be complicated by delayed wound healing, wound infection, and the development of lymphedema or seromas. Complications occur more frequently after inguinal lymphadenectomy than after axillary lymphadenectomy.

3. Management of in-transit metastases

  a. If the patient does not have evidence of disseminated disease, in-transit metastases (single or multiple) could be resected with curative intent, but only 18% to 28% patients will remain free of disease at 5 years. Patients with unresectable in-transit metastasis or for whom surgery would not provide a meaningful control of the disease should be managed as patients with metastatic disease.

  b. Few patients are treated with isolated limb perfusion (ILP) or isolated limb infusion (ILI); most patients are treated with systemic therapy in the same way as patients with stage IV disease. ILP is a procedure in which vasculature is separated surgically and chemotherapy (e.g., melphalan in high concentrations) can be perfused through the affected limb without exposing the rest of the body. Complete responses can be achieved in approximately 50% of cases, and about half of them are durable. ILI is a less-invasive procedure in which the vein and the artery are accessed percutaneously and is similarly efficacious.

4. Surgical management of metastases. Patients with solitary metastases, oligometastatic melanoma (limited number of metastatic sites), or residual lesions after successful systemic therapy may benefit from metastasectomy.

B. Radiation therapy. In the adjuvant setting, RT to the primary site can be considered for patients with positive surgical margins. RT to the regional nodal basin can be considered for patients who had multiple positive lymph nodes (at least four), bulky disease (lymph nodes >3 cm), extranodal soft tissue extension, involvement of cervical lymph nodes, or recurrence. RT decreases the rate of local recurrence by 30% to 50%, but it does not prolong survival. Adjuvant RT may decrease the risk of local recurrence for desmoplastic melanoma. Patients with metastatic melanoma are rarely treated with RT. Radiation to pain-causing tumor or tumor-invading vital structures can be used as palliation. Management of brain metastasis includes RT (see Section VII.A).

C. Systemic therapy. Systemic therapy in patients with melanoma can be divided into three distinct groups: (*1*) immunotherapy, (*2*) targeted therapy, and (*3*) chemotherapy (see Fig. 17-1). Chemotherapy targets dividing cells or their environment; it can rarely lead to durable remissions but almost never results in cure.

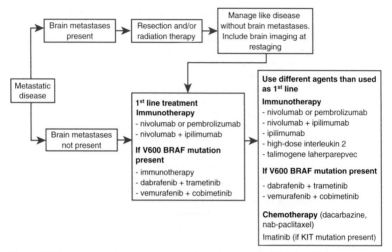

Figure 17-1 Algorithm of the management of patients with metastatic melanoma.

Targeted therapy uses small molecules that target known molecular alterations. Immunotherapy alters the patient's own immune system to reject tumor. Although the response rate to immunotherapy is frequently lower than with the use of targeted therapy, it can result in cure in some patients. The combination of chemotherapy and immunotherapy is called *biochemotherapy*, and since introduction of active targeted therapies and immunotherapeutic agents, it is used very rarely.

1. **Adjuvant systemic therapy.** Patients who present with the involvement of regional lymph nodes (high-risk group) and patients with localized thick tumors (i.e., thickness >4 mm without ulceration or thickness >2 mm with ulceration) may benefit from adjuvant therapy. Multiple agents have been tested in the adjuvant setting: interferon alpha (IFN-α), pegylated IFN-α, and ipilimumab have shown potential benefit.

   a. **Interferon alpha-2b.** Patients enrolled in the large, randomized ECOG 1648 trial were treated with high doses of IFN-α2b. The schedule consisted of IV therapy at maximal tolerated doses of 20 mU/m^2 5 d/wk for 4 weeks followed by 10 mU/m^2 subcutaneously three times a week for additional 48 weeks. After a median follow-up of 7 years, the treatment resulted in a prolonged relapse-free and overall survival of approximately 10% at 5 years. Another large, randomized trial confirmed these results. Trials using low or intermediates doses of IFN have showed decreased or no benefit. When patients were followed for a longer time, and when the pooled analysis of three high-dose IFN-α2b clinical trials was performed, the difference in overall survival was not statistically significant. Most patients required dose adjustment because of toxicity. Side effects of INF therapy included fatigue, nausea, fever, depression, neutropenia, and reversible elevation of liver enzymes. Some patients develop clinical autoimmune syndromes (hyperthyroidism, hypothyroidism, hypopituitarism, vitiligo, antiphospholipid syndrome) or autoantibodies (antithyroid microsomal, antithyroglobulin, antinuclear, anti-DNA, antiplatelet, or anti–islet cell antibodies) and it correlates with a decreased risk of melanoma recurrence.

b. Pegylated interferon alpha-2b is a long-acting formulation of IFN-α. In the EORTC 18991 trial, patients with resected stage III melanoma were treated with subcutaneous injections of pegylated interferon at the dose of 6 mcg/kg/wk for 8 weeks followed by injections at the dose of 3 mcg/kg/wk for total of 5 years. At 4 years, a 7% improvement in relapse-free survival (RFS) was reported (46% vs. 39%). No improvement in overall survival was seen at 7.6 years. The benefit was seen mainly in patients with ulcerated primary melanoma who had microscopic lymph node involvement only.

c. Ipilimumab (CTLA-4 blocking antibody). CTLA-4 is a molecule on the surface of activated T lymphocytes that is responsible for inhibiting immune responses. Blocking this molecule can potentially result in the enhancement of antitumor responses. Ipilimumab at the dose of 10 mg/kg every 3 weeks for 4 doses, then every 3 months for up to 3 years, was studied in patients with resected stage III melanoma with melanoma deposit in lymph nodes of more than 1 mm. When compared to placebo, the treatment with ipilimumab resulted in a 12% improvement in RFS at 3 years and 9-month improvement in median RFS. The therapy was complicated by frequent immune-related adverse events: 40% of patients discontinued the therapy during the induction phase and five patients died of side effects (colitis with bowel perforation, complications of Guillain-Barré syndrome, myocarditis).

2. **Immunotherapy for metastatic melanoma**

a. Pembrolizumab is a PD-1–blocking antibody. PD1 is an inhibitory molecule present on T cells and it is responsible for late regulation of immune responses. The treatment with pembrolizumab in 655 patients resulted in a 33% response rate and 66% 12-month and 49% 24-month overall survival. The treatment with pembrolizumab was also superior to ipilimumab with a 20% improvement in PFS at 6 months and 12-month overall survival 68% to 74% versus 58%. Significant side effects (diarrhea, colitis, hepatitis, pneumonitis, hypo/hyperthyroidism, type 1 diabetes) were seen in 13% to 15% of patients.

b. Nivolumab is also a PD-1–blocking antibody. The treatment with nivolumab resulted in a 32% response rate and 63% 12-month and 48% 24-month overall survival in the phase 1 trial. Similarly to pembrolizumab, the treatment with nivolumab resulted in the improved response rate, progression-free survival, and overall when compared to chemotherapy or ipilimumab.

c. Ipilimumab. Treatment with ipilimumab, a human CTLA4-blocking antibody, resulted in improvement in overall survival when compared to a vaccine treatment (10 vs. 6 months). The treatment can be complicated by the development of myriad autoimmune side effects including dermatitis, colitis, hepatitis, and endocrinopathies.

d. Combination of nivolumab and ipilimumab. This treatment is associated with an increased antimelanoma activity, but it also results in a significantly higher toxicity. The randomized trial of 945 treatment-naive in which patients were randomly assigned to nivolumab (1 mg/kg every 3 weeks) plus ipilimumab (3 mg/kg every 3 weeks) for 4 doses followed by nivolumab (3 mg/kg every 2 weeks), nivolumab (3 mg/kg every 2 weeks), or ipilimumab (3 mg/kg every 3 weeks for four doses) showed an improvement in PFS of 11.5 versus 7 versus 3 months, respectively, and similarly, an improved response rate of 58%, 44%, and 19%. In the combination group, serious adverse events were seen in 55% of patients, and 36% discontinued the therapy because of the adverse events.

e. **Talimogene laherparepvec** is a form of intralesional therapy in which an oncolytic herpes virus that was modified to proliferate in the injected tumor but not normal cells and that contains granulocyte–macrophage colony-stimulating factor (GM-CSF) gene is injected directly into the tumor. The treatment effect was also seen in the uninjected lesions and visceral metastasis most probably through eliciting systemic immune responses. The responses lasting more than 6 months were significantly more common in patients injected with talimogene laherparepvec than in patients injected with GM-CSF alone (16% vs. 2%).

f. **IL-2** given in high doses (600,000 to 720,000 U/kg every 8 hours for a maximum of 15 doses/cycle) resulted in a 16% response rates. Responses were higher in patients with stages M1a and M1b melanoma compared with patients with other visceral metastasis. Of responders, 44% were alive at 6-year follow-up. The treatment is associated with extensive toxicity and can be administered only in experienced centers.

g. **Adoptive cell transfer immunotherapy.** Adoptive cell transfer of *ex vivo* expanded tumor-infiltrating lymphocytes followed by treatment with high-dose IL-2 to 93 patients who received a nonmyeloablative lymphocyte-depleting conditioning regimen with fludarabine and cyclophosphamide resulted in 56% responses, including 20% complete responses. Adoptive transfer of lymphocytes that were transduced *ex vivo* with a retrovirus encoding a T-cell receptor for a melanoma-specific peptide led to response in 2 of 18 patients.

3. **Molecularly targeted therapy for metastatic melanoma**

a. **BRAF inhibitors**. The V600 BRAF mutation is present in about 40% to 50% of melanomas, and the treatment with two BRAF inhibitors, vemurafenib and dabrafenib, showed a response rate of 50% to 60% and a clinical benefit rate of 70% to 80%. The median duration of the response was 7 months.

b. **MEK inhibitors** are another category of agents that block MAPK pathway by inhibiting the activity of MEK, a downstream kinase from BRAF. Trametinib showed activity in patients with BRAF-mutated melanoma, but it is very rarely used as a single agent in this patient population. The treatment with binimetinib resulted in 20% response rate in NRAS-mutated melanomas.

c. **BRAF and MEK inhibitor combinations.** Dual inhibition of MAPK pathway with a combination of a BRAF inhibitor and an MEK inhibitor is more efficacious than the treatment with a single agent. The treatment with dabrafenib 150 mg twice a day and trametinib 2 mg daily when compared to the treatment with dabrafenib alone showed an improved progression-free survival (11 vs. 9 months), improved overall survival (25 vs. 19 months), and improved response rate (69% vs. 53%). Similarly, the treatment with vemurafenib 960 mg twice a day and cobimetinib 60 mg daily for 21 days followed by 7 days of break resulted in improved PFS (12 vs. 7 months) and response rate (70% vs. 50%). These trials established that patients with V600 BRAF–mutated melanoma should be offered the combination therapy.

    d. Kit inhibitors (imatinib) revolutionized the treatment of patients with GIST. Occasionally, the same kit mutations are present in patients with melanoma. The treatment with imatinib resulted in 33% to 50% response rates in c-kit–mutated melanomas.

  4. Chemotherapy for metastatic melanoma remains a treatment option for patients whose disease progressed on immunotherapy and targeted therapy.

    a. Dacarbazine (DTIC) is a well-tolerated agent when 250 mg/m^2 is given IV daily for 5 days, or 850 to 1,000 mg/m^2 once every 2 to 4 weeks. The response rates to dacarbazine are 6% to 12%.

    b. Temozolomide is an oral analog of dacarbazine that degrades to MTIC, the active metabolite of DTIC. It does penetrate the blood–brain barrier, so it can be used in patients with brain metastasis. When compared with DTIC, treatment with temozolomide resulted in no significant improvement in median survival. The drug is used at the doses of 200 mg/m^2/d orally for 5 days every 28 days or 75 mg/m^2/d for 6 weeks every 8 weeks.

    c. Nab-paclitaxel at 150 mg/m^2 on days 1, 8, and 15 every 4 weeks when compared to DTIC improved PFS (5 vs. 2.5 months), but there was improvement in neither overall survival nor response rate.

    d. Other single agents. Platinum-containing agents (cisplatin, carboplatin), nitrosoureas (carmustine, lomustine, fotemustine), microtubule toxins (vinblastine, vindesine), and other taxanes (paclitaxel, docetaxel) resulted in modest responses. None of these agents has been proved to be superior to dacarbazine in a randomized clinical trial.

VII. BRAIN METASTASES OF MALIGNANT MELANOMA

  A. Prognostic factors. Brain metastases are a common development in patients with malignant melanoma. Patients at especially high risk for the development of brain metastases are males with primary lesions located on mucosal surfaces or on the skin of the trunk or head and neck, with thick or ulcerated primary lesions, or with acral lentiginous or nodular lesions. These metastases contribute to death in 95% of these patients. The median survival from the time of diagnosis of brain metastasis is 4 months, and only 14% to 19% patients survive 1 year.

    Favorable prognostic factors include good performance status, younger age, absence of extracranial metastases, and the presence of a solitary brain metastasis.

  B. Local treatment. All patients with a new diagnosis of brain metastasis from melanoma should be evaluated for possible surgical resection or stereotactic irradiation utilizing convergent radiation beams. Control of progression in >90% of lesions can be achieved with these methods.

    With multiple simultaneous metastasis (>5), whole brain radiation therapy may be the only feasible treatment approach.

  C. Systemic therapy. The new improved immunotherapeutic agents and targeted therapies can have also activity against brain metastasis. The response rate to ipilimumab, when used alone or in combination with stereotactic radiosurgery, was similar in the brain and outside the brain in patients who were asymptomatic or minimally symptomatic and who were not on steroids or were on a low dose of steroids. It is unclear if symptomatic patients who require high-dose steroids to control their symptoms would have a chance to benefit from immunotherapy.

    BRAF inhibitors have also activity against brain metastases of V600E BRAF–mutated melanomas. The treatment with dabrafenib resulted in a 39% and 31% response rate in the brain in patients who were treatment naive and previously treated with radiation therapy, respectively. When a V600K mutation was present, the response rate was 15%.

It is questionable whether chemotherapy with agents that can penetrate through the blood–brain barrier, such as temozolomide or fotemustine (not available in the United States), can enhance the response to radiation.

VIII. FOLLOW-UP

The goal of a follow-up is to identify potentially curable recurrence and to screen for secondary primary tumors. At least one annual skin examination by a dermatologist is recommended. Patients with high-risk factors (including family history of melanoma, skin type, and presence of dysplastic nevi or non-melanoma skin cancers) may require more frequent examination.

Patients with stage IA melanoma should be seen every 3 to 12 months, and the examination of regional lymph nodes should be emphasized. For patients with stage IB to III melanomas, history and physical should be performed every 3 to 6 months for 3 years, then every 4 to 12 months for 2 years, and annually thereafter. Patients with stage IV disease who are rendered disease-free are followed as are patients with stage III disease. The regular follow-up should last between 5 and 10 years.

At clinician discretion, a chest x-ray study, LDH, LFT, and CBC may be obtained. Imaging studies (CT scan, PET scan) are ordered if clinically indicated. Abdominal or chest CT scans should be considered in patients with node-positive disease.

BASAL CELL AND SQUAMOUS CELL CARCINOMAS

I. EPIDEMIOLOGY AND ETIOLOGY

A. **Incidence.** Nonmelanoma skin cancers (NMSC), mainly basal cell carcinoma (BCC) and squamous cell carcinoma (SCC), are the most common type of malignancy, but they account for <0.1% of cancer-related deaths. BCC is four to five times more common than SCC. The exact incidence is unknown, because these cancers are not reported to the registry; estimate is that there are 1.3 million cases a year.

B. **Risk factors**

1. **UV light exposure.** Excessive UV light exposure is the main risk factor. NMSC are >50 times less common in non-white population than in white persons. Of these cancers, 90% develop in sun-exposed areas of the body. Blue-eyed, fair-skinned, and blond and red-haired people and those who are easily sunburned are at increased risk.

2. **Exposure to ionizing radiation.** Individuals who were exposed to ionizing radiation (uranium miners, individuals treated with radiation, cancer survivors) have a higher risk of NMSC.

3. **Chronic immunosuppression and chronic use of glucocorticoids.** Organ transplant recipients have 60- to 250-fold higher risk of development of SCC than the general population.

4. **Inorganic arsenic** exposure predisposes to the development of Bowen disease, multiple BCC, and SCC and is also associated with a higher incidence of intestinal carcinoma.

5. **Other environmental risk factors** include smoking and phototherapy combined with psoralens.

6. **Infection**

   a. **Epidermodysplasia verruciformis,** which is primarily caused by human papillomavirus (HPV) types 5 and 8, results in *in situ* and invasive SCC synergistically with other carcinogens, such as sunlight.

    b. SCC of the genitals and anal regions are strongly associated with HPV serotypes 16 and 18. Infection, usually through sexual transmission, increases the risk for regional SCC. **Verrucous carcinoma** (Buschke-Lowenstein tumor) is typically a slow-growing, HPV-associated (usually serotypes 6 and 11) neoplasm of the anogenital region that may deeply invade underlying structures.

    c. Periungual SCC is associated with HPV type 16.

7. **Chronic inflammation.** SCC can occasionally originate from the site of chronic ulcers or scars, sites of thermal burns, chronic draining osteomyelitis, and sinus tracts.

8. **Hereditary factors**

    a. Basal cell nevus syndrome (Gorlin syndrome) is a rare autosomal dominant disorder caused by mutations in the human-patched gene (PTCH1). Under normal conditions, the PTCH1 protein is in complex with another protein called smoothened (SMO) and they are in an inactive state. When the hedgehog (HH) protein binds to PTCH1, SMO is released and activates transcription factors that results in cell proliferation. In patients with Gorlin syndrome, PTCH1 is mutated and therefore cannot form complexes with SMO; it results in constant pathway activation. Multiple BCC lesions appear over the face, arms, and trunk during the late teenage years. Individuals also present with macrocephaly, frontal bossing, bifid ribs, bone cysts, palmar and plantar pitting, kyphoscoliosis, spina bifida, short metacarpals, hyporesponsiveness to parathyroid hormone, medulloblastoma, and ovarian fibromata.

    b. Xeroderma pigmentosum is a multigenic, autosomal recessive disorder in which DNA repair ability is impaired. Homozygotes have severe skin and eye sensitivity to sunshine. They develop SCC, BCC, and melanomas in the early childhood. Eye abnormalities include keratitis, iritis, opacification of the cornea, and choroidal melanoma. Frequently, they also suffer from neurologic disorders (seizures, mental and speech disturbances). A severe form (De Sanctis-Cacchione syndrome) includes microcephaly, mental deficiency, dwarfism, and failure of gonadal development.

    c. Oculocutaneous albinism is a group of genetic disorders characterized by generalized decrease in pigmentation.

II. PATHOLOGY AND NATURAL HISTORY

    A. BCC originates in the basal cell layer of the epidermis. Distant metastases from BCC are extremely rare. It has several recognized subtypes:

      1. Nodular BCC is the most common type (approximately 60% of cases). It arises predominantly on the head and neck as a well-circumscribed nodule with pearly or rolled borders and telangiectasias. Some lesions are pigmented and clinically indistinguishable from melanoma. Larger tumors may develop central necrosis and ulcerate, forming a so-called rodent ulcer.

      2. Superficial BCC represents 30% of cases. Lesions usually arise on the trunk, are often multiple, and appear as red, scaly patches with areas of brown or black pigmentation. They spread over the skin surface and may have areas of nodularity.

      3. Sclerosing (morpheaform) BCC represents 5% to 10% of cases. Lesions usually affect the face. The tumors resemble scars and may have an ivory-colored, ill-defined, indurated border. Histologically, the cancer cells are surrounded by a dense bed of fibrosis ("morphealike").

      4. Other subtypes: cystic, linear, and micronodular are less common.

B. **SCC** usually presents as a hyperkeratotic papule, plaque, or nodule. Hyperkeratosis is an important feature of SCC. In 60% of cases, SCC arises from actinic keratoses.

1. **Cutaneous horns** usually represent a premalignant process of hyperkeratosis on an erythematous base but occasionally may be an SCC.

2. **Bowen disease** is a form of intraepithelial SCC *in situ*, but invasion may occur. It appears as a red-brown eczematoid plaque. It usually occurs on sun-damaged areas in older persons, but it may arise in mucous membranes. Bowenoid papulosis is an intraepithelial neoplasia of the genital area caused by HPV.

3. **Keratoacanthoma** is a hyperkeratotic nodule with a central keratin plug. It grows rapidly, distinguishing it from other forms of SCC. It may regress spontaneously, but it should be treated because it may further invade the dermis and involve deeper soft tissue.

4. **Basosquamous carcinoma** has features of both BCC and SCC, but it is usually grouped with SCC because of its more aggressive behavior and metastatic capacity.

5. **Metastases.** Tumors that metastasize are usually poorly differentiated. The incidence of metastasis is <3% for actinically induced SCC and 35% for nonactinically induced SCC. The draining lymph nodes are the most frequent sites of metastases, although distant organs are eventually involved.

III. DIAGNOSIS AND WORKUP

Patients with suspicious lesions are offered a complete skin examination. If the lesion suggests SCC, examination of the regional lymph nodes should be performed. All suspicious lesions must be biopsied.

IV. STAGING SYSTEM AND PROGNOSTIC FACTORS

A. **TNM system** of staging was modified by the AJCC for NMSC in its seventh (2010) edition. More than 95% of BCC and SCC involve only local disease, and the staging system is rarely used.

B. **Prognostic factors.** Several prognostic factors are associated with inadequate treatment of primary tumors.

1. NMSC occurring on the head and neck and tumors >2 cm in diameter are more likely to recur.

2. SCC in the genital area, on mucosal surfaces, or on the ear has a higher propensity to metastasize.

3. Tumors that recur more frequently are those that are characterized by ill-defined clinical borders or perineural involvement and those that present as recurrent disease or develop in chronically immunosuppressed individuals (especially, organ transplant recipients).

4. BCC with micronodular, infiltrative, sclerosing, or morpheaform features and SCC with desmoplastic histologic features are also more likely to recur.

5. Basosquamous carcinoma has a higher capacity to metastasize than BCC or SCC.

6. High-risk features for SCC: Size ≥20 mm on trunk or extremities; size ≥10 mm on cheeks, forehead, scalp, neck, or pretibia; size ≥6 mm on the central face, eyelids, eyebrows, periorbital nose, lips, chin, mandible, preauricular and postauricular skin/sulci, temple, ear, genitalia, hands, and feet; poorly defined borders; recurrent tumors; immunosuppression; tumor in the site of previous radiation therapy or inflammation; rapid growth; neurologic symptoms; moderate or poor differentiation; adenoid, adenosquamous, and desmoplastic histology; depth ≥2 mm; and perineural/perivascular invasion.

V. PREVENTION

Primary prevention is largely achieved by encouraging patients and other responsible parties to minimize sunlight exposure and other reducible risk factors. Skin erythema from solar exposure, even from UV light on cloudy days, represents skin damage that is cumulative over the years. Sunscreens with an SPF of ≥15 and protective clothing, including hats, are helpful. Those who fastidiously avoid sunlight exposure to decrease their risk for skin cancer should meet their vitamin D requirement through diet or dietary supplements.

Successful *secondary prevention* is dependent on a regular follow-up. About 40% of patients with NMSC will develop another NMSC within 5 years. These individuals are also at higher risk for development of melanoma. Nicotinamide at the dose of 500 mg twice a day given for 12 months led to the 23% reduction in the relative risk for the development of another NSMC in patients who had at least 2 NSMCs in the past.

VI. MANAGEMENT

A. **Actinic keratoses** (precancerous lesions for SCC) are treated with cryosurgery, surgery, photodynamic therapy, or topical treatment with 5% 5-fluorouracil, 3.75% or 5% imiquimod, 0.015% or 0.05% ingenol mebutate, or 3% diclofenac sodium. Cryotherapy is associated with the risk of scarring, infection, and pigmentary changes; topical therapies are associated with application site irritation.

B. **BCC and SCC** can be treated with surgical techniques, radiation therapy, and topical therapies. It is important to customize therapeutic approaches to the particular factors and the individual needs of patients.

  1. **Mohs micrographic surgery** is the surgical method with the highest primary tumor cure rate (99% for BCC and 96% for SCC) and excellent cosmetic effects. Other techniques may require less training and be less costly, less invasive, or less time consuming. Therefore, Mohs surgery is recommended mainly for high-risk lesions and for recurrent tumors wherein the success rates are 95% for BCC and 93% for SCC.

  2. **Excision with postoperative margin evaluation.** The rate of cure is about 90% for primary tumors <2 cm in diameter when a 4- to 6-mm margin is applied. Larger or recurrent tumors require 10-mm margins that may result in significant cosmetic or functional deficits; cure rates range from 50% to 85%.

  3. **Curettage and electrodessication** is effective for low-risk tumors. It should not be used for tumors in the hair-bearing areas, and it should be followed by surgical excision if the subcutaneous layer is reached.

  4. **Cryosurgery using liquid nitrogen** may be considered for patients with small, clinically well-defined primary tumors. It is especially useful for debilitated patients with medical conditions that preclude other types of surgery.

  5. **Radiation therapy** is indicated in patients requiring extensive surgery or whose tumors are in surgically difficult locations. It should be avoided in young individuals (younger than 40 to 50) because of the risk of secondary malignancies, if tumors are located on the hands, feet, or nose and if the tumor recurred after previous RT. RT is also relatively contraindicated in patients with xeroderma pigmentosum, epidermodysplasia verruciformis, or the basal cell nevus syndrome, because RT may induce more tumors in the treated field. RT is not used as a sole method of treatment in patients

with high-risk SCC, but adjuvant RT should be considered after surgery for SCC demonstrating perineural invasion in large-caliber nerves or invasion into muscle or periosteum owing to increased risk for local recurrence and nodal metastases.

6. **Topical therapies** with 5-fluorouracil, imiquimod, or photodynamic therapy are used in patients with low-risk shallow cancers and in those who have contraindications for surgery and radiation therapy.

7. **Chemotherapy.** Experience in treating metastatic skin cancers is extremely limited. Response has been reported for advanced cases of SCC and BCC treated with cisplatin in combination with either a 5-day infusion of 5-fluorouracil (dosages similar to those used for head and neck cancers) or doxorubicin.

8. **Molecularly targeted agents.** Vismodegib and sonidegib are oral agents that inhibit the sonic hedgehog pathway by inactivation of surface receptor smoothened (SMO). The treatment with vismodegib resulted in a 67% and 38% response rate in patients with locally advanced and metastatic BCC, respectively. Similarly, sonidegib gave responses of 43% and 15%.

C. **Management of enlarged lymph nodes.** Occasionally, SCC can spread to the regional lymph nodes. Enlarged regional lymph nodes should undergo fine needle aspiration (FNA) or be biopsied. If lymph nodes are involved by tumor, an ELND followed by radiation therapy is recommended.

MERKEL CELL CARCINOMA

I. EPIDEMIOLOGY

Merkel cell carcinoma (MCC) is a rare type of skin cancer with the estimated incidence in the United States of 0.44 per 100,000 and 33% mortality, which is the highest mortality rate among cutaneous malignancies. The median age at presentation is 65 years.

A. **Risk factors.** Sun exposure, advanced age, and chronic immunosuppression (previous solid organ transplantation, concomitant B-cell malignancies, HIV positivity, chronic immunosuppressive therapy for rheumatologic disorders) are important risk factors.

B. **Prognostic factors.** The extent of the disease is the most important prognostic factor. Patients with localized disease have a 65% to 85% 5-year survival, with disease metastatic to regional lymph nodes 35% to 45%, and with distant metastases 20% to 25%.

II. PATHOLOGY AND NATURAL HISTORY

These cells, first discovered by Merkel in the snout skin of voles in 1875, are thought to originate from the neural crest and to act as mechanoreceptors. Tumors are assumed to be derived from the large, oval neuroendocrine Merkel cells that are located in the basal layer of the epidermis and are associated with terminal axons.

A new polyoma virus associated with MCC has been recently identified and may play a role in the pathogenesis of MCC. It is present in 80% of MCC samples.

Initially, tumor cells spread from the primary site through the lymphatic system to local lymph nodes, and then, they can disseminate throughout the whole body. The most common sites of distant metastases are liver, brain, lungs, bones, and skin.

III. DIAGNOSIS

A. **Signs.** MCC manifests as a rapidly growing, painless, indurated, and erythematous to violaceous nodule. The lesions appear mainly in the sun-exposed areas. Head and neck (30% to 45%) and the extremities (35%) are the most common sites for the primary tumor, but the tumor can occur on the trunk, the buttocks, or genitalia. Most patients (75%) present with the disease localized to the primary skin site. Involvement of regional lymph nodes occurs in 25% of cases and distant metastases develop in 2% to 4%. Some patients (approximately 2%) are diagnosed with the metastatic disease in the setting of the carcinoma of unknown primary site.

B. **Diagnosis.** Biopsy of the growing lesion is required for diagnosis. The three histologic types are trabecular, intermediate cell, and small cell, but histologic subtypes do not carry prognostic value. It is often difficult to differentiate MCC from other "small blue cell tumors" (see immunohistochemical phenotypes in Appendix C4.II).

C. **Staging.** Physical examination, concentrating especially on regional lymph nodes and computerized tomography scan of the chest, abdomen and pelvis, should be used as a part of staging investigations.

IV. MANAGEMENT

A. **Surgery.** Patients who have no evidence of metastatic disease should be considered for wide excision of the primary tumor with 1 to 2 cm margins; SNLB is routinely performed at the same time. Patients who are unfit for surgery can be treated with primary radiation therapy.

B. **Assessment of the regional lymph nodes.** Individuals who had negative lymph nodes on surgical assessment of their status by SNLB, ELND, or therapeutic nodal staging had a 97% 5-year disease-free survival (DFS) compared with a 75% 5-year DFS for individuals whose lymph nodes were assessed only clinically. Patients who have a positive SNLB or have clinically or radiographically demonstrable nodal involvement are treated with total lymphadenectomy.

C. **Radiation therapy.** Adjuvant RT to the primary site improves local tumor control. Patients treated with surgery alone are 3.7 times more likely to develop a local recurrence and 2.7 times more likely to develop a regional recurrence than patients who received combination surgery and RT. The rate of distant metastasis is similar between the groups. Adjuvant RT to nodes is recommended when SNLB has not been performed or when clinically or pathologically evident nodal disease is present. Delays before commencement of RT should be minimized because they may result in disease progression.

D. **Chemotherapy.** The role of adjuvant chemotherapy is controversial and most studies suggest that, although it may improve the locoregional control, it does not prolong survival. In a study performed by Trans-Tasman Radiation Oncology Group, patients with high-risk features (size of the primary tumor >1 cm, lymph node involvement, recurrence after primary therapy, or gross residual disease after resection) received synchronous RT and chemotherapy with carboplatin and etoposide; this approach resulted in an excellent overall survival at 3 years of 76%. In a subsequent follow-up study, a greater number of patients were compared with historical controls, and this comparison revealed no benefit in overall survival for individuals receiving chemotherapy.

Currently, chemotherapy is not recommended for patients with node-negative disease but can be considered for high-risk patients. Individuals with metastatic disease should be treated with chemotherapy.

No standard chemotherapy regimen has been established, but in regimens commonly used for the treatment of small cell lung cancer, such as CAV (cyclophosphamide, doxorubicin, vincristine), CEV (cyclophosphamide, etoposide, vincristine) with or without prednisone, and EP (etoposide, cisplatin), topotecan have been prescribed most frequently. Use of CAV or CEV resulted in 75% response rate, including 35% complete responses; EP resulted in 60% response rate and 35% complete responses. Median overall survival for patients treated with any type of chemotherapy is 22 months (ranging from 1 to 118 months), and at 2 years, 36% individuals remain alive.

E. Treatment of recurrent disease. Locally and regionally recurrent disease is treated with surgery and RT or chemoradiation therapy. Systemic recurrence is treated with chemotherapy.

F. Immunotherapy. Both anti-PD1 antibodies (pembrolizumab) and anti PD-L1 antibodies (avelumab) showed significant activity with response rates 30–56%.

Suggested Readings

Malignant Melanoma

Eggermont AM, Chiarion-Sileni V, Grob JJ, et al. Adjuvant ipilimumab versus placebo after complete resection of high-risk stage III melanoma (EORTC 18071): a randomised, double-blind, phase 3 trial. *Lancet Oncol* 2015;16(5):522.

Kirkwood JM, Strawderman MH, Ernstoff MS, et al. Interferon alfa-2b adjuvant therapy of high-risk resected cutaneous melanoma: the Eastern Cooperative Oncology Group Trial EST 1684. *J Clin Oncol* 1996;14(1):7.

Larkin J, Ascierto PA, Dréno B, et al. Combined vemurafenib and cobimetinib in BRAF-mutated melanoma. *N Engl J Med* 2014;371(20):1867.

Larkin J, Chiarion-Sileni V, Gonzalez R, et al. Combined nivolumab and ipilimumab or monotherapy in untreated melanoma. *N Engl J Med* 2015;373:23.

Long GV, Stroyakovskiy D, Gogas H, et al. Dabrafenib and trametinib versus dabrafenib and placebo for Val600 BRAF-mutant melanoma: a multicentre, double-blind, phase 3 randomised controlled trial. *Lancet* 2015;386(9992):444.

Morton DL, Thompson JF, Cochran AJ, et al. Final trial report of sentinel-node biopsy versus nodal observation in melanoma. *N Engl J Med* 2014;370(7):599.

Robert C, Schachter J, Long GV, et al. Pembrolizumab versus ipilimumab in advanced melanoma. *N Engl J Med* 2015;372:2521.

Basal Cell and Squamous Cell Carcinomas

Basset-Seguin N, Hauschild A, Grob JJ, et al. Vismodegib in patients with advanced basal cell carcinoma (STEVIE): a pre-planned interim analysis of an international, open-label trial. *Lancet Oncol* 2015;16(6):729.

Kauvar AN, Arpey CJ, Hruza G, et al. Consensus for nonmelanoma skin cancer treatment. Part II: squamous cell carcinoma, including a cost analysis of treatment methods. *Dermatol Surg* 2015;41(11):1214.

Migden MR, Guminski A, Gutzmer R, et al. Treatment with two different doses of sonidegib in patients with locally advanced or metastatic basal cell carcinoma (BOLT): a multicentre, randomised, double-blind phase 2 trial. *Lancet Oncol* 2015;16(6):716.

Merkel Cell Carcinoma

Becker JC. Merkel cell carcinoma. *Ann Oncol* 2010;21(suppl 7):vii81.

Feng H, Shuda M, Chang Y, et al. Clonal integration of a polyomavirus in human Merkel cell carcinoma. *Science* 2008;319(5866):1096.

Gupta SG, et al. Sentinel lymph node biopsy for evaluation and treatment of patients with Merkel cell carcinoma. The Dana-Farber experience and meta-analysis of the literature. *Arch Dermatol* 2006;142:685.

Lemos BD, Storer BE, Iyer JG, et al. Pathologic nodal evaluation improves prognostic accuracy in Merkel cell carcinoma: analysis of 5823 cases as the basis of the first consensus staging system. *J Am Acad Dermatol* 2010;63(5):751.

18 Sarcomas

Charles A. Forscher

I. EPIDEMIOLOGY AND ETIOLOGY

Primary mesenchymal tumors localized outside the skeleton, parenchymatous organs, or hollow viscera are generally designated as soft tissue sarcomas (STSs). Sarcomas of the mediastinum, heart, and blood vessels are discussed in Chapter 20.

A. **Incidence.** Sarcomas constitute about 1% of all cancers and will account for an estimated 12,310 new cases of STS and 3,000 cases of bone sarcoma in the United States in 2016. These will be associated with 4,990 and 1,500 deaths, respectively.

1. STSs outnumber bone sarcomas by a ratio of 3:1. In children, most STSs are rhabdomyosarcomas or undifferentiated tumors originating in the head and neck regions. In adults, STSs occur most frequently on the extremities or retroperitoneum and least frequently in the head and neck region.

2. Bone sarcomas occur mostly between 10 and 20 years of age (osteogenic sarcoma) or between 40 and 60 years of age (chondrosarcoma).

3. Most sarcomas show no sexual predilection. Incidence peaks during childhood and in the fifth decade.

B. **Etiology.** Certain kinds of sarcomas are associated with exposure to specific agents or with underlying medical conditions:

1. **Lymphangiosarcoma.** Prolonged postmastectomy arm edema (Stewart-Treves syndrome).

2. **Angiosarcoma and other STSs.** Polyvinyl chloride, thorium dioxide, dioxin, arsenic, and androgens.

3. **Osteosarcoma.** Radium (watch dials) exposure, postmastectomy irradiation, Paget disease of the bone.

4. **Fibrosarcoma.** Postirradiation: Paget disease of the bone.

5. **Kaposi sarcoma.** Human herpesvirus 8 and human immunodeficiency virus type 1 (HIV-1; discussed in Chapter 37).

6. **Leiomyosarcoma.** HIV-1 in children.

7. **Genetic diseases and syndromes.**

   a. **Li-Fraumeni syndrome.** Various sarcomas (especially rhabdomyosarcoma) and carcinomas of the breast, lung, and adrenal cortex (*p53* gene)

   b. **Neurofibromatosis.** Schwannomas and malignant peripheral nerve sheath tumor (*NF1* gene)

   c. **Familial retinoblastoma.** Osteosarcoma (*RB1* gene)

8. **Chromosomal aberrations** are found in nearly all sarcomas. Some of these may be limited aberrations such as specific translocations (e.g., the X;18 translocation in synovial sarcoma, the 11;22 translocation in Ewing sarcoma, and the 12;16 translocation in myxoid liposarcoma). Other sarcomas have complex chromosomal abnormalities as occurs in myxofibrosarcoma and pleomorphic liposarcoma.

II. PATHOLOGY AND NATURAL HISTORY

A. **Histology and nomenclature.** The multipotential capacities of the mesenchymal tissue and the appearance of several histologic elements in the same tumor often make clear-cut histologic diagnosis difficult.

1. **Sarcomas are named for the tissue of origin** (e.g., osteosarcoma, chondrosarcoma, schwannoma, liposarcoma).

2. **Tumors are also named for special histologic characteristics** or given a nondescriptive name because the tissue of origin is unknown (alveolar soft parts sarcoma, Kaposi sarcoma, Ewing sarcoma).

3. **Pathologists recognize several features in determining the grade of a sarcoma.** These include the degree of cellular differentiation, the presence (or absence) of mitotic activity, spontaneous necrosis, and vascular invasion.

4. **The presence of osteoid formation** by the tumor cells suggests the diagnosis of osteogenic sarcoma. This must be distinguished from reactive or metaplastic bone formation by the pathologist.

5. **Immunohistochemistry** may be helpful in confirming the tissue of origin.

6. **Cytogenetics** can be useful in the diagnosis of Ewing sarcoma, synovial sarcoma, and rhabdomyosarcoma. Techniques such as fluorescent *in situ* hybridization (FISH) analysis are useful, especially in translocation sarcomas.

B. **Natural history.** Generally, sarcomas arise *de novo* and not from preexisting benign neoplasms. Tumors can "dedifferentiate," however, from a lower grade to a higher grade. Sarcomas spread without interruption along tissue planes; they invade local nerve fibers, muscle bundles, and blood vessels. Histologic sections usually show much greater local extension than is apparent on gross examination.

1. **Histologic grade.** The biologic behavior of sarcomas can usually be predicted by their histologic grade. Low-grade tumors tend to remain localized; high-grade tumors (especially those with a marked degree of necrosis) have a greater propensity to metastasize. Most osteogenic sarcomas, rhabdomyosarcomas, Ewing sarcomas, and synovial sarcomas are high-grade malignancies.

2. **Site of origin.** The site of origin of the sarcoma may suggest the cell type as follows:

   a. **Head and neck:** rhabdomyosarcoma (in a child), angiosarcoma (in an elderly person), osteogenic sarcoma (jaw)

   b. **Distal extremity:** epithelioid sarcoma, synovial sarcoma, clear cell sarcoma, osteogenic sarcoma (femur)

   c. **Proximal tibia or humerus:** osteogenic sarcoma

   d. **Abdomen, retroperitoneum, and mesentery:** leiomyosarcoma, gastrointestinal stromal tumor (GIST), liposarcoma, desmoplastic small round cell tumor

   e. **Genitourinary tract:** rhabdomyosarcoma (in a child), leiomyosarcoma (in an adult)

   f. **Skin:** angiosarcoma, lymphangiosarcoma, Kaposi sarcoma, epithelioid sarcoma, dermatofibrosarcoma protuberans (on trunk)

3. **Metastases.** Sarcomas typically spread hematogenously. Lung metastases occur most commonly. Hepatic metastases can be seen from primary gastrointestinal or gynecologic sarcomas. The retroperitoneum can be a site of metastasis for extremity liposarcomas. Other sites, such as bone, subcutaneous tissue, and brain, are less common and are often detected only after pulmonary metastases have developed (tertiary metastases). An exception is myxoid liposarcoma, which can metastasize to extrapulmonary sites before appearing in the lung.

    a. Sarcomas that metastasize to lymph nodes: rhabdomyosarcoma, synovial sarcoma, epithelioid sarcoma

    b. Sarcomas that rarely metastasize and are associated with a favorable survival: liposarcoma (well-differentiated types), fibrosarcoma (infantile and well-differentiated types), myxofibrosarcoma (superficial type), dermatofibrosarcoma protuberans, and parosteal osteosarcoma.

C. Clinical aspects of specific STSs

  1. Alveolar soft part sarcoma

    a. Tissue of origin (incidence). Unknown (rare).

    b. Features. Unique histology with no benign counterpart; often indolent even with lung metastases, which are common. This sarcoma is most frequently associated with brain metastases. Commonly affects the thigh in adults and the head and neck in children. The 5-year survival rate exceeds 60%.

  2. Angiosarcoma (hemangiosarcoma, lymphangiosarcoma)

    a. Tissue of origin (incidence). Blood or lymph vessels (2% to 3%).

    b. Features of hemangiosarcoma. Affects the elderly; aggressive. Arises in many organs, notably the head and neck region, breast, spleen, and liver; especially affects the skin and superficial soft tissues (whereas most STSs are deep). Dedifferentiation from a hemangioma is rare. The 5-year survival rate is <20%.

    c. Features of lymphangiosarcoma. Affects older adults; aggressive. Arises in areas with chronic lymphatic stasis (especially postmastectomy). The 5-year survival rate is 10%.

  3. Clear cell sarcoma

    a. Tissue of origin (incidence). Tumor of deep soft tissues with melanocytic differentiation. EWSR1-ATF1 fusion gene is commonly detected.

    b. Features. Affects adults <40 years of age; painless, firm, spherical masses on tendon sheaths and aponeurotic structures of distal extremities. The 5-year survival rate is about 50%.

  4. Epithelioid sarcoma

    a. Tissue of origin (incidence). Unknown (rare).

    b. Features. Affects young adults; aggressive; typically appears on distal extremities. Epithelioid sarcoma and synovial sarcoma are the most common tumors of the hand and foot. Differs from other STSs by having a greater tendency to spread to noncontiguous areas of the skin, subcutaneous tissue, fat, draining lymph nodes, and bone. The 5-year survival rate is about 30%.

  5. Fibrosarcoma

    a. Tissue of origin (incidence). Fibrous tissue (5% to 20%).

    b. Features. Affects all age groups; arises in many mesenchymal sites; usually involves the abdominal wall or extremities. Ninety percent are well differentiated (desmoid). Dermatofibrosarcoma protuberans (rare) develops on the skin of the trunk and almost never metastasizes. Fibromyxosarcoma affects any soft tissue site but usually develops on the extremities. Ten percent are poorly differentiated (high grade). Survival is directly related to tumor grade (also see Section II.D.5).

  6. Pleomorphic sarcoma, not otherwise specified (NOS) (previously named malignant fibrous histiocytoma [MFH])

    a. Tissue of origin (incidence). Unknown (10% to 23%).

    b. Features. Age >40 years (<5% of affected patients are <20 years of age). It is a common histologic diagnosis. Develops in extremities (especially legs), trunk, and retroperitoneum. Superficial version develops close to the skin surface and is often low grade; the 5-year survival rate is 65%. Deep pleomorphic sarcoma is high grade; the 5-year survival rate is 30% to 60%.

7. **Solitary fibrous tumor**
   a. **Tissue of origin (incidence).** Blood vessels or fibrous tissue (<1%).
   b. **Features.** Affects all ages. Develops under fingertips (glomus tumors), on lower extremities or pelvis, in the retroperitoneum, and elsewhere. Benign and malignant versions. The 5-year survival rate is about 50%.

8. **Kaposi sarcoma (KS).** All varieties of KS are associated with human herpesvirus type 8 (HHV-8). KS typically presents as purplish blotches or nodules that may be painful or pruritic. Treatment of KS in patients with AIDS is discussed in Chapter 37.
   a. **Tissue of origin (incidence).** Controversial (varied).
   b. **Features of classic KS.** Classically affects older adults with Mediterranean ancestry; extremely indolent lesions arise on lower extremities (occasionally on the hands, ears, and nose) and rarely cause death.
   c. **Features of epidemic KS.** The epidemic and aggressive variety is associated with AIDS, African children, renal transplant recipients, immunosuppressed nontransplantation patients, and Eskimos. These patients develop a widely disseminated, aggressive, and usually fatal form of the disease. Generalized cutaneous involvement, generalized lymphadenopathy, and visceral or gastrointestinal involvement are typical.

9. **Leiomyosarcoma, gastrointestinal stromal tumor (GIST), and metastasizing leiomyoma**
   a. **Tissue of origin (incidence).** Smooth muscle for leiomyoma and leiomyosarcoma; interstitial cell of Cajal for GIST (7% to 11%).
   b. **Features.** Affects all age groups. Develops in the gastrointestinal tract, uterus, retroperitoneum, and other soft tissues. GIST tumors are refractory to chemotherapy and radiotherapy. The 5-year survival rate is 30%.
   c. **Gastrointestinal stromal tumors (GISTs)** are morphologically similar to leiomyosarcoma but have different immunohistochemical staining characteristics. GISTs do not stain for actin (as leiomyosarcomas do), and most express CD117 (*c-kit* protein). Treatment of GIST is presented in Section VII.C.7.
   d. **Leiomyoma peritonealis disseminata (LPD).** A condition in women, usually in reproductive years. Myriads of asymptomatic benign leiomyomas are usually scattered throughout the peritoneal cavity and range from 1 to 10 cm in size; they are stimulated by estrogen. LPD causes occasional mechanical problems with bowel or pain. Generally, no treatment is required; when symptomatic, treatment is with estrogens or antiestrogens.
   e. **Leiomyoma, benign metastasizing.** Histologically benign, these leiomyomas are typically discovered as persistent pulmonary nodules and possibly as a variant of LPD. Associated nodules in the pelvis are mostly in round ligaments of uterus and not as diffuse as in LPD. Treatment is surgical for symptomatic or progressive lesions.

10. **Liposarcoma**
    a. **Tissue of origin (incidence).** Fat tissue (15% to 18%).
    b. **Features.** Affects middle and older age groups, mostly men. Develops in the thigh, groin, buttocks, shoulder girdle, and retroperitoneum. Does not arise from benign lipomas. Low grade lipomatous tumors are termed atypical lipomatous tumor in the extremities and are designated as well-differentiated liposarcoma in the retroperitoneum. Well-differentiated

liposarcomas may have dedifferentiated elements with the tumor. The 5-year survival rate is 80% for low-grade liposarcomas and 20% for high-grade liposarcomas of an extremity. Survival rates are lower, and local recurrence rates are high for abdominal/retroperitoneal liposarcomas. Myxoid liposarcoma has genetic profile distinct from well-differentiated/dedifferentiated liposarcoma.

11. **Schwannoma and malignant nerve sheath tumor (MPNST)**
    a. **Tissue of origin (incidence).** Nerve (5% to 7%).
    b. **Features.** Affects young and middle-aged adults and patients with neurofibromatosis type 1 (von Recklinghausen disease; about 10% develop sarcomatous changes during lifetime). Presents with thickening of nerves and without anatomic predilection. Superficial variety is low grade, spreads extensively along nerve sheaths without metastasizing, and has a 5-year survival rate of >90%. MPNST is a malignant counterpart of schwannoma, and it often originates from a plexiform neurofibroma. Schwannomas do not transform into MPNST. A 5-year survival of MPNST patients is <20%.

12. **Rhabdomyosarcoma**
    a. **Tissue of origin (incidence).** Striated muscle (5% to 19%).
    b. **Features.** By definition in the G-TNM staging system, all are grade 3. All types can occur in any age group, but the typical onset and distribution are noted below (see Chapter 19).
    c. **Features of embryonal rhabdomyosarcoma.** Affects infants and children; sites are head and neck (70%) and genitalia (15% to 20%). Includes sarcoma botryoid. The 5-year survival rate is about 70%.
    d. **Features of alveolar rhabdomyosarcoma.** Affects teenagers at any site; highly aggressive; histology resembles lung alveoli. The 5-year survival rate is about 50%.
    e. **Features of pleomorphic rhabdomyosarcoma.** Affects patients >30 years of age, is rare, and develops in extremities. Often is highly anaplastic; microscopically confused with MFH. The 5-year survival rate is about 25%.

13. **Synovial sarcoma**
    a. **Tissue of origin (incidence).** Unknown. Recent data suggest that these tumors may arise from primitive muscle cells. Although these tumors can arise near joints, they are not composed of cells with synovial differentiation. The name is a misnomer that persists. They rarely arise within a joint space.
    b. **Features.** Affects young adults but may occur from the second to fourth decade. Monophasic and biphasic subtypes are distinguished. Presents with firm masses, often painful, near tendons in the vicinity of joints of the hands, knees, or feet. Synovial and epithelioid sarcomas are the most common tumors of the hand and foot. Often calcified, with characteristic radiographic appearance. The majority of synovial sarcomas are high grade. Lymph node involvement may be seen in up to 20% of cases. The 5-year survival rate is from 30% to 50%.

D. **Clinical aspects of specific bone sarcomas**
   1. **Adamantinoma**
      a. **Tissue of origin (incidence).** Unknown; nonosseous (<1%).
      b. **Features.** Osteolytic tumor; often develops on the upper tibia; resembles ameloblastoma of mandible. Indolent behavior; the 5-year survival rate is >90%.

   2. **Chondrosarcoma**
      a. **Tissue of origin (incidence).** Cartilage (30%).

b. Features. Age 40 to 60 years; <4% of patients are <20 years of age. Usually develops in the shoulder girdle (15%), proximal femur (20%), or pelvis (30%). Chondrosarcomas are the most common malignant tumors of the sternum and scapula. Most tumors are grade 1 or 2; higher-grade tumors metastasize frequently; however, tumor grade does not appear to affect prognosis. Local recurrence is a major problem in management. Usually refractory to both radiation therapy (RT) and chemotherapy. Dedifferentiated chondrosarcomas may, however, respond to chemotherapy. Complete surgical removal is the main determinant of recurrence and survival. The 5-year survival rate is about 50%.

   (1) Central chondrosarcomas (75%) arise within a bone; peripheral chondrosarcomas (25%) arise from the surface of a bone. Peripheral lesions can become quite large without causing pain; central lesions present with a dull pain but rarely with a mass. Pain means that the apparently "benign" cartilage tumor on radiographs is probably a central chondrosarcoma.

   (2) About 25% of chondrosarcomas represent malignant transformation of a preexisting endochondroma or osteocartilaginous exostosis. The presentation of multiple benign cartilaginous tumors has a higher rate of malignant transformation than the corresponding solitary lesions.

3. Chordoma

   a. Tissue of origin (incidence). Primitive notochord cells (5%).

   b. Features. Develops in the midline of the neural axis at base of the skull or sacrococcygeal area. The physaliferous (bubble-bearing) cells are pathognomonic histologically. Indolent tumor with almost universal tendency for local recurrence. Low grade but eventually fatal after many years because of complications associated with invasion into neural tissues. Treated with surgery and RT. The 5-year survival rate is 50%.

4. Ewing sarcoma

   a. Tissue of origin (incidence). Unknown; nonmesenchymal elements of bone marrow (15%)

   b. Features. Affects children 10 to 15 years of age; rare in blacks; highly aggressive; arises in many bones, but especially the femoral diaphysis (see Chapter 19)

5. Fibrosarcoma of bone

   a. Tissue of origin (incidence). Fibrous tissue (2%).

   b. Features. Affects middle-aged patients in major long bones; develops occasionally in conjunction with an underlying disease (bone infarcts, osteomyelitis, benign giant cell tumor, Paget disease, after RT). Resembles fibrosarcoma, but osteoid is detected in parts of the lesion. Often high grade, which correlates with metastatic potential and survival (see Section II.C.5).

6. Malignant fibrous histiocytoma of bone

   a. Tissue of origin (incidence). Fibrous and primitive mesenchymal tissue (5%).

   b. Features. Affects older patients; arises *de novo* or as a complication of Paget disease. Most common sites are metaphyses of long bones, especially around the knee. In contrast to osteogenic sarcoma, serum alkaline phosphatase levels are normal. Pathologic fracture is often the first manifestation. Aggressive with high rate of dissemination to the lungs (also see Section II.C.6).

7. **Giant cell tumor of bone**
   a. **Tissue of origin (incidence).** Primitive mesenchymal stromal cell, which expresses RANKL. Giant cells are reactive.
   b. **Features.** Patients usually >20 years of age. Most common sites are around the knee, radius, and sacrum. Tumor is usually benign but can be locally aggressive. Rare malignant transformation can occur.

8. **Osteogenic sarcoma**
   a. **Tissue of origin (incidence).** Bone (40% to 50%).
   b. **Features of classic osteogenic sarcoma.** Affects any age, but the onset is usually between 10 and 20 years; more common in boys and men. Most tumors originate in the metaphysis of long bones, the region of highest growth velocity. Tender, bony masses in the distal femur, proximal tibia, and proximal humerus account for 85% of cases. Nearly always high grade.
   c. **Features of low-grade osteogenic sarcoma.** Rare; central lesions can occur.
   d. **Features of osteogenic sarcoma of the jaw.** Affects patients between the ages of 20 and 40 years; men are more commonly affected; frequently detected during dental examinations. These tumors often have a cartilaginous component. High- and low-grade varieties are treated with hemimaxillectomy or hemimandibulectomy and reconstruction. Local control can often be a major problem if less than radical surgery is performed.
   e. **Features of telangiectatic osteogenic sarcoma.** Affects younger patients; a purely lytic tumor that can be confused with an aneurysmal bone cyst. Highly malignant; metastasizes early.
   f. **Features of multifocal sclerosing osteogenic sarcoma.** Rare; affects children <10 years of age. Develops multiple simultaneous primary sites in metaphyses; rapidly metastasizes to lung and soft tissues.
   g. **Features of periosteal osteogenic sarcoma.** Rare. Affects patients between the ages of 15 and 25 years; arises on external bone surface growing into the overlying soft tissues as an enlarging painless mass with minimal involvement of medullary canal. Histologically confused with chondrosarcomas. More than 50% metastasize (also see Section II.D.9).

9. **Parosteal (juxtacortical) sarcoma**
   a. **Tissue of origin (incidence).** Bone surface (<2%).
   b. **Features.** A distinct clinical entity (see Section II.D.8.g). Onset from 20 to 30 years of age. Characteristic exophytic lesion that is often on the posterior aspect of the distal femur or medial aspect of the proximal humerus. Presents as a fixed painless mass. Usually low grade with an indolent course; rarely involves medullary canal. Infrequently metastasizes; the 5-year survival rate is 80%.

10. **Sarcomas of bone associated with other conditions**
    a. **Paget disease of the bone.** Affects patients >60 years of age; the risk for sarcoma is 1,000-fold greater than in the general population at this age. Sarcomatous transformation occurs in 0.7% of patients with Paget disease and accounts for 5% to 14% of osteogenic sarcomas. The histologic form varies among reported series but is usually osteogenic sarcoma, MFH, or fibrosarcoma; chondrosarcoma, giant cell tumor, and other forms occur infrequently. Tends to affect the pelvis and proximal femur; frequently presents as pathologic fracture of the femur. Highly malignant.

   b. After high-dose RT. Sarcoma develops within the irradiated field (bone or adjacent soft tissue structures) about 10 years after treatment. Highly malignant.

   c. Familial or bilateral retinoblastoma. A tumor suppressor gene (*RB*) has been identified on the 13q chromosome in some patients with retino-blastoma. Patients who have a 13q deletion are at increased risk for later development of osteogenic sarcoma, not only in the irradiated field but also in long bones distant from irradiated sites about 10 to 20 years later. Highly malignant.

III. DIAGNOSIS

   A. Symptoms and signs are summarized in Sections II.C and D. Patients with STS typically present with a painless, progressive swelling in an extremity; all such swellings are suspect for malignancy. Head and neck sarcomas manifest as proptosis, masses, or neurologic abnormalities. Retroperitoneal sarcomas present with back pain, lower extremity edema, and abdominal masses. Bone sarcomas usually result in visible enlargement of bone and pathologic fractures.

   B. Biopsy. An accurate biopsy diagnosis is essential.

   C. Radiographic studies

   1. Plain radiographs of soft tissues may demonstrate bone involvement. Stippled calcification may be present within the mass. Patients with painful or enlarged bones should have radiographic study of these areas. The following findings are helpful for making the diagnosis of osteogenic sarcoma:

   a. An osteoblastic appearance is often seen in osteosarcoma.

   b. Periosteal reaction with elevated periosteum forming a triangle (*Codman triangle*) with bone cortex. Any periosteal elevation in an apparent bone lesion is an indication for biopsy.

   c. Sunray-like spiculation of bones

   d. Onion-skin appearance (a common finding in Ewing sarcoma)

   2. CT scans are most useful for evaluating retroperitoneal or head and neck regions. CT scanning of the extremities appears to be effective in delineating the extent of the tumor.

   3. Magnetic resonance imaging (MRI) is comparable to CT scans in defining the relation of the tumor to neurovascular and skeletal structures, but MRI might be better for predicting resectability.

   4. Radionuclide scans. Bone scan is performed in patients with bone sarcomas to search for multifocal disease. PET scanning is useful both for determining sites of disease and for assessing response to therapy.

   5. CT of the thorax is necessary for all patients with sarcoma to detect lung metastases, which may be resected after the primary tumor is managed. An "old calcified granuloma" is an untenable radiologic diagnosis in a young person with sarcoma.

   6. Serum alkaline phosphatase levels are elevated in 60% of patients with osteogenic sarcoma and rarely in other bone sarcomas. When elevated at the time of diagnosis, this result is an important tumor marker to evaluate response to therapy.

IV. STAGING SYSTEM AND PROGNOSTIC FACTORS

   A. Staging system. Refer to the current AJCC Cancer Staging atlas for TNM staging system. Tumor grade is the single most important prognostic factor in sarcomas and is incorporated into the staging system.

TABLE 18-1	Stage Grouping and Survival for Soft Tissue Sarcomas	
Stage	**Grade**	**5-yr Survival Rate**
Stage I	Low	85%–90%
Stage II	High	70%–80%
Stage III	High	45%–55%
Stage IV	Any	0%–20%

B. **Prognostic factors**
   1. **Histologic grade** (the degree of differentiation, the amount of necrosis, and the number of mitoses per high-power microscopic field) is the single most important prognostic factor, especially for STS. The shortcoming of this system is less-than-ideal reproducibility.
   2. **Local recurrence** predisposes to further recurrences. The absence of clear surgical margins, with or without postoperative RT, increases the rate of local recurrence in patients with STS but does not affect survival. The development of distant metastases after local recurrence may be either directly related to the recurrence or only a reflection of the more aggressive tumor biology.
   3. **Site of disease.** Half of deaths in patients with STS occur in the 8% of patients with retroperitoneal lesions.
C. **Stage groupings and survival for STS** are shown in Table 18-1. The rate of progression for GIST depends both on the mitotic rate, size and the site of the primary tumor.
D. **Long-term survival.** About 80% of all STSs that recur do so within 2 years. Patients with osteogenic sarcoma who survive 3 years without evidence of disease appear to be cured.

V. PREVENTION AND EARLY DETECTION
The physician must suspect and biopsy all soft tissue masses, *de novo* bony abnormalities, and periosteal elevations with an apparent bone lesion.

VI. MANAGEMENT OF BONE SARCOMAS
A. **Surgery.** Treatment of osteogenic sarcomas results in a 65% to 80% 10-year, disease-free survival. Relapse after 3 years of disease-free survival is unusual.
   1. **Limb-salvage surgery** is now the standard treatment for most patients with osteogenic sarcomas of the extremities, where nearly 90% of these tumors originate. The historical fear of "skip metastases" (within the same bone of involvement) has proved excessive; the occurrence rate of skip metastases appears to be <10%. Only occasionally do patients require amputation. The widespread, successful use of limb-salvage therapy has been made possible by the following advances:
      a. **Significant progress in the development of modern prostheses** that are available immediately after surgery. For example, young children who would have had unacceptable leg-length discrepancy with limb-salvage procedures can now be given a prosthesis that can be lengthened as the patient grows (expandable prosthesis).
      b. **The use of preoperative (neoadjuvant) chemotherapy**
         (1) Preoperative chemotherapy can result in enough tumor shrinkage to permit the use of prosthesis for limb-sparing surgery.
         (2) Preoperative chemotherapy provides an *in vivo* drug trial to determine the drug sensitivity of an individual tumor. Patients who have

an excellent response to preoperative chemotherapy (>90% necrosis) have the most favorable long-term prognosis.

2. **Amputation** provides definitive surgical treatment in patients in whom a limb-sparing resection is not a prudent option. The procedures include hip disarticulation, hemipelvectomy, and forequarter resection. Although these procedures were once used for technically difficult resections and proximal tumors, most sarcomas of the shoulder girdle or knee can now be resected rather than amputated.

B. **Adjuvant RT** is usually not utilized for osteogenic sarcomas of the extremities. Tumors of the jaw, facial bones, and axial skeleton require combined RT and limited surgery.

C. **Chemotherapy**

1. **Preoperative (neoadjuvant) chemotherapy** provides a response rate of 60% to 85% with combination regimens, including high-dose methotrexate (HDMTX) with leucovorin rescue. Response to preoperative chemotherapy is the single most important prognostic variable in predicting relapse-free survival.

2. **Adjuvant chemotherapy** is standard practice in the management of all patients with osteogenic sarcoma. Prospective, randomized, controlled studies demonstrated improvement in relapse-free survival for patients treated adjuvantly with chemotherapy compared with those treated with surgery alone (17% vs. 65% to 85% at 2 years). A steep dose–response curve has been repeatedly observed for chemotherapy of sarcomas: the higher the dose, the higher the response rate. HDMTX, ifosfamide, doxorubicin, and cisplatin have all demonstrated activity as single agents in osteosarcoma. The most recent trials of combination chemotherapy have shown that the addition of ifosfamide to a three-drug combination of HDMTX, doxorubicin, and cisplatin does not improve survival. However, ifosfamide appears to be the most active agent in patients with recurrent disease. As the cure rates for chemotherapy have plateaued with the currently available drugs, new approaches are necessary for progress to occur against this disease.

D. **Treatment of other bone sarcomas.** Cryosurgery—using liquid nitrogen after curettage of a tumor cavity—can decrease local recurrence for aggressive benign bone tumors and low-grade sarcomas.

1. **Chondrosarcoma.** Complete surgical excision with limb-sparing procedures where applicable. Adjuvant RT or chemotherapy is not helpful but may be tried in cases of dedifferentiated chondrosarcoma.

2. **MFH of bone.** Radical surgical resection. Because of the poor prognosis, adjuvant chemotherapy along the lines of treatment for osteosarcoma can be considered.

3. **Fibrosarcoma of bone.** Surgery alone.

4. **Chordoma.** The first surgical procedure has the best chance for cure. Inadequate surgery results in local recurrence and ultimate death. RT is also used adjuvantly with disappointing results. Heavy-particle irradiation appears promising for improving local control. Recent studies have shown activity for tyrosine kinase inhibitors such as sunitinib or imatinib.

5. **Ewing sarcoma** is discussed in Chapter 19, "Ewing Sarcoma."

6. **Giant cell tumor of bone.** Surgical removal cures 90% of these tumors when benign. Amputation is reserved for massive recurrence or malignant transformation. RANK ligand inhibition with agents such as denosumab has shown activity against this entity.

VII. MANAGEMENT OF STS

A. **Surgery.** Wide, adequate surgical resection with pathologically proven clear margins is the most effective therapeutic approach. Soft part resection can be accomplished without amputation in at least 80% of patients.

1. **Extent of resection.** Surgical exploration of the tumor demonstrates apparent encapsulation; this is actually a *pseudocapsule*. Local recurrences develop in 80% of patients treated only by enucleation of the pseudocapsule. The surgeon must remove the localized sarcoma *within a complete envelope of normal tissue*; normal structures must be sacrificed if necessary to encompass the tumor. The biopsy site, skin, and most of the subcutaneous tissue, fibrous tissue, and (often) the adjacent muscle group should be included in the resection.

2. **Regional lymph node dissection.** Node dissection is not done routinely for soft tissue or bone sarcomas and is only performed if nodal involvement is suspected clinically.

3. **Amputation of painful extremities.** Removal of a painful, functionless extremity that is the site of an eroding, necrotic tumor may be palliative, even in patients with metastatic disease. Surgery may be attempted after chemotherapy and RT have failed to control progressive disease.

4. **Resection of pulmonary metastasis** is a reasonable measure in selected patients with resectable pulmonary metastasis and no other evidence of disease.

B. **RT** is administered to the tumor bed before or after surgery (depending on the treatment center) for high-grade or large STSs to improve local control rates.

1. **Microscopically positive surgical margins** increase the risk for local failure. The presence of microscopically positive surgical margins or the occurrence of local failure, however, does not affect overall survival. Adjuvant RT may be most important when achieving clear margins that would require amputation or significant functional compromise of the extremity.

2. **For lesions distal to the elbow or knee,** postoperative RT raised the ability rate to perform limb-salvage surgery to 95% and reduced the local recurrence rate to 10%. These results were the same as if radical amputation or muscle group excision were performed.

3. **Palliation.** RT can provide palliation to sites of painful bony disease or to sites of unresectable local soft tissue disease.

C. **Treatment of STS for specific presentations**

1. **Grade 1 and small grade 2 lesions** are treated with surgery alone; the relapse rate is <10% with surgery alone. Adjuvant RT is not required.

2. **Grade 2 lesions that are proximal and large** are treated with surgery and postoperative RT.

3. **Grade 3 lesions.** RT is advisable before or after surgery.

4. **Head and neck STS.** Appropriate therapy is not defined. Wide surgical excision and RT before or after surgery is advisable.

5. **Childhood rhabdomyosarcoma** is treated intensively with chemotherapy, RT, and surgery (see Chapter 19).

6. **Retroperitoneal STS** (mostly leiomyosarcomas and liposarcomas) must be radically extirpated. Complete resection is possible in about 65% of patients and strongly predicts outcome. Median survival with complete resection is 80 months for low-grade STS and 20 months for high-grade disease. Median survival with incomplete resection for all STSs is only 24 months. The survival rate is not affected by tumor type or size.

7. **GIST.** Imatinib has demonstrated activity in advanced GIST in up to 70% of cases with doses ranging from 400 to 800 mg/d. Sunitinib has demonstrated an improvement in time to progression and progression-free survival at a dose of 50 mg/d in those who have progressed after or were intolerant to imatinib. Regorafenib is now approved for use as a third-line agent in GIST.

Trials in the adjuvant setting have shown both a decreased rate of recurrence and an improved overall survival with the use of imatinib for 3 years compared with 1 year following complete surgical resection. Sensitivity of GIST to the treatment with imatinib is dependent on the type of oncogenic mutation, for example, GIST with KIT exon 11 mutation is very sensitive to imatinib, and with PDGFRA D842V, appears to be resistant to imatinib.

8. **Kaposi sarcoma**
   a. **KS in AIDS.** Highly active antiretroviral therapy (HAART) has markedly decreased the incidence of KS and is effective in the treatment of early KS. Management of KS in AIDS patients is discussed in Chapter 37.
   b. **Classic KS.** A topical treatment for cutaneous KS, 0.1% alitretinoin gel, should be tried first for local control; however, local erythema and dermatitis may limit its use. Liquid nitrogen can be used for the destruction of localized nodular lesions. RT, including electron beams, is useful for local disease; KS is very radiosensitive. Chemotherapy is inconsistently effective; taxanes, liposomal doxorubicin appear to be the most active agents.

D. **Chemotherapy for STS.** Currently used combination chemotherapy regimens for sarcoma are shown in Table 18-2.
   1. **Single agents.** The response rates of STS to doxorubicin, ifosfamide, or dacarbazine used as single agents range from 10% to 25%, depending on a study. Other drugs have response rates of <15%. Pazopanib is now approved for advanced STS (excluding liposarcoma) following progression on standard therapy. Trabectedin is approved for use in metastatic STS (leiomyosarcoma and liposarcoma) after progression following doxorubicin. Eribulin

---

TABLE 18-2 | **Combination Chemotherapy Regimens for Sarcoma**

Regimen (Cycle: 21–28 d)	Drug	Daily Dose (mg/m²)	Days Given in Cycle (route)
Ifosfamide, high dose	Ifosfamide	Age ≥ 50 yr: 2,000	For 5 d (CIV)
	Mesna	Age < 50 yr: 2,000	For 5–7 d (CIV)
		Age ≥ 50 yr: 2,000	For 5 d (CIV)
		Age < 50 yr: 2,000	For 5–7 d (CIV)
D + C	Doxorubicin	75	Over 48–96 h (CIV)
	Cisplatin	90–120	1 (IV)
G + D	Gemcitabine	900[a]	1 and 8 (IV)
	Docetaxel	100	8 (IV)[b]
MAID	Mesna	1,500–2,500	1, 2, and 3 (CIV)
	Doxorubicin	15–20	1, 2, and 3 (CIV)
	Ifosfamide	1,500–2,500	1, 2, and 3 (CIV)
	Dacarbazine	250	1, 2, 3, and 4 (CIV)
Temozolomide	Temozolomide	150	1–7, 15–21
Bevacizumab (for solitary fibrous tumor)	Bevacizumab	5 mg/kg	8, 22

[a]Gemcitabine dose reduced to 675 mg/m² if patient received prior pelvic RT.
[b]Support with granulocyte colony-stimulating factor.
CIV, continuous intravenous infusion; IV, intravenously.

has been approved for advanced liposarcoma. Taxanes, both paclitaxel and docetaxel, have demonstrated activity in angiosarcoma. Published data support the use of temozolomide and bevacizumab in solitary fibrous tumor.

2. **Adjuvant chemotherapy** is standard practice in the management of rhabdomyosarcoma in children. Adjuvant chemotherapy for STS in adults with high-grade tumors remains controversial. Meta-analyses have suggested a beneficial role for the use of adjuvant chemotherapy in STSs. However, the most recent trials performed by the EORTC (European Organization for Research and Treatment of Cancer) failed to demonstrate a benefit in overall survival with the use of adjuvant chemotherapy, although a benefit was seen in relapse-free survival.

3. **Combination chemotherapy regimens** appear to provide no advantage over single agents for palliation or survival but are more toxic. Pulmonary and soft tissue metastases are more responsive than liver and bone metastases. The most recent trial by the EORTC comparing doxorubicin alone with doxorubicin and ifosfamide failed to show a significant difference in overall survival for the combination. Response rates and toxicity were greater in the combination chemotherapy group. Their conclusion was that doxorubicin alone remains the standard for treatment of advanced STS, but combination regimens may be considered if the goal is tumor shrinkage.

   a. The combination of vincristine, actinomycin D, and cyclophosphamide (VAC) in children with rhabdomyosarcoma produces a response rate of 90% even with disseminated disease.

   b. The combination of gemcitabine and docetaxel has shown promising activity in advanced leiomyosarcomas.

   c. Dose intensity probably correlates with response rates in the treatment of sarcomas. High-dose combinations of ifosfamide (with mesna uroprotection), doxorubicin, and dacarbazine (MAID regimen) result in a higher response rate (45%) than single agents but at the expense of substantial myelosuppression. Comparison studies of lower doses of ifosfamide (6 g/m^2) versus higher doses ifosfamide (12 g/m^2), both given with doxorubicin at 60 mg/m^2, have not shown a clear benefit for the higher-dose regimens in terms of either disease-free or overall survival at 1 year.

ACKNOWLEDGMENT

The author would like to acknowledge Dr. Dennis A. Casciato, who significantly contributed to earlier versions of this chapter.

Suggested Readings

Duffaud F, Maki RG, Jones RL. Treatment of advanced soft tissue sarcoma: efficacy and safety of trabectedin, a multitarget agent, and update on other systemic therapeutic options. *Expert Rev Clin Pharmacol* 2016;9:501.

Goorin AM, Schwartzentruber DJ, Devidas M, et al. Presurgical chemotherapy compared with immediate surgery and adjuvant chemotherapy for nonmetastatic osteosarcoma: pediatric Oncology Group Study POG-8651. *J Clin Oncol* 2003;21:1574.

Jaffe N. Osteosarcoma: review of the past, impact on the future. The American experience. *Cancer Treat Res* 2009;152:239.

Joensuu H, Eriksson M, Sundby Hall K, et al. Adjuvant imatinib for high-risk GI stromal tumor: analysis of a randomized trial. *J Clin Oncol* 2015;62:9170.

Judson I, Verweij J, Gelderblom H, et al. Doxorubicin alone versus intensified doxorubicin plus ifosfamide for first-line treatment of advanced or metastatic soft-tissue sarcoma: a randomized controlled phase 3 trial. *Lancet Oncol* 2014;4:415.

Kattan MW, Leung DH, Brennan MF. Postoperative nomogram for 12-year sarcoma-specific death. *J Clin Oncol* 2002;20:627.

Le Cesne A, Ouali M, Leahy MG, et al. Doxorubicin-based adjuvant chemotherapy in soft tissue sarcoma: pooled analysis of two STBSG-EORTC phase III clinical trials. *Ann Oncol* 2014;25:2425.

Maki RG, et al. Randomized phase II study of gemcitabine and docetaxel compared with gemcitabine alone in patients with metastatic soft tissue sarcoma. *J Clin Oncol* 2007;19:2755.

Miettinen M, Sobin LH, Lasota J. Gastrointestinal stromal tumors of the stomach: a clinicopathologic, immunohistochemical, and molecular genetic studies of 1765 cases with long-term follow-up. *Am J Surg Pathol* 2005;29:52.

Park MS, Patel SR, Ludwig JA, et al. Activity of temozolomide and bevacizumab in the treatment of locally advanced, recurrent and metastatic hemangiopericytoma and solitary fibrous tumor. *Cancer* 2011;117:4939.

Pervaiz N, Colterjohn N, Farrokhyar F, et al. A Systematic meta-analysis of randomized controlled clinical trials of adjuvant chemotherapy for localized, respectable soft-tissue sarcoma. *Cancer* 2008;113:573.

Schoffski P, Chawla S, Maki RG, et al. Eribulin versus dacarbazine in previously treated patients with advanced liposarcoma or leiomyosarcoma: a randomized, open-label, multicenter, phase 3 trial. *Lancet* 2016;387:1629.

Thomas D, Henshaw R, Skubitz K, et al. Denosumab in patients with giant cell tumor of bone: an open label phase 2 study. *Lancet Oncol* 2010;11:275.

Van der Graaf WT, Blay JY, Chawla SP, et al. Pazopanib for metastatic soft-tissue sarcoma (PALETTE): a randomized, double-blind, placebo-controlled phase 3 trial. *Lancet* 2012;379:1879.

Whelan JS, Bielack SS, Marina N, et al. EURAMOS-1, an international randomized study for osteosarcoma: results from pre-randomisation treatment. *Ann Oncol* 2015;26:407.

Worden FP, Taylor JM, Biermann JS, et al. Randomized phase II evaluation of 6 g/m^2 of ifosfamide plus doxorubicin and granulocyte colony-stimulating factor (G-CSF) with 12 g/m^2 of ifosfamide plus doxorubicin and G-CSF in the treatment of poor-prognosis soft tissue sarcoma. *J Clin Oncol* 2005;23(1):105.

19 Cancers in Childhood

Carole G. H. Hurvitz and Theodore B. Moore

INCIDENCE AND SURVEILLANCE

I. INCIDENCE AND OVERVIEW

Although cancer is the second leading cause of death in children (12% of deaths), it is still relatively uncommon. The incidence of cancer is increasing, however. Fortunately, with modern aggressive multidisciplinary therapy, 5-year survival rates for children with cancer exceed 75%.

A. Cooperative groups. The treatment of children with cancer is highly specialized. Whenever possible, patients younger than 18 to 21 years of age should be treated in specialized centers related to one of the major pediatric cooperative groups. More than 90% of children younger than 10 years of age are treated in such centers, and their mortality has decreased proportionally. Only about 30% of teenagers are enrolled in such centers, however, and the mortality rates in this group have not shown the same improvement.

B. Incidence. Leukemia and lymphoma make up almost half of the cases of malignancy in childhood, followed by central nervous system (CNS) tumors. The mortality rate for CNS cancers now exceeds that for acute lymphocytic leukemia.

There is no formal reporting system for malignant tumors in children in the United States. SEER (Surveillance, Epidemiology, and End Results) reports from the National Cancer Institute indicate that approximately 164 cases of cancer occur per 1 million population <20 years of age in the following incidences per million:

Leukemia—43	Neuroblastoma—8	Bone tumors—9
CNS tumors—29	Wilms tumor—6	Retinoblastoma—3
Lymphomas—22	Soft tissue sarcomas—11	

II. LONG-TERM SURVIVAL AND SURVEILLANCE

Now that more or most children with cancer are cured, the complications of the disease and its management are becoming increasingly important. The most significant complications are as follows:

A. Neurocognitive development. Radiation to the brain and CNSs leads to learning disabilities and school problems. Fortunately, RT has been almost eliminated from leukemia treatment plans. Chemotherapy, especially methotrexate, but other agents also, can lead to learning difficulties.

B. Growth retardation. Radiation to the spine or limbs causes reduced growth in the affected area. Steroids and brain irradiation lead to endocrine and growth problems.

C. Second malignances. Breast cancer is a very significant problem in girls who have had radiation to the chest, especially for Hodgkin lymphoma. The incidence reaches almost 40% by age 40 years. Even the newer reduced-dose regimens are still associated with an increased incidence of breast cancer. Brain tumors were frequently seen in leukemia patients after CNS radiation. Having one cancer may put patients at risk of a second cancer. Cancer survivors are at risk of developing colon and skin cancers, leukemia, and lymphoma.

D. **Fertility.** High-dose chemotherapy can reduce oogenesis and spermatogenesis. Radiation to the pelvis, as in Wilms tumor, causes increased fetal losses due to damage to the uterus.

E. **Cardiovascular and respiratory systems.** Anthracyclines cause damage to the heart. Recent studies are showing that even lower doses, thought to be safe, can have long-term effects. The younger the child and the greater the dose, the greater the risk. Pregnant women who were treated for cancer as children may develop heart failure during delivery. Radiation to the lungs and drugs such as bleomycin and cyclophosphamide can damage the lungs and cause decreased respiratory reserve.

F. **Recommended surveillance**

1. **Mammograms**, or preferably breast MRI, and breast examination are recommended annually for girls with RT to the chest, especially for Hodgkin lymphoma. They should begin screening at 8 years after irradiation or age 25 years, whichever is first.

2. **Echocardiograms** are recommended every 2 to 5 years, depending upon the age at treatment and the dose. These recommendations are subject to change.

3. **Colonoscopy** is recommended beginning age 25 or 10 years after RT for those who have received radiation therapy to the pelvis and abdomen.

4. **Skin examinations** annually are recommended for patients following radiation and stem cell transplantation.

LEUKEMIA AND LYMPHOMA

I. ACUTE LEUKEMIA

A. **Pathology.** Acute lymphoblastic leukemia (ALL) accounts for 80% to 85% of leukemias in childhood. Acute myelogenous leukemia (AML) accounts for 15%, and chronic myelogenous leukemia accounts for 5% of cases.

In ALL, 15% to 25% of cases are T-cell, <5% are B-cell, and the remainder are precursor B-cell leukemias. Of the precursor B-cell leukemias, 70% possess the common acute lymphoblastic leukemia antigen (CALLA, CD10). They are usually also terminal deoxynucleotidyl transferase positive. Almost all are also CD19 positive.

B. **Treatment** of ALL in childhood involves induction of remission, prophylaxis to the CNS, a phase of consolidation and reinduction, and maintenance therapy. Standard treatment for ALL leads to long-term remission in >85% of cases. Induction therapy employs vincristine, prednisone, dexamethasone, and L-asparaginase with the addition of daunomycin or doxorubicin, depending on risk stratification. Intensification therapy includes CNS prophylaxis. During maintenance therapy, oral mercaptopurine is given daily and methotrexate weekly for 2 to 3 years. Many patients receive monthly pulses of vincristine plus prednisone or dexamethasone. One or two cycles of a reinduction regimen are often added in ALL.

1. **Favorable prognostic factors for ALL.** Average-risk factors include initial white blood cell (WBC) count of <50,000/μL and age 1 to 9 years. Favorable features include pre-B subtype, L1 morphology, hyperploidy, lack of organomegaly, low bone marrow blasts on day 7 of induction therapy, trisomy

of chromosomes 4 and 10, and t(4;11) or Tel/AML1 translocations now known as ETV/RUNX1. It has been shown that lack of minimal residual disease (MRD) at the end of induction gives a better prognosis or at least a positive MRD carries a much poorer prognosis.

2. **Poor prognostic factors** include WBC > 50,000/μL, age <1 year or >10 years, massive organomegaly, lymphoma-like features, CNS involvement at diagnosis, mediastinal mass, failure to achieve remission by day 14 or 28, and certain chromosomal translocations, especially hypodiploidy, *MLL* gene rearrangements (11q23) in infants, the presence of the Philadelphia chromosome, and positive MRD at the end of induction or at any other time.

3. **AML** (acute myeloid leukemia) accounts for 15% to 25% of leukemias in childhood.

   In AML, high-risk features include monosomy 7, monosomy 5, 5q deletions, and FLT3 mutations. FLT3/ITD (internal tandem duplication) is a poor prognostic factor. In adults, 20% to 30% are FLT3 positive. Secondary AML is particularly difficult to treat and carries a poor prognosis. In children, only 5% to 17% are positive. Positivity increases with age. Good risk features include inv (16)/t(16;16), t(15;17), and t(8;21) conferring survival exceeding 70%.

   Treatment of AML requires intensive chemotherapy. At the present time, hematopoietic stem cell transplantation (HSCT) is recommended for high-risk patients, preferably matched family donor (MFD) if available. MFD is recommended for intermediate risk if available and chemotherapy alone for low-risk patients.

C. **Survival.** The 5-year survival rate is >85% in children with "good-prognosis" ALL following standard therapy. Even children with poorer risk factors who receive intensive therapy have an overall long-term survival of at least 70%. Sites of relapse include the CNS, testes, and bone marrow. The risk for relapse after 2 years off therapy is very low.

   The 5-year survival rate with the best available regimens for children with AML is 65% to 70% in first remission with favorable prognostic factors or when consolidated with a sibling donor HSCT and about 50% for those without. HSCT (allogenic, autologous, or matched unrelated) is also often recommended for patients with ALL and AML who relapse.

II. LYMPHOMA

A. **Non-Hodgkin lymphoma** (see Chapter 22). In pediatrics, lymphomas can be considered to be lymphoblastic or nonlymphoblastic and localized or nonlocalized. Lymphoblastic lymphomas are usually T cell and, when nonlocalized, may be the same entity as T-cell leukemia; these illnesses are usually treated in the same way. Nonlymphoblastic lymphomas are usually B cell and frequently were previously called Burkitt (or Burkitt-like) lymphoma.

   Different combination chemotherapeutic regimens are necessary for the subtypes of lymphoma. Localized lymphomas respond very well to chemotherapy even when bulky and have a cure rate of >90%. The prognosis for disseminated T-cell lymphomas is the same as for T-cell ALL. The outlook for disseminated nonlymphoblastic or B-cell lymphoma is about 50%.

B. **Hodgkin lymphoma** (see Chapter 22). There is no consensus on the treatment of Hodgkin lymphoma in children. Chemotherapy is used for all stages of disease. The alternation of the COPP and ABVD regimens (**see Appendix C**) or a hybrid of them is frequently recommended rather than either regimen alone. In children, local-field rather than extended-field radiation is preferred in an effort to reduce long-term side effects, such as growth retardation and second cancers, especially breast cancer in girls.

BRAIN TUMORS

I. EPIDEMIOLOGY

Brain tumors in children may be associated with certain underlying diseases including neurofibromatosis, tuberous sclerosis, and von Hippel-Lindau angiomatosis. Family clusters of CNS tumors have occasionally been reported.

II. PATHOLOGY AND NATURAL HISTORY

A. Pathology. Most CNS neoplasms in children are primary tumors of the brain. Astrocytomas are the most frequent type (about 50% of all cases). Medulloblastomas account for 25% of cases, ependymomas for 9%, and glioblastomas for 9%.

B. Sites of disease. Brain tumors in children tend to occur along the central neural axis (i.e., near the third or fourth ventricle or along the brainstem). Most brain tumors that occur during the first year of life are supratentorial. In patients between 2 and 12 years of age, 85% are infratentorial. In patients >12 years of age, the relative incidence of supratentorial tumors increases.

III. SYMPTOMS AND SIGNS

A. Symptoms. The most common symptoms include headaches, irritability, vomiting, and gait abnormalities. Morning headaches are most characteristic, but drowsiness and abnormal behavior are also common. Symptoms may be intermittent, particularly in very young children who have open fontanelles. A head tilt is a common finding and often missed.

B. Physical findings include enlarged or bulging fontanelles in very young children and cerebellar abnormalities, papilledema, and sixth cranial nerve abnormalities in older children.

IV. TREATMENT AND SURVIVAL

Survival rates for patients with low-grade astrocytomas are high if the tumor can be surgically removed (>90% at 5 years) and low if the tumor is high grade (<10% at 5 years). Survival for medulloblastoma depends on both local recurrence (<25% with surgery and radiotherapy) and spinal metastases (about 35% incidence without prophylactic spinal irradiation); this tumor is invariably recurrent when treated with surgery alone, but average-risk patients have approximately 80% survival when treated with surgery, radiation, and chemotherapy.

Chemotherapy is now being used more frequently in children with brain tumors in an attempt to improve survival and to reduce the use of radiation, which has devastating effects in young children. RT is deferred in children <3 years of age and preferably in children <10 years whenever possible. Unlike childhood leukemia, relatively little improvement in survival has been obtained over the years. High-dose therapy with autologous HSCT support has shown promising results in certain disease types.

NEUROBLASTOMA

I. EPIDEMIOLOGY AND ETIOLOGY

Neuroblastoma is the most common congenital tumor and the most common tumor to occur during the first year of life. It rarely occurs in patients >14 years of age. About 40% occur in the first year of life, 35% from 1 to 2 years of age, and 25% after 2 years of age. Rarely, family clusters are reported.

II. PATHOLOGY AND NATURAL HISTORY

Neuroblastoma has the highest incidence of spontaneous regression of any tumor in humans.

A. Histology. Neuroblastoma closely resembles embryonic sympathetic ganglia. The tumors partially differentiate into rosettes or pseudorosettes, mature ganglion cells, or immature chromaffin cells. The most primitive histologic type of neuroblastoma is composed of small round cells with scant cytoplasm. The ganglioneuroma is composed of larger, more mature ganglion cells with more abundant cytoplasm.

Homogeneously staining regions and double minute chromosomes seen in poor-prognosis neuroblastomas represent amplified *N-myc* segments. Amplification of *N-myc* is an intrinsic property of poor-prognosis tumors and can be rapidly detected by fluorescent *in situ* hybridization (FISH) concordant with Southern blot analysis.

B. Sites. The most common primary site is the adrenal gland (40% of cases); a tumor of the adrenal gland produces an abdominal mass. Involvement of posterior sympathetic ganglion cells results in both intrathoracic and intra-abdominal masses, the so-called *dumbbell tumor* that causes compression of the spinal cord.

C. Mode of spread. Most cases of neuroblastoma present with widespread metastatic disease. The most common metastatic sites include the bone, bone marrow, liver, skin, and lymph nodes.

III. DIAGNOSIS

A. Symptoms. The most common symptoms include abdominal pain and distention, bone pain, anorexia, malaise, fever, and diarrhea. Exophthalmos and "raccoon eyes" are a rare but typical presentation.

B. Physical findings include hepatomegaly, hypertension, orbital mass and ecchymosis, subcutaneous nodules (particularly in infancy), intra-abdominal mass, and Horner syndrome.

C. Laboratory studies
1. Complete blood count (CBC), serum chemistry panel
2. Urine for total catecholamines and metabolites, including vanillylmandelic acid (VMA) and homovanillic acid (HVA)
3. CT or PET–CT scan of the abdomen or thorax (possibly preceded by abdominal and renal ultrasound)
4. Bone scan
5. Bone marrow aspiration and biopsy to look for tumor cells
6. ^{131}I-metaiodobenzylguanidine, which is specific for neuroblastoma and pheochromocytoma
7. Examination of tumor for amplification of the *N-myc* gene

IV. PROGNOSTIC FACTORS

A. Survival and prognostic factors. The prognosis for neuroblastoma is closely related to the age of the patient and stage of disease.
1. **Age.** Patients with congenital tumors have the most favorable prognosis, even with widespread disease, and they also have the highest rate of spontaneous regression without treatment. Patients who are between 1 and 5 years of age do worse than patients younger than 1 year or older than 5 years of age.
2. **Stage.** Patients with advanced disease, except for stage IVS, have a poor survival rate. The overall 2-year survival is >80% for stages I and II and <40% for stage IV. Stage IVS has a 90% survival rate. Patients with stage III and IV disease who have amplification of the *N-myc* gene do worse.

3. **The urinary VMA:HVA ratio** is an indirect measure of dopamine hydroxylase. Absence of this enzyme may convey a poorer prognosis (i.e., if the VMA:HVA ratio is <1.5) and may cast doubt on the diagnosis of neuroblastoma.

V. MANAGEMENT

A. **Surgery.** Localized disease is managed primarily by surgical resection. For metastatic disease, biopsy or excision of the primary tumor is important for *N-myc* gene assessment. Complete resection is usually delayed until after chemotherapy is administered but may be done at the time of diagnosis.

B. **RT** is used for bulky tumor in combination with chemotherapy.

C. **Chemotherapy**
   1. **Residual localized or advanced disease.** Aggressive multimodal chemotherapy with active agents such as doxorubicin, cyclophosphamide, etoposide, cisplatin, vincristine, and topotecan combined with surgical resection and bone marrow transplantation has improved survival in stage III and IV disease.
   2. **Congenital disease.** In patients with congenital disease, specifically for stage IVS, chemotherapy is not used unless the tumor causes significant symptoms.

D. **HSCT** (usually autologous) after intensive radiation and chemotherapy appears to improve the outlook for patients with advanced disease, especially when used in conjunction with posttransplant 13-*cis*-retinoic acid. The most recent treatment protocol within the COG examined whether consolidation with tandem high-dose therapy with autologous hematopoietic stem cell support yields superior outcome to a single consolidation. This study is now closed and in follow-up.

E. **Dinutuximab** is a chimeric antibody against GD2 (disialoganglioside), and it is approved for the treatment of patients with a high-risk neuroblastoma who achieved at least a partial response to prior chemotherapy.

WILMS TUMOR (NEPHROBLASTOMA)

I. EPIDEMIOLOGY AND ETIOLOGY

A. **Incidence.** Wilms tumor most frequently affects children between 1 and 5 years of age and rarely those >8 years of age. The incidence is about 7 per 1 million in the childhood age group. Familial clusters have been described, particularly in patients with bilateral Wilms tumors.

B. **Associated abnormalities.** Wilms tumor has been associated with certain congenital anomalies, including genitourinary anomalies, aniridia (absence of an iris), and hemihypertrophy (Beckwith-Wiedemann syndrome). Deletion of the short arm of chromosome 11 has been associated with a syndrome of Wilms tumor, mental retardation, microcephaly, bilateral aniridia, and ambiguous genitalia.

II. PATHOLOGY AND NATURAL HISTORY

A. **Histopathologic classification** is most accurate for determining the prognosis.
   1. **Wilms tumor.** Tumors that display mature elements and few anaplastic cells have the most favorable prognosis and are termed *favorable histology.* *Unfavorable histology* concerns tumors that have focal or diffuse anaplasia, rhabdoid sarcoma, or clear cell sarcoma. Unfavorable histology accounts for 12% of Wilms tumors but almost 90% of deaths.
   2. **Congenital mesoblastic nephroma** is a rare benign tumor that is common in infancy (the most common renal neoplasm during the first month of life) and can be histologically confused with Wilms tumor.

B. **Sites.** About 7% of Wilms tumors are bilateral at the time of diagnosis.

C. **Mode of spread.** The lungs are the principal sites of metastases; liver and lymph nodes are the next most common sites. Bone marrow metastases are extremely rare and tend to be associated with clear cell subtypes of sarcomatous Wilms tumor.

D. **Paraneoplastic syndromes.** Wilms tumors have been associated with increased erythropoietin (erythrocytosis) and increased renin (hypertension).

III. DIAGNOSIS

A. **Symptoms.** The most common symptoms include enlarged abdomen, abdominal pain, and painless hematuria.

B. **Physical findings.** A palpable abdominal mass is the most common finding. Hypertension is sometimes present.

C. **Laboratory studies**
1. CBC, serum chemistries, urinalysis
2. Plain radiographs of the chest and abdomen
3. CT or, preferably, MRI scan of the abdomen
4. Abdominal/pelvic ultrasound

IV. PROGNOSTIC FACTORS

A. **Survival and prognostic factors.** The most important prognostic factors are the histopathologic classification and the clinical and surgical staging. Age at diagnosis is of minor importance, although younger patients appear to have a slightly better outcome. The overall 2-year survival rate is >95% for stage I, II, and III disease, with favorable histology, and about 50% for stage IV disease.

V. MANAGEMENT

A. **Surgery.** All patients must have surgery for both staging and removal of as much tumor as possible. A transabdominal incision is mandatory to examine the vessels of the renal pedicle and the noninvolved kidney. The tumor bed and any residual tumor should be outlined with metallic clips at the time of surgery.

B. **RT** is useful for treating stage III disease and metastatic disease to the bone, liver, or lung.

C. **Chemotherapy.** Multiple courses of combination chemotherapy are the preferred treatment. The major active chemotherapeutic agents are actinomycin D, vincristine, and doxorubicin. Cyclophosphamide is an effective second-line drug. Cisplatin is active against Wilms tumor and is being used in investigational protocols. The youngest patients are particularly susceptible to serious toxic effects from chemotherapy, particularly hematologic, and drug dosages should be reduced 50% for patients <15 months of age.

D. **Treatment according to stage of disease.** Surgery and chemotherapy are used for all stages of disease.
1. **Stage I.** Tumor is limited to the kidney. RT is not necessary.
2. **Stages II** (tumor extends beyond the kidney, but it was completely removed) **and III** (residual tumor is present after surgery). RT is not needed for stage II with favorable histology but is used for unfavorable histology and stage III.
3. **Stage IV** (metastases are present) **or recurrent disease.** If possible, surgery can be used. Chemotherapeutic agents can be restarted if they were discontinued or changed if relapse occurred during treatment. RT is useful for metastatic disease. Intensive chemotherapy with autologous HSCT may be beneficial in recurrent disease.
4. **Stage V** (bilateral tumor). Bilateral Wilms tumor necessitates a special effort to preserve as much renal tissue as possible. Initially, biopsy is done and

then chemotherapy followed by judicious resection of the remaining tumor. Bilateral nephrectomy followed by chemotherapy, and renal transplantation is a last resort. The 3-year survival rate is 75% for these patients.

RHABDOMYOSARCOMA

I. EPIDEMIOLOGY

Rhabdomyosarcoma (RMS) is the most common soft tissue sarcoma in children; there are about eight cases per million.

II. PATHOLOGY AND NATURAL HISTORY

A. **Histology.** Four major histologic categories of this striated muscle neoplasm have been described: embryonal (including sarcoma botryoid), alveolar, pleomorphic, and mixed. Rhabdomyoblasts have acidophilic cytoplasm, which is often periodic acid–Schiff stain (PAS) positive. There are characteristic genetic alterations that can be observed. Embryonal RMS may have a characteristic loss of heterozygosity at the 11p15 locus. The majority of alveolar RMS have a characteristic t(2;13) resulting in a chimeric *PAX3* and *FKHR* fusion gene product with a smaller percentage having t(1;13) involving *PAX7* and *FKHR*.

B. **Sites.** The head and neck are involved in 35% of cases, the trunk and extremities in 35%, and the genitourinary tract in 30%.

C. **Mode of spread.** These tumors have a great tendency to recur locally and to metastasize early through the venous and lymphatic systems. Any organ may be involved with metastases, but the lungs are most frequently affected.

III. DIAGNOSIS

A. **Symptoms.** The most common presenting symptom is a painless, enlarging mass. Hematuria and urinary tract obstruction are seen with primary tumors of the genitourinary tract. The painless swelling is often noticed after minor trauma that calls attention to the enlarging mass.

B. **Physical findings** include mass lesions, urinary tract obstruction, and a "cluster of grapes" protruding through the vaginal canal (sarcoma botryoid). Exophthalmos or proptosis occurs with head and neck primaries.

C. **Laboratory studies**
   1. CBC, liver function tests
   2. Plain radiographs and MRI or CT scans of involved areas
   3. Bone marrow aspiration and biopsy for high-risk patients
   4. PET–CT
   5. CSF examination in parameningeal tumors

IV. PROGNOSTIC FACTORS

A. **Survival and prognostic factors.** Survival is closely correlated with stage and pathologic subtype. The 5-year survival rate with the standard VAC chemotherapy regimen (vincristine, actinomycin D, and cyclophosphamide) is almost 100% for stage I and II disease, >60% for stage III disease, and about 40% for stage IV disease. The overall survival rate is 70%. Survival is higher for younger ages and embryonal subtype.

V. MANAGEMENT

The treatment of RMS should be aggressive, even with localized disease. Surgery, RT, and chemotherapy should be used for all cases with any residual disease.

A. **Surgery** should include total excision, if possible, but radical surgery is unnecessary and unwarranted. Lymph node dissection is useful for staging in extremity or genitourinary tract tumors.

   B. RT usually consists of 5,000 to 6,000 cGy given over 5 to 6 weeks to the primary tumor site with wide ports to include margins of all dissected tumors.
   C. Chemotherapy. The VAC regimen is most commonly given. Studies that compared doxorubicin, etoposide, and ifosfamide with VAC for advanced disease showed no survival advantage, although the combination may be useful in recurrent or resistant disease.

EWING SARCOMA AND PRIMITIVE NEUROECTODERMAL TUMOR (EWING FAMILY TUMORS)

I. EPIDEMIOLOGY AND ETIOLOGY

The incidence of Ewing family tumors (EFT), Ewing sarcoma, and primitive neuroectodermal tumor (PNET) is about 1.5 cases per 1 million. The disease is very rare among black children. Seventy percent of patients are <20 years of age. The peak incidence is at 11 to 12 years of age for girls and 15 to 16 years of age for boys. The male-to-female incidence ratio is 2:1. A reciprocal translocation between chromosomes 11 and 22 in about 85% of tumors creates a chimeric *ews-fli1* fusion gene.

II. PATHOLOGY AND NATURAL HISTORY

   A. Histology. EFT is a small cell tumor of bone or soft tissue characterized by islands of anaplastic, small, round blue cells. The spectrum of EFT includes Ewing sarcoma of bone, extraosseous Ewing sarcoma, and PNET. Ewing sarcoma and PNET carry the same chromosomal translocation.
   B. Sites of disease. These tumors occur predominantly in the midshaft of the humerus, femur, tibia, or fibula, but they also occur in the ribs, scapula, pelvis, or extraosseous sites. PNETs in the chest are called *Askin tumors.*
   C. Mode of spread. At the time of diagnosis, 20% to 30% of these tumors have metastasized. Most metastases are to the lung. Metastases to other bones or lymph nodes can also occur. CNS metastases, particularly meningeal, have been reported but are rare.

III. DIAGNOSIS

   A. Symptoms. Pain that is followed by localized swelling is the most frequent manifestation.
   B. Physical findings include tenderness and a palpable mass over the tumor site.
   C. Preliminary laboratory studies may show an elevated erythrocyte sedimentation rate and lytic bone lesions on radiograph (frequently, the lesions have an "onion-skin appearance"). A chest radiograph and CT should be obtained in all patients.
   D. Special diagnostic studies
      1. Bone scan
      2. MRI or CT scans of involved sites
      3. Bone marrow biopsy
      4. PET–CT

IV. STAGING AND PROGNOSTIC FACTORS

   A. Staging. The two major stages for Ewing sarcoma and PNET are simply
      1. Localized disease
      2. Metastatic disease
   B. Survival and prognostic factors. Patients with a primary tumor in a central location have a higher incidence of local recurrence and a generally poorer prognosis than do patients with tumors in other primary sites. The prognosis

for patients with metastatic disease at the time of diagnosis remains grave; bone metastases have the worst prognosis. High WBC count and fever at diagnosis also are associated with a poor prognosis. The disease-free survival depends on the response to chemotherapy.

V. MANAGEMENT
A. **Treatment according to stage of disease**
   1. **Localized disease.** All patients with localized disease should receive intensive chemotherapy followed by complete surgical resection, if possible. If resection is not feasible or complete, RT is given. RT is not needed if the tumor can be removed with >1 cm margin.
   2. **Metastatic disease** is treated with intensive chemotherapy followed by surgical resection (if possible) or RT.
B. **Chemotherapy** involves multiple drugs given in multiple cycles. The most active agents include vincristine, actinomycin D, cyclophosphamide, doxorubicin, ifosfamide, and etoposide; combinations of these drugs are effective. Patients with recurrent disease are often treated with combination of topotecan and cyclophosphamide or irinotecan and temozolomide.
C. **Surgery.** The initial procedure should be biopsy only. Open biopsy is preferred in children. Control of the primary tumor site is essential. Surgery is used in selected patients with localized disease and in patients with bulky metastatic disease. The total removal of tumor is not necessary in instances in which severe disabilities could result. Concerted efforts at limb preservation should be made.
D. **RT** is aimed at eradicating all disease while preserving limb function. The optimal volume of bone to be irradiated has not been determined.
   1. **Nonbulky lesions.** When combined with chemotherapy, delivering 4,000 to 5,000 cGy of RT to the entire bone with an additional 1,000 to 1,500 cGy coned down to the involved site yields good results.
   2. **Leg-length discrepancies.** In the past, when the probabilities for leg-length discrepancies were excessive (e.g., for younger children with lesions near the knee), patients underwent primary amputation plus chemotherapy. Expandable endoprosthetic reconstruction now makes surgical resection an option for younger children. This regimen usually results in better extremity function than limbs treated with orthovoltage irradiation. Limb-salvage procedures using chemotherapy are also frequently performed when appropriate.
   3. **Pelvic primaries.** Moderate doses of RT (4,000 cGy) with limited surgery are used for pelvic primary tumors because excessive morbidity is associated with large doses of radiation delivered to bowel and bladder. Chemotherapy must be used as well.

RETINOBLASTOMA

I. EPIDEMIOLOGY AND ETIOLOGY
A. **Incidence.** Retinoblastoma occurs in about 3 per 1 million children annually. The average age of patients is 18 months, and >90% are <5 years old. The incidence in Asians is four times that in Whites. Patients have a high risk for other neoplasms, particularly radiation-induced osteosarcomas that arise in treatment portals.
B. **Familial retinoblastoma.** About 40% of cases are hereditary. These have bilateral multifocal involvement, early age at diagnosis, secondary tumors, and a positive family history. Siblings have a 10% to 20% chance of developing

retinoblastoma if the affected child has bilateral disease and about 1% if unilateral. The offspring of a patient who survived bilateral retinoblastoma have about a 50% chance of developing the disease.

II. PATHOLOGY AND NATURAL HISTORY

A. **Histology.** Retinoblastoma is a malignant neuroectodermal tumor. It appears histologically as undifferentiated small cells with deeply stained nuclei and scant cytoplasm. Large cells are sometimes seen forming pseudorosettes, particularly in bone marrow aspirates.

B. **Mode of spread.** Multiple foci of tumor in the retina are typical at the outset. Most patients die from CNS extension through the optic nerve or widespread hematogenous metastases.

III. DIAGNOSIS

A. **Symptoms.** The disease typically presents with a "cat's eye" (white pupil or leukokoria). A squint or strabismus is occasionally noted. Orbital inflammation or proptosis rarely occurs.

B. **Physical findings** are usually limited to the eye, but patients must have a complete neurologic examination. Ophthalmologic examination under anesthesia is essential for infants and small children, for both those with symptoms and those at high risk for developing the disease. Two pathognomonic features are as follows:
   1. The typical pattern of fluffy calcifications in the retinas
   2. The presence of vitreous seeding by tumor cells

C. **Preliminary laboratory studies**
   1. CBC, liver function tests
   2. MRI or CT scans of head and orbit (both scans performed with contrast)

D. **Special diagnostic studies**
   1. Lumbar puncture with cerebrospinal fluid by cytocentrifuge
   2. Bone marrow aspiration and biopsy
   3. Serum levels of carcinoembryonic antigen and α-fetoprotein, which are frequently elevated in this disease
   4. Urinary catecholamine levels, which are infrequently elevated

IV. PROGNOSTIC FACTORS

A. **Survival and prognostic factors.** The prognosis is related to both stage and the interval between discovery of clinical signs and the initiation of treatment. The survival rate is virtually 100% for groups I to IV and 83% to 87% for group V patients with a large tumor involving half the retina or the optic nerve, or spreading into the vitreous. After disease has invaded the orbit, the mortality rate exceeds 80% despite aggressive chemotherapy.

V. MANAGEMENT

A. **Surgery is the primary modality of treatment.** Prompt enucleation in unilateral disease and enucleation of the most extensively involved eye in bilateral disease are most commonly employed. Another approach has been to enucleate only those eyes with optic nerve involvement and to treat the remaining disease with RT. When enucleation is performed, as long a segment of the optic nerve as possible should be removed. Chemotherapy, photocoagulation, cryotherapy, and plaque radiotherapy may be used in selected cases.

B. **External beam RT** is given, in most cases, to either the tumor bed or the non-removed involved eye. Usually, the dose given is about 3,500 cGy in nine fractions over a 3-week period to the posterior retina. This technique, particularly when using megavoltage irradiation, is used to attempt to spare the anterior chamber and avoid cataract formation; it is unsuitable for tumors at or beyond the midpoint of the eye.

RT without surgery is usually reserved for patients with advanced disease in both eyes, residual tumor after surgery, or tumors involving the optic nerve.

C. **Brachytherapy** with I-125 radioactive plaque inserted in the site of the tumor can be used as the primary therapy or in combination with chemotherapy and results in better visual outcomes. It is an appropriate tumor for smaller and unifocal tumors.

D. **Laser coagulation and cryotherapy** have been used for discrete lesions, particularly for small recurrences.

E. **Chemotherapy** is useful for metastatic disease. Adjuvant therapy for localized disease has not been shown to increase longevity. Many chemotherapeutic agents are active (vincristine, actinomycin D, cyclophosphamide, and doxorubicin).

Suggested Readings

Arndt CA, Hawkins DS, Meyer WH, et al. Comparison of results of a pilot study of alternating vincristine/doxorubicin/cyclophosphamide and etoposide/ifosfamide with IRS-IV in intermediate risk rhabdomyosarcoma: a report from the Children's Oncology Group. *Pediatr Blood Cancer* 2008;50:33.

Baker DL, Schmidt ML, Cohn SL, et al.; Children's Oncology Group. Outcome after reduced chemotherapy for intermediate-risk neuroblastoma. *N Engl J Med* 2010;363(14):1313.

Children's Oncology Group. Long Term Follow-Up Guidelines & Survival of Childhood and Adolescent Cancer. http://ww.survivorshipguidelines.org.

Hawkins DS, Gupta AA, Rudzinski ER. What is new in the biology and treatment of pediatric rhabdomyosarcoma. *Curr Opin Pediatr* 2014;26:50.

Hunger SP, Mulligan CG. Acute lymphoblastic leukemia in children. *N Engl J Med* 2015;373(16):1541.

Maris JM. Recent advances in neuroblastoma (Review). *N Engl J Med* 2010;362(23):2202.

Mullighan CG, Su X, Zhang J, et al.; Children's Oncology Group. Deletion of IKZF1 and prognosis in acute lymphoblastic leukemia. *N Engl J Med* 2009;360(5):470.

Panosyan EH, Ikeda AK, Chang VY, et al. High-dose chemotherapy with autologous hematopoietic stem-cell rescue for pediatric brain tumor patients: a single institution experience from UCLA. *J Transplant* 2011;2011:740673.

Pizzo PA, Poplack DG. *Pediatric Oncology, Principles and Practice*. 5th ed. Philadelphia, PA: Lippincott Williams & Wilkins, 2006.

Pui CH, Evans WE. Treatment of acute lymphoblastic leukemia. *N Engl J Med* 2006;354:166.

Pui CH, Campana D, Pei D, et al. Treating childhood acute lymphoblastic leukemia without cranial irradiation. *N Engl J Med* 2009;360(26):2730.

Rubnitz JE, Razzouk BI, Lensing S, et al. Prognostic factors and outcome of recurrence in childhood acute myeloid leukemia. *Cancer* 2007;109:157.

Siegel MJ, Finlay JL, Zacharoulis S, et al. State of the art chemotherapeutic management of pediatric brain tumors. *Expert Rev Neurother* 2006;6:765.

Yu AL, Gilman AL, Ozkaynak MF, et al.; Children's Oncology Group. Anti-GD2 antibody with GM-CSF, interleukin-2, and isotretinoin for neuroblastoma. *N Engl J Med* 2010;363(14):1324.

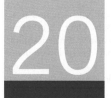

Miscellaneous Neoplasms

Bartosz Chmielowski

I. PRIMARY TUMORS OF THE MEDIASTINUM

A. General features

1. **Anatomy.** The mediastinum is bounded by the sternum anteriorly, the thoracic vertebral bodies posteriorly, the diaphragm inferiorly, and the first thoracic vertebrae superiorly. Its lateral boundaries are the parietal and pleural surfaces of the lungs. The mediastinum is arbitrarily divided into anterior, middle, and posterior segments by the heart and great vessels.

2. **Etiology.** 75% of mediastinal tumors are benign. Many are detected serendipitously in chest radiographs obtained for other reasons.

   a. **The most common mediastinal masses** are thymoma, teratoma, goiter, and lymphoma. In the mediastinum, metastatic cancers are more common than the primary mediastinal tumors.

   b. **Lymphomas** most typically involve the anterior or middle mediastinum. Hodgkin lymphoma is the most common cause of isolated mediastinal disease among the lymphomas; the nodular sclerosing subtype has a predilection for the anterior mediastinum. Other lymphomas are infrequently limited to the mediastinum at the time of diagnosis. Lymphomas are discussed in Chapter 22.

   c. **Mediastinal goiters** without a cervical component are rare. They usually descend into the left anterosuperior mediastinum. Infrequently, they descend behind the trachea into the middle and posterior mediastinum.

3. **Age and sex.** Most of the tumors show no sexual predilection. Mediastinal teratomas usually arise after the age of 30 years. Benign thymomas may occur in any age group. Thymic carcinomas are more common in elderly men. Tumors of nerve tissue origin may occur at any age but are more common in children.

4. **Symptoms and signs.** Presenting symptoms depend on the tumor location, type, and rate of growth. Symptoms are more likely to be present with rapidly growing, malignant tumors. Hypertrophic osteoarthropathy can occur with any primary mediastinal tumor.

   a. **Anterior mediastinal tumors** can present with retrosternal pain, dyspnea, upper airway obstruction, and development of collateral venous circulation over the chest. Dullness to percussion may be observed over the upper sternum.

   b. **Posterior mediastinal tumors** can cause tracheal compression (cough and dyspnea), phrenic nerve compression (hiccups or diaphragm paralysis), involvement of left recurrent laryngeal nerve (hoarseness), esophageal compression (dysphagia), vena cava obstruction, Horner syndrome or pain, or palsies in the brachial or intercostal nerve distribution.

B. Tumors of the anterior and middle mediastinum

1. **Thymomas** represent 20% of all mediastinal tumors and are the most common cause of anterior mediastinal masses. The peak frequency of the diagnosis is between 40 and 60 years of age. They are composed of both

445

nonneoplastic lymphocytes and neoplastic epithelial cells. Thymomas are benign in 70% of cases and are locally invasive in 30%. Only 1% of thymic tumors are thymic carcinomas. Invasive thymomas involve the pericardium, myocardium, lung, sternum, and large mediastinal vessels. Disseminated metastases are uncommon (Table 20-1).

According to histologic classification, thymic epithelial tumors are divided into six subtypes.

a. **Paraneoplastic immunologic syndromes** associated with both benign and malignant thymomas occur in 50% to 60% of patients, do not affect prognosis, and may not reverse following thymectomy. These syndromes include the following:

(1) **Myasthenia gravis** occurs in more than half of patients with thymoma; manifestations are improved in about 70% of patients who undergo thymectomy. About 20% of patients with myasthenia gravis have thymomas. Patients suspected of having thymoma should have an assay of serum anti–acetylcholine-receptor antibody.

(2) **Pure red-cell aplasia** (PRCA, <5% of thymomas). About 10% of patients with PRCA have a thymoma in contemporary series. The pathophysiology of this complication is poorly understood. Thymectomy results in remission of PRCA in <20% of patients. Various immunosuppressive treatments have been attempted with variable success (cyclosporine, antithymocyte globulin).

(3) **Immunodeficiency.** Acquired hypogammaglobulinemia with low to absent levels of B cells and CD4+ T lymphocytopenia (Good syndrome) occurs in about 10% of patients with thymoma. Patients experience recurrent sinopulmonary infections secondary to encapsulated organisms, skin or urinary tract infections, and bacterial diarrheas. Therapy with intravenous immunoglobulins (IVIG) should be helpful in reducing the occurrence of infections.

(4) **Rare paraneoplastic syndromes** associated with thymoma: ectopic Cushing syndrome, polymyositis, dermatomyositis, granulomatous myocarditis, systemic lupus erythematosus, Churg-Strauss syndrome, microscopic polyangiitis, isolated pauci-immune necrotizing crescentic glomerulonephritis, optic neuritis, limbic encephalitis, hypertrophic osteoarthropathy, thymoma-associated multiorgan autoimmunity (TAMA).

TABLE 20-1	Histologic Subtypes of Thymoma	
Subtype	**Histologic Features**	**Clinical Behavior**
A	Bland spindle cells, few lymphocytes	Usually noninvasive
AB	Mixture of type A and type B	Either noninvasive or minimally invasive
B1	Epithelial cells and extensive lymphocytic infiltrates	Invasion of surrounding structures in 12% of patients
B2	Predominance of lymphocytes and scattered epithelial cells	Invasion of surrounding structures in majority of patients. It can metastasize.
B3	Well-differentiated thymic carcinoma, mild atypia present in epithelial cells	Invasion of surrounding structures in 83% of patients. It can metastasize
C	Thymic carcinoma, significant cellular atypia present	Invasion of surrounding structures and high metastatic potential, 5-year survival 40%

b. Therapy

(1) **Surgery.** Thymectomy and complete surgical tumor excision result in a cure rate that exceeds 95% for encapsulated, noninvasive thymomas. Less than 10% of complete resected encapsulated thymomas recur, sometimes years after excision. Minimally invasive procedures are not recommended.

(2) **Radiation therapy**, 4,500 to 5,000 cGy given postoperatively for locally invasive or incompletely excised thymomas, reduces the local recurrence rate from about 30% to 5% in 10 years. Thymomas rarely spread to the local lymph nodes, and therefore, nodal RT is unnecessary. If the disease is not resectable, the recommended dose of RT is 6,000 to 7,000 cGy. The recurrence rate for locally invasive thymomas treated with RT alone is 20% to 30%.

(3) **Combination chemotherapy** regimens for locally advanced or metastatic disease usually involve cisplatin, doxorubicin, and cyclophosphamide. These combinations consistently result in response rates that are >50%, less than half of those are complete responses. The median duration of complete responses in widespread disease is about 12 months. The 5-year survival rate for these patients is about 30%. For patients with locally advanced disease (for whom there is no standard therapy), it is reasonable to use induction chemotherapy first, followed by resection and RT. Other regimens such as cisplatin/etoposide and carboplatin/paclitaxel have been used too, and the latter is the preferred regimen against thymic carcinoma.

(4) **Somatostatin analogs**, such as lanreotide (30 mg intramuscular [IM] every 14 days), combined with prednisone, are effective therapy in thymic tumors refractory to standard chemotherapeutic agents as long as the tumor is positive on an octreotide scan.

(5) **Molecularly targeted therapy.** Sunitinib may have activity in patients with thymic carcinoma. Thymomas may rarely have mutations in KIT, and in these cases, KIT inhibitors could be used.

2. **Thymic carcinomas** are obviously malignant histologically and are usually not associated with paraneoplastic syndromes. Neoplasms that are well circumscribed and low grade with a lobular growth pattern have a relatively favorable prognosis for survival (90% 5-year survival rate). High-grade thymic carcinomas are locally invasive; they are frequently associated with pleural or pericardial effusions and frequently metastasize to regional lymph nodes and distant sites. Cisplatin-based chemotherapy plus RT for high-grade tumors is associated with a 5-year survival rate of 15%.

3. **Thymic carcinoids** are rare. About half have endocrine abnormalities, especially ectopic production of adrenocorticotropic hormone and multiple endocrine neoplasia syndrome, but carcinoid syndrome rarely occurs. Regional lymph node metastases and osteoblastic bone metastases develop in most patients. Metastases are often refractory to therapy.

4. **Germ cell tumors** (see Chapter 13). Teratomas (or dermoids) represent 10% of mediastinal neoplasms. About 10% of these are malignant. Malignant germ cell tumors of the mediastinum are usually large and solid.

a. **Benign (mature) teratoma** accounts for about 70% of mediastinal germ cell tumors, especially in children and young adults. They appear as a round, dense mass (often with a calcified capsular shell and occasionally with teeth). They are usually small with multilocular cysts and asymptomatic, but they can attain a large size. The serum of a patient with benign teratoma contains no α-fetoprotein (AFP) or β-human chorionic gonadotropin (β-hCG). These characteristics often differentiate benign teratoma from germ cell malignancy. The treatment is surgical excision.

  b. Seminoma constitutes only 2% to 4% of mediastinal masses, but it is the most common malignant germ cell neoplasm of the mediastinum, occurring most frequently in men 20 to 40 years of age. The lesions are rarely calcified. Less than 10% of cases have an elevated β-hCG, and none has an elevated AFP. Treatment of mediastinal seminoma is surgical excision if the tumor is small, followed by irradiation of the mediastinum and the supraclavicular nodes. For locally advanced disease, combination chemotherapy, followed by resection of residual disease, is preferred. The 5-year survival rate for these patients is >80%.

  c. Mediastinal nonseminomatous germ cell tumors are malignant, aggressive, and usually symptomatic. The prognosis is worse than for patients with mediastinal seminoma. They are usually associated with elevations of serum levels of β-hCG, AFP, or lactate dehydrogenase (LDH). Choriocarcinoma in the mediastinum presents with gynecomastia and testicular atrophy in half of all male patients. Embryonal or yolk sac tumors of the mediastinum are highly aggressive cancers that are large and bulky at the time of diagnosis.

    Surgery may be required initially to establish the histologic diagnosis. Definitive treatment consists of aggressive chemotherapy as outlined for testicular cancer followed by resection of residual masses.

 5. Other anterior mediastinal masses: goiter and thyroid cysts (10% of mediastinal masses), lymphomas, parathyroid adenoma (10% are ectopic), thymic cysts, thymolipoma, lymphangioma (cystic hygroma), soft tissue sarcomas, plasmacytoma.

 6. Middle mediastinal masses

  a. Lymphomas

  b. Goiter

  c. Aortic aneurysm (10% of mediastinal masses in surgical series)

  d. Congenital foregut cysts (20% of mediastinal masses). About 50% of foregut cysts are bronchogenic, 10% are enterogenous (including esophageal duplication), and 5% are neurenteric.

  e. Pericardial cysts

C. Tumors of the posterior mediastinum

 1. Neurogenic tumors are the most common cause of a posterior mediastinal mass and constitute 75% of neoplasms in the posterior mediastinum; about 15% are malignant, and half of these are symptomatic. Among mediastinal neoplasms, neurogenic tumors constitute 20% of cases in adults and 35% of cases in children.

  a. Neurofibromas and schwannomas are most common. *Malignant tumor of nerve sheath origin* is their malignant counterpart.

  b. Sympathetic ganglia tumors originate from nerve cells rather than nerve sheath. They are rare and range from benign ganglioneuroma to malignant ganglioneuroblastoma to highly malignant neuroblastoma. Some produce a syndrome identical to pheochromocytoma.

 2. Mesenchymal tumors, including lipomas, fibromas, myxomas, mesotheliomas, and their sarcomatous counterparts, are rare mediastinal tumors; more than half are malignant. Therapy necessitates surgical debulking. RT, chemotherapy, or both are used as a surgical adjuvant for treating sarcomas.

 3. Other posterior mediastinal masses: lymphomas, goiter, lateral thoracic meningocele.

II. RETROPERITONEAL TUMORS

A. **Etiology.** Excluding renal tumors, 85% of primary retroperitoneal neoplasms are malignant. About one-sixth of cases are Hodgkin lymphoma, and one-sixth are non-Hodgkin lymphoma. Sarcomas often appear in the retroperitoneum, particularly rhabdomyosarcoma (in children), leiomyosarcoma, and liposarcoma. Germ cell tumors, adenocarcinomas, and rare neuroblastomas account for most of the remainder of cases. Carcinomas of the breast, lung, and gastrointestinal tract can metastasize to retroperitoneal structures by way of the bloodstream or the spinal venous plexus.

B. **Evaluation**

1. **Symptoms.** Back pain, upper urinary tract obstruction, and leg edema caused by lymphatic or vena cava obstruction frequently are manifestations of retroperitoneal malignancies; arterial insufficiency does not appear to occur.

2. **Laboratory studies.** History, physical examination, and routine blood studies are performed. Uremia can result from entrapment of the ureters. Intravenous pyelography, barium contrast study of the colon, and abdominal CT scanning are performed to evaluate the extent of tumor.

C. **Management.** Biopsy should be performed to establish diagnosis. En bloc surgical excision of the tumor is most important for most nonlymphomatous tumors especially soft tissue sarcomas. RT is used to treat residual disease. Chemotherapy as the first-line treatment is used for patients with lymphomas or with tumors that cannot be removed surgically and are not responsive to RT. The specific chemotherapy selected depends on the tumor type.

III. CARDIOVASCULAR TUMORS

Primary cardiac tumors are exceedingly rare. Metastasis to the heart (see Chapter 30) is more than 20 times as frequent as primary cardiac tumors. Tumors of blood vessels are mostly sarcomas, which are discussed in Chapter 18. Symptoms are largely dependent on the location of the tumor and not on the histologic type. The patients may present with symptoms of congestive heart failure because of the blood flow obstruction, arrhythmias and heart blocks secondary to direct invasion of the myocardium, pericardial effusion, or pulmonic or peripheral embolization.

A. **Malignant heart tumors** include rhabdomyosarcoma, fibrosarcoma, angiosarcoma, leiomyosarcoma, and sarcoma otherwise nonspecified. Tumors usually arise in the right auricle and extend into the heart substance and valves. Their aggressive course is characterized by heart failure, angina, life-threatening arrhythmias, or cardiac rupture. They are treated with resection and frequently chemotherapy. The prognosis is generally poor; patients with low-grade sarcomas have a better prognosis.

B. **Benign heart tumors**

1. **Myxoma** is most frequently located in the left atrium. It grows into the lumen of the left atrium and leads to symptoms of mitral regurgitation and can cause a syndrome resembling microbial endocarditis with heart murmur, fever, joint pain, and systemic emboli. If myxoma is located in the right atrium, it will present like tricuspid stenosis. Patients with these findings and sterile blood cultures should have an echocardiogram, which is highly accurate for diagnosing myxoma of the heart. Some patients may require a cardiac MRI to differentiate between a tumor and thrombus. Occasionally, the diagnosis is established by the finding of myxomatous tissue in arterial embolectomy specimens. Myxomas are treated surgically, usually with a good outcome.

2. **Papillary fibroelastoma** usually grows as a pedunculated, mobile tumor on a heart valve. The growth is frequently complicated by a thrombotic event (i.e., cerebrovascular event, myocardial infarction, angina pectoris, peripheral or pulmonary embolism).

3. **Rhabdomyoma, teratoma, fibroma, and lipoma** are less common types of cardiac tumors.

C. **Hemangiopericytomas**, in the past, were considered to originate from pericytes. Currently, it is believed that they originate from fibroblasts and that they belong to the same spectrum of tumors as solitary fibrous tumor. They are characterized by the presence of NAB2-STAT6 fusion protein that can be detected by FISH. Histologic appearance and grade do not closely correlate with the metastatic potential; 15% to 20% of tumors develop distant metastases.

These highly vascular tumors are treated by resection after embolic therapy. Postoperative RT may reduce local recurrence. Metastatic tumors are treated with doxorubicin-based chemotherapy; they can also respond to antiangiogenic treatments such as the combination of bevacizumab and temozolomide or sunitinib.

D. **Primary intravascular sarcomas** are rare tumors that present with signs of focal vascular obstruction. Venous sarcomas, particularly leiomyosarcomas, are the most common IV sarcomas. Vena cava tumors can produce Budd-Chiari syndrome, renal failure, or pedal edema; patients may present with poorly defined back or abdominal pain. CT scan or venography suggests the diagnosis. Treatment is surgical resection, when technically feasible.

IV. CARCINOSARCOMAS

Carcinosarcomas are rare tumors, which have a histologic appearance of combined sarcomatous and epithelial elements. Conceptually, they represent carcinomas that develop sarcomatous elements via metaplasia of the epithelial element. Typically, they arise in the myometrium, prostate, or lung, but can occur elsewhere.

Surgical resection is the treatment of choice. The role of postoperative irradiation is not clear. Recurrent or metastatic disease is associated with a dismal prognosis. Since these tumors represent carcinomas, standard chemotherapy applicable to the organ of origin is currently used.

V. ADENOID CYSTIC CARCINOMAS

Adenoid cystic carcinomas (ACC or *cylindromas*) are rare epithelial tumors that most often arise in salivary glands or the large airways but also can develop in the external auditory canal, nasopharynx, lacrimal glands, breast, vulva, esophagus, and other sites. The term cylindroma describes also a benign adnexal tumor that has a very different clinical behavior from ACC. These tumors have tendency to perineural spread, and local recurrence after surgery is common. Lymphatic spread is much less common than hematogenous spread, especially to the lungs. Pulmonary metastases are radiologically dramatic but often have an indolent course over several years.

Primary tumors are treated surgically. Local recurrences may respond to RT. Symptom-free patients with lung metastases do not need specific treatment. Patients with symptomatic disease may respond to imatinib and occasionally to standard chemotherapy such as fluorouracil, paclitaxel, cisplatin, vinorelbine, or doxorubicin.

VI. DENTAL TUMORS

A. **Ameloblastomas** appear to originate in odontogenic rests (remnants from the embryologic process of odontogenesis). Eighty percent occur in the mandible

(70% in the molar areas). The remaining 20% of histologically similar tumors arise in other bones and, occasionally, soft tissues. Ameloblastomas are locally invasive and have a high risk for local recurrence after surgery.

Peripheral (extraosseous) ameloblastomas arise from the gingiva or mucosa and do not involve the bone. Malignant ameloblastoma does not differ histologically from benign ameloblastoma, but it is characterized by development of distant metastasis (mainly in the lungs), even years after the treatment of the primary tumor.

Therapy is by surgical resection. Some surgeons use intraoperative cauterization or cryotherapy for better local control. RT has no role in managing the tumor or recurrences.

B. **Cementoma** is probably an area of calcified fibrous dysplasia and not a neoplasm.

C. **Other dental tumors.** Ameloblastic adenomatoid tumors, calcifying epithelial odontoma, ameloblastic fibroma, dentinoma, ameloblastic odontoma, and complex odontoma are all benign tumors of the embryologic precursors of teeth. Surgical removal is the therapy of choice. Transformation into malignancy may occur, but rarely.

VII. ADAMANTINOMA

Adamantinoma is a rare tumor of long bones of the epithelial origin. The name originates from the histologic resemblance to ameloblastoma. Eighty percent of cases occur in the tibia. Although it is a low-grade neoplasm, it can recur locally and can rarely metastasize to the lungs. Both primary and metastatic adamantinoma are treated surgically. The responses of metastatic adamantinoma to chemotherapy (cisplatin and etoposide) or sunitinib are anecdotal.

VIII. ESTHESIONEUROBLASTOMA

Olfactory neuroblastoma (ONB or *esthesioneuroblastoma*) is an uncommon malignancy of the sensory epithelium of the nasal cavity close to the cribriform plate. This tumor is considered in the differential diagnosis of poorly differentiated, small, blue round cell neoplasms. The tumor's immunophenotype is that of a neuroendocrine tumor.

A. **Presenting features** are unilateral nasal obstruction, anosmia, epistaxis, rhinorrhea, sinus pain, headache, diplopia, or proptosis. It may be an incidental finding during polypectomy or nasal septoplasty. Metastases to neck nodes develop in about 30% of patients. Intracranial extension and orbital involvement are independent factors affecting outcome.

B. **Multimodality therapy** has improved survival for these patients. Five-year overall survival is more than 80%. Aggressive surgical resection is the treatment of choice. Postoperative or neoadjuvant RT improves local control and survival. The results of salvage therapy on relapse are very good. The use of chemotherapy is anecdotal.

IX. PARAGANGLIOMAS

These neoplasms originate from chromaffin cells of the neural crest and develop from paraganglia tissues, which are themselves chemoreceptor organs that are distributed throughout the body in association with the sympathetic chain. Nearly half originate in the head and neck region (particularly, at the carotid bifurcation and in the temporal bone), and the remainder develop in the mediastinum, retroperitoneum, abdomen, and pelvis. A conventional concept is that pheochromocytoma is simply a paraganglioma confined to the adrenal gland (see Chapter 16).

A. **Occurrence.** These uncommon neoplasms are either familial (predominantly men) or nonfamilial (predominantly women). Familial paragangliomas are usually associated with mutations in succinate dehydrogenase complex subunit B, C, or D. They are multiple at several locations in 25% to 50% of the familial type and in 10% of the nonfamilial type.

B. Natural history. Paragangliomas, which are usually considered to be benign, are characterized by slow and inexorable growth from the site of origin. Clinical course and not histology is the indicator of tumor behavior. Manifestations depend on the cellular characteristics and tumor location. About 5% of tumors are functional, manifest excessive secretion of neuropeptides and catecholamines, and produce a syndrome identical to pheochromocytoma. Metastases, which are the exception rather than the rule, develop in organs that do not contain paraganglia tissue (lungs, lymph nodes, liver, spleen, and bone marrow).

C. Evaluation. Paragangliomas must always be considered as potentially multiple, especially in patients with a family history of such tumors. Patients should be screened for evidence of excessive catecholamine secretion.

Computed tomography or MRI is useful in delineating the tumors. Arteriography may be useful for tumor embolization done just before surgery or for evaluating contralateral crossover blood supply. Radionuclide scintigraphy using ^{131}I-metaiodobenzylguanidine (MIBG) may be helpful in localizing both paragangliomas and pheochromocytomas. These tumors have a rich blood supply; caution must be exerted not to cause hemorrhage during biopsy. Fine needle aspiration cytology is often useful if performed carefully.

D. Treatment. Surgical extirpation is the treatment of choice, particularly for small head and neck lesions, but technical expertise in vascular surgery is mandatory. RT is effective in local control and is probably the treatment of choice for lesions that are large or erode bone, particularly in older patients. Chemotherapy is generally ineffective in patients with benign paraganglioma. Metastatic malignant paraganglioma may respond to chemotherapy; the combination of cyclophosphamide, vincristine, and dacarbazine has been used most frequently. Some patients respond to the treatment with sunitinib. High doses of MIBG, a radionuclide that is used in lower doses in diagnosis of catecholamine-secreting tumors, have generated interest as a therapeutic modality.

Suggested Readings

Esthesioneuroblastoma

Jethanamest D, et al. Esthesioneuroblastoma: a population-based analysis of survival and prognostic factors. *Arch Otolaryngol Head Neck Surg* 2007;133:276.

Rimmer J, et al. Olfactory neuroblastoma: a 35-year experience and suggested follow-up protocol. *Laryngoscope* 2014;124:1542.

Tajudeen BA, Arshi A, Suh JD, et al. Esthesioneuroblastoma: an update on the UCLA experience, 2002–2013. *J Neurol Surg B Skull Base* 2015;76:43.

Paraganglioma

Ayala-Ramirez M, Chougnet CN, Habra MA, et al. Treatment with sunitinib for patients with progressive metastatic pheochromocytomas and sympathetic paragangliomas. *J Clin Endocrinol Metab* 2012;97:4040.

Gedik GK, Hoefnagel CA, Bais E, et al. ^{131}I-MIBG therapy in metastatic phaeochromocytoma and paraganglioma. *Eur J Nucl Med Mol Imaging* 2008;35:725.

Goffredo P, Sosa JA, Roman SA. Malignant pheochromocytoma and paraganglioma: a population level analysis of long-term survival over two decades. *J Surg Oncol* 2013;107:659.

Huang H, Abraham J, Hung E, et al. Treatment of malignant pheochromocytoma/paraganglioma with cyclophosphamide, vincristine, and dacarbazine: recommendation from a 22-year follow-up of 18 patients. *Cancer* 2008;113:2020.

Thymoma

Hamaji M, Kojima F, Omasa M, et al. A meta-analysis of surgical versus nonsurgical management of recurrent thymoma. *Ann Thorac Surg* 2014;98:748.

Omasa M, Date H, Sozu T, et al. Postoperative radiotherapy is effective for thymic carcinoma but not for thymoma in stage II and III thymic epithelial tumors: the Japanese Association for Research on the Thymus Database Study. *Cancer* 2015;121:1008.

Thomas A, Rajan A, Berman A, et al. Sunitinib in patients with chemotherapy-refractory thymoma and thymic carcinoma: an open-label phase 2 trial. *Lancet Oncol* 2015;16:177.

Thompson CA, Steensma DP. Pure red cell aplasia associated with thymoma: clinical insights from a 50-year single-institution experience. *Br J Haematol* 2006;135:405.

Other Neoplasms

DeLair D, et al. Ameloblastic carcinosarcoma of the mandible arising in ameloblastic fibroma: a case report and review of the literature. *Oral Surg Oral Med Oral Pathol Oral Radiol Endod* 2007;103:516.

Dudek AZ, Murthaiah PK, Michael Franklin M, et al. Metastatic adamantinoma responds to treatment with receptor tyrosine kinase inhibitor. *Acta Oncol* 2010;49(1):101.

Gondikvar SM, Gadbail AR, Chole R, et al. Adenoid cystic carcinoma: a rare clinical entity and literature review. *Oral Oncol* 2011;47:231.

Hall WA, Ali AN, Gullett N, et al. Comparing central nervous system (CNS) and extra-CNS hemangiopericytomas in the Surveillance, Epidemiology, and End Results program: analysis of 655 patients and review of current literature. *Cancer* 2012;118:5331.

McClary AC, West RB, McClary AC, et al. Ameloblastoma: a clinical review and trends in management. *Eur Arch Otorhinolaryngol* 2016;273(7):1649–1661.

Park MS, Araujo DM. New insights into the hemangiopericytoma/solitary fibrous tumor spectrum of tumors. *Curr Opin Oncol* 2009;21(4):327.

Perchinsky MJ, Lichtenstein SV, Tyers GFO. Primary cardiac tumors: forty years' experience with 71 patients. *Cancer* 1997;79:1809.

Schweizer L, Koelsche C, Sahm F, et al. Meningeal hemangiopericytoma and solitary fibrous tumors carry the NAB2-STAT6 fusion and can be diagnosed by nuclear expression of STAT6 protein. *Acta Neuropathol* 2013;125:651.

Strollo DC, Rosado-de-Christenson ML, Jett JR. Primary mediastinal tumors. *Chest* 1997;112:511 (Part I), 1344 (Part II).

21

Cancer of Unknown Primary Site

Bartosz Chmielowski

The definition of cancer of unknown primary (CUP). CUP is a heterogenous group of diseases consisting of metastatic solid tumors for which the site of origin is not suggested by thorough history, physical examination, imaging and laboratory studies, and thorough histologic evaluation.

The predicament of CUP. The detection of CUP usually represents the discovery of a far-advanced malignancy that is rarely curable. Most patients are symptomatic and present with decreased performance status. Tumors that are potentially responsive to systemic treatment are found in only about 20% of all patients with CUP. The diagnostic evaluations inflicted on these patients in pursuit of the primary site are typically excessive and futile. The primary site is found in <30% of cases, and that discovery rarely affects the prognosis or treatment. All efforts to manage patients who meet the criteria defined above should be guided by the understanding that there are two basic categories of CUPs: (1) those that are treatable and (2) those that are not (Fig. 21-1).

I. EPIDEMIOLOGY AND BIOLOGY

A. **Incidence.** About 2% to 3% of patients with cancer present with CUP. The percentage of cancers diagnosed as CUP has been decreasing over time. CUP is the seventh most frequent malignancy, ranking below only cancers of the lung, prostate, breast, cervix, colon, and stomach. About 75% of tumors in the CUP syndrome originate below the diaphragm. The average age at onset is 60 years. Patients who present with a midline distribution of poorly differentiated carcinoma (10% of all CUP patients) have a median age of 39 years.

B. **Prognosis.** The median survival is approximately 3 to 4 months with <25% and 10% of patients alive at 1 and 5 years, respectively. Patients can have tumors with favorable or unfavorable presentation. If only lymph node metastases are present, the prognosis is better than when extranodal metastases are detected. The list of poor prognostic factors include male gender, poor performance status, adenocarcinoma involving multiple organs, malignant ascites, and brain metastases. The good prognostic factors are women with adenocarcinoma of the peritoneal cavity, women with adenocarcinoma in axillary lymph nodes only, squamous cell carcinomas (SCC) involving cervical lymph nodes only, poorly differentiated neuroendocrine carcinomas, men with elevated PSA and bone metastases, and potentially resectable tumor.

C. **Manifestations.** At the time of diagnosis, multiple sites are involved in more than 50% of patients. Symptoms of metastasis are present in nearly all patients with CUP syndrome. The most frequent presenting features are the following:
   1. Pain (60%)
   2. Liver mass or other abdominal manifestations (40%)
   3. Lymphadenopathy (20%)
   4. Bone pain or pathologic fracture (15%)
   5. Respiratory symptoms (15%)

METASTATIC SITE   **HISTOLOGY**   **TREATMENT**

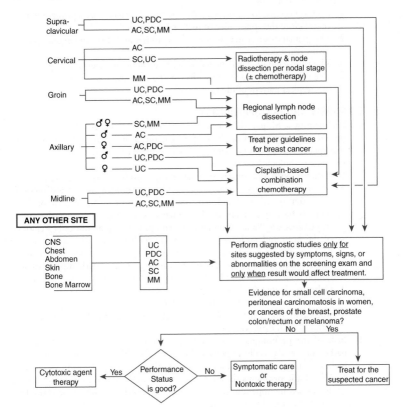

Figure 21-1 An algorithm of the treatment of patients with cancer of unknown primary. AC, adenocarcinoma; PDC, poorly differentiated carcinoma; SC, squamous cell carcinoma; UC, undifferentiated carcinoma; MM, malignant melanoma; CNS, central nervous system.

   6. Central nervous system abnormalities (5%)
   7. Weight loss (5%)
   8. Skin nodules (2%)
   D. Aberrant natural history of CUPs compromises the ability to predict the primary site of disease. By definition of CUP, the primary site is asymptomatic and not easily detected on imaging studies. This shows that CUPs are a group of cancers characterized by atypical clinical behavior, including patterns of dissemination. The observation represents the distinct biology of these malignancies wherein the metastatic behavior predominates unpredictably, while the primary tumor remains occult. Occasionally the pattern of spread can facilitate identification of the primary site: lung metastases are seen twice as often when

primary site is above the diaphragm; liver metastases are more commonly seen when primary is below the diaphragm.

E. **Mechanisms** that could explain the presence of occult primary neoplasms include the following:

1. Excision or electrocautery may have removed unrecognized primary lesions years before the appearance of metastatic lesions.

2. The primary cancer may have shed metastases and then undergone spontaneous regression.

3. The primary tumor may be too small to be detected, even at autopsy.

4. The site of origin may be obscured by the extensiveness of metastases or by the atypical pattern of dissemination.

II. DIAGNOSIS AND HISTOPATHOLOGY

A. **Performing a biopsy** should be the first order of business. The pathologist should be informed before the biopsy that the primary site is not evident so that special studies can be planned. The less differentiated the tumor, the more complex pathologic evaluation takes place.

1. **Patients with metastases to neck lymph nodes only.** Suspicious cervical nodes should *not undergo excisional biopsy* until a complete diagnostic evaluation of the head and neck has been performed. About 35% of these patients have potentially curable cancers of the upper aerodigestive tract. Approximately 2% to 5% of patients with primary squamous cell carcinoma of the head and neck region will present with cervical adenopathy as the primary disease manifestation; about 10% of this group will present with bilateral adenopathy. This is not the case for patients with supraclavicular lymph nodes, which may be directly excised for histologic examination.

2. **Other patients who have suspected metastatic cancer.** Biopsy of *the most accessible site* should be performed *before* specialized blood or radiologic studies are done; the histologic findings provide an invaluable guide for a rational diagnostic workup.

B. **Role of the pathologist** Close communication between the clinician and the pathologist is especially important in cases of CUP. Morphologic clues may make certain anatomic sites more likely and direct the sequence of investigation.

1. **Histologic problems** (histologic and immunohistochemical clues for origin are shown in Appendix B1). These cancers can be usually characterized as one of five histologic subtypes.

   a. **Well or moderately differentiated adenocarcinoma** (60%). When a primary site is determined, the sites of origin and relative frequencies are as follows: pancreas (25%), lung (20%), stomach, colorectum, hepatobiliary tract (8% to 12% each), kidney (5%), breast, ovary, and prostate (2% to 3% each).

   b. **Poorly differentiated adenocarcinoma or undifferentiated carcinoma** (29%). The distinction between a poorly differentiated tumor of epithelial, hematopoietic, or neuroectodermal origin is very important.

   c. **Squamous cell carcinoma** (5%). Most squamous cancers that appear as CUP originate in the head and neck or lung. Other squamous cell cancer primary sites include the uterine cervix, penis, anus, rectum, esophagus, and, occasionally, urinary bladder. Acanthocarcinomas (squamoid tumors) may develop in the gastrointestinal (GI) tract, notably in the pancreas and stomach. Squamous skin cancer that arises in a chronic osteomyelitis fistula may not be apparent until regional draining lymph nodes become involved.

d. **Poorly differentiated malignant neoplasm** (5%). Patients who are younger than 50 years, who have a tumor of midline tumor distribution, multiple pulmonary nodules or lymph nodes, elevated serum levels of beta human chorionic gonadotropins (hCG) or alpha-fetoprotein (AFP), whose tumors have cell positive for beta hCG or AFP by immunohistochemical stain or neuroendocrine granules can be possible cured with chemotherapy and/or radiation therapy (RT).

e. **Neuroendocrine tumor of unknown primary (NUP)** (1%). Small cell neoplasms or "oat cell" carcinomas can develop in the entire alimentary canal, upper aerodigestive tract, thymus, breast, prostate, urinary bladder, uterine cervix, endometrium, and skin, as well as in the lung. About 2% of small cell carcinomas originate in extrapulmonary sites. Although this subtype constitutes only a small percentage of the patients who present with CUP, it represents one of the treatable varieties.

   (1) **NUPs.** Low-grade NUPs are usually recognizable by light microscopy, have features of islet cell or carcinoid tumors, and often have an indolent behavior. Pheochromocytoma, paragangliomas, and medullary thyroid carcinoma are other examples of indolent NUPs.

   Anaplastic small cell carcinomas and poorly differentiated NUPs behave aggressively and require immunohistochemical analysis of biopsies for synaptophysin and chromogranin. Merkel cell tumors and neuroblastomas are other types of aggressive NUPs.

   (2) **Undifferentiated small cell neoplasms** may also represent a number of cancers that can be simply recalled with the mnemonic *MR. MOLSEN* (*m*yeloma, *r*habdomyoblastoma, *m*elanoma [amelanotic], *o*at cell carcinoma, *l*ymphoma, *s*eminoma [anaplastic], *E*wing sarcoma, *n*euroblastoma).

f. **Other types.**

   (1) About 5% of malignant **melanoma** cases present as CUP. It is important to distinguish melanoma from other histologies because melanoma can respond to BRAF/MEK inhibitors (if BRAF mutation is present) or immunotherapy. Amelanotic melanoma may be mistaken as undifferentiated carcinoma.

   (2) **Clear cell tumors** are characterized by polygonal cells with clear cytoplasm that can represent artifactual changes, benign neoplasms, or malignancies. Seminomas, nonseminomatous germ-cell carcinomas, lymphomas, and benign tumors can be clear cell tumors with a virtually identical clear cell appearance. Differentiation requires detailed analysis of clinical, histologic, immunohistochemical, and, occasionally, electron microscopic features.

2. **Immunohistochemistry** improves the chances of the diagnosis of a tissue of origin. Excessive ordering of immunohistochemical testing is rarely beneficial. Staining for keratins, leukocyte common antigen, and S100 is usually most helpful. A stepwise approach is recommended:

   a. Markers to determine the lineage, for example, sarcoma, carcinoma, lymphoma, melanoma

   b. Markers suggestive of the putative site

   c. Tumor biomarkers that can help with treatment decisions: EGFR, BRAF, ROS, ALK, Her2

3. **Immunohistochemistry diagnostic algorithms** are included in Appendix B. These markers are stains attached to antibodies that must be *interpreted* for positivity, negativity, and relevance; none of these results is perfect.

The most useful immunohistochemical stains in the evaluation of patients with CUP syndrome are cytokeratins (CK) and those for lymphoma (CD45, leukocyte common antigen) and for melanoma (S100 protein, HMB45, Melan-A/Mart-1). Immunohistochemical stains for neuron-specific enolase, synaptophysin, chromogranin, CD56, and CD57 are helpful in patients who could have neuroendocrine tumors.

A few immunohistochemical markers have enough tissue-type specificity that allows for their use in trying to establish a primary tumor. These include
   a. PSA (prostatic adenocarcinoma and benign prostatic epithelium)
   b. Thyroglobulin (thyroid follicular epithelium and nonmedullary thyroid carcinomas)
   c. Thyroid transcription factor-1 (TTF-1; thyroid and lung cancers and carcinoid tumors)
   d. Gross cystic disease fluid protein-15 (breast carcinoma and tumors of apocrine sweat glands or salivary glands)
   e. RCC (renal cell carcinoma) and HepPar-1 (hepatocellular carcinoma)
   4. Gene expression testing. Tests based on gene expression profiling have been developed, and they can facilitate identification of a tissue of origin (the accuracy rate is 85% to 90% when tested on tumor of known origin). The tests can be based on the analysis of mRNA, RNA, or DNA. It remains unclear if this knowledge changes the clinical outcome.
   5. Polymerase chain reaction (PCR) analysis. If nasopharyngeal carcinoma is suspected, PCR for Epstein-Barr virus can be performed. Detection of i(12p) is helpful with diagnosis of midline germ-cell tumors.
   6. Electron microscopy is rarely needed and helpful. Occasionally, it can help with detection of desmosomes and bundles of tonofilaments in SCC, core granules in neuroendocrine tumors, microacinar spaces in adenocarcinoma, or early melanosomes in melanoma.
 C. Imaging CT scans remain the standard imaging modality. PET scans or PET–CT scans may be helpful when local therapy is planned. Imaging identifies the primary site in 20% to 40% of patients. A diagnostic mammogram is indicated if adenocarcinoma is found in the axillary and mediastinal lymph nodes.

III. SITES OF METASTASES AND PROGNOSIS
 A. Survival according to sites of metastases
   1. Patients with metastases to lymph nodes alone have 5-year survival rates according to sites of involvement, which are as follows:
      a. Upper or middle cervical nodes alone (30% to 50%)
      b. Axillary nodes alone in women (>65%)
      c. Axillary nodes alone in men (25%)
      d. Groin nodes alone (50%, perhaps)
      e. Midline lymph node distribution with poorly differentiated adenocarcinoma, particularly in young men (30%)
   2. Patients with metastases to sites other than peripheral lymph nodes alone. Except for peritoneal carcinomatosis in females, the median survival time for all patients ranges between <1 and 5 months. More than 75% of patients die within 1 year of diagnosis. Bone marrow and epidural metastases have the worst prognosis (median survival time of <1 month).
   3. Particularly unfavorable prognostic features in patients with CUP include the following:
      a. Multiple metastatic sites, particularly the liver
      b. Supraclavicular lymph node involvement

    c. Well-differentiated or moderately differentiated adenocarcinoma histology

    d. Elevated serum alkaline phosphatase or lactic dehydrogenase levels; lower serum albumin levels or lymphocyte counts

    e. Older age

    f. Lower performance status

B. Neck lymph node metastasis. Neck masses in adults, other than thyroid nodules, are malignant in 80% of cases. After 50 years of age, 90% of neck masses are malignant. About 35% of patients with CUP to upper and middle cervical lymph nodes can potentially be cured. However, CUP to lower cervical or supraclavicular lymph nodes is associated with an ominous prognosis.

C. Axillary lymph node metastasis. Axillary lymphadenopathy that is excised for diagnosis is found to have benign disease in 75% of cases, lymphoma in 15%, and solid tumors (particularly adenocarcinoma) in 10%.

    1. The most likely sites of origin of a solid tumor metastasizing to the axilla are the breast, lung, arm, and regional trunk. In patients with isolated malignant axillary lymphadenopathy, the primary site is detected in only half of the cases.

    2. Breast cancer. About 0.5% of all breast cancer patients present with masses palpable in the axilla and not in the breast. Breast cancer accounts for 70% of cases of CUP involving axillary lymph nodes in women when the primary site is eventually diagnosed. Ultimately, 30% to 50% of female patients develop evidence of a primary breast cancer; the primary tumor becomes evident in <20% of these patients if the breast is treated with RT, most likely emanating from the upper outer quadrant of the ipsilateral breast.

D. Groin lymph node metastasis. The primary tumor is detectable in 99% of patients having malignant groin lymphadenopathy. Metastases are most likely to arise from the skin (especially the lower extremities and lower half of the trunk), vulva, vagina, cervix, penis, scrotum, rectum, anus, or urinary bladder.

E. Midline lymphadenopathy (anterior mediastinal or retroperitoneal with or without peripheral lymphadenopathy) represents a highly treatable presentation of CUP when it is associated with poorly differentiated carcinomas (including undifferentiated carcinomas and poorly differentiated adenocarcinomas). Most patients are men, with a median age of 39 years and rapidly growing tumor masses. Many patients have achieved excellent responses to cisplatin-based combination chemotherapy (most commonly combination of vinblastine, bleomycin, and cisplatin).

F. Other sites of metastases

    1. Bone and bone marrow metastases

        a. Bone cortex. When a primary site is found, carcinoma of the lung accounts for most patients with CUP who have bone metastases. When presenting as a CUP, pancreatic carcinoma frequently involves the skeleton (in contrast to its usual behavior). The median survival time of patients presenting with CUP and predominantly bone metastases is 3 months.

        b. Bone marrow is shown to be involved by aspiration or biopsy techniques in 10% to 15% of CUP cases during life, particularly in patients who prove to have lung, breast, or prostate cancer. Leukoerythroblastic peripheral blood smears are the most accurate barometers of bone marrow involvement in patients with solid tumors. The median survival time of patients presenting with CUP as marrow metastases is <1 month.

2. **Intrathoracic metastases**
    a. **Pulmonary metastases** may be solitary, and primary lung cancer lesions may be multiple.
    b. **Pleural effusion**, when caused by malignant disease, is associated with an unknown primary tumor in 20% of cases.
3. **Intra-abdominal metastases** most frequently involve the liver and originate in the GI tract, but the primary site is determined during life in only about 30% of cases.
    a. **Liver metastases.** Carcinomas of the prostate or ovary metastasize to the liver more frequently when they present as CUP than when they occur as known primaries. The median survival time of patients presenting with CUP and, predominantly, liver metastases is <4 months.
    b. **Ascites**, when caused by malignant disease, is associated with CUP in 10% of cases. The median survival time is <1 month, except for women with peritoneal carcinomatosis, which is considered to be a variant of ovarian carcinoma with similar associated survival. Approximately 55% of women who present with malignant ascites have a primary site identified in the ovary.
4. **Central nervous system metastases**
    a. **Brain metastases** are most frequently associated with bronchogenic carcinoma, melanoma, breast cancer, but also with CUP. In 80% of patients, development of brain metastasis follows the diagnosis of metastatic cancer, and in 20% of patients, they present at the time of diagnosis or precede the diagnosis of metastatic disease. In case of CUP, the primary site eventually becomes evident during life in 40% of cases, and 60% of these are lung carcinomas. Patients with favorable prognosis and a limited number of metastasis can be offered surgery or stereotactic radiosurgery. Patients with poor prognosis are offered supportive care only or the whole brain RT. The median survival time of patients presenting with CUP and single brain metastasis that is resected is 3 to 6 months.
    b. **Spinal cord compression** is occasionally a manifestation of CUP. In these cases, laminectomy has been traditionally recommended as the first step to establish the histopathologic diagnosis. The median survival time of patients presenting with CUP and epidural metastasis is <2 months.
5. **Cutaneous metastases** are associated with carcinomas of the breast and lung in most cases. When skin metastases represent the initial manifestation of cancer, renal adenocarcinoma or bronchogenic carcinoma is the most likely possibility. The region of the skin near the primary tumor is most often involved. **Umbilical nodules** (*Sister Joseph nodules*) represent intra-abdominal carcinomatosis. The median survival time of patients presenting with CUP and predominantly skin metastases is 7 months if the primary site does not prove to be the lung.

IV. SEARCHING FOR THE PRIMARY TUMOR SITE

When the primary site of cancer is evident, the biopsy is performed, and the number of diagnostic tests ordered is significantly fewer than when patients present with CUP. The pursuit of the occult primary site through a prolonged investigative pathways is unnecessary, expensive, time consuming, and potentially dangerous.

Even if all patients undergo exhaustive evaluation with barium enema, upper GI series, skeletal survey, mammography (women), whole-body CT scans, endoscopy, and a variety of radionuclide scans, *<15% of patients* with CUP (excluding those who have disease only in cervical nodes) have the primary site established before death. Searching for the primary tumor site should be guided by the following questions:

A. **What is the effect on outcome of finding the primary site?** The prognosis in patients with CUP is unaffected by whether the primary lesion is ever found. This observation applies not only to metastases involving visceral or skeletal sites but also to metastases involving lymph nodes alone at any site (including the neck) with any histology (carcinoma or melanoma).

B. **What are the clinical clues?**
   1. **Histology.** The finding of squamous carcinoma obviates the need to investigate organs in which adenocarcinomas develop. If the pathologist is not certain of the diagnosis because of the morphology or quality of the specimen, special studies or another biopsy may be in order.
   2. **Presentation.** The history, physical examination, and screening studies should be reviewed with awareness of the natural histories of the potentially causal malignancies.

C. **Which advanced malignancies are treatable?** They are
   1. **Metastases to unilateral lymph nodes alone**
      a. Melanoma to peripheral lymph nodes in a single region
      b. Squamous cell or undifferentiated carcinoma in the upper two-thirds of the cervical chain
      c. Adenocarcinoma in the axillary chain in women
      d. Carcinoma in unilateral groin nodes
   2. **Metastases that are sensitive to systemic therapy**
      a. Small cell carcinomas or NUPs.
      b. Peritoneal carcinomatosis in women.
      c. Poorly differentiated carcinoma metastatic to retroperitoneum and/or mediastinum, with or without involvement of peripheral lymph nodes, particularly in younger men.
      d. Adenocarcinomas that are treatable in advanced stages (breast, ovary, prostate, colon, and thyroid).
      e. Lymphomas should be considered in any patient with a poorly differentiated or undifferentiated neoplasm or with tumors that respond exquisitely to chemotherapy.
   3. **Cancers that harbor targetable mutations**, such as mutations in BRAF, EGFR, ALK, ROS, and KIT, may respond quickly to targeted therapies. The term *Lazarus effect* has been recently used, and it reflects a rapid and significant improvement in patient's symptoms after targeted therapy has been started.

D. **What are the limitations of diagnostic studies?** Despite subjection to an alarming battery of tests, >85% of patients with CUP do not have the primary site determined while they are alive. Postmortem examination, the ultimate diagnostic test, fails to detect the primary site in 25% to 40% of CUP cases.

E. **Should I order tumor markers?** Serum tumor markers, including CEA, CA-125, CA 15-3, CA 19-9, and β-hCG, used as a screening method, are generally of little use in determining the primary site because of their lack of specificity. All five of these markers are commonly elevated in patients with CUP. PSA should be ordered in men older than 40 with an adenocarcinoma of unknown primary site unless metastatic disease is limited to the liver or brain. CA-125 can be ordered only if ovarian primary, CA 19-9 if pancreatic or biliary tract primary are suspected. Even **estrogen receptor** determination has not been helpful in identifying the primary site or in prescribing therapy for patients with CUP.

V. MANAGEMENT

A. **Discussion with the patient** must not be underestimated. Patients when they receive the diagnosis of CUP frequently consider it a failure of the diagnostic workup and are in a significant emotional distress. They must be counseled on the natural history of these diseases and prognosis. End-of-life discussions should be started early.

B. **Symptom management** is more important than exposure to toxicities of chemotherapy, especially in poor-prognosis patients.

C. **Malignant melanoma involving peripheral lymph nodes only.** Inquire about skin lesions that may have been removed previously. Search the skin carefully for a possible primary lesion; biopsy any suspect lesion. Exclude visceral metastases. Recommended treatment for malignant melanoma involving lymph nodes alone is radical lymphadenectomy of the affected nodal region. The procedure is repeated if the tumor recurs and the patient has no other evidence of disease. The prognosis with lymphatic metastasis is affected neither by knowing the primary site nor by having a history of a pre-existing lesion. The prognosis is best if the metastasis involves only one node, and not the cervical chain, and if surgical intervention is prompt and aggressive.

D. **Metastatic disease in neck lymph nodes only**, particularly in the upper and middle cervical nodes, is potentially curable with RT, concomitant chemotherapy and RT, or node dissection under appropriate circumstances. If SCC involves the mid or upper cervical lymph nodes, a direct laryngoscopy, nasopharyngoscopy under anesthesia, and upper esophagoscopy should be performed.

E. **Metastatic disease in unilateral axillary lymph nodes only.** The major treatable malignancies presenting as CUP in axillary lymph nodes are occult breast carcinoma, amelanotic melanoma mistaken as undifferentiated carcinoma, and malignant lymphoma mistaken as carcinomas. If the diagnosis can be established, it should be managed as the diagnosed disease; if no primary site is found, axillary node dissection is performed, attempting to achieve local control and long-term survival. RT to the axilla is frequently given, but there is no evidence to indicate that survival is improved over that achieved with resection of the involved nodes alone.

F. **Metastatic disease in unilateral groin lymph nodes only.** If the diagnosis can be established, it should be managed as the diagnosed disease; if no primary site is found, a superficial groin node dissection affords local control with less morbidity than radical dissection. If SCC is present in the lymph nodes, gynecologic exam and anal endoscopy are recommended. RT does not appear to be necessary. Chemotherapy has been useful for carcinomas of the anus and cervix. Half of patients treated with excisional biopsy or superficial groin dissection alone appear to survive >2 years.

G. **Poorly differentiated carcinomas with midline lymphadenopathy** (especially in young men with elevated serum levels of β-hCG and α-FP) are managed as extragonadal germ-cell tumors. Testicular ultrasound should be considered.

   1. **Recommended treatment.** Administer four cycles of cisplatin-based combination chemotherapy using regimens recommended for testicular cancer.

   2. **Results of treatment.** The response rate with disease confined to the mediastinum, retroperitoneum, or peripheral lymph nodes is 60% to 75%, with complete remissions observed in 50% of patients. In some series, the median

survival time for patients achieving a complete remission is >4 years; the 5-year survival rate is 35% for patients with disease confined to the retroperitoneum and peripheral lymph nodes and 15% for those with disease affecting predominantly the mediastinum. For patients with this histology and metastases to other sites, the response rate to cisplatin-based chemotherapy is 20%, and the 5-year survival rate is about 5%.

H. **Peritoneal carcinomatosis in women**

1. **Recommended treatment.** If no extraovarian primary site is evident, perform exploratory laparotomy. If peritoneal carcinomatosis is confirmed without an extraovarian primary site, treat the patient as if she had ovarian carcinoma by performing total abdominal hysterectomy, bilateral salpingo-oophorectomy, omentectomy, and cytoreductive debulking of metastases. Thereafter, treat with a platinum-based combination chemotherapy regimen for six to eight cycles. Second-look laparotomy is not a consideration in these patients.

2. **Results of treatment.** The median survival rates are 1.5 to 2 years for all patients, 2.5 years for patients with limited residual disease after surgery, and 1 year for patients with extensive residual disease after surgery. About 10% to 25% of patients survive 3 years. Most long-term remissions have been observed in patients who had successful cytoreduction before receiving chemotherapy.

I. **Neuroendocrine tumors of unknown primary**

1. **Recommended treatment**

a. **Low-grade NUPs** are relatively resistant to chemotherapy. Aggressive regimens should be avoided. For patients with localized disease, the treatment with RT or dissection alone is recommended.

b. **Poorly differentiated NUPs** are often highly sensitive to chemotherapy. The most commonly used regimens are cisplatin (or carboplatin) plus etoposide or paclitaxel, carboplatin, and etoposide. If a complete remission is obtained, consider administering RT to the known previous sites of disease.

2. **Results of treatment.** The response rate of poorly differentiated NUPs to chemotherapy is 35% to 70%, and the 2-year survival rate is about 40%. Long-term survival can be seen in patients who achieve a complete response after treatment for limited disease. Prolonged survival also occurs in patients presenting with cervical node metastases from occult primary small cell tumors of the minor salivary glands or paranasal sinuses after treatment with RT or neck dissection alone.

J. **All other patients with CUP.** All patients should receive a complete history and physical examination (including the breasts, rectum, and pelvis), CT scans, and routine laboratory tests. Because of the low frequency of detecting the primary site in patients with CUP and the frequently misleading results of radiologic studies, radiologic or radionuclide studies are justified only in the presence of either specific abnormalities in the screening evaluation or possibilities suggested by review of histopathology.

When the initial database does not suggest a primary organ site, further evaluation is usually fruitless and is not indicated. It is important to recognize that these patients have incurable cancer that is usually refractory to treatment. With the exception of treatable malignancies, documenting a site is more important to the patient (or physician) psychologically than therapeutically.

1. **For possible breast or prostate cancer.** Treat according to the principles established for those malignancies, especially considering hormonal manipulations.

2. **Patients with a "colon cancer profile"** (predominant metastatic sites in the liver and/or peritoneum; adenocarcinoma with histology typical of GI origin; immunohistochemistry pattern CK20 positive/CK7 negative and CDX2 positive) may respond to chemotherapy with modern regimens developed for metastatic colorectal carcinoma. A regimen such as FOLFOX-6 may be tried. These regimens have resulted in substantial improvement in survival for patients with metastatic colorectal cancer compared with earlier regimens.

3. **For all other patients with CUP metastatic to viscera.** Nearly 80% of these patients have CUP metastases from cancers of the pancreas, GI tract, lung, and other or never-to-be-known sites that are usually refractory to chemotherapy. When patients with malignancies that are poorly differentiated or metastases that are restricted to lymph nodes are excluded, <20% of patients experience partial tumor regression after treatment with cytotoxic agents (used singly or in combination). Responses are associated with only a minimal (if any) improvement in survival. Median survival is reported to be improved by 4 to 6 months in patients who respond to therapy compared with those who do not, but this form of reporting data is largely discredited. One must be very cautious when reading about chemotherapy results in this heterogeneous group of patients because differences may be due to patient selection factors.

   The most optimistic reports of response of adenocarcinomas to therapy were with the combinations of carboplatin plus paclitaxel, carboplatin (or cisplatin) plus gemcitabine, carboplatin (or cisplatin) plus docetaxel, irinotecan plus gemcitabine, oxaliplatin plus gemcitabine, or gemcitabine plus docetaxel. SCCs responded to cisplatin plus 5-fluorouracil (most frequently used) and platinum plus taxane (especially if head-and-neck primary is suspected). Taxanes show a slight advantage over platinum-based regimens. Response rates to these combinations are reported to be 25% to 35%, with median survivals being 5 to 10 months; combinations using three drugs result in more toxicity without improvements in response.

4. **Recommended treatment.**
   a. **Patients with good performance status**
      (1) **Adenocarcinoma presenting as a single metastatic lesion.** Most patients who present with a single metastatic lesion manifest other metastatic sites within a relatively short period of time. However, definitive local treatment (surgical excision or RT) sometimes produces long disease-free intervals.
      (2) **Multiple metastatic sites.** An empiric trial of combination chemotherapy as discussed above may be offered.
   b. **Patients with poor performance status.** Best supportive care without chemotherapy. If chemotherapy is started, the regimen should be least toxic possible to spare the patient from unnecessary side effects.

ACKNOWLEDGMENT

The author would like to acknowledge Dr. Dennis A. Casciato, who significantly contributed to earlier versions of this chapter.

Suggested Readings

Amela EY, Lauridant-Philippin G, Cousin S, et al. Management of "unfavourable" carcinoma of unknown primary site: synthesis of recent literature. *Crit Rev Oncol Hematol* 2012;84:213.

Chen KW, Liu CJ, Lu HJ, et al. Evaluation of prognostic factors and the role of chemotherapy in unfavorable carcinoma of unknown primary site: a 10-year cohort study. *BMC Res Notes* 2012;5:70.

Conner JR, Hornick JL. Metastatic carcinoma of unknown primary: diagnostic approach using immunohistochemistry. *Adv Anat Pathol* 2015;22:149.

Greco FA, Navlidis N. Treatment of patients with unknown primary carcinoma and unfavorable prognostic factors. *Semin Oncol* 2009;36:65.

Hainsworth JD, Fizazi K. Treatment for patients with unknown primary and favorable prognostic factors. *Semin Oncol* 2009;36:44.

Lee J, Hahn S, Kim DW, et al. Evaluation of survival benefits by platinums and taxanes for an unfavourable subset of carcinoma of unknown primary: a systematic review and meta-analysis. *Br J Cancer* 2013;108(1):39.

Pavlidis N, Pentheroudakis G. Cancer of unknown primary site. *Lancet* 2012;379:1428.

Pentheroudakis G, Lazardis G, Pavlidis N. Axillary nodal metastases from carcinoma of unknown primary (CUPAx): a systematic review of published evidence. *Breast Cancer Res Treat* 2010;119:1.

Riihimäki M, Thomsen H, Hemminki A, et al. Comparison of survival of patients with metastases from known versus unknown primaries: survival in metastatic cancer. *BMC Cancer* 2013;13:36.

Urban D, Rao A, Bressel M, et al. Cancer of unknown primary: a population-based analysis of temporal change and socioeconomic disparities. *Br J Cancer* 2013;109(5):1318.

Varadhachary GR, Raber MN. Cancer of unknown primary site. *N Engl J Med* 2014;371:757.

Varadhachary GR, Spector Y, Abbruzzese JL, et al. Prospective gene signature study using microRNA to identify the tissue of origin in patients with carcinoma of unknown primary. *Clin Cancer Res* 2011;17:4063.

III Hematopoietic Malignancies

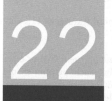

22 Hodgkin and Non-Hodgkin Lymphoma

Lauren C. Pinter-Brown

I. SYMPTOMS AND SIGNS

A. History

1. **Painless lymphadenopathy,** involving any of the superficial lymph nodes, is the most common chief complaint of patients with Hodgkin lymphoma (HL) and non-Hodgkin lymphoma (NHL).

2. **Systemic symptoms.** Fevers, night sweats, and weight loss are characteristic in advanced presentations of HL and aggressive NHL but may be encountered in all stages and pathologic types of lymphoma. Marked fatigue and general weakness may also be reported, not always correlating with the degree of anemia.

   a. Pruritus, often intense, may be the presenting symptom in HL, particularly the nodular sclerosis subtype, and may antedate diagnosis by months or years.

   b. Pel-Ebstein fever is periodic and uncommon but characteristic of HL.

3. **Pain**

   a. Alcohol-induced pain in areas of involvement is infrequent but is characteristic of HL.

   b. Abdominal pain or discomfort may be due to splenomegaly, bowel dysfunction due to adenopathy or bowel involvement, or hydronephrosis.

   c. Bone pain may reflect localized areas of bone destruction or invasion or diffuse marrow infiltration.

   d. Neurogenic pain is caused by spinal cord compression, plexopathies, nerve root infiltration, meningeal involvement, and complicating varicella zoster.

   e. Back pain suggests massive retroperitoneal nodal involvement, often with psoas muscle invasion.

B. Physical examination should evaluate for hepatosplenomegaly, the presence of effusions, evidence of neuropathy, and signs of obstruction (e.g., extremity edema, superior vena cava syndrome, spinal cord compression, hollow viscera dysfunction). Lymph node chains must be carefully examined, including the cervical, supraclavicular, axillary, epitrochlear, inguinal, femoral, and popliteal nodes.

1. **The lymph nodes** are examined for size, multiplicity, consistency, and tenderness. Lymphomatous involvement typically imparts a rubbery consistency, not the rock-hard quality of carcinoma.

2. **The tonsils and oropharynx** are thoroughly examined. Waldeyer ring involvement mandates complete evaluation of the nasopharynx, oropharynx, and hypopharynx by endoscopy.

II. DIFFERENTIAL DIAGNOSIS (Table 22-1) compares clinical features of HL and NHL.

 A. **Lymphadenopathy**

  1. **Infections.** Patients, particularly young children with apparent viral or other infections, may develop striking lymphadenopathy. Such patients should be evaluated for infectious processes and observed for clear-cut resolution. Microorganisms associated with prominent lymphadenopathy include Epstein-Barr virus (EBV; infectious mononucleosis), cytomegalovirus (CMV), human immunodeficiency virus (HIV), hepatitis virus, secondary syphilis, mycobacteria, some fungi, and *Toxoplasma*, *Brucella*, and *Rochalimaea* species infection. In some cases, biopsy is required for diagnosis of specific infectious diseases.

  2. **Systemic immune disorders,** such as rheumatoid arthritis, Sjögren syndrome, and systemic lupus erythematosus, are associated with both benign lymphadenopathy and lymphoma. Progressive or asymmetric lymphadenopathy mandates biopsy.

  3. **Patients at risk for HIV infection** present problems requiring individualization in management. Persistent generalized lymphadenopathy is a part of the acquired immunodeficiency syndrome (AIDS) spectrum, but lymphadenopathy can also be caused by opportunistic infections, Kaposi sarcoma, or lymphoma.

  4. **Lymph nodes that are usually benign.**
   a. **Occipital.** Consider scalp infection
   b. **Posterior auricular.** Usually viral or scalp infection
   c. **Shotty inguinal nodes.** Often present with no obvious cause but may suggest external genital or lower extremity infections

  5. **Cervical nodes.** Patients with isolated enlargement of high or middle cervical lymph nodes often harbor occult primary carcinoma of the head and neck. The special approach required for these patients is discussed in Chapter 8, Section X.

 B. **Midline masses**

  1. **Retroperitoneal masses** (see Chapter 20, Section II).

  2. **Mediastinal masses** may occur in a variety of nonneoplastic and neoplastic (both primary and metastatic) conditions (see Chapter 20, Section I).

TABLE 22-1	Comparison of Hodgkin and Non-Hodgkin Lymphomas		
		In Non-Hodgkin Lymphoma	
Characteristic	**In Hodgkin Lymphoma**	**Low Grade**	**Others**
Site of origin	Nodal	Extranodal (~10%)	Extranodal (~35%)
Nodal distribution	Centripetal (axial)	Centrifugal	Centrifugal
Nodal spread	Contiguous	Noncontiguous	Noncontiguous
CNS involvement	Rare (<1%)	Rare (<1%)	Uncommon (<10%)
Hepatic involvement	Uncommon	Common (>50%)	Uncommon
Bone marrow involvement	Uncommon (<10%)	Common (>50%)	Uncommon (<20%)
Marrow involvement adversely affects prognosis	Yes	No	Yes
Curable by chemotherapy	Yes	No	Yes

3. **Hilar masses.** Isolated symmetric bilateral hilar lymphadenopathy (without mediastinal mass) is strongly suggestive of sarcoidosis, and many experts believe that observation alone could suffice in this clinical setting. Unilateral hilar masses are frequently secondary to lung cancer; metastatic disease must also be considered. Coccidioidomycosis and histoplasmosis enter the differential diagnosis in the appropriate clinical and geographic milieu.

C. **Splenomegaly.** The diagnosis can usually be made with careful history taking and physical examination, laboratory evaluation, CT scans of the abdomen, bone marrow biopsy or aspiration with flow cytometric analysis, and, occasionally, liver biopsy. When a diagnosis cannot be established by these means, careful follow-up of the patient is warranted. Splenectomy should be considered for diagnosis in patients with massive or progressive isolated splenomegaly.

1. **Normal.** A palpable spleen is occasionally seen in otherwise healthy young adults of thin body habitus.

2. **Infections** include most pathogens listed in Section II.A.1, bacterial endocarditis, malaria, and abscess.

3. **Secondary to portal hypertension** (congestive splenomegaly). Patients with chronic liver disease or portal or splenic vein thrombosis may have no other findings to direct the diagnostic search. Portal hypertension may be documented by ultrasound of the abdomen with Doppler or by liver–spleen scanning, which reveals redistribution of the radionuclide to the spleen and marrow.

4. **Storage diseases,** particularly Gaucher disease, may produce prominent splenomegaly; characteristic cells are seen in the bone marrow in most cases.

5. **Tumors** are predominantly hematologic, including lymphomas and leukemias. Metastases, particularly from melanoma and breast cancer, and primary splenic sarcomas may also occur.

6. **Myeloproliferative disorders** such as polycythemia vera, chronic idiopathic myelofibrosis, and chronic myelogenous leukemia may cause marked splenomegaly.

7. **Autoimmune disorders.** Rheumatoid arthritis (Felty syndrome), systemic lupus erythematosus, and autoimmune hemolytic anemia may produce splenomegaly (not isolated autoimmune thrombocytopenia) and can usually be diagnosed by history and associated laboratory findings.

8. **Miscellaneous.** Splenic cysts, thyrotoxicosis, sarcoidosis, chronic nonimmune hemolysis, and amyloidosis are unusual causes of splenomegaly.

III. BIOPSY PROCEDURES

A. **Sites and methods of diagnostic biopsy.** Tissues or organs that are suspected of involvement are subjected to generous biopsy for primary diagnosis wherever possible. Fine needle aspiration cytology is mainly used for staging evaluation or for proving recurrence but may sometimes allow cytologic diagnosis *if expertise in interpretation is available. Excisional, incisional, or core biopsy is strongly encouraged.*

1. **Peripheral node biopsy.** One of the largest accessible lymph nodes is excised or sampled whenever peripheral lymphadenopathy is present. Small lymph nodes may be more readily removed but may be uninvolved.

2. **Inguinal lymph nodes** are frequently enlarged because of benign chronic inflammatory processes in the lower extremities. These nodes should be biopsied only when other sites are not suspected or when pathologic involvement is clearly anticipated.

3. **Bone marrow biopsy** combined with aspiration is used for staging and may lead to diagnosis, particularly in the presence of abnormal circulating cells or cytopenias.

4. **Mediastinoscopy or limited thoracotomy** (e.g., Chamberlain procedure) for definitive diagnosis is required for a substantial proportion of patients with mediastinal masses.

5. **Laparotomy** is used to diagnose some cases of lymphoma restricted to the abdomen and may include biopsies of the liver and random lymph nodes, as well as the primary area in question.

6. **Laparoscopy** assesses the liver and peritoneum and allows extensive biopsy, obviating the need for laparotomy in some patients.

7. **Endoscopic gastric biopsy** with staining for *Helicobacter pylori* may be helpful in the diagnosis of gastric MALToma. Repeated attempts with deeper biopsies and immunoperoxidase staining for leukocyte common antigen and keratin intermediate filaments may be helpful in the differential diagnosis between lymphoma and carcinoma. Small bowel involvement beyond the duodenum usually requires open biopsy, although capsule endoscopy may be suggestive of lymphoma in some cases.

8. **Retroperitoneal and mesenteric masses** may be evaluated by imaging-guided Tru-Cut biopsy obviating the need for laparotomy.

B. **Handling the biopsy material.** The procured biopsy specimen is submitted to the pathologist directly and *not placed in a fixative* by the operating surgeon to ensure the best use of the available tissue. Prior communication with the pathologist is advantageous. Pathology tissue processing includes the following procedures:

1. **Touch preparations** (imprints), which provide cytologic detail and material for immunologic phenotyping.

2. **Immunologic phenotyping** with monoclonal antibodies can be crucial to diagnosis. Lymphoid cells are characterized immunologically using flow cytometry or immunohistochemistry. Discriminatory immunophenotypes in lymphoma are shown in Appendix C5. A common NHL panel should include assessment of expression of CD2 or CD3, CD5, CD19 or CD20, and CD23 in blood, bone marrow, or biopsy specimens. Classic Reed-Sternberg (RS) cells are usually CD15 positive and CD30 positive. More surface markers may need to be analyzed if this screening is inconclusive or if rare entities (such as natural killer [NK] cell or hairy cell leukemia) are considered.

3. **Special handling of tissues for additional studies:** Tissue should be obtained to allow for additional studies such as cytogenetics, molecular analysis, and electron microscopy that can allow for further characterization of the disorder, aid in difficult diagnostic problems, and help in treatment decisions.

4. **Microbial culture** of submitted material when the clinical picture or tissue suggests infection.

IV. CLINICAL EVALUATION

The extent of the staging evaluation is determined by the individual case presentation, the histopathologic diagnosis, and the effect of the stage on treatment planning.

A. **Evaluation of blood tests**

1. **Hematologic manifestations** are discussed in Chapter 35.

2. **Diagnostically abnormal circulating lymphoid cells or lymphocytosis** is seen in some patients with either indolent or aggressive forms of NHL. Lymphoid cells are characterized immunologically using flow cytometry, and monoclonality may be established by kappa:lambda ratios (B cell) or

gene rearrangement technology (T and B cell); these techniques are capable of detecting minute clones of circulating lymphoma cells not detectable by inspection of the blood smears.

3. **Acute-phase reactants,** such as the erythrocyte sedimentation rate (ESR), fibrinogen, haptoglobin, and serum copper levels, may parallel disease activity, especially in HL.

4. **Liver function tests** are unreliable in predicting lymphomatous involvement of the liver. Marked elevation of alkaline phosphatase and occasionally frank cholestatic jaundice may complicate HL as a paraneoplastic event without direct liver involvement. Extrahepatic biliary obstruction may also occur with lymphoma caused by enlarged nodes in the porta hepatis.

5. **Renal function tests.** Elevated creatinine and blood urea nitrogen levels suggest ureteral obstruction and, less commonly, direct renal involvement. Uric acid nephropathy or hypercalcemia may contribute to renal insufficiency. Frank nephrotic syndrome as a paraneoplastic phenomenon may complicate HL and other lymphomas (see Chapter 32).

6. **Serum uric acid.** Hyperuricemia is a common manifestation of high-turnover-rate (aggressive) NHL and may also be seen with extensive lower-grade lymphomas. Treatment of high-grade NHL or treatment of sensitive bulky low-grade lymphoma may provoke brisk tumor lysis, leading to further elevation of uric acid and renal shutdown (see Chapter 28, Section IX). Hypouricemia may be seen in HL.

7. **Hypercalcemia** has been noted in some cases of lymphoma and may be secondary to production of parathyroid hormone–related peptide or activation of vitamin D by lymphoma tissue.

8. **Serum lactate dehydrogenase (LDH) levels** reflect tumor bulk and turnover, particularly in the aggressive NHL, and are considered an independent prognostic factor.

9. **Serum immunoglobulins.** Polyclonal hypergammaglobulinemia is commonly seen in HL and NHL. Hypogammaglobulinemia is particularly common in the small lymphocytic lymphomas (SLLs) and late in the disease. Monoclonal spikes or paraproteins are seen occasionally in NHL patients.

B. **Evaluation of the chest**

1. **Chest radiographs** may demonstrate mediastinal and hilar lymphadenopathy, pleural effusions, and parenchymal lesions. A cavitating lesion is more typical of infection than lymphomas.

2. **CT scans** tend to replace chest x-rays because they can demonstrate parenchymal and mediastinal abnormalities in more detail.

3. **Thoracentesis and pleural biopsy** may demonstrate direct lymphomatous involvement of the pleura. Obstruction of mediastinal lymphatic–venous drainage may result in cytologically negative or chylous effusions.

C. **Evaluation of the abdomen and retroperitoneum**

1. **CT scans** are useful in delineating abnormal enlargement of nodes in retroperitoneal, mesenteric, portal, and other lymph node sites. The CT scan also detects splenomegaly and, with constant enhancement, may define space-occupying lesions in the liver, spleen, and kidneys.

2. **Abdominal ultrasonography** is too insensitive to be useful in routinely assessing abdominal lymphadenopathy. It is occasionally helpful in distinguishing hepatic or splenic lesions (cystic vs. solid) and in excluding an obstructive basis for renal insufficiency and jaundice.

3. **MRI** with contrast may be useful in distinguishing benign from malignant hepatic lesions.

D. Evaluation of the gastrointestinal (GI) tract. Direct involvement of the GI tract is uncommon in HL but is common in NHL. Patients with Waldeyer ring lymphoma, suggestive GI symptoms, extensive abdominal nodal involvement, unexplained iron deficiency, or GI bleeding may be evaluated with upper GI series and complete small bowel follow-through. Barium enema may be necessary. Endoscopic examination and biopsy of accessible abnormalities are performed. Routine GI tract evaluation for patients with mantle cell lymphoma (MCL) is performed in some centers.

E. Evaluation of the central nervous system (CNS). Spinal fluid examination is routinely used to exclude occult lymphomatous involvement of the meninges in patients with Burkitt lymphoma (BL) or lymphoblastic lymphoma and is often performed in patients with intermediate-grade or high-grade lymphoma involving the testes or paranasal sinuses (B-cell histology), with extensive bone marrow involvement, or with multiple sites of extranodal involvement and elevated LDH. In these cases, the incidence of CNS disease is in the 5% range. Patients with AIDS-related lymphoma may require CT or MRI scans of the brain and spinal fluid analysis. Symptoms suggestive of intracranial, spinal cord, or peripheral nerve involvement require immediate diagnostic evaluation.

F. Nuclear scans

1. **Positron emission tomography (PET)** using ^{18}F-fluorodeoxyglucose scans has replaced gallium scans. It is more sensitive in detecting unsuspected areas of involvement or in differentiating active versus uninvolved nodes with accuracy approaching 95% depending on nodal histology. Similar to gallium scans, PET is somewhat less reliable in indolent lymphoma. False-positive results can be produced by any inflammation, whereas faint normal uptake of muscles, the bowel, and bone marrow recovering from chemotherapy should be differentiated from involvement. The advent of combined PET/CT scan is thought to increase the accuracy of the procedure.

HODGKIN LYMPHOMA

I. EPIDEMIOLOGY AND ETIOLOGY

A. Incidence. HL accounts for about 1% of new cancer cases annually in the United States, or 7,000 cases per year.

1. **Age.** HL demonstrates a bimodal age–incidence curve in the United States and some industrialized European nations. The first peak, constituting predominantly the nodular sclerosis subtype, occurs in the 20s, and the second peak occurs after 50 years of age. In Third World countries, the first peak is absent, and there is a significant incidence of mixed cellularity (MC) and lymphocyte-depleted (LD) HL in men.

2. **Sex.** About 85% of children with HL are boys. In adults, the nodular sclerosing (NS) subtype of HL shows a slight female predominance, whereas the other histologic subtypes are more common in men.

B. Risk factors. In Western countries, the first peak of HL is associated with a higher social class, advanced education, and small family size; a delayed exposure to a common infectious or other environmental agent has been suggested. HL may be associated with EBV infection, but the significance of this association is unclear. A slightly increased incidence of HL has been demonstrated with HIV infection; HIV-associated HL (see Chapter 37, Section III) often presents with constitutional symptoms, advanced stage, and unusual sites of involvement (e.g., marrow, skin, leptomeninges).

II. PATHOLOGY AND NATURAL HISTORY

A. **Histology.** The pathologic diagnosis of HL depends on the presence of RS cells and their variants in *an appropriate pathologic milieu*. The bulk of lymphatic tissue involved by HL is not composed of neoplastic cells but rather a variety of normal-appearing lymphocytes, plasma cells, eosinophils, neutrophils, and histiocytes existing in different proportions in the various histologic subtypes. Important variants of RS cells include L&H (lymphocyte and histiocyte) cells, lacunar cells, and RS-like cells (see Appendix B3. Discriminatory Immunophenotypes for Lymphoid Neoplasms).

1. **The Rye classification** for HL relates the histopathologic subtypes to clinical behavior. This older classification system comprises lymphocyte-predominant (LP), NS, MC, and the uncommon LD varieties of HL. The LP subtype was further divided into nodular LP and diffuse LP subtypes. Immunohistochemistry, however, has resulted in deletion of the diffuse LP subtype and redefinition of the nodular LP subtype as nonclassical HL (see Section II.A.2).

2. **The World Health Organization (WHO) classification** divides HL into *nodular LP HL* and *classical HL*. Classical HL in this newer classification system comprises the lymphocyte-rich, NS, MC, and LD varieties (Appendix B4).

   a. **Nodular LP HL** with its L&H cells, which are not classical RS cells, is now clearly recognized to be most like an indolent B-cell NHL and not true HL. For that reason, nodular LP HL is distinguished from classical HL in the WHO classification. Table 22-2 shows this classification system with distinguishing histopathologic features, clinical correlates, and immunophenotypes.

   b. **Diffuse LP HL in the Rye classification** has disappeared as an entity. In the new WHO classification of lymphocytic neoplasms, what was thought to be diffuse LP HL is now classified as lymphocyte-rich classical HL (with true RS cells that are CD30 positive), Lennert lymphoma (lymphoepithelioid peripheral T-cell lymphoma [PTCL]), T-cell–rich B-cell lymphoma, or other entities.

3. **RS cells and their variants**

   a. **RS cells** are giant cells that have more than one nucleus and large, eosinophilic, inclusion-like nuclei. Single-cell polymerase chain reaction analysis has shown that the RS cells are B cells that originate in the germinal centers of lymph nodes. RS cells and the accompanying mononuclear *Hodgkin cell* variants are the neoplastic cells in HL and are surrounded by a reactive cellular infiltrate. Classic RS cells usually express CD15 and CD30. CD30 (Ki-1) is an antigen that is also expressed in anaplastic large cell lymphoma (ALCL) and occasionally in other forms of NHL (e.g., large B-cell lymphoma [LBCL], PTCL). RS cells express CD20 infrequently, but not CD45 (leukocyte common antigen).

   b. **The lacunar cell** is a variant of the RS cell and has the *same* immunophenotype. It characterizes NS HL and is often far more plentiful than classic RS cells in that subtype.

   c. **L&H cells** are RS-like but have a *different* immunophenotype. L&H cells manifest B-cell markers (CD20, CD45, and CD79a), but not CD15 or CD30. Although the L&H cells are believed to be of monoclonal origin, the surrounding B-cell infiltrates may be polyclonal. L&H cells were identified in nodular LP HL, which is now considered a separate entity because of its distinct immunophenotype.

TABLE 22-2	Pathologic and Clinical Features of Hodgkin Lymphoma Subtypes[a]			
Histologic Subtype	Frequency (%)	Histopathology	Clinical Characteristics	Common Stages
Nodular lymphocyte predominant HL[b]	5	L&H ("popcorn cells") intermingled with polymorphous infiltrate; nodular or nodular and diffuse patterns	Males; usually localized to peripheral nodes; frequent relapses; excellent prognosis	I–IIA
Lymphocyte-rich CHL[c]	5	RS scattered in background of small lymphocytes; nodular and diffuse patterns; absent eosinophils and neutrophils	Older males; localized to peripheral nodes; fewer relapses; excellent prognosis	I–IIA
Nodular-sclerosing CHL[c]	70	RS variable; nodular growth pattern with collagen bands and "lacunar cells"; heterogeneous cellularity with numerous eosinophils and neutrophils	Females; mediastinal masses and peripheral nodes	I–IIIA or B
Mixed-cellularity CHL[c]	20–25	RS more frequent in a mixed inflammatory background without NS fibrosis	Frequently retroperitoneal; often symptomatic	II–IVA or B
Lymphocyte-depleted CHL[c]	<5	RS predominant in variable patterns, including diffuse fibrosis; depleted of nonneoplastic lymphocytes	Aggressive course; liver and marrow involved with relative sparing of peripheral nodes	III–IVB

[a]World Health Organization classification system.
[a]L&H cells immunophenotype: CD15⁻, CD30⁻, CD20⁺, CD45⁺, EMA⁺, CD79a⁺.
[c]Classical HL—RS immunophenotype: CD15⁺, CD30⁺, CD20⁺, CD45⁻, EMA⁻, ALK-1⁻.
HL, Hodgkin lymphoma; L&H, lymphocytic and histiocytic cells; CHL, classical HL; RS, Reed-Sternberg cells; EMA, epithelial membrane antigen; ALK-1, anaplastic lymphoma kinase.

    d. RS-like cells are found in a variety of infectious, inflammatory, and neoplastic disorders, including infectious mononucleosis, lymphoid hyperplasia associated with phenytoin therapy, and high-grade NHLs.

B. Mode of spread (see Table 22-1). HL almost always originates in a lymph node. Whenever a primary diagnosis of HL is made in an extranodal site without contiguous nodal involvement, the diagnosis should be highly suspected with the exception of HIV-infected individuals. For much of its natural history, HL appears to spread in an orderly fashion through the lymphatic system by contiguity. Histologic types other than NS, however, often skip the mediastinum, and disease appears in the neck and upper abdomen. The axial lymphatic system is almost always affected in HL, whereas distal sites (e.g., epitrochlear and popliteal nodes) are rarely involved. Hematogenous dissemination occurs late in the course of disease and is characteristic of the LD subtype.

C. Sites of involvement

    1. Peripheral lymph nodes. Cervical or supraclavicular lymphadenopathy occurs in >70% of cases. Axillary and inguinal lymph nodes are less frequently involved. Generalized lymphadenopathy is atypical of HL. Left supraclavicular lymphadenopathy is more strongly associated with abdominal involvement (specifically, splenic involvement) than is right-sided disease.

    2. Thorax

        a. The anterior mediastinum is a prime location for NS HL. Mediastinal precedes hilar lymph node involvement.

        b. Lung involvement may occur by direct contiguity with hilar involvement in HL as well as by hematogenous dissemination. Pulmonary involvement by HL may produce discrete nodules and irregular, interstitial, or even lobar infiltrates.

        c. Pleural effusion may occur secondary to mediastinal compression of vascular–lymphatic drainage and by direct pleural involvement. Chylous effusions occasionally occur.

        d. Pericardial involvement may be found on CT scans, but overt cardiac tamponade is uncommon.

        e. Superior vena cava syndrome is more frequent in NHL than in HL.

    3. Spleen, liver, and upper abdomen

        a. The spleen, splenic hilar nodes, and celiac nodes are the earliest abdominal sites of involvement in infradiaphragmatic HL. Mesenteric lymph nodes are rarely involved in HL.

        b. At least 25% of spleens not clinically enlarged harbor occult HL at laparotomy, and as many as half of spleens believed to be enlarged on physical examination or radiologic assessment are histologically normal.

        c. Liver involvement is uncommon at diagnosis and is almost always associated with infiltration of the spleen.

    4. Retroperitoneal lymph node involvement tends to occur relatively late in the course of supradiaphragmatic HL and after spleen, splenic hilar, and celiac nodal involvement. Periaortic involvement without splenic involvement is uncommon. The retroperitoneal nodes are, however, affected early in the course of inguinal presentations of HL.

    5. The bone marrow is rarely involved at the time of diagnosis of HL. Patients with advanced-stage disease, systemic symptoms, and MC or LD histologies have a higher risk for bone marrow involvement. A marrow biopsy is mandatory to evaluate the bone marrow because HL is difficult to diagnose on marrow aspirates. Granulomatous changes or fibrosis may be seen, which is not diagnostic of HL involvement.

6. **Bone.** Osseous involvement of HL usually produces an osteoblastic reaction mimicking prostatic carcinoma. Extradural masses may result in spinal cord compression. Sternal erosion by mediastinal NS HL may occur.

7. **Other extranodal sites** are rarely involved in HL. Liver or skin involvement is rare and usually a late manifestation of disease. CNS involvement is very uncommon with the exception of extrinsic spinal cord compression. Clinical involvement of meninges, brain, Waldeyer ring, GI tract, kidney, and other extranodal sites usually suggests an alternative diagnosis.

III. STAGING SYSTEM AND PROGNOSTIC FACTORS

A. **Staging** is the most crucial determinant of prognosis and treatment in HL. The modified system is called the *Cotswolds Staging Classification* and is shown in Table 22-3.

B. **Prognostic factors**

1. **Stage** is clearly the single most important prognostic factor in HL. Within each stage, the presence of B symptoms confers a poorer prognosis. About 60% of patients with HL in the United States have stage I or II disease at the time of diagnosis. The percentage of patients with stage III or IV disease is generally higher in Third World countries and in lower socioeconomic enclaves.

2. **Histopathology.** With advances in therapy, the value of histopathologic subtype as an independent prognostic variable (apart from stage) is less clearly defined than it was in the past.

3. **Adverse prognostic factors** were evaluated by an international group in a multivariate retrospective analysis of 4,695 patients, mostly with extensive disease (see Hasenclever et al. 1998 in "Suggested Readings"). Patients with

TABLE 22-3	Cotswolds Staging Classification of Hodgkin Lymphoma
Stage	**Description**
I	Involvement of a single lymph node region or lymphoid structure
II	Involvement of two or more lymph node regions on the same side of the diaphragm (the mediastinum is considered as a single site, whereas hilar lymph nodes are lateralized). The number of anatomic sites should be indicated by a subscript (e.g., II_3).
III	Involvement of lymph node regions or structures on both sides of the diaphragm
	III_1 With involvement of splenic hilar, celiac, or portal nodes
	III_2 With involvement of para-aortic, iliac, and mesenteric nodes
IV	Involvement of one or more extranodal sites in addition to a site for which the designation "E" has been used

Designations Applicable to any Disease Stage	
A	No symptoms
B	Fever (temperature higher than 38°C), drenching night sweats, or unexplained loss of >10% of body weight within the preceding 6 mo
X	Bulky disease (a mediastinal mass exceeding one-third the maximum transverse diameter of the chest or the presence of a nodal mass with a maximal dimension >10 cm)
E	Involvement of a single extranodal site that is contiguous or proximal to a known nodal site
CS	Clinical stage
PS	Pathologic state (as determined by laparotomy or biopsy)

no adverse factors had an 84% freedom from progression, whereas the presence of *each factor* depressed the freedom from progression curve plateau by about 8%. Interestingly, neither tumor bulk nor histology emerged as independent factors. The seven independent prognostic factors identified were as follows:

Adverse Factor	Relative Risk of Relapse
Male sex	1.35
Age ≥45 yr	1.39
Stage IV disease	1.26
Hemoglobin < 10.5 g/dL	1.35
White blood cell (WBC) count > 15,000/μL	1.41
Lymphocyte count < 600/μL or <8% of WBC	1.38
Serum albumin < 4 g/dL	1.49

4. **Independent adverse prognostic factors for NS HL** include eosinophilia, lymphocyte depletion, and RS cell atypia.
5. **Adverse prognostic factors in early-stage HL** include ESR ≥ 50 mm/hr, four or more separate sites of nodal involvement, bulky mediastinal mass (defined as >33% of the maximum intrathoracic diameter) or any mass ≥10 cm, or extranodal sites of disease.

IV. DIAGNOSIS
A. **Clinical evaluation.** See "Evaluation of Suspected Lymphoma," Sections I through IV.
B. **Staging evaluation**
   1. Adequate surgical biopsy reviewed by experienced hematopathologist. Fine needle aspiration is not an adequate means of initial diagnosis.
   2. Thorough history and physical examination.
   3. Laboratory tests: CBC with differential and platelet count, serum chemistries including LDH, ESR, urinalysis.
   4. CT scan of the neck, chest, abdomen, and pelvis with contrast.
   5. Bone marrow aspiration and biopsy (bilateral iliac crest) unless clinical stage IA to IIA with no anemia or other blood count depression.
   6. Bone scan in the presence of bone pain or elevated serum alkaline phosphatase or calcium level.
   7. PET scans are useful in follow-up of residual masses on chest radiograph or CT scan after therapy, given the propensity of treated HL nodes to remain visible on CT scans.
   8. HIV testing should be considered in patients whose disease presentation is primarily extranodal.
   9. Pregnancy test and fertility counseling in patients of childbearing age should be performed with staging evaluation.

V. MANAGEMENT: PRIMARY THERAPY
A. **Treatment philosophy.** More than one treatment approach may be used in the management of cases of HL. The challenge is to determine a course of therapy that preserves cure while minimizing long-term complications.
B. **Surgery** is limited to diagnosis, possibly laparotomy, and laminectomy for the diagnosis of cause of spinal cord compression.
C. **RT alone** is still used in the United States to treat many patients with stage IA or possibly IIA disease nonclassical HL. However, it is increasingly replaced in the treatment of classical HL with combined-modality treatment.

1. **Radiation dose.** HL may be locally sterilized in almost all cases with 3,000 to 4,400 cGy given at a rate of about 1,000 cGy per week. Lesser doses may be adequate as consolidation after chemotherapy.

2. **Radiation fields**

   a. **Involved-site radiation therapy** (ISRT) consists of irradiation to original sites of known disease only and is used with curative intent in combination with chemotherapy. It has become the most common use of RT in HL with other fields such as mantle field, or inverted Y field, or spade field (Fig. 22-1) of mostly historical interest. Doses given in combined-modality therapy range from 2,000 to 3,600 cGy. The treatment plan is designed using conventional, 3D conformal, or IMRT techniques using CT-based simulation techniques.

D. **Combination chemotherapy** is the mainstay modality for all stages of classical HL and possibly for advanced stages of nonclassical HL. Chemotherapy, often in combination with RT, is also preferable for patients with early-stage disease and/or bulky disease. The selection among the available regimens is often guided by the desire to avoid long-term toxicities associated with specific treatments. The advent of the nonleukemogenic, gonadal-sparing ABVD chemotherapy regimen expanded the use of chemotherapy to patients with earlier stages and obviated the need for laparotomy; it has replaced the historic MOPP. More aggressive regimens such as BEACOPP (Appendix C1, Section II) may improve on ABVD (see Section V.D.3), especially in patients with advanced disease. Maintenance therapy is not recommended.

1. **Useful chemotherapy regimens for HL** are shown in Appendix C1. These regimens must be strictly followed because delays in therapy or reduction in dosages not indicated by the protocol can clearly compromise results. The total dose and dose rate (dose intensity) are important in achieving cure. Regimens used as salvage therapy in HL are shown in Appendix C3.

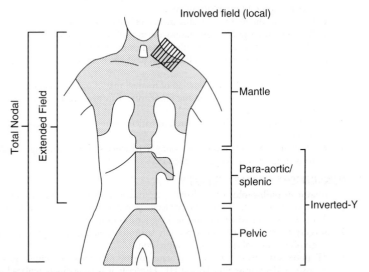

Figure 22-1 Radiation fields used in Hodgkin lymphoma. *Stippled area* is the area irradiated.

2. **ABVD regimen** (Appendix C1, Section I) is superior to the MOPP regimen and causes much less leukemia and infertility. Potential cardiac toxicity caused by doxorubicin and pulmonary toxicity caused by bleomycin (particularly with the concomitant use of granulocyte growth factors) have been occasional problems using this schedule. The concern is heightened when combined with mediastinal RT. ABVD-based treatment has replaced MOPP as the standard regimen for HL.

   a. Generally, the same therapeutic rules as with the MOPP regimen apply: 6 to 8 monthly cycles are usually administered and at least two cycles beyond maximum response.

   b. Pulmonary function should be monitored. If dyspnea, pneumonitis, or significant reduction to <40% of predicted lung diffusion capacity is noted, bleomycin should be discontinued. Bleomycin pneumonitis usually responds to corticosteroids and mandates discontinuation of bleomycin. As there is a concern that the use of myeloid growth factors may increase the risk for bleomycin pulmonary toxicity, their use has been discouraged.

   c. Cardiac function should be monitored in patients with pre-existing heart disease and in those receiving high cumulative doses of doxorubicin. A baseline measurement of left ventricular ejection fraction is suggested before beginning doxorubicin administration.

3. **MOPP or COPP regimen** (Appendix C1, Section I). The National Cancer Institute (NCI) recommends that vincristine should not be limited to a 2-mg maximum dosage in this regimen, but most clinicians sustain the 2-mg limit. Treatment is administered in 28-day cycles for two additional cycles beyond the attainment of a restaged complete response (CR) and a minimum of six cycles (6 months).

   a. The CR rate using the MOPP regimen is between 70% and 80% for stages III and IV HL. About 60% to 70% of CR cases are durable, with relapses rare after 42 months. More than 80% of patients with stage IIIA or IVA disease survive 10 years without recurrence of disease. Histologic subtype appears to have little effect on results with MOPP.

   b. The MOPP regimen is particularly emetogenic, and it is associated with myelosuppression, neuropathy, leukemogenesis, and infertility. It is believed that COPP (replacing mechlorethamine with cyclophosphamide) may be better tolerated.

4. **MOPP and ABVD in alternating cycles and the MOPP/ABV hybrid** have both been found to be less satisfactory than ABVD alone. While MOPP/ABV and ABVD were equally efficacious, the hybrid regimen was associated with increased acute toxicity, myelodysplastic syndrome, and leukemia in a randomized trial. While MOPP/ABVD and ABVD were both superior regimens to MOPP alone, ABVD was less myelotoxic than the combined regimen.

5. **Dose-intense regimens** have been developed with the hope of improving outcome, especially in patients with high-risk HL. The value of these regimens remains unclear.

   a. **BEACOPP.** This aggressive 3-week cycle regimen has been compared favorably to COPP–ABVD in randomized prospective and mature studies. Higher response rates and progression-free survival are reported with dose escalation and mandatory use of growth factors, possibly with a higher risk for secondary leukemia. The effect on sterility is not fully evaluated.

b. **Stanford V** (Appendix C1, Section II). Excellent results achieved with this weekly regimen in phase II studies at a single institution have not yet been confirmed in multicenter randomized trials.

c. **High-dose chemotherapy** followed by autologous stem cell transplantation (SCT) for patients in first remission is not generally recommended.

6. **Compared effectiveness**

a. A large, randomized trial conducted by a cooperative group showed that ABVD alone may be as effective as MOPP plus ABVD and more effective than MOPP alone in the management of most patients with advanced HL. ABVD is considered the standard first-line treatment for most patients and is superior to MOPP in efficacy and toxicity profile.

b. A three-arm randomized clinical study compared COPP–ABVD with standard-dose BEACOPP and escalated-dose BEACOPP (see Diehl et al. 2003, in "Suggested Readings"). The 5-year relapse-free rates were 69% for COPP–ABVD, 76% for standard BEACOPP, and 87% for escalated BEACOPP. The 5-year survival rate was 83% for the COPP–ABVD arm, 88% for the standard-dose BEACOPP arm, and 91% for the escalated-dose BEACOPP arm. Patients with advanced HL and adverse prognostic factors appear to derive benefit from dose escalation. BEACOPP in one of its forms can clearly be considered the treatment of choice for selected patients with high-risk HL.

7. **Combined-modality treatment** is becoming popular in the management of early-stage disease. The advantage of this approach is the limitation of radiation to the involved site only (and thus the reduction of the total dose), reducing long-term radiation-related complications.

a. ISRT can complement an abbreviated course of chemotherapy in patients with clinical stage I or II and nonbulky disease.

b. ISRT may be prescribed after a full course of chemotherapy to consolidate previously bulky areas of disease, especially those that respond only partially to chemotherapy. ISRT to prior sites of disease, however, may not be helpful for patients who achieve a CR with chemotherapy.

E. **Treatment controversies and recommendations in classical HL** (Table 22-4)

1. **Stages IA and IIA**

a. **Supradiaphragmatic disease.** Traditionally, most patients used to undergo staging laparotomy and, if found to have pathologic stage I or II disease, would receive subtotal nodal irradiation. This approach resulted in an 80% probability of disease-free survival. Overall survival, on the other hand, may not be affected because most patients who relapse after RT can be salvaged by chemotherapy.

Excellent disease-free survival, however, has been documented after treatment with an abbreviated course of chemotherapy (two to four cycles) followed by ISRT. ABVD regimen or the Stanford V regimen (Appendix C1, Sections I and II) is often used. In a randomized study using four cycles of ABVD, there was no difference in outcome between groups irradiated with 2,000 or 4,000 cGy, suggesting that the dose of radiation can also be reduced.

b. **Infradiaphragmatic disease.** Generally, similar principles apply for early disease. Most patients could be treated with a combined-modality approach or full-course combination chemotherapy.

c. **Current studies** intend to assess the minimum number of cycles of a first-line regimen, such as ABVD, that can be given without

TABLE 22-4	Hodgkin Lymphoma: Recommended Treatment According to Clinical Presentation

Presentation	Recommended Treatment
Early Stages	
Classical HL, IA–IIA	ABVD × 4 cycles with IFRT or Stanford V for 2 cycles with IFRT
NLP HL, IA–IIA	IFRT alone; observation (if patient cannot tolerate RT); chemotherapy followed by IFRT can be used in CS IIA
IB, IIB	Full-course chemotherapy
Advanced Stages	
Bulky disease stage I–II	ABVD × 6 cycles or Stanford V for 3 cycles with RT to bulky site
Clinical stage III–IV and/or presence of B symptoms	ABVD × 6–8 cycles (or Stanford V or BEACOPP)

HL, Hodgkin lymphoma; IFRT, involved field radiation therapy; NLP, nodular lymphocyte predominant; RT, radiation therapy; CS, clinical stage.

compromising outcome. Less aggressive chemotherapy may suffice for patients with no risk factors, such as anemia, elevation of ESR, or bulky disease.

2. **Stages IB and IIB** management is somewhat controversial. Early-stage B disease has a nearly 50% relapse rate when treated with radiation monotherapy. It is preferable to treat such patients with a full course of chemotherapy, although a combined-modality approach may be considered.

3. **Bulky mediastinal presentations.** About 60% of patients with stage IA to IIB disease and bulky mediastinal masses fail treatment with RT alone; relapses occur predominantly in the mediastinum and lungs. Full-course combination chemotherapy and IFRT are recommended for these patients. Patients with bulky mediastinal disease and more advanced stages (IIIA to IVB) may also receive mediastinal RT at the end of chemotherapy. Using both modalities, results approaching the cure rate for patients without large mediastinal masses may be attained.

4. **Stage IIIA.** The 10-year disease-free survival rate using chemotherapy alone is 80%. Such results are superior to RT alone and probably cannot be improved by combined-modality therapy.

5. **Stage IIIB or IV.** The ABVD regimen is probably adequate management for most patients, although medically fit patients with adverse features may benefit from BEACOPP.

6. **E (extranodal) presentations.** Patients with contiguous limited extranodal disease (such as a single bone involved adjacent to an involved lymph node) can sometimes be managed by radiation alone or more frequently in combination with chemotherapy. Multiple E lesions and extensive E disease (such as a large pulmonary lesion) are best managed with chemotherapy or a combined approach.

7. **HIV and HL.** Patients with HIV usually present with stage IV disease involving the bone marrow or other extranodal sites. The desired intensity of the treatment should be weighed against the patient's tolerance. Full-course chemotherapy should be tried with curative intent in patients with good performance status and controlled viremia (see Chapter 37, Section III).

VI. MANAGEMENT AFTER PRIMARY THERAPY

A. **Restaging.** All CRs resulting from either irradiation or chemotherapy must be verified by a restaging evaluation that consists of the repetition of all examinations that were initially abnormal.

1. The initial restaging occurs 2 to 3 months after completion of radiation and traditionally after three or four cycles of chemotherapy, provided that all palpable and radiographic disease has disappeared.

2. Restaging mandates repeat biopsy of previously involved and accessible stage IV sites, such as liver or bone marrow.

3. Persistent and stable abnormalities on chest radiograph or CT scan in the mediastinum are not uncommon (particularly in patients treated for NS). Occasionally, persistent stable abdominal masses or palpable nodal masses may also occur. These abnormalities demand close follow-up. In most cases, however, these findings represent only fibrosis and do not require biopsy. PET scanning is useful in distinguishing viable HL from fibrosis.

B. **Follow-up.** Most relapses after therapy occur within the first 2 to 5 years, although later recurrences have been observed.

1. Follow-up should occur every 2 to 4 months for the first 2 years and every 3 to 6 months for the next 3 to 5 years. Follow-up examinations include
   a. History and physical examination
   b. CBC, chemistry panel, ESR, chest radiograph
   c. CT scans every 6 to 12 months for the first 2 years
   d. Thyroxine and thyroid-stimulating hormone (TSH) levels at least annually (see Section VII.A.1) if radiation to the neck has been administered

2. Health maintenance counseling and cancer screening are imperative for long-term survivors of HL (Chapter 7). Smoking cessation and avoidance of additional practices associated with increased risk for cancer should be encouraged. If irradiation above the diaphragm was administered, women should be encouraged to start annual mammograms 8 to 10 years after treatment, or earlier if 40 years of age (whichever comes first). Some groups have suggested the addition of breast MRI especially for those women receiving irradiation to the chest between ages 10 to 30 for screening in this high-risk population.

3. PET scanning is not recommended for surveillance due to the high false-positive rate. Any management decisions should not be based on PET scanning alone but require clinical or pathologic correlation. PET scanning after two cycles of treatment is currently being investigated as a possible determinant in decision making for continued treatment (e.g., total number of cycles of ABVD, escalation of ABVD to BEACOPP, de-escalation of BEACOPP).

C. **Salvage therapies**

1. **RT failures** are generally treated with combination chemotherapy with results at least as successful as with *de novo* chemotherapy.

2. **Chemotherapy failures**
   a. **Failure to achieve a CR** with effective combination chemotherapy is associated with a poor prognosis. Although alternate combinations may be temporarily useful, long-term disease control is unlikely. Such patients should be referred for autologous SCT or less likely for allogeneic SCT. The decision depends on the age of the patient, the availability of a donor, bone marrow status, and responsiveness to a salvage chemotherapy regimen.

b. **Relapses after chemotherapy-achieved CR.** The initial combination can be used again (provided there is no cardiotoxicity risk) if the unmaintained CR lasts >1 year, but it should not be used again if the CR lasts <1 year. No known available regimen is capable of producing long-term disease-free survival in >10% to 20% of chemotherapy relapsed cases. Patients who respond to salvage chemotherapy should be referred for consideration of autologous SCT.

c. **Patients who are resistant to MOPP and ABVD** may experience brief (although occasionally long) responses to alternate chemotherapy. Single-agent therapy with a nitrosourea, vinca alkaloid, etoposide (possibly the oral form), or combinations of these and other agents may be helpful. Gemcitabine is an active agent, particularly in combination with vinorelbine or platinum. Gemcitabine-based salvage regimens are shown in Appendix C3. Other second-line and third-line combination chemotherapy regimens are also shown in Appendix C3. The use of bendamustine containing combinations has also been explored for the use in treatment of patients with relapsed/refractory HL. Brentuximab vedotin (a CD30 antibody-drug conjugate) can also be considered. Chemotherapy failures with predominantly nodal relapses may benefit from extended-field irradiation, which results in some long-term disease-free survival. Allogeneic SCT can be considered for young patients. Experimental trials would also be appropriate to consider for the treatment of this patient population.

3. **Intensive chemoradiotherapy with autologous SCT** has undergone extensive study. High doses of chemotherapy (potentially myeloablative), often combined with total-body irradiation, are administered ("conditioning regimen"), and either autologous bone marrow or peripheral stem cells (mobilized by growth factors) are used to rescue the patient from prolonged myelosuppression. This procedure is performed in most experienced centers with a mortality rate of <5%; the hospital stay averages 3 weeks. Candidates include patients who have either relapsed after a CR or never achieved a CR with adequate combination chemotherapy. About 60% of chemosensitive candidates and 40% of patients failing induction chemotherapy achieve prolonged disease-free survival.

4. **Other therapies.** Immunoconjugates, such as anti-CD30 conjugated to a chemotherapeutic agent, have been tested in patients with HL in phase II studies, with promising results so far. Rituximab is being used for nodular LP HL. Several agents with activity in the relapsed setting are currently being examined in the front-line setting in combination with ABVD or as maintenance therapy after autologous SCT in high-risk patients and include the immunoconjugate brentuximab vedotin. PD-1 inhibitor agents, such as nivolumab, have also been found to be useful in the relapsed/refractory setting. MTOR pathway inhibitors such as everolimus have also been of use in these situations.

VII. SPECIAL CLINICAL PROBLEMS IN HL

A. **Sequelae and complications of therapy**

1. **Hypothyroidism.** Overt hypothyroidism can be expected in 10% to 20% of patients and elevation of serum TSH in up to 50% of patients treated with mantle-field RT or neck irradiation. Replacement therapy corrects the problem.

2. **Sterility.** RT poses problems for female patients who receive pelvic irradiation without oophoropexy and appropriate gonadal shielding. The

testes are shielded during irradiation. MOPP and similar therapies produce near-universal sterility in male patients and can be anticipated to produce sterility in women in their late 20s or older. ABVD is not associated with sterility. BEACOPP is expected to cause sterility in many patients, although the incidence is unknown. Sperm banking is encouraged in male patients about to receive MOPP, BEACOPP, autologous SCT, or similar therapies.

3. **Lung damage**
    a. **Radiation pneumonitis.** Mantle-field irradiation routinely produces a paramediastinal fibrosis that is usually not clinically significant. When large ports are necessitated by large mediastinal–hilar masses, the potential for more severe reaction exists. In addition, patients given MOPP who have a prior history of mantle-field irradiation may experience an abrupt episode of pneumonitis, presumably secondary to steroid withdrawal. Therefore, prednisone is avoided after mantle-field irradiation, even if the radiation was administered years earlier.

    b. **Bleomycin pulmonary toxicity.** Almost all patients treated with bleomycin (in ABVD and the like) experience a reduction in their lung diffusion capacity. This reduction is usually asymptomatic and slowly improves after treatment. Severe idiopathic pulmonary toxicity is occasionally seen at bleomycin doses of >50 mg, although it usually does not occur until cumulative doses exceed 200 mg/m^2.

    Even more severe pulmonary toxicity (pulmonary infiltrates, restrictive defects, exertional dyspnea) is reported when bleomycin is given in combination with mediastinal RT. These adverse effects depend partly on the total dose of bleomycin and the radiation field. Caution is needed in patients who already have compromised lung function.

4. **Cardiac damage**
    a. **Radiation.** The risk for radiation pericarditis is relatively small when modern anteroposterior weighted radiation ports are used and when large portions of the heart are not radiated. Radiation pericarditis with or without pericardial effusion or tamponade can develop, however. Constrictive pericarditis is a rare complication of RT.

    b. **Chemotherapy.** Doxorubicin, which is a component of ABVD and related regimens, is a well-known cardiotoxic agent. The incidence of cardiotoxicity is related to the cumulative dose and probably to peak serum levels. The cumulative dose of doxorubicin in ABVD is usually 300 mg/m^2, below the clinically significant cardiotoxic level when given without radiation. Administration of mediastinal and/or neck RT, however, increases the chance of cardiomyopathy, pericarditis, or coronary artery disease and other accelerated atherosclerotic disease and valvular disorders as well as the potential for delayed cardiomyopathy.

5. **Aseptic necrosis of the femoral heads** has been reported and is probably secondary to prednisone therapy in MOPP.

6. **Depressed cellular immunity.** Progressive loss of cell-mediated immunity with the development of cutaneous anergy, lymphocytopenia, and increased susceptibility to a variety of organisms is associated with advancing HL, even in the absence of therapy. Treatment with chemotherapy, corticosteroids, and RT accentuates these abnormalities. Late in the course of HL, hypogammaglobulinemia may also develop.
    a. **Infections associated with depressed cell-mediated immunity and therapy** (particularly corticosteroids) include *Listeria*, *Toxoplasma*, and

Mycobacterium spp., fungi, and slow viruses (such as progressive multifocal leukoencephalopathy). Patients treated with corticosteroids are at particularly increased risk for infections with *Pneumocystis carinii* and CMV.

  b. **Herpes zoster** appears in >25% of patients, particularly in patients with irradiated dermatomes and in those undergoing splenectomy. Generalized cutaneous involvement is not uncommon, but visceral involvement is rare.

  c. **Splenectomy-related infections** involve encapsulated microorganisms, particularly pneumococci, and less commonly *Haemophilus influenzae* and *Salmonella* sp., especially in children. Pneumococcal infection in an asplenic host can be rapidly fatal. Vaccination with polyvalent pneumococcal vaccine, *haemophilus*, and meningococcus is recommended before splenectomy, although its effectiveness in this population is not certain. Early, aggressive treatment with antibiotics of all febrile patients after splenectomy is mandatory.

7. **Secondary neoplasms**

  a. **Acute myelogenous leukemia,** often preceded by a prodrome of myelodysplastic syndrome, develops in 2% to 10% of patients treated with MOPP or similar combined-modality therapy containing alkylating agents. The problem appears to be greatest in patients older than 40 years of age and may be increased in patients undergoing splenectomy. The leukemia generally occurs between 3 and 10 years after treatment, is often associated with total or partial deletion of chromosomes 5 and 7, and has an extremely poor prognosis. Acute leukemia is extremely uncommon in patients treated with RT alone and appears to be rare in patients treated with ABVD.

  b. **NHL** may occur during the course of HL and may represent an evolution of the natural history of disease rather than a treatment complication. Most reported cases are high-grade B-cell tumors, with a particularly high incidence in cases of nodular LP HL. As previously noted, LP HL may be a B-cell lymphoma (see Section II.A.2). High-grade PTCLs and mycosis fungoides (MF) have also complicated HL, particularly the NS type.

  c. **Epithelial tumors and sarcomas** are being increasingly reported as complications of RT and possibly of combined-modality therapy, and actuarial statistics suggest a rate of second neoplasms exceeding 20% with prolonged follow-up. Tumors may include breast cancer, sarcoma, melanoma, lung cancer, and other solid tumors. The relative risk for cancer appears to be higher for younger patients and synergistic to other predisposing factors. This significant risk applies to a patient population treated in the 1960s and 1970s; modern strategies limiting radiation exposure may reduce this risk.

8. **Neurologic complications**

  a. **Lhermitte sign,** which follows thoracic irradiation for HL, is an innocuous but worrisome finding for the patient. It consists of shock-like sensations down the back and legs, often precipitated by flexing the neck, and it gradually disappears.

  b. **Transverse myelopathy** is a rare but serious complication of RT that is usually caused by failure to leave an appropriate gap between the mantle and abdominal ports.

9. **Retroperitoneal fibrosis** has been described as a complication of HL treatment.

B. **Synchronous neoplasms.** HL is said to be associated with an increased risk for simultaneous Kaposi sarcoma, leukemia, NHL, and myeloma.

C. **Nephrotic syndrome** (Chapter 32, Section VI), as a remote effect of malignancy, occurs most often in patients with HL. Lipoid nephrosis is typical. **Other paraneoplastic phenomena** that have been described in the setting of HL include autoimmune hemolysis, immune thrombopenia, neurologic deficits, and jaundice.

D. **Pregnancy in HL.** See Chapter 27.

E. **Ichthyosis.** Adult-onset ichthyosis is associated with HL in 75% of cases (see Chapter 29, Section II.I).

NON-HODGKIN LYMPHOMA

I. EPIDEMIOLOGY AND ETIOLOGY

A. **Incidence.** NHL occurs with increasing frequency, with about 60,000 new cases annually in the United States. The incidence is rising dramatically for unknown reasons.

B. **Age and sex.** SLLs occur in the elderly. Lymphoblastic lymphoma has a predilection for male adolescents and young adults. Follicular lymphomas occur mainly in middle-adult life. BL occurs in children and young adults.

C. **Etiology.** Viral etiology and abnormal immune regulation have been implicated in the development of lymphomas. The two mechanisms may be interrelated. An etiologic agent, however, can be identified in only a minority of cases.

1. **Pathogens**
   a. **RNA viruses.** The human T-cell lymphotrophic virus type 1 (HTLV-1) is associated with adult T-cell leukemia–lymphoma (ATLL). HIV produces AIDS, and the resultant immune deficiency is associated with high-grade B-cell lymphomas. Chronic hepatitis C virus infection has been associated with indolent B-cell lymphoma.
   b. **DNA viruses.** EBV has been found in the genome of African BL cells. EBV is also detected in biopsies of nasal T-cell and NK-cell lymphoma. This virus has also been associated with lymphomas in situations characterized by reduced immune surveillance, such as in patients with the X-linked lymphoproliferative syndrome, organ transplantation, the elderly, and, in many instances, HIV-associated lymphoma.
   c. **Chronic *H. pylori* infection** of the gastric mucosa is clearly associated with gastric lymphoma. Eradication of the infection produces remission in more than two-thirds of patients.

2. **Immunodeficiency or immune dysregulation** states associated with development of lymphomas include the following:
   a. AIDS
   b. Organ transplant recipients
   c. Congenital immunodeficiency syndromes (e.g., agammaglobulinemia, ataxia–telangiectasia, Wiskott-Aldrich syndrome)
   d. Autoimmune disorders (e.g., Sjögren syndrome, rheumatoid disease, lupus erythematosus, Hashimoto thyroiditis)
   e. Phenytoin may cause a spectrum from benign lymphoproliferation to frank lymphoma.
   f. Elderly patients with "senescent" immune systems

3. **Treatment related.** The potential role of chemotherapy or RT in the development of NHL after HL and myeloproliferative disorders remains uncertain.

4. **Toxins.** Exposure to toxins such as Agent Orange utilized during the Vietnam War is associated with increased lymphoma risk.

5. **Genetics.** Approximately 10% of patients with SLL/chronic lymphocytic leukemia (CLL) will have more than one family member with that or other lymphoproliferative disorders.

II. PATHOLOGY AND NATURAL HISTORY

A. **Two complementary classification systems for NHL** have been used: the Working Formulation (WF) and the WHO classification, which were based on the Revised European American Lymphoma (REAL) classification. The WF captures and describes the most common lymphomas in terms of biologic behavior or "grades." The REAL then WHO classifications intend to distinguish lymphoma entities based on their unique clinical, pathologic, immunologic, and/or genetic characteristics and include the uncommon lymphomas. Because of its dependence on immunophenotypic and cell lineage analysis, the WHO system is more reproducible.

B. The WF was previously the most commonly used system for the classification of NHL in the United States. This scheme was developed in 1982 as the result of a consensus panel made up of distinguished hematopathologists, each previously espousing his or her own classification. The WF attempts to associate clinical behavior with descriptive histopathologic features of NHL and for that reason is still a helpful concept to the student of NHL. However, it does not incorporate accepted information regarding B-cell or T-cell origin of lymphomas and does not recognize a large variety of newly described clinicopathologic entities. Table 22-5 shows the WF with the frequencies, some clinical correlates, and median survival rates for the various types of NHL using prerituximab chemotherapeutic regimens.

1. **Grades.** The WF divides NHLs into low, intermediate, and high grades that reflect their biologic aggressiveness. The dividing lines between these categories are sometimes arbitrary.

   a. In general, small cell size, round or cleaved nuclei, and a low mitotic rate characterize low-grade NHLs. The intermediate-/high-grade NHLs usually manifest larger cell size, prominent nucleoli, and a higher mitotic rate.

   b. Clinically, it is useful to consider low-grade NHLs as being indolent or nonaggressive, whereas the intermediate-grade and high-grade NHLs are aggressive diseases with a short, natural history if untreated. Most clinicians consider lymphoblastic lymphomas and the small noncleaved NHLs, particularly the Burkitt variant, as high-grade NHLs requiring special management.

2. **Survival curves** based on the WF are shown in Figure 22-2.

C. **The WHO/REAL classification** was established after a consensus meeting of hematopathologists in 1993. It incorporates immunophenotypic characteristics to determine cell lineage and to define subtypes by a more scientific method. It continues to evolve, recognizing several less common entities that were unclassifiable by the WF. The WHO accepted the REAL proposal with some additions and should be the current classification standard. The WHO classification, which serves as a common language among hematologists, is shown in Appendix B4 and B5.

1. WHO entities may include lymphomas of various clinical behaviors, provided that they originate from the same cell type. Leukemias are considered to be an extreme of the spectrum where blood involvement typifies the condition of certain lymphoproliferative disorders.

2. Acute lymphocytic leukemias and lymphoblastic lymphomas are grouped together.

3. CLL is classified together with SLL because they both consist of small, round, B lymphocytes that are positive for CD5 and CD23.

TABLE 22-5	The Working Formulation Classification of Non-Hodgkin Lymphoma[a]				
Type of Lymphoma	Frequency (%)	Median Age (y)	Stage III or IV (%)	Marrow Involved (%)	Median Survival (y)
Low Grade					
A—Small lymphocytic; plasmacytoid	3.6	60	89	71	5.0
B—Follicular, small cleaved cell	22.5	54	82	51	7.2
C—Follicular, mixed (small cleaved and large cell)	7.7	56	73	30	5.1
Intermediate Grade					
D—Follicular, large cell	3.8	55	73	34	3.0
E—Diffuse, small cleaved cell	6.9	58	72	32	3.4
F—Diffuse, mixed (small cleaved and large cell)	6.7	58	55	14	2.7
G—Diffuse, large cell	19.7	57	54	10	1.5
High Grade					
H—Immunoblastic (large cell)	7.9	51	49	12	1.3
I—Lymphoblastic	4.2	17	73	50	2.0
J—Small, noncleaved (Burkitt, non-Burkitt)	5.0	30	66	14	0.7
Total	88.0				

[a]The Working Formulation was based on a study of 1,014 patients. It does not include cutaneous T-cell lymphomas, adult T-cell leukemia–lymphoma, diffuse intermediately differentiated lymphocytic lymphoma, and malignant histiocytosis, which constitute 12% of cases.

Extracted from Rosenberg SA, Berard CW, Braun BW Jr, et al. National Cancer Institute sponsored study of classifications of non-Hodgkin's lymphomas. Summary and description of a working formulation for clinical usage. *Cancer* 1982;49:2112, with permission from Wiley.

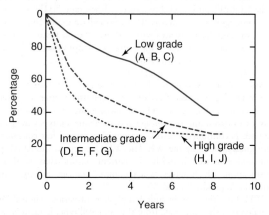

Figure 22-2 Actuarial Survival Curves For The National Cancer Institute's Working Formulation subtypes of lymphomas. Each of the three major prognostic categories (grades) is significantly different from the other ($p < 0.0001$). Table 22-5 defines the histopathologic subtypes A through J for the grades. (From Rosenberg SA, et al. National Cancer Institute sponsored study of classifications of non-Hodgkin lymphomas. Summary and description of a working formulation for clinical usage. *Cancer* 1982;49:2112, with permission from Wiley.)

4. All follicular lymphomas constitute one group with grade designation (grades 1 to 3).

5. MCL is recognized as a separate entity with its distinct features and clinical aggressiveness. MCL was previously described as SLL, diffuse small cleaved cell lymphoma, or at times follicular lymphoma in the WF.

6. Detailed classification of T-cell and NK-cell malignancies is attempted in this system. Such lymphomas were not recognized by the WF.

7. Because about two-thirds of the NHL histologies are follicular or diffuse large cell, clinical decisions often rely on WF principles.

D. **Pathogenesis**

1. **Monoclonal antibodies** can identify epitopes on lymphoid cells characteristic of developmental stages of B-cell and T-cell ontogeny. The antibodies are used with flow cytometry in cell suspensions and with indirect immunoperoxidase labeling in frozen sections. Some of the most useful antibodies are shown in Appendix B3. Monoclonality of B-cell lymphomas is usually established by showing marked dominance of a single light chain (kappa or lambda) type.

2. **Gene rearrangements.** B cells and T cells must rearrange DNA to assemble antigen-specific receptors. Each clone rearranges its genes in a unique way that can be differentiated from the germ line pattern by Southern blot techniques. Identification of gene rearrangements for immunoglobulin and T-cell receptor loci can help establish cellular lineage and sometimes monoclonality for lymphoid neoplasms. The application of the polymerase chain reaction method may enable detection of down to one clonal cell in one million using amplification of breakpoint regions by specific primers.

3. **Specific chromosomal translocations** (Table 22-6) have been associated with histologically distinct lymphoma types. The genetic material found at or near the breakpoint of each translocated chromosome is frequently

TABLE 22-6	Chromosomal Translocations in Lymphoma	
Lymphoma type	**Translocation**	**Genes at Breakpoint**
B-cell lymphoma		
Small lymphocytic	t(14;19)(q32;q13)	Heavy chain; *BCL-3*
Plasmacytoid	t(9;14)(p13;q32)	Heavy chain; —
Mantle cell	t(11;14)(q13;q32)	Heavy chain; *BCL-1*
Follicular	t(14;18)(q32;q21)	Heavy chain; *BCL-2*
Small noncleaved (including Burkitt)	t(8;14)(q24;q32)	Heavy chain; *MYC*
	t(2;8)(p12;q24)	Kappa; *MYC*
	t(8;22)(q24;q11)	Lambda; *MYC*
Large cell	t(3;14)(q27;q32)	*BCL-6*
	t(3;22)(q27;q11)	
	t(2;3)(p12;q27)	
T-cell lymphoma		
Lymphoblastic	Variable involvement of T-cell receptor genes	—
Anaplastic large cell (Ki-1)	t(2;5)(p23;q35)	—

Key: CD5, Leu-1, or T-101; CD10, common acute lymphocytic leukemia antigen (CALLA); Sig, surface immunoglobulin; Cig, cytoplasmic immunoglobulin; TdT, terminal deoxynucleotidyl transferase. See Appendix C4 for leukocyte differentiation antigens and Appendix A for glossary of cytogenetic nomenclature.

highly informative and provides clues regarding pathogenesis. For example, in BL, the transforming c-*myc* cellular oncogene found on chromosome 8 is involved in a translocation within or adjacent to the heavy chain gene on chromosome 14 or to one of the light chain genes (κ on chromosome 2 or λ on chromosome 22).

In the follicular lymphomas, the translocation also involves the heavy chain gene on chromosome 14, which is this time juxtaposed with the so-called *BCL-2* gene on chromosome 18. The *BCL-2* gene appears to be significantly involved in the abrogation of *apoptosis* (programmed cell death). Thus, the activation of the *BCL-2* gene by translocation in follicular lymphomas may result in the excessive longevity or accumulation of lymphoma cells, implying a defect in cell death rather than a pure problem of proliferation in that disease. In MCL, the heavy chain gene on chromosome 14 and the *BCL-1* gene on chromosome 11 are brought into proximity. The *BCL-1* gene encodes cyclin-D1, which is involved in the cell cycle.

Such cytogenetic abnormalities can be demonstrated with the use of florescence *in situ* hybridization techniques to analyze specific genetic abnormalities that a tumor may possess.

4. **Production of lymphokines** by tumor cells may be related to the symptoms or manifestations of specific lymphomas. For example, production of interleukin (IL)-4 by T cells in Lennert lymphoma may explain the exuberant proliferation of histiocytes in that disease, whereas in angioimmunoblastic lymphomas, IL-6 production may result in plasmacytosis and hypergammaglobulinemia.

5. **The pattern of surface antigens** (Appendix B3) found on lymphoma cells when flow cytometry or immunohistochemical staining is used may help identify or corroborate certain lymphoma types. For example, the CD5 antigen, a pan T-cell antigen expressed by a small minority of B lymphocytes, is found on the neoplastic cells of patients with small cell lymphocytic lymphoma and MCL but is absent from the cells of follicular lymphomas and monocytoid B-cell lymphoma.

III. NATURAL HISTORY

NHL exhibits a remarkable range of natural histories, with doubling times varying between days (e.g., BL) and years (some low-grade NHLs). Treatment tends to have a much more dramatic effect on intermediate-/high-grade NHLs (collectively also called *aggressive*) than on low-grade NHLs. Early bone marrow involvement and hematogenous and noncontiguous dissemination characterize NHL, particularly the low-grade types, in sharp contrast to the distribution in HL. Extra-axial nodes, including epitrochlear and mesenteric nodes, are often involved, again in distinction to HL (Table 22-1). Intermediate-grade and high-grade NHLs often present in extranodal sites, including Waldeyer ring, GI tract, skin, bone, and CNS.

A. **B-cell lymphomas: low grade** (see Appendixes B3 and B4)

1. **Small lymphocytic lymphoma** (SLL) is the tissue or nodal counterpart of CLL and classically presents with diffuse lymphadenopathy and marrow involvement. Cells are positive for CD5, CD20, and CD23. CLL and chronic B-cell prolymphocytic leukemia are discussed in Chapter 24, in "Chronic Lymphocytic Leukemia."

2. **Lymphoplasmacytic lymphomas,** including Waldenström macroglobulinemia, may manifest monoclonal IgM spikes in the serum. The cellular composition of plasmacytoid lymphocytic lymphoma is made up of

lymphocytes, plasma cells, and hybridized forms with features of both. Cells are usually CD20 positive, in contrast to frank plasma cells. Hyperviscosity syndrome caused by the IgM protein that forms asymmetric pentamers or neuropathy may dominate the clinical picture in Waldenström macroglobulinemia, which is discussed in detail in Chapter 23.

3. **Follicular lymphoma.** The follicular lymphomas include lymphocytic infiltrates that are composed mostly of small cleaved cells with increasing numbers of large cells with increasing grade. Cells are positive for CD10 and CD20 and negative for CD5.

   a. **Cytogenetics.** Follicular lymphomas bear the t(14;18) translocation that results in up-regulation of *BCL-2* expression. The *BCL-2* gene product is considered a potent inhibitor of apoptosis.

   b. **Follicular lymphoma subtype,** according to the WHO classification, is defined by the average number of large cells (centroblasts) in a high-power field (hpf):

   > Grade 1, if <5 large cells/hpf
   > Grade 2, if 5 to 15 large cells/hpf
   > Grade 3, if >15 large cells/hpf

   c. **Aggressiveness.** Follicular lymphomas grades 1 and 2 are generally considered to be low grade. The rarer follicular large cell type, or grade 3, is considered by most as intermediate grade, although it is not clear that the natural history is distinct. In the WHO classification, A and B subtypes are suggested. Cytologic transformation to intermediate-grade or high-grade NHL may occur at any point in the disease and is often characterized by *p53* mutation. A similar transformation may take place in other forms of low-grade NHL.

   d. **Behavior.** The follicular lymphomas tend to present as nodal disease. About 85% of cases are stage III or IV at presentation, with frequent bone marrow involvement (>50% of cases). The liver, spleen, and mesenteric nodes are often involved. Follicular lymphomas often progress slowly and may not require immediate therapy. Temporary spontaneous regressions are observed in up to 30% of cases. Follicular lymphomas are highly responsive to therapy, but few patients are cured. Average survival times vary between 6 and 10 years in the past, with possible increases in median survival times in the "rituximab era."

4. **Marginal-zone lymphoma** is believed to be derived from parafollicular or marginal-zone cells that surround the mantle zone. Cells are negative for CD10 and CD5 and positive for CD20.

   a. **MALTomas** (MALT: mucosa-associated lymphoid tissue) are a group of extranodal lymphomas that frequently present as localized tumors in the stomach, lung, ocular adnexa, thyroid, skin, and other extranodal sites where they are often incited by an immune reaction to another comorbid condition.

   (1) In some cases, a pre-existing organ-associated autoimmune disease is noted (e.g., Sjögren syndrome in the case of lacrimal or parotid gland or Hashimoto thyroiditis in the case of thyroid lymphoma). Many of these were designated *pseudolymphomas* in the past.

   (2) The natural history includes prolonged survival without widespread dissemination and suggests a role for RT or surgery in management.

   (3) Gastric MALToma is clearly associated with *H. pylori* infection and regresses in two-thirds of the patients after eradication of the infection.

    b. Splenic lymphomas are an uncommon form of marginal-zone lymphomas. These are characterized by pronounced splenic enlargement, often without systemic disease, and with blood and/or bone marrow involvement. Cells often have villi (splenic lymphoma with villous lymphocytes).

    c. Nodal marginal zone lymphomas may also be called **monocytoid lymphomas** because of their appearance.

5. Hairy cell leukemia is characterized by an indolent course, splenomegaly and hypersplenism, and neutropenia. Characteristic lymphocytes may be seen with the tartrate-resistant acid phosphatase (TRAP) stain. Cells are characteristically positive for CD103, CD22, CD11c, and often CD25. This disease is discussed in Chapter 24, in "Hairy Cell Leukemia."

B. B-cell lymphomas: intermediate grade and high grade (see Appendixes B3 and B4)

1. Mantle cell lymphoma (MCL) is a unique B-cell lymphoma with an adverse prognosis. It is derived from CD5-positive, CD20-positive, and CD23-negative lymphocytes surrounding the germinal center. It is associated with the t(11;14) translocation, which results in up-regulation of cyclin D1, a promoter of cell cycling.

    a. MCL may present with a variety of histologic variations ranging from a pseudofollicular pattern to a blastic form. The most common appearance is a diffuse, small cell, slightly irregular infiltrate.

    b. MCL usually presents at advanced stage with B symptoms and involvement of the GI tract and bone marrow. Conventional chemotherapy usually produces disappointingly short remissions and a median survival of about 2.5 years, but novel therapies are now available.

    c. Mantle-zone lymphoma with a "mantle zone pattern" is an uncommon indolent variety of MCL without invasion of the follicular center of the involved lymph nodes.

2. Diffuse large B-cell lymphomas (DLBCL). About 30% of cases originate in extranodal sites, such as the GI tract and Waldeyer ring, sinuses, bone, or CNS. In contrast to most low-grade NHLs, localized presentations (stage I and II disease) are more common, and bone marrow involvement is less frequent (<25% of cases). Localized presentations (stage I and II disease) may be curable in up to 80% of cases, whereas disseminated disease (stage III and IV disease) is curable 50% of the time.

    a. AIDS-related NHLs are almost universally intermediate-grade or high-grade B-cell lymphomas (see Chapter 37, Section II). Most patients present with extranodal disease, often including the GI tract, bone, jaw, and CNS (as parenchymal involvement), but almost any organ can be involved. Dissemination to bone marrow and meninges is characteristic.

    b. Posttransplantation lymphoproliferative disorders describe a spectrum of oligoclonal lymphoproliferation following intense, often iatrogenic, immunosuppression in organ transplant recipients and also occurring in other immunocompromised patients. It is believed that polyclonal or oligoclonal B-cell proliferation is initially driven by EBV infection escaping immune surveillance. Ongoing proliferation results in true malignant transformation and development of monoclonal aggressive NHL (Chapter 37).

The disease can manifest with hectic fever, malaise, and cytopenias. Nodal involvement may or may not be noted at presentation. These lymphomas share similar histology and a proclivity for extranodal involvement with AIDS lymphomas. This disorder may respond to withdrawal of immunosuppression in early stages, but systemic chemotherapy and/or monoclonal antibody therapy may be required. The prognosis depends largely on comorbid conditions and the length of the time from transplant to diagnosis of the lymphoma.

  c. **Primary effusion lymphoma** is an aggressive lymphoma originating in serosa and presenting with effusions. Dissemination of disease is the rule. It has been strongly associated with presence of the human herpes virus type 8 (HHV-8) and HIV infection.

3. **The "high-grade" B-cell lymphomas** are rapidly proliferating lesions with an extremely high mitotic rate and doubling times as brief as 24 hours. Many lymphomas associated with AIDS or organ transplantation are of this type.

  a. **Burkitt lymphoma** has a distinctive morphology, natural history, and behavior and is divided into African (endemic), sporadic, and immunosuppressive types. The cells are all nearly equal in size and contain prominent small nucleoli and cytoplasmic lipid vacuoles. In the non-Burkitt type of small noncleaved lymphoma, the cells have a less homogeneous cellular size and composition. BL is discussed later in Section VIII.E.

  b. **B-cell lymphoblastic lymphoma** is classified with B-lineage acute lymphoblastic leukemia (ALL) and is approached similarly (see Chapter 26, "Acute Leukemia" section).

C. **T-cell NHLs** constitute about 20% of NHLs in Western societies. T-cell lymphomas have been analyzed in detail by the WHO classifications (see Appendix B4), despite the difficulty arising from the rarity of certain categories.

  1. **Precursor T-cell lymphoblastic leukemia/lymphomas** (including T-cell ALL) are malignancies of immature T cells that occur predominantly in male adolescents and young adults. The nuclei are often convoluted in appearance, and the mitotic rate is high.

  a. **Terminal deoxynucleotidyl transferase (TdT)** activity is characteristically positive in these patients. TdT positivity is generally restricted to lymphoblastic lymphoma, ALL (pre-B, T, and null subtypes), and the lymphoid blast crisis of chronic myelogenous leukemia; it is not seen in other NHLs.

  b. **Clinical aspects.** Patients usually present with anterior mediastinal masses and often manifest pleural effusion, pericardial effusion, or superior vena cava syndrome. Bone marrow and peripheral blood involvement are frequent, and the syndrome then merges with T-cell ALL. Meningeal involvement is anticipated unless CNS prophylaxis is used. Therapy that is similar to that used for ALL may cure half of the cases of lymphoblastic lymphoma.

  2. **Peripheral T-cell and NK-cell neoplasms** refer to all NHLs of T-cell or NK-cell origin except precursor T-cell lymphoblastic leukemia/lymphoma. The spectrum includes low-grade disorders, such as MF, the most common cutaneous T-cell lymphoma, and a variety of other more aggressive clinicopathologic syndromes. With the exception of MF and large granular lymphocytic leukemia, T-cell lymphomas tend to be clinically aggressive even if the morphology suggests a low-grade behavior. It appears that

the noncutaneous PTCLs have a poorer prognosis than intermediate-/high-grade B-cell NHLs stage for stage. Occasionally, hemophagocytic syndrome can occur.

   a. The pathologic manifestations of PTCL often include infiltration of T-cell lymph node regions (paracortical) and increased atypical epithelioid venules. The pleomorphic tumor cells often exhibit clear cytoplasm and occasionally resemble RS cells. These tumors frequently contain an admixture of interdigitating cells, epithelioid cells, eosinophils, and plasma cells. Many PTCLs would be placed in the *diffuse mixed* category of the WF.

   b. Clinical aspects of PTCL. PTCLs often develop in middle-aged to elderly patients, who present with constitutional symptoms (B symptoms). Most patients have nodal-based stage III or IV disease with frequent hepatosplenomegaly. Pulmonary and skin involvement are not uncommon. Eosinophilia and polyclonal hypergammaglobulinemia develop in some cases.

D. Peripheral T-cell and NK-cell entities (see Appendixes B3 and B4)

   1. Adult T-cell leukemia–lymphoma (ATLL) was initially described in southwestern Japan but has been subsequently seen throughout the world, including the United States. The HTLV-1 virus apparently causes the disease. Cutaneous involvement, lymphadenopathy, organomegaly, a leukemic blood picture, hypercalcemia with osteolytic bone lesions, and pulmonary involvement characterize the acute phase of ATLL. The cells frequently show a remarkable "knobby" configuration of the nuclei. Immunologically, the cells are CD4 positive. The response to treatment has been poor; combinations of zidovudine and interferon (IFN) may be useful, and newer monoclonal antibody treatments are in development. A prodromal, less aggressive chronic and smoldering phase is also recognized, which may clinically appear indistinguishable from MF, but with positive serology for the causative agent, HTLV-1.

   2. Aggressive NK-cell leukemia–lymphoma is a rare and rapidly fatal NK-cell malignancy. It is more prevalent among Asians than whites. The immunophenotype is identical to extranodal nasal-type NK-/T-cell lymphomas.

   3. T-cell prolymphocytic leukemia is discussed in Chapter 24, Section VI.B of "Chronic Lymphocytic Leukemia."

   4. T-cell or NK-cell large granular lymphocytic leukemia is an indolent disease with subtle lymphocytosis of the blood or bone marrow and paraneoplastic neutropenia. It usually does not require treatment. Responses to cyclosporine have been reported. This is also discussed in Chapter 24, Section III.D.8 of "Chronic Lymphocytic Leukemia."

   5. Anaplastic large cell lymphoma (ALCL) is usually of T-cell origin. Occasional cases appear to be of undefined lineage (null cell). The large anaplastic cells are positive for Ki-1 (CD30), an antigen initially described in HL but later found to be present in some neoplastic cells in a variety of aggressive NHLs. It is often associated with t(2;5), which results in fusion of the nucleophosmin gene *NPM* to a tyrosine kinase, ALK (anaplastic lymphoma kinase) causing overexpression of the ALK protein. The presence of t(2;5) and ALK positivity is believed to confer a better prognosis.

      Pathologically, the cases are frequently confused with epithelial tumors (carcinomas) or melanoma. The confusion is sometimes compounded by positive staining for epithelial membrane antigen and by a sinusoidal distribution, which is characteristic of carcinomas or melanomas. Pathologically, it can be confused with HL, with lymphomatoid papulosis (a relatively benign cutaneous condition with similar histology and spontaneous regressions), or with cutaneous anaplastic lymphoma, which has an excellent prognosis with local treatment despite almost always being ALK negative. Treatment of ALK-positive ALCL is similar to that of large cell B-cell lymphoma and is believed to have a slightly better outcome.

6. **Angioimmunoblastic T-cell lymphoma.** Immunoblastic lymphadenopathy and angioimmunoblastic lymphadenopathy with dysproteinemia (AILD) were originally described as abnormal immune reactions clinically characterized by fever, skin rash, autoimmune hemolytic anemia, polyclonal hypergammaglobulinemia, and generalized lymphadenopathy. Pathology revealed diffuse effacement of lymph node architecture, involvement by immunoblasts and plasma cells, and often an abnormal vascular network. Immunohistochemistry and gene rearrangement studies have indicated that many of these patients have underlying T-cell lymphomas from the onset. The course may vary in aggressiveness, with occasional spontaneous remissions. Satisfactory and prolonged responses to corticosteroids or cyclosporine can be seen. More often, patients require treatments similar to aggressive NHL.

7. **Nasal-type NK-cell and T-cell lymphomas** include the former angiocentric lymphoma and lethal midline granuloma (malignant midline reticulosis). The neoplastic cells in these disorders involve vessels and lead to an angiodestructive necrotizing process. Nasal NK-/T-cell lymphoma involves the palate and sinuses, but involvement of other sites, such as skin, can occur. The course can be indolent but is more commonly aggressive, particularly if disseminated. It is uncommon in the United States and more common in Asia. In contrast to aggressive diffuse large cell B-cell lymphoma of the nasal cavity, nasal NK-/T-cell lymphoma does not usually extend to the CNS. Cells usually are positive for T-cell markers and CD56. Chemotherapy and RT can be curative for localized disease. Chemotherapeutic regimens that include the use of L-asparaginase (i.e., combination of *s*teroid, *m*ethotrexate, *i*fosfamide, *L*-asparaginase, *e*toposide: SMILE) can be quite effective in this disorder even when extranasal.

8. **Hepatosplenic T-cell lymphoma** is characterized by sinusoidal infiltration of the liver by cytotoxic T cells expressing the γ-δ rather than the most common αβ T-cell receptor complex. The bone marrow is nearly always involved, and lymph nodes are rarely involved. This rare form of NHL is often associated with a hemophagocytic syndrome. Despite the bland appearance of the cells, the clinical course is usually relentless. A possible relationship between treatment of adolescents and young adults with TNF blocking agents, azathioprine, and 6-mercaptopurine is being further investigated.

9. **Enteropathy-type T-cell lymphoma** presents with ulcerative intestinal lesions in patients with gluten-sensitive (celiac disease) or other enteropathy most commonly. Patients present with abdominal pain, often associated with perforation. It is uncommon in the United States.

10. **Subcutaneous panniculitis-like T-cell lymphoma** is rare and is characterized by infiltration of the subcutaneous tissue with cytotoxic T cells, expressing the αβ T-cell receptor complex. Patients present with multiple subcutaneous nodules, usually in the absence of other sites of disease. A hemophagocytic syndrome is a possible complication and often the harbinger of an aggressive clinical course.

11. **Mycosis fungoides and the Sézary syndrome** are described separately (see Section VIII.B).

E. **Histiocytic and dendritic cell neoplasms** represent a rather confusing category of ill-defined very rare diseases. The cells of origin, histiocytes and accessory cells, have a major role in the processing and presentation of antigen to both T and B cells.

1. **Malignant histiocytosis–hemophagocytic syndrome** (fever, jaundice, hepatosplenomegaly, coagulopathy, and hemophagocytosis) has been described and most often represents a complication of T-cell lymphoma. Etoposide and sometimes cyclosporine have been reported to control this syndrome (see Chapter 35 Cytopenia, Section III).

2. **Langerhans cell histiocytosis** is a condition caused by clonal proliferation of Langerhans cells. Most cases occur in childhood. Langerhans cell histiocytosis is associated with both HL and NHL. It may be localized or generalized with variable aggressiveness. Unifocal disease occurs in a majority of cases (eosinophilic granuloma), usually involving bone. Multifocal, unisystem disease (Hand-Schüller-Christian disease) involves several sites in one organ system (usually the bone). Combination chemotherapy may be necessary for multiple system involvement.

F. **Immunologic abnormalities**

1. Hypogammaglobulinemia is typically seen in SLL but may develop in other lymphomas, particularly after treatment with rituximab.

2. Paraprotein spikes, often IgM, are seen particularly in lymphoplasmacytic lymphomas but are also noted in other B-cell malignancies and in AILD.

3. Warm or cold antibody immune hemolytic anemias may be seen with any B-cell malignancy, particularly in the small lymphocytic type and sometimes with AILD.

4. Additional autoimmune phenomena, such as circulating anticoagulants (e.g., acquired von Willebrand disease) or angioedema (associated with C'1 esterase deficiency), may occur, especially in the SLLs.

5. Polyclonal hypergammaglobulinemia is commonly observed in patients with AIDS or PTCL.

6. Defects in T-cell function are prominent in ATLL even before treatment and in other lymphomas after treatment.

IV. STAGING SYSTEM AND PROGNOSTIC FACTORS

A. **The Ann Arbor staging system** is applied to NHL, but histopathologic subtype is the prime determinant of survival in NHL. MF has a different staging system (see Section VIII.B).

B. **Survival** (see Fig. 22-2 and Table 22-5)

1. **Low-grade lymphomas** are rarely curable and appear to cause a steady percentage of deaths annually. It is possible that the rare, early stages of low-grade NHL (stage I or II) may be curable in some cases, but even this is uncertain. Survival time averaged between 6 and 10 years for follicular lymphomas in the prerituximab era but is likely longer at this time.

2. **Intermediate-grade and high-grade lymphoma** survival curves generally display two components: a rapid falloff in the first 1 to 2 years followed by an eventual plateau representing a presumptively cured population. About 80% to 90% of patients with stage I or early stage II disease and 50% with stage III or IV intermediate-/high-grade lymphomas may be curable.

3. MCL survival curve shows a rapid and steady decline, with no survival plateau, and a median survival time of 2 to 2.5 years with conventional chemotherapy; survival is likely longer with more aggressive treatment and with the use of novel agents.

C. Prognostic factors. Extent of disease at presentation and survival rates are shown in Table 22-5.

1. Low-grade lymphomas

a. Sensitivity to therapy is a prognostic sign in that the attainment of a CR or an excellent partial response (PR) with duration of over 1 year identifies patients who are likely to do well.

b. Early stage. Stage I and II cases constitute <15% of all patients with low-grade lymphoma. In one small series, 80% of stage I and II patients younger than 40 years of age who were treated with RT were disease-free 10 years after diagnosis.

c. Follicular mixed (grade 2) lymphomas. It is unclear whether there is a difference in long-term outcome based on grade.

d. The FLIPI scale (*F*ollicular *L*ymphoma *I*nternational *P*rognostic *I*ndex) may be helpful to determine prognosis of patients with follicular lymphoma. Variables (score one point per variable) included in this score are as follows (mnemonic: *NOLASH*):

> Greater than 4 **No**dal areas of involvement
> Abnormal **L**DH
> **A**ge > 60 years
> **S**tage III or IV
> **H**emoglobin < 12 g/dL

Those with a low FLIPI score (0 to 1) have a 5-year survival of 90%, and those with a high score (3 or greater) have a 53% 5-year survival in the prerituximab era.

e. The international prognostic index (IPI) described in Section IV.C.2.a is also useful in stratifying patients with indolent lymphoma.

2. Intermediate-/high-grade lymphomas. Stage I or II presentations, constituting 30% to 40% of these lymphomas, are highly curable (about 80%), although tumor bulk (>10 cm in largest diameter) adversely affects outcome.

a. The IPI has established *five independently important prognostic factors*. The 5-year survival rate was 73% for patients manifesting none or one of the adverse risk factors and 26% for patients with four or five risk factors in the prerituximab era. In the postrituximab era, even those with 3 to 5 points have a 4-year progression-free survival of 55%. These important **adverse risk factors** are as follows (mnemonic: *APLES*):

(1) Age older than 60 years

(2) Performance status (ECOG > 1; see Chapter 6, Table 6-1)

(3) LDH abnormal

(4) Extranodal sites more than one

(5) Stage III or IV

b. Gene profiling. Retrospective microarray analysis of gene expression has identified subgroups of DLBCL with distinct gene cluster expression patterns. Recognized subgroups may resemble the expression profile of the follicular center cells, which confer better prognosis, or the expression pattern of activated lymphocytes, which confer a worse outcome even with the use of rituximab. This association is independent of the IPI and may explain why treatment fails in certain patients who have a favorable IPI score. In addition to prognostic information, the evolution of gene profiling is expected to offer significant insight into the pathophysiology of the disease and in the identification of putative therapeutic targets.

c. **Gene overexpression.** Overexpression of *c-myc* in patients with diffuse LBCL appears to confer a worse prognosis as well as the detection of cmyc translocations with/without translocation of bcl-2 and bcl-6 (so-called double- or triple-hit lymphomas)

V. STAGING EVALUATION

A. **Clinical evaluation.** See "Evaluation of Suspected Lymphoma," Sections I through IV.

B. **Initial staging evaluation**

1. The staging evaluation as outlined in "Hodgkin Lymphoma" Section IV.B is generally applicable in NHL. Laboratory evaluation should also include uric acid, serum protein electrophoresis, hepatitis B and C testing, and HIV if diagnosis is high-grade B-cell malignancy. β_2-Microglobulin may be substituted for ESR.

2. Flow cytometry on the peripheral blood and bone marrow in low-grade lymphomas may define a clonal excess and suggest hematogenous involvement, even when circulating lymphoma cells are not seen.

3. Diagnostic spinal tap is indicated in lymphoblastic lymphoma, lymphomas occurring in AIDS, BL, and probably in intermediate-/high-grade lymphomas with extensive marrow, sinus, or testicular involvement or with any parameningeal focus.

4. Upper GI and small bowel series should be performed in patients with GI symptoms, unexplained iron deficiency, and/or Waldeyer ring involvement. Endoscopic evaluation is performed as indicated, particularly in MCL.

C. **Restaging evaluation** is performed to verify CR (all lymph nodes that were ≥1.5 cm). All abnormal studies are repeated, including biopsies of accessible previously involved sites, particularly with potentially curable histologies.

Patients with intermediate-grade or high-grade lymphomas and residual masses on CT scans or radiographs should be followed closely with serial studies; stable residual masses usually do not contain lymphoma. PET is often used to ensure negativity of the presumed inert residual mass. The frequent presence of residual masses when using CT scanning has resulted in the definition of "unconfirmed CR" (CRu), whereby all the requirements for CR exist except that a residual lymph node may be >1.5 cm, provided it has been reduced by >75% in the bidimensional product. This designation has been largely eradicated by the use of PET scanning in staging.

VI. THERAPY FOR INDOLENT LYMPHOMAS

A. **True stage I and II disease** (15% cases): RT to a dose of 2,400 to 3,600 cGy may be administered to all known sites of disease (including draining lymph nodes in E presentation). Large RT fields do not increase the cure rate and may decrease tolerance to chemotherapy later. Prolonged disease-free survival has been reported in some patients. Observation in select patients may also be a reasonable option.

B. **Stage III and IV disease**

1. **No treatment.** Most patients with advanced indolent disease may be observed with no therapy and without adverse influence on survival. Spontaneous remissions may occur during the period of no therapy. Therapy

is instituted in the presence of any systemic symptoms, rapid nodal growth, or imminent complications of the disease, such as significant cytopenias, obstructive phenomena, or effusions. The median times for "requiring therapy" vary from 16 months for the follicular mixed group, to 48 months for the follicular small cleaved group, and to 72 months for the small lymphocytic group.

2. **Single-agent chemotherapy while not utilized with as great as frequency as in past** with chlorambucil or cyclophosphamide gives good responses in indolent NHL. Cyclophosphamide has the disadvantages of alopecia and hemorrhagic cystitis. The purine analogs, fludarabine and cladribine, exhibit activity rivaling the alkylating agents; up to 50% of patients with previously treated low-grade lymphomas respond to these purine analogs. Dosages are as follows:

   a. Chlorambucil, 2 to 6 mg/m^2 PO daily
   b. Fludarabine, 25 mg/m^2 IV daily for 5 days every 4 weeks
   c. Cladribine, 0.14 mg/kg/d IV over 2 hours for 5 days every 4 weeks or 0.1 mg/kg/d by continuous IV infusion for 7 days every 4 weeks
   d. Bendamustine, 90 mg/m^2 IV, on day 1 and 2 when combined with rituximab every 3 to 4 weeks

3. **Combination chemotherapy.** Multiagent therapy may be used if a more rapid response is required. Chlorambucil or cyclophosphamide plus corticosteroids in pulse doses and fludarabine plus mitoxantrone combinations are regimens that have been utilized (see CVP in Appendix C2, Section I for regimens and dosages).

   Single-agent or combination chemotherapy produces CRs or excellent PRs in 60% to 80% of patients. Doxorubicin-containing regimens have no clear advantages for low-grade NHL and are often reserved for later stages of the disease or adverse presentations. Treatment is generally continued until a maximum response is achieved. Maintenance chemotherapy does not prolong survival, may compromise further treatment, and is potentially leukemogenic.

4. **Rituximab** is a chimeric humanized anti-CD20 monoclonal antibody approved for the treatment of refractory or relapsed indolent B-cell lymphoma and the first-line therapy of follicular lymphoma when combined with CVP. It is believed to mediate cytotoxicity through activation of antibody-dependent cytotoxic T cells, possibly by activation of complement, and by mediating direct intracellular signaling.

   a. An overall 50% response rate with a median duration of about 1 year is expected for indolent B-cell lymphomas with rituximab monotherapy. SLL may be less responsive than follicular NHL because of lower expression of CD20 antigen. Responses of about 30% have been reported in large cell lymphoma that is relapsed or refractory to treatment or occurs in patients that have not been treated but are over age 60. Combinations of rituximab with a variety of chemotherapy regimens are feasible and are believed to be synergistic, with documented increased disease-free survival. Rituximab allows for flexibility in its coadministration with chemotherapy, with no particular schedule known to be more advantageous. Combinations with novel agents such as lenalidomide also appear to be synergistic.
   b. The established dose of rituximab is 375 mg/m^2 IV weekly for 4 or 8 weeks. The maximum tolerated dose has not been defined, but it is doubtful that higher doses improve outcome. There are no criteria for

choosing the 4- or 8-week dosing. Retreatment on progression is feasible with an expected response rate of 40%. Given its lack of cytotoxicity, maintenance regimens have been investigated and usually demonstrate considerable delay of progression; however, given the frequently successful retreatment on progression, it is unclear whether maintenance with rituximab really delays the time to refractoriness to this agent.

  c. Mild infusion-related fever or rigors are common, particularly during the first infusion. Cytopenias develop occasionally. Reactions resulting in death (anaphylaxis, tumor lysis syndrome, adult respiratory distress syndrome) have also been seen, mainly in patients with circulating lymphoma cells or the elderly; slow escalation of the dose as tolerated is recommended for such patients. Reactivation of latent viruses has been reported (such as hepatitis B and slow virus), as well as immune phenomena such as serum sickness and lupus-like syndromes. The resulting B-cell depletion for 6 months or more seems to be well tolerated but may contribute to ongoing hypogammaglobulinemia. Precipitation of hyperviscosity on lymphoplasmacytoid lymphomas has been seen.

5. Radioactive monoclonal antibodies offer the advantage of targeted radioimmunotherapy. Responses rates of 50% to 80% have been reported in previously treated patients. ^{131}I-labeled anti-CD20 (tositumomab [Bexxar]) and ^{90}Y-labeled anti-CD20 (ibritumomab tiuxetan [Zevalin]) are available.

  a. A randomized study of Zevalin versus rituximab demonstrated a higher response rate (80% vs. 55%) and a higher CR rate (30% vs. 15%) for the radioimmunoconjugate.

  b. The treatment is given once and is well tolerated with the exception of cytopenias. Grade IV cytopenia occurs in one-third of the patients. Nadirs occur during the 6th and 7th weeks following therapy. Patients are excluded from this treatment with >25% involvement or hypocellularity in the bone marrow, with platelets <100,000/µL, or with neutrophil counts <1,500/µL.

  c. Radiation hazard with Zevalin is negligible, whereas lead shielding and more stringent release instructions are needed for Bexxar.

6. IFN-α has been used in several randomized studies as part of either induction or maintenance therapy for previously untreated patients. No clear-cut dose schedule is superior, and doses as low as two to three million units three times weekly may produce responses in up to 40% to 60% of patients.

  The place of IFN-α in the routine management of follicular lymphoma is not clear. Results of some series suggest a potentiation of response rates, a prolongation of remission duration, and possibly an effect of IFN-α on survival.

7. Palliative RT is used for sites of bulky disease and to relieve obstruction or pain. RT alone may be used when most of the disease sites do not require treatment but one or two areas are troublesome. However, multiple courses of RT exhaust the marrow and are discouraged when chemotherapy is an effective alternative.

8. Pathway inhibition is a mechanism of action of the newer drugs such as idelalisib, a oral PI3 kinase inhibitor.

C. Histologic conversion. Indolent lymphomas that transform to an aggressive cell type usually have a poor prognosis. Limited, relatively asymptomatic presentations, however, may respond well to treatment used for intermediate-/high-grade NHL. The CNS can be involved (particularly the meninges) in transformed NHL and is rarely affected in low-grade NHL. High-dose chemotherapy and stem cell support for cases of transformed chemosensitive low-grade NHL may be considered.

D. Primary cutaneous B-cell lymphoma (CBCL) is defined as having no extracutaneous dissemination at presentation and for 6 months thereafter. They are most commonly follicular or marginal zone lymphomas that are indolent and have a good prognosis. Localized CBCL is treated with RT, even for multifocal disease. Polychemotherapy or monoclonal antibody therapy is reserved for noncontiguous anatomic sites or extracutaneous spread. The diagnosis of primary cutaneous LBCL, leg type, confers a poorer prognosis and may mandate a different treatment approach.

E. Experimental therapies
   1. **Monoclonal antibodies** of several types, in addition to rituximab, have been used in the treatment of low-grade (and some aggressive) NHL. Targets include B-cell antigens (e.g., CD23, CD19, CD20, CD22) or more generalized common antigens (CD5, CD25, CD80, CD40).
      a. **Alemtuzumab** is a humanized antibody against CD52 (present in B cells, T cells, and monocytes) and is believed to have satisfactory activity in CLL, prolymphocytic leukemia, and certain T-cell lymphomas but modest action against indolent NHL.
      b. **Immunotoxins** have been under investigation.
      c. **Novel agents.** Lenalidomide (an immunomodulatory agent) has demonstrated single-agent activity in follicular lymphomas and mantle zone lymphoma. Bortezomib and temsirolimus have some activity in MCL.
   2. **Autologous bone marrow or peripheral stem cell support** following high-dose chemotherapy has undergone extensive study in patients with relapsed low-grade NHL. Although no convincing data support high-dose therapy in the routine management of low-grade NHL, it can be used in relatively young patients with adverse presentations in an effort to prolong remissions.
   3. **Allogeneic SCT** is proposed by certain centers for the treatment of refractory young patients with related donors and should probably be reserved for isolated cases. The use of nonmyeloablative, less toxic preparative regimens has been shown to be a particularly useful allogeneic transplant approach in patients with indolent lymphoma with excellent early disease-free survival.

VII. THERAPY FOR AGGRESSIVE NHL

Therapy for special lymphoma subtypes is discussed in Section VIII. Therapy for AIDS-associated lymphoma is discussed in Chapter 37, Section II. Useful combination chemotherapy regimens for these malignancies are shown in Appendixes C2 and C3.

A. Localized presentations of intermediate-/high-grade NHL. Nonbulky (<10 cm) stages IA and IIA cases, including extranodal (E) presentations, can be successfully managed by three or four cycles of a doxorubicin-containing regimen (i.e., CHOP) followed by ISRT (equivalent to 3,000 cGy in 10 fractions). Virtually all patients achieve CR, and the actuarial relapse-free survival exceeds 80%. Another approach is full-course chemotherapy with or without subsequent RT.

B. Stage I to II (bulky), III, and IV disease is treated with full-course CHOP chemotherapy (Appendix C2, Section II) with the addition of rituximab if the lymphoma is CD20 positive. For areas of bulky disease, ISRT may benefit the patient if all bulky disease that was present before giving chemotherapy can be safely encompassed by the radiation ports.

Pursuant to the results of the randomized Groupe d'Etude des Lymphomes de l'Adulte (GELA) study in which elderly patients with aggressive NHL demonstrated a survival advantage (see Coiffier et al. 2002 in "Suggested Readings"), rituximab is added to each cycle of CHOP. The addition of rituximab to CHOP increased the overall survival at 3 years from 49% to 62% when compared with treatment with CHOP alone. One can expect long-term disease control ("cure") in roughly 50% of patients with advanced-stage, intermediate-/high-grade NHL treated with R-CHOP and similar programs.

Despite claims to the contrary, there is no proof that any of the more complex and more toxic regimens are superior to CHOP. The results of an intergroup trial comparing CHOP with three of the purportedly more effective combinations showed CHOP to be equally active and less toxic. The claims for improved outcome reported in single-institution trials using other regimens are likely the result of incomplete follow-up and selection bias. A recent study comparing RCHOP with R dose adjusted EPOCH has been completed with results pending.

1. **Complete restaging** to assess completeness of response is mandatory. Restaging is usually done after three to four cycles of CHOP and again after six cycles. Patients are generally given at least two additional cycles of therapy after attainment of CR (usually a total of six to eight cycles). Ideally, patients should be in CR after the fourth cycle.

2. **CNS prophylaxis** using intrathecal chemotherapy appears to be indicated in situations associated with a high risk for meningeal relapse. This strategy is particularly advised in cases of involvement of the paranasal sinuses, when there is contiguous spread to the CNS, and in BL. Other indications may include lymphoblastic lymphoma, primary testicular lymphoma, and intermediate-/high-grade lymphomas that involve the bone marrow extensively, and those with multiple extranodal sites and elevated LDH, although the latter indications are more controversial.

3. **Autologous SCT** has been proposed as consolidation during first remission for high-risk patients but is of no proven efficacy in multiple randomized trials.

4. **Maintenance therapy** does not enhance survival and thus is not advised.

C. **Refractory or relapsed intermediate-/high-grade lymphomas**

1. **Refractory patients** failing to achieve a CR may be salvaged with consolidation RT if the involved area is not extensive. Salvage chemotherapy, followed by autologous SCT, is the preferred approach, if feasible. Patients achieving a PR may have a 20% to 40% chance of cure, but the long-term survival rate of truly refractory patients is in the 10% range, so that high-dose chemotherapy is not generally recommended. Allogeneic SCT can be considered for these patients.

2. **Salvage chemotherapy regimens** often employ high-dose cytosine arabinoside or gemcitabine, corticosteroids, and platinum-containing chemotherapeutic agents with or without etoposide (see ESHAP in Appendix C3). Combinations employing ifosfamide (ICE, MINE) and other potentially helpful regimens (infusional EPOCH) are also shown in Appendix C3. Any of these regimens could be combined with rituximab, but the impact of this practice is unclear. These programs generally produce significant but short-lasting remissions in 40% to 50% of patients. A small proportion of patients, probably fewer than 10%, have prolonged responses.

3. **High-dose chemotherapy with or without RT with autologous bone marrow or stem cell support.** A similar strategy to that employed in HL has been adopted for intermediate-grade NHL after relapse from standard CHOP-like chemotherapy. A conditioning regimen based on high-dose chemotherapy, sometimes combined with total-body irradiation, is used and followed by reinfusion of cryopreserved peripheral blood progenitor cells (stem cells) mobilized by growth factors. The results of this strategy are best in chemosensitive recurrences, in which about 40% of patients may derive long-term, disease-free survival. The results are far less optimistic in patients whose disease is chemoresistant or in patients who have never achieved remission. The relative merits of salvage chemotherapy followed by autologous SCT have been convincingly proved in a multicenter randomized European study (the PARMA study).

4. **Allogeneic SCT** differs from autologous SCT in that a potential graft versus lymphoma immune reaction may complement the effects of the conditioning regimen. The degree to which this effect exists in lymphoma is subject to debate and may vary with the type of lymphoma. Allogeneic SCT may be most reasonable in young patients who have a suitable donor match and who do not fall into the favorable categories for benefit from autologous transplantation.

5. **Experimental therapies.** Newer therapies being given with a palliative intent include lenalidomide and ibrutinib in certain patient populations.

D. **Therapy for MCL** with standard chemotherapy regimens has generally been ineffective at achieving long-term remissions. The hyper-CVAD regimen (see Appendix C2, Section III) alternated with high-dose methotrexate plus high-dose cytarabine has been proposed for treatment of MCL by the M.D. Anderson Cancer Center. Rituximab has been supplemented to the regimen. Allogeneic or autologous transplantation after two or four rounds of chemotherapy is considered for patients younger than 65 years of age. Aggressive approaches to MCL such as this may have shifted the survival curve to the right, but it still remains unclear if long-term remission is possible. Rituximab maintenance following autologous transplantation has also been studied. Bendamustine with rituximab is also utilized with or without rituximab maintenance as front-line therapy. Patients who relapse may receive palliative treatment with agents such as rituximab, bortezomib, and/or radioimmunotherapy. New agents such as idelalisib, ibrutinib, or lenalidomide have been approved for use in the relapsed/refractory setting.

E. **Therapy for lymphoblastic lymphoma** is patterned after therapy for the closely related ALL. Overall results of therapy indicate a 40% long-term, disease-free survival, with the best prognosis seen in patients who have minimal or no marrow involvement, no CNS involvement, and normal serum LDH levels. Patients with poor prognostic presentations of lymphoblastic lymphoma can be considered for early allogeneic SCT or more intensive primary chemotherapy programs.

Stanford University researchers reported a 94% freedom-from-relapse rate at 5 years for patients without the previously named adverse prognostic factors with a regimen that involves 1 month of induction therapy, 1 month of CNS prophylaxis, 3 months of consolidation, and, finally, 7 months of maintenance therapy, as follows:

Cyclophosphamide, 400 mg/m^2 PO for 3 days, on weeks 1, 4, 9, 12, 15, and 18

Doxorubicin, 50 mg/m^2 IV, on weeks 1, 4, 9, 12, 15, and 18

Vincristine, 2 mg IV, on weeks 1, 2, 3, 4, 5, 6, 9, 12, 15, and 18

Prednisone, 40 mg/m² daily for 6 weeks (tapered off); then for 5 days on weeks 9, 12, 15, and 18

CNS prophylaxis consists of whole-brain RT (WBRT) (2,400 cGy in 12 fractions) and intrathecal methotrexate (12 mg for each of six doses) given between weeks 4 and 9.

L-Asparaginase, 6,000 units/m² IM (maximum, 10,000 units) for five doses at the beginning of CNS prophylaxis.

Maintenance therapy consists of methotrexate (30 mg/m² PO weekly) and 6-mercaptopurine (75 mg/m² PO daily) during weeks 23 to 52.

F. **Therapy for ATLL** with polychemotherapy has been largely ineffective. A combination of zidovudine (AZT) and IFN-α has been stated to show promise. Occasionally, patients may benefit briefly from combination chemotherapy programs used in intermediate-/high-grade NHL or from 2-deoxycoformycin, a purine analog. Investigational agents, such as anti-CCR4 antibodies, are attractive treatment options for this group of patients.

G. **Therapy of peripheral T-cell lymphomas.** Patients with non–B-cell aggressive lymphomas usually relapse after aggressive chemotherapy and fare worse than patients with B-cell NHL. Often, the remissions may last only for a few weeks (kinetic failure). Aggressive approaches with autologous or allogeneic SCT are justified. Participation in clinical trials is highly recommended for this group of patients. Histology-specific treatments are being developed such as that described for enteropathy type T-cell lymphoma (see Sieniawski et al. 2010 in *Suggested Readings*) as well as lineage-specific drugs such as pralatrexate and/ or histone deacetylase inhibitors (HDI). Anti-CD30 antibodies conjugated to chemotherapy have been utilized to treat CD30 overexpressing lymphomas such as ALCL.

1. **Angioimmunoblastic lymphoma (AILD)** has been managed with generally poor results by conventional chemotherapy or corticosteroids, although occasional long-term responses or spontaneous regressions have occurred. More recently, responses to IFN-α, cyclosporine, or high-dose chemotherapy with stem cell support have been described in small series or case reports.

2. **T/NK lymphoma, nasal type** with localized involvement of the palate and sinuses ("lethal midline granuloma") may benefit from RT followed by chemotherapy. Specific chemotherapy regimens, such as the SMILE regimen employing L-asparaginase and non–multidrug-resistant drugs, are especially attractive in this patient group (see Yamaguchi, et al. 2008 in *Suggested Readings*).

3. **Primary cutaneous CD30 (Ki-1)-positive T-cell disorders** comprise a spectrum of closely related skin lesions that, although they may look identical microscopically, can be distinguished on physical examination of the patient's skin.

   a. **Lymphomatoid papulosis** has the best prognosis and is often a self-limited disease. It appears as crops of <2-cm nodules that may have central ulceration and leave scars but spontaneously resolve within 6 to 8 weeks.

   b. **Cutaneous anaplastic large cell lymphoma** (C-ALCL), which appears as single >2-cm skin lesions often with ulcerative centers, can be treated with local irradiation or surgery or, if multiple, single-agent chemotherapy (cyclophosphamide or weekly low-dose methotrexate) with or without corticosteroids or RT. Spontaneous remission can occur in up to

30% of cases within 6 to 8 weeks. It can often be confused with ALCL, which is treated as a common aggressive lymphoma.

VIII. SPECIAL LYMPHOMA SYNDROMES

A. **Systemic Castleman disease.** Initially, Castleman disease refers to *localized giant lymph node hyperplasia,* usually involving the mediastinum or abdomen. The disease is associated with infection with HHV-8 and probably promoted by viral IL-6 production. A disorder exhibiting the histopathologic features of the plasma cell type of Castleman disease but with a generalized presentation has been described.

1. **Clinical features**
   a. Fever, malaise, and weakness
   b. Lymphadenopathy, usually generalized
   c. Organomegaly
   d. Edema, anasarca, and effusions
   e. Pulmonary and CNS involvement
   f. Anemia, thrombocytopenia, polyclonal hypergammaglobulinemia, and elevated ESR

2. **Histopathology** shows preservation of lymph node architecture, but with prominent germinal centers, either hyperplastic or hyalinized, and diffuse marked plasma cell infiltration.

3. **Clinical course** is either persistent or episodic with remissions and exacerbations. Lymphoma or Kaposi sarcoma occasionally develops. The median survival time is 30 months.

4. **Treatment.** Corticosteroids and antitumor agents used in NHL have met with occasional responses. IL-6 has been implicated in the pathogenesis of this disorder, with a reported clinical response to treatment with an anti–IL-6 antibody.

B. **Mycosis fungoides (MF) and Sézary syndrome (SS)** are CTCLs (see Appendix B4). Both are malignant cutaneous lymphoproliferative disorders usually of helper T cells (CD4 positive). Approximately 15% to 20% transform to CD30-positive or CD30-negative large cell lymphoma.

1. **Dermatologic presentation** is in localized patches or plaques, which may evolve into tumor nodules in MF and diffuse exfoliative erythroderma associated with abnormal circulating cells in SS.

2. **Histopathology** shows atypical T cells with irregular cerebriform nuclei (MF cells) infiltrating the epidermis and the upper dermis, forming characteristic Pautrier microabscesses. Enlarged lymph nodes do not always show overt lymphomatous infiltration, but techniques such as T-cell–receptor gene arrangement may be positive.

3. **Natural history.** A long history of undiagnosed skin disease often precedes the specific diagnosis.
   a. **Cutaneous stages of MF**
      (1) Patch stage
      (2) Plaque stage
      (3) Tumor stage
   b. **Lymph node involvement** occurs with increasing skin involvement. Histologically confirmed lymph node involvement with complete lymph node effacement on microscopic examination conveys a poor prognosis.
   c. **Visceral involvement.** Almost any organ can be involved late in the disease, particularly the liver, spleen, lung, and GI tract, but

the marrow is relatively spared. A peculiar epitheliotropic pattern of dissemination may be observed.

4. **Prognosis.** About 90% of patients with stage IA survive >15 years with treatment; median survival is not different from age-matched controls. Median survival time is 2 to 4 years from onset of tumor stage or lymph node involvement and <2 years from visceral involvement.

5. **Topical treatment**

   a. **Topical corticosteroids** frequently achieve good responses.

   b. **Topical nitrogen mustard** is useful in the patches or plaque stages. It can be used for involved skin only or in a total body application. Cutaneous allergic reactions may develop.

   c. **Psoralen with ultraviolet light A (PUVA) or narrow-band UVB** repeated two to three times a week is effective for the patch or plaque phase. Long-term benefits and side effects are poorly defined.

   d. **Bexarotene** gel is a retinoid that selectively binds to the retinoid X-receptor (RXR) family of retinoid receptors. The response rate of localized patch or plaque disease to the gel is >60%. Bexarotene is the only retinoid that has been approved for this indication.

   e. **Electron-beam RT** to the total skin is technically demanding but has produced durable remissions, particularly in early stages of disease. Local electron-beam RT can be used in the treatment of tumors, especially if they are few in number.

6. **Systemic chemotherapy and investigational approaches** have resulted in short-term responses without an effect on survival.

   a. **Systemic chemotherapy** is recommended only for patients with advanced disease. A variety of single agents (e.g., methotrexate, corticosteroids, alkylating agents, gemcitabine, etoposide, doxorubicin, pegylated liposomal doxorubicin) achieve temporary responses in 30% of patients. The purine analogs 2-deoxycoformycin (pentostatin), cladribine, and fludarabine have all also shown response rates of about 30%. Combination chemotherapy is sometimes advocated for those with disease transformation to large cell lymphoma.

   b. **Bexarotene** is an oral rexinoid that is approved in the treatment of CTCL. The most common side effects are hypertriglyceridemia, central hypothyroidism, and myelosuppression.

   c. **IFN-α** has response rates of 15% to 50% in MF/SS.

   d. **Denileukin diftitox** (DAB$_{389}$-IL-2) is a fusion protein between IL-2 and diphtheria toxin that was approved for the treatment of CTCLs failing other treatments. Most common side effects include vascular capillary leak syndrome, abnormal liver function tests, and infusion reactions.

   e. **Antibody therapy.** Transient responses to monoclonal T-cell antibodies, such as alemtuzumab, have been observed in CTCL, especially in SS.

   f. **Extracorporeal photophoresis (ECP),** a systemic form of PUVA therapy, is an effective immunoadjuvant therapy for CTCL. The procedure involves exposure of leukapheresed mononuclear cells to a psoralen-photoactivating agent and UVA *ex vivo* followed by reinfusion of the treated cells. ECP induces an anti-idiotype cytotoxic T-cell response against circulating tumor cells. ECP is most effective with the erythrodermic phase (SS) of CTCL.

   g. **Histone deacetylase inhibitors** (HDI). Vorinostat, an oral HDI, and romidepsin, an IV HDI, have been approved for the treatment of the skin manifestations of CTCL. The most common side effects are GI, thrombopenia, and constitutional.

C. **Primary CNS lymphoma (PCNSL)** is essentially always of high histologic grade (large cell, immunoblastic) and of B-cell origin. Lesions are primarily parenchymal and involve deep periventricular structures. Multiple lesions occur in 20% to 40% of cases. The leptomeninges are involved in 30% of cases at diagnosis and in most cases at autopsy.

1. **Etiology and epidemiology**

   a. PCNSL accounts for about 1% of brain tumors and 1% of extranodal lymphomas. The disease is associated with advanced age (>60 years), AIDS, drug-induced immunosuppression (e.g., for transplantation), and congenital immunodeficiency syndromes.

   b. PCNSL accounts for roughly 50% of all lymphomas seen in transplant recipients and occurs at a somewhat lower frequency in AIDS. In AIDS cases, PCNSL appears in a setting of severe CD4 depression, with counts frequently <50/μL.

   c. Relationship to EBV infection is suggested by discovery of the *EBV* genome in some cases of PCNSL arising in transplant recipients and AIDS patients.

2. **Clinical presentations** include headache, personality changes, and hemiparesis. Symptoms of meningeal infiltration or spinal cord compression are less common. Associated systemic lymphoma is rare. Ocular lymphoma (appearing as uveitis or vitritis) may precede or follow the diagnosis of CNS lymphoma. PCNSL complicating AIDS is associated with a median survival time of <3 months.

3. **Evaluation.** The diagnosis can usually be made with stereotactic biopsy and without formal surgical exploration.

   a. **Brain CT scan.** Deep periventricular lesions often involve the corpus callosum, basal ganglia, or thalamus and often appear hyperdense before contrast dye injection. Contrast often produces generalized intense enhancement, unlike the picture of gliomas and metastases. In AIDS patients, the precontrast scan may be hypodense.

   b. **Brain MRI** may reveal additional lesions not seen by CT scan.

   c. **Lumbar puncture.** Nonspecific elevation of cerebrospinal fluid (CSF) protein is common. Abnormal cells may be found in 25% to 35% of patients undergoing lumbar puncture at diagnosis. Identification of malignant cells may be enhanced by immunofluorescent techniques with monoclonal antibodies.

   d. **Ophthalmologic examination,** including slit-lamp examination.

   e. **HIV antibody; HIV viral load if positive.

   f. **Enumeration of the CD4 count.

   g. **Abdominal CT scan, chest radiograph or CT chest (often accompanied by PET scan).

   h. **Bone marrow biopsy.

4. **Therapy**

   a. **Corticosteroids** are extremely effective in PCNSL. Lesions may disappear on steroids alone and preclude histologic diagnosis after steroids are given.

   b. **Whole-brain RT (WBRT)** was previously the preferred treatment for PCNSL. Doses of 4,000 to 5,000 cGy appear necessary, with 1,000 to 1,500 cGy focal boost to the tumor bed. However, WBRT is associated with severe delayed neurotoxicity. Up to 90% of patients over 60 years of age develop totally debilitating dementia, gait ataxia, and urinary dysfunction within 1 year of treatment, if they survive. Delayed treatment-related cerebrovascular disease, alone or in combination with progressive leukoencephalopathy, has been observed in younger patients 7 to 10 years after WBRT.

   c. **Chemotherapy** with high doses of methotrexate (>3 g/m^2) and/or high-dose Ara-C has become the preferred treatment because it improves disease-free survival significantly and because it is not associated with the high rate of neurotoxicity from combined-modality treatment. The response rate to high doses of methotrexate is 70% to 95%, with an expected 2-year survival rate of 60% and median survival of 32 months. Relapses are treated with WBRT and/or salvage chemotherapy. Intrathecal chemotherapy is not given unless CSF cytology is positive. Approaches utilizing high-dose methotrexate, cytarabine, and autologous stem cell transplant are being investigated.

D. **Primary gastrointestinal lymphoma** (PGL) is the most common form of solitary extranodal disease and may occur in the stomach, small bowel, and large bowel.

   1. **Associated diseases.** The incidence of enteropathy-type T-cell lymphoma is increased in patients with ulcerative colitis, regional enteritis, or celiac disease. α-Heavy chain disease is present in some patients with the Mediterranean type of PGL. MALToma of the stomach is associated with *H. pylori* infection.

   2. **Histopathology.** PGL may originate from either T cells or B cells. MALToma, follicular lymphoma, MCL, or other aggressive lymphomas may be found anywhere along the GI tract. B-cell PGL tends to present at lower stages, have fewer complications, and have a better prognosis than T-cell PGL.

   3. **Symptoms and physical findings.** Anorexia, nausea, vomiting, weight loss, GI bleeding, or abdominal pain is present in most patients. An abdominal mass may be present, but peripheral lymphadenopathy is not common.

   4. **Complications.** Obstruction may complicate the course of PGL. Perforation or hemorrhage may be either a presenting sign or a complication of treatment for PGL. Therapy can cause perforation by the lysis of the lymphoma's involvement of the full thickness of the wall of the organ involved.

   5. **Diagnosis.** Endoscopy or barium contrast radiographs usually show large mucosal folds, ulceration, masses, lumen narrowing, or annular strictures. Gastric lymphomas may be indistinguishable from peptic ulcer by both radiologic and endoscopic criteria. Undifferentiated carcinoma or adenocarcinoma of the GI tract may be confused with intermediate-/high-grade lymphoma even after expert histologic evaluation; immunohistochemical verification of diagnosis is mandatory. Multiple sites of involvement should be excluded by barium follow-through or endoscopy.

   6. **Management of PGL**

      a. **Surgical management.** Laparotomy may be needed to establish the diagnosis or treat complications. Resection of bowel should be considered in cases with solitary lesions, intractable bleeding, or high risk of perforation. Subtotal gastrectomy for gastric lymphoma is rarely performed.

      b. **Medical management** should be based on histologic subtype and extent of disease. Intermediate-/high-grade lesions are treated primarily with combination chemotherapy, such as CHOP. The 2-year survival after CHOP is better than 90% for B-cell PGL and 25% to 35% for T-cell PGL.

7. **Gastric MALToma.** *H. pylori*–associated MALToma of the stomach usually has low-grade histology. Occasionally, transformation to a large cell lymphoma may occur. Significant mucosal thickening may be present before spread to regional or distant nodes. *H. pylori* can usually be found in endoscopic biopsies.

   a. **Treatment of *H. pylori*.** MALToma usually regresses after eradication of *H. pylori*. At least a 70% CR is expected but may be observed up to 6 months after treatment. A t(11;18) translocation is a predictor for no response to antibiotic therapy. The following 2-week regimen can be used for *H. pylori* (amoxicillin may be used instead of metronidazole in case of intolerance):

   Clarithromycin (Biaxin), 500 mg b.i.d.
   Metronidazole (Flagyl), 500 mg b.i.d.
   Omeprazole (Prilosec), 20 mg b.i.d.

   b. **Antineoplastic therapy.** Patients with a large cell component, deeply penetrating disease, or with metastatic disease, are not expected to respond to antimicrobial therapy. IFRT is used for disease localized to the stomach (3,000 to 3,300 cGy). Gastrectomy is probably not superior to RT for local control and has been abandoned. Rituximab can also be used if RT is contraindicated. Systemic chemotherapy is used for more advanced disease that is symptomatic, bulky or with areas of transformation.

E. **Burkitt lymphoma (BL)** is a specific subtype of the small, noncleaved cell, high-grade NHL. The cells in BL are very uniform with round or oval nuclei, two to five prominent nucleoli, and cytoplasm rich in RNA. The cells are of B lineage, expressing monoclonal surface IgM with *c-myc* overexpression. A consistent series of cytogenetic translocations (Table 22-6) and explosive growth characterizes BL.

   1. **Epidemiology and etiology**
      a. BL is endemic in certain regions of equatorial Africa and other tropical locations. A sporadic form of BL occurs in the United States and throughout the world. The disease occurs predominantly in childhood but can be seen in young adults, particularly in the sporadic form.
      b. EBV has been found in the genome of endemic BL but rarely in the sporadic form. Very high EBV antibody titers are seen in the endemic form.

   2. **Clinical features** of BL are shown in Table 22-7.

TABLE 22-7	**Clinical Features of Burkitt Lymphoma**	
Feature	**Endemic (Africa)**	**Sporadic**
Association with EBV	Yes	Rarely
Chromosomal translocation	t(8;14), common	t(8;14), common
Sites of involvement	Jaw, orbit	Abdomen, GI tract, marrow
Lymph node involvement	Rarely	Not infrequently
Therapy	50% prolonged survival rate with cyclophosphamide	Requires multiple agents
Relapse	Survival possible	Guarded prognosis

3. **Staging system.** A variety of systems have been proposed. The NCI system is as follows:

Stage	Disease Distribution
A	Single solitary extra-abdominal site
AR	Intra-abdominal: >90% of tumor resected
B	Multiple extra-abdominal sites
C	Intra-abdominal tumor
D	Intra-abdominal plus one or more extra-abdominal sites

4. **Prognosis.** Before effective treatment, only 30% of sporadic cases survived. Using combination chemotherapy and CNS prophylaxis, the survival rate is at least 60%. Children and young adults with limited-stage (A, AR, B) disease have an excellent prognosis with a 90% survival rate. Bone marrow and CNS involvement carry a poor prognosis. Adult cases of BL, particularly those of advanced stage, do more poorly than childhood cases. So-called double-hit BL that contains both 8;14 and 14;18 translocations or triple hit that also contain bcl-6 rearrangements have a worse prognosis.

5. **Treatment**

   a. Cyclophosphamide therapy alone has been curative for many localized presentations in Africa.

   b. Multiagent, aggressive regimens are necessary for the sporadic form as well as for Burkitt-like NHL. One such program would be hyper-CVAD with or without rituximab. Another appropriate treatment alternates two cycles of CODOX-M with two cycles of IVAC (see Appendix C2, Section III) in patients with Burkitt-like NHL, with excellent results. Low-risk patients (those with normal LDH and complete resection of an abdominal tumor or single extra-abdominal mass) may be treated with CODOX-M alone combined with intrathecal prophylaxis. Dose-adjusted R-EPOCH has been utilized in this patient population. *CHOP is not adequate therapy for this group of patients.*

   c. Because of the extremely rapid growth rate, massive acute destruction of tumor with initial chemotherapy usually results in tumor lysis syndrome and mandates prophylaxis for tumor lysis syndrome when the patient is initially treated (see Chapter 32, VII.A).

ACKNOWLEDGMENT

The author would like to acknowledge Dr. Dennis A. Casciato who significantly contributed to earlier versions of this chapter.

Suggested Readings
Hodgkin Lymphoma

Aleman BMP, et al. Involved-field radiotherapy for advanced Hodgkin's lymphoma. *N Engl J Med* 2003;348:2396.

Bonnadonna G, et al. ABVD plus subtotal nodal versus involved–field radiotherapy in early-stage Hodgkin's disease: long-term results. *J Clin Oncol* 2004;22:2285.

Borchmann P, et al. Combined modality treatment with intensified chemotherapy and dose-reduced involved field radiotherapy in patients with early unfavorable Hodgkin lymphoma (HL): final analysis of the German Hodgkin Study Group (GHSG) HD11 trial. *Blood* 2009;114:299.

Canellos GP, et al. Chemotherapy of advanced Hodgkin's disease with MOPP, ABVD, or MOPP alternating with ABVD. *N Engl J Med* 1992;327:1478.

Diehl V, et al. Standard and increased-dose BEACOPP chemotherapy compared with COPP–ABVD for advanced Hodgkin's disease. *N Engl J Med* 2003;348:2386.

Dores GM, et al. Second malignant neoplasms among long-term survivors of Hodgkin's disease: a population-based evaluation over 25 years. *J Clin Oncol* 2002;20:3484.

Engert A, et al. Reduced treatment intensity in patients with early stage Hodgkin lymphoma. *N Engl J Med* 2010;363:640.

Hasenclever D, et al. A prognostic score for advanced Hodgkin's disease. *N Engl J Med* 1998;339:1506.

Hutchings M, et al. FDG-PET after two cycles of chemotherapy predicts treatment failure and progression-free survival in Hodgkin lymphoma. *Blood* 2006;107:52.

Meyer RM, et al. Randomized comparison of ABVD chemotherapy with a strategy that includes radiation therapy in patients with limited-stage Hodgkin's lymphoma: National Cancer Institute of Canada Clinical Trials Group and the Eastern Cooperative Oncology Group. *J Clin Oncol* 2005;23:4634.

Oki Y, Younes A. Current role of gemcitabine in the treatment of Hodgkin lymphoma. *Leuk Lymphoma* 2008;49:883.

Non-Hodgkin Lymphoma

Armitage JO, et al. New approaches to classifying non-Hodgkin lymphomas: clinical features of the major histologic subtypes. *J Clin Oncol* 1998;16:2780.

Browne WB, et al. The management of unicentric and multicentric Castleman's disease: a report of 16 cases and a review of the literature. *Cancer* 1999;85:706.

Coiffier B, et al. CHOP chemotherapy plus rituximab compared with CHOP alone in elderly patients with diffuse large-B-cell lymphoma. *N Engl J Med* 2002;346:235.

DeAngelis LM, Iwamoto FM. An update on therapy of primary central nervous system lymphoma. *Hematology Am Soc Hematol Educ Program* 2006:311.

Feugier P, et al. BCL2 expression is a prognostic factor for the activated B-cell like type of diffuse large B-cell lymphoma: a study by the Groupe d'Etude des Lymphomes de l'Adulte. *J Clin Oncol* 2005;23:4117.

Fisher RI, et al. New treatment options have changed the survival of patients with follicular lymphoma. *J Clin Oncol* 2005;23:8447.

Habermann TM, et al. Rituximab-CHOP with or without maintenance rituximab in patients 60 years of age or older with diffuse large B-cell lymphoma (DLBCL). An update. *J Clin Oncol* 2006;24:3121.

Iqbal J, et al. BCL2 expression is a prognostic factor for the activated B-cell-like type of diffuse large B-cell lymphoma. *J Clin Oncol* 2006;24:961.

Khouri IF, et al. Hyper-CVAD and high-dose methotrexate/cytarabine followed by stem-cell transplantation: an active regimen for aggressive mantle-cell lymphoma. *J Clin Oncol* 1998;16:3803.

Liu Q, et al. Improvement of overall and failure-free survival in stage IV follicular lymphoma: 25 years of treatment experience at the University of Texas M.D. Anderson Cancer Center. *J Clin Oncol* 2006;24:1582.

Marcus R, et al. CVP chemotherapy plus rituximab compared with CVP as first-line treatment for advanced follicular lymphoma. *Blood* 2005;105:1417.

Montoto S, et al. Risk and clinical implications of transformation of follicular lymphoma to diffuse large B-cell lymphoma. *J Clin Oncol* 2007;25:2426.

Sehn LH, et al. The revised International Prognostic Index (R-IPI) is a better predictor of outcome than the standard IPI for patients with diffuse large B-cell lymphoma treated with R-CHOP. *Blood* 2007;109:1857.

Sieniawski M, et al. Evaluation of enteropathy-associated T-cell lymphoma comparing standard therapies with a novel regimen including autologous stem cell transplantation. *Blood* 2010;115:3664.

Staudt LM, Dave S. The biology of human lymphoid malignancies revealed by gene expression profiling. *Adv Immunol* 2005;87:163.

Swerdlow SH, et al. *World Health Organization Classification of Tumours of Hematopoietic and Lymphoid Tissues.* 4th ed. Lyon, France: IARC Press; 2008.

Van Oers MHJ, et al. Chimeric anti-CD20 monoclonal antibody (rituximab; mabthera) in remission induction and maintenance treatment of relapsed/resistant follicular non-Hodgkin's lymphoma. Final analysis of a Phase III randomized intergroup clinical trial. *Blood* 2005;106:107a.

Wilson WH, et al. Dose-adjusted EPOCH chemotherapy for untreated large B-cell lymphomas: a pharmacodynamic approach with high efficacy. *Blood* 2002;99:2685.

Winter JN, et al. Prognostic significance of Bcl-6 protein expression in DLBCL treated with CHOP or R-CHOP: a prospective correlative study. *Blood* 2006;107:4207.

Witzig TE, et al. Randomized controlled trial of Yttrium-90-labeled ibritumomab tiuxetan radioimmunotherapy versus rituximab immunotherapy for patients with relapsed or refractory low-grade, follicular, or transformed B-cell non-Hodgkin's lymphoma. *J Clin Oncol* 2002;20:2453.

Yamaguchi M, et al. Phase I study of dexamethasone, methotrexate, ifosfamide, L-asparaginase, and etoposide (SMILE) chemotherapy for extranodal natural killer (NK)/T-cell lymphoma and leukemia. *Cancer Sci* 2008;99:1016.

23 Plasma Cell Dyscrasias and Waldenström Macroglobulinemia

Sarah M. Larson

Immunoglobulins are produced by B lymphocytes and plasma cells. Properties of normal serum immunoglobulins are shown in Table 23-1. A clone of cells producing immunoglobulins may proliferate to sufficient mass that a monoclonal protein (M-protein or paraprotein) is detectable as a peak or "spike" on serum protein electrophoresis (PEP). The "M" in M-protein can stand for monoclonal, myeloma, macroglobulinemia, or the M-like appearance of the serum PEP (SPEP) graph. These disorders are included in the World Health Organization's classification of neoplastic diseases of lymphoid tissues (Appendix B4). Their immunohistochemistry phenotypes are shown in Appendix B3.

I. EPIDEMIOLOGY AND ETIOLOGY

  A. **Classification** of diseases associated with monoclonal paraproteinemia
   1. **Plasma cell neoplasms**
     a. Multiple myeloma (MM)
     b. Smoldering multiple myeloma (SMM)
     c. Monoclonal gammopathy of undetermined significance (MGUS)
     d. Amyloidosis
     e. Heavy chain disease
     f. Papular mucinosis
   2. **Other neoplastic diseases**
     a. Waldenström macroglobulinemia (WM)
     b. Malignant B-cell non-Hodgkin lymphoma, chronic lymphocytic leukemia (CLL)
     c. Neoplasms of cell types not known to synthesize immunoglobulins (solid tumors, monocytic leukemia, myelodysplastic syndromes)
   3. **Nonneoplastic disorders**
     a. Autoimmune diseases (e.g., systemic lupus erythematosus)
     b. Hepatobiliary disease
     c. Chronic inflammatory diseases
     d. Immunodeficiency syndromes
     e. Miscellaneous diseases (e.g., Gaucher disease)
     f. Pseudoparaproteinemia (see Section IX.C)
  B. **Incidence.** MGUS, SMM, MM, and WM are the most common disorders associated with M-proteins. The median age of diagnosis is 69 years, and the incidence increases with age.
   1. **MGUS** (formerly *benign monoclonal gammopathy*). The approximate incidence of MGUS is 0.2% for patients 25 to 49 years of age, 2% for those 50 to 79 years of age, and 10% for those 80 to 90 years of age.
   2. **SMM** progresses to MM at a rate of about 10% per year during the first 5 years and the rate of progression decreases after that time.

TABLE 23-1	Normal Human Serum Immunoglobulins			
Ig (Heavy Chain)	MW (×1,000)	$T_{1/2}$ (days)	Portion of Ig (%)	IV (%)
IgG[a] (γ)	150	20	75	52
IgA (α)	160	6	15	55
IgM (μ)	900	5	10	75
IgD (δ)	180	3	0.2	75
IgE (ε)	190	3	0.005	40

Ig, immunoglobulin; IV, proportion of Ig distributed intravascularly; MW, molecular weight; $T_{1/2}$, half-life.
[a]Four subclasses comprise IgG. About 70% of IgG is IgG_1, 17% is IgG_2, 8% is IgG_3, and 5% is IgG_4. The data shown apply to all subtypes except IgG_3. IgG_3 differs from the other subclasses in that 65% is distributed IV, its serum half-life is 7 days, and it is not affected by high serum concentrations; it most avidly binds complement (other subclasses do so weakly, if at all), and it is most likely to produce hyperviscosity.

3. **MM** develops in 3 per 100,000 population and constitutes 1% of new cancer cases in the United States. The median age at diagnosis is 69 years and many patients are >70 years of age. Men are affected slightly more often than women. MM is the second most common hematologic malignancy.

4. **WM** has an incidence that is about 5% to 10% of that of MM. Two-thirds of cases occur in men.

5. **Lymphomas.** Excluding MGUS, MM, and WM, about half of the patients with a monoclonal gammopathy have lymphocytic lymphoma or CLL. The M-protein is nearly always either IgM or IgG and usually causes no symptoms. Patients with other types of lymphoma do not have an increased incidence of monoclonal proteins.

C. **Etiology.** No specific etiologic agent for the plasma cell dyscrasias has been found. Predisposing factors in humans appear to be the following:

1. **Radiation exposure** increases the risk of MM. Survivors of the atomic bomb in Japan have been shown to have a higher risk of developing monoclonal gammopathies.

2. **Chronic antigen stimulation.** Many M-proteins have been shown to be antibodies directed against specific antigens, such as microbial antigens, red blood cell antigens, neural antigens, lipoproteins, rheumatoid factors, and coagulation factors. Chronic antigenic stimulation (e.g., chronic osteomyelitis or cholecystitis) may predispose to the development of MM or MGUS. Patients with autoimmune disease may be at high risk for MM.

3. **Environmental exposure.** Exposure to pesticides and benzene in the workplace are associated with an increased incidence of MM. Farmworkers have been shown to be at high risk for MM in several epidemiologic studies.

4. **Human herpesvirus 8 (HHV8)** has been found in the nonmalignant bone marrow dendritic cells of patients with myeloma. It remains to be determined if HHV8 contributes to the growth of the malignant plasma cells in these patients.

5. **Family history of a monoclonal gammopathy** is a risk factor for the development of a plasma cell dyscrasia.

D. **Cytogenetics**

1. **MM.** Multiple, complex karyotypic changes are observed in the malignant plasma cells of most patients. Fluorescent *in situ* hybridization (FISH) analysis has shown that most patients with MM have malignant cells with translocations involving chromosome 14 at the site of the immunoglobulin heavy chain gene locus and a limited number of nonimmunoglobulin

partner chromosomes. Unlike the site of translocation in other B-cell malignancies that involves the joining region JH, the location of the breakpoint in myeloma usually occurs in the switch regions that are involved in heavy chain class switching from Cµ to another heavy chain class.

Hyperdiploidy is observed in approximately 40% of cases of MM and associated with an improved survival. In contrast, patients with hypodiploidy have a worse outcome as this is commonly associated with chromosomal translocations associated with poor survival.

  a. **Chromosomal alterations:** The most common sites of the nonimmunoglobulin breakpoints include chromosomes 11 at the site of cyclin D, chromosome 16 at the site of the c-*MAF* protooncogene, and chromosome 4 at the site of the fibroblastic growth factor receptor 3. Loss of material on the long arm of chromosome 13 occurs in nearly 20% of patients. Loss of 17p is observed in approximately 10% of patients. Addition of material at 1q21 also commonly occurs in MM.

  Prior to bortezomib- and lenalidomide-based therapies (see below), specific translocations such as t(4;14) were associated with poor outcomes, whereas patients with 11;14 translocations had improved outcomes. However, following the introduction of these agents in combination therapies, patients with t(4;14) showed an improvement in outcome.

  b. **Mutations** of *ras* genes occur in about 20% of myelomas and are associated with a poor prognosis. Similarly, mutations of *p53* are found in 15% to 20% of cases and are associated with more advanced and clinically aggressive disease. Abnormalities in the c-*MYC* protooncogene occur in the majority of cases

  These studies have led to a new classification of myeloma based on these results. Recent studies suggest that clinical features such as the presence of bone disease are associated with specific gene expression profiles. In addition, single nucleotide polymorphism and comparative genomic hybridization studies have identified patients with different outcomes in MM.

  c. **Gene expression profiling** has identified specific subgroups of patients with MM. These studies have suggested a markedly different outcome depending on the expression of specific genes. These profiles also may predict responsiveness to specific therapies.

2. **MGUS and SMM.** Studies have shown that patients with MGUS and SMM have similar karyotypic abnormalities to patients with MM.

3. **WM.** Complex karyotypes are also commonly observed in WM. Occasional patients have translocations involving the immunoglobulin heavy chain locus on chromosome 14 and either c-*MYC* on chromosome 8 or *BCL-2* on chromosome 18.

II. PATHOLOGY AND NATURAL HISTORY

  A. **Bone marrow pathology** is usually distinctive in MM and WM. Plasma cells that constitute ≥10% of the nucleated marrow cells (*excluding erythroblasts*) are characteristic but not diagnostic of MM.

  1. **MGUS.** By definition, patients have <10% light chain–restricted plasma cells and a serum monoclonal protein <3 g/dL.

  2. **SMM.** Monoclonal protein ≥3 g/dL and/or 10% to 60% bone marrow involvement of clonal plasma cells, in the absence of end organ damage (hypercalcemia, anemia, renal insufficiency, lytic lesions). As well as lack of a biomarker associated with accelerated progression to end organ damage including ≥60% bone marrow involvement of clonal plasma cells, >1 bone lesion on MRI, or involved/uninvolved free light chain ratio of ≥100.

3. **MM.** Plasma cells usually constitute 10% to 100% of the marrow cells; they have abundant basophilic cytoplasm and eccentric nuclei with paranuclear clear zones. Immaturity of the plasma cells is evident with the presence of prominent nucleoli ("myeloma cells"). The presence of large, homogeneous infiltrates or nodules of plasma cells is highly suggestive of MM. Early in its course, however, marrow involvement is patchy, and normal marrow particles may be obtained from sampling effects. End organ damage or a biomarker indicating an increased risk of progression to end organ damage is necessary for the diagnosis of MM.

4. **WM** may closely resemble CLL. Bone marrow in WM contains 10% to 90% plasmacytoid lymphocytes or small mature lymphocytes; mast cells are often prominent.

5. **Reactive plasmacytosis.** Peripheral blood plasmacytosis occurs in many viral illnesses (including human immunodeficiency virus [HIV] infection), serum sickness, and plasma cell leukemia (which is rare). Bone marrow plasmacytosis, when not caused by myeloma, is characterized by a diffuse distribution (not infiltrative) and alignment of mature plasma cells along blood vessels or near marrow reticulum cells. Since reactive plasmacytosis is not a malignant clonal disorder, the plasma cells do not show kappa or lambda light chain restriction. Reactive bone marrow plasmacytosis is commonly seen in many disorders, including the following:
   a. Viral infections
   b. Serum sickness
   c. Collagen vascular disease
   d. Granulomatous disease
   e. Liver cirrhosis
   f. Neoplastic disease
   g. Marrow hypoplasia

B. **Natural history of MGUS.** MGUS occurs in nearly 5% of individuals over the age of 70. Although these individuals are symptom-free at diagnosis, nearly 25% of cases progress to a malignant disorder (usually MM) by 25 years of follow-up.

Importantly, the risk for malignancy remains constant over time (approximately 1% per year). The presence of a high ratio of abnormal to normal plasma cells as characterized by immunofluorescence has been shown to predict a higher risk of developing MM. Some studies suggest that patients with MGUS are at higher risk of developing accelerated bone loss and fractures, especially of the vertebral bodies. In addition, these patients appear to be at higher risk of developing thromboembolic events.

1. **Karyotypic abnormalities** in these patients are similar to those seen with MM.

2. **The presence of depressed normal immunoglobulin levels** occurs in many patients with MGUS, but is not associated with a higher risk for infection and does not predict a higher risk for malignancy.

3. **Peripheral neuropathy** is seen and may be associated with a monoclonal antibody with reactivity to a myelin-associated glycoprotein (MAG) (see Section IX.B).

C. **Natural history of WM.** WM originates from clones of lymphocytes or plasma cells that synthesize μ heavy chains. The natural history of WM resembles lymphocytic lymphoma much more than MM. Many patients do not require therapy for more than a decade of follow-up. Separating WM from MGUS, CLL, or lymphocytic lymphoma with IgM spikes can be done with FISH and molecular testing for the MYD88 (L265P) mutation, which is present in almost all WM patients.

Lymphadenopathy, splenomegaly, and hyperviscosity are hallmarks of WM; skeletal lesions and impaired renal function are unusual. Concomitant macroglobulinemia and osteolytic lesions usually signify malignant lymphoma or solid tumor rather than primary WM. Glomerular lesions are frequent in WM, but renal failure is uncommon. Low levels of light chains in the urine occur in about 25% of patients.

D. Natural history of MM. Three to twenty years of clonal growth may pass before MM becomes clinically evident. The disease may be localized (5% of cases), indolent (10%), or disseminated and progressive (85%). Nearly all cases of MM originate as MGUS. Manifestations of disease progression arise from bone marrow and skeletal involvement, plasma protein abnormalities, and the development of renal disease.

1. **Hematopoiesis** is often impaired. At the time of diagnosis, 60% of patients have anemia; 15%, leukopenia; and 15%, thrombocytopenia. Nucleated red blood cells and immature granulocytes may be present in the peripheral blood (leukoerythroblastic reaction).

2. **Plasmacytomas** (plasma cell tumors) may develop anywhere in the skeleton or, rarely, in extraosseous sites, with the most common locations being the head and neck. Localized plasmacytomas produce a monoclonal spike in the serum or urine PEP in only half of the cases. The median survival is 10 years. Most plasmacytomas that appear to be solitary become generalized in about 3 years, particularly those involving the skeleton. Extramedullary plasmacytomas have a better prognosis than plasmacytomas of bone and less frequently progress to MM.

3. **Skeletal disease in MM**

    a. **Osteolytic lesions.** Multiple osteolytic lesions are present in about 70% of patients at diagnosis, single osteolytic lesions or diffuse osteoporosis in 15%, and normal skeletal radiographs in 15%. Lesions are most commonly seen in the skull, vertebrae, ribs, pelvis, and proximal long bones. The use of MRI indicates that skeletal abnormalities exist in nearly all patients with myeloma.

    Previously, it was thought that the demineralization and lytic lesions occur as a result of osteoclastic-activating factors and osteoblastic inhibitory factors produced by neoplastic plasma cells and activated by inflammatory cytokines. The loss of bone in these patients, however, now appears to be a complex interplay involving the tumor cells, stromal cells in the bone marrow, and both the osteoblasts and osteoclasts. The factors responsible involve other important molecules, including macrophage colony-stimulating factor, vascular endothelial growth factor, specific matrix metalloproteinases, macrophage inflammatory protein-1α (MIP1-α), dickkopf1 (DKK1), secreted frizzled protein-3, and the receptor activator of nuclear factor-kB (RANK).

    (1) **RANK–RANKL proteins** play a key role in the development of myeloma bone disease. Increased levels of RANKL have been found in myeloma bone marrow and are associated with enhanced bone loss.

    (2) **Osteoprotegerin (OPG)**, the natural soluble decoy inhibitor of RANKL–RANK signaling, is decreased in MM bone marrow and blood. Blockade of RANKL prevents skeletal lesions in animal models of MM. The ratio of circulating RANKL/OPG predicts bone disease in MM patients.

    (3) **The chemokine macrophage inflammatory protein (MIP1-α)** also appears to play a key role in myeloma bone disease. MIP1-α

is elevated in myeloma bone marrow; it is associated with increased bone loss and may stimulate myeloma cell growth.

(4) **DKK1**, an inhibitor of osteoblast development and function, also has an important role in myeloma bone disease. Levels of DKK1 are elevated in the blood and bone marrow from patients with myeloma compared with normal subjects. The inhibition of osteoblast function ultimately leads to a loss of bone formation and enhanced bone loss.

b. **Osteoblastic lesions** occur in <2% of patients, often in association with neuropathy and the POEMS syndrome. Because of their rarity, the diagnosis of MM should be suspect in the presence of osteoblastic lesions.

c. **POEMS syndrome** is a multisystem disorder usually associated with osteosclerotic myeloma. It is characterized by the combination of **p**olyneuropathy (chronic inflammatory demyelinating neuropathy), **o**rganomegaly, **e**ndocrinopathy, **M**-protein (mainly IgG-γ or IgA-γ), and **s**kin changes (hyperpigmentation, thickening, hypertrichosis). Various other signs, such as cachexia, fever, edema, clubbing, and telangiectasia, can also occur. Autoantibodies to peripheral nerve components are absent. The syndrome appears to be the result of marked activation of the proinflammatory cytokines. Patients with POEMS syndrome, particularly those associated with Castleman disease, have been found to contain HHV8.

d. **Hypercalcemia.** About 10% of patients with MM present with hypercalcemia, and another 10% develop it during the course of their disease. This complication results from enhanced bone resorption, resulting in the release of calcium into the circulation. Hypercalcemia is a major cause of renal failure among patients with MM, and normalization of the serum calcium often reverses these renal dysfunction. Avoid bed rest and immobilization because these factors can contribute to both the development and worsening of hypercalcemia. Serum alkaline phosphatase levels are usually normal but may be increased with recalcification of fractures. It is important to remind patients who are on calcium and vitamin D supplements to discontinue these supplements until the calcium level is under control.

4. **Protein abnormalities**

a. **Frequency.** The incidence of monoclonal immunoglobulins in MM and in comparison to MGUS is shown in Table 23-2.

b. **Increased excretion of κ or λ light chains in the urine** depends on the rate of unbalanced synthesis of excess light chains, plasma volume, degradation rate, renal catabolism, and urine volume. Monoclonal light

TABLE 23-2	Frequency of Monoclonal Immunoglobulins in MM and MGUS	
M-protein	**MM**	**MGUS**
IgG	52%	69%
IgA	21%	14%
IgD	2%	<1%
IgM	Very rare	17%
Light chains only	25%	62% kappa
		38% lambda
Nonsecretory	<1%	—

MM, multiple myeloma; MGUS, monoclonal gammopathy of undetermined significance.

chains in the urine are present in two-thirds of all patients with MM and present without an M-protein in the serum in 25%.

c. **Serum-free light chains** are identified in MM patients and, importantly, in many patients with otherwise "nonsecretory" disease.

d. **Normal immunoglobulins** are usually decreased in the serum of patients with MM and are occasionally decreased in patients with MGUS. The mechanism of inhibition of their synthesis is unknown. Older series showed a high rate of infection with encapsulated organisms that was thought to be related to patients' marked decrease in normal serum immunoglobulins. The risk for infection, however, largely occurs during chemotherapy-induced neutropenia or during the terminal stages of the disease.

e. **Other plasma alterations** (see Section IX.A). Hyperviscosity is unusual in MM (<5% of patients).

5. **Renal dysfunction,** both acute and chronic, occurs at diagnosis in 15% to 20% of cases and develops during their course in most patients with MM. Many patients have renal dysfunction from causes other than MM owing to comorbid diseases such as diabetes mellitus or hypertension, urinary tract infections, nephrotoxic medications, or dehydration. Patients with MM secreting urinary light chains commonly present with renal failure. The most important causes of renal dysfunction in these MM patients are hypercalcemia and myeloma kidney.

a. **Myeloma kidney** is generally attributed to the deposition of κ and λ light chains in the distal and collecting tubules, which is where the light chains are catabolized. The tubules dilate, apparently obstructed by casts surrounded by multinucleated giant cells, and undergo cellular atrophy. Glomerular basement membrane disease also occurs in most patients with myeloma kidney. In most instances, proteinuria contains monoclonal light chains only. These abnormalities occur slightly more commonly in MM associated with lambda light chain production.

Malignant myeloma is the most common cause of the **adult Fanconi syndrome** (aminoaciduria, glycosuria, phosphaturia, and electrolyte loss in the urine). Fanconi syndrome may precede the recognition of MM by many years.

b. **Amyloidosis** also develops commonly in MM. It affects the glomeruli and results in nonselective proteinuria.

c. **Inconstant findings** that may aggravate renal function include pyelonephritis, metabolic abnormalities in addition to hypercalcemia (nephrocalcinosis and hyperuricemia), glomerulosclerosis, and focal myeloma cell infiltration. Renal tubular acidosis occasionally occurs. Nephrotic syndrome is rare in MM unless amyloidosis supervenes. Recent studies suggest, however, that chronic administration of IV pamidronate may also be associated with nephrotic syndrome (see below).

d. **Intravenous contrast dye studies** should be done with caution (if at all) because patients with MM are more susceptible to renal dysfunction after such studies, particularly if they are dehydrated.

6. **Neurologic dysfunction** often develops in MM and is the result of several pathogenetic mechanisms.

a. **Central nervous system (CNS).** Spinal cord and nerve root compression develops in about 15% of patients and is usually caused by epidural plasmacytoma. Amyloidosis is a rare cause of epidural masses. Collapse of vertebral bodies can also cause spinal cord compression but, more likely, produces radicular symptoms secondary to nerve root compression.

Cranial nerve palsies can develop from tumor occlusion of calvarial foramina. Intracerebral and meningeal plasmacytomas are rare.

With the longer survival of myeloma patients, meningeal myeloma seems to be occurring more frequently than had been previously observed.

Many of the newer anti-MM agents are recognized to cause fatigue and cognitive dysfunction.

b. Peripheral neuropathy. The carpal tunnel syndrome, which is usually the result of amyloid infiltration of the flexor retinaculum of the wrist (causing entrapment of the median nerve), is a common peripheral neuropathy in MM. Infiltration of nerve fibers and vasa nervorum with amyloid can also produce peripheral neuropathy. Additionally, peripheral neuropathy may be associated with monoclonal immunoglobulins to MAGs (see Section IX.B). Rarely, patients with MM and POEMS syndrome develop a characteristic peripheral neuropathy. The most common cause of peripheral neuropathy in patients with MM is from treatment with drugs such as thalidomide and bortezomib.

c. Neurologic paraneoplastic syndromes (see Chapter 33, Section V)

III. DIAGNOSIS

A. Symptoms. Fatigue, weakness, and weight loss are common in both MM and WM.

1. **Skeletal pain** occurs in 70% of patients with MM at the time of diagnosis but is rare in patients with WM.

2. **Symptoms of hypercalcemia** (see Chapter 28, Section I) are present in about 10% of patients with MM at the time of diagnosis and develop in another 10% later in the course of the disease.

3. **Hyperviscosity syndrome symptoms** (bleeding, neurologic dysfunction, visual disturbances, or congestive heart failure) are present in about 50% of patients with WM and in <5% of patients with MM (see Section IX.A.1).

4. **Cold sensitivity** may occur in patients with cryoglobulins, especially in WM (see Section IX.A.2).

B. Physical findings

1. **Hepatosplenomegaly** is present in 40% of patients with WM at the time of diagnosis and is uncommon in MM except with the POEMS variant.

2. **Lymphadenopathy** occurs in 30% of patients with WM but is rare in patients with MM except late in the disease.

3. **Bone tenderness** in patients with MM often signifies recent fracture or subperiosteal infiltration with malignant cells.

4. **Neurologic abnormalities** are frequent in MM; neurologic abnormalities in WM are caused by hyperviscosity or demyelination.

5. **Purpura** signifies thrombocytopenia in MM and hyperviscosity syndrome in WM. Occasionally, patients with MM will develop coagulopathies associated with purpura.

C. Laboratory studies. The following studies should be obtained in the investigation of patients with suspected plasma cell neoplasms:

1. **Routine studies.** CBC, blood urea nitrogen, creatinine, electrolytes, calcium, albumin, and total protein.

2. **Serum proteins** evaluated with SPEP, immunofixation (IFE), and quantitative immunoglobulins (QIG). Because of the inherent variability of results of these tests, it is critical to perform all of these tests in diagnosing and following response to therapy. The following assays are also useful:

a. **Serum β_2-microglobulin (β2m)** reflects tumor mass and is a standard measure of tumor burden in MM.

b. **C-reactive protein (CRP)** is a surrogate marker for interleukin-6 (IL-6), which is a prime stimulator of myeloma growth.

c. **Lactic dehydrogenase (LDH)** may be a measure of tumor burden.

d. **Serum viscosity,** if hyperviscosity is suspected.

e. **Serum-free light chains.**

3. **Urine light chains.** Twenty-four–hour excretion of protein and urinary PEP (UPEP) and IFE of a specimen concentrated 100- to 200-fold (urine dipsticks are usually not sufficiently sensitive to detect light chains, and Bence-Jones protein assays are unreliable). About 20% of patients with MM have urinary M-proteins only, and 20% to 30% of patients will show the presence of both serum and urine M-protein. It is important to measure both the urine and the serum M-proteins on an ongoing basis to determine the patient's response to treatment.

Approximately 1% to 2% of patients with myeloma do not show the presence of serum or urine M-protein. This occurrence appears to result largely from aberrant rearrangements of the immunoglobulin genes that normally produce antibodies in the malignant plasma cells.

4. **Bone marrow aspiration and biopsy** are necessary to establish the diagnosis. Bone marrow findings are discussed in Section II.A. Flow cytometry may help confirm the diagnosis, but should not be used to evaluate the percentage of plasma cell involvement. Conventional cytogenetic studies frequently do not detect abnormalities given the low proliferative rate of MM. Biopsy of a solitary osteolytic lesion, masses, skin nodules, or enlarged lymph nodes may be necessary in selected cases.

5. **Evaluation of the skeleton**

a. **Complete skeletal radiographic survey,** including skull and long bones, is required in all patients suspected of having MM.

b. **MRI** of the spine may be necessary in some patients if there is a paraspinal mass or signs of cord or nerve root compression or solitary plasmacytoma of bone. This will determine if there is spinal cord involvement and can help to determine the extent of myeloma involvement in the spine. It has become more important to evaluate the spine accurately because of the development of several surgical techniques that help immensely in controlling back pain caused by compression fractures from bone loss in patients with MM.

c. **Computed tomography scan** (avoiding the use of contrast dyes) for evaluation of suspected bone involvement or plasmacytoma.

d. **Positron emission tomography (PET) scans** may be helpful to evaluate extent of disease. The routine use of PET scans is being evaluated to stage at diagnosis and to follow patients with MM.

e. **Bone scans** are of limited use in MM because most lesions are osteolytic, and bone scans require perilesional osteoblastic activity to be positive. Positive bone scans in MM usually indicate regions of fracture or arthritis, except in the rare event of osteoblastic myeloma.

f. **Bone densitometry** studies may be useful at diagnosis and are especially useful among MM patients without obvious osteolytic disease on plain films but who manifest osteopenia or osteoporosis. These assessments may identify patients who could benefit from bisphosphonate therapy. Patients with MGUS appear to be at high risk for osteopenia and osteoporosis; one should strongly consider baseline assessment of bone density in this high-risk group.

g. **Bone formation and resorption markers** may predict risk of skeletal complications but should not be performed routinely.

6. **Special studies.** Serum viscosity, cryoglobulins, and rectal biopsy or analyses of joint effusions for amyloid are obtained when indicated.

D. **Protein studies.** Serum immunoglobulin properties that have clinical relevance are listed in Table 23-1. Kinetic studies of protein synthesis in animals and humans show tumor burden to be closely correlated with the quantity of M-protein in the blood (approximately 1 g/dL corresponds to 100 g of tumor and 1×10^{11} plasma cells).

1. **Protein electrophoresis** is valuable for recognizing cases of monoclonal gammopathies and for following quantitative changes in spikes. SPEP will quantify the protein, but will not provide the heavy and/or light chain. The IFE will provide this information and is more sensitive for detection of a monoclonal protein than is the SPEP. Examples of serum and urine PEP patterns are shown in Figure 23-1.

   a. **M-proteins** appear as tall, narrow, sharply defined peaks (spikes) that reflect their structural homogeneity. They are usually located in the γ or γβ region. Monoclonal peaks in the α or αβ region are usually not caused by M-proteins but by reactant proteins (see Section IX.C).

   b. **IgG spikes** are usually tall, narrow, and located in the β region. **IgA spikes** are usually broader because the molecule tends to form polymers of different sizes; they are located in the β region. **IgM spikes** are usually located near the point of origin. **IgD spikes** usually cause only slight deflections in the pattern because the protein is present in a relatively small concentration.

   c. **Light chains** are not ordinarily found in the serum because light chains are rapidly catabolized by the kidney or excreted in the urine. Light chain spikes may be found in the serum of patients with renal insufficiency or in instances in which polymerization of light chains has occurred. Recent studies have used this assay to establish a more stringent complete response among MM patients.

      (1) The normal ratio of κ-to-λ chains in humans is 0.26 to 1.65. This normal ratio is usually maintained when excretion of light chains is owing to renal disease but is significantly altered when the excretion is caused by malignant gammopathies.

      (2) Urinary excretion of monoclonal light chains is found in 50% to 60% of patients with MM and in 10% to 20% of patients with WM. Patients with MGUS may also show light chains in the urine, but the amount of monoclonal urinary protein is usually <1 g/24 hr.

      (3) The serum-free light chains can be used, in addition to the urinary studies, to follow the extent.

2. **IFE** determines the exact heavy chain class (γ, α, μ, δ, ε) and light chain type (κ, λ) of the M-protein and distinguishes polyclonal and monoclonal increases in gamma globulins. IFE is more sensitive than PEP for low-concentration or heterogeneous globulin mixtures.

3. **QIG** estimations are excellent for measuring normal or decreased immuno-globulin levels. QIG are unreliable, however, if levels are markedly increased or if protein aggregation has occurred. The variability in QIG estimation with assays measured in the same laboratory over time limits the use of QIG for following response to therapy.

4. **Serum viscosity.** The rate of descent of serum at 37°C through a calibrated capillary tube is compared with that of distilled water. Plasma is not used because elevated levels of fibrinogen can markedly affect the results. Normal values for serum viscosity ratios range from 1.4 to 1.9. Symptoms usually do not develop unless the serum viscosity >4.

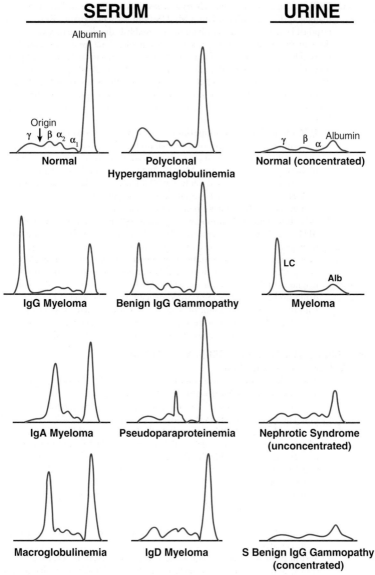

Figure 23-1 Electrophoresis patterns. Alb, albumin. **SERUM.** Normal: The point of application of serum is indicated. Polyclonal hypergammaglobulinemia: occurs in many conditions. Benign immunoglobulin G (IgG) gammopathy: normal levels of albumin and gamma globulins plus a peak in the γ region. Pseudoparaproteinemia: small peaks in β or α regions (see Section IX.C). **URINE.** Myeloma: typical homogeneous peak of light chains (LC) in γ region. Nephrotic syndrome: panproteinuria. Benign IgG gammopathy: normal pattern in urine.

E. **Differentiation of plasma cell dyscrasias.** In the absence of biopsy proof of malignant disease, differentiating MGUS from early malignant disease may be impossible at the initial examination. To establish the diagnosis, serial evaluations of the patient and M-protein level must be done for several months or years. These data predict benign or malignant monoclonal gammopathy, but none is diagnostic by itself; patients with MGUS may slowly progress to MM. About 25% of patients with MGUS progress to MM or a related B-cell malignancy (WM, lymphoma, or amyloidosis). The most important findings that suggest malignant disease are significant and progressive increases in the serum M-protein or urinary light chain concentration.

1. **IgM monoclonal gammopathies** may be benign or owing to WM, lymphoproliferative disorders, or epithelial tumors that can present with a serum abnormality years before the neoplasm becomes evident. Thus, the division of IgM gammopathies into MGUS, WM, and secondary macroglobulinemia is at times arbitrary. Only 0.05% of patients with myeloma present with an IgM monoclonal gammopathy; these patients have typical features of myeloma with osteolytic bone disease, renal dysfunction, or both.

2. **IgG, IgA, and IgD monoclonal gammopathies: diagnostic criteria for MM.** To establish the diagnosis of MM, there must be evidence of end organ damage or a biomarker predicting progression to end organ damage in the near future. High concentrations of monoclonal serum immunoglobulins (≥ 3 g/dL) are consistent with SMM, but are not alone sufficient for the diagnosis of MM. If the diagnosis of MM cannot be proved, the working diagnosis becomes MGUS or SMM depending on the level of the monoclonal protein and the amount of bone marrow involvement by clonal plasma cells. These patients must be monitored at very regular intervals to detect clinical or laboratory changes that may signal progression to MM.

IV. STAGING SYSTEMS AND PROGNOSTIC FACTORS

A. **Staging systems for MM**

1. **The classic Salmon-Durie staging system** for MM is shown in Table 23-3.

2. **The International Staging System** (ISS) has replaced the Salmon-Durie system and was recently revised to include LDH and cytogenetic abnormalities. The revised ISS (R-ISS) is now used for prognosis in the era of novel agents and utilizes LDH and cytogenetics by FISH in addition to β2m and albumin. For this system, del(17p), translocation t(4;14), and translocation t(14;16) are considered high risk. The absence of these factors is considered standard risk. The R-ISS consists of the following stages in the order of worsening prognosis:

   a. **Stage I:** serum β2 m < 3.5 mg/L and serum albumin $\geq$3.5 g/L with normal LDH and standard risk cytogenetics

   b. **Stage II:** neither stage I nor III

   c. **Stage III:** serum β2 m $\geq$ 5.5 mg/L and either high-risk cytogenetics or elevated LDH

3. **Serum β2m** is the light chain moiety of classic human leukocyte antigens (HLA) and is found on the surface membranes of most nucleated cells. Patients with MM and higher initial values of β2m appear to have a worse prognosis. Despite the high correlation of β2m levels with renal function, β2m has emerged as an important independent prognostic factor.

   a. Elevated β2m levels are also found in patients with acute or chronic myelocytic leukemia, lymphoproliferative disorders, myeloproliferative disorders, myelodysplastic syndromes, benign or malignant liver diseases, and autoimmune diseases.

TABLE 23-3	Salmon-Durie Staging System for Multiple Myeloma

Stage	Extent of Disease
I	**Low tumor mass** (<0.6 × 10^{12} plasma cells/m^2). Patients must have *all* of the following: Hemoglobin >10 g/dL Serum calcium: normal or ≤12 mg/dL Low M-component production rates 　IgG < 5 g/dL 　IgA < 3 g/dL 　UPEP M-component light chain < 4 g/24 hr Skeletal x-ray: normal or with a solitary plasmacytoma
II	**Intermediate tumor mass** (0.6–1.2 × 10^{12} plasma cells/m^2). Patients who qualify for neither stage I nor III
III	**High tumor mass** (>1.2 × 10^{12} plasma cells/m^2). Patients having *any one* of the following: Hemoglobin <8.5 g/dL Serum calcium >12 mg/dL High M-component production rates 　IgG > 7 g/dL 　IgA > 5 g/dL 　UPEP M-component light chain > 12 g/24 hr Extensive lytic bone lesions
Substage A	Serum creatinine < 2 mg/dL
Substage B	Serum creatinine ≥ 2 mg/dL

UPEP, urine protein electrophoresis.

    b. Serum albumin also is decreased among patients with poor outcome and represents an assessment of nutritional status as well as pro-MM cytokine activity.

B. Prognostic factors

    1. MGUS. Patients with MGUS progress to MM at a rate of 1% per year. There has been significant focus placed on attempting to identify which patients are at a higher risk of progression to MM. Three factors have been identified including non-IgG MGUS, serum monoclonal protein level ≥1.5 g/dL, and abnormal serum-free light chain. The risk for progression to MM at 20 years is 58% for patients with 3 risk factors, 37% for patients with 2 risk factors, and 21% with one risk factor.

    2. SMM. The risk of progression to MM is highest during the first 5 years at 10% per year and then decreases to 3% per year for the next 5 years. It further decreases to 2% per year after 10 years. Patients with increased bone marrow involvement (>10%), abnormal serum-free light chain ratio, or serum monoclonal protein >3 g/dL have an increased risk of progression. Studies are ongoing to determine if using these characteristics along with cytogenetic and molecular studies should be used to treat high-risk SMM before it progresses to MM.

    3. WM. Median survival has dramatically improved among these patients with median overall survival close to 10 years. The development of complications, such as hyperviscosity, hemorrhage, or infection, contributes to death. In fact, studies are now showing that many deaths may be attributed to myelodysplasia and secondary leukemias from drugs, especially purine analogs, that are used to treat WM. Age > 60 years, male gender, reduced IgM levels, and hemoglobin < 10 g/dL are associated with shortened survival time.

4. **MM.** The overall median survival of MM patients has dramatically improved during the past decade. The prognosis in MM is improving with the wide array of new agents available to treat patients.

a. **Labeling index (LI).** The LI is indicative of the percentage of cells undergoing mitosis. A high LI (>3%) is associated with a poor prognosis in MM.

b. **Cytogenetic abnormalities**

(1) **Abnormalities associated with a poor prognosis**

(a) Abnormalities involving loss of chromosome 17p remain a poor prognostic factor.

(b) Gains on the long arm of chromosome 1.

(c) Translocations t(14;16) and t(14;20).

(d) Translocation t(4;14) was formerly considered a poor prognostic factor; however, the use of novel agents, and proteasome inhibitors in particular, has moved this to an intermediate-risk factor.

(e) The absence of chromosome 13 is no longer considered an independent prognostic factor in MM. It is considered intermediate-risk factor.

(2) **Abnormalities associated with standard risk disease**

(a) Translocation t(11;14)

(b) Translocation t(6;14)

(c) Hyperdiploidy

c. **Renal function** previously was thought to be an important prognostic factor. Increasing degrees of azotemia were associated with progressively shorter life expectancies. Advances in plasmapheresis, dialysis, and supportive care have diminished this prognostic factor. The outcome for patients whose renal function normalizes with initial therapy is not different from that for patients who present with normal renal function.

d. **Response to therapy.** The depth of response has increasingly been noted as an important prognostic factor. Patients who show progressive disease during initial therapy have a worse outcome. In contrast, long-term maintenance of a complete disappearance of the M-protein is associated with an improved outcome. For this reason, measurement of minimal residual disease (MRD), performed by multiparametric flow cytometry or polymerase chain reaction (PCR), is being evaluated as a prognostic factor. It is currently being done in the context of clinical trials and is not routinely used as standard of care.

e. **Immunoglobulin class.** Although earlier studies suggested that patients with IgD or λ light chain disease had a worse prognosis, analyses of prognostic factors in large MM trials have not shown the paraprotein type to be a prognostic factor.

f. **Other prognostic factors.** The presence of a *p53* deletion, plasmablastic morphology, higher numbers of circulating monoclonal plasma cells, higher serum levels of LDH, or cytogenetics can predict for a more aggressive disease course. In early-stage disease, the pattern and number of MRI abnormalities predict both progression to symptomatic disease and overall survival. The gene expression profiling pattern may predict outcome as well.

V. PREVENTION AND EARLY DETECTION

The availability of PEP and of screening chemistry panels has probably resulted in earlier detection of monoclonal gammopathies. If IFE were used for screening populations, the incidence of MGUS might well double, but it is not clear that survival would be impacted.

VI. MANAGEMENT OF WM

A. Diagnosis

1. **Diagnostic criteria for WM**
   a. IgM monoclonal gammopathy of any concentration.
   b. Bone marrow infiltration by small lymphocytes, plasmacytoid lymphocytes, and plasma cells in a diffuse, interstitial, or nodular pattern.
   c. The immunophenotype is positive for surface immunoglobulin, CD19, and CD20 and is negative for CD5, CD10, and CD23.
   d. The MYD88 mutation L265P is present in 91% of cases.

2. **Additional workup at presentation**
   a. Chest x-ray study and CT scan of chest, abdomen, and pelvis
   b. Serum viscosity, cold agglutinins, and cryocrit
   c. Hepatitis serology

B. Treatment.
Patients with asymptomatic disease, without anemia, hyperviscosity, renal insufficiency, or neurologic abnormalities, should be monitored for clinical status and by PEP and IgM levels until disease progression is confirmed.

1. **Indications for treatment**
   a. Anemia or pancytopenia
   b. Symptomatic hyperviscosity, cryoglobulinemia, or neuropathy
   c. Bulky lymphadenopathy or symptomatic organomegaly
   d. Amyloidosis
   e. Cryoglobulinemia
   f. Cold agglutinin disease
   g. Transformation to another aggressive B-cell malignancy

2. **Treatment alternatives.** Patients are treated similarly to low-grade lymphomas (see Chapter 22). Hyperviscosity is relieved by plasmapheresis because >70% of the IgM protein is in the plasma rather than the tissues (see Section IX.A), but it is required only in a few patients with very high IgM levels.
   a. Treatment options for WM patients have changed dramatically during the past several years. Although alkylating agents were considered the initial therapy of choice, this is no longer the case. Current treatment options include monoclonal antibodies, chemoimmunotherapy, novel inhibitors, and chemotherapy. If patients have a low disease burden and severe cytopenias, single-agent rituximab is a reasonable option. Patients with a larger disease burden will often receive a bortezomib-based regimen, such as bortezomib, rituximab, and dexamethasone.
   b. Patients with WM should be treated with only several courses of these agents because decreases in M-protein can occur for many months after discontinuing therapy. In addition, treatment with rituximab may be associated with an initial rise in IgM, the so-called "flare" response, followed by a drop in serum IgM levels and tumor burden. Plasmapheresis should be considered for patients showing a very high pretreatment IgM level or a significant increase in IgM during the first 2 months of anti-CD20 treatment. Treatment of hyperviscosity with urgent plasmapheresis should always be the first step if the hyperviscosity syndrome is present. However, plasmapheresis alone is not sufficient to control the disease and should be followed with more definitive therapy.
   c. For progressive or relapsed disease, the first drug approved for WM, ibrutinib, is available. It is an oral medication that is an irreversible inhibitor of Bruton's tyrosine kinase (BTK). If patients have already received ibrutinib, they should be considered for a clinical trial.

VII. MANAGEMENT OF MGUS AND SOLITARY, SMOLDERING, OR STAGE I MM

A. MGUS. The optimal monitoring schedule for patients with MGUS is not clear, but most experts agree that patients should have a clinical and laboratory evaluation every 6 months. Patients with MGUS should not be treated with cytotoxic agents. Only patients showing significant rises in M-protein levels, new laboratory findings, or new symptoms should have additional diagnostic studies (bone marrow aspirate and biopsy, skeletal survey). It may be useful to obtain periodic bone density studies on these patients because of their higher risk to develop bone loss and fractures.

B. Solitary plasmacytoma of bone is potentially curable and is treated with at least 4,000 to 5,000 cGy of RT to the involved field. It is important to recognize that many patients treated for a solitary plasmacytoma of bone actually have systemic disease. These patients may benefit from PET–CT scan to identify possible additional disease that may require systemic therapy; the presence of additional lesions suggests that these patients are at high risk to develop MM. This should be taken into consideration before an attempt is made at curative local RT. The M-protein is measured every 3 to 6 months as indicated. Radiologic skeletal survey is performed annually or when symptoms develop.

C. Solitary extramedullary plasmacytoma is also potentially curable and is treated with 4,000 to 5,000 cGy of radiation therapy. The patients should undergo imaging and laboratory evaluation 3 to 4 months after completion of therapy. After this evaluation, most patients are followed every 3 months for the first 2 years, and then the visits are spaced. However, there is not a single accepted follow-up schedule, and there are institutional differences.

D. Smoldering MM

   1. Definition of smoldering MM
      a. M-protein $\geq$ 3 g/dL.
      b. Plasma cell infiltration of bone marrow is >10% but <60%.
      c. No anemia, lytic lesions (including MRI), renal failure, or hypercalcemia.
      d. Involved/uninvolved free light chain ratio <100.

   2. Clinical course. The majority of patients that progress will do so with a median time of 4.8 years. The risk factors for progression are outlined in Section IV.B.

   3. Treatment. Patients are observed without treatment until the disease progresses to MM (anemia, hypercalcemia, renal insufficiency, bone lesions) or associated amyloidosis. Several clinical trials are underway attempting to slow the progression of disease. In a study where patients with high-risk SMM were randomized to receive lenalidomide and dexamethasone versus observation, the patients in the lenalidomide and dexamethasone arm demonstrated a longer progression-free survival and overall survival rate at 3 years. At this point, treatment of SMM should occur only in the context of a clinical trial. Among patients with severe bone loss demonstrated on bone densitometry, it is certainly reasonable to consider treatment with bisphosphonates.

VIII. MANAGEMENT OF MM

The management of MM has changed substantially with the onset of the novel agents, specifically the proteasome inhibitors, immunomodulatory agents, and monoclonal antibodies. These in combination with stem cell transplantation have tripled the survival for patients with newly diagnosed MM. The first step in the decision process for patients with newly diagnosed MM is whether or not they are eligible for high-dose melphalan and autologous stem

TABLE 23-4	International Myeloma Working Group (IMWG) Response Criteria
Response	**Definition**
sCR = Stringent Complete Response	Negative immunofixation of blood and urine, disappearance plasma-cytoma, <5% plasma cells in the bone marrow, no evidence by flow cytometry
CR = Complete Response	Negative immunofixation of the blood and urine, disappearance plasmacytoma, <5% plasma cells in the bone marrow
VGPR = Very Good Partial Response	≥90% reduction in blood and urine M-protein, urine M-protein <100 mg/24 hr
PR = Partial Response	≥50% reduction in M-protein, ≥50% decrease in difference between light chains, ≥50% decrease in bone marrow involvement
SD = Stable Disease	Does not meet criteria for any of the above

cell transplantation (ASCT). For patients that are transplant eligible, they will undergo induction therapy followed by consolidation with stem cell transplantation and maintenance therapy. Transplant-ineligible patients undergo induction therapy followed by maintenance. The response to treatment is determined by the International Myeloma Working Group (IMWG) criteria, which is outlined in Table 23-4.

A. Common frontline (induction) regimens. Both doublet and triplet options are available for patients with newly diagnosed MM. There is not a standard of care for frontline treatment of MM and treatment regimens should be chosen based on patient and disease characteristics. Patients who are transplant eligible should have minimal exposure to cytotoxic agents. In general, melphalan-containing regimens are rarely used due to the availability of the novel agents, but should specifically be avoided in patients for whom a transplant is planned.

1. Immunomodulatory drugs (IMIDs). The mechanisms of action of the IMIDs (thalidomide, lenalidomide, and pomalidomide) include immunomodulatory and antiangiogenic properties. The agents are very active in MM but differ in their toxicity profile. The dose-limiting side effects are neurologic (somnolence, peripheral neuropathy) for thalidomide and myelosuppression for lenalidomide and pomalidomide. All three are teratogenic and thrombophilic. Venous thromboembolism prophylaxis with aspirin is recommended in all patients receiving IMIDs. Pomalidomide is only approved in the relapsed and refractory setting.

    a. Thalidomide (with dexamethasone or other steroids): a dose of 100 mg PO daily at night is as effective, but with fewer neuropathic effects, than higher doses.

    b. MPT (cycle frequency is every 4 weeks)
    Melphalan: 4 mg/m^2 daily on days 1 through 7
    Prednisone: 40 mg/m^2 daily on days 1 through 7
    Thalidomide: 100 mg daily at night

    c. MPR (cycle frequency every 28 days)
    Melphalan: 9 mg/m^2 (0.18 mg/kg) PO daily on days 1 through 4
    Prednisone: 2 mg/kg PO daily on days 1 through 4
    Revlimid (lenalidomide): 10 mg PO daily on days 1 through 21

    d. Rev/Dex (cycle frequency is every 4 weeks)
    Revlimid (lenalidomide): 25 mg PO daily for 21 days followed by a 7-day rest period
    Dexamethasone: 40 mg PO weekly

e. **Response rates**

   (1) **Thalidomide** as a single agent leads to durable responses in one-third of relapsing patients. The response rate to thalidomide plus dexamethasone is 60% with a 15% complete response rate. The side effects of this medication limit its use, and the second- and third-generation IMIDs, lenalidomide and pomalidomide, respectively, are used instead.

   (2) **Lenalidomide** with dexamethasone is also associated with a 60% response rate and approximately 20% complete response. The number of lenalidomide combination therapies is rapidly increasing, and they demonstrate higher response rates with some of these new regimens approaching 100% (e.g., RVD below).

2. **Proteosome inhibitor regimens.** The currently available proteasome inhibitors include bortezomib, carfilzomib, and ixazomib. Bortezomib is frequently used as part of a two- or three-drug regimen for front-line therapy. Dose-limiting side effects of bortezomib are peripheral neuropathy (predominantly sensory) and myelosuppression (especially thrombocytopenia). Carfilzomib is approved after two lines of therapy, and ixazomib is approved for patients who have received 1 to 3 prior lines of therapy. These medications are presently being studied in combinations in the frontline setting. Shingles reactivation occurs with this drug class, and patients should receive antiviral prophylaxis. The regimens listed below are potential first-line therapies for patients with MM.

   a. **Bortezomib/Dex** (cycle frequency is every 3 weeks)
      Bortezomib: 1.3 mg/m^2 SC days 1, 4, 8, and 11
      Dexamethasone: 40 mg PO weekly

   b. **BMP** (cycle frequency is every 6 weeks)
      Bortezomib: 1.3 mg/m^2 SC on days 1, 4, 8, 11, 22, 25, 29, and 32
      Melphalan: 9 mg/m^2 PO daily on days 1 through 4
      Prednisone: 60 mg/m^2 PO daily on days 1 through 4

   c. **CyBorD** (cycle frequency every 4 weeks)
      Cyclophosphamide: 300 mg/m^2 PO on days 1, 8, 15, and 22
      Bortezomib: 1.3 mg/m^2 SC on days 1, 4, 8, and 11
      Dexamethasone: 40 mg PO on days 1 through 4, 9 through 13, 17 through 20, and 11

   d. **RVD** (cycle frequency every 3 weeks)
      Revlimid: 25 mg PO daily on days 1 through 14
      Velcade (bortezomib): 1.3 mg/m^2 SC on days 1, 4, 8, and 11
      Dexamethasone: 40 mg PO on days 1, 8, and 15

   e. **Response rates.** Although bortezomib as a single agent shows a 30% response rate, adding steroids increases the response rate to >50%. The three-drug combination of RVD is associated with response rates of well over 90%.

B. **Older chemotherapy regimens for MM.** These regimens are rarely used, but are listed here for historical purposes. The overall response rates were around 30% with increased myelosuppression and side effects compared to the current treatment regimens.

   1. **Dexamethasone alone:** 40 mg PO daily for 4 days every other week

   2. **M&P** (cycle frequency is 4 to 6 weeks)
      Melphalan: 10 mg/m^2 PO on days 1 through 4
      Prednisone: 60 mg/m^2 PO on days 1 through 4

3. **VAD** (cycle frequency is 4 weeks)
   Vincristine: 0.4 mg/d for 4 days by continuous IV infusion
   Doxorubicin (Adriamycin): 9 mg/m^2/d for 4 days by continuous IV infusion
   Dexamethasone: 40 mg PO on days 1 through 4, 9 through 13, and 17 through 21
4. **EC** (cycle frequency is every 4 weeks)
   Etoposide: 100 mg/m^2 IV on days 1 through 3
   Cyclophosphamide: 1,000 mg/m^2 IV on day 1
5. **DVD** (cycle frequency every 4 weeks)
   Doxil (liposomal doxorubicin): 30 to 40 mg/m^2 IV on day 1
   Vincristine: 2 mg IV on day 1
   Dexamethasone: 40 mg PO on days 1 through 4
C. **Duration of therapy.** Transplant-eligible patients should receive 4 to 6 cycles of therapy followed by mobilization of the peripheral blood progenitor cells if a partial response (PR) or better is achieved. This would be followed by high-dose melphalan and reinfusion of the previously cryopreserved progenitor cells. For transplant-ineligible patients, they should receive 6 to 8 cycles of therapy followed by maintenance. The optimal time to continue therapy is unclear and depends on the patient and disease characteristics as well as the tolerability of the regimen. Several studies have demonstrated the efficacy and tolerability of prolonged administration of the novel agents, specifically bortezomib and lenalidomide.
   1. **Maintenance therapy** with bortezomib and lenalidomide has been studied in the transplant-eligible and transplant-ineligible population. One trial demonstrated a benefit of bortezomib maintenance over thalidomide maintenance with respect to progression-free survival and overall survival. However, this trial used a conventional chemotherapy induction regimen as well as tandem ASCT. The most widely used maintenance after ASCT is lenalidomide. In two large, randomized, placebo-controlled trials, maintenance with lenalidomide was compared to observation (placebo arm.) In both studies, patients received a novel induction regimen followed by ASCT. After ASCT, the patients were randomized to receive lenalidomide maintenance with one trial administering lenalidomide for 2 years and the other giving lenalidomide until disease progression or side effects that limited further administration. Both trials showed a progression-free survival benefit of lenalidomide over observation. Only the trial that continued lenalidomide until disease progression showed a survival benefit. The long-term follow-up from this trial has not yet presented. Given these findings, the length of maintenance therapy is controversial, but most recommend at least 2 years of maintenance therapy after ASCT.
D. **High-dose regimens and transplantation**
   1. **High-dose therapy with ASCT** in some studies is associated with increased rates of complete remission, improved event-free survival, and increased overall survival. Other studies, however, have not shown a difference in overall survival despite the higher complete remission rate among patients who have high-dose therapy. It remains a standard of care for patients with newly diagnosed MM who are eligible.
   Stem cells are harvested from the peripheral blood of patients at the time of maximal response to induction therapy. Autologous peripheral blood stem cell transplantation (SCT) is not curative. Improvements in supportive care have reduced the treatment-related mortality (TRM) rate to 1% in most centers.
   2. **Allogeneic SCT** is associated with high TRM rates (nearly 40%); thus, the use of this procedure has been reduced to primarily clinical trials for younger patients who have a compatible donor and have progressed on all

other available therapies. Studies have used donor leukocyte infusions with some reduction in M-protein levels but also with significant graft versus host disease toxicity. Some studies attempted to decrease the TRM by using reduced intensity conditioning regimens or T-cell depletion. However, the increased relapsed rate associated with these approaches has not been able to demonstrate a clear benefit over autologous SCT.

3. **Autologous bone marrow transplantation.** Because many tumor cells are found in the autograft, attempts have been made to *purge* autografts of tumor using stem cell selection. Although this procedure successfully eliminates tumor cells in the autograft, it does not improve overall survival, probably because of the relatively high tumor burden remaining in the patient even after myeloablative chemotherapy.

E. **Relapsed and refractory disease.** There are a number of new therapeutics approved for these patients including proteasome inhibitors, immunomodulatory agents, epigenetic modifiers, and monoclonal antibodies. The choice of regimen for patients should be based on disease and patient characteristics. For disease characteristics, previous therapies, number of previous therapies, ability to tolerate therapy, goals of therapy, and trajectory of disease should be considered. The patient characteristics to consider include age, performance status, comorbidities, organ function, and residual side effects from previous therapies (i.e., peripheral neuropathy). Table 23-5 lists several of the potential treatment options for relapsed and refractory patients based on the number of previous therapies.

1. **Proteosome inhibitors.** As mentioned previously, there are three available proteasome inhibitors: bortezomib, carfilzomib, and ixazomib.

   a. **Bortezomib.** In relapsed and refractory patients, bortezomib has been combined with dexamethasone, lenalidomide and dexamethasone, bendamustine and dexamethasone, and cyclophosphamide and dexamethasone. Patients who have not previously received bortezomib or patients in whom bortezomib produced a favorable response followed by a different treatment regimen or period of observation are ideal candidates for this medication in the relapsed setting.

   b. **Carfilzomib** is approved in the relapsed and refractory setting in combination with dexamethasone and in combination with dexamethasone and lenalidomide. The combination of carfilzomib and dexamethasone showed a doubling of progression-free survival compared to bortezomib and

TABLE 23-5	Therapeutic Options for Patient With Relapsed and Refractory Multiple Myeloma	
1–3 Prior Lines	**>2 Prior Lines**	**>3 Prior Lines**
Daratumumab, lenalidomide, dexamethasone		
Daratumumab, bortezomib, dexamethasone		
Elotuzumab, lenalidomide, dexamethasone	Pomalidomide, dexamethasone	Daratumumab
Bortezomib, dexamethasone	Carfilzomib, dexamethasone	Bendamustine, bortezomib, dexamethasone (off label)
Bortezomib, lenalidomide, dexamethasone	Carfilzomib, lenalidomide, dexamethasone	
Ixazomib, lenalidomide, dexamethasone	Carfilzomib, pomalidomide, dexamethasone (off label)	
Lenalidomide, dexamethasone		
CyBorD		

dexamethasone in patients with relapsed MM. It is given as a twice-weekly infusion for three weeks followed by one week off therapy. A weekly dosing schedule is being evaluated. Severe cardiotoxicity has been reported in 3% to 5% and should be used with caution in patients with severe underlying cardiovascular disease. Peripheral neuropathy is rare with carfilzomib.

  c. Ixazomib is an oral proteasome inhibitor that is given once weekly for three weeks, followed by one week off therapy. It is approved for relapsed and refractory patients who have received 1 to 3 previous lines of therapy. GI toxicity and thrombocytopenia are the most notable side effects, but can be managed with appropriate dose reductions. Similar to carfilzomib, peripheral neuropathy is rare with this medication.

2. **Epigenetic modifier.** The first pan-histone deacetylase inhibitor to be studied in MM was vorinostat in combination with a proteasome inhibitor, but no benefit was seen. The more potent inhibitor, panobinostat (Farydak), was then evaluated in combination with bortezomib and dexamethasone in relapsed and refractory patients. A progression-free survival benefit was seen, and the combination of bortezomib, panobinostat, and dexamethasone is approved for patients who have received 1 to 3 prior lines of therapy. GI toxicity is the main side effect, and panobinostat is packaged with loperamide.

3. **Monoclonal antibodies.** Given the immune dysfunction present in MM and loss of surface markers with terminal B-cell maturation, effective monoclonal antibodies were not developed until very recently. The two approved monoclonal antibodies are elotuzumab (Empliciti) and daratumumab (Darzylex).

  a. Elotuzumab is an anti-CS1 monoclonal protein that works through antibody-dependent cellular cytotoxicity (ADCC) and has the unique mechanism of Fc receptor binding to CD16 to further activate natural killer cells and augment ADCC. Elotuzumab does not have single-agent activity, but does have activity in combination with an immunomodulatory agent. The combination of elotuzumab, lenalidomide, and dexamethasone produced a progression-free survival benefit compared to lenalidomide and dexamethasone alone in patients with relapsed and refractory MM. Elotuzumab is very well tolerated and is approved in combination with lenalidomide and dexamethasone for patients who have received 1 to 3 prior lines of therapy.

  b. Daratumumab is an anti-CD38 monoclonal antibody that has single-agent activity in heavily pretreated patients with MM. It was initially approved as a single agent for patients who have received >3 lines of therapy. Currently it is also approved in combination with dexamethasone plus lenalidomide or bortezomib for the treatment of patients who have received at least 1 prior therapy. Addition of daratumumab to lenalidomide and dexamethasone reduced the risk of disease progression or death by 63% and to bortezomib, and dexamethasone reduced the risk of progression or death by 61%. The most prominent side effect is infusion reactions, which are usually only present on the first infusion. Patients require significant premedication and slow infusions. The monoclonal antibody also interferes with type and screen testing for packed red blood cell transfusion and will cause false-positive antibody results. Type and screen samples should be treated with dithiothreitol (DTT) and transfused K-units.

4. **IMIDS.** Lenalidomide and pomalidomide are used in combination with dexamethasone in the relapsed and refractory setting. Pomalidomide in combination with dexamethasone has shown response rates as high as 60% in patients with relapsed MM. It is approved for patients who have received as leave 2 prior therapies.

F. **Supportive care** is extremely important in MM. Mobility is frequently limited due to the pain from lytic lesions and due to fractures. Patients should be referred for physical and occupational therapy. Bed rest further promotes bone demineralization, which may lead to hypercalcemia.

1. **Bisphosphonates** (pamidronate, 90 mg IV over >2 hours, or zoledronic acid, 4 mg IV over 15 minutes) given monthly are indicated for all patients with stage II or III MM (and perhaps stage I as well). These agents have significantly decreased the incidence of skeletal complications in this disease. Bisphosphonates reduce pain and analgesic usage and prevent the deterioration of quality of life compared with placebo. Bisphosphonates are also discussed in Chapter 34.

   a. A large randomized study showed that monthly zoledronic acid not only reduced skeletal complications but also improved overall survival compared to a weaker oral bisphosphonate, clodronate, administered daily among previously untreated MM patients who also required anti-MM treatment.

   b. It is important to recognize that these agents occasionally are associated with renal dysfunction. Pamidronate more often will cause a glomerular lesion initially associated with proteinuria, which may be at nephrotic levels. By contrast, zoledronic acid more often causes tubular dysfunction and, thus, is not often associated with albuminuria.

   c. Bisphosphonates are associated with an increased risk of **osteonecrosis of the jaw** (ONJ). This complication occurs more frequently among patients who have had recent dental surgery or trauma, poor dental hygiene, or who abuse alcohol or use tobacco. Before initiating bisphosphonate treatment, patients should have a complete dental examination, and any dental extractions or removal of jawbone(s) should be completed several months before initiating these drugs to reduce the risk of ONJ.

      The course of ONJ is variable, and many patients do not show worsening of the condition, although this can occur. No studies have evaluated whether discontinuing these drugs among patients with this complication affects the course of ONJ. It is clear that surgical intervention to treat this problem should be kept to a minimum and undertaken only by dental professionals experienced with this problem.

   d. Reports of **atypical fractures** of the femurs and of the metatarsal bones of the feet have been made among patients who receive long-term bisphosphonate treatment.

2. **Skeletal complications**

   a. **Surgery** for MM is restricted to orthopedic procedures (also see Chapter 34). Fractures of long bones usually require fixation with a medullary pin and postoperative irradiation. Sometimes, impending fractures with large osteolytic lesions of the femoral head are internally fixed prophylactically. If the diagnosis of the underlying disease is in doubt, acute spinal cord compression or vertebral fracture may make laminectomy necessary. Either vertebroplasty or kyphoplasty should be considered for symptomatic vertebral compression fractures. Kyphoplasty may reverse the compression fracture and can lead to immediate and sustained pain relief for patients with symptomatic vertebral compression fractures, especially when they occur in either the thoracic or the lumbar spine. The risk of leakage of the cement appears to be lower with this procedure than with vertebroplasty, although these procedures have not been compared with one another in any randomized trials. However, a recent randomized study shows the superiority of immediate kyphoplasty to nonsurgical management for cancer patients with vertebral compression fractures, and myeloma was the most common type of cancer among enrolled patients.

b. **RT** in low doses is useful for palliation of lesions that are localized or that cause spinal cord or nerve root compression. Small subcutaneous tumors or small painful lesions in bone may be treated with only a single dose of 800 cGy. Large osteolytic lesions in long bones should be irradiated before a fracture occurs. Large lytic lesions or paraspinous masses rarely need >2,000 cGy given over 5 days. Many patients, however, will have significant pain relief with effective treatment of their underlying myeloma. In some patients, it may be prudent to wait before initiating RT to relieve pain. Because of the radiosensitizing effects of several anti-MM agents including anthracyclines (such as doxorubicin and its liposomal formulation) and bortezomib, use of these drugs may have to be delayed during the period of time that the patient undergoes RT.

c. **Back pain** is relieved by RT unless the pain is caused by compression fracture. Because spinal cord compression is a common complication in MM, the physician should not hesitate to order an MRI or CT myelogram in patients with MM who have new or changing back pain. This should be treated emergently if it occurs (see Chapter 33, Section III).

The use of RT to the spine should be done judiciously. The spine represents a large reservoir for the production of normal bone marrow, and thus, its compromise with RT must be taken into consideration among patients who will require myelotoxic treatment for their underlying disease. Given the high response rates approaching 100% with some of the newer anti-MM regimens, treating patients with cord compression with systemic therapy alone is being done with increasing frequency.

d. **Pain relief** may be achieved with focal RT. Analgesics should be prescribed in a regimen that gives the most consistent pain relief. Nonsteroidal anti-inflammatory drugs (NSAIDs) should be avoided to decrease the chances of renal dysfunction. However, often, systemic myeloma therapy effectively relieves bone pain rapidly without subjecting patients to the side effects of RT.

e. **Ambulation** should be maximized as early as possible after the onset of fractures or pain. Corsets and braces may be effective in relieving back pain by stabilizing the spine, but often, patients will do just as well with well-designed physical therapy regimens.

f. **Calcium and vitamin D deficiencies** occur in many patients with myeloma, and serum calcium levels may also be reduced with bisphosphonate treatment. Thus, oral calcium (1,000 mg daily) is recommended. Monitoring of serum calcium is necessary, however, because occasionally patients may develop hypercalcemia.

All patients with MM should have baseline vitamin D levels assessed and their dose of vitamin D adjusted accordingly. Regardless, patients should receive 800 to 1,200 IU daily. It is important to discontinue both calcium and vitamin D supplementation should the patient become hypercalcemic.

g. **Fluoride** is not effective in increasing bone remineralization in patients with MM; fluoride treatment results only in increased bone density because of fluorosis.

3. **Infections** are the foremost cause of death in patients with MM. Infections must be investigated and treated urgently. These patients have similar infections to other cancer patients treated with chemotherapy. In fact, the risk for infection is primarily during periods of chemotherapy-induced neutropenia or in the terminal stages of the disease. Patients receiving proteasome inhibitors should receive antiviral prophylaxis as herpes zoster infections occur commonly among patients receiving this drug.

Although the use of prophylactic antibiotics and intravenous immunoglobulins (IVIG) may be attempted in patients with recurrent infections, most patients do not require these interventions. IVIG therapy should be considered in cases of recurrent, life-threatening infections.

Pneumococcal and influenza vaccine should also be considered. Because it is a live vaccine, vaccination with the herpes zoster vaccine should be avoided in MM patients.

4. **Renal failure** is best prevented by hydration, treatment of hyperuricemia and hypercalcemia, and avoidance of both IV contrast media and NSAID. Recent randomized studies have not demonstrated the benefit of plasmapheresis. When renal failure becomes severe, some patients may be candidates for hemodialysis treatment, especially if they have a reasonable prognosis and have not failed initial therapy. Azotemia may improve slowly in these patients; it may take several months for these patients to discontinue dialysis treatment.

IX. SPECIAL CLINICAL PROBLEMS IN PATIENTS WITH PLASMA CELL DISORDERS

A. **Plasma alterations in patients with M-proteins**
1. **Hyperviscosity syndrome.** The blood cells normally contribute more to the whole blood viscosity than do plasma proteins. The development of hyperviscosity with M-proteins depends on their concentration and their ability to aggregate or polymerize. WM is typically associated with hyperviscosity. Symptoms usually do not occur unless the serum M-protein concentration exceeds 4 g/dL and the serum viscosity index exceeds 4.
   a. **Complications** of hyperviscosity include the following:
      (1) **Bleeding diathesis** is manifested by spontaneous bruising, purpura, retinal hemorrhages, epistaxis, or mucosal bleeding. The hemorrhagic diathesis is compounded by thrombocytopenia. Bleeding in the hyperviscosity syndrome appears to be a result of the following:
         (a) **Interference with coagulation,** especially the third stage of coagulation (polymerization of fibrin monomer), resulting in prolongation of clotting times
         (b) **Impaired platelet function** resulting in abnormalities of bleeding times, clot retraction, and other platelet functions
      (2) **Retinopathy** is manifested by venous dilation and segmentation ("link-sausage" appearance), retinal hemorrhages, and papilledema.
      (3) **Neurologic symptoms,** which develop in about 25% of patients, include malaise, focal neurologic defects, stroke, and coma.
      (4) **Hypervolemia** develops with an increase of M-protein concentration, resulting in distention of peripheral blood vessels and increased vascular resistance. Plasma volume expansion may actually lessen the viscosity but may also precipitate congestive heart failure (which occurs in about 10% of patients who have hyperviscosity).

    b. Management. Hyperviscosity syndrome is treated by reducing the quantity of M-protein in the serum. Reduction of M-protein concentrations with cytotoxic agent therapy takes several weeks or months. Symptomatic patients should be treated with plasmapheresis, 4 to 6 units daily, until the viscosity index is <3. Patients with hyperviscosity caused by monoclonal IgM usually respond to plasmapheresis more rapidly than those with IgG or IgA gammopathies because IgM has a predominantly intravascular distribution (Table 23-1). Additionally, an exponential relationship exists between serum viscosity and IgM level so that, for example, a 20% decrease in IgM concentration results in a 100% decrease in serum viscosity. Improvement should be monitored by noting changes in clinical findings, coagulation tests, and serum viscosity determinations.

  2. Cold sensitivity may afflict patients with M-proteins (especially IgM) that have physicochemical properties that permit cold precipitation. The cryoglobulins in plasma cell dyscrasias and lymphoproliferative disorders are monoclonal. The cryoglobulins in other disorders (e.g., collagen vascular diseases and viral infections) are circulating soluble immune complexes (IgM–IgG, IgA–IgG, IgG–IgG). Manifestations include cold urticaria, Raynaud phenomenon, and vascular purpura in the absence of severe thrombocytopenia.

  3. Cold agglutinins are IgM with a specificity for specific red blood cell antigens (usually Ia) at temperatures <37°C. These proteins may be responsible for a mild extravascular complement-dependent hemolysis and acrocyanosis, but not for other symptoms of cold sensitivity unless cryoglobulins are also present.

  4. Pseudohyponatremia may be observed with high levels of M-proteins (plasma water is displaced by the M-protein).

  5. Pseudo-low HDL cholesterol (HDL-C). Low levels of HDL-C may be found because paraproteins can interfere with HDL-C measurements in various automated analyzers.

  6. Anion gaps, noted with measurement of serum electrolytes (serum concentration of sodium chloride bicarbonate), may be decreased in patients with cationic monoclonal proteins. The decreased gap is produced by the increase of chloride and bicarbonate anions.

B. Peripheral neuropathy (PN)

  1. PN associated with gammopathy occurs especially in patients with IgM monoclonal gammopathies. About 5% of patients with a sensorimotor neuropathy have an associated monoclonal gammopathy. Nearly 10% of patients with WM or with MGUS and an IgM paraprotein develop a demyelinating PN. Sural nerve biopsies demonstrate monoclonal IgM deposition on the outer myelin sheath. The antibody can be shown to react with MAG in half of the cases. These patients usually have a mostly sensory or ataxic polyneuropathy, whereas patients with non–MAG-reactive antibodies usually have both a sensory and a motor component to their neuropathy. Treatment with plasmapheresis may be effective in some cases. Other forms of treatment have included high doses of glucocorticosteroids, IVIG, and rituximab.

  2. PN associated with treatment. PN more often results from treatment of plasma cell disorders with agents such as thalidomide or bortezomib. Most patients receiving thalidomide will develop irreversible neuropathy after 6 months of treatment. Approximately half of patients treated with bortezomib develop treatment-related neuropathy, which occasionally may be painful but is reversible in most cases. The risk of neuropathy with these two agents is directly related to the dose used. Also, longer cycles, changes in schedule (weekly compared to twice weekly), and subcutaneous route of administration are also associated with a reduction in the occurrence and severity of PN with bortezomib administration. Drugs such as gabapentin (Neurontin), pregabalin (Lyrica), duloxetine (Cymbalta), doxepin, and over-the-counter alpha-lipoic acid may be helpful to reduce the severity of this complication.

C. **Pseudoparaproteinemia.** The PEP can detect serum proteins when the concentration is >200 mg/dL. In certain situations, a nonimmunoglobulin homogeneous protein concentration may be >300 mg/dL and appears as a spike on PEP. The location of these spikes usually are in the α and β regions but may be in the β–γ region. The differential diagnosis is clarified by review of the clinical picture, the location of the PEP spike, and IEP. Conditions that may produce pseudoparaproteinemia include the following:

1. Hyper-α_1-globulinemia (acute-phase reactant in many inflammatory and neoplastic diseases)
2. Hyper-α_2-globulinemia (nephrotic syndrome or hemolysis)
3. Hemoglobin–haptoglobin complexes (intravascular hemolysis)
4. Hyperlipidemia
5. Hypertransferrinemia (iron deficiency)
6. Bacterial products
7. Desiccated serum
8. Fibrinogen (if plasma is measured)

D. **Pseudomyeloma.** Several malignancies, including lymphoma and cancer of the breast, bowel, or biliary tract, can be associated with the production of an M-protein. These same malignancies may produce lytic lesions in the skeleton and induce marrow plasmacytosis. Pseudomyeloma must be distinguished from true myeloma.

E. **Therapy-linked acute leukemia** is discussed in Chapter 35, Section I.C in "Cytopenia."

F. **Heavy chain diseases** (HCD) are rare plasma cell lymphocytic neoplasms characterized by secretion of abnormal heavy chains (γ, α, or μ) without light chains (κ, λ). α-HCD is the most common, and μ-HCD is the rarest. The heavy chains may also be excreted in the urine and detected by urine PEP. Normal immunoglobulin levels are usually suppressed. Diagnosis of these disorders necessitates detailed immunochemical investigation. IEP is the crucial test; it should demonstrate reaction of antisera with the appropriate heavy chain but not with light chains.

1. α-**HCD** nearly always involves only the α_1 subtype of heavy chain and is associated with GI lymphomas.
2. γ-**HCD** usually affects elderly patients. Generalized lymphadenopathy, hepatosplenomegaly, involvement of Waldeyer ring, fever, pancytopenia, and eosinophilia are common features of the disease. The illness initially resembles granulomatous disease or Hodgkin disease. Biopsies of lymph nodes and bone marrow are rarely diagnostic. The disease has a variable course, developing over a few months to several years. A satisfactory treatment plan has not been established.
3. μ-**HCD** nearly always occurs in patients with CLL, and the two disorders are treated in the same manner. In μ-HCD, however, lymphadenopathy is infrequent, and in contrast to other HCDs, large amounts of κ light chains

are excreted in the urine. The rare disease may be suspected when a patient with CLL has unusual vacuolated plasma cells (characteristic of μ-HCD) in the bone marrow.

G. **Amyloidosis** may be primary (with or without associated plasma cell or lymphoid neoplasms), secondary to a variety of chronic inflammatory diseases or hereditary disorders (familial Mediterranean fever), or associated with the aging process. The disease is characterized by organ deposition of fibrillar substances of many different types. The fibrils are mostly or exclusively composed of immunoglobulin light chains (especially the l type) in amyloidosis associated with primary amyloidosis and myeloma, but the fibrils are composed of substances other than light chains in secondary amyloidosis.

1. **Organ distribution of amyloid.** The various forms of amyloidosis overlap considerably. **Secondary amyloidosis** affects the kidneys, spleen, liver, or adrenal glands and rarely involves the heart, GI tract, or musculoskeletal system. **Primary amyloidosis and amyloidosis associated with MM** mostly affect the heart, GI tract, skeletal muscle, ligaments (carpal tunnel syndrome), and periarticular and synovial tissue (articular manifestations) as well as the tongue (macroglossia) and skin. Skin involvement most commonly is located in the periorbital and skinfold regions and is manifested by spontaneous purpura and ecchymoses, which may be aggravated by coagulation factor X deficiency, which occasionally accompanies amyloidosis; postproctoscopic eyelid ecchymoses are characteristic. Involvement of the respiratory tract, endocrine glands, and peripheral and autonomic nervous systems also occurs.

2. **Diagnosis**

   a. **Biopsy** of an involved organ (especially the bone marrow, carpal ligament, sural nerve, rectum, or gingivae) must be performed to establish the diagnosis of amyloidosis; liver or renal biopsy may result in hemorrhage. Amyloid deposits have a homogenous eosinophilic appearance on light microscopy. Confirmation is made by the demonstration of specific birefringence by polarized microscopy of specimens stained with Congo red.

   b. **Monoclonal light chains** in the urine are found in both the primary type and in amyloidosis associated with MM. Many patients with primary amyloidosis are found to have developed a plasma cell dyscrasia, if they survive sufficiently long. On the other hand, patients with MM or WM may develop amyloidosis.

3. **Prognosis.** The prognosis of patients with amyloidosis has improved to 3 to 4 years with the introduction of many new agents, although the prognosis varies greatly depending on the type of amyloid, the sites and extent of organ involvement, and other possible associated plasma cell disease. Patients with primary amyloidosis generally have the worst outcome. Those with cardiac involvement have the worst prognosis, whereas patients with renal disease have a better outcome. Newer prognostic factors include serum uric acid, troponin, and brain-type natriuretic peptide levels.

4. **Treatment** of amyloidosis is directed at both the affected organs and the underlying process producing the amyloid deposits. Data are insufficient to identify optimal therapy for this plasma cell disorder. Treatment options are similar to MM and include CyBorD, bortezomib and dexamethasone, IMIDs, and high-dose melphalan with autologous SCT. Results of a randomized study, however, showed no overall survival advantage with high-dose therapy compared with conventional treatment despite the increase in

progression-free survival with the more intensive treatment. Recent studies show that thalidomide and lenalidomide, with or without the addition of glucocorticoids and bortezomib, are very effective for patients with amyloidosis and may lead to long-term remissions. The significant neurotoxic side effects of both thalidomide and bortezomib must be considered in choosing these agents for patients with amyloidosis-associated neuropathy.

H. Papular mucinosis (lichen myxedematosus) is a dermatologic condition characterized by cutaneous papules and plaques that result from the deposition of a mucinous material. The disease is often preceded by chronic pyoderma. It demonstrates an M-protein, usually IgG-l, with a characteristic mobility (slower than any other gamma globulin component), and a strong affinity for normal dermis. Other manifestations of MM (plasmacytosis, osteolysis, and excretion of light chains) are rare. Treatment with melphalan is often beneficial.

ACKNOWLEDGMENTS

The authors would like to acknowledge Drs. James R. Berenson and Dennis A. Casciato, who significantly contributed to earlier versions of this chapter.

Suggested Readings

Multiple Myeloma

Attal M, et al. Single versus double autologous stem-cell transplantation for multiple myeloma. *N Engl J Med* 2003;349:2495.

Attal M, et al. Lenalidomide maintenance after stem-cell transplantation for multiple myeloma. *N Engl J Med* 2012;366:1782.

Berenson J, et al. Balloon kyphoplasty versus non-surgical fracture management for treatment of painful vertebral body compression fractures in patients with cancer: a multicenter, randomized controlled trial. *Lancet Oncol* 2011;12:225.

Cavo M, et al. International Myeloma Working Group consensus approach to the treatment of multiple myeloma patients who are candidates for autologous stem cell transplantation. *Blood* 2011;117:6063.

Dimopoulos MA, et al. Renal impairment in patients with multiple myeloma: A consensus statement on behalf of the International Myeloma Working Group. *J Clin Oncol* 2010;28:4976.

Korde N, et al. Monoclonal gammopathy of undetermined significance (MGUS) and smoldering multiple myeloma (SMM): novel biological insights and development of early treatment strategies. *Blood* 2011;117:5573.

Kumar SK, et al. Safety and tolerability of ixazomib, an oral proteasome inhibitor, in combination with lenalidomide and dexamethasone in patients with previously untreated multiple myeloma: an open label phase ½ study. *Lancet Oncol* 2014;15:1503.

Kyle RA, et al. Review of 1027 patients with newly diagnosed multiple myeloma. *Mayo Clin Proc* 2003;78:21.

Kyle RA, et al. Clinical course and prognosis of smoldering (asymptomatic) multiple myeloma. *N Engl J Med* 2007;356:2582.

Lokhorst HM, et al. Targeting CD38 with daratumumab monotherapy in multiple myeloma. *N Engl J Med* 2015;373:1207.

Lonial S, Cavanaugh J. Emerging combination treatment strategies combining novel agents in newly diagnosed multiple myeloma. *Br J Haematol* 2009;145:681.

McCarthy PL, et al. Lenalidomide after stem-cell transplantation for multiple myeloma. *N Engl J Med* 2012;366:1770.

Morgan G, et al. First-line treatment with zoledronic acid as compared with clodronic acid in multiple myeloma (MRC Myeloma IX): a randomized controlled trial. *Lancet Oncol* 2010;376:1989.

Palumbo A, Anderson K. Multiple myeloma. *N Engl J Med* 2011;364:1046.

Palumbo A, et al. Revised international staging system for multiple myeloma: a report from the international myeloma working group. *J Clin Oncol* 2015;33:2863.

Raje N, Roodman GD. Advances in the biology and treatment of myeloma bone disease. *Clin Cancer Res* 2011;17:1278.

Richardson PG, et al. Lenalidomide, bortezomib, and dexamethasone combination therapy in patients with newly diagnosed multiple myeloma. *Blood* 2010;116:679.

San Miguel JF, et al. Bortezomib plus melphalan and prednisone for initial treatment of multiple myeloma. *N Engl J Med* 2008;359:906.

San Miguel JF, et al. Panobinostat plus bortezomib and dexamethasone versus placebo plus bortezomib and dexamethasone in patients with relapsed or relapsed and refractory multiple myeloma: a multicenter, randomized, double-blind phase 3 trial. *Lancet Oncol* 2014;15:1195.

Shah JJ, Orlowski RZ. Proteasome inhibitors in the treatment of multiple myeloma. *Leukemia* 2009;23:1964.

Sonneveld P, et al. Bortezomib induction and maintenance treatment in patients with newly diagnosed multiple myeloma: results of the randomized phase III HOVON-65/GMMG-HD4 trial. *J Clin Oncol* 2012;30:3654.

Weber D, et al. Thalidomide alone or with dexamethasone for previously untreated multiple myeloma. *J Clin Oncol* 2003;21:16.

Van de Donk NW, et al. Clinical efficacy and management of monoclonal antibodies targeting CD38 and SLAMF7 in multiple myeloma. *Blood* 2016;127:681.

Zhou Y, et al. The molecular characterization and clinical management of multiple myeloma in the post-genome era. *Leukemia* 2009;23:1941.

Other Topics

Comenzo R. How I treat amyloidosis. *Blood* 2009;114:3147.

Merlini G, et al. Amyloidosis: pathogenesis and new therapeutic options. *J Clin Oncol* 2011;29:1924.

Migliorati CA, et al. Osteonecrosis of the jaw and bisphosphonates in cancer: a narrative review. *Nat Rev Endocrinol* 2011;7:34.

Rajkumar SV, et al. Monoclonal gammopathy of undetermined significance, Waldenstrom macroglobulinemia, AL amyloidosis, and related plasma cell disorders: diagnosis and treatment. *Mayo Clin Proc* 2006;81:693.

Treon SP, et al. CD20-directed antibody-mediated immunotherapy induces responses and facilitates hematologic recovery in patients with Waldenstrom's macroglobulinemia. *J Immunother* 2001;24:272.

Vijay A, Gertz MA. Waldenstrom macroglobulinemia. *Blood* 2007;109:5096.

Chronic Leukemias

Herbert Eradat and Ronald L. Paquette

CHRONIC LYMPHOCYTIC LEUKEMIA

I. EPIDEMIOLOGY AND ETIOLOGY

A. **Incidence.** Chronic lymphocytic leukemia (CLL) is the most common type of leukemia in Western countries, accounting for one-third of cases. The incidence in the United States is 3.5 per 100,000. Ninety percent of patients are >50 years of age, and the median age at diagnosis is approximately 71 years. Men are affected more often than women by a ratio of 2:1.

B. **Etiology**

1. **Genetic factors.** The vast majority of cases are sporadic. Familial clusters of CLL have been described. Indeed most important risk factor for the development of CLL is a family history of CLL. 8% to 10% of patients with newly diagnosed CLL have a family history of CLL. The relative risk among first-degree relatives of persons with CLL is between 7.0 and 8.5. This suggests an inherited, rather than environmental, basis for familial CLL. Some CLL kindreds suggest a dominant inheritance. Genome-wide linkage studies in familial CLL have identified chromosome 2q21.2 as associated with inheritance of CLL. However, no causative genes have been identified at this locus. The etiology in the majority of cases is unknown.

2. **Immunologic factors.** Inherited and acquired immune deficiency is often associated with CLL and other lymphoproliferative neoplasms. This observation supports a concept that defective immune surveillance may result in proliferation of malignant cell clones and increased susceptibility to potential leukemogenic transduction, such as by viruses.

3. **Molecular and cytogenetic aberrations.** Somatic mutations of the immunoglobulin gene take place in the germinal center of secondary lymphoid follicles after antigen exposure. IgV_H hypermutations are detected in approximately half of the cases of CLL, indicating that the cells are derived from postgerminal center or memory B cells and do not express ZAP-70, a molecule usually required for selective activation of T cells but aberrantly expressed in some cases of (B-cell) CLL. Some cases of CLL show characteristics of naive B cells with unmutated antigen receptors and are ZAP-70 positive.

   Chromosomal abnormalities are detected in >80% of cases of CLL by use of interphase fluorescence *in situ* hybridization (FISH). CLL is characterized by loss or gain of chromosomal genetic material rather than by translocations. Conventional cytogenetics typically miss these abnormalities. Incidence, genes involved, and clinical features of the most common chromosome abnormalities are shown in Table 24-1.

4. **Radiation and cytotoxic agents.** Populations exposed to ionizing radiation or cytotoxic chemotherapy are not associated with an increased incidence of CLL.

TABLE 24-1	Chromosomal Abnormalities in Chronic Lymphocytic Leukemia		
Chromosome	Frequency (%)	Involved Genes	Clinical Characteristics
Del 13q14.3	>50	Telomeric to *RB1*	Good prognosis, low CD38, mutated V$_H$ genes
Del 11q22–q23	19	*ATM*	Poor prognosis, extensive lymphadenopathy
Trisomy 12	15	*MDM-2*	Intermediate prognosis, high CD38, unmutated V$_H$ genes, atypical morphology
Del 17p13.3	15	*p53* (deleted)	Poor prognosis, >10% prolymphocytosis, Richter transformation

II. PATHOLOGY AND NATURAL HISTORY

A. Pathology. CLL had been considered a disease of accumulation, due to a defect in programmed cell death. Another proposed model CLL pathogenesis suggests that in a genetically susceptible host, there is tonic stimulation of B cells by a stereotyped antigen, likely a low-affinity autoantigen. This initiates expansion of a premalignant clone, and through a combination of tonic antigenic stimulation, acquisition of somatic genetic mutations, and support from the tumor microenvironment, the potentially autoreactive clone escapes immune surveillance and begins to expand.

1. **Loss of apoptosis.** 13q14 deletion is the most common genetic abnormality in CLL. MicroRNAs are small nonprotein coding RNAs that modulate the levels of certain proteins by biding sequence complimentary mRNAs. In CLL, the 13q14 deletion results in a deletion of microRNA miR15/16 cluster with consequent up-regulation of antiapoptotic BCL2 proteins.

2. **B-cell receptor signaling.** Approximately half of CLL cases show immunoglobulin heavy chain (IGH) mutations, and the other half show an unmutated IGH. The former group typically has a more indolent disease course. Both groups of B cells are derived from memory B cells. The IGH unmutated CLL cells have the capacity for proliferation in response to B-cell receptor stimulation. These IGH unmutated cells may be autoreactive and normally would be targeted for apoptosis, but avoid cell death through either tonic BCR stimulation or transforming genetic events. On the other hand in the IGH mutated cells, B-cell receptor signaling favors an anergic and antiapoptotic response.

3. **Tumor microenvironment.** In lymphoid organs, nurse-like cells (NLCs), large CD14$^+$ mononuclear cells, constitutively express the chemokines CXCL12 (stromal-derived factor-1α [Sdf-1]) and CXCL13. CLL cells express CXCR4 (the receptor for Sdf-1), and this interaction promotes cell survival through activation of STAT3 and MAPK pathways. NLCs also secrete B-cell activating factor (BAFF) and a proliferation-inducing ligand (APRIL). Engagement of these ligands with CLL cells induces intracellular NF-κB1 and MCL-1. NLCs can deliver multiple prosurvival signals that utilize distinct signaling pathways. CD4+ T cells express CD40L, which engages CD40 expressed on the surface of CLL cells thus inducing the NF-κB pathway. The tumor microenvironment thus enhances CLL cell resistance to apoptosis and chemotherapy.

4. **Acquired genetic factors.** Acquired chromosomal abnormalities involving chromosomes 11, 12, 13, and 17 are common in CLL. In addition,

a number of recurrently mutated genes have been identified, including NOTCH1, MYD88, TP53, and SF3B1. The mutations can coexist with some of the chromosomal abnormalities analyzed by FISH.

   a. Patients with trisomy 12 follow a somewhat more aggressive course than those patients with normal FISH. The genes that contribute to CLL pathogenesis in trisomy 12 remain unknown. There appears to be an association between tri12 and the presence of mutations in the *NOTCH1* gene, which extends the half-life of the protein.

   b. Patients with 11q22-23 deletion (approximately 15% of CLL patients) experience an aggressive clinical course with shorter survival. This deletion involves the radixin (*RDX*) and ataxia telangiectasia mutated (*ATM*) genes, crucial for DNA repair. Deletion of this region likely leads to enhanced clonal aggressiveness and evolution due to the acquisition of novel genomic variants.

   c. Patients with 17p deletion (approximately 7% of CLL patients) almost invariably have an aggressive clinical course because of loss of *TP53*. More than 80% of cases with del(17p13) have single nucleotide somatic mutations of the TP53 allele on the other chromosome 17 (the allele in trans), thereby causing near complete loss of TP53 function. This deletion is a prime facilitator of clonal evolution to a more aggressive disease. The number of leukemic cells with del(17p) often increases in patients who do not respond to therapy or who relapse after chemotherapy.

   d. NOTCH1 mutations. There is a clear relationship between the *NOTCH1* mutation and poor patient outcome, resistance to therapy, and transition to Richter transformation.

5. **Expression of cell surface or intracellular markers.** Expression of CD38 and ZAP-70 plays critical roles in the pathogenesis of CLL.

   a. Cell surface CD38 has a pivotal role in initiating and modulating a series of input signals from the microenvironment. CD38 is localized in close contact with the BCR complex (CD19/CD81) and with molecules regulating homing (CXCR4 and CD49d). Once in contact with accessory cells such as NLCs, its engagement triggers activation of intracellular signaling pathways that include ZAP-70 and ERK1/2. These signals increase chemotaxis and proliferation of neoplastic B cells.

   b. Intracellular ZAP-70 retards internalization of surface membrane IgM and CD79b from the cell membrane, leading to prolonged BCR pathway signaling. ZAP-70⁺ CLL cells are more likely to express adhesion molecules such as CD49d and chemokine receptors. These promote migration toward a series of chemokines and inhibit apoptosis.

B. **Natural history**
   1. **Immunologic abnormalities in CLL**
      a. **Hypogammaglobulinemia.** Advanced disease is associated with hypogammaglobulinemia and an increased risk of infection with encapsulated bacterial organisms.

      b. **Abnormal T-cell repertoire and function.** A variety of *in vitro* lymphocyte function tests are abnormal. T-cell numbers may be elevated but the T-cell repertoire may be contracted. The numbers of circulating T cells are elevated 2.5 to 4 times normal, at least pretherapy. The T-cell repertoire is significantly contracted in CLL, with oligoclonal and monoclonal subsets. Suppressive regulatory T cells (T_{reg}) are increased in patients with CLL. Immunomodulatory cytokines such as IL-6, IL-10, and TGF-β shift the helper T-cell response from a Th1 response to an anergic Th2 response.

   c. **Monoclonal paraproteins** may not be routinely identified; however, most patients with CLL secrete small amounts of paraproteins (usually immunoglobulin M [IgM]). These paraproteins almost never produce symptoms of hyperviscosity.

   d. **Coombs-positive warm antibody hemolytic anemia** occurs in about 10% of CLL patients and immune thrombocytopenia in about 5%. Immune neutropenia and pure red blood cell aplasia are rare.

   e. **Skin cancers.** Compared with the general population, the incidence of skin carcinoma is increased eightfold and visceral epithelial cancers twofold in patients with CLL.

2. **Clinical course.** The natural history of CLL is highly variable. Because most patients are elderly, >30% die of diseases unrelated to leukemia.

   a. **Manifestations.** In most patients, CLL is first recognized at routine physical examination (showing adenopathy or hepatosplenomegaly) or by a routine CBC (with evidence of lymphocytosis). Clinical manifestations develop as the leukemia cells accumulate in the lymph nodes, spleen, liver, and bone marrow.

     (1) **Pulmonary infiltrates and pleural effusions** are common late in the course of disease.

     (2) **Renal involvement** is common in CLL, but functional impairment is unusual in the absence of obstructive uropathy, pyelonephritis, autoimmune nephropathy, or hyperuricemia secondary to tumor lysis from therapy.

     (3) **Transformation** into a diffuse large cell lymphoma (Richter syndrome) or prolymphocytic leukemia occurs in <5% of all patients with CLL; however, this is estimated to be higher in patients who have required therapy for their disease.

     (4) **Skin involvement** is rare.

     (5) **Osteolytic lesions and isolated mediastinal involvement** are unusual and suggest a diagnosis other than CLL.

   b. **Progressive disease** is accompanied by deterioration of both humoral and cell-mediated immunity. As the disease progresses, patients develop progressive pancytopenia, persistent fever, and inanition. Death is usually caused by infection, bleeding, or other complications of the disease.

     (1) **Herpes zoster** is the cause of 10% of infections in CLL patients.

     (2) **Bacterial pathogens** associated with hypogammaglobulinemia include *Streptococcus pneumoniae*, *Haemophilus influenzae*, and *Legionella* sp.

     (3) ***Pneumocystis jiroveci*** may be the causative infectious agent in patients with pulmonary infiltrates, especially in those who have had therapy with corticosteroids, purine nucleoside analogues, or PI3 kinase inhibitors.

III. DIAGNOSIS

A. **Symptoms and signs.** Patients with CLL that was discovered incidentally are usually asymptomatic. Chronic fatigue and reduced exercise tolerance are the first symptoms to develop. Advanced disease and progressive disease are manifested by severe fatigue out of proportion to the degree of the patient's anemia and by fever, bruising, and weight loss.

   Lymphadenopathy, splenomegaly, and hepatomegaly should be carefully assessed. Edema or thrombophlebitis may result from obstruction of lymphatic or venous channels by enlarged lymph nodes.

B. **Laboratory studies**
1. **Hemogram**
   a. **Erythrocytes.** Anemia may be caused by lymphocyte infiltration of the bone marrow, hypersplenism, autoimmune hemolysis, and other factors. Red blood cells are usually normocytic and normochromic in the absence of prominent hemolysis.
   b. **Lymphocytes.** The absolute lymphocyte count is typically elevated. It may exceed 500,000/mL. Lymphocytes are usually mature appearing with scanty cytoplasm and clumped nuclear chromatin. When blood smears are made, the cells are easily ruptured, producing typical "basket" or "smudge" cells.
   c. **Granulocytes.** Absolute granulocyte counts are normal until late in the disease.
   d. **Platelets.** Thrombocytopenia may be produced by bone marrow infiltration, hypersplenism, or immune thrombocytopenia.
2. **Other useful studies** that should be obtained in patients with CLL include the following:
   a. Biologic markers of the disease. FISH for trisomy 12, del(11q), del(13q), and del(17p). Metaphase karyotype analysis for complex karyotypes. TP53 sequencing.
   b. Molecular analysis to detect IGH (variable region) mutation status.
   c. CD38 and ZAP-70 expression by flow cytometry.
   d. Flow cytometry of the peripheral blood lymphocytes for typical markers of CLL. (positive for CD5, CD19, CD20, CD23; negative for CD10) (See Appendix B3).
   e. Renal and liver function tests.
   f. Hepatitis B testing (hepatitis B surface antibody, hepatitis B surface antigen, and hepatitis B core antibody), if therapy with an anti-CD20 monoclonal antibody is planned.
   g. Direct antiglobulin (Coombs) test, reticulocyte count, fractionated bilirubin, and haptoglobin.
   h. Serum protein electrophoresis and serum quantitative immunoglobulins.
   i. Computed tomography (CT) scans, which can be used to evaluate mediastinal, retroperitoneal, abdominal, and pelvic lymph nodes. PET CT is useful to assess for hypermetabolic nodes and directing lymph node biopsy if there is suspicion of Richter transformation.
3. **Bone marrow examination** is usually not necessary to establish the diagnosis in patients with persistent lymphocytosis. The pattern of bone marrow infiltration is prognostic factor (see Section IV.A.2). The indications for bone marrow aspiration and biopsy may include the following:
   a. Thrombocytopenia, to distinguish immune thrombocytopenia from severe bone marrow infiltration
   b. Coombs-negative, unexplained anemia
4. **Lymph node biopsy** in patients with CLL shows malignant lymphoma of the small lymphocytic type. A lymph node biopsy is not indicated in CLL unless Richter transformation is suspected.
C. **Establishing the diagnosis of CLL.** The National Cancer Institute (NCI) Working Group on CLL has established useful guidelines for the minimum diagnostic requirements for this disease, which are as follows:
1. Absolute peripheral blood lymphocytosis ($\geq$5,000/μL) that is sustained, with mature-appearing lymphocytes

2. **Characteristic immunophenotype**
   a. Monoclonal (kappa or lambda light chain restricted) B cells
   b. Expression of pan–B-cell antigens (CD19, CD20, and CD23)
   c. Coexpression of CD5 on the leukemic B cells
   d. Exclusion of Mantle cell lymphoma via cyclin D1 or FISH for t(11;14)
   e. Surface immunoglobulin of low intensity (most often IgM)

D. **Differential diagnosis**
   1. **Benign causes of lymphocytosis in adults:** The lymphocytes are polyclonal and tend to appear activated.
      a. Viral infections, especially hepatitis, cytomegalovirus, and Epstein-Barr virus (EBV). Lymphadenopathy and hepatosplenomegaly are absent or mild in elderly patients with infectious mononucleosis. The presence of fever, LFTs compatible with hepatitis, and positive EBV serologies should distinguish mononucleosis from CLL. Other viral serologies should also be evaluated.
      b. Brucellosis, typhoid fever, paratyphoid, and chronic infections.
      c. Autoimmune diseases; drug and allergic reactions.
      d. Thyrotoxicosis and adrenal insufficiency.
      e. Postsplenectomy state.
   2. **Monoclonal B-cell lymphocytosis** can have the characteristic immunophenotype identical to CLL, with monoclonal B cells with B-cell antigens CD19, CD20, and coexpression of CD5 and CD23. This entity however presents with absolute monoclonal B lymphocyte <5,000/μL. Adenopathy and other clinical features of a lymphoproliferative disorder are absent. This can be seen in about 5% of normal adults over age 40; a small percentage of these patients however can progress to CLL.
   3. **Mantle cell lymphoma** must be differentiated from CLL. The natural history and management of the two disorders are different. Circulating lymphocytes in Mantle cell lymphoma have a characteristic immunophenotype of monoclonal (kappa or lambda light chain restricted) B cells with expression of B-cell antigens (CD19, CD20) and coexpression of CD5 on the leukemic B cells, but typically lack expression of CD23. The cells are positive by immunohistochemistry for cyclin D1, and FISH is positive for t(11;14).
   4. **Hairy cell leukemia** must be differentiated from CLL. Management of the two disorders is different. Diagnosis depends on recognizing the pathognomonic hairy cells by immunophenotyping (see Appendix B3). This entity is also positive for the *BRAF* V600E mutation.
   5. **Cutaneous T-cell lymphomas** are suspected if skin involvement is extensive. Differentiation from CLL is made by identifying the convoluted nuclei and helper T cells phenotype (by immunohistochemistry and flow cytometry) that are characteristic of this disease (see Appendix B3).
   6. **Leukemic phase of non-Hodgkin lymphoma** (NHL) is usually distinguished from CLL morphologically and immunologically. Follicular lymphoma, marginal zone lymphoma, Mantle cell lymphoma, hairy cell leukemia, and diffuse large B-cell lymphoma may all present with circulating monoclonal B lymphocytes. NHL cells are often cleaved, whereas CLL cells are never cleaved. In addition, NHL cells demonstrate intense surface immunoglobulins without the CD5 and CD23 antigens, and the opposite is generally true for CLL cells.
   7. **Prolymphocytic leukemia** has large lymphocytes with prominent nucleoli. Lymphadenopathy is minimal; splenomegaly is massive (see Section VI.B).

8. **Large granular lymphocytic leukemia/lymphoma** (LGLL) has a characteristic morphology with abundant pale to clear, sharply defined cytoplasm and multiple distinct azurophilic granules of varying size. The cells are either T cells or NK cells, and most correspond to natural killer cells. The immunophenotype is positive for CD3, CD8, CD16, and CD57. LGLL is indolent and almost uniformly associated with neutropenia. Rheumatoid arthritis is present in about one-third of patients.

IV. STAGING SYSTEM AND PROGNOSTIC FACTORS

A. **Prognostic factors.** Routine CBC may detect asymptomatic cases of CLL, but this has no bearing on the overall survival of these patients.

1. **Clinical staging** is helpful for determining prognosis and deciding when to initiate treatment. Anemia and thrombocytopenia adversely affect prognosis when they are due to leukemic infiltration ("packing") of the bone marrow but not when they are due to autoimmune destruction of red blood cells or platelets.

2. **The pattern of bone marrow infiltration** also appears to affect prognosis. Patients with nodular or interstitial patterns of bone marrow involvement have longer survival than patients with diffuse ("packed") involvement.

3. **IgV genes.** Two subsets of CLL are defined by the IgV_H mutational status. Patients with somatic mutations of the V_H genes generally have a better prognosis than those with unmutated V_H genes.

4. **CD38 expression** on CLL cells (>30%) generally is associated with a poorer prognosis than absent or low-level expression of CD38.

5. **Chromosome abnormalities.** The presence of del(11q) and/or del(17p) is associated with short progression-free survival despite chemotherapy and chemoimmunotherapy approaches. Presence of del(17p) maintains its unfavorable effect even in patients treated with B-cell receptor signaling inhibitors. Complex karyotype with >2 unrelated chromosome abnormalities, in more than one cell on karyotyping of stimulated CLL cells, is also associated with an unfavorable prognosis. In contrast, del(13q) as the sole abnormality on FISH is associated with a favorable prognosis. Trisomy 12 is generally thought to carry an unfavorable prognosis.

6. **Other adverse prognostic factors** include a lymphocyte doubling time of <12 months and an elevated serum β_2-microglobulin level.

B. **Staging system.** Two staging systems are utilized. The *modified Rai classification* of CLL as well as Binet staging system. For patients with cytopenias, immune-mediated cytopenias are not used as the basis for these stage systems. (Table 24-2) (see Section III.C for differences with the NCI Working Group criteria).

TABLE 24-2	The Modified Rai Classification of Chronic Lymphocytic Leukemia		
Stage	**Extent of Disease**	**Risk**	**Median Survival (yr)**
0	Lymphocytosis of bone marrow (40% lymphocytes) and blood (>5,000/mL)	Low	10
I	Stage 0 plus lymphadenopathy	Intermediate	7
II	Stage 0 or I plus splenomegaly and/or hepatomegaly	Intermediate	7
III	Stage 0, I, or II plus anemia (hemoglobin < 11.0 g/dL)[a]	High	2
IV	Stage 0, I, or II plus thrombocytopenia (platelets < 100,000/mL)[a]	High	2

[a]Excluding anemia or thrombocytopenia caused by immunologic destruction of cells.

V. MANAGEMENT

A. Indications for treatment. CLL is usually an indolent disease. Treatment of asymptomatic stable disease is not warranted. The magnitude of the blood lymphocyte count does not indicate the need to start therapy. The initiation of therapy should be timed according to the clinically assessed pace of disease. Complete remission has traditionally not been the goal, although as more effective treatment strategies have become available, complete remission and minimal residual disease are becoming more important. The indications for instituting therapy in CLL are as follows:

1. Persistent or progressive systemic symptoms related to CLL, including fever, sweats, weight loss, sever fatigue.
2. Lymphadenopathy that is symptomatic causes mechanical obstruction or threatens end organ function.
3. Progressive enlargement of the lymph nodes, liver, or spleen.
4. Stage III or IV (high-risk) disease that results from the replacement of bone marrow with lymphocytes.
5. Immune hemolysis or immune thrombocytopenia.
6. Rapid lymphocyte doubling time.

B. Treatment options

1. **Nucleosides.** Purine nucleoside analogues (**fludarabine, cladribine** [2-chlorodeoxyadenosine, 2 CdA], or **pentostatin**) may be the initial treatment of choice for patients who would benefit from a rapid and sustained remission, such as those designated for further aggressive therapy. Fludarabine is superior to alkylating agents, and it is associated with an increased complete response rate and duration of response but not in overall survival. Prolonged treatment with this class of drugs is associated with marked immunosuppression and an increased risk of opportunistic infections, autoimmune hemolysis, and myelodysplasia. Typically, these nucleosides are combined with an alkylating agent and/or anti-CD20 monoclonal antibodies.

2. **Alkylating agents** remain useful and effective for palliative therapy. Patients with del(11q) benefit from this class of compounds in their regimen of therapy. **Chlorambucil** is effective for palliative therapy. **Cyclophosphamide** is typically combined with nucleoside analogues and anti-CD20 monoclonal antibodies. **Bendamustine** is an alkylating agent with purine-like benzimidazole ring. It has low cross-resistance with other alkylating agents. It is also typically combined with anti-CD20 monoclonal antibodies.

3. **Monoclonal antibodies** are highly useful for CLL particularly in the context of chemoimmunotherapy.

   a. Rituximab is an anti-CD20 chimeric monoclonal antibody. In the frontline setting, rituximab monotherapy has modest activity with an overall response rate of approximately 50%, but complete remission rates are relatively low. This is a highly tolerable regimen of therapy with no significant myelosuppression. It may be an appropriate option for patients who have substantial comorbidities or decreased performance status. For CLL, by convention, the standard dose is different from doses of 375 mg/m^2 given in NHL. The standard dose in patients with CLL is 375 mg/m^2 on week 1, followed by 500 mg/m^2 at subsequent infusions. Remission rate with single-agent therapy is low. However, rituximab is not typically associated with myelosuppression. Primary toxicity is infusion-related cytokine release syndrome that is typically associated with the first infusion.

  b. **Obinutuzumab** is a glycoengineered humanized type II anti-CD20 monoclonal antibody. Data suggest that in combination with chlorambucil, it is superior in efficacy to chlorambucil alone and chlorambucil with rituximab.

  c. **Ofatumumab** is another anti-CD20 monoclonal antibody, fully human. It is effective as single agent for the treatment of CLL refractory to fludarabine and alemtuzumab. In treatment of patients with previously untreated CLL who are inappropriate candidates for fludarabine-based regimens, it, in combination with chlorambucil, has established superiority to chlorambucil alone, in terms of overall response rate and complete response rate.

  d. **Alemtuzumab** is a humanized anti-CD52 monoclonal antibody whose antigen is expressed on more than 95% of mature B and T lymphocytes and may be used for the treatment of fludarabine-refractory CLL. Alemtuzumab preferentially eliminates CLL cells from the blood, bone marrow, and spleen but is less effective in nodal sites of disease. Approximately one-third of the patients will have a partial response to alemtuzumab; complete responses are rare. Alemtuzumab can cause cytokine release syndrome, immunosuppression, and neutropenia. The acute infusion reactions following intravenous administration are markedly reduced with subcutaneous injection. The immunosuppression has resulted in opportunistic infections so that trimethoprim/sulfamethoxazole (Bactrim) and acyclovir are recommended for prophylaxis.

4. **Immunomodulatory agents. Lenalidomide** is modestly active in CLL. As a single agent, it has an overall response rate of approximately 56% with no complete remissions. Major morbidity associated with the drug is tumor flare reaction occurring in more than 85% of patients. It is also associated with neutropenia, thrombocytopenia, anemia, or febrile events. There are data suggesting that a subgroup of patients with unmutated IgV_H, and in older patients with 11q abnormality, may have a higher overall response rate and a higher complete remission rate with this class of agents. Due to noted significant toxicity associated with this agent, its use outside of clinical trials is not recommended.

5. **B-cell receptor signaling inhibitors.** A number of novel small molecule inhibitors targeting Phosphoinositide-3 (PI3) kinase and Bruton's tyrosine kinase (BTK) are effective in CLL.

  a. **Ibrutinib** is a covalent binding reversible inhibitor of BTK. It is administered via continuous daily dosing of 420 mg, until progression or toxicity is noted. Ibrutinib causes a "compartment shift" with rapid improvement of adenopathy and concomitant early mobilization of lymphocytes into the blood. This lymphocytosis can be dramatic, but clinical sequelae including leukostasis are extremely rare. If there is evidence for overall clinical improvement, this should not be mistaken for progressive disease. Resolution of lymphocytosis may be protracted and incomplete; however, this does not appear to impact progression-free survival. Ibrutinib is effective for previously untreated patients as well as those with relapsed or refractory disease. In patients with del(17p) ibrutinib is also highly active with nodal response rate >80%. It is well tolerated. Bleeding events have been observed, especially with concomitant warfarin. It is also associated with atrial fibrillation.

  b. **Idelalisib** is an oral inhibitor of PI3 kinase delta isoform. It has been approved, in combination with rituximab for treatment of relapsed refractory CLL. Also, in combination with bendamustine and rituximab (BR), there is improvement in overall survival, in comparison to BR alone, for patients with relapsed refractory CLL. Its toxicity profile includes hepatotoxicity, especially in the first 3 months of therapy; rash; diarrhea/colitis and pneumonia/pneumonitis; CMV reactivation; and PJP pneumonia.

C. **Treatment considerations.** CLL is a disease of older adults, with a median age of 72 at diagnosis, and comorbidities are often present in this patient population. Comorbidities including performance status, age, renal function, marrow reserves, and physical fitness should be considered in selection of therapy for patients with CLL. In addition, del(17p) should be assessed before initiation of therapy as these patients may benefit from regimes other than cytotoxic chemotherapy. Del(11q) should be assessed before initiation of therapy as well, as these patients may benefit from alkylators in their regimen of therapy.

D. **Modern combination therapies** have resulted in high response rates (70% to 95%) and high complete response rates (20% to 65%) in previously untreated patients. **Prophylaxis** with fluconazole, acyclovir, and Bactrim is recommended for all chemoimmunotherapy strategies.

1. **Chemoimmunotherapy**
   a. **Fludarabine, cyclophosphamide, and rituximab (FCR)** combination is associated with an overall response rate in excess of 90% with complete remission rate of approximately 44%. This combination is superior to FC in terms of PFS and OS.
   b. **Pentostatin, cyclophosphamide, and rituximab (PCR)** combination has demonstrated similar significant clinical activity to FCR.
   c. **Bendamustine and rituximab (BR)** combination, in previously untreated patients, showed an overall response of 88% and complete remission rate of 23%, with a reasonable durability response.

      FCR and BR have been compared as frontline therapy for CLL patients without 17p deletion. The overall response rate was similar in both treatment groups, with no difference in overall survival; however, the FCR regimen resulted in a higher complete remission rate, more minimal residual disease–negative status, and consequently longer immediate progression-free survival. As such, FCR remains the standard frontline therapy for previously untreated fit patients. FCR is however associated with significantly more frequent severe infection, especially in the older patient population.
   d. **Rituximab with high-dose methylprednisolone** has an overall response rate >95% with a complete remission rate of about 32%, progression-free survival of 30.5 months. Prophylaxis with fluconazole, acyclovir, and Bactrim is recommended.
   e. **Obinutuzumab and chlorambucil** or **rituximab and chlorambucil** combinations are other options with high response rates of around 80% and complete remission rates of 10% to 15%. This combination with rituximab is somewhat inferior to chlorambucil with obinutuzumab but is recommended if the patient cannot tolerate obinutuzumab.

2. **B-cell receptor signaling inhibitors**
   a. **Ibrutinib** as single-agent continuous therapy is another option for adults with previously untreated CLL. This agent has demonstrated efficacy in CLL, including, but not limited to, disease characterized by del(17p), in the frontline and relapsed setting. Overall response rates were 86%, with few CR rates (4%).

b. Idelalisib and **rituximab** combination is a reasonable therapeutic choice for patients with relapsed CLL who have comorbidities and are not candidates for chemoimmunotherapy options. Overall response was 81%, with majority of the patients achieving a PR.

E. Treatment of relapsed or refractory disease. A number of highly effective therapeutic options are available for patients with relapsed disease, as enumerated in the sections above; however, the ideal treatment of these patients is not known. Ibrutinib continuous dosing monotherapy or the combination of idelalisib and rituximab is a reasonable option. Retreatment with chemoimmunotherapy is also an option, especially for those who have had a durable response from prior chemoimmunotherapy courses (e.g., an initial response duration greater than the median progression-free survival for a particular treatment regimen).

F. Radiation therapy (RT). Local irradiation is recommended only for reduction of lymph node masses that threaten vital organ function and that respond poorly to chemotherapy. Splenic irradiation may result in improvement of disease elsewhere and may temporarily improve signs of hypersplenism; however, the clinical usefulness of splenic irradiation has not been established.

G. Surgery. Splenectomy is seldom indicated in CLL. It is sometimes considered in patients who have immune hemolytic anemia or immune thrombocytopenia that either fails to respond to IVIG, corticosteroid, or rituximab therapy or must be treated with corticosteroids chronically. Splenectomy may also be considered in patients with symptomatic splenomegaly or functional hypersplenism.

VI. SPECIAL CLINICAL PROBLEMS IN CLL

A. Richter syndrome. About 5% to 10% of patients with CLL develop a diffuse large cell lymphoma with rapid clinical deterioration. The clinical features include fever, weight loss, increasing localized or generalized lymphadenopathy, lymphocytopenia (as well as other cytopenias), and dysglobulinemia. Combination chemotherapy with R-CHOP or R-EPOCH is usually initiated. Patients should be considered for postremission autologous or allogeneic transplantation.

B. Prolymphocytic leukemia is a rare variant of CLL. The main clinical feature is massive splenomegaly without substantial lymph node enlargement. Leukocytosis usually exceeds $100,000/\mu L$ and is characterized by large lymphoid cells with single prominent nucleoli. Tissue sections show almost no mitotic figures despite the immature appearance of the leukemic cells.

1. Eighty percent of cases involve B cells that have different surface markers than typical CLL (the B cells of prolymphocytic leukemia show intense surface immunoglobulin, the CD19 and CD20 B-cell antigens, but typically not the CD5 antigen). Twenty percent of cases are T cell, usually with a T-helper phenotype (CD3 and CD4 positive).

2. A small percentage of CLL patients develop a "prolymphocytoid" transformation, whereby more than 30% of the peripheral blood cells are prolymphocytic. This differs from *de novo* prolymphocytic leukemia in that the cells maintain the immune features of CLL, and the clinical course resembles typical CLL, albeit in a late stage of the disease.

3. Single-agent therapy with fludarabine, cladribine, or alemtuzumab or combination therapy with CHOP may be useful.

HAIRY CELL LEUKEMIA

I. EPIDEMIOLOGY AND ETIOLOGY

Hairy cell leukemia (HCL; leukemic reticuloendotheliosis) accounts for about 2% of all leukemia. The disease occurs more frequently in men than women by a ratio of 5:1. The median age of patients is 55 years; patients <30 years of age are unusual. The etiology is unknown.

II. PATHOLOGY AND NATURAL HISTORY

A. **Pathology.** The pathognomonic cells with irregular cytoplasmic projections can be identified in the peripheral blood, bone marrow, liver, and spleen of affected patients. HCL is a chronic disorder of B lymphocytes.

B. **Natural history.** The natural history is characterized by neutropenia. The time course can be variable, ranging from a relatively fulminant course to a waxing and waning course of exacerbations and spontaneous improvements, and to prolonged survival measured in decades. Patients with HCL usually present with an insidious development of nonspecific symptoms, splenomegaly, neutropenia or pancytopenia, and infections. Classic HCL is usually responsive to therapies (see below) and may have a normal life expectancy. A variant disorder (HCLv) represents a more aggressive disease with distinct immunophenotypic and molecular profiles and is less responsive to the standard therapies.

III. DIAGNOSIS

A. **Symptoms and signs.** Weakness and fatigue are the presenting symptoms in about 40% of cases. Bleeding, recent infection, or abdominal discomfort is present in about 20% of patients. Splenomegaly is usually present ± hepatomegaly. Peripheral adenopathy is rare.

B. **Laboratory studies**

1. **CBC.** Anemia and thrombocytopenia occur in 85% of patients. About 60% of patients have neutropenia; 20% have increased hairy cells with leukocytosis but an absolute neutropenia. Monocytopenia is common.

2. **Blood chemistries.** Only 10% to 20% of patients have abnormal liver or renal function tests. Polyclonal hyperglobulinemia or decreased normal immunoglobulin concentrations occur in 20% of patients.

C. **Special diagnostic studies.** The diagnosis of HCL is made by identifying the pathognomonic mononuclear cells in the peripheral blood or bone marrow, but an immunophenotype characteristic of HCL is required. The cells have irregular and serrated borders with characteristic slender, hair-like cytoplasmic projections, and round, eccentric nuclei with spongy chromatin. The cytoplasm is sky blue without granules.

1. **Immunophenotype and molecular characterization:** Classic HCL cells express CD20, CD19, CD11c, CD25, CD103, and CD123. About 10% of HCL patients have a more aggressive variant disease (HCLv) with cells positive for CD20, CD19, and CD11c, but negative for CD25 and CD123. Classic HCL cells have a mutation in BRAF p.V600E. HCLv cells express the wild-type BRAF.

2. **Phase-contrast microscopy** with supravital staining of fresh preparations is valuable for demonstrating the cellular characteristics because the cytoplasm of hairy cells is often poorly preserved in films mixed with Wright stain.

3. **Tartrate-resistant acid phosphatase** (TRAP). HCL cells have a strong acid phosphatase activity, which is resistant to inhibition by 0.05 M tartaric acid. A strongly positive TRAP study is present in most patients with HCL but is not required for the diagnosis and can be detected in other lymphoid malignancies.

4. **Bone marrow aspiration** frequently is unsuccessful ("dry tap"). Marrow biopsy shows a characteristic loose and spongy arrangement of cells, even with extensive infiltration with hairy cells. Fibrosis of the marrow with reticulin fibers is also characteristic in areas of HCL infiltration and accounts for the high frequency of dry taps.

5. **Splenic morphology.** The spleen is the most densely infiltrated organ in HCL. The red pulp may contain a unique vascular lesion: pseudosinuses lined by hairy cells.

D. **Differential diagnosis.** It is important to distinguish HCL from other diseases because management is substantially different. HCL is most often confused with CLL, Malignant lymphomas, myelofibrosis, or monocytic leukemia. Differentiation is made by identifying the pathognomonic cell, the characteristic immune profile, and pathologic findings of the bone marrow biopsy.

IV. MANAGEMENT

A. **The decision to treat.** Many cases tend to have an indolent course, and these patients have excellent survival without therapy. Therapy may be deferred for asymptomatic patients until the patient develops symptomatic anemia or clinically worrisome granulocytopenia and/or thrombocytopenia, or infections. Prior to starting therapy, it is important to differentiate classical from variant HCL since HCLv has poor response to the purine nucleoside analogues but respond to antibody therapy.

B. **Purine nucleosides.** Because of significant lymphodepletion, prophylaxis with acyclovir and Bactrim should be considered.

1. **Cladribine** is the treatment of choice for classical HCL. The drug can be given by continuous intravenous infusion at a dose of 0.1 mg/kg/d for 7 days. Other regimens have been published, including a 5-day bolus IV treatment, or a 5-day subcutaneous bolus injection (0.14 mg/kg/d). Virtually, all patients with classical HCL respond, and 95% achieve complete response. Relapse occurs in 35% of patients, usually after 3 years, and most respond to an additional course of cladribine. Toxicity has been limited to transient fever, usually associated with neutropenia. Survival at 9 years exceeds 95%.

2. **Pentostatin** (Nipent) is also a highly effective therapy for classical HCL. Most patients not only have normalization of their CBC but also have a complete response with disappearance of hairy cells from their bone marrow. Complications include skin rash and neurotoxicity. The dosage is 4 mg/m^2 IV every 2 weeks for 3 to 6 months.

C. **Biologic therapies**

1. Rituximab has activity but is not as effective as a single agent as the purine analogues. It can be effective when combined with purine analogues to improve the response in patients with HCLv.

2. BRAF inhibitors, B-cell receptor inhibitors, and anti-CD22 immunoconjugate have shown some activity in HCL and are presently being evaluated in clinical trials.

CHRONIC MYELOGENOUS LEUKEMIA

I. EPIDEMIOLOGY AND ETIOLOGY

Chronic myelogenous leukemia (CML) is a myeloproliferative disorder with a characteristic cytogenetic abnormality and a propensity to evolve from a chronic phase (CP) into a blast phase (BP) with features similar to acute leukemia.

A. **Incidence.** CML has an incidence of approximately 1 case in 100,000 population and comprises 20% of adult leukemias in Western countries. The median age at onset is in the mid-50s, but children can infrequently be affected.

B. **Etiology.** The cause of most cases of CML is unknown, although radiation exposure is a known risk factor. There is no familial predisposition to this disorder.

II. PATHOGENESIS AND NATURAL HISTORY

A. **Clonality.** CML is a clonal disease of an abnormal stem cell. Myeloid, erythroid, megakaryocytic, and B-lymphoid cells are involved in the malignant clone.

B. **The Philadelphia chromosome (Ph¹)** is the diminutive chromosome 22 produced by an unbalanced translocation between chromosomes 9 and 22. This translocation, designated t(9;22), fuses the 3′ portion of the *c-ABL* gene on the long arm of chromosome 9 (band q34) to the 5′ end of the breakpoint cluster (*BCR*) gene on the long arm of chromosome 22 (band q11). The resultant fusion gene encodes a chimeric protein of 210 kDa (p210) with constitutive tyrosine kinase activity. The *BCR-ABL* protein stimulates the proliferation and enhances the survival of CML hematopoietic progenitor cells.

1. **Ph¹ chromosome in acute leukemia.** The Ph¹ chromosome can occur in approximately 30% of adults with acute lymphoblastic leukemia (ALL) and rarely in acute myelogenous leukemia (AML). Some of these cases represent CML in *de novo* blast crisis that was never diagnosed in the CP.

C. **Clinical course.** Three stages of CML are recognized: CP, accelerated phase (AP), and blast phase (or blast crisis, BP). Most patients are diagnosed while in CP. All stages of disease can present with fatigue, low-grade fevers, night sweats, and early satiety or abdominal pain from splenomegaly. Symptoms tend to be more severe when advanced disease is present. Evolution to accelerated or BP from the CP can be suggested by the development of thrombocytopenia or progressive splenomegaly, leukocytosis with increased numbers of blasts (≥10%), basophilia (≥20%), or recurrent constitutional symptoms, including bone pain, while on a stable dose of therapy. The disease status should be re-evaluated in this setting.

Cytogenetic changes other than the Ph¹ abnormality are commonly observed in association with blast crisis evolution. Approximately 70% of blast crises are myeloid, in which the blasts display a phenotype indistinguishable from acute myeloid leukemia. The remaining cases of blast crisis are lymphoid, in which the blasts have immunophenotypic characteristics of pre-B cells or have biphenotypic features (myeloid and B lymphoid).

III. CLINICAL MANIFESTATIONS

A. **Symptoms and signs**

1. CML can be asymptomatic and be discovered incidentally by routine blood counts.

2. The excessive numbers of metabolically active myeloid cells can cause fevers and sweats. Fatigue and malaise are also commonly present.

3. Bone pain and tenderness can result from the expanding leukemic mass in the marrow.

4. Splenomegaly is present in the majority of cases, and it may be massive. It can be manifested as early satiety, abdominal fullness, or pain. Hepatomegaly is less common and is usually asymptomatic.

5. Marked leukocytosis (particularly white blood cell counts [WBCs] exceeding 100,000/μL) can be associated with symptoms of leukostasis.

Manifestations may include visual changes, seizures, cerebral or myocardial infarctions, and priapism.

B. **Laboratory studies**

1. **Leukocytes.** The WBC usually exceeds 30,000/mL and usually ranges from 100,000 to 300,000/μL at the time of diagnosis. The peripheral blood smear in the CP is often described as appearing like a bone marrow aspirate smear due to presence of all stages of myeloid cell maturation. Myeloblasts constitute <10% of the leukocytes in the peripheral blood, and promyelocytes plus blasts combined compose <30% in the CP. Eosinophil and basophil counts are often elevated, but basophils constitute <20% of the peripheral blood leukocytes in the CP.

2. **Platelets.** Thrombocytosis is common, and the platelet count may exceed 1,000,000/μL at presentation. Uncommonly, CML can present with isolated thrombocytosis. Thrombocytopenia is unusual in the CP.

3. **Erythrocytes.** The hemoglobin level is usually normal, but a mild normocytic, normochromic anemia can be present. A few nucleated red blood cells can be seen on the peripheral blood smear.

4. **Bone marrow aspiration and biopsy** should be performed on all patients as part of the diagnostic evaluation. This is necessary to stage the disease at presentation. In all cases, the marrow is markedly hypercellular as a result of massive myeloid hyperplasia, resulting in a markedly increased myeloid-to-erythroid ratio. Megakaryocyte numbers are frequently increased. Fibrosis may be present but is rarely profound in the CP.

5. **Cytogenetic analysis** should be performed at the time of bone marrow examination on all patients. The characteristic t(9;22) is identified in the majority of patients. However, complex translocations infrequently occur that can mask the *BCR-ABL* translocation. In this situation, FISH or polymerase chain reaction (PCR) for *BCR-ABL* can identify the characteristic abnormality. It is best to order all three tests initially to ensure that an occult translocation is not missed. Cytogenetics are particularly important to determine if additional chromosomal abnormalities associated with advanced disease are present.

6. **FISH** for the *BCR-ABL* gene rearrangement can be performed on peripheral blood or bone marrow. This assay uses fluorochrome-labeled DNA probes to detect rearrangement of *ABL* to the *BCR* locus and does not require dividing cells, so can be performed on peripheral blood or bone marrow. It can be useful if complex chromosomal translocations are present.

7. **PCR** is a molecular assay performed on the peripheral blood RNA that detects the *BCR-ABL* translocation. Like the FISH test, it is capable of detecting *BCR-ABL* in the setting of complex or occult chromosomal rearrangements. The **quantitative PCR (QPCR)** assay is the most sensitive method to follow residual disease during the treatment of CML. When adjusted according to the International Scale (IS), the results should be comparable across all laboratories using that methodology. It also permits the evaluation of an individual patient's results according to currently recommended response landmarks.

8. **Leukocyte alkaline phosphatase** activity in circulating granulocytes is decreased or absent in CML and was previously helpful diagnostically. This test has been replaced by FISH and PCR assays for *BCR-ABL*.

9. **Uric acid.** Hyperuricemia is often present at diagnosis.

IV. DIAGNOSTIC CRITERIA AND PROGNOSTIC VARIABLES

A. **World Health Organization (WHO) diagnostic criteria for chronic phase (CP) CML** include:

1. Peripheral blood leukocytosis due to increased numbers of mature and immature neutrophils
2. No significant dysplasia
3. Promyelocytes, myelocytes, and metamyelocytes >10% of WBCs
4. Blasts <10% of WBCs
5. Monocytes usually <3% of WBCs
6. Bone marrow hypercellularity with granulocytic proliferation and often expansion of small megakaryocytes with hypolobated nuclei
7. Less than 10% blasts in the bone marrow

B. **WHO criteria for diagnosis of accelerated phase (AP) CML require one or more of the following:**

1. Blasts 10% to 19% in the blood or bone marrow
2. Basophils ≥20% of peripheral blood leukocytes
3. Platelets ≥1,000,000/mL unresponsive to therapy or ≤100,000/mL unrelated to therapy
4. Increasing spleen size and/or increasing WBC count unresponsive to therapy
5. Cytogenetic evidence of clonal evolution (cytogenetic abnormalities in addition to the Ph^1 chromosome)

C. **WHO criteria for diagnosis of blast phase CML (blast crisis, BP)**

1. Blasts ≥20% of bone marrow cells or peripheral WBC
2. Extramedullary blasts (e.g., osteolytic bone lesions, lymphadenopathy)

D. **Differential diagnosis**

1. **Leukemoid reactions** rarely show the full spectrum of myeloid cells (especially myelocytes, promyelocytes, or blasts) in the peripheral blood and lack the *BCR-ABL* translocation.
2. **Other myeloproliferative disorders** may present with leukocytosis and thrombocytosis but will not have the *BCR-ABL* translocation.
3. **Atypical (Ph¹-negative) CML.** Approximately 1% to 2% of cases that appear clinically to be CML are Ph^1 negative by bone marrow cytogenetics, FISH, and PCR assays. The peripheral blood demonstrates a leukocytosis with >10% metamyelocytes, myelocytes, or promyelocytes. Dysgranulopoiesis is prominent, often with pseudo–Pelger-Huet cells. Monocytes are <10% of leukocytes and basophilia is absent. Blasts may be increased but are <20% of leukocytes in the blood or bone marrow. The bone marrow is hypercellular and myeloid predominant with prominent dysgranulopoiesis. Anemia, thrombocytopenia, and splenomegaly are common clinical features. Cytogenetics are most often normal but trisomy 8 or deletion 20q can be observed. Rearrangement of PDGFRA, PDGFRB, or FGFR1 is absent. Activating mutations of the granulocyte colony-stimulating factor receptor (CSF3R) occur in up to 40% of these patients. Other reported molecular abnormalities include mutations of SETB1, NRAS, or CBL. Hydroxyurea can be used to treat the leukocytosis and splenomegaly. Because CSF3R signals through the JAK/STAT pathway, inhibition of JAK kinase activity is a promising potential treatment for patients with the CSF3R T618I mutation, and this approach is currently under clinical investigation.
4. **Chronic neutrophilic leukemia** is a rare disorder characterized by mature neutrophilia (WBC ≥ 25,000/µL with >80% segmented neutrophils and bands). Unlike atypical CML, immature myeloid cells comprise <10% of leukocytes in the blood, and myeloid dysplasia is not present. Blasts are not

increased in the blood or bone marrow. Cytogenetics are typically normal, and there is no *BCR-ABL* translocation or rearrangement of *PDGFRA, PDGFRB,* or *FGFR1.* Like atypical CML, mutations of the CSF3R gene, especially T618I, occur frequently.

E. **Prognostic variables.** The Sokal score (www.roc.se/Sokal.asp) and Hasford score (www.pharmacoepi.de/cgi-bin/cmiscore.cgi) use variables including age, spleen size, platelet count, peripheral blood blast percentage, and peripheral blood basophil and eosinophil percentages to calculate the likelihood of achieving a remission in chronic phase patients, but are not currently used to select treatment. Ongoing assessment of response during therapy has emerged as a more important predictor of progression-free survival. Advanced phase disease, especially blast crisis, conveys a very adverse prognosis and warrants referral to a tertiary center capable of hematopoietic stem cell transplant evaluation.

V. MANAGEMENT

A. **Imatinib** competitively interferes with ATP binding to the kinase domain of *ABL,* thus acting as a tyrosine kinase inhibitor (TKI). Use of this drug in CML has led to survival rates that approach those of age-matched controls. Long-term progression-free survival of CML patients on imatinib therapy correlates with the depth of response to treatment.

1. **Imatinib dosing.** The standard dose of imatinib is 400 mg/d for CP and 600 mg/d for advanced disease. Suboptimal response (Table 24-3) may warrant a dose increase to 600 mg/d or 800 mg/d administered in divided doses as (400 mg b.i.d.). Potential side effects include fluid retention, nausea, diarrhea, muscle cramps, skin rash, fatigue, and myelosuppression. If moderate toxicity warrants dose reduction, re-escalation to a standard dose should be attempted once side effects abate. When compared to imatinib as initial treatment for CP CML, the second-generation TKIs, dasatinib or nilotinib, induce more rapid achievement of therapeutic milestones and reduce the risk of disease progression, but are associated with similar long-term survival.

TABLE 24-3	European Leukemia Net Recommendations for the Management of CML (2013)		
Time from Start	**Optimal Response**	**Warning**	**Treatment Failure**
3 mo	BCR-ABL ≤10% and/or Ph+ <65%	BCR-ABL >10% and/or Ph+ 65%–95%	No CHR or Ph+ >95% or new mutations
6 mo	BCR-ABL ≤10% and/or Ph+ <35%	Ph+ 35%–65%	BCR-ABL >10% and/or Ph+ >65% and/or new mutations
12 mo	BCR-ABL ≤1% and/or Ph+ 0	BCR-ABL 1%–10% and/or Ph+ 1%–35%	BCR-ABL >10% and/or Ph+ >35% and/or new mutations
Then, and at any time	BCR-ABL ≤0.1%	CCA/Ph− (−7 or 7q−) or BCR-ABL >1%	Loss of CHR Loss of CCyR or PCyR New mutations Confirmed loss of MMR CCA/Ph+

CHR, complete hematologic response; CCyR, complete cytogenetic response; PCyR, partial cytogenetic response; MMR, major molecular response; Ph+, Philadelphia chromosome–positive metaphases; CCA/Ph−, clonal chromosome abnormalities in Ph− cells.

2. **Acquired imatinib resistance** is defined as loss of a previous hematologic or cytogenetic response. A confirmed increase in the QPCR *BCR-ABL* level by 10-fold or more can also be indicative of drug resistance. The best understood mechanisms of resistance are point mutations of *BCR-ABL* that impair the binding of imatinib to the *ABL* kinase domain or alter the ability of the protein to enter an inactive conformation in response to drug. *BCR-ABL* mutation analysis should be sent if acquired resistance develops. CML with most of the common *BCR-ABL* mutations that occur under imatinib treatment can be effectively treated by the second-generation kinase inhibitors dasatinib, nilotinib, or bosutinib. The V299L and F317I *BCR-ABL* mutations confer relative resistance to dasatinib, the V299L is bosutinib resistant, and the Y253H, E255V/K, and F359V/C mutations are resistant to nilotinib. The T315I mutation is highly resistant to all of the TKIs but the third-generation drug, ponatinib. Another mechanism of resistance to all of the TKIs is amplification of *BCR-ABL* copy number, as detected by FISH.

B. **Additional drugs. Second-generation *BCR-ABL* TKIs, dasatinib, nilotinib, and bosutinib**, were developed and approved to treat CML patients with resistance or intolerance to imatinib. These agents are more potent inhibitors of the *BCR-ABL* kinase than imatinib. Randomized trials subsequently demonstrated that the rates of CCyR and MMR after a year of treatment with dasatinib or nilotinib were significantly higher than with imatinib. Therefore, they are also FDA approved as initial therapy for newly diagnosed chronic phase CML patients.

1. **Dasatinib** is a *SRC* and *ABL* kinase inhibitor that is administered once a day with a meal. Starting dose is 100 mg/d for CP and 140 mg/d for advanced disease. Common side effects include myelosuppression, fluid retention (especially pleural effusion), diarrhea, rash, and bone pain. Dasatinib impairs platelet function and can cause serious gastrointestinal or intracranial bleeding in patients with severe thrombocytopenia.

2. **Nilotinib** is an imatinib analogue administered at a dose of 300 mg twice daily for newly diagnosed patients and 400 mg twice daily after imatinib failure or for AP disease. Patients must fast for 2 hours before and 1 hour after each dose to prevent increased drug absorption, which can result in QT prolongation. Nilotinib prolongs the QT interval, and sudden deaths were reported in early clinical trials. Common side effects include myelosuppression, arthralgias and myalgias, rash, and nausea. Additional laboratory abnormalities caused by nilotinib include elevated lipase, hyperglycemia, hyperbilirubinemia, and transaminase elevations. Arterial occlusive events also appear to occur more commonly with nilotinib than with imatinib.

3. **Bosutinib** is an *SRC* and *ABL* kinase inhibitor that is approved for treating CML patients who have not responded to, or are intolerant of, a prior TKI. Dosing is initiated at 500 mg/d with food. Gastrointestinal side effects including diarrhea, nausea, and vomiting are very common and should be managed with antimotility agents, antiemetics and dose modification, as clinically indicated. Additional side effects that require monitoring include myelosuppression and liver function abnormalities.

4. **Ponatinib** is a third-generation TKI that was developed specifically to address the T315I mutation of *BCR-ABL*, which confers high-level resistance to all of the other TKIs. Remarkably, it is active clinically against every mutation that arises during treatment with all of the other TKIs, and it induces the highest response rate after failure of any second-generation drug. Unfortunately, it was found to cause arterial occlusions and venous

thromboses in at least 27% of patients, including fatal myocardial infarctions, strokes, TIAs, and severe peripheral vascular occlusions requiring urgent revascularization procedures. These events occurred even in patients without known cardiovascular risk factors. Although not evaluated clinically, use of prophylactic antiplatelet therapy should be considered for every patient without thrombocytopenia who is receiving ponatinib. Additional serious side effects include heart failure, so it is recommended to monitor cardiac function. Severe hepatotoxicity has also been observed, which warrants liver function monitoring when the drug is initiated. These risks must be weighed against the potential benefits of ponatinib in the individual patient. It is perhaps best used as a bridge to transplant in a patient resistant to all of the other TKIs. The recommended starting dose of 45 mg/d may not be appropriate for older patients or those with comorbidities that could increase the risks associated with this drug.

5. **Omacetaxine** is a drug with a novel mechanism of action; it inhibits RNA synthesis. As a result, its activity is not affected by mutations of *BCR-ABL*. This makes it less selectively myelosuppressive, and blood counts must be closely monitored. It can also cause hyperglycemia. Dosing is 1.25 mg/m^2 twice daily as a subcutaneous injection for 14 days of a 28-day cycle for induction. In responding patients, maintenance therapy is 1.25 mg/m^2 twice daily for 7 days of a 28-day cycle. It is approved for CML patients who have not responded to at least 2 TKIs. It can be used as a bridge to transplant in patients who do not respond or tolerate any of the TKIs.

C. **Efficacy monitoring. Close monitoring of response is essential to optimize patient outcomes.** Guidelines for adequacy of response to imatinib as initial therapy for chronic phase CML have been established by the European Leukemia Net (Table 24-3) and the National Comprehensive Cancer Network. Patients with suboptimal responses to initial therapy should be considered for dose escalation or therapy with an alternative TKI. A bone marrow biopsy with cytogenetics and *BCR-ABL* mutation analysis should be performed before switching therapy due to failure to achieve response landmarks, especially during the first 2 years of therapy when most progression events occur.

1. **Complete hematologic response** (CHR) is defined as a normalization of the peripheral blood counts. Failure to achieve this end point by 3 months is considered a primary treatment failure and a change in treatment.

2. **Cytogenetic responses**—bone marrow cytogenetic testing has been largely supplanted by peripheral blood PCR monitoring. However, if PCR testing is not available, cytogenetic testing should be performed every 3 months until a complete cytogenetic response is achieved. Otherwise, bone marrow biopsy with cytogenetics can be used to evaluate what appears to be an inadequate response by PCR testing.

a. **Partial cytogenetic response** (PCyR) is reduction of the Ph^1 chromosome to ≤35% of bone marrow metaphases. Ideally, a PCyR should be observed by 3 months. Lack of a PCyR at 6 months indicates the need to evaluate and address the cause of treatment failure, and possibly by changing the TKI.

b. **Complete cytogenetic response** (CCyR) is defined as normalization of the bone marrow cytogenetics. A CCyR is ideally achieved by 6 months and at the latest by 12 months.

c. **Major cytogenetic response** (MCyR) combines PCyR and CCyR.

3. **QPCR testing for *BCR-ABL*** performed on the peripheral blood is a highly sensitive method of assessing response to therapy. QPCR should be

performed at baseline and every 3 months. A confirmed 10-fold increase in QPCR is considered to be clinically significant. A bone marrow biopsy should be considered if there is an unexplained progressive increase in the QPCR assay (>10-fold).

a. **BCR-ABL ≤ 10%** at 3 months has emerged as an important predictor of long-term success of TKI therapy. Patients who do not meet this landmark by 3 months should do so by 6 months.

b. **Major molecular response** (MMR) or ≤0.1% on the IS is a ≥3-log (1,000-fold) reduction in the level of disease compared to a reference control of untreated patient samples. Patients who achieve this end point by 1 year have minimal risk of disease progression to AP or BP at 5 years.

c. **PCR undetectable** (PCR-U) or <0.0032% IS represents the limit of sensitivity of the PCR assay. Imatinib-treated patients who maintained a stable PCR-U response for at least 2 years were taken off treatment and monitored closely for relapse. Approximately 40% of patients remained PCR-U without treatment for at least 5 years. Similar results have been observed for persistently (>2 years) PCR-U patients receiving the second-generation TKIs. Therefore, PCR-U should be the goal of treatment for any "younger" patient who would otherwise require lifelong therapy.

4. **FISH** is somewhat more sensitive than routine cytogenetics (evaluates 200 to 300 cells vs. 20 cells, respectively), and it can be performed on peripheral blood, but it has not been used to assess response in any clinical trial and it has not been validated prospectively as a surrogate end point for outcome.

D. **Therapeutic goal** should be to prevent progression to advanced disease using a dose and schedule of TKI with acceptable side effects. Because achievement of a MMR appears to be associated with minimal chance of disease progression, it should be the goal of treatment for most patients. The lifespan of most CML patients treated with TKIs is dictated more by their comorbidities than their CML, so for older patients or those with multiple comorbidities, less aggressive cytoreduction may be adequate to prevent disease progression during their lives. In contrast, younger patients could be expected to require treatment for many years. Although not validated by prospective clinical trials, it is reasonable to attempt to achieve PCR-U status in younger patients with the prospect for TKI discontinuation sometime in the future. Every effort should be made to encourage compliance, especially in young patients. Selecting a TKI with acceptable side effects is of critical importance given the prolonged duration of therapy required for CML.

E. **Safety monitoring** for myelosuppression is similar for all of the TKIs. At the initiation of therapy, all peripheral blood cells are derived from the CML clone. Therefore, cytopenias are anticipated during the transition to normal hematopoiesis induced by TKI therapy. Most other laboratory side effects of the TKIs are observed within the first few weeks after initiating therapy. Close initial monitoring of potential clinical and laboratory abnormalities is essential.

1. CBC with differential, liver function tests, and electrolyte assessment must be performed before starting therapy and every 2 weeks until blood counts have normalized. Electrolyte abnormalities should be corrected prior to initiating therapy. Indications for holding drug include ANC < 1,000/μL, platelets < 50,000/μL, AST/ALT greater than fivefold above upper limit of normal (ULN), or bilirubin greater than threefold above ULN.

2. For patients taking dasatinib, physical examinations should routinely evaluate for development of a pleural effusion. This complication can even occur after many months on therapy.

3. For patients taking nilotinib, an ECG must be performed prior to initiating therapy. The baseline QTcF should be <450 ms prior to starting drug to minimize the risk of clinically significant QT prolongation. A repeat ECG is done after 1 week of therapy to ensure QTcF is <450 ms on therapy.

4. Nilotinib and ponatinib can cause pancreatitis, so amylase and lipase should be checked periodically after initiating therapy. Asymptomatic elevations of these assays is common, but drug should be held for levels exceeding 2.5-fold above the ULN.

5. All of the TKIs are metabolized by the CYP3A4 hepatic microsomal enzyme, so grapefruit juice and drugs that induce or inhibit this enzyme should be avoided.

6. **Pregnancy must be avoided with all the TKIs as they are teratogenic.**

F. **Bone marrow transplantation (BMT)** is the only therapy that is unquestionably curative for CML, but its role in the management of this disease has been diminished by the marked success of the TKIs. The disadvantage of transplantation is that there is approximately 20% risk of mortality at 1 year. In comparison, the risk of death from CML on a TKI is <10% in 10 years, and the prior use of a TKI before transplantation does not appear to adversely affect outcome. Therefore, BMT is primarily reserved for patients who are in second CP from blast crisis, have T315I mutation, or have experienced treatment failure to two or more TKIs.

Outcomes of BMT for CML include:

1. Long-term (5 to 10 years) disease-free survival is reported in 60% to 80% of patients in chronic phase CML who are treated with BMT using related donors. Allogeneic transplants using 10/10 matched unrelated donors produce survival results that are slightly inferior to those patients receiving transplants from matched related donors. Survival rates after BMT appear to plateau after 3 to 7 years.

2. Patients undergoing BMT face a 20% risk of transplant-related death within 1 year of the procedure. Significant graft versus host disease (GVHD) occurs in 10% to 60% of cases and is the major risk. The incidence of severe GVHD and mortality increases with age and with degree of HLA disparity between the donor and recipient.

3. Survival rates decrease by half when performing BMT in the AP and by half again when used in the BP.

4. Relapses of CP CML can be effectively treated with lymphocyte infusions from the original donor (donor lymphocyte infusions, or DLI) without additional chemotherapy. CCyR can be expected in approximately 60% of patients with chronic phase CML treated with DLI. The predominant risk of this therapy is worsening GVHD. Patients who relapse with AP or BP disease should ideally be returned to CP before the use of DLI.

G. **Management of the accelerated phase (AP) or blast phase (BP).** Randomized studies are not available to guide the choice of TKI in these patients. It is suggested that dasatinib 140 mg/d, nilotinib 400 mg twice daily, or imatinib 600 to 800 mg/d be used as initial therapy in AP patients. Patients who evolve AP on one TKI should be switched to a different second-generation agent and be referred to a transplant center. The AP patients who achieve a CCyR can maintain stable benefit from TKI therapy. Patients who present with or evolve BP would be best managed on a clinical trial or be considered for therapy with combination TKI and chemotherapy. Treatment regimens for Ph^1-positive ALL can be used to treat lymphoid blast crisis. Because of its ability to penetrate the CNS, dasatinib may have particular benefit in patients at risk for this complication, such as those with lymphoid blast crisis. AML induction regimens can be combined with a TKI for myeloid blast crisis. Should a second chronic or AP be achieved, allogeneic stem cell transplantation is the only option that confers a chance of long-term survival. Side effects of all TKIs are more common and are potentially more severe in patients who present with advanced disease. Patients who experience severe cytopenias (neutrophils < 500/µL or platelets < 20,000/µL) on treatment should have a bone marrow biopsy to determine if the low counts are due to the drug or the disease. If the bone marrow is hypocellular without increased blasts, then treatment should be held until the neutrophils are ≥1,000/µL, and the platelets are ≥20,000 to 50,000/µL. If increased numbers of blasts persist in the bone marrow, treatment should be continued, and the bone marrow biopsy should be repeated in 2 to 4 weeks if the cytopenias persist.

H. Other treatment modalities

1. **Allopurinol**, 300 mg/d, is given to all patients at diagnosis and is continued until the WBC normalizes.

2. **Leukapheresis** rapidly decreases the leukocyte count for short periods of time but should be considered in patients with central nervous system or pulmonary symptoms or priapism from leukostasis. Leukostasis can develop when the WBC count exceeds 100,000/µL, especially with significant proportions of blasts in the blood. Leukapheresis should be implemented emergently in combination with cytoreductive therapy with hydroxyurea or a TKI.

3. **Interferon alpha** can induce hematologic and cytogenetic responses in CML patients and was the standard therapy for many years. This drug has been supplanted by TKIs. However, it can be useful in pregnant patients who require cytoreductive therapy, as it is not believed to be teratogenic.

4. **Hydroxyurea** (up to 2 g t.i.d.) has been used for many years to rapidly reduce the blood counts of CML patients. It is well tolerated, but it does not induce cytogenetic responses. The rapid effectiveness of the TKIs has relegated hydroxyurea to a minor role in therapy, except in the setting of marked leukocytosis before a diagnosis is certain.

5. **Chemotherapy** is used in conjunction with a TKI in blast crisis CML as noted above.

CHRONIC MYELOMONOCYTIC LEUKEMIA

I. TERMINOLOGY

Chronic myelomonocytic leukemia (CMML) is classified as a "myelodysplastic/myeloproliferative syndrome" in the WHO system (Appendix B). It is divided into two subtypes (CMML-1 and CMML-2), depending on the percentage of blasts in the bone marrow.

II. DIAGNOSIS

A. Clinical features. CMML most commonly affects the elderly. Splenomegaly is often present and tends to increase as the disease progresses. Hepatomegaly is uncommon, and lymphadenopathy is rare.

B. Diagnosis according to the WHO classification requires all of the following:

1. A persistent, unexplained monocytosis (>1,000/µL) must be present.

2. The Ph^1 chromosome or *BCR-ABL* fusion gene must be absent.

3. Fewer than 20% blasts (myeloblasts, monoblasts, and promonocytes) must be present in the bone marrow, and dysplasia must involve one or more myeloid lineages.

4. If dysplasia is not evident, there must be a clonal cytogenetic abnormality, the monocytosis must have been present for at least 3 months, and other potential causes of the monocytosis must have been excluded.

C. **Additional laboratory abnormalities** are commonly observed.

1. **Leukocytosis** in the range of 11,000 to 50,000/mL (because of increased numbers of both granulocytes and monocytes) is present in most patients, but leukopenia occasionally occurs. The morphology of the leukocytes is characteristically abnormal. Cells with nucleoli in the peripheral blood are uncommon. Eosinophilia is observed in CMML harboring a rearrangement of the PDGFRB gene (Section II.E).

2. **Mild anemia**, often macrocytic.

3. **Thrombocytopenia** is mild in most patients and severe in 15%. Some patients have normal platelet counts. Rarely, thrombocytosis is observed.

D. **Bone marrow aspirates** in CMML are very hypercellular. Granulocytic hyperplasia with monocytoid features is typical, but pure monocytic hyperplasia is unusual. Blasts account for <10% of the nucleated cells in CMML-1 and for 10% to 19% in CMML-2. Dysplastic features are typically present in one or more cell lines.

E. **Cytogenetic abnormalities** occur in approximately 20% to 40% of cases, but the Ph[1] chromosome is absent. It is important to evaluate whether there is rearrangement of the *PDGFRB* gene on chromosome 5q33 by FISH or PCR when eosinophilia is present. *PDGFRB* can partner with ETV6 on chromosome 12p13, HIP1 on chromosome 7q11, RAB5 on chromosome 17p13, and others. The fusion gene created by these translocations encodes a protein in which the tyrosine kinase activity of *PDGFRB* is constitutively active. Treatment of patients with *PDGFRB* gene rearrangements with imatinib has induced hematologic and cytogenetic remissions due to the ability of the drug to inhibit the kinase activity of *PDGFRB*.

F. **Molecular abnormalities** include point mutations of the *KRAS, NRAS, ASXL1, CBL, EZH2, TET2, JAK2,* and *RUNX1* genes, predominantly in patients without cytogenetic abnormalities. These genetic alterations are not unique to CMML, as they are also observed in other myeloproliferative disorders, myelodysplastic syndromes, and AML (Chapter 26). The encoded proteins can be categorized functionally into those involved in growth factor signaling pathways (*KRAS, NRAS, ASXL1, CBL, JAK2*) and epigenetic DNA regulation (*EZH2, TET2*).

III. CLINICAL COURSE

Distinguishing CMML from acute myelomonocytic leukemia is essential. CMML-1 often has an insidious onset and an indolent course. Most of these patients live ≥2 years, and many survive >5 years. Patients with CMML-2 have a high risk of AML evolution and should be treated to improve peripheral blood counts and prevent AML evolution.

IV. MANAGEMENT

A. **Allogeneic stem cell transplantation** remains the only curative option for CMML. The criteria for determining the appropriateness of this therapy should be extrapolated from the experience with myelodysplastic syndrome (Chapter 25).

B. **Imatinib** should be administered to patients with rearrangement of the *PDGFRB* gene on chromosome 5q33. Complete remissions have been observed with imatinib 400 mg/d in this uncommon subset of CMML patients.

C. **Hypomethylating agents,** including azacitidine or decitabine, have been reported to induce partial or complete remissions in 30% to 60% of CMML patients. An additional 10% to 20% of patients experience some hematologic improvement. The randomized trials of these drugs versus supportive care in MDS patients included small numbers of CMML patients. These studies demonstrated a superior response rate and progression-free survival for study patients treated with hypomethylating agents versus best supportive care.

Indications for treatment include high-risk disease (CMML-2) to prevent AML evolution or cytopenias that are severe or unresponsive to supportive care measures. The drugs should be dosed as for MDS, and at least four cycles should be given before assessing response, unless there is evidence of progressive disease. Treatment is typically continued for as long as there is clinical benefit, unless transplant is planned. There appears to be little long-term toxicity other than myelosuppression.

D. **Hydroxyurea** can be used to reduce the leukocytosis or splenomegaly in CMML, but it does not induce remissions.

E. **Induction chemotherapy,** as for acute myeloid leukemia, should be reserved for disease progression as it has not been shown to improve survival.

F. **Erythropoiesis-stimulating agents** may be considered for patients with low-risk disease (bone marrow blasts <5%) and symptomatic anemia. As in MDS, a serum erythropoietin level of <200 U/L and minimal or absent transfusion requirements are associated with a higher likelihood of response.

G. **Blood product transfusions** are standard supportive care measures in CMML patients with symptomatic anemia and/or thrombocytopenia.

ACKNOWLEDGMENTS

The authors would like to acknowledge Drs. Gary Schiller and Dennis A. Casciato, who significantly contributed to earlier versions of this chapter.

Suggested Readings

Chronic Lymphocytic Leukemia

Chiorazzi N, Rai KR, Ferrarini M. Chronic lymphocytic leukemia. *N Engl J Med* 2005;352:804.

Damle RN, et al. B-cell chronic lymphocytic leukemia cells express a surface membrane phenotype of activated, antigen-experienced B lymphocytes. *Blood* 2002;99:4087.

Dighiero G, et al. Chlorambucil in indolent chronic lymphocytic leukemia. French Cooperative Group on Chronic Lymphocytic Leukemia. *N Engl J Med* 1998;338:1506.

Dohner H, et al. Genomic observations and survival in chronic lymphocytic leukemia. *N Engl J Med* 2000;343:1910.

Hamblin TJ, et al. Unmutated Ig V(H) genes are associated with a more aggressive form of chronic lymphocytic leukemia. *Blood* 1999;94:1848.

Mavromatis B, Cheson BD. Monoclonal antibody therapy of chronic lymphocytic leukemia. *J Clin Oncol* 2003;21:1874.

O'Brien SM, et al. Rituximab dose-escalation trial in chronic lymphocytic leukemia. *J Clin Oncol* 2001;19:2165.

Rai KR, et al. Fludarabine compared with chlorambucil as primary therapy to chronic lymphocytic leukemia. *N Engl J Med* 2000;343:1750.

Shanafelt TD, et al. Pentostatin, cyclophosphamide, and rituximab regimen in older patients with chronic lymphocytic leukemia. *Cancer* 2007;109:2291.

Van Den Neste E, et al. Chromosomal translocations independently predict treatment failure, treatment-free survival and overall survival in B-cell chronic lymphocytic leukemia patients treated with cladribine. *Leukemia* 2007;21:1715.

Weiss MA, et al. Pentostatin and cyclophosphamide: an effective new regimen in previously treated patients with chronic lymphocytic leukemia. *J Clin Oncol* 2003;21:1278.

Hairy Cell Leukemia

Chadha P, et al. Treatment of hairy cell leukemia with 2-chlorodeoxyadenosine (2-CdA): long-term follow-up of the Northwestern University experience. *Blood* 2005;106:241.

Cheson BD, et al. Treatment of hairy cell leukemia with 2-chlorodeoxyadenosine via the group C protocol mechanism of the National Cancer Institute: a report of 979 patients. *J Clin Oncol* 1998;16:3007.

Goodman GR, et al. Extended follow-up of patients with hairy cell leukemia after treatment with cladribine. *J Clin Oncol* 2003;21:891.

Kreitman RJ, et al. Efficacy of the anti-CD22 recombinant immunotoxin BL22 in chemotherapy-resistant hairy-cell leukemia. *N Engl J Med* 2001;345:241.

Chronic Myelogenous Leukemia

Baccarani M, et al. European LeukemiaNet recommendations for the management of chronic myeloid leukemia: 2013. *Blood* 2013;122:872–884.

Cortes JE, et al. A phase 2 trial of ponatinib in Philadelphia chromosome-positive leukemias. *N Engl J Med* 2013;369:1783–1796.

Hochhaus A, et al. Six-year follow-up of patients receiving imatinib for the first-line treatment of chronic myeloid leukemia. *Leukemia* 2009;23:1054–1061.

Hochhaus A, et al. Long-term benefits and risks of frontline nilotinib vs imatinib for chronic myeloid leukemia in chronic phase: 5-year update of the randomized ENESTnd trial. *Leukemia* 2016;30(5):1044–1054. doi: 10.1038/leu.2016.5.

Hughes T, et al. Impact of baseline BCR-ABL mutations on response to nilotinib in patients with chronic myeloid leukemia in chronic phase. *J Clin Oncol* 2009;27:4204.

Jabbour E, et al. Early response with dasatinib or imatinib in chronic myeloid leukemia: 3-year follow-up from a randomized phase 3 trial (DASISION). *Blood* 2014;123:494–500.

Kantarjian HM, et al. Bosutinib safety and management of toxicity in leukemia patients with resistance or intolerance to imatinib and other tyrosine kinase inhibitors. *Blood* 2014;1309–1318.

Müller MC, et al. Dasatinib treatment of chronic-phase chronic myeloid leukemia: analysis of responses according to preexisting BCR-ABL mutations. *Blood* 2009;114:4944.

O'Brien S, et al. Chronic myelogenous leukemia, version 1.2014. Featured updates to the NCCN guidelines. *JNCCN* 2013;11:1327–1340.

Swerdlow SH, et al. *WHO Classification of Tumours of Haematopoietic and Lymphoid Tissues*. 4th ed. Lyon, France: International Agency for Research on Cancer, 2008.

Weisdorf DJ, et al. Allogeneic bone marrow transplantation for chronic myelogenous leukemia: comparative analysis of unrelated versus matched sibling donors. *Blood* 2002;99:1971.

Atypical CML/Chronic Neutrophilic Leukemia

Gotlib J, et al. The new genetics of chronic neutrophilic leukemia and atypical CML: implications for diagnosis and treatment. *Blood* 2013;122:1707.

Chronic Myelomonocytic Leukemia

Aribi A, et al. Activity of decitabine, a hypomethylating agent, in chronic myelomonocytic leukemia. *Cancer* 2007;109:713.

Costa R, et al. Activity of azacitidine in chronic myelomonocytic leukemia. *Cancer* 2011;117(12):2690–2696.

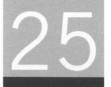

25 Myeloproliferative Neoplasms

Ronald L. Paquette

COMPARABLE ASPECTS

The World Health Organization (WHO) classification of the chronic myeloproliferative neoplasms (MPNs) includes polycythemia vera (PV), chronic idiopathic myelofibrosis (MF), essential thrombocythemia (ET), chronic eosinophilic leukemia (CEL)/hypereosinophilic syndrome (HES), chronic myelogenous leukemia (CML), chronic neutrophilic leukemia, and unclassifiable chronic MPN. Chronic myelomonocytic leukemia (CMML) has features of both an MPN and a myelodysplastic syndrome (MDS). Details on CML and CMML are presented in Chapter 24. This chapter focuses on PV, ET, MF, CEL/HES, and systemic mastocytosis (SM).

The MPNs each result from a genetic alteration within a pluripotent hematopoietic progenitor cell that induces the excessive production of one or more cell lineages. The individual diseases are distinguished by the predominant lineage that is overproduced. Table 25-1 compares important clinical and distinguishing features of the MPNs. There is considerable overlap between several of the MPNs. Long-term observation may be required to clarify the diagnosis.

Erythrocytosis, granulocytosis, eosinophilia, basophilia, and thrombocytosis may be due to disorders other than MPNs, as discussed in Chapter 35 in "Increased Blood Cell Counts." Similarly, bone marrow fibrosis may be secondary to a variety of other etiologies, as discussed in Chapter 35, Section I.B, in "Cytopenia."

I. PATHOGENESIS

The MPNs are clonal neoplastic disorders that arise from a single pluripotential hematopoietic stem cell. The molecular abnormalities occurring in the MPNs have overlap.

A. Molecular and cytogenetic abnormalities

1. ***JAK2* mutations.** A mutation of the Janus kinase 2 (*JAK2*) gene has been identified in PV, ET, and MF (>95%, 55%, and 65%, respectively). The JAK2 protein is a tyrosine kinase that is phosphorylated by the receptors for erythropoietin (EPO), thrombopoietin, granulocyte colony-stimulating factor, granulocyte–macrophage colony-stimulating factor, and interleukin-3 in response to ligand binding. Activation of *JAK2* in this way initiates a signaling cascade that induces cell proliferation in response to these growth factors. The most commonly observed *JAK2* mutation results in the replacement of valine by phenylalanine at position 617 (V617F) in exon 14. The mutated protein enables hematopoietic cells to survive in the absence of growth factors and to have enhanced proliferation when exposed to low growth factor concentrations. The *JAK2* V617F mutation occurs in approximately 95% of PV, 50% of ET or MF, 20% of unclassifiable MPN, and 2% of HES. The mutation is homozygous in approximately 40% of PV due to mitotic recombination. Mutations involving exon 12 of *JAK2* have been identified in about 4% of PV patients. The rare *JAK2* V625F and F556V mutations have been reported in ET.

TABLE 25-1 Clinical Features of the Myeloproliferative Neoplasms and Chronic Myelogenous Leukemia

Feature	PV	ET	MF	U-MPN	CML
Degree of Cellular Proliferation[a]					
Erythrocytosis	2+	N	N or D	N	N
Thrombocytosis	1+ → 2+	4+	2+ → 4+	1+	1+ → 2+
Granulocytosis	1+ → 2+	N → 2+	D → 2+	1+ → 2+	4+
Marrow fibrosis	1+	N → 1+	3+ → 4+	N → 1+	N → 1+
Extramedullary hematopoiesis	Late	A → 1+	2+ → 4+	A → 1+	N → 1+
Proportion of Patients with					
Splenomegaly	75%	30%	95%	Variable	95%
Hepatomegaly	40%	A	75%	A	50%
Cytogenetics					
Ph[1] chromosome	A	A	A	A	80%
Abnormal karyotypes	10%–20%	A	35%	Unknown	Ph[1], *bcr/abl*
JAK2 mutations	95%	50%	50%	20%	A
Preeminent Clinical Features	Hyperviscosity, thrombosis	Thrombosis, hemorrhage	Poikilocytosis, splenomegaly	Leukoerythroblastosis	Leukemic infiltration
Transition to Acute Leukemia	Uncommon	Rare	5%–10% at 10 yr	Unknown	6% at 5 yr

[a]The designations 1+ → 4+ indicate relative degrees of prominence.
PV, polycythemia vera; ET, essential thrombocythemia; MF, myelofibrosis with myeloid metaplasia; U-MPN, unclassifiable myeloproliferative disorder; CML, chronic myelogenous leukemia; N, normal; D, decreased; A, absent.

2. **MPL mutations.** Point mutations at position 515 (exon 10) of the thrombopoietin receptor (MPL) have been identified in 5% to 10% of patients with MF or ET. Rare mutations outside exon 10 have also been reported (T119I, S204P, S204F, Y591N, Y591D). The mutated MPL protein is hypersensitive to thrombopoietin, or it activates the *JAK2* signaling pathway in the absence of thrombopoietin.

3. **Calreticulin (CALR) mutations.** Calreticulin is a chaperone protein in the endoplasmic reticulum that regulates protein folding. It normally plays no known role in growth factor signaling, but it is mutated in 70% of ET and MF patients without a JAK2 mutation. CALR mutations are mutually exclusive with JAK2 or MPL mutations, suggesting that the mutated protein acts in a novel manner that intersects with JAK2 signaling. The numerous different CALR mutations occur in exon 9 of the gene and all cause a 1 base pair frame shift that produces a novel sequence in the carboxyl terminus of the CALR protein. The mutant C-terminus has numerous positively charged amino acid residues that replace negatively charged residues in the normal protein. This mutated C-terminus of CALR binds specifically to MPL and activates downstream signaling from the receptor in the absence of ligand.

4. **Mutations** have been identified in additional genes that encode proteins involved in critical cell processes. Mutations of these genes are also observed in myeloid malignancies.

   a. **Kinase signaling**: CBL ubiquitinates receptor tyrosine kinases, leading to their inactivation. Loss-of-function CBL mutations have been observed in MF. LNK inhibits JAK2 signaling. Inactivating mutations of LNK have been reported in ET and MF.

   b. **Epigenetic regulation**: TET2 transfers a hydroxyl group to methylcytosine of DNA. Mutations of TET2 have been reported in 5% to 20% of MPNs. ASXL1 participates in histone demethylation and is mutated in <10% of MPN patients. EZH2 plays a role in histone methylation and is mutated in approximately 13% of MF cases.

5. **Chromosome abnormalities** are found in about 20% of PV cases at the time of diagnosis, with deletions of 20q or 13q, or trisomies of 8 or 9 being most common. In MF, abnormal karyotypes are found in 35% of cases; deletions of 20q or 13q or trisomy 1q account for 70% of the abnormal karyotypes found. In some cases of CEL, a very small interstitial deletion on chromosome 4q12 fuses the *FIP1L1* and platelet-derived growth factor receptor alpha *(PDGFRA)* genes, producing a novel transforming fusion gene. The t(5;12)(q33;p13) occurs in other CEL cases and fuses the *PDGFR* beta *(PDGFRB)* gene to the *ETV6* gene.

B. **Familial MPNs** are associated with single nucleotide polymorphisms in noncoding regions of the JAK2, MECOM, TERT, or HBS1L-MYB genes. These genetic variants cannot be routinely tested at this time.

C. **Hematopoiesis in the MPNs** is generally characterized by autonomous growth of progenitor cells in the absence of growth factors and hypersensitivity to the proliferative effects of growth factors.

   1. **Erythropoiesis** *in vitro* in semisolid media normally requires exogenous EPO. Bone marrow progenitor cells from patients with PV form colonies *in vitro* without exogenous EPO and proliferate in response to very low EPO concentrations. Serum EPO levels are usually low in PV and are normal or elevated in most cases of secondary polycythemia.

2. **Granulocytopoiesis** is frequently increased in all MPNs to varying degrees and is manifested by neutrophilia (and in some cases eosinophilia or basophilia) and myeloid hyperplasia in the marrow.

3. **Megakaryocytopoiesis.** Megakaryocyte progenitors from ET patients are able to grow autonomously *in vitro* without added thrombopoietin.

4. **Extramedullary hematopoiesis** occurs in the liver and spleen in patients with MF and contributes to organ enlargement.

D. **Bone marrows in MPNs** demonstrate hypercellularity that is often trilineage but are diagnostic of a specific disorder only in MF. Megakaryocytes are greatly increased in number and size in ET and MF at all stages of disease and to a lesser degree in PV. Clustering of megakaryocytes is a common histopathologic feature of the MPNs.

1. **Reticulin fibrosis of the marrow** develops in all patients with MF and in many patients with PV or ET over time. The fibrosis is caused by the release of cytokines, including transforming growth factor β and basic fibroblast growth factor, from clonal megakaryocytes or monocytes. The growth factors act on nonclonal fibroblasts and stromal cells and induce increased deposition of various interstitial and basement membrane glycoproteins, including collagen types I, III, IV, and V. Type III collagen is uniformly and preferentially increased. The fine reticulin fibers that are visible with silver stains are principally type III collagen and do not stain with trichrome dyes.

2. **MF.** Marrow fibrosis is prominent in MF. Megakaryocytes are increased in number, and they are atypical, enlarged, and immature. Neutrophilic granulopoiesis is hyperplastic. A marked neovascularization is also present, even in the early proliferative phase of the disease.

3. **PV.** Trilineage hyperplasia in the marrow is the hallmark of PV. Erythroid hyperplasia is most prominent. Megakaryocytes are enlarged, clustered, mature, and pleomorphic with multilobulated nuclei. Iron stores are absent or decreased in most untreated patients. In secondary erythrocytosis, erythroid hyperplasia may be present, but megakaryocytes remain small and normal with no tendency to cluster.

4. **ET.** The bone marrow demonstrates increased numbers of enlarged megakaryocytes with mature cytoplasm, multilobulated nuclei, and a tendency to cluster. Cellularity is variably increased. In reactive thrombocytosis, increased numbers of megakaryocytes may be present, but they have normal size and morphology, and no tendency to cluster.

II. COMPLICATIONS OF THE MPNs

A. **Thrombotic phenomena,** both venous and arterial, can complicate PV, ET, and MF. Myocardial and cerebrovascular ischemias occur more commonly in patients with MPN compared to age-matched controls. Thrombosis in atypical locations such as the cerebral venous sinuses, mesenteric vein, or portal or hepatic veins is characteristic of MPNs. A patient with such a clotting event should be ruled out for MPN in the absence of a prior diagnosis.

1. **Thrombosis risks and prevention.** Major risk factors for thrombosis in PV, ET, and MF include age >60 years and history of a prior thrombotic event. Additional risk factors for thrombosis include hypertension, hyperlipidemia, diabetes, and smoking history. In ET and MF, the JAK2V617F mutation conveys an increased risk of thrombosis. The International Prognostic Score of thrombosis in Essential Thrombocythemia (IPSET-thrombosis) assigns 1 point for age >60 years, 2 points for thrombosis history, 1 point for cardiovascular risk factors, and 2 points for JAK2V617F mutation. Low-risk

patients (<2 points) generally do not need therapy. Aspirin is considered for intermediate-risk patients (2 points), provided there are no contra-indications. Cytoreductive therapy is recommended for high-risk disease (>2 points). Patients who experience thrombosis in spite of optimal medical management may require anticoagulation in addition to cytoreduction, with or without antiplatelet therapy.

In PV, the risk of thrombosis increases with the hematocrit, so phle-botomy is performed to keep the hematocrit <45% in men and <42% in women. All PV patients should also take a baby aspirin daily. Higher-risk patients (age >60 or prior thrombosis) should be considered for cytoreduc-tive therapy in addition to the other measures. PV patients should receive hydroxyurea when cytoreduction is clinically indicated, but the drug of choice in ET is not clear. One randomized trial demonstrated that hydroxy-urea (HU) was more effective than anagrelide (AG) in preventing arterial thrombotic events in high-risk ET patients. A smaller randomized study comparing HU and AG showed no significant difference in the incidence of arterial or venous thromboses in high-risk ET. The concern with long-term HU administration is a small, but significantly higher, risk of acute myeloid leukemia in patients receiving HU, which has not been observed with AG. Young ET patients who require long-term cytoreduction for thrombocytosis should probably receive AG as a result.

2. **Microvascular arterial thrombosis.** Erythromelalgia, localized painful ery-thema and warmth in the distal extremities, is a characteristic vasoocclusive manifestation of MPNs. It can be controlled by low-dose aspirin, but may require cytoreductive therapy.

B. **Bleeding risk in ET.** The level of the platelet count does *not* correlate with the risk of thrombosis in ET. In fact, higher platelet counts (over 1 million/µL) can be associated with increased bleeding risk due to sequestration of large von Willebrand multimers by the platelets. This condition, **acquired von Willebrand syndrome** (aVWS), should be evaluated by checking ristocetin cofactor activity prior to starting antiplatelet therapy in ET patients. Activity <20% would be a contraindication to aspirin administration. Careful assess-ment of risk/benefit should be undertaken before administering aspirin to patients with platelet counts over 1 million/µL. No characteristic platelet dys-function has been identified in ET.

C. **Pregnancy in ET and PV** is associated with a 20% to 30% risk of spontane-ous abortion in the first trimester, and the risk declines thereafter. Premature delivery occurs in about 6% of pregnancies. Maternal complications including thrombosis, hemorrhage, and pre-eclampsia appear to be higher in PV than in ET patients. Known risks include JAK2V617F mutation (in ET), platelet count >1 million, age >35 years, and especially history of previous complications with pregnancy. There are limited data from case series regarding use of prophylactic treatment in pregnancy. Low-dose aspirin could be considered for most patients as long as no bleeding diathesis is present (platelets > 1 million or acquired vWD). Aspirin appears to be safe during pregnancy, but its benefit is unknown. It is usu-ally discontinued 1 to 2 weeks before anticipated delivery. Low molecular weight heparin can be started after discontinuation of aspirin or initiated at the begin-ning of pregnancy for higher-risk patients. It is usually stopped 12 hours before anticipated delivery. Interferon alpha is reserved for the highest risk ET patients who require platelet-lowering therapy. Because thrombotic risk is very high post-partum, restarting aspirin and low molecular weight heparin could be considered for most patients without clinical contraindications, continuing for 6 weeks.

D. **Hyperuricemia** is often present in patients with active MPN. Treatment with allopurinol can prevent gouty arthritis, uric acid nephropathy, and nephrolithiasis.

E. **Progression to myelofibrosis** can occur in patients with ET or PV many years after diagnosis. Falling hemoglobin and platelet counts, progressive splenomegaly, and development of constitutional symptoms are clinical signs of this process.

F. **Transformation to acute myelogenous leukemia (AML).** The risk of progressing to AML is approximately 2% for ET, 5% for PV, and 30% for MF within 10 years of diagnosis.

G. **Cytoreductive therapy** can be indicated in PV, MF, or ET patients at high risk for thrombosis. It can also be used to reduce symptoms related to panmyelosis or splenomegaly.

   1. **Hydroxyurea (HU) or hydroxycarbamide** is a ribonucleotide reductase inhibitor that interferes with DNA synthesis. HU is the initial drug of choice for treating panmyelosis associated with PV. It is less beneficial than ruxolitinib in MF. In ET, HU may be more effective than AG in reducing arterial thrombotic events and progression of MF. Side effects of HU include myelosuppression, macrocytic anemia, fever, rash, stomatitis, leg ulcers, nausea, diarrhea, and renal dysfunction. Hydroxyurea has a low risk of leukemogenesis, which should be a concern in younger patients who require long-term cytoreductive therapy.

   2. **Anagrelide** is a selective inhibitor of platelet production that controls thrombocytosis in MPN patients within 1 to 6 weeks. The maintenance dosage is usually 2 to 2.5 mg/d in two divided doses. The main side effects of AG are headache, palpitations, fluid retention, liver function abnormalities, nausea, diarrhea, and abdominal pain. It can also cause tachycardia, torsades de pointes, and congestive heart failure, so it should be used cautiously in patients with cardiac problems. Interstitial pneumonitis is an uncommon but potentially serious side effect. Its safety in pregnancy has not been established so it should be avoided in this setting. Chronic administration may cause progressive anemia. It may be more likely than HU to be associated with progressive marrow fibrosis.

   3. **Ruxolitinib** is a JAK1/JAK2 inhibitor initially approved to reduce constitutional symptoms and splenomegaly in intermediate- or high-risk MF that is either primary or secondary to other MPNs. It also appears to improve survival in MF, so it is the initial treatment of choice. Its activity against JAK2 is not specific for the V617F mutant, and it conveys similar benefit regardless of mutational status. Ruxolitinib also alleviates the need for phlebotomy, reduces splenomegaly, and reduces constitutional symptoms in PV patients who are refractory or intolerant to HU. Approved dosing for MF is 20 mg b.i.d. for baseline platelet count >200,000/μL and 15 mg b.i.d. for platelets 100,000 to 200,000/μL; in PV, it is 10 mg b.i.d. However, these dosing schedules can induce a profound and rapid decline in blood counts. Therefore, **it is best to initiate therapy at 5 mg b.i.d. and titrate the dose up gradually as tolerated**. The median dose capable of controlling symptoms in MF patients is 10 mg b.i.d., but higher doses may be required to optimize reduction of splenomegaly. Side effects include anemia, thrombocytopenia, dizziness, diarrhea, fever, weight gain, and increased risk of herpes zoster.

   4. **Interferon α** suppresses hematopoietic progenitor and bone marrow fibroblast proliferation and reduces levels of fibrogenic cytokines including platelet-derived growth factor and transforming growth factor β. Interferon α, when

given at a dose of 500,000 to 3 million units SQ three times weekly, can reduce blood counts, eliminate phlebotomy requirements (in PV), reduce splenomegaly, ameliorate pruritus, and possibly delay MF. Its effect on thromboembolic risk is unknown. In ET and PV, it can reduce the percentage of cells with *JAK2*V617F mutation slowly over several months, and complete molecular remissions can be achieved, but its impact on the natural history of MPN is unclear. Its use is limited by side effects including flu-like symptoms, fatigue, weight loss, altered mental status, depression, peripheral neuropathy, and autoimmune disease. Interferon α is not leukemogenic or teratogenic, so it can be used in pregnant patients. Pegylated interferon α is a better tolerated preparation that requires less frequent (once weekly) dosing and has less severe side effects. Pegylated interferon α is started at a dose of 90 mg SQ weekly for 2 weeks and then escalated as tolerated every 2 weeks up to 180 mg/week.

5. **Radioactive phosphorus (^{32}P) and alkylating agents** can control panmyelosis and reduce the incidence of thrombosis, but they unacceptably increase the incidence of AML.

POLYCYTHEMIA VERA

See "Comparable Aspects" at the beginning of this chapter for pathogenesis and complications of PV.

I. DIAGNOSIS

PV is a clonal MPN that harbors a *JAK2* V617F mutation in >95% of cases. Exon 12 *JAK2* mutations are present in most of the remaining patients. Therefore, mutation analysis of the *JAK2* gene will segregate PV from secondary causes of erythrocytosis.

A. WHO criteria (2008). The diagnosis of PV requires both major criteria plus any minor criterion, or the A1 criterion plus any two minor criteria.

  1. Major criteria

  A1. Hemoglobin (Hg) >18.5 g/dL in men, >16.5 g/dL in women, or Hg >99th percentile of method-specific reference range for age, sex, and altitude of residence

  Hg >17 g/dL in men or >15 g/dL in women if a sustained increase of >2 g/dL from baseline that is not due to correction of iron deficiency

  Red cell mass >25% above mean predicted

  A2. Presence of *JAK2* V617F or exon 12 mutation

  2. Minor Criteria

  B1. Bone marrow biopsy hypercellular for age with trilineage growth (panmyelosis) with prominent erythroid, granulocytic, and megakaryocytic proliferation

  B2. Serum EPO level below the reference range for normal

  B3. Endogenous erythroid colony formation *in vitro*

B. Laboratory studies

  1. Red blood cell mass (RBCM). Autologous RBCs are ^{51}Cr labeled and injected intravenously, and then a blood sample is drawn to quantitate the dilution of the labeled cells and calculate the circulating RBCM. RBCM using ^{51}Cr is rarely available today.

  2. Clonal genetic abnormality. The presence of the *JAK2* V617F or exon 12 mutation in the blood or bone marrow is adequate to demonstrate a clonal etiology for the erythrocytosis. Absence of a *JAK2* mutation suggests a secondary cause for the erythrocytosis.

3. **Erythroid colony-forming assay.** PV bone marrow cells proliferate without EPO in culture. This assay is not routinely performed by clinical laboratories.

4. **Supportive studies**
   a. **CBC.** Erythrocytes are usually normocytic and normochromic unless iron deficiency is present. Poikilocytosis and anisocytosis accompany the transition into MF late in the disease course. Granulocytosis in the range of 12,000 to 25,000/µL occurs in two-thirds of patients at presentation. Early forms may be present but are not frequent. Two-thirds of patients have basophilia. Platelet counts usually are in the range of 450,000 to 800,000/µL, occasionally with abnormal morphology.
   b. **Serum EPO levels** can be normal or reduced in PV. Although autonomous expansion of the RBCM would be expected to suppress EPO production, this assay cannot reliably distinguish between PV and EPO-driven erythrocytosis. Furthermore, a normal serum EPO level is common in hypoxic erythrocytosis unless the hypoxemia is extreme.
   c. **Abdominal ultrasonography, CT, or MRI scanning** can rule out renal or hepatic causes of erythrocytosis and quantitate spleen size.
   d. **Bone marrow examination** can be used to demonstrate panmyelosis and abnormal megakaryocyte morphology consistent with PV or quantitate the extent of reticulin fibrosis if transition to MF is suspected.

C. **Differential diagnosis** includes the other MPNs and relative or secondary erythrocytosis (see Chapter 35, Section I, in "Increased Blood Cell Counts"). Reduced plasma volume, hypoxemia (e.g., altitude, emphysema, sleep apnea), renal cysts or carcinoma, hepatic neoplasms, or uterine myomata can cause secondary erythrocytosis.

II. CLINICAL COURSE

The survival of patients with PV approaches that of a matched otherwise healthy population with modern therapy. The median survival exceeds 12 years.

A. **Predominant signs and symptoms** early in the disease are caused by increased RBCM that results in plethora and hyperviscosity. Hyperviscosity results in decreased blood flow and causes tissue hypoxia. Manifestations include headache, dizziness, vertigo, tinnitus, visual disturbances, claudication, stroke, angina pectoris, and myocardial infarction. Modest splenomegaly is present in 75% of cases and hepatomegaly in 40%. Splenomegaly is initially caused predominantly by increased splenic red blood cell pooling and not by extramedullary hematopoiesis. Pruritus, urticaria, and gout are relatively common in PV.

B. **Phases of disease**
   1. **Erythrocytic phase.** The phase of persistent erythrocytosis that necessitates regular phlebotomies lasts from 5 to 25 years.
   2. **Spent phase.** Eventually, the patient enters a "spent" or "burned-out" phase; the need for phlebotomies is greatly reduced, and the patient enters a period of apparent remission. Anemia eventually supervenes, but thrombocytosis and leukocytosis usually persist. The spleen increases in size, and marrow fibrosis can be present.
   3. **Myelofibrotic phase.** MF develops in 5% to 10% of patients with PV. Anemia and often thrombocytopenia evolve in this phase. Constitutional symptoms and progressive splenomegaly develop. Reticulin fibrosis with or without osteosclerosis is present in the bone marrow. When cytopenias and progressive splenomegaly develop, the clinical manifestations, course, and treatment are the same as for primary MF.

III. MANAGEMENT

A. **Principles of treatment** (see "Complications of the MPNs" above)

1. **Phlebotomy** to reduce the hematocrit (<45 for males, <42 for females)

a. Initially, 500 mL of blood may be removed every other day (only 250 mL of blood should be removed in patients with serious vascular disease).

b. About 200 mg of iron is removed with each 500 mL of blood (the normal total body iron content is about 5 g). Iron deficiency to reduce erythropoiesis is a goal of chronic phlebotomy, so do not replace iron.

2. **Low-dose aspirin** to reduce thrombotic risk and manage erythromelalgia.

3. **Cytoreductive therapy** should be given to high-risk patients.

4. **Cardiovascular risk factors** should be modified when possible.

5. Supportive care

a. **Hyperuricemia** is treated with allopurinol, 100 to 600 mg/d PO.

b. **Anticoagulation** for acute thrombotic complications is managed as for patients without PV.

c. **Pruritus** can be treated with the following:

(1) Histamine blockers, such as hydroxyzine (25 mg PO q.i.d.).

(2) Selective serotonin reuptake inhibitors, including paroxetine 20 mg/d or fluoxetine 10 mg/d.

(3) If the above measures fail, HU or ruxolitinib can be tried.

d. **Symptomatic splenomegaly** may be addressed with HU or ruxolitinib.

B. **Surgery**

1. **Elective surgery** should be avoided if PV is inadequately controlled, due to a high risk of hemorrhagic or thrombotic complications. If surgery is required, the following approaches are recommended:

a. **Phlebotomy.** The hematocrit should be reduced to <45%. The blood obtained by phlebotomy may be saved for autologous transfusion.

2. **Emergency surgery.** Aggressive phlebotomy should be performed prior to surgery, if HCT is not controlled. Assess the need for clotting factor replacement if >4 units are removed.

3. **Splenectomy** is occasionally performed for massive splenomegaly in the myelofibrotic phase of PV. Unfortunately, a high rate of perioperative mortality may be expected for elderly or frail patients. In addition, splenomegaly unresponsive to therapy is often an indicator of disease progression, which may become evident shortly after the procedure.

ESSENTIAL THROMBOCYTHEMIA

See "Comparable Aspects" at the beginning of this chapter for pathogenesis, bone marrow findings, and complications of ET.

I. DIAGNOSIS

A. **WHO criteria (2008).** The diagnosis of ET requires all four major criteria (A1 to A4):

A1. Platelet count sustained >450,000/µL.

A2. Bone marrow shows primarily megakaryocytic proliferation with increased numbers of large, mature megakaryocytes. Granulopoiesis and erythropoiesis are not increased or left shifted.

A3. Does not meet WHO criteria for CML, PV, MF, MDS, or other myeloid neoplasm.

A4. Presence of JAK2 or MPL mutation, or other clonal marker; no evidence of reactive thrombocytosis.

B. **Laboratory studies**
1. **Platelet counts** always exceed 450,000/μL and are often present as clumps, giant platelets, or megakaryocytic fragments.
   a. **Erythrocytes.** Hypochromic, microcytic anemia can be present. Howell-Jolly bodies may indicate splenic atrophy from repeated infarctions.
   b. **Granulocytosis** is present in half of cases, usually in the range of 15,000 to 30,000/μL. Myelocytes and earlier forms are rare, and basophilia is mild, if present.
2. **Iron studies** including iron, TIBC, and ferritin should be done to exclude iron deficiency as the cause for thrombocytosis.
3. **Markers of inflammation** such as Westergren sedimentation rate, ANA, and rheumatoid factor should be ordered if clinically indicated to rule out inflammation as a cause of thrombocytosis.
4. **Bone marrow examination** shows hypercellularity, markedly increased numbers of megakaryocytes, often occurring in clusters (see "Comparable Aspects," Section I.C). Iron stores should be adequate. Cytogenetic studies show no Philadelphia chromosome or *BCR/ABL* gene rearrangement (observed in CML) and no 5q deletion (observed in MDS).
C. **Differential diagnosis** of ET includes reactive thrombocytosis (splenectomy, iron deficiency, malignancy, infection, inflammation, or GI bleeding as discussed in Chapter 35, Section VII, in "Increased Blood Cell Counts"), familial thrombocytosis related to increased levels of thrombopoietin, the other MPNs, CML, and MDS. The MDS subtypes that are most frequently associated with thrombocytosis include refractory anemia with the deletion 5q chromosomal abnormality or refractory anemia with ringed sideroblasts.

II. CLINICAL COURSE

A. **Signs and symptoms.** Most patients do not have symptoms when ET is discovered. The spleen may be enlarged, normal, or atrophic. Hepatomegaly is absent. Extramedullary hematopoiesis is not a major feature of ET. Pruritus develops in 10% to 15% of patients.
B. **Thrombotic or hemorrhagic events.** These are addressed above in "Complications of the MPNs."
C. **Survival** approaches that of age matched, otherwise healthy controls. The median survival exceeds 10 years, and the 5-year survival rate is >80%. Transformation of ET into MF is a late event, and acute myeloid leukemia is rare if leukemogenic agents have not been used.

III. MANAGEMENT

A. **Prevention of thrombosis** is addressed in detail above in "Complications of the MPNs."
1. **Low-dose ASA** for intermediate- or high-risk ET.
2. **Cytoreductive therapy** for high-risk disease.
3. **Platelet pheresis** is indicated for emergency treatment of life-threatening complications of severe thrombocytosis.
4. **Cardiovascular risk factors** should be modified when possible.

PRIMARY MYELOFIBROSIS

See "Comparable Aspects" at the beginning of this chapter for pathogenesis, bone marrow findings, and complications of the MPNs. Radiation exposure is associated with an increased incidence of MF but accounts for only a small percentage of cases. Familial genetic factors can predispose to MF.

I. DIAGNOSIS

A. **WHO criteria (2008).** The diagnosis of MF requires all three major criteria and two minor criteria.

1. **Major criteria**

   A1. Bone marrow shows megakaryocyte proliferation and atypia (small to large megakaryocytes with aberrant nuclear/cytoplasmic ratio; hyperchromatic, irregularly folded nuclei; and dense clustering) accompanied by reticulin and/or collagen fibrosis. In the absence of reticulin fibrosis, the megakaryocyte changes must be accompanied by increased bone marrow cellularity, granulocytic proliferation, and decreased erythropoiesis (prefibrotic MF).

   A2. Does not meet WHO criteria for CML, PV, ET, MDS, or other myeloid neoplasm.

   A3. JAK2 V617F mutation, or other clonal marker; no evidence of reactive fibrosis.

2. **Minor criteria**

   B1. Leukoerythroblastic blood smear (nucleated red blood cells and granulocytosis) with anisocytosis and poikilocytosis

   B2. Increased serum LDH

   B3. Anemia

   B4. Palpable splenomegaly

B. **Laboratory studies**

1. **Mutations of *JAK2, CALR,* or** *MPL* occur in 50%, 30%, and 5% of MF patients, respectively, and are mutually exclusive. Triple-negative patients have an adverse prognosis. The presence of a mutation excludes secondary causes of fibrosis but does not exclude other MPNs.

2. **Erythrocytes.** Anemia is moderate in two-thirds of patients at presentation. Dacrocytes ("teardrop" cells), ovalocytes, pronounced anisocytosis, polychromasia, and nucleated red blood cells make up the characteristic blood picture of MF. Reticulocytosis can be present.

3. **Granulocytes** usually range from 10,000 to 30,000/μL. Blasts and promyelocytes constitute <10% of the granulocytes. Granulocytopenia occurs in a minority of patients. Basophils are only slightly increased.

4. **Platelets** are increased in one-third, normal in one-third, and decreased in one-third of patients with MF, depending on the stage of disease. Thrombocytopenia is indicative of advanced disease.

5. **Bone marrow examination** shows hypercellularity, granulocytic hyperplasia, and markedly increased numbers of atypical megakaryocytes. Fibrosis is patchy and variable in distribution; reticulin is always increased.

6. **Immunologic abnormalities** such as monoclonal antibodies (10%), positive direct Coombs tests (20%), polyclonal hyperglobulinemia, RF, ANA, antiphospholipid antibodies, or circulating immune complexes can be found in patients with MF. Anemia in such patients may respond favorably to a trial of glucocorticoids.

C. **Differential diagnosis of MF** includes the other MPNs, CML, MDS, AML of the megakaryoblastic (M7) subtype, hairy cell leukemia, Hodgkin lymphoma, metastatic carcinoma associated with marrow fibrosis (desmoplastic reaction), autoimmune diseases (especially systemic lupus erythematosus), and disseminated mycobacterial infection. Secondary MF is discussed in Chapter 35, Section I.B, in "Cytopenia."

II. CLINICAL COURSE

A. **Symptoms** can be due to excessive production of inflammatory cytokines such as interleukin-6, anemia, or splenomegaly. Virtually all patients have splenomegaly, which may be massive, and three-fourths of patients have hepatomegaly. Progression to AML is commonly manifested by fever, weight loss, and debilitating bone pain.

B. **Thrombotic events.** MF patients are at increased risk of thrombotic complications, as described above under "Complications of the MPNs."

C. **Survival.** The clinical course of MF is extremely variable. Death is due to heart failure, infection, hemorrhage, or transformation to AML. Development of AML occurs in approximately 30% of MF patients. Several prognostic scoring systems have been published. These were validated prior to the use of ruxolitinib, the use of which is likely to significantly prolong median survival for MF.

1. **Dynamic International Prognostic Scoring System (DIPSS)** can be used at diagnosis or anytime thereafter.
   a. **Variables**
      (1) Hemoglobin < 10 g/dL (2 points)
      (2) WBC > 25,000/μL (1 point)
      (3) Peripheral blood blasts ≥1% (1 point)
      (4) Constitutional symptoms (1 point)
      (5) Age ≥65 years (1 point)
   b. **Scoring**
      Score 0: low risk (median survival not reached)
      Score 1–2: intermediate-1 risk (median survival 9.8 years)
      Score 3–4: intermediate-2 risk (median survival 4.8 years)
      Score 5–6: high risk (median survival 2.3 years)

2. **DIPSS Plus** further refines prognosis
   a. **Variables**
      (1) DIPSS intermediate-1 (1 point)
      (2) DIPSS intermediate-2 (2 points)
      (3) DIPSS high risk (3 points)
      (4) Unfavorable karyotype (1 point) (complex with ≥3 abnormalities or 1 to 2 abnormalities that include +8, –7/7q, i(17)q, –5/5q–, 12p–, inv(3), or 11q23 rearrangement)
      (5) Platelets < 100,000/μL (1 point)
      (6) Red cell transfusion dependent (1 point)
   b. **Scoring**
      Score 0: low risk (median survival 185 months)
      Score 1: intermediate-1 risk (median survival 78 months)
      Score 2–3: intermediate-2 risk (median survival 35 months)
      Score 4–6: high risk (median survival 16 months)

D. **Associated syndromes**

1. **Portal hypertension and varices in MF** are caused by massive increases in splenoportal blood flow and decreased hepatic vascular compliance. The decreased compliance is due to extramedullary hematopoiesis and its secondary collagen deposition.

2. **Extramedullary hematopoietic tumors** can develop in any location. Foci of these tumors on serosal surfaces can cause effusions containing immature hematopoietic cells. Biopsy should be performed to rule out conversion to acute myeloid leukemia (myeloid sarcoma).

III. MANAGEMENT

A. **Medical management** (see "Complications of the MPNs" above)

1. **Low-dose aspirin** should be given unless contraindicated by thrombocytopenia to prevent thrombosis.

2. **Ruxolitinib** should be considered for patients with constitutional symptoms or symptomatic splenomegaly. Although it can improve symptoms and prolong survival, it can exacerbate anemia and thrombocytopenia.

3. **Hydroxyurea** can reduce splenomegaly in MF, but it is less effective than ruxolitinib, and it is myelosuppressive.

4. **Interferon α** use in MF is complicated by intolerable side effects and worsening cytopenias.

5. **Lenalidomide** in doses of 10 mg daily can improve anemia, thrombocytopenia, in a minority of patients, but it is more likely to exacerbate cytopenias instead.

6. **Glucocorticoids,** such as prednisone (starting 20 mg/d), can ameliorate systemic symptoms and anemia in a minority of MF patients.

7. **Androgens,** such as fluoxymesterone 10 mg PO b.i.d. or danazol 200 to 400 mg PO b.i.d., may improve anemia in a minority of MF patients. Several months of treatment are necessary before improvement is evident.

8. **Erythropoiesis-stimulating agents** can improve the anemia in some MF patients, but their efficacy would likely be reduced by ruxolitinib, as EPO signals through JAK2.

B. **Bone marrow or peripheral blood stem cell transplantation** is potentially curative for MF, but it is associated with 10% to 20% risk of nonrelapse mortality at 1 year. Selecting the optimal timing for transplant is difficult because the long-term impact of ruxolitinib on survival has not yet been fully evaluated. However, it is critical to transplant a suitable patient before AML evolution occurs. Therefore, transplant should be considered for intermediate-2 or high-risk disease or intermediate-1 risk patients who have not benefitted from ruxolitinib. Reduced intensive conditioning regimens can extend the use of transplantation to older patients by decreasing nonrelapse mortality, albeit at the cost of increasing risk of relapsed disease.

C. **Splenectomy** can provide relief from symptoms of massive splenomegaly and can unpredictably improve anemia and thrombocytopenia. There is a perioperative mortality risk of approximately 10%. Peripheral blood cytopenias may persist or worsen if a significant amount of extramedullary hematopoiesis is carried out in the spleen prior to splenectomy. There is no reliable preoperative test to predict the contribution of splenic hematopoiesis. Conversely, marked thrombocytosis can follow splenectomy in approximately 20% of patients and be associated with an increased risk of postoperative thrombosis. Progressive hepatomegaly may follow splenectomy in approximately 16% of patients. Because progressive splenomegaly often is an indicator of disease progression, development of AML occurs in approximately 16% of patients within a year after surgery. There is no clear benefit of routine splenectomy prior to allogeneic transplantation other than earlier hematopoietic recovery.

D. **Radiation therapy (RT)**

Small doses (20 to 300 cGy per course given in daily fractions of 20 cGy) of RT to the spleen can relieve pain and early satiety secondary to massive splenomegaly in MF, usually for a few months. RT can be considered when ruxolitinib is ineffective and splenectomy is contraindicated.

CHRONIC EOSINOPHILIC LEUKEMIA AND HYPEREOSINOPHILIC SYNDROME

I. DEFINITION AND MANIFESTATIONS

A. **CEL and HES** are characterized by blood eosinophilia (eosinophils $\geq$ 1,500/µL) and by tissue infiltration with relatively mature eosinophils, resulting in multisystem organ dysfunction. CEL is distinguished from HES by the former having evidence of clonality, such as a cytogenetic or molecular abnormality, or increased blasts (>2% in blood or >5% in bone marrow). In addition, the WHO classification distinguishes CEL from myeloid neoplasms with eosinophilia and abnormalities of *PDGFRA, PDGFRB,* or *FGFR1* based on the characteristic chromosomal translocations observed in the latter conditions. HES, on the other hand, is idiopathic and not clonal. Because CEL and HES have overlapping clinical manifestations, they can be difficult to distinguish, and HES is a diagnosis of exclusion. CEL and HES occur predominantly in men, usually between the ages of 20 and 50 years.

B. **Etiology and pathogenesis.** CEL is associated most commonly with a small interstitial deletion of the *CHIC2* gene on chromosome 4q12 that fuses the *PDGFRA* gene to the *FIP1L1* gene, producing a novel transforming fusion gene. This deletion is too small to be detected by routine cytogenetics, but it can be identified by fluorescence *in situ* hybridization (FISH) or reverse transcriptase polymerase chain reaction (PCR) for the *FIP1L1–PDGFRA* fusion. These patients often have increased mast cells (MCs) in the bone marrow. CEL also can be associated with a translocation involving the *PDGFRB* gene on chromosome 5q31–33 and the *ETV6* gene on chromosome 12p12–13, or numerous other partners, resulting in the formation of another novel fusion gene. These patients often have eosinophilia accompanying CMML. Other rare cases of CEL can occur as a result of translocations involving *FGFR1, ABL1,* or *JAK2.* Next-generation sequencing has identified mutations commonly occurring in other myeloid malignancies, in approximately 27% of patients otherwise thought to have HES, thus reclassifying them as CEL. These mutations include ASXL1, TET2, EZH2, SETBP1, CBL, and NOTCH1. These patients have a clinical course that is similar to other CEL patients.

   The etiology of HES is idiopathic by definition. In some cases, there may be overproduction of cytokines that stimulate eosinophil production, such as granulocyte–macrophage colony-stimulating factor, interleukin-3, or interleukin-5.

C. **Organ system involvement**

   1. **Hematopoietic system involvement.** The absolute eosinophil count must be >1,500/µL in the absence of other causes of eosinophilia and usually ranges from 3,000 to 25,000/µL. The eosinophils are usually mature but often contain decreased numbers of granules that are small in size. Half of the patients have a normocytic, normochromic anemia. Bone marrow cytology shows myeloid hyperplasia with 25% to 75% of these cells being eosinophils, which have left-shifted maturation. Increased numbers of myeloblasts and cytogenetic abnormalities are absent.

   2. **Cardiac involvement** (55% to 75% of cases). Myocardial necrosis is associated with the presence of increased numbers of eosinophils seen on endomyocardial biopsy. Thrombi develop in the ventricles or atria and can embolize. Mitral or tricuspid valvular regurgitation and restrictive cardiomyopathy due to endomyocardial fibrosis develop after about 2 years of eosinophilia.

3. **Neurologic involvement** can include cerebral thromboembolism originating in the heart, encephalopathy, and peripheral sensory polyneuropathy.

4. **Lung involvement** usually manifests as a chronic nonproductive cough. Initially, the chest radiograph can be clear, or pleural effusions can be present. Pulmonary function test abnormalities are rare in the absence of congestive heart failure or pulmonary emboli arising from the right ventricle. Diffuse or focal infiltrations develop in 20% of patients. Bronchial asthma is a rare occurrence in CEL or HES.

5. **Cutaneous involvement.** Skin rashes develop in >50% of cases. Urticarial or angioedematous lesions, erythematous papules and nodules, or mucosal ulcers may develop.

6. **Involvement of other organs.** Splenomegaly develops in 40% of cases. Rheumatologic manifestations include arthralgias, effusions, and Raynaud phenomenon. Eosinophilic gastritis, enterocolitis, chronic active hepatitis, and Budd-Chiari syndrome have been observed in CEL and HES. Visual blurring caused by microemboli or microscopic hematuria may occur.

II. DIFFERENTIAL DIAGNOSIS

See Chapter 35, Section III, in "Increased Blood Cell Counts" for eosinophilia.

A. **Other chronic MPNs.** Patients with CEL or HES rarely have expansions of other cell lines besides eosinophils to the extent seen in the other chronic MPNs and do not develop severe MF.

B. **Other hematopoietic malignancies,** especially acute myelomonocytic leukemia with inv(16) cytogenetics, T-cell lymphoma, Hodgkin lymphoma, and SM.

C. **Eosinophilic syndromes limited to specific organs** lack the multiplicity of organ involvement often found in CEL or HES.

D. **Churg-Strauss syndrome** is the major vasculitis associated with eosinophilia. It is characterized by asthma, pulmonary infiltrates, eosinophilia, paranasal sinus abnormalities, neuropathy, and blood vessels showing extravascular eosinophils. Asthma is usually absent in HES, which distinguishes it from Churg-Strauss syndrome.

III. DIAGNOSIS

A. **Diagnostic criteria for HES**

1. Persistently increased absolute eosinophil count >1,500/μL for longer than 6 months

2. Absence of parasites, allergies, or other causes of eosinophilia

3. Evidence of organ system involvement

4. Absence of clonal chromosome or molecular abnormalities, which would justify the diagnosis of CEL

B. **Helpful studies**

1. Complete history and physical examination, CBC, liver and renal function tests, and urinalysis

2. Immunoglobulin E levels and serologic tests for collagen vascular disorders

3. Chest radiograph

4. Electrocardiogram, echocardiogram, and serum troponin T assay to assess cardiac involvement

5. Bone marrow aspirate and biopsy with chromosome analysis

6. FISH and PCR assays for *PDGFRA, PDGFRB,* and *FGFR1* gene rearrangements

7. T-cell receptor gene rearrangement assay to rule out clonal T-cell disorder

8. Next-generation genome sequencing for myeloid neoplasm-associated gene mutations

9. Biopsy of skin lesions

10. Serum tryptase level and *c-KIT* mutation analysis to rule out SM

    11. Several stool samples for ova and parasites
    12. Serology to exclude *Strongyloides* sp. infection

IV. PROGNOSIS

Historically, >75% of patients survived for at least 5 years and 40% survived at least 10 years, depending on the ability to manage the effects of end-organ damage. Congestive heart failure or a WBC count >90,000/µL at presentation is associated with a poor prognosis.

V. MANAGEMENT

  A. Imatinib. All patients with CEL or HES should be given a trial of imatinib 400 mg daily because even patients without identifiable *PDGFRA* or *PDGFRB* gene rearrangement have been reported to respond to this therapy. Doses as low as 100 mg/d are effective to treat some patients. When *PDGFRA* and *PDGFRB* translocations are present, monitoring of disease status every 3 months while on therapy by quantitative PCR (if available) or FISH should be performed. In patients with baseline cardiac abnormalities, serial monitoring of troponin T levels should be performed after initiating imatinib therapy to monitor for exacerbation of cardiac dysfunction. This potential complication may be reduced by pretreatment with glucocorticoids of at-risk patients.

  B. Glucocorticoids. Most patients benefit from glucocorticoid therapy. Treatment is usually reserved for symptomatic disease. Moderately high doses of prednisone (1 mg/kg/d) should be started and tapered as tolerated to minimum effective dose.

  C. Cytoreductive therapy with HU of interferon alpha can sometimes be beneficial for symptomatic patients. Hypomethylating agents could be considered for patients with increased blasts.

MASTOCYTOSIS

I. PATHOGENESIS

Mastocytosis includes a heterogeneous group of diseases characterized by abnormal growth and accumulation of MCs in one or more organ systems. Although not classically listed as a myeloproliferative syndrome, MCs are myeloid cells and are clonally derived from CD34+ progenitors; thus, mastocytosis is included in this chapter.

    MCs express stem cell factor receptor (CD117), CD2, and CD25. *KIT* is the protooncogene that encodes the tyrosine kinase receptor for stem cell factor. KIT mutations occur in the tyrosine kinase domain and are associated with autonomous phosphorylation and activation of the receptor. More than 80% of patients with SM have the point mutation of *KIT* at codon 816 (mostly D816V) detected by PCR.

II. WHO CLASSIFICATION OF MC DISEASE is as follows (note that the D816V mutation has been found in all of these categories):

Cutaneous mastocytosis (CM)
Indolent systemic mastocytosis (ISM)
Aggressive systemic mastocytosis (ASM)
Systemic mastocytosis with associated clonal, hematologic non-MC lineage disease (SM-AHNMD; e.g., AML, CML, MDSs, MPNs, and CEL)
MC leukemia
MC sarcoma and extracutaneous mastocytoma (very rare localized phenomena)

III. CLINICAL FEATURES

CM affecting children accounts for >85% of cases of MC disease. It presents as urticaria pigmentosa or diffuse CM and usually has a benign course that resolves before puberty.

SM is an uncommon disease, affects mostly adults and is most frequently reported in Israelis and light-skinned Caucasians. MCs infiltrate any organ that contains mesenchymal tissue (particularly the lymph nodes, liver, spleen, and bone marrow) and produce local destructive or fibrotic changes. Organ infiltration often indicates acceleration of the disease.

A. **Skin changes.** Urticaria pigmentosa is the most common early manifestation of systemic disease. Brownish skin nodules diffusely infiltrated with MCs may be localized or diffuse, flat or raised, bullous, or erythematous. Mild skin trauma may produce urticaria or dermatographia.

B. **Organ infiltration** may develop years after skin lesions have appeared and is manifested by hepatomegaly, lymphadenopathy, bone pain, bone marrow fibrosis, and, occasionally, MC leukemia. Osteosclerotic lesions on radiographs are common. Extracutaneous organ infiltration often indicates acceleration of the disease. Hyperchlorhydria occasionally occurs and can result in peptic ulcers and malabsorption.

C. **Hyperhistaminemia symptoms** may be precipitated by exposure to cold, alcohol, narcotics, fever, or hot baths and include the following:
1. Erythematous flushing, urticaria, edema, and pruritus
2. Abdominal pain, nausea, vomiting (occasionally diarrhea), flatulence, and steatorrhea
3. Sudden hypotension

IV. DIAGNOSIS

The histopathologic diagnosis of SM is made using immunostaining against tryptase, CD117, CD2, and CD25. Bone marrow, rather than blood, should be assayed for the *KIT* D816V mutation.

A. **CM** is confirmed by skin biopsy; bone marrow biopsy is not needed. Serum tryptase levels are normal.

B. **SM** is diagnosed by biopsies of both skin and bone marrow. Because of its implications regarding treatment, the *KIT* mutation variant should be determined. The diagnosis of SM is established with the major criterion plus one minor criterion or at least three minor criteria.
1. **Major criterion for diagnosis:** multifocal dense MC infiltrates (>15 MCs per infiltrate) in the bone marrow or other extracutaneous organ
2. **Minor criteria**
   a. In biopsy specimens of bone marrow or other extracutaneous lesions, >25% of MCs are spindle shaped or have an atypical morphology.
   b. Expression of CD2 and/or CD25 on blood, marrow, or organ MC.
   c. *KIT* point mutation at codon 816 in marrow or extracutaneous organ.
   d. Serum tryptase level >20 ng/mL.

V. MANAGEMENT

In the vast majority of patients with SM, the condition is very stable over many years. Results of various treatments have been unsatisfactory.

A. **Histamine antagonism** by H_1 and H_2 receptor blockade may help flushing, itching, and gastric distress. Cyclooxygenase inhibition may prevent prostaglandin D_2–induced hypotension when indicated. Oral cromolyn (200 mg PO q.i.d.) may prevent GI symptoms and bone pain.

B. **Cytoreduction** is considered when the patient develops evidence of decreased organ function such as anemia (hemoglobin <10 g/dL), neutropenia (<1,000/μL), thrombocytopenia (<100,000/μL), abnormal liver function tests, ascites, hypersplenism, malabsorption with weight loss, or large osteolytic lesions and/or severe osteoporosis.

1. **Cladribine** (2-CdA) is associated with a major response rate of about 50%. The dosing schedule is 0.1 to 0.15 mg/kg/d given IV over 2 to 3 hours for 5 consecutive days every 2 to 6 months for one to six cycles.

2. **Interferon α** is associated with a major response rate of about 20%, as well as significant morbidity from the drug. Doses have ranged from 9 to 42 million units per week, usually given with glucocorticoids.

3. **Tyrosine kinase inhibitors,** which have activity against *KIT*, including imatinib and dasatinib, are not active against the D816V mutation. Imatinib is very effective in patients with SM and eosinophilia who harbor the *FIP1L1–PDGFRA* fusion. Midostaurin, active in FLT-3–mutated AML, has activity in SM, but has not yet been approved by the Food and Drug Administration.

C. **Treatment approach**

1. **CM and SM.** Patients are treated with drugs targeting only histamine mediators unless they have severe osteopenia or recurrent shock-like episodes. Patients with smoldering SM are observed expectantly; cytoreduction can be considered with progression.

2. **SM with slow progression** can be treated with 2-CdA or interferon alpha. In the absence of D816V, consider imatinib.

3. **SM with rapid progression** or MC leukemia is treated with multiagent chemotherapy. Stem cell transplantation can also be considered.

ACKNOWLEDGMENT

The author would like to acknowledge Dr. Dennis A. Casciato who significantly contributed to earlier versions of this chapter.

Suggested Readings

Myeloproliferative Neoplasms

Griesshammer M, Struve S, Barbui T. Management of Philadelphia negative chronic myeloproliferative disorders in pregnancy. *Blood Rev* 2008;22:235.

Swerdlow SH, et al. *WHO Classification of Tumours of Haematopoietic and Lymphoid Tissues.* 4th ed. Lyon, France: International Agency for Research on Cancer; 2008.

Polycythemia Vera

Landolfi R, Marchioli R, Kutti J, et al. Efficacy and safety of low-dose aspirin in polycythemia vera. *N Engl J Med* 2004;350:114.

Essential Thrombocythemia

Barbui T, Finazzi G, Carobbio A, et al. Development and validation of an International Prognostic Score of thrombosis in World Health Organization-essential thrombocythemia (IPSET-thrombosis). *Blood* 2012;120:5128.

Gisslinger H, Gotic M, Holowiecki J, et al. Anagrelide compared with hydroxyurea in WHO-classified essential thrombocythemia: the ANAHYDRET study, a randomized controlled trial. *Blood* 2013;121:1720.

Griesshammer M, Heimpel H, Pearson TC. Essential thrombocythemia and pregnancy. *Leuk Lymphoma* 1996;22:57.

Harrison CN, Campbell PJ, Buck G, et al. Hydroxyurea compared to anagrelide in high-risk essential thrombocytopenia. *N Engl J Med* 2005;353:33.

Passamonti F, Randi ML, Rumi E, et al. Increased risk of pregnancy complications in patients with essential thrombocythemia carrying the *JAK2 (617V>F)* mutation. *Blood* 2007;110:485.

Myelofibrosis

Ballen KK, Shrestha S, Sobocinski KA, et al. Outcome of transplantation for myelofibrosis. *Biol Blood Marrow Transplant* 2010;16:358.

Gangat N, Caramazza D, Vaidya R, et al. DIPSS Plus: a refined dynamic international prognostic scoring system for primary myelofibrosis that incorporates prognostic information from karyotype, platelet count, and transfusion status. *J Clin Oncol* 2010;29:392.

Passamonti F, Cervantes F, Vannucchi AM, et al. A dynamic prognostic model to predict survival in primary myelofibrosis: a study by the IWG-MRT (International Working Group for Myeloproliferative Neoplasms Research and Treatment). *Blood* 2010;115:1703.

Hypereosinophilic Syndrome

Cools J, DeAngelo DJ, Gotlib J, et al. A tyrosine kinase created by fusion of the PDGFRA and FIP1L1 genes as a therapeutic target of imatinib in idiopathic hypereosinophilic syndrome. *N Engl J Med* 2003;348:13.

Gotlib J, Cools J, Malone JM III, et al. The FIP1L1-PDGFRa fusion tyrosine kinase in hypereosinophilic syndrome and chronic eosinophilic leukemia: implications for diagnosis, classification, and management. *Blood* 2004;103:2879.

Kilon AD. How I treat hypereosinophilic syndromes. *Blood* 2015;126:1069.

Wang SA, Tam W, Tsai AG, et al. Targeted next-generation sequencing identifies a subset of idiopathic hypereosinophilic syndrome with features similar to chronic eosinophilic leukemia, not otherwise specified. *Mod Pathol* 2016;29(8):854–864. doi: 10.1038/modpathol.2016.75.

Mastocytosis

Garcia-Montero AC, Jara-Acevedo M, Teodosio C, et al. KIT mutation in mast cells and other bone marrow hematopoietic cell lineages in systemic mast cell disorders: a prospective study of the Spanish Network on mastocytosis (REMA) in a series of 113 patients. *Blood* 2006;108:2366.

Kluin-Nelemans HC, Oldhoff JM, Van Doormaal JJ, et al. Cladribine therapy for systemic mastocytosis. *Blood* 2003;102:4270.

Orfao A, Garcia-Montero AC, Sanchez L, Escribano L, et al. Recent advances in the understanding of mastocytosis: the role of KIT mutations. *Br J Haematol* 2007;138:12.

Pardanani A, Elliott M, Reeder T, et al. Imatinib for systemic mast-cell disease. *Lancet* 2003;362:535.

Pauls JD, Brems J, Pockros PJ, et al. Mastocytosis: diverse presentations and outcomes. *Arch Intern Med* 1999;159:401.

26 Acute Leukemia and Myelodysplastic Syndromes

Mira Kistler and Gary Schiller

ACUTE LEUKEMIA

Acute leukemia includes acute myeloid leukemia (AML) and acute lymphoblastic leukemia (ALL).

I. EPIDEMIOLOGY AND ETIOLOGY

A. Incidence. AML is the most common adult acute leukemia with an incidence of 4 per 100,000 population per year. ALL has an incidence of 1.7 per 100,000 population and is the most common childhood leukemia.

1. **Cell type.** Of cases of ALL, 80% occur in children, and 90% of cases of AML occur in adults.

2. **Age.** In adults, AML rates begin to rise exponentially after 50 years of age; the age-specific incidence rate is 3.5/100,000 in adults 50 years of age, and increases significantly to 15 at age 70 and 35 at age 90. The median age at diagnosis for AML in the United States is 67 years. A peak incidence of ALL occurs at 3 to 4 years of age; the incidence steadily decreases after 9 years of age and rises in incidence after 40 years of age. Despite being considered a childhood cancer, the age-related increase in incidence of most cancers also pertains to ALL.

3. **Sex.** Acute leukemia shows a male predilection only in very young and elderly patients.

B. Etiology

1. **Hereditary**

   a. **Hereditary syndromes** that are associated with chromosomal abnormalities, a high risk of acute leukemia, and excessive chemosensitivity include the following: Bloom syndrome, Fanconi congenital pancytopenia (Fanconi anemia), Down syndrome, and ataxia telangiectasia.

   b. **Siblings** of younger patients with acute leukemia have a fivefold increased risk of developing leukemia. There is about a 15% concordance if one member of a pair of monozygotic twins develops AML, although this may be due to placental metastasis.

2. **Radiation** is a well-documented leukemogenic factor in humans. Increased incidence of leukemia proportional to the cumulative radiation dose has been demonstrated in populations exposed to atomic bombs, in patients irradiated for ankylosing spondylitis and in radiologists (before current protective precautions). Doses <100 cGy are not believed to be associated with the development of leukemia. The types of leukemia induced by radiation are ALL, AML, and chronic myelogenous leukemia (CML) but not chronic lymphocytic leukemia.

3. **Viruses** have not been shown to be etiologic for acute leukemia in humans, although an association is seen with Epstein-Barr virus with ALL-L3

(Burkitt leukemia). HTLV-1 is discussed in Chapter 22, in "Non-Hodgkin Lymphoma."

4. **Chemicals.** The ability of chemicals to produce acute leukemia and pancytopenia is likely related to their ability to mutate or ablate the bone marrow stem cells.

   a. **Benzene and toluene** were identified as carcinogens associated with acute leukemia a century ago. Acute leukemia develops 1 to 5 years after exposure and is often preceded by bone marrow hypoplasia, dysplasia, and pancytopenia.

   b. **Drugs.** Drug-induced acute leukemia is usually preceded by myelodysplasia. Alkylating agents and topoisomerase II inhibitors given for prolonged periods are associated with a markedly increased risk of AML when compared with the general age-matched population. Exposure to arsenicals has also been implicated as an increased risk factor for leukemia development. Secondary AML currently accounts for 10% to 20% of all AML cases.

5. **Hematologic diseases.** Transformation into acute leukemia ("blast crisis") is seen in >80% of cases of CML and is part of its natural history. Patients with myelodysplastic syndromes (MDS) clearly have an increased likelihood of evolution to AML. The incidence of AML in myeloproliferative disorders (MPD), myeloma, and certain solid tumors is increased by the use of chemotherapy.

6. **Smoking.** Cigarette smoking is associated with approximately 50% increase in leukemia risk.

II. PATHOLOGY, CLASSIFICATION, AND NATURAL HISTORY OF ACUTE LEUKEMIA

A. Classification

1. **Morphologic features of acute leukemia**

   a. **The French–American–British (FAB) histopathologic classification** of acute leukemia was originally proposed in 1976. This system has been supplanted by the World Health Organization (WHO) classification below. The FAB defined the M1–M7 and L1–L3 subtypes of acute leukemia as follows (Table 26-1) but is frequently left out in modern interpretations of AML.

   b. **Auer rods** are abnormal condensations of cytoplasmic granules. Their presence in the immature cells distinguishes AML from ALL; their absence is not diagnostically helpful.

TABLE 26-1	FAB Classification of Acute Leukemia
FAB Subtype	**Acute Leukemia Type**
M0:	Myeloblastic without maturation
M1:	Myeloblastic with minimal maturation
M2:	Myeloblastic with maturation
M3:	Promyelocytic; M3v: promyelocytic ("microgranular")
M4:	Myelomonocytic; M4 Eos: myeloblastic with abnormal eosinophils (Eos)
M5:	Monocytic: poorly (M5a) or well differentiated (M5b)
M6:	Erythroleukemia
M7:	Megakaryoblastic
L1:	ALL, childhood form
L2:	ALL, adult form
L3:	ALL, Burkitt type

    c. Cytologic features of the acute leukemia subtypes, particularly the nuclear configurations, cytoplasm granularity, and prevalence of Auer rods, are shown in Appendix B5.

    d. Cytochemistry. Identifying the type of early cell may be difficult, but it is facilitated by flow cytometry. Traditionally used histochemical techniques, particularly for myeloperoxidase and nonspecific esterase (see Appendix B5), are seen in AML. Myeloperoxidase activity can be assessed by both cytochemistry and flow cytometry.

    e. Immunologic markers assessed by flow cytometry usually distinguish ALL from AML as well as identify their subtypes. These markers are also summarized in Appendix B5. Antibodies against platelet glycoproteins (CD41 or CD61) are useful in distinguishing megakaryocytic (M7) leukemia. Flow cytometry has largely replaced cytochemistry for classification of acute leukemia in most centers. Flow cytometry is most useful when using antibodies against panmyeloid antigens (CD13 and CD33), monocyte antigens (especially CD11b and CD14), and hematopoietic progenitor cell antigens (CD34 and HLA-DR).

2. The WHO classification has replaced the FAB classification. The FAB classification, which provided a consistent morphologic and cytochemical framework, did not reflect the cytogenetic or clinical diversity of the disease. The WHO classification system takes into account the developing knowledge of the biology of AML and its distinct subtypes divided into diseases characterized by proliferative biology and diseases characterized by disorders of maturation. The WHO classification of AML is as follows (see also Appendix B5):

    a. AML with recurrent cytogenetic abnormalities

        (1) AML with inv(16)(p13;q22) or t(16;16)(p13;q22), CBFB-MYH11

        (2) Acute promyelocytic leukemia (APL) and variants; t(15;17)(q21;q11) and its variants

        (3) AML with t(8;21)(q22;q22); RUNX1-RUNX1T1

        (4) AML with 11q23 (MLL) abnormalities

        (5) AML with inv(3)(q21q26.2) or t(3;3)(q21;q26.2); RPN1-EVI1

        (6) AML with t(6;9)(p23q34) DEK-NUP214

        (7) AML (megakaryoblastic) with t(1;22)(p13;q13); RBM15-MKL1

        (8) AML with mutated NPM1 (provisional entity)

        (9) AML with mutated CEBPA (provisional entity)

    b. AML with myelodysplasia-related changes

    c. AML and MDS, therapy related (alkylating agents, topoisomerase inhibitors, other types)

    d. AML not otherwise categorized

        (1) AML minimally differentiated

        (2) AML without maturation

        (3) AML with maturation

        (4) Acute myelomonocytic leukemia

        (5) Acute monoblastic and monocytic leukemia

        (6) Acute erythroid leukemia

        (7) Acute megakaryoblastic leukemia

        (8) Acute panmyelosis with myelofibrosis

        (9) Acute basophilic leukemia (very rare)

    e. Myeloid sarcoma ("chloroma," "granulocytic sarcoma"; extramedullary masses of monoblasts or myeloblasts)

    f. Myeloid proliferations related to Down syndrome

    g. Blastic plasmacytoid dendritic cell neoplasm

    h. Acute lymphocytic leukemia is now included in the WHO classification of lymphoid tissues as "precursor B-cell lymphoblastic leukemia/lymphoma" and "precursor T-cell lymphoblastic leukemia/lymphoma" (see Appendix B4). These were designated as L1, L2, or L3 subtypes of ALL in the FAB system.

  3. The two most significant differences between the FAB and the WHO classifications are

    a. A lower blast threshold for the diagnosis of AML: The WHO defines AML when the blast percentage reaches **20%** in the bone marrow (rather than 30% as defined by FAB).

    b. Patients with recurring clonal cytogenetic abnormalities should be considered to have AML regardless of the blast percentage: t(8;21)(q22;q22), t(16;16)(p13;q22), inv(16)(p13;q22), or t(15;17)(q22;q12).

B. Pathology. Bone marrow examination in acute leukemia demonstrates hypercellularity with a monotonous infiltration of immature cells. Normal marrow elements are markedly decreased. Erythroblast maturation is commonly megaloblastoid in all types of AML, especially subtype M6. Cytologic features of the AML subtypes are shown in Appendix B5.

C. Natural history. In acute leukemia, immature and malfunctioning leukocyte progenitors progressively replace the normal bone marrow and infiltrate other tissues. Relapse is inevitable in most patients unless complete remission after induction and consolidation therapy persists at least 4 years. Relapse is associated with progressively poorer response to therapy, and if second or subsequent remission is achieved, it is generally of shorter duration. Unsuccessful therapy is usually followed by death within 2 months. Death in acute leukemia is usually caused by either infection or hemorrhage.

D. Biology of acute promyelocytic leukemia (APL)

  1. Morphology. Classified as M3 in the FAB classification, APL is characterized morphologically by the presence of blasts cells with heavy azurophilic granules, bundles of Auer rods, and a bilobed or reniform nucleus. Although most APL cases fit the description of hypergranular blasts, a cytologic microgranular variant (M3v) has been identified. The blasts in M3v have a bilobed, multilobed, or reniform nucleus and, under the usual staining, are devoid of granules or contain only a few fine azurophilic granules. The apparent paucity of granules is a result of their submicroscopic size. M3v is commonly associated with hyperleukocytosis and accounts for 15% to 20% of APL cases.

  2. Immunophenotyping. APL blasts are positive for CD33 and CD13 but negative for HLA-DR and usually have a low-level expression of CD34. M3v blasts tend to be positive for CD34, CD2, and CD19.

  3. Cytogenetics. Both the classic and the M3v forms of APL are associated with a specific cytogenetic abnormality, t(15;17)(q22;q21). This translocation disrupts the PML gene on chromosome 15 and the retinoic acid receptor *a* (RAR*a*) on chromosome 17, resulting in a fusion gene (PML/RAR*a*). The protein product of PML/RAR*a* retains the retinoic acid (RA) ligand-binding domain and plays a key role in leukemogenesis, as well as in mediating the response to retinoids.

    a. Four other alternative translocations associated with APL have been characterized:

      (1) t(11;17)(q23;q21) involving the *PLZF* gene on chromosome 11.

      (2) t(5;17)(q35;q21) involving the *NPM* gene on chromosome 5.

      (3) t(11;17)(q13;q21) involving the *NuMA* gene on chromosome 11.

      (4) t(1;17) occurs but is rare.

    b. PML/RAR*a*-mediated APL is sensitive to retinoids, as are the variants *NPM*/RAR*a*- and *NuMA*/RAR*a*-mediated APL. In contrast, *PLZF*/RAR*a*-associated APL is considered resistant to retinoids as well as to arsenic trioxide.

III. DIAGNOSIS

A. Symptoms

1. **Nonspecific fatigue and weakness** are the most common symptoms. Bruising, fever, and weight loss are frequent.

2. **Central nervous system (CNS) involvement** may be manifested by headaches, nausea, vomiting, blurred vision, or cranial nerve dysfunction.

3. **Abdominal fullness** usually reflects hepatosplenomegaly, which is more frequent in ALL or the monocytic subtype of AML.

4. **Oliguria** may result from dehydration, uric acid nephropathy, or disseminated intravascular coagulation (DIC).

5. **Obstipation** may signify disorders of hypercalcemia or hypokalemia; potassium wasting may occur in monocytic leukemia.

B. Physical findings

1. **General examination**

    a. Pallor, petechiae, and purpura are the most frequent findings in acute leukemia.

    b. Sternal tenderness to palpation, lymphadenopathy, and hepatosplenomegaly are much more common in ALL than in AML.

    c. Meningismus may indicate CNS involvement. CNS leukemia is most common in ALL. When seen in patients with AML, M4 (particularly with abnormal bone marrow eosinophils) and M5 subtypes are commonly involved. It is far less common in the remaining AML subtypes but can be seen at relapse.

    d. Leukemia infiltrates in the optic fundus appear like Roth spots with flame hemorrhages.

2. **Extramedullary infiltration or masses of blasts,** especially involving the skin, orbits, breasts, gingivae, or testes, are most likely to occur in acute monocytic leukemia (M5) and ALL.

3. **Bleeding** out of proportion to the degree of thrombocytopenia suggests the presence of DIC, which is particularly common in APL.

4. **Signs of infection** should be carefully elicited.

C. Laboratory studies.
Evaluation of the peripheral blood smear should be done in every case where leukemia is in the differential diagnosis. Finding circulating leukemia blasts establishes the diagnosis, but this should be confirmed by the evaluation of the bone marrow from which successful cytogenetic analysis is more likely. Fluorescent *in situ* hybridization (FISH) for common, recurring molecular abnormalities may identify distinct clonal abnormalities not easily elicited by conventional cytogenetics.

1. **Hemogram**

    a. Leukocytes. The WBC count is elevated in about 60% of cases, normal in 15%, and decreased in 25%, depending on the referral base of the treatment center. Circulating blasts are demonstrated in virtually every case of acute leukemia; however, some patients present with a very low percentage of circulating blasts.

    b. Erythrocytes. Ninety percent of patients have a normocytic, normochromic anemia, which is usually severe. Reticulocytes are nearly always decreased. Macrocytosis usually reflects megaloblastic maturation and suggests a history of prior MDS. Circulating nucleated red blood cells should always prompt further evaluation of the bone marrow.

    c. Platelets are decreased in 90% of cases and are <50,000/μL in about 40%.

2. **Biochemical tests** that should be obtained include the following:
   a. Serum uric acid, ionized calcium, phosphorus, magnesium, and lactic dehydrogenase (LDH) levels
   b. Serum renal and liver function tests
   c. Coagulation tests for DIC
3. **Bone marrow findings** are discussed earlier, in Section II. Blasts in excess of 20% establish the diagnosis of acute leukemia.
4. **Flow cytometry** results for AML are shown in Appendix B5. Results for ALL are shown in Appendix B3.
5. **Cytogenetic testing** is essential in every new patient because of its prognostic significance. Standard banded chromosome evaluation as well as FISH using a panel of the common acute leukemia probes should be obtained. Cytogenetic abnormalities distinguish unique types of AML and are the single most predictive factor for response to treatment, duration of response, and relapse. The abnormalities are categorized as "favorable-," "standard,- or intermediate-," and "unfavorable- or poor-" risk cytogenetics (Table 26-2).
6. **Molecular studies.** Molecular markers identified through genomic analysis serve as independent prognostic factors for AML and are used to guide treatment. These markers help to stratify normal karyotype AML (45% of AML patients) into subgroups. **All newly diagnosed AML patients should be tested for FLT3 (Fms-like tyrosine kinase 3), NPM1 (nucleophosmin 1), and CEBPA (CCAAT enhancer–binding protein-alpha).**

   The NPM1 and CEBPA biallelic mutations confer favorable prognosis. FLT3-ITD (internal tandem duplications) mutations occur in 30% of AML patients and confer a less favorable prognosis. These and other molecular markers are used to group patients into the favorable-, intermediate-, and poor-risk categories to guide treatment and transplant recommendations (Table 26-2).

   Newer mutations identified through gene sequencing include DNMT3A and IDH1 and 2, TET2, and ASLX1. Studies have identified prognostic associations with these mutations; however, they are still under investigation

TABLE 26-2	Cytogenetic Abnormalities and Prognostic Risk Category of Acute Myelogenous Leukemia in Adults
Prognostic Risk Category	**Cytogenetic and Molecular Classification**
Favorable	t(8;21)(q22;q22); RUNX1-RUNX1T1
	inv(16)(p13.1q22) or t(16;16)(p13.1q22); CBFB-MYH11
	NPM1 mutation without FLT3-ITD mutation
	CEBPA biallelic mutation
Intermediate	Normal karyotype
	NPM1 mutation with FLT3-ITD mutation
	FLT3-ITD mutation
	Core binding factor with c-kit mutation
	t(9;11)(p22;q23); MLLT3-MLL
	Cytogenetic abnormalities not classified as favorable or adverse
Poor	Complex cytogenetics
	Monosomal karyotype (−5,−7, 5q−)
	Abnormal 17p
	inv(3)(p21;q26.2) or t(3;3)(q21;q26.2); RPN1-EVI1
	t(6;9)(p23;q34); DEK-NUP214
	t(v;11)(v;q23); MLL rearrangements

Adapted from Döhner H, Estey EH, Amadori S, et al. Diagnosis and Management of acute leukemia in adults: Recommendations from an international expert panel, on behalf of the European Leukemia Net. *Blood* 2010;115:453.

both as prognostic markers and therapeutic targets and have not been incorporated into standard-risk criteria and recommendations for transplantation or treatment.

7. **Radiographic studies** that should be obtained include the following:
   a. **Chest radiograph** to look for leukemic or infectious infiltrates
   b. **Bone radiographs** of painful or tender areas to look for periosteal elevation or bony destruction from extramedullary bone masses
   c. **CT scans** of the chest and abdomen/pelvis should be obtained on patients with ALL to evaluate lymphadenopathy and organomegaly.

8. **Cerebrospinal fluid (CSF) examination** should be performed at some time in all patients with ALL, where it is usually part of the induction therapy. CSF evaluation should be done in patients with acute monocytic leukemia and in those patients with AML who have meningismus or CNS abnormalities. Cytarabine or methotrexate may be instilled into the CSF at the completion of the examination because of the possibility of leukemic contamination from the blood (see Section IX.B).

   Meningeal involvement with leukemia is associated with decreased sugar and increased protein concentrations in the CSF, along with pleocytosis, and leukemia cells identified by cytologic examination.

IV. PROGNOSTIC FACTORS AND SURVIVAL

Complete remission (CR) is the paramount prognostic factor in all forms of acute leukemia. A CR is defined as all of the following:
- Bone marrow contains fewer than 2% to 5% blasts, and these should not be clonal.
- Granulocyte and platelet counts have recovered.

A. **AML prognostic factors.** The most important factors portending a **poor prognosis** in AML are as follows:
1. Advanced age (typically described as age >60)
2. Antecedent myelodysplasia
3. Therapy-related AML
4. High WBC count at presentation
5. Unfavorable cytogenetics and molecular markers

B. **APL Prognostic Factors**
1. Low-risk disease is defined as WBC count ≤10,000/μL and platelets >40,000/μL.
2. Intermediate-risk disease is defined as WBC count ≤10,000/μL and platelets ≥40,000/μL.
3. High-risk disease is defined as WBC count >10,000/μL.

C. **ALL prognostic factors.** ALL is not a uniform disease but consists of subtypes with distinct biologic, clinical, and prognostic features. The most important prognostic factors are age, initial WBC count, immunophenotype, and cytogenetic features.
1. **Favorable prognostic factors in adult ALL.** The Cancer and Leukemia Group B (CALGB) identified the following clinical and biologic features that correlate with favorable long-term outcome:
   a. Younger age
   b. WBC count (≤30,000/μL)
   c. Absence of the Philadelphia chromosome (Ph[1])
2. **Adverse prognostic factors in ALL**
   a. **Clinical characteristics**
      (1) Older age
      (2) WBC count >30,000/μL
      (3) Late achievement of CR (occurring after >3 to 4 weeks)

b. Immunophenotype
   (1) Pre–B-cell ALL
   (2) Pre–T-cell ALL
   (3) Mature T-cell ALL

c. Cytogenetics and molecular genetics
   (1) t(9;22)(p34;q11) [Ph[1]]; *BCR/ABL* fusion gene: occurs in 25% of adults with ALL
   (2) t(1;19)(q23; p13); *PBX/E2A:* occurs in 25% of children with ALL
   (3) Abnormal 11q23; *MLL* gene rearranged: poor prognosis in adults and in infants <1 year of age.
   (4) t(4;11)/ALL1-AF4; common clinical features of this subtype include the following:
      (a) High WBC count (median 180,000/μL)
      (b) L1 or L2 morphology with B-cell lineage
      (c) Unfavorable immunophenotype (CD10–, CD19+, HLA-DR+) with frequent coexpression of myeloid markers (CD15+, CDw65+)
   (5) Expression of multidrug resistance (rarely assayed)

3. Response rates and survival
a. AML.
Forty to seventy percent of patients achieve a CR to standard induction chemotherapy. The median survival is 12 to 24 months for patients who achieve CR; the median duration of first remission is 10 to 12 months. Twenty to forty percent of patients who achieve CR (5% to 30% of all patients) survive >5 years, and many of these patients may be cured. Most relapses occur within 3 years.

Approximately 50% of patients with "favorable" cytogenetics who achieve CR survive. Only 5% to 15% of patients in CR achieve long-term survival if they are >60 years or develop AML following primary or secondary MDS.

b. ALL (also see Acute Leukemia in Chapter 19)
   (1) **"Standard-risk" children** (1 to 9 years of age, WBC count <50,000/μL, precursor B-cell subtype, and without adverse prognostic factors). Of cases, <20% relapse if properly treated, and >80% have a 5-year disease-free survival. Relapse or death is unusual in these patients after 4 years of continuous CR.
   (2) **"High-risk" children** (those with adverse prognostic factors) have remission duration and survival similar to those of adults, yet some series report 70% of patients surviving disease free for 4 years. The survival time for infants is <2 years.
   (3) **Adolescents and adults** have a median first CR duration of 12 to 24 months and a median survival time of 24 to 30 months. Late adolescents (17 to 21 years of age) appear to have a substantially improved survival time if treated with aggressive pediatric protocols. The median survival time is <18 months for patients >60 years of age with an elevated WBC count at presentation.

V. MANAGEMENT OF EVERY PATIENT WITH ACUTE LEUKEMIA WHO MAY UNDERGO ALLOGENEIC HEMATOPOIETIC STEM CELL TRANSPLANTATION (HSCT)

The following precautions are very important in all patients (generally, <70 years of age) who are eligible for allogeneic HSCT when initially diagnosed with acute leukemia:

A. Leukocyte reduction and irradiation of all administered blood products
B. Obtain HLA typing of the patient for both class I and class II antigens on admission and before giving any treatment that will suppress blood counts.
C. Assess cytomegalovirus (CMV) antibody titers on admission. All blood products should be screened and negative for CMV until titers become available. CMV-seronegative patients should probably receive CMV-negative products if allotransplant is ever contemplated, whereas CMV-positive patients can receive CMV-safe products (positive but leukofiltered).

VI. MANAGEMENT OF AML

A. Remission induction. Standard treatment consists of infusional cytarabine plus an anthracycline. Cytarabine has been given in doses ranging from 100 to 6,000 mg/m^2, but it is not clear that higher dosages in induction give better results. Daunorubicin, idarubicin, and mitoxantrone at equipotent doses also appear to give similar results. Daunorubicin at 45 mg/m^2 is definitely considered to be inadequate; higher dosages (60 to 90 mg/m^2) are associated with better overall survival and no increase in grade 3 to 5 toxicities or early death. Idarubicin may induce higher remission rate, but overall survival compared to higher dose daunorubicin is similar. A typical regimen is as follows:

Cytarabine, 200 mg/m^2/d by continuous IV infusion for 7 days
Daunorubicin, 60 to 90 mg/m^2 (or idarubicin, 12 mg/m^2; or mitoxantrone, 12 mg/m^2) IV push on days 1, 2, and 3

If the blasts are not cleared from the blood and bone marrow after the first course of treatment, and if the patient can tolerate another such intensive treatment, the combination therapy is repeated again. A CR usually is achieved about 1 month after initiating treatment. More than 95% of CR is achieved with one or two courses of induction chemotherapy.

1. Toxicity of induction therapy
  a. Tumor lysis syndrome can occur with its associated hyperuricemia, hyperphosphatemia, hypocalcemia, and hyperkalemia. Patients with acute leukemia should be given allopurinol (300 to 600 mg daily), if possible beginning 12 to 48 hours before starting chemotherapy. Patients at high risk for tumor lysis such as WBC >100 × 10^9/L or uric acid >7.5 should receive a dose of rasburicase.
  b. Cardiac abnormalities. Anthracyclines may be associated with electrocardiographic changes, arrhythmias, or congestive heart failure. All patients must have a nuclear heart scan or an echocardiogram to assess the left ventricular ejection fraction before starting an anthracycline.
  c. Tissue necrosis. Anthracyclines are vesicants and, if infiltrated out of the veins into the tissues, will cause severe tissue necrosis. A safer approach would be to use a well-secured central venous access catheter (i.e., Hickman catheter), which should be checked for position and good blood return before infusing the anthracycline.
  d. Pancytopenia secondary to bone marrow suppression is both caused by the disease and a goal of therapy. This results in infectious and hemorrhagic complications. Patients will also become dependent on transfusions until remission is achieved and normal hematopoiesis is restored.
  e. Nausea and vomiting tend to be minimal with an effective antiemetic regimen. The emetic potential of cytarabine is low, but patients need effective antiemetics during the anthracycline administration. A typical regimen involves serotonin antagonist and dexamethasone (10 mg PO daily) for the 3 days of anthracycline administration.

f. Alopecia is the rule and is usually reversible.

g. Toxicity of high-dose cytarabine. When used at high dose (2 to 3 g/m² over 1 to 3 hours), cytarabine can be associated with cerebellar, ophthalmologic, and GI toxicity, particularly in patients >60 years of age. These toxicities occur in much lower frequency when given in lower dosages (1.5 g/m²) or when a much lower dose of drug is infused over longer periods of time (100 to 400 mg/m² by continuous IV infusion).

2. **Elderly patients.** The treatment of patients >60 years of age is controversial. Older patients often cannot tolerate the toxic effects of intensive induction therapy as well as can younger patients; the treatment-related mortality during induction is between 10% and 30% with intensive regimens. Furthermore, elderly patients often develop AML with adverse disease features, following antecedent MDS or with high-risk cytogenetics. Remission rates are low. Yet, several studies have shown that aggressive treatment results in improved survival and quality of life when compared to palliative care alone.

   a. Unfavorable risk factors that portend a grave prognosis and short survival are as follows:

   (1) Age ≥ 75 years
   (2) Antecedent hematologic disorder for more than 1 year
   (3) Poor-risk cytogenetics
   (4) WBC > 50,000/µL
   (5) LDH > 600 IU/L
   (6) Poor performance status (ECOG > 2)

   b. Patients who do not have the above unfavorable risk factors can be treated with the following regimen (more intensive daunorubicin dosage has not been shown to be beneficial in this age group):
   Cytarabine, 100 mg/m²/d by continuous IV infusion for 7 days
   Daunorubicin, 60 to 90 mg/m² (or idarubicin, 12 mg/m²) IV push on days 1, 2, and 3

   c. Less intensive regimens, which have been associated with less myelosuppression and fewer early deaths, for elderly patients who are in good general medical condition include the following:

   (1) Cytarabine 100 mg/m²/d for 5 days given by continuous IV infusion and idarubicin 12 mg/m² IV for one dose only.
   (2) The hypomethylating agents azacitidine and decitabine have shown improved overall survival compared to best supportive care and have minimal toxicity.
   (3) "Low-dose cytarabine" (10 mg/m² SC once or twice daily or 20 mg SC twice daily for 10 days every 4 to 6 weeks).
   (4) Clofarabine is an acceptable intermediate intensity alternative to standard induction.

   d. The use of supportive care alone is a reasonable option for some elderly patients with AML, particularly for those who are not in good general medical condition, although survival is typically measured in weeks.

B. **Postremission therapy.** After CR is achieved, the goal is to prevent recurrence. Leukemia cells that are not clinically apparent are nearly always present in the bone marrow. Therapy to eradicate residual leukemia is required, or recurrence is inevitable. The best form of postremission therapy, however, remains controversial.

1. **Patients <60 years of age** are usually presented three potential postremission options.

    a. Intensive chemotherapy consolidation. Relatively high doses of drugs are given shortly after the patient has achieved CR, have regained normal hematologic function, and have recovered clinically from any complications of prior therapy. Three or four cycles of high-dose cytarabine (HDAC) are given to patients with favorable-risk AML or those patients not proceeding to transplantation after induction chemotherapy.

    b. Autologous HSCT may offer a lower risk of relapse compared with intensive chemotherapy, but relapse remains higher than that associated with allogeneic transplantation. The major cause of death remains disease recurrence.

    c. Allogeneic HSCT. Most prospective studies have failed to show a survival advantage for allogeneic transplantation in good-risk patients (those with favorable cytogenetics) in first remission. On the other hand, reduced relapse and improved disease-free survival was demonstrated in standard-risk patients. Poor-risk patients with unfavorable cytogenetics seem to derive the maximal benefit from allogeneic HSCT.

  2. Patients older than 60 years. Although all large studies have included postremission therapy in these patients, there is no standard postremission strategy. Older patients did not benefit from any dosage of cytosine. A single cycle of HDAC adjusted for the patient's age and comorbidities is a reasonable choice for these patients. With reduced-intensity conditioning regimens, allogeneic HSCT has become a valid option.

C. Treatment of relapses. Relapses in AML are typically systemic (i.e., in the marrow and elsewhere). Occasionally, extramedullary relapse (e.g., chloromas in skin or lymph nodes) may precede systemic relapse. Up to half of those with recurrent AML achieve a second CR with treatment. Eligible patients with an available histocompatible stem cell donor should be strongly considered for allogeneic HSCT.

D. Targeted therapy. Tyrosine kinase inhibitors have shown activity in patients with FLT3 mutated AML. A phase II study evaluated **sorafenib** in combination with 5-azacytidine in relapsed FLT3-ITD AML. The study evaluated response in 37 patients and reported a response rate of 46% with 27% complete response with incomplete count recovery, 16% with complete response, and 3% partial response. Sorafenib is a consideration for relapsed/refractory AML.

    The RATIFY Trial is a randomized phase III placebo-controlled trial that evaluated **midostaurin,** a multitargeted small molecule FLT3 inhibitor plus standard induction and consolidation in patients with FLT3-ITD and FLT3-TKD mutations. This study showed that the addition of midostaurin to chemotherapy and then continued maintenance therapy improved both event-free survival (8 vs. 3 months) and overall survival (74.7 vs. 26 months for placebo). Midostaurin has not yet been approved for use at the time of this writing.

VII. MANAGEMENT OF ACUTE PROMYELOCYTIC LEUKEMIA

A. Induction. Patients suspected of having APL should be started on All-trans-retinoic acid (ATRA) immediately pending confirmatory cytogenetics in an attempt to control life-threatening coagulopathy. If the diagnosis is not APL, then ATRA can be discontinued. Both ATRA and arsenic trioxide (ATO) act as differentiation agents in APL.

    In the Intergroup APL0406 trial, ATRA plus ATO was compared to ATRA plus idarubicin in a phase III trial. The CR rates were similar in both arms, but the 2-year EFS was 97% for ATRA-ATO and 86% for the ATRA-idarubicin group. Overall survival was better for the ATRA-ATO group. This study demonstrated that ATRA-ATO was noninferior to ATRA plus chemotherapy. The ATRA plus ATO combination has been shown to have less toxicity.

1. **Low- and intermediate-risk patients** may be treated with ATRA plus arsenic trioxide, ATRA plus idarubicin, or ATRA plus daunorubicin and cytarabine for induction therapy.

2. **High-risk patients** receive treatment with ATRA plus chemotherapy. Regimens include ATRA plus daunorubicin and cytarabine, ATRA plus idarubicin, and ATRA plus ATO and idarubicin.

B. **Consolidation.** Following CR in APL, it is mandatory to administer consolidation therapy to avoid relapse. Treatment consists of continuing ATRA plus ATO or ATRA with an anthracycline with or without cytarabine.

C. **Maintenance.** Following consolidation and confirmation of molecular remission, patients proceed to maintenance therapy. The role of maintenance for low- and intermediate-risk patients treated with ATRA and ATO has recently been questioned. The SO521 noninferiority study randomized patients with low- and intermediate-risk disease treated with standard induction with ATRA plus chemotherapy and consolidation that included ATO. Patients who achieved molecular remission were then randomized to observation or maintenance with ATRA, 6-mercaptopurine, and methotrexate. After 36 months of follow-up, there were no relapses in either arm of the study suggesting that patients treated with ATRA and ATO may not require maintenance.

1. Patients should proceed to the maintenance regimen associated with the induction and consolidation protocol that the patient has been treated on.

2. Patients should be monitored at regular intervals by PCR to assess continued molecular remission.

D. **APL differentiation syndrome (APLDS)** is a cardiorespiratory syndrome manifested by fever, weight gain, respiratory distress, interstitial pulmonary infiltrates, pleural and pericardial effusion, episodic hypotension, and acute renal failure. The disorder is attributed to rapid differentiation of blasts to (clonal) neutrophils with subsequent vascular complications and can be induced by either ATRA or arsenic trioxide. The incidence is 25% when ATRA is used alone. The concurrent administration of chemotherapy and ATRA may reduce the incidence to below 10%, but this has not been clearly established. Corticosteroids can be effective as prophylaxis and therapy of the differentiation syndrome. The mortality rate with APLDS has declined from 30% to 5%, likely reflecting earlier recognition and earlier institution of dexamethasone therapy. No factors are clearly predictive of APLDS.

E. **DIC.** Coagulopathy exacerbated by cytotoxic chemotherapy was previously seen in >90% of patients with APL and resulted in severe hemorrhagic manifestations in excess of that expected for the degree of thrombocytopenia. Both the incidence and severity of DIC have substantially decreased with differentiation therapy. Laboratory abnormalities include not only features associated with DIC (decreased fibrinogen and increased fibrin and fibrinogen degradation products) but also evidence of increased fibrinolysis (acquired deficiency of the fibrinolysis inhibitor, α_2-antitrypsin).

Patients should be monitored closely for the development of DIC and treated at its first sign. Transfusions with platelets and cryoprecipitate (to sustain fibrinogen levels) are the mainstays of therapy. Heparin is now rarely used. Antifibrinolytic agents, such as epsilon-aminocaproic acid, may be useful in the setting of excess fibrinolysis.

VIII. MANAGEMENT OF ACUTE LYMPHOBLASTIC LEUKEMIA

A. Remission induction

1. **Children** (also see Chapter 19 for discussion of treatment of children). The combination of vincristine with prednisone (V + P) or dexamethasone produces CR in 85% to 90% of cases of childhood ALL. Asparaginase is typically added. Daunorubicin or doxorubicin is added for higher-risk patients. Most children achieve CR within 4 weeks of therapy; if CR is not achieved within 6 weeks, alternative treatments are started, no value is found in continuing the initial drugs unless under unusual circumstances such as in ataxia telangiectasias. Children often achieved CR without prolonged myelosuppression.

   a. **Standard-risk patients** are treated with V + P plus asparaginase for 4 to 6 weeks.

   > Vincristine, 1.5 mg/m^2 (maximum 2 mg) IV push weekly
   > Prednisone, 40 mg/m^2 PO daily
   > Peg-asparaginase 2,500 units/m^2 IV

   b. **High-risk patients** are treated with V + P, Peg-asparaginase, and daunorubicin (25 mg/m^2) IV weekly for two doses.

2. **Adults.** The V + P regimen results in CR in 45% to 65% of adults with ALL. The addition of an anthracycline (with or without asparaginase) increases the CR rate to 75%. Regimens with five drugs may further increase the CR rate to 85%; an example regimen is the following (see Larson RA, et al. in *Suggested Readings*):

   > Cyclophosphamide, 1,200 mg/m^2 IV on day 1
   > Daunorubicin, 45 mg/m^2 IV on days 1, 2, and 3
   > Vincristine, 2 mg IV on days 1, 8, 15, and 22
   > Prednisone, 80/m^2 IV or PO on days 1 through 21

   In our practice, we give peg-asparaginase 2,500 units/m^2 IV for adults younger than age 40 and consider 1,500 units/m^2 for adults aged 40 to 60 years, and we do not give peg-asparaginase to adults older than age 60.

3. **Toxicity of induction therapy**

   a. **V + P**

   (1) Intestinal colic and constipation (bulk laxatives should be used prophylactically)

   (2) Peripheral neuropathy (usually reversible)

   (3) Bone marrow suppression

   (4) Alopecia (uncommon)

   b. **V + P plus an anthracycline.** Same as above, in Section VIII.A.3.a, along with nausea, vomiting, stomatitis, alopecia, myelosuppression, and possibly cardiac toxicity.

   c. **V + P and peg-asparaginase.** Same as above, in Section VIII.A.3.a, with the addition of coagulation defects with decreased fibrinogen level, allergic reactions, and encephalopathy, hyperbilirubinemia, elevated hepatic transaminases, pancreatitis, phlebitis, or thrombosis. We use reduced doses of peg-asparaginase in older adults due to increasing severity of toxicities with age, and generally hold the medication after age 60.

B. CNS prophylaxis after induction chemotherapy prevents early CNS relapse and is mandatory in ALL. The CNS is the initial site of relapse in more than half of children unless prophylaxis is given and it is also a frequent site of relapse in adults.

1. **Regimens.** The form of CNS prophylaxis is controversial. Many authorities recommend intrathecal methotrexate (6 to 12 mg/m^2 of preservative-free methotrexate up to a maximum of 15 mg/dose is given twice weekly for

five to eight doses). Intrathecal methotrexate is often combined with cranial irradiation (approximately 2,400 cGy in 12 fractions over 2.5 weeks) for patients >1 year of age. Intrathecal methotrexate alone is recommended by some authorities for patients at low risk for relapse (age 2 to 9 years, WBC count <10,000/μL, and CD10+). Triple intrathecal therapy (methotrexate, hydrocortisone, cytarabine) with or without high-dose systemic methotrexate or cytarabine may substitute for cranial irradiation, which can lead to late intellectual disabilities when used in children. For adults, prophylactic intrathecal chemotherapy alone is considered sufficient.

2. **Toxicities associated with CNS prophylaxis** include transient encephalopathy, alopecia after cranial irradiation, chemical arachnoiditis, leukoencephalopathy, and neuropsychologic effects.

C. Intensive postremission therapy

1. **Consolidation treatment** with an intensive multidrug regimen has been shown to improve survival in children and is considered standard treatment. A retrospective analysis in adults showed a superior outcome among trials implementing multidrug intensive consolidation, but randomized trials are inconclusive. High-dose cytarabine may be beneficial for T-cell ALL and some high-risk subgroups. High-dose methotrexate may be useful in B-cell lineage ALL.

2. **Allogeneic HSCT** in first CR has been demonstrated to improve survival for adults with ALL in all age categories. It is not recommended for first CR for children with standard-risk ALL, but HSCT may be important for specific subgroups of ALL (perhaps for patients with the Philadelphia chromosome positive ALL) or for those who relapse after initial remission.

D. Maintenance therapy for 2 to 3 years is mandatory in childhood ALL and is typically used in adults as well.

1. **Effective drugs.** Methotrexate (20 mg/m^2 PO to a maximum of 35 mg weekly) plus mercaptopurine (50 to 75 mg/m^2 PO daily) are the cornerstones of maintenance therapy in ALL. It is important that the drugs be given in dosages sufficient to produce myelosuppression to produce an impact on disease-free survival. Monthly pulses of V + P are also given. Intrathecal chemotherapy is typically administered every 90 days.

2. **Toxicity of maintenance therapy**
   a. Therapy is interrupted if any of the following occurs:
      (1) Significant myelosuppression (which is dose limiting but a necessary goal)
      (2) Abnormal LFT
      (3) Stomatitis, diarrhea
      (4) Renal tubular necrosis secondary to the methotrexate (renal function is closely monitored)
   b. Immunosuppression (increased susceptibility to infection, particularly varicella and *Pneumocystis jirovecii*)
   c. Growth inhibition
   d. Skin disorders
   e. Osteoporosis with long-term methotrexate treatment

3. **When to stop maintenance therapy**
   a. **Children.** Prolonged chemotherapy is of greatest consequence in children because adverse, late side effects may develop. Most children in remission are treated for 30 to 36 months; 20% of children taken off treatment relapse, most within the first year. Elective testicular biopsy of boys before stopping maintenance therapy has been shown to be of no clinical value.

 b. Adults. Most adults with ALL relapse despite maintenance therapy. The question of how long adults with ALL should continue maintenance is yet to be answered, but it seems that prolonged and more dose-intensive regimens lead to better results. We recommend maintenance therapy for at least 2 years in adults with ALL based on the experience with children.

E. **Treatment of relapses.** ALL may relapse systemically or in sanctuary sites (testicle or CNS).

 1. **Extramedullary relapse.** Without CNS prophylaxis, relapse only in the CNS is common. Relapse in the testis occurs, but less commonly. Patients who have solitary extramedullary relapse and normal bone marrow may be treated with local therapy alone (i.e., CNS irradiation plus intrathecal chemotherapy for CNS relapse or irradiation of the testicle for testicular relapse). Frequently, relapse in these sites predicts for systemic relapse.

 2. **Systemic relapse** may be successfully treated with the agents used to induce the original remission in half of the cases, but any relapse should prompt consideration of allogeneic transplantation.

  a. Blinatumomab is a bispecific T-cell engager (BiTE) monoclonal antibody directed at anti-CD19 and the anti-CD3 moiety of cytotoxic T cells and is approved for relapsed/refractory Ph negative B-ALL. A multicenter phase II study evaluated 189 patients with relapsed/refractory disease and reported a complete remission or complete remission with incomplete hematologic recovery in 43% of patients. Blinatumomab is administered as a continuous intravenous infusion for 4 weeks. Significant toxicities associated with the drug include neurologic toxicities including seizures and encephalopathy and cytokine release syndrome.

  b. Liposomal vincristine is approved for relapsed Ph-negative B-ALL.

F. **Targeted therapy**

 1. **Ph-Positive ALL.** The addition of a BCR-ABL tyrosine kinase inhibitor has improved response rates in Ph-positive ALL and allowed for greater numbers of these patients to proceed to allogeneic transplant. The UKALLXII/ECOG2993 study evaluated patients prior to introduction of imatinib and then with late and early administration of imatinib. The study found the CR rate was 92% in the imatinib cohort compared to 82% in the preimatinib cohort. The overall survival at 4 years of patients in the imatinib cohort was 38% versus 22% in the preimatinib cohort. More patients who received imatinib proceeded to allogeneic stem cell transplant.

  In Ph-positive ALL, tyrosine kinase inhibitors are added to standard induction therapy and continued after transplant or during maintenance if the patient does not proceed to transplant in first CR.

 2. **CD20-positive ALL.** The anti-CD20 monoclonal antibody rituximab has shown benefit when added to standard ALL chemotherapy regimens. The GRAALL-R 2005 study is a multicenter randomized trial that compared the GRAALL protocol with and without rituximab in patients aged 18 to 59 with CD20-positive, Ph-negative B-ALL. The study randomized 220 patients and reported that the patients treated with rituximab had a lower incidence of relapse of 18% versus 30.5% and a 2-year EFS of 65% versus 52%. When allogeneic transplant patients were censored, there was a significant overall survival benefit at 2 years of 74% versus 63%.

IX. MANAGEMENT OF ACUTE LEUKEMIA: OTHER ISSUES

A. **Supportive care**

1. **Indwelling tunneled central venous catheters** are used during the induction phase to facilitate the administration of IV therapies and the sampling of blood for laboratory tests.

2. **Blood component therapy**

a. **Platelet transfusions** are clearly indicated for patients with severe thrombocytopenia when there is active bleeding, fever, or infection. Without petechiae or bleeding, platelets are transfused prophylactically when counts are $\leq 10,000/\mu L$ unless the patient is febrile, at which point platelets should be kept at a slightly higher level of $20,000/\mu L$ owing to enhanced platelet consumption.

b. **Packed red blood cell transfusions** are used to treat symptomatic anemia and active hemorrhage. The hemoglobin concentration is generally kept ≥ 8 g/dL because these patients have aregenerative bone marrows. If the patient is actively bleeding or has a medical history, transfusion is given to target a higher hemoglobin level.

c. **Granulocyte transfusions** are not generally recommended. They can be used, however, in certain settings such as an overwhelming fungal sepsis, when the patient is expected to recover within a short period of time. In the absence of a reasonable chance of recovery, granulocyte transfusions are not typically used.

3. **Infections.** It is critical to initiate prompt empiric IV antibiotics in the event of fever. The choice of antibiotics is institution dependent but should always contain adequate coverage of gram-negative bacteria and also *Staphylococcus aureus* in patients suspected of having a catheter-related infection. For persistently febrile patients, empiric coverage with antifungal agents has been demonstrated to improve survival.

a. **Management of neutropenic fever** is thoroughly discussed in Section II of Chapter 36.

b. **Prophylaxis against infection** (see Chapter 36)

4. **Tumor lysis syndrome** (see Chapter 32)

B. **Treatment of meningeal leukemia**

1. **Manifestations.** Meningeal leukemia should be considered in the setting of cranial neuropathy, other neurologic signs, or altered mental status. Blast cells identified by cytologic evaluation of the CSF are diagnostic, but evaluation of the CSF is not sensitive.

2. **Treatment.** Optimal treatment has not been determined. Most patients are given cranial or craniospinal irradiation over a 3-week period plus intrathecal chemotherapy. Intrathecal therapy alone may be insufficient.

a. **Drugs.** Preservative-free methotrexate (6 to 12 mg/m^2 to a maximum of 15 mg) or cytarabine (50 to 100 mg) is used for intrathecal therapy. Methotrexate should be avoided in the setting of renal failure. The concomitant use of methotrexate during CNS irradiation can be associated with increased CNS toxicity. Toxic effects of methotrexate in the periphery may be prevented by giving IV or oral leucovorin.

b. **Diluents.** Artificial spinal fluid (Elliotts B solution) is available at some institutions to dilute the cytotoxic agents.

c. **Technique.** Intrathecal chemotherapy is given isovolumetrically and gradually by serial withdrawal and injection of spinal fluid with a syringe containing the chemotherapeutic agents. The drugs can be administered by lumbar or cisternal puncture, or through an inserted intraventricular (Ommaya) reservoir.

    d. Duration. Intrathecal chemotherapy is given at 2- to 7-day intervals until abnormal cells and excess protein are cleared from the spinal fluid. Therapy is often continued at 1- to 2-month intervals for a period thereafter.

C. Special clinical problems

    1. Leukostasis is more common in AML than in ALL and frequently occurs in patients with WBC count >100,000/µL. Sludging impairs circulation and results in organ dysfunction. The circulating blast count can be rapidly reduced with leukapheresis, thereby reducing the risks of leukostasis, DIC, and metabolic abnormalities associated with tumor lysis. Hydroxyurea (3 g/d) or alternative chemotherapy should be instituted with leukapheresis.

    2. Ocular and gingival involvement. Irradiating eyes involved with leukemic infiltrates may prevent blindness. Gingival enlargement in patients with monocytic leukemia does not require special treatment because it should resolve with induction chemotherapy.

    3. Patients exposed to varicella zoster infections should be given acyclovir and zoster immune globulin (see Chapter 36).

    4. Acute leukemia during pregnancy (see Chapter 27, Section III)

MYELODYSPLASTIC SYNDROMES

Myelodysplastic syndromes (MDS) are a group of malignant disorders affecting hematopoietic stem cells that result in dysplastic changes and ineffective hematopoiesis. MDS can be considered as a preleukemic condition, and patients are at increased risk of transformation to AML. The diagnosis of primary MDS may be made only in the absence of conditions that produce secondary myelodysplasia, which include drug and toxin exposure, growth factor therapy, viral infections, immunologic disorders, congenital disorders, vitamin deficiencies, copper deficiency, and excessive zinc supplementation. Notably, folic acid and vitamin B_{12} deficiencies are reversible disorders that may have bone marrow morphologic changes that can be confused with myelodysplasia.

I. CLINICAL FEATURES

MDS usually affects patients >65 years of age, with the incidence increasing further with older age. Men are affected more than women. It is usually diagnosed when a cytopenia, especially a macrocytic anemia, is noted on laboratory studies. Symptoms are nonspecific and usually reflect the degree of cytopenias. Physical examination is usually normal. The bone marrow frequently shows dysplastic changes.

II. DYSHEMATOPOIESIS

Dyshematopoiesis is manifested by cytopenias in the presence of a normocellular or hyper cellular bone marrow. Components and features of dyshematopoiesis, which occur in various combinations for each syndrome, are as follows:

A. Dyserythropoiesis

    1. Peripheral blood. Anemia and reticulocytopenia from ineffective erythropoiesis; anisocytosis, poikilocytosis, basophilic stippling; macrocytosis (when megaloblastoid maturation is present); and dimorphic (normo-cytic, normochromic, and microcytic, hypochromic) red blood cell populations.

2. **Bone marrow.** Erythroid hyperplasia or hypoplasia, ringed sideroblasts, and megaloblastoid maturation (multinucleation, nuclear fragments, karyor-rhexis, or cytoplasmic vacuoles).

3. **Other assays.** Decreased CD55 and CD59 expression on granulocytes or erythrocytes define paroxysmal nocturnal hemoglobinuria. Periodic acid–Schiff (PAS)-positive cytochemistry and increased fetal hemoglobin levels may be detected in some cases of myelodysplasia.

B. **Dysgranulocytopoiesis**

1. **Peripheral blood.** Neutropenia, decreased or abnormal neutrophil granules, neutrophil hyposegmentation (pseudo-Pelger-Huët anomaly), hypersegmen-tation, or bizarre nuclei

2. **Bone marrow.** Granulocytic hyperplasia, abnormal or decreased granules in neutrophil precursors, increased numbers of blast cells

3. **Other assays.** Decreased neutrophil alkaline phosphatase score and myelo-peroxidase activity

C. **Dysmegakaryopoiesis**

1. **Peripheral blood.** Thrombocytopenia, large platelets with abnormal and decreased granularity

2. **Bone marrow.** Reduced numbers of megakaryocytes, micromegakaryocytes, and megakaryocytes with large, single nuclei or multiple, small separated nuclei

3. **Other assays.** Abnormal platelet function tests

III. CLASSIFICATION

A. **The French–American–British classification of MDS** initially categorized patients based entirely on morphology and dysplastic changes in at least two of the three hematopoietic cell lines into six subtypes:

1. Refractory anemia (RA): <5% marrow blasts

2. RA with ringed sideroblasts (RARS): <5% blasts plus >15% ringed sideroblasts

3. RA with excess blasts (RAEB): 5% to 20% marrow blasts

4. RAEB in transformation (RAEB-T): 21% to 30% marrow blasts

5. Chronic myelomonocytic leukemia (CMML): ≤20% marrow blasts plus peripheral blood monocytosis >1,000/μL

6. AML: >30% marrow blasts

B. **The WHO guidelines** revised and restructured the traditional FAB classifica-tion and incorporated cytogenetic data. The blast percentage threshold for the definition of AML was lowered from 30% to 20%. The category of RAEB-T was eliminated. The WHO classification for MDS is shown in Appendix B.6.

IV. GENE ABNORMALITIES

A. **Cytogenetics are important in both diagnosis and prognostication of MDS.**

1. Patients with cytopenias and a clinical presentation of MDS, but no significant dysmorphology on bone marrow exam, may be diag-nosed presumptively with MDS if they have the following cytogenetic abnormalities.

   a. Unbalanced Abnormalities: −7 or del(7q), −5 or del(5q), i(17p) or t(17p, i(17q) or t(17p, Del(11q), Del(12p), Del(9q), Idic(x)(q13)

  b. Balanced Abnormalities: t(11;16)(q23;p13.3), t(3;21)(q26.2;q22.1), t(1;3)(p36.3;q21.1), t(2;11)(p21;23), inv(3)(q21q26.2), t(6;9)(p23;q34)

2. The following cytogenetic abnormalities are diagnostic of AML regardless of blast count: t(8;21) (q22;q22), inv(16)(p13.1q22) or t(16;16)(p12.1;q22), and t(15;17)(q22;q21.1).

3. The 5q– syndrome is recognized as a distinct clinical entity that predominantly affects females and has a favorable prognosis with a low risk of transformation to AML. This entity is to be distinguished from AML characterized by a deletion of chromosome 5 or deletion of 5q with other chromosomal abnormalities. The 5q– syndrome is associated with response to lenalidomide.

B. Molecular genetics. Recurrent gene mutations have been identified in MDS patients. Some of the most frequently mutated genes include SF3B1, TET2, ASXL1, SRSF2, and RUNX1. The mutated genes are involved in epigenetic regulation, RNA splicing, transcription, and signaling pathways. Many of these mutations are also found in AML. Prognostic information is associated with some of the gene mutations. However, gene mutation data have not yet been incorporated into standard prognostic or treatment regimens.

V. PROGNOSIS

Life expectancy in MDS ranges from several months to 10 years, depending on the initial presentation, cytopenias, cytogenetics, and age. The IPSS was the original prognostic system introduced in 1997 and is a weighted grouping based on cytopenias, cytogenetics, and blast percentage in the bone marrow. The IPSS-R was introduced in 2012 and adds more cytogenetic data and uses different cutoffs for cytopenias. Patients are classified into very low-, low-, intermediate-, high-, or very high-risk categories. The IPSS-R and associated median survivals are shown in Table 26-3. The IPSS and the IPSS-R were developed using de novo MDS cases. Patients with secondary MDS generally have a worse prognosis than those with de novo disease.

VI. MANAGEMENT OF MDS

Because treatment for MDS is unsuccessful in most patients, patients should be encouraged to enroll into clinical trials. Treatment selection should be based on the patient's age, performance status, and IPSS-R subgroup categorization. Following are some of the therapeutic options available to patients.

A. Supportive care is a mainstay of treatment for MDS.

1. Transfusions. Patients receive supportive transfusions of red blood cells and platelets. Patients with low-risk disease may only require supportive care.

2. Erythropoietin (EPO) increases hemoglobin levels in approximately 15% of patients; 5% to 10% of patients may have a decrease in red blood cell transfusion requirements. Responses usually occur within 2 to 3 months, if they are to occur. Pretreatment serum EPO concentrations are inversely correlated with probability of response. **High doses of EPO** (40,000 to 60,000 U weekly) may be helpful. Dosage is adjusted if the drug is effective. Response is more likely if the patient has ringed sideroblasts and serum EPO levels of <500 mU/mL.

3. The combination of EPO and G-CSF (1 mg/kg/d) may increase the response rate of the anemia, producing synergistic erythropoietic activity in patients who fail to respond to erythropoietin alone.

B. Remittive therapies

1. DNA-hypomethylating agents are used for low- and intermediate-risk patients, and for high-risk patients who are not candidates for intensive

TABLE 26-3	Revised International Scoring System (IPSS-R) for Myelodysplastic Syndromes

	IPSS-R Score						
	0	0.5	1.0	1.5	2.0	3.0	4.0
Cytogenetics	Very good		Good		Intermediate	Poor	Very poor
Bone marrow blast (%)	≤2		>2 to <5		5 to 10	>10	
Hemoglobin (g/dL)	≥10		8 to <10	<8			
Platelets (x 10³/μL)	≥100	50 to 100	<50				
Absolute neutrophil count (per/μL)	≥0.8	<0.8					

IPSS-R Risk:
Very good, del(11q), −Y; Good, normal cytogenetics, del(5q), del(12p), del(20q), double including del(5q); Intermediate, del(7q), +8, +19, iso(17q), and any other single or double independent clones; Poor, −7, inv(3)/t(3q)/del(3q), double including −7/del(7q), 3 abnormalities; very poor, >3 abnormalities

Total Score	IPSS-R Risk Category	Median Survival (Years)	Median Time to 25% AML Development (Years)
≤1.5	Very low	8.8	NR
>1.5 to 3.0	Low	5.3	10.8
>3 to 4.5	Intermediate	3.0	3.2
>4.5 to 6	High	1.6	1.4
>6	Very high	0.8	0.7

therapy. A randomized phase III trial of azacitidine (75 mg/m²/d SC for 7 days every 28 days) compared with supportive care alone identified the value of azacitidine to improve blood cell counts, decrease or eliminate transfusion requirements, and improve both survival and quality of life. Decitabine produced a similar spectrum of improvement in a randomized phase III trial.

2. **Lenalidomide** is approved for treatment of patients with low- or intermediate-risk MDS and the 5q deletion. Treatment with lenalidomide results in improved anemia and reduced transfusion requirements and improvement in cytogenetics. Patients who respond to lenalidomide may have longer overall survival and reduced risk of progression to AML.

3. **Immunosuppressive therapy.** Low marrow cellularity and absence of blasts increase the likelihood of response of MDS to immunosuppressive agents such as prednisone, antithymocyte globulin (ATG), and cyclosporine.

C. **Curative therapies for high-risk MDS.** Induction chemotherapy followed by allogeneic HSCT may lead to complete resolution of myelodysplasia. Although commonly believed that HSCT is the only curative option for MDS, the projected 3-year disease-free survival for patients <60 years of age is dependent on the risk category of disease. Allogeneic HSCT should only be offered in inter-mediate- or advanced-disease settings.

Standard chemotherapy for MDS or MDS-related AML is associated with lower response rates than in *de novo* AML. This disparity is owing to advanced age in patients with MDS, poor-risk cytogenetics, and increased expression of multidrug resistance.

D. Management of CMML is discussed in Chapter 24, "Chronic Myelomonocytic Leukemia."

ACKNOWLEDGMENTS

The authors would like to acknowledge Drs. Mary Territo and Dennis A. Casciato, who significantly contributed to earlier versions of this chapter.

Suggested Readings

Acute Leukemia

Cashen AF, Schiller GJ, O'Donnell MR, et al. Multicenter, phase II study of decitabine for the first-line treatment of older patients with acute myeloid leukemia. *J Clin Oncol* 2010;28:556.

Döhner H, Estey EH, Amadori S, et al. Diagnosis and management of acute myeloid leukemia in adults: recommendations from an international expert panel, on behalf of the European LeukemiaNet. *Blood* 2010;115:453.

Dombret H, Gardin C. An update of current treatments for adult acute myeloid leukemia. *Blood* 2016;127:53.

Fielding AK, Rowe JM, Buck G, et al. UKALLXII/ECOG2993: addition of imatinib to a standard treatment regimen enhances long-term outcomes in Philadelphia positive acute lymphoblastic leukemia. *Blood* 2014;123:843.

Juliusson G, Antunovic P, Derolf A, et al. Age and acute myeloid leukemia: real world data on decision to treat and outcomes from the Swedish Acute Leukemia Registry. *Blood* 2009;113:4179.

Larson RA, Dodge RK, Burns CP, et al. A five-drug remission induction regimen with intensive consolidation for adults with acute lymphoblastic leukemia: cancer and leukemia group B study 8811. *Blood* 1995;85:2025.

Lo-Coco F, Avvisati G, Vignetti M, et al. Retinoic acid and arsenic trioxide for acute promyelocytic leukemia. *N Engl J Med* 2013;369:111.

Luskin MR, Lee JW, Fernandez HF, et al. Benefit of high-dose daunorubicin in AML induction extends across cytogenetic and molecular groups. *Blood* 2016;127:1551.

Rowe JM, Buck G, Burnett AK, et al. Induction therapy for adults with acute lymphoblastic leukemia: results of more than 1500 patients from the international ALL trial: MRC UKALL XII/ECOG E2993. *Blood* 2005;106:3760.

Schiller GJ. High-risk acute myelogenous leukemia: treatment today … and tomorrow. *Hematol Am Soc Hematol Educ Program* 2013;2013:201.

Shiller GJ. Evolving treatment strategies in patients with high-risk acute myeloid leukemia. *Leuk Lymphoma* 2014;55:2438.

Topp MS, Gökbuget N, Stein AS, et al. Safety and activity of blinatumomab for adult patients with relapsed or refractory B-precursor acute lymphoblastic leukaemia: a multicenter, single-arm, phase 2 study. *Lancet Oncol* 2015;16:57.

Myelodysplastic Syndromes

Greenberg PL, Tuechler H, Schanz J, et al. Revised International Prognostic Scoring System for Myelodysplastic Syndromes. *Blood* 2012;120:2454.

Guillermo Garcia-Manero. Myelodysplastic syndromes: 2015 Update on diagnosis, risk-stratification and management. *Am J Hematol* 2015;90:832.

Haferlach T, Nagata Y, Grossman V, et al. Landscape of genetic lesions in 944 patients with myelodysplastic syndromes. *Leukemia* 2014;28:241.

Malcovati L, Hellstrom-Lindberg Eva, Bowen D, et al. Diagnosis and treatment of primary myelodysplastic syndromes in adults: recommendations from the European LeukemiaNet. *Blood* 2013;122:2943.

Swerdlow SH, et al. *World Health Organization Classification of Tumours of Haematopoietic and Lymphoid Tissues.* Lyon, France: IARC Press; 2008.

IV Complications

27 Sexual Function, Fertility, and Cancer During Pregnancy

Jordan E. Rullo, Kathryn J. Ruddy, and Alison W. Loren

I. SEXUAL HEALTH

The impact of cancer on sexual health and the patient's sexual relationship is an important aspect of the patient's quality of life. It is imperative that health care providers share with their patients the impact treatment options may have on sexual function in order to assist in treatment planning.

A. Breast cancer

1. **Surgery**
   a. **Lumpectomy** may cause a change in breast sensation, scarring, and breast malformation.
   b. **Mastectomy** may result in a worse body image compared to lumpectomy. Mastectomy may cause feelings of reduced femininity and grieving the loss of breasts, as well as scarring.
   c. **Reconstruction** may improve sexual function and body image. However, breast and nipple sensation continue to be altered.

2. **Radiation therapy** causes fatigue, which may result in low sexual desire. Radiation can also cause skin damage, skin discoloration, and pain at the radiation site.

3. **Chemotherapy** with an alkylating agent may cause premature ovarian insufficiency (POI). This causes treatment-induced menopause and may lead to low sexual desire, genitourinary syndrome of menopause (GSM), dyspareunia, decrease in genital sensations, urinary incontinence, and vasomotor symptoms. Women experiencing vasomotor symptoms are twice as likely to experience sexual dysfunction.

4. **Endocrine manipulation**
   a. **Tamoxifen** has a mild estrogenic effect on the vaginal mucosa and may cause an increase in vaginal lubrication.
   b. **Aromatase inhibitors** (AIs) result in more sexual concerns compared to tamoxifen. These include vaginal dryness, dyspareunia, and low sexual desire.

B. Prostate cancer

1. **Radical prostatectomy (RP)** causes erectile dysfunction (ED) in up to 85% of men postsurgery. This is usually permanent after RP and temporary, lasting up to 24 months, in nerve-sparing radical prostatectomy (NS-RP). Ejaculation is impossible. RP may cause penile shortening of 1 to 3 cm in most men by 1 year postsurgery, but the nerve-sparing approach protects against penile shortening.

2. **External beam radiation and brachytherapy** may cause similar rates of ED as compared to RP. Longitudinally, brachytherapy may pose a reduced risk of ED compared to external beam radiation. Radiation is also known to cause anejaculation.

3. **Cryosurgery** causes ED. It is estimated that erectile function is preserved in >60% of men who undergo focal ablation, compared to 25% to 47% of those who undergo whole gland.

4. **Androgen deprivation therapy (ADT)** may cause ED, change in orgasmic function, low sexual desire, body feminization, and genital atrophy/shrinkage. ADT administered intermittently, versus continuously, has been shown to have better sexual function outcomes.

C. **Cervical cancer**

1. **Simple hysterectomy** causes vaginal shortening, dyspareunia, reduced genital sensation and vaginal lubrication, and orgasmic difficulties. Long-term impact of hysterectomy includes decreased sexual desire and vaginal lubrication.

2. **Radical hysterectomy (RH)** causes greater sexual dysfunction compared to simple hysterectomy. RH commonly causes reduced vaginal lubrication, length, elasticity, orgasmic dysfunction, and bowel and bladder dysfunction. How a woman reaches orgasm (vaginal, cervical, or clitoral stimulation) may predict the impact of type of surgery on orgasmic function.

3. **Radiation therapy,** compared to surgery, causes more difficulty with sexual arousal, orgasmic function, vaginal lubrication, dyspareunia, vaginal length, and overall sexual satisfaction.

4. **Total pelvic exenteration** with construction of neovagina may allow for vaginal penetration for approximately half of women by 1 year postsurgery. Common concerns include pain, small size of neovagina, and vaginal dryness. Natural vaginal lubrication is no longer possible.

D. **Colorectal cancer**

1. **Radiation therapy (RT)** for colorectal cancer causes ED, orgasmic dysfunction, and ejaculatory dysfunction in men and dyspareunia in women.

2. **Surgery**

   a. **Total mesorectal excision (TME)** performed robotically (R-TME) results in better sexual function recovery than does laparoscopic TME (L-TME).

   b. **Anterior resection (AR) and abdominoperineal resection (APR)** cause ED in men and dyspareunia in women. Sexual function difficulties are less common after AR compared to APR.

   c. **Pelvic exenteration** causes permanent ED and anejaculation.

   d. **Colostomy and ileostomy** and the resulting stoma are associated with sexual dysfunction in many patients. Sexual dysfunction may continue even after ostomy reversal.

E. **Bladder cancer**

1. **Radical cystectomy (RC)** may cause dyspareunia and vaginal narrowing/shortening and may impair vaginal lubrication and orgasm. In men, RC can cause ED and low sexual desire. Nerve-sparing radical cystectomy (NS-RC) may result in better sexual function preservation than RC.

F. **Testicular cancer**

1. **Surgery**

   a. **Hemiorchiectomy and orchiectomy** are associated with decreased sexual desire, sexual discomfort, and ED. ED rates range from 18% to 25%.

   b. **Retroperineal lymph node dissection (RPLND)** increases likelihood of ejaculatory dysfunction and usually leads to retrograde ejaculation. Nerve-sparing RPLND leads to retrograde ejaculation in 10% to 15% of patients.

2. **Radiation** adjuvant to surgery may lead to greater ED, as compared to other treatment options.

3. **Chemotherapy** combined with surgery may lead to temporary low sexual desire and erection and ejaculatory difficulties. Cisplatin-based chemotherapy may cause testicular shrinkage and localized reduction in blood flow.

G. **Ovarian cancer**

1. **Oophorectomy** commonly causes decreased sexual desire, vaginal dryness, and dyspareunia in premenopausal women who enter menopause early as a result. Oophorectomy may cause vaginal dryness and dyspareunia in recently postmenopausal women.

H. **Endometrial cancer**

1. **Vaginal brachytherapy and external beam radiotherapy** cause similar rates of vaginal dryness and low sexual desire 5 years post radiation.

I. **Hematologic cancers**

1. **Hematopoietic stem cell transplant**

   a. **Total body irradiation (TBI)** may cause long-term vaginal dryness and dyspareunia in women and low sexual drive, ED, and azoospermia in men. For women, another side effect is POI, which impacts 40% to 100% of women.

   b. **Chronic genital graft versus host disease (GVHD)** may cause vaginal dryness, stenosis, and adhesions and dyspareunia and affect 29% to 49% of women with chronic GVHD. For men, genital GVHD may cause phimosis, urethral scarring, stenosis, and ED and may affect up to 20% of men with chronic GVHD.

J. **Treatment of sexual problems**

1. **Assessment:** It is important that sexual function is assessed prior to treatment and at regular intervals. This can be accomplished by direct questioning, such as: "Do you have any sexual health concerns?" in combination with a brief screener (see Figure 27-1).

2. **Brief counseling:** Give the patients validation that they are not alone. Provide information about the impact of cancer treatment on sexual function. Pamphlets on sexual health and cancer are free on the American Cancer Society Web site (www.cancer.org). Patients may need to be informed that this is their new normal for now. Patients may need specific suggestions to

---

Single-item Screener for Self-Reported Sexual Problems

In the past 12 months, has there ever been a period of 3 months or more when you had any of the following problems or concerns? Check all that apply.

☐ You wanted to feel more interest in sexual activity
☐ You had difficulty with erections (penis getting or staying hard)—MEN ONLY
☐ Your vagina felt too dry—WOMEN ONLY
☐ You had pain during or after sexual activity
☐ You had difficulty having an orgasm
☐ You felt anxious about sexual activity
☐ You did not enjoy sexual activity
☐ Some other sexual problem or concern
☐ No sexual problems or concerns

Figure 27-1 Brief, validated, assessment of sexual problems. Reprinted from Flynn K, Lindau ST, Lin L, et al. Development and validation of a single-item screener for self-reporting sexual problems in U.S. adults. *J Gen Intern Med* 2015;30(10):1468–1475, with permission of Springer.

alleviate or navigate sexual dysfunction, including when it is safe to return to penetrative sexual activity, not to engage in any painful sexual activity, and to remember to engage in nonsexual physical touch. Including the patient's partner in this conversation may be beneficial. If needed, refer the patient to a sexual medicine specialist or sex therapist, who can be found at www.ISSWSH.org and www.aasect.org.

3. **Interventions**
   a. **Vasomotor symptoms** are most effectively treated with systemic hormone therapy (HT). For patients with hormone receptor–sensitive cancers, a thorough discussion of risks and benefits is necessary before any hormonal intervention.
   b. **GSM/vaginal dryness** is effectively treated with low-dose vaginal estrogen and results in minimal serum estrogen elevation. Still, for patients with hormone receptor–sensitive cancers, discussion of risks and benefits is necessary beforehand. A moisturizer used three times per week for at least 12 weeks, such as Replens or Hyalo GYN, is a nonhormonal option.
   c. **Dyspareunia** can be reduced with the use of a lubricant during sexual activity. Choose a glycerine-free, water-based lubricant, such as Jo. Ospemifene is an FDA-approved selective estrogen receptor modulator for the treatment of dyspareunia, but it has not been studied in cancer survivors, and there is some theoretical risk of interaction with endocrine therapies and/or causation of uterine cancer. Lidocaine applied to the vulvar vestibule prior to penetrative sexual activity may be a palliative option.
   d. **Vaginal stenosis** is treated with use of vaginal dilators and lubricant, as guided by a physical therapist specializing in pelvic health. Regular penetrative sexual activity may act as a substitute for dilator use.
   e. **Pelvic floor myalgia,** experienced as pain with deep (versus initial) penetration, commonly co-occurs with dyspareunia and is most effectively treated by a physical therapist specializing in the pelvic floor. Providers can be found at www.apta.org and www.hermanwallace.com.
   f. **Mastectomy-related** poor body image may be at least partly alleviated by use of a prosthesis. The American Cancer Society Reach to Recovery program can assist in this process.
   g. **Chronic genital GVHD** treatment for women involves first treating estrogen deficiency and then topical glucocorticoid therapy, topical genital tract cyclosporine, and prophylactic dilator use weekly.
   h. **Erectile dysfunction** is treated first line by PDE5 inhibitors. However, these will not work for most men within 6 months after RP. RP requires penile rehabilitation (PR), which involves medically induced erections (by penile injections) two to three times per week to maintain tissue health. Fifty-two to sixty-seven percent of men will regain erectile functioning with PR. Erections may also be induced with a vacuum device. If none of the above are effective by 24 months, penile implant surgery is the last option.
   i. **Retrograde ejaculation and anejaculation** are treated with sympathomimetic or anticholinergic agents such as ephedrine, midodrine, imipramine, or pseudoephedrine, which may restore antegrade ejaculation in 50% to 100% of men.
   j. **Low sexual desire/arousal** is multifactorial and may not be due primarily to cancer diagnosis or treatment. Psychological, relational, and

sociocultural factors need to be assessed to determine causal factors. Common factors include fatigue, depression, poor body image, and discord in relationship. Mindfulness-based cognitive behavioral therapy has been found to be effective for low sexual desire in cancer patients. Flibanserin is FDA approved to treat low sexual desire in premenopausal women, but has not been studied in cancer populations.

k. Orgasm difficulties may be due to inadequate stimulation, selective serotonin reuptake inhibitors, or reduced genital sensation due to hormonal changes or may have a multifactorial etiology. For orgasm due to decreased genital sensation, use of vibratory stimulation with a lubricant may be beneficial.

l. Ostomy bags should be emptied prior to sexual activity, and an ostomy cover can be used during sexual activity.

II. FERTILITY

Consultation with a fertility specialist is advised as soon as possible after a cancer diagnosis (ideally before antineoplastic therapy is given) for men and women who are interested in preserving fertility. Reproductive technologies are rapidly evolving, and timely reproductive endocrinology referrals facilitate optimal fertility preservation with minimal delay of oncologic therapy. There is no evidence that pregnancy is unsafe in cancer survivors, nor that past antineoplastic treatments cause germ cell abnormalities that lead to an increased rate of birth defects in progeny of cancer survivors (though preterm deliveries and low birth weights are slightly more common in cancer survivors). With the exception of familial cancer syndromes and cases of radiation exposure to the fetus, there is no increased risk of cancer in offspring of cancer survivors. Referrals to a genetic counselor are appropriate when inherited predisposition to cancer is suspected. Importantly, all cancer patients should be counseled about contraception during cancer treatment.

MEN

A. Pretreatment hypogonadism. Low sperm counts prior to cancer treatment are common with germ cell tumors, probably due to the disease itself and to irregularities of the malignancy-prone testis. It is also common for men with other cancers including Hodgkin lymphoma and leukemia to have low sperm counts prior to treatment. Metastatic cancer and malnutrition can also reduce hormone levels and limit reproductive capability of male cancer patients before treatment. Disease-associated stressors may make it difficult for men to bank sperm.

B. Effects of radiation therapy (RT). The testes are extremely radiation sensitive. Testicular doses as low as 15 cGy result in transient suppression of spermatogenesis, with prolonged azoospermia seen at higher doses, and permanent sterility following >600 cGy. Once treatment begins, it may take 2 to 3 months for sperm counts to decline, but DNA damage to formed spermatozoa occurs almost immediately. Thus, cancer patients should use effective contraception immediately upon initiating radiation.

C. Effects of chemotherapy. Spermatogenesis can also be impaired by gonadotoxic chemotherapy, and higher doses are more problematic. As with radiation, DNA damage occurs rapidly after chemotherapy exposure although there is a delay in reduction in sperm counts. Hence, contraceptive counseling is essential.

1. **Alkylating agents** such as cyclophosphamide cause germ cell depletion in a dose-dependent fashion. The odds of azoospermia increase by 22% and of oligospermia by 14% for every 1,000 mg/m^2 increase in cyclophosphamide equivalent dose. Sperm recovery may occur in 20% to 25% of patients after even the most intensive therapies including myeloablative hematopoietic cell transplantation (HCT), although recovery may be delayed by years after therapy.

2. **Other drugs** that are probably associated with reduced sperm count include doxorubicin, vinblastine, and cisplatin.

3. **Combination regimens.** About half of all patients treated with cisplatin, etoposide, and bleomycin for nonseminomatous testicular cancer recover sperm production within 3 years. Many combination regimens used to treat hematologic and nonhematologic malignancies will not result in permanent azoospermia, though it is always safest to offer fertility preservation techniques before chemotherapy to any man who desires future biologic children.

4. **Hematopoietic cell transplantation (HCT).** Myeloablative transplant regimens (both allogeneic and autologous) typically include very high doses of alkylators (cyclophosphamide and/or busulfan), TBI at doses >800 cGy, or both. Patients undergoing myeloablative HCT have a nearly 100% chance of azoospermia.

D. **Measures to protect reproductive function in men**

1. **Sperm banking** should be offered to all men who are interested in future fertility before receipt of potentially gonadotoxic therapy. Typically, sperm banking requires self-stimulation to produce three samples 48 to 96 hours apart. The efficacy of sperm banking may be limited in some men because of low sperm counts (<20 million/mL) with poor motility (<50%) even before treatment begins. For men who are unable to produce a sperm sample for banking (due to young age, discomfort, or azoospermia), microsurgical epididymal sperm aspiration, testicular sperm extraction, and electroejaculation are options to collect sperm before antineoplastic therapy begins. Perhaps the greatest barrier to sperm banking is the failure of oncologists to counsel and to refer these patients, with fewer than half of oncologists reporting that they consistently make these referrals.

2. **Artificial insemination** may be tried in women whose partner's posttreatment sperm quality is good despite low sperm count. Rates of sperm aneuploidy increase immediately after chemotherapy or radiation, so a man should ideally wait at least 12 months after treatment before he tries to impregnate his partner with sperm that were not banked before treatment.

3. **In vitro fertilization (IVF)** can be performed before cancer therapy to create embryos to freeze. This can be successful even in men who have few sperm, and intracytoplasmic sperm injection can facilitate fertilization even in some apparently azoospermic men (requiring only a single viable sperm).

4. **Oncologic treatment decision-making** may be impacted by fertility concerns. For men with low-risk testicular cancer (or other low-risk cancers), chemotherapy and radiation may be omitted in favor of surveillance in order to optimize fertility. For men with prostate cancer, nerve-sparing prostatectomies, modified lymph node dissections to minimize retrograde ejaculation, and testicular shielding during radiation may be considered.

WOMEN

Both chemotherapy and radiation are toxic to the ovaries, resulting in diminished ovarian reserve and premature ovarian failure in a dose-, class-, and age-dependent fashion. Even when cancer therapy does not cause immediate permanent amenorrhea, it may result in accelerated ovarian aging, a shortened "fertility window," and early menopause. For example, women who receive 300 cGy of radiation to the pelvis at age 20 can expect to enter menopause at approximately age 35; women who receive 1,200 cGy at that age can expect to enter menopause almost immediately.

A. **Effects of RT.** As with the testes, ovaries are exquisitely sensitive to radiation. Approximately 50% of oocytes are lost at doses of 200 cGy to the ovaries, and doses of >500 cGy to the ovaries usually result in permanent ovarian failure.

B. **Effects of chemotherapy.** The likelihood of permanent ovarian failure after chemotherapy increases with age and is dependent on class and dose of cytotoxic agents, with alkylating agents most strongly associated with risk of amenorrhea. Chemotherapy exerts differential effects on the ovarian cortex and on the oocytes, depending on their stage of maturation. Chemotherapy is directly toxic to mature ovarian follicles by inducing apoptosis of the surrounding, nourishing granulosa cells. In addition, chemotherapy may diminish blood supply to the primordial follicles, cause fibrosis of the ovarian cortex, and cause recruitment of additional primordial follicles into mature follicles, which are then susceptible to direct toxicity.

1. **Alkylating agents:** These drugs are the most toxic to the ovaries and cause oocyte destruction in a dose-dependent fashion. Importantly, the risk of permanent amenorrhea rises with increasing age at the time of treatment. Women in their 40's treated with significant doses of alkylating agents almost never recover menstrual function. The gonadotoxicity of the alkylators is attributed to these drugs' direct cytotoxicity, which may occur independently of the cell cycle.

2. **Other drugs:** Platinum-based drugs are also toxic to ovaries. Newer and targeted agents have unknown effects on fertility and require further study. At least one such drug, bevacizumab, has been reported to result in increased rates of amenorrhea, which may be permanent.

3. **Combination regimens:** At age 40, there is an approximately 50% chance of permanent menopause during standard multiagent chemotherapy for early-stage breast cancer. Even for women who regain menses after chemotherapy, menopause is likely to occur earlier than it would have otherwise. Counseling women about the likelihood of premature ovarian failure and early menopause is essential. Women with hematologic malignancies are typically treated with multiagent therapies that have <20% chance of immediate permanent amenorrhea, although more intensive alkylator-based regimens (such as dose-escalated BEACOPP for high-risk Hodgkin lymphoma) can cause higher rates of permanent ovarian failure.

4. **Hematopoietic stem cell transplantation:** As noted above, myeloablative HSCT (both allogeneic and autologous) is conditioned with high-dose alkylating agents and/or total body radiation at doses that are expected to result in a 100% chance of immediate, permanent amenorrhea. Although reduced-intensity approaches use lower doses and are associated with markedly less toxicity, it appears that ovarian function and fertility are still significantly impacted. Therefore, reduced-intensity transplants should also

be considered highly gonadotoxic. The presence of chronic graft versus host disease may also impact fertility.

C. Surgery. Ovarian, cervical, and uterine surgeries can cause infertility in women. Cancer patients who need hysterectomy without oophorectomy sometimes opt to use surrogates to carry their future pregnancies if finances and state laws allow.

D. Measures to protect fertility in women

1. **Embryo cryopreservation** is the gold standard for fertility preservation prior to cancer treatment.

2. **Oocyte cryopreservation.** In experienced centers, cryopreservation of oocytes (for patients without a male partner who do not want to use donor sperm) is just as successful as embryos. Oocyte cryopreservation is considered standard of care, on par with embryo cryopreservation. Both embryo and oocyte cryopreservation usually require a 10- to 14-day period of hormonal stimulation and a minimally invasive transvaginal procedure to retrieve the stimulated oocytes. Alternative stimulation protocols that minimize estrogen exposure may be desirable in women with hormonally sensitive cancers.

3. **Ovarian tissue cryopreservation** is currently experimental in the United States and is contraindicated in women with hematologic malignancies, as tissue contamination with malignant cells has been documented.

4. **Gonadotropin-releasing hormone analogues (GnRHa).** There are several prospective randomized trials with conflicting data about the efficacy of GnRHa for fertility preservation. Most of the evidence suggests that administration of GnRHa before and during chemotherapy can reduce the risk of permanent amenorrhea and premature ovarian failure. GnRHa have additional advantages including:

   a. Potential to preserve ovarian function, not just fertility, which has positive health effects in terms of menopausal symptoms, bone mineral density, and cardiovascular risk reduction.

   b. Lack of the 10- to 14-day "waiting period" (for GnRH antagonists) required for methods requiring oocyte stimulation and retrieval.

   c. Avoidance of menses and/or menorrhagia during treatment, although some women do experience vaginal bleeding following the first dose of GnRHa.

   d. If other, standard-of-care options such as oocyte or embryo cryopreservation are feasible and appropriate, GnRHa should not be relied upon as the sole method of fertility preservation. However, for women who require urgent or immediate antineoplastic therapy, or who are deemed too high risk to undergo hormonal stimulation and/or oocyte retrieval, a careful discussion of risks, side effects, and expectations from the use of GnRHa is appropriate as this approach may represent the only option for these patients.

5. **Oncologic treatment decision-making.** Some cancer therapies can be modified to reduce the risk of subsequent infertility. For example, patients may decide not to receive chemotherapy to reduce risk of recurrence of early-stage breast cancer. For cervical cancer, radical trachelectomy may be considered for early-stage cervical cancer to preserve future reproductive function.

6. **Hematologic malignancies.** These patients may present acutely, with significant cytopenias, infections, disseminated intravascular coagulation, venous thromboembolism, or cardiopulmonary compromise. Hence, some special considerations apply:

a. The patients' clinical status may preclude consideration of standard fertility preservation options. They may require urgent or emergent therapy that precludes a period of hormonal stimulation or an invasive retrieval procedure, and they are not eligible for ovarian tissue cryopreservation due to concern for malignant contamination. Hence, hormonal therapy with GnRHa may be the only option available to them.

b. It is essential for the provider to be able to identify patients who are not eligible for standard fertility preservation methods. The oncologist's first priority should always be to treat potentially curable patients with optimal therapy without unnecessary delays.

c. Although the chemotherapy regimens used for acute leukemias and Hodgkin lymphoma may be associated with <20% chance of permanent amenorrhea, they will likely result in diminished ovarian reserve over the longer term. It is possible to harvest oocytes after completion of therapy, and this may be an appropriate consideration given the shortened fertility window these patients may face.

d. There is a substantial chance of relapse for many of these patients, which is typically managed with HCT; as noted above, HCT is associated with a nearly 100% chance of permanent ovarian failure. Given these considerations, referral to a reproductive specialist even after completion of therapy is a reasonable consideration.

7. Chronic myelogenous leukemia (CML) requires lifelong therapy with oral tyrosine kinase inhibitors (TKIs). These agents are associated with an increased risk of spontaneous abortion and congenital anomalies and are thus contraindicated in pregnancy. Women on a TKI who desire pregnancy should first achieve a complete molecular response (>4.5 log reduction in quantitative bcr/abl transcripts by IS) for at least 2 years' duration, after which time they may temporarily discontinue TKI to permit conception and gestation. The TKI should be resumed immediately after delivery; breast-feeding is contraindicated. If an unplanned pregnancy occurs while taking a TKI, the drug should be stopped immediately. Close monitoring of blood counts and molecular monitoring of bcr/abl by quantitative PCR is essential. A new diagnosis of asymptomatic CML in chronic phase during pregnancy may be managed expectantly, with watchful waiting, until delivery. In all cases, if CML progression occurs during pregnancy, interferon may be used safely prior to delivery.

III. CANCERS DURING PREGNANCY

A. Background

1. Incidence. Cervical cancer, breast cancer, and melanoma are the most commonly diagnosed cancers during pregnancy (affecting 1 in 1,000 pregnancies overall). Hematologic malignancies are rare (0.02% of pregnancies) with Hodgkin lymphoma most common among these.

2. Natural history. The incidence of malignancy is not increased during pregnancy, though breast cancer incidence does increase for a few years after each pregnancy. Pregnancy is not detrimental to prognosis unless it impedes recommended treatment, and even hormonally sensitive breast cancer has not been shown to be more likely to recur due to pregnancy.

3. Teratogenesis. First trimester exposure to chemotherapy or radiation can cause birth defects and/or spontaneous abortion. Many women have delivered healthy babies after treatment with chemotherapy during the second and third trimesters, though there is still a risk of intrauterine growth retardation and associated developmental delays. Maternal–fetal medicine specialists with experience with cancer during pregnancy should care for these patients.

B. **Diagnostic studies during pregnancy**

1. **Biopsies** under local anesthesia are almost completely safe for a fetus. Even biopsies under general anesthesia are low risk.

2. **Studies to avoid** unless absolutely necessary for the health of the mother: radionuclide scans, GI/GU contrast studies, abdominal or chest CTs, FDG-PET, and pelvic and lumbosacral spine films. Ultrasound is the preferred alternative to CTs and radionuclide scans, and MRI is also likely safe at least in the second and third trimesters.

3. **Mammograms** have a low negative predictive value in pregnancy and during lactation due to breast engorgement.

4. **Chest, spine, and long bone radiographs** are usually possible with use of proper abdominal shielding. The dose of ionizing radiation to the fetus is <0.5 cGy with these x-rays.

5. **Sentinel node imaging** can safely be performed as the ^{99}mTc dose to the fetus is negligible.

6. **Bone marrow aspirates and biopsies** can be performed safely with the patient in the lateral decubitus position.

C. **Principles of managing cancer during pregnancy**

The overarching goals of cancer management during pregnancy are (a) to prioritize and to optimize the curability of the cancer by avoiding cancer treatment delays or modifications and (b) to attempt to deliver at term when possible.

1. **Pregnancy prevention** should be emphasized in all women of childbearing age who are on active treatment. Contraceptive options should be addressed, and referrals to appropriate family planning specialists are essential. All options, including pregnancy termination, should be discussed when a pregnant woman requires cancer treatment; therapeutic abortion (TAB) may be performed up to the 24th week of gestation.

2. **Determination of gestational age** is an essential first step when cancer and pregnancy coincide to inform the safety of diagnostic studies and therapy.

3. **Chemotherapy.** If delays do not compromise curability, chemotherapy during the first trimester should be avoided. If that is not possible, pregnancy termination should be strongly considered. Chemotherapy has been safely administered during the second and third trimester, but risks are greater in the second trimester. A full discussion of the management of the pregnant cancer patient is beyond the scope of this chapter. It is absolutely essential that a multidisciplinary team of experienced hematologist–oncologists, maternal–fetal medicine specialists, and neonatologists are involved in the management of these patients.

4. **Specific drugs.** Trastuzumab should never be administered during pregnancy due to a >70% risk of oligohydramnios/anhydramnios when given in the 2nd or 3rd trimester. Endocrine therapy (such as tamoxifen) is almost never given during pregnancy due to teratogenicity, with the greatest risk during the first trimester. Methotrexate is contraindicated early in pregnancy, and rituximab has been shown to cross the placenta and result in miscarriage, preterm delivery, and cytopenias in the fetus. As discussed above, TKI therapy for CML patients is contraindicated during pregnancy, as are many other oral agents such as thalidomide and its derivatives.

5. **Acute leukemia management.** Acute leukemias present particular challenges given the associated profound cytopenias and infectious risks as well

as the need for an indwelling central catheter. In general, acute leukemia diagnosed before week 20 should be managed with TAB followed by standard therapy; after week 20, standard therapy may be attempted without pregnancy termination, but substantial risks of bleeding, clotting, and infection remain major concerns. One particular subtype of AML, acute promyelocytic leukemia (APL), is often associated with disseminated intravascular coagulation. APL is highly curable when treated appropriately; standard of care dictates emergent institution of ATRA (all-trans retinoic acid) therapy, which is teratogenic in the first trimester. Hence, APL patients in the first trimester should undergo TAB, but ATRA can be given safely in the 2nd trimester or later. Arsenic, another highly potent agent for APL, is highly teratogenic and contraindicated throughout pregnancy.

6. **Radiation.** Radiation during the first 15 weeks of gestation is generally contraindicated; if required, consultation with a medical physicist to estimate fetal dose is essential. Proton therapy holds promise as a safer alternative to traditional radiation. Late effects of fetal radiation exposure include an increased incidence of thyroid cancer and leukemia, as well as mental retardation, growth delays, cataracts, and infertility; these risks are dose dependent.

7. **Surgery.** Surgery is usually safe during pregnancy except for cervical or uterine cancer (colposcopy can be done, but endocervical curettage biopsy is contraindicated, and cervical conization should be avoided if possible due to an increased risk of cervical hemorrhage and a high incidence of incomplete resection).

8. **Watchful waiting.** Consideration may be given to expectant management of early-stage cervical cancer (stage IA with <3 mm invasion), early-stage Hodgkin lymphoma, and indolent non-Hodgkin lymphomas (until after delivery).

9. **Breast-feeding** is usually contraindicated because chemotherapeutic agents are excreted into human milk and have caused neutropenia in infants.

Suggested Readings

Sexual Function

Huffman LB, Hartenbach EM, Carter J, et al. Maintaining sexual health throughout gynecologic cancer survivorship: a comprehensive review and clinical guide. *Gynecol Oncol* 2016;140(2):359.

Chung E, Brock G. Sexual rehabilitation and cancer survivorship: a state of art review of current literature and management strategies in male sexual dysfunction among prostate cancer survivors. *J Sex Med* 2013;10(suppl 1):102.

Traa MJ, De Vries J, Roukema JA, et al. Sexual (dys)function and the quality of sexual life in patients with colorectal cancer: a systematic review. *Ann Oncol* 2012;23(1):19.

Fertility

Loren AW, Mangu PB, Beck LN, et al. Fertility preservation for patients with cancer: American Society of Clinical Oncology clinical practice guideline update. *J Clin Oncol* 2013;31(19):2500.

Meirow D, Biederman H, Anderson RA, et al. Toxicity of chemotherapy and radiation on female reproduction. *Clin Obstet Gynecol* 2010;53:727.

Meistrich ML. Effects of chemotherapy and radiotherapy on spermatogenesis in humans. *Fertil Steril* 2013;100:1180.

Practice Committee of American Society for Reproductive Medicine. Fertility preservation in patients undergoing gonadotoxic therapy or gonadectomy: a committee opinion. *Fertil Steril* 2013;100:1214.

Ruddy KJ, Partridge AH. Fertility (male and female) and menopause. *J Clin Oncol* 2012;30 (30):3705.

Wallace WH, Thomson AB, Saran F, et al. Predicting age of ovarian failure after radiation to a field that includes the ovaries. *Int J Radiat Oncol Biol Phys* 2005;62:738.

Cancer During Pregnancy

Andersson TM, Johansson AL, Fredricksson I, et al. Cancer during pregnancy and the postpartum period: a population-based study. *Cancer* 2015;121(12):2072.

Lishner M, Avivi I, Apperley JF, et al. Hematologic malignancies in pregnancy: management guidelines from an international consensus meeting. *J Clin Oncol* 2016;34(5):501.

Palani R, Milojkovic D, Apperley JF. Managing pregnancy in chronic myeloid leukaemia. *Ann Hematol* 2015;94(suppl 2):S167.

Web Sites

Fertile hope: fertility resources for cancer patients. **www.fertilehope.org**.

Referrals to sexual medicine or sex therapist. **www.ISSWSH.org and www.aasect.org**.

Physical therapy referrals for pelvic floor. **www.apta.org and www.hermanwallace.com**.

I. HYPERCALCEMIA

A. Mechanisms. Cancer is the most common cause of hypercalcemia in hospitalized patients.

1. **Bone metastases.** Most tumors capable of bone metastasis can also produce hypercalcemia. Local production of various substances by tumor cells stimulates osteoclastic bone resorption. This occurs most commonly in breast cancer and multiple myeloma.

2. **Humoral hypercalcemia of malignancy** is caused by production of a PTH-like substance called PTH-related peptide (PTH-RP) by a variety of carcinomas (squamous tumors of many organs, renal cell carcinoma, breast cancer). PTH-RP has bone-resorbing activity and interacts with the renal PTH receptor to stimulate renal calcium resorption.

3. **Vitamin D metabolites** (e.g., 1,25-dihydroxyvitamin D) may be produced by some lymphomas; these metabolites promote intestinal calcium absorption.

4. **Prostaglandins and interleukin-1** produced by various tumors may occasionally cause hypercalcemia, perhaps by enhancing bone resorption.

5. **Ectopic parathyroid hormone** (PTH) secretion appears to be rare.

B. Diagnosis

1. **Symptoms of hypercalcemia** depend both on the serum level of ionized calcium and on how fast the level rises. Rapidly rising serum calcium levels tend to produce obtundation and coma with only moderately elevated serum calcium levels (e.g., 13 mg/dL). Slowly rising serum calcium levels may produce only mild symptoms, even with serum levels exceeding 15 mg/dL.

   a. **Early symptoms:** polyuria, nocturia, polydipsia, anorexia, easy fatigability, weakness

   b. **Late symptoms:** apathy, irritability, depression, decreased ability to concentrate, mental obtundation, coma, profound muscle weakness, nausea, vomiting, vague abdominal pain, constipation, obstipation, pruritus, abnormalities of vision

2. **Differential diagnosis of hypercalcemia.** The possible etiologies of hypercalcemia include the following:

   a. Malignancy

   b. Primary hyperparathyroidism

   c. Thiazide diuretic therapy

   d. Vitamin D or vitamin A intoxication

   e. Milk–alkali syndrome

   f. Familial benign hypocalciuric hypercalcemia

   g. Others: immobilization of patients with accelerated bone turnover (e.g., Paget disease or myeloma), sarcoidosis, tuberculosis, and other granulomatous diseases, hyperthyroidism, lithium administration, adrenal insufficiency, diuretic phase of acute renal failure, severe liver disease

3. **Laboratory studies.** All patients with cancer and polyuria, mental status changes, or gastrointestinal symptoms should be evaluated for hypercalcemia.
   a. **Routine studies**
      (1) **Serum calcium, phosphorus, and albumin levels**
         (a) Ionized calcium constitutes about 47% of the serum calcium and is in equilibrium with calcium bound to proteins, especially to albumin. Roughly 0.8 mg of calcium is bound by 1 g of serum albumin. When serum albumin is low, the measured serum calcium can be corrected (to a normal albumin concentration of 4 g/dL) using the following formula:

$$\text{Corrected serum calcium (mg/dL)} =$$
$$\text{measured calcium} + 0.8 \times (4.0 - \text{measured albumin}).$$

         (b) Long-standing hypercalcemia with hypophosphatemia suggests primary hyperparathyroidism.
      (2) **Serum alkaline phosphatase.** Elevated levels may be due to either hyperparathyroidism or metastatic disease to the bone or liver.
      (3) **Serum electrolytes.** Serum chloride concentrations are frequently elevated in primary hyperparathyroidism. Renal tubular acidosis may complicate chronic hypercalcemia.
      (4) **Blood urea nitrogen (BUN) and serum creatinine.** The direct effect of hypercalcemia on the kidneys can result in nephrogenic diabetes insipidus with defective renal tubular water conservation (i.e., symptoms of polyuria) leading to dehydration and azotemia.
      (5) **Electrocardiogram (ECG).** Hypercalcemia results in relative shortening of the QT interval and prolongation of the PR interval. The T wave widens at blood levels above 16 mg/dL, paradoxically lengthening the QT interval.
      (6) **Radiographs of the abdomen and bones**
         (a) **Nephrocalcinosis** and other ectopic calcifications are common in long-standing hypercalcemia.
         (b) **Subperiosteal bone resorption** is pathognomonic of hyperparathyroidism, but diffuse osteopenia is the most common radiologic finding in this condition.
   b. **Further studies.** Results from preliminary evaluation may indicate the need for measuring serum PTH levels or for performing other tests.
      (1) **Evidence for concomitant primary hyperparathyroidism**
         (a) Documented long history of hypercalcemia or renal stones
         (b) Radiographic evidence of hyperparathyroid bone disease (subperiosteal reabsorption, osteitis fibrosa cystica, or salt-and-pepper skull)
         (c) Hyperchloremic acidosis, particularly with a serum chloride-to-phosphate ratio ≥ 34
         (d) Elevated serum PTH level in the presence of hypercalcemia
         (e) Absence of hypocalciuria; if the ratio of calcium clearance to creatinine clearance in a 24-hour urine specimen is <0.01, the patient probably has familial hypocalciuric hypercalcemia, which can otherwise mimic primary hyperparathyroidism. Note, however, that vitamin D deficiency must first be corrected in order to accurately assess urinary calcium excretion.

(2) Evidence for humoral hypercalcemia of malignancy

  (a) Low or low-normal serum PTH levels in the presence of hypercalcemia

  (b) Elevated serum level of PTH-RP

  (c) Metabolic alkalosis

  (d) Low serum level of 1,25-dihydroxyvitamin D

C. Management

  1. Acute, symptomatic hypercalcemia should be treated as an emergency.

  a. Hydration and saline diuresis. Achieving and maintaining normal intravascular volume and hydration are the cornerstones of promoting urinary calcium excretion. Isotonic saline is given initially at high rates, e.g., 200 to 300 mL/hr, and then tapered.

  (1) Fluid intake and output and body weight are carefully monitored. If necessary, loop diuretics may be given to treat volume overload in patients with cardiac or renal disease.

  (2) Blood levels of calcium, potassium, and magnesium are measured every 8 to 12 hours, and concentrations of cations in the IV solutions are adjusted.

  (3) Treatment is continued until the blood calcium concentration is below 12 mg/dL. Central nervous system manifestations in elderly or comatose patients may not improve until normal blood calcium levels are maintained for several days.

  b. Bisphosphonates are potent inhibitors of osteoclast activity and are effective in the treatment of hypercalcemia of malignancy. Zoledronic acid is the most effective of the available drugs; it is given as a single IV infusion of 4 mg in 100 mL of normal saline over 15 minutes. Pamidronate is given as a single IV infusion of 60 to 90 mg in 250 to 500 mL of normal saline over 2 to 4 hours. With either drug, significant reductions in serum calcium occur in 2 to 4 days and generally persist for several weeks. Caution should be used in giving these agents to patients with renal impairment. Patients should be well hydrated both before and after administration of IV bisphosphonates. Doses may be repeated every 7 to 30 days. A potential adverse effect of bisphosphonates is osteonecrosis of the jaw (see Chapter 34). Atypical subtrochanteric fractures of the femur have also been rarely reported with prolonged use.

  c. Calcitonin is useful for rapid reduction of blood calcium levels. Blood calcium levels are decreased within 2 to 3 hours of administration. The drug inhibits bone resorption and increases renal calcium clearance. The effect is transient and generally only limited to 48 hours due to rather rapid development of tachyphylaxis. Allergy is the only important complication of therapy. Synthetic salmon calcitonin is given in a dose of 4 units/kg SC or IM every 8 to 12 hours; the dose may be increased to 8 units/kg every 8 to 12 hours if needed. Calcitonin can be given when diuresis or other drugs are contraindicated or ineffective (e.g., renal failure, congestive heart failure).

  d. Denosumab, a monoclonal antibody with affinity for nuclear factor-kappa ligand (RANKL), is a potent inhibitor of osteoclast action and is used for hypercalcemia that is refractory to bisphosphonates. It may be of most benefit in patients for whom bisphosphonates are contraindicated due to renal insufficiency. The optimal dose of denosumab for treating hypercalcemia has not been established, but it is recommended to give lower doses such as 0.3 mg/kg SC initially, as higher doses may result in prolonged hypocalcemia. This effect may be attenuated by establishing adequate vitamin D levels prior to treatment. As with bisphosphonate therapy, osteonecrosis of the jaw as well as atypical femoral fractures have been reported as adverse effects from prolonged exposure to denosumab.

  e. **Dialysis.** Peritoneal dialysis and hemodialysis rapidly lower blood calcium levels but are rarely used and are generally considered an option of last resort.

  f. **Other therapies** such as gallium nitrate and mithramycin can be used to reduce serum calcium levels in the acute setting; concern for various toxicities and superior potency of bisphosphonates and calcitonin make these agents second line, and rarely used.

2. **Chronic hypercalcemia.** Ambulation is encouraged to minimize bone resorption that accompanies immobilization. Liberal fluid intake (2 to 3 L/d) is prescribed. Foods containing large amounts of calcium, such as milk products, are avoided. Thiazide diuretics aggravate hypercalcemia and should not be taken. Treatment of the underlying malignancy may be beneficial.

  a. **Glucocorticoids.** Prednisone, 20 to 40 mg PO daily, or hydrocortisone, 100 to 150 mg IV every 12 hours, may be used for patients with tumors that are sensitive to glucocorticoids (e.g., lymphoma, multiple myeloma, and granulomatous disease). Glucocorticoids also increase renal calcium excretion.

  b. **Bisphosphonates.** Zoledronic acid (4 mg IV) or pamidronate (60 to 90 mg IV) may be given every 7 to 30 days as needed to control hypercalcemia.

  c. **Denosumab** 0.3 mg/kg, or up to 120 mg SC every 4 weeks.

  d. **Calcimimetics** such as cinacalcet are used to treat PTH–related hypercalcemia such as in parathyroid carcinoma, tertiary hyperparathyroidism, and, to a lesser extent, in primary hyperparathyroidism.

3. **When should neck surgery for primary hyperparathyroidism be considered?**
   Parathyroid surgery is justified if all of the following apply:

  a. Clinical and laboratory findings (see earlier) suggest hyperparathyroidism.

  b. The malignancy is under control, and the patient's expected survival is reasonably long.

  c. The general condition of the patient makes the surgical risk acceptable.

  d. The hypercalcemia is severe enough to warrant treatment. Surgery may be considered if serum calcium levels are only mildly elevated, but there is evidence of complications such as recurrent nephrolithiasis or decreased bone mineral density that is thought to be due to the increased PTH level.

  e. Parathyroid scanning with technetium-99m sestamibi or neck sonography demonstrates a probable parathyroid adenoma.

II. HYPOCALCEMIA

A. Mechanisms

1. **Paraneoplasia.** Hypocalcemia is an extremely rare paraneoplastic syndrome.

  a. **Rapid uptake of calcium.** Patients with osteoblastic bone metastases may occasionally develop hypocalcemia due to uptake of calcium in the bone lesions. In addition, patients with bone metastases from prostate or breast cancer who are treated with hormonal agents may develop hypocalcemia, supposedly because of rapid bone healing. Calcifying chondrosarcoma is a rare tumor that has been associated with hypocalcemia.

  b. **Calcitonin** production by medullary carcinoma of the thyroid rarely causes hypocalcemia.

2. **Magnesium deficiency.** Magnesium is necessary both for the secretion of PTH and for its peripheral action. Hypomagnesemia results in hypocalcemia that does not respond to calcium replacement therapy. Magnesium deficiency occurs in the following circumstances:

   a. Patients who have prolonged nasogastric drainage

   b. Patients who receive parenteral hyperalimentation without magnesium replacement

   c. Cisplatin therapy–induced renal tubular dysfunction with urinary magnesium loss

   d. Chronic diuretic therapy or diuresis due to glycosuria

   e. Chronic alcoholism (alcohol interferes with renal conservation of magnesium)

   f. Chronic diarrhea

   g. Therapy with EGFR-blocking antibodies: cetuximab (6% to 55%) and panitumumab (7%)

3. **Other causes of hypocalcemia:** therapy for hypercalcemia, especially if using IV bisphosphonates or denosumab, hypoalbuminemia (pseudohypocalcemia), hyperphosphatemia (see Section III), pancreatitis, renal disease, hypoparathyroidism, pseudohypoparathyroidism (PTH resistance), rickets and osteomalacia, sepsis, calcium chelator exposure (citrate, EDTA) from large volume blood transfusion, gadolinium, when used for MRI imaging, can cause spurious, asymptomatic hypocalcemia that resolves within hours.

B. **Diagnosis**

1. **Symptoms and signs** are aggravated by hyperventilation or other causes of alkalosis.

   a. Tetany is the most prominent symptom of hypocalcemia and is manifested by paresthesias (especially numbness and tingling of the face, hands, and feet), muscle cramps, laryngospasms, or seizures. Other problems include diarrhea, headache, lethargy, irritability, and loss of recent memory. Chronic hypocalcemia may be well tolerated, however, with few symptoms.

   b. Dry skin, abnormal nails, cataracts, and papilledema may develop in long-standing cases.

   c. Chvostek sign: twitching of muscles around the mouth, nose, or eyes after tapping the facial nerve.

   d. Trousseau sign: spasm of the hand during 3 to 4 minutes of exercise while a blood pressure cuff on the arm is inflated midway between systolic and diastolic pressures.

2. **Laboratory studies.** Serum levels of calcium, phosphorus, magnesium, electrolytes, BUN, creatinine, albumin, intact PTH, and 25-hydroxy-vitamin D should be obtained. The ECG may show a prolonged QT interval; the ECG is monitored during therapy.

C. **Management**

1. **Severe, acute, symptomatic hypocalcemia** (blood calcium < 6 mg/dL) is generally managed in an intensive care setting with ECG monitoring.

   a. **Calcium gluconate or calcium chloride**, 1 g, diluted in 50 mL of either D5W or normal saline, is given over 10 to 20 minutes. This is then followed by a slow infusion of calcium, which is prepared by combining 11 g calcium gluconate in D5W or normal saline, to reach final volume of 1,000 mL. This is then infused at a rate of 50 mL/hr.

   b. **Magnesium sulfate**, 1 g IV or IM every 8 to 12 hours, is also administered if the blood magnesium level is unknown or <1.5 mg/dL until the calcium or magnesium blood levels have normalized.

   c. **Hyperventilating** patients should breathe into a paper bag to decrease respiratory alkalosis.
   d. **Serum calcium levels** are obtained every 1 to 2 hours until the serum calcium level exceeds 7 mg/dL.
2. **Moderate hypocalcemia** (blood calcium between 6 and 8 mg/dL)
   a. **Calcium** may be given either PO or, if the patient is severely symptomatic, IV.
      (1) Calcium carbonate, 2.5 g/d, or calcium citrate, 4 to 5 g/d PO in divided doses: either form, will provide about 1,000 mg of elemental calcium daily.
      (2) Calcium gluconate, 2 g IV in 500 mL of 5% dextrose in water, is given every 8 hours.
   b. **Hypomagnesemia** (<1.5 mg/dL) is treated with magnesium sulfate, 1 g IM or IV once or twice daily, until the blood level is normal. Persistent hypomagnesemia can be treated with oral magnesium, 300 mg daily in divided doses.
   c. **Patients recovering from hypercalcemia** who were treated with IV bisphosphonates or denosumab are in jeopardy of recurrent life-threatening hypocalcemia for as long as 4 days after treatment is stopped.
   d. **Patients with postthyroidectomy hypoparathyroidism** are discussed in Chapter 16, Section III.G.1.

III. HYPERPHOSPHATEMIA

A. **Mechanisms.** Hyperphosphatemia (>4.5 mg/dL) is a rare complication of treatment of certain tumors, notably leukemia and lymphoma (especially Burkitt lymphoma). Rapid tumor lysis releases large amounts of potassium, phosphate, and nucleic acids (which are metabolized to uric acid).
B. **Diagnosis.** The serum phosphate level itself does not cause symptoms. Renal damage or acute renal failure results from precipitation of calcium phosphate in the kidneys. Tetany and seizures may develop if the ionized calcium concentration becomes inordinately reduced (e.g., with alkalosis from bicarbonate administration or vomiting).
   1. **Laboratory studies.** Serum phosphate, calcium, and other electrolyte levels should be measured regularly in susceptible patients during the initial course of antitumor therapy.
   2. **Differential diagnosis**
      a. Hypoparathyroidism
      b. Renal failure
      c. Rapid tissue breakdown after muscle trauma or burn (rhabdomyolysis)
      d. Tumor lysis syndrome (see Chapter 32)
      e. Large oral or rectal doses of phosphates
C. **Management**
   1. **Acute.** High phosphate levels must be lowered rapidly to avoid or reverse renal damage. Volume expansion with normal saline increases phosphate excretion, but must be used with caution as hydration will worsen hypocalcemia. Intravenous insulin in combination with dextrose can be used to drive phosphate into cells. Serum chemistries are monitored every 4 to 6 hours. Hemodialysis is often needed in refractory cases, in those with severe hyperphosphatemia (>14 mg/dL), and in patients with renal insufficiency.
   2. **Chronic.** In addition to a low-phosphate diet, oral phosphate binders are given to bind phosphate in the intestine.
      a. Sevelamer hydrochloride, 800 to 1,600 mg orally t.i.d. with meals
      b. Lanthanum carbonate, 500 to 1,000 mg orally t.i.d. with meals

IV. HYPOPHOSPHATEMIA

A. Mechanism. Hypophosphatemia (<3 mg/dL) is occasionally associated with rapidly growing tumors (such as acute leukemia), presumably because tumor cells consume phosphate. Severe hypophosphatemia (<1 mg/dL) may result in rhabdomyolysis or hemolysis. Hypokalemia may be associated with hypophosphatemia, the reasons for which are unclear. In patients with cancer, hypophosphatemia more commonly accompanies marked nutritional deprivation or cachexia.

B. Diagnosis

1. **Laboratory studies.** Hypophosphatemia is usually recognized by routine serum electrolyte studies in patients with nutritional disturbances.

2. **Differential diagnosis of hypophosphatemia**

   a. Renal phosphate wasting accompanies certain syndromes associated with malignancies, including myeloma (Fanconi syndrome), multiple endocrine neoplasia (hyperparathyroidism), and oncogenic osteomalacia.

   b. Therapy with phosphate-binding antacids or other phosphate binders

   c. Starvation or malabsorption (decreased phosphate intake)

   d. Cachexia

   e. Alcoholism

   f. Recovery from malnutrition without adequate phosphate supplementation (refeeding syndrome)

   g. Massive, rapid tumor growth

   h. Alkalosis

   i. Treatment of diabetic ketoacidosis

   j. Use of IV bisphosphonates

   k. Use of imatinib, sunitinib, sorafenib, or temsirolimus

C. Management

1. Patients with phosphorus levels <1.5 mg/dL are given 0.25 to 0.5 mmol/kg of neutral sodium phosphate or sodium potassium phosphate administered IV over 8 to 12 hours. Intravenous phosphorous treatment carries the risk of causing hypocalcemia, calcium phosphate precipitation in the kidneys, and arrhythmia. Close monitoring of serum phosphate levels (every 6 hours) should be done, with conversion to oral supplementation once serum phosphate concentration is >1.5 mg/dL, if feasible.

2. Patients with blood phosphorus levels of >1.5 mg/dL may be given oral inorganic phosphate supplements, which come in various forms, often in combination with sodium and potassium. Care must be taken to avoid overrepletion of these elements.

3. Patients with *simultaneous hypokalemia* are treated with 20 mEq of KCl in 10% solution three times daily or with potassium-containing phosphate preparations. Neutra-Phos-K and Phos-Tabs both contain 50 to 57 mEq of potassium per gram of phosphate.

V. HYPERNATREMIA

A. Mechanisms. Hypernatremia nearly always is due to a loss of water from the body fluids. Any hypotonic fluid loss (e.g., sweating, hyperventilation, fever, vomiting, nasogastric suction) causes mild hypernatremia if not treated. Extreme elevations of plasma sodium concentrations (>160 mEq/L) are usually encountered in only three clinical situations:

1. **Decreased or absent fluid intake** is the most common cause of hypernatremia, especially in patients who have disabilities that impair normal fluid intake.

2. **Diabetes insipidus** (insufficient production of antidiuretic hormone [ADH]) is usually caused by head trauma (accidental or neurosurgical) or pituitary or hypothalamic neoplasms (primary or metastatic). Although there are other rare causes of diabetes insipidus, nearly half of the cases are idiopathic. Nephrogenic diabetes insipidus occurs when the kidney is unable to respond to normal circulating levels of ADH and may be the result of hypercalcemia, hypokalemia, or medications. Patients with even severe diabetes insipidus (either central or nephrogenic) will generally maintain normal or close to normal serum sodium levels so long as the thirst mechanism is intact, and there is free access to water.

3. **Osmotic diuresis** and often osmotic diarrhea are encountered in obtunded patients who receive a massive urea load from high-protein nasogastric tube feedings. Other high urea states include patients with increased tissue catabolism and those in recovery from azotemia. Progressive dehydration develops, and the osmotic diuresis produces an apparently normal urine output.

B. **Diagnosis**

1. **Signs and symptoms.** Most patients with severe hypernatremia are already seriously ill. The specific contribution of hypertonicity is frequently difficult to distinguish from the underlying disease.

2. **Laboratory studies**. To make a diagnosis of diabetes insipidus, a water-deprivation test is performed. Baseline body weight, serum sodium concentration, serum osmolality, and urine osmolality are measured. Water intake is completely restricted; however, these patients should *never* be deprived of water without continuous observation. Beginning in the morning, urine volume and the baseline studies are determined hourly. The test should be terminated if the patient's weight decreases by >3% or when serum osmolality exceeds 300 mOsm/kg. Pending results of direct measurement, the serum osmolality can be rapidly and accurately estimated from serum concentrations of sodium, urea nitrogen, and glucose by the following formula:

$$\text{Serum osmolality} = 2 \text{ (sodium)} + \text{BUN}/2.8 + \text{glucose}/18.$$

a. **Criterion for diagnosing diabetes insipidus.** Urine osmolality is <600 mOsm/kg when serum osmolality is >300 mOsm/kg.

b. **Differentiating pituitary diabetes insipidus.** Significant diabetes insipidus is excluded if the urine osmolality is >600 mOsm/kg after water deprivation in the absence of glycosuria or recently injected contrast media. Urine osmolality between 200 and 600 mOsm/kg suggests partial diabetes insipidus. It is necessary to distinguish pituitary (central) diabetes insipidus from nephrogenic diabetes insipidus. To do this, the kidney's response to ADH is assessed. Desmopressin, 4 mcg, is given SC at the conclusion of the water-deprivation test, and hourly urine specimens are collected for an additional 3 hours. After desmopressin injection, urine osmolality exceeds 400 mOsm/kg in patients with ADH deficiency and 800 mOsm/kg in normal persons; values are lower in patients with nephrogenic diabetes insipidus.

C. **Management**

1. **Severe hypernatremia** is life threatening and must be carefully managed. Correcting the water deficit too rapidly may precipitate fatal cerebral edema. It is important to determine, if possible, the timing of the onset of hypernatremia, as acute hypernatremia (onset <48 hours) can, and should, be more rapidly corrected than chronic hypernatremia.

a. **Acute hypernatremia** should be corrected with 5% dextrose in water with the goal to decrease serum sodium concentration by 1 to 2 mmol/L/hr to a goal concentration of 145 mmol/L. It is essential to monitor the sodium concentration closely (every 2 to 3 hours) and to adjust fluid rate accordingly. It is also important to identify the source of ongoing fluid loss, if present, and to resolve or minimize the problem, as is possible.

b. **Chronic hypernatremia** should be corrected at a much slower rate to avoid irreversible brain injury from cerebral edema as well as seizures. The goal serum sodium concentration of 145 mmol/L remains the same; however, the rate of correction should not exceed 10 mmol/L/d.

c. Hypernatremia in a patient who is also **hypovolemic** and requires plasma volume expansion must be managed very carefully. In this setting, normal saline should be used initially, with close monitoring of serum sodium concentration, until hemodynamic stability is attained, at which time fluids can be changed to 5% dextrose in water.

d. **Therapy for chronic ADH deficiency** usually involves administration of desmopressin (desamino-D-arginine vasopressin [DDAVP]), 5 to 10 μg intranasally or 1 to 2 μg by SC injection, which produces 6 to 18 hours of antidiuresis. To avoid water intoxication, the next dose is not given until thirst and polyuria redevelop. Oral desmopressin is also available for chronic therapy; doses of 0.05 to 1.2 mg/d are given.

VI. HYPONATREMIA: SYNDROME OF INAPPROPRIATE ANTIDIURETIC HORMONE (SIADH)

A. **Mechanisms**

1. **ADH** is normally released from the posterior pituitary gland in response to increased osmolality or decreased plasma volume. The release of ADH is normally inhibited by decreased plasma osmolality and increased plasma volume. The hormone acts by increasing water resorption from the renal collecting ducts.

2. **SIADH.** Unregulated production of ADH results in increased water retention by the kidney, increased total body water, and moderate expansion of plasma volume. Plasma hypotonicity fails to suppress the secretion of ADH. Hyponatremia, plasma hypo-osmolality, and inability to excrete maximally diluted urine are the consequences of SIADH.

3. **Associated tumors.** Ectopic production of ADH may occur with any malignancy but is most frequently associated with bronchogenic carcinoma, especially the small cell type, and mesothelioma.

4. **Central nervous system disease** (e.g., mass lesions, hemorrhage, infection) and pulmonary infection (e.g., pneumonia, tuberculosis, abscess) may result in excessive ADH release from the posterior pituitary.

5. **Cerebral salt wasting** may occur in patients with intracranial trauma or hemorrhage. This syndrome resembles SIADH and manifests hyponatremia and increased urinary sodium excretion. However, in contrast to SIADH, plasma volume contraction is seen with cerebral salt wasting, and BUN and serum creatinine may be high–normal or mildly decreased. Therapy is directed at salt and volume replacement.

6. **Drugs associated with hyponatremia**

   a. **Diuretics** commonly produce hyponatremia, particularly in patients with unrestricted fluid intake.

   b. **Carbamazepine and oxcarbazepine** induce ADH secretion.

   c. **Intravenous narcotics** have been associated with SIADH.

    d. Antidepressants and antipsychotics have occasionally been associated with SIADH.

    e. Vincristine and vinblastine may produce SIADH and profound hyponatremia. Manifestations develop 1 to 2 weeks after treatment.

    f. Cyclophosphamide, when given intravenously, may produce SIADH. Mild hyponatremia develops 4 to 12 hours after a dose, persists for about 20 hours, and is usually asymptomatic.

    g. Cisplatin, high-dose melphalan, and thiotepa have been associated with SIADH.

    h. Nausea, which is a common side effect of many of the above chemotherapeutic drugs, is also a potent stimulus for ADH release.

B. Diagnosis

    1. Symptoms and signs. Lethargy, nausea, anorexia, and generalized weakness are common symptoms in patients with hyponatremia. Confusion, convulsions, coma, and death may ensue if the hyponatremia is severe or rapid in onset.

    2. Laboratory studies. Laboratory results in conditions associated with hyponatremia are shown in Table 28-1. Measurements that should be obtained in patients with hyponatremia are as follows:

        a. In all patients with hyponatremia:

            (1) Serum electrolytes, creatinine, urea nitrogen, calcium, phosphate, glucose, total protein, and triglycerides

            (2) Urine sodium

        b. In patients with hyponatremia and without an elevated BUN:

            (1) Serum and urine osmolality

            (2) Chest radiograph or CT scan to look for evidence of lung cancer and brain CT or MRI to look for CNS lesions

TABLE 28-1   Hyponatremia: Differential Diagnosis and Laboratory Results

Condition	BUN	Osmolality S	Osmolality U	Urine Sodium Concentration
SIADH	D, (N)	D	I	N, I
Edematous states	D, N, I	D	I	D
Myxedema	N	D	N, I	(D), N, I
Salt-wasting states				
Mineralocorticoid deficiency	I	D	I	I
Glucocorticoid deficiency	N	D	(N), I	N, I
Diuretics	N, I	D	I	(D), N, I
Chronic renal failure	I	D	D, N, I	D, N, I
Cerebral salt wasting	N, I	D	I	N, I
GI loss with hypotonic replacement	N, I	D	D	D
Compulsive water drinking	N, D	D	D	N
Hypothalamic osmoregulatory defect	N	D	N	D, N, I
Pseudohyponatremia				
Hyperglycemia	N, I	I	D, N, I	N
Mannitol	N, I	N	D, N	D, N
Marked hyperlipidemia or paraproteinemia	N	N	N	N

BUN, blood urea nitrogen; S, serum; U, urine; SIADH, syndrome of inappropriate antidiuretic hormone; D, decreased; N, normal; I, increased; GI, gastrointestinal. Parentheses indicate slight or occasional amount.

   c. In patients with evidence of endocrine hypofunction:
   (1) Thyroid function tests
   (2) Adrenal function tests
   (3) Pituitary gland function tests, as necessary
   3. Diagnostic criteria for SIADH include *all five* of the following:
   a. Hyponatremia with a disproportionately low BUN (often (<10 mg/dL)
   b. Absence of intravascular volume contraction. Persistent urinary excretion of sodium constitutes indirect evidence of volume expansion (urine sodium concentration >30 mEq/L; fractional excretion of sodium >1).
   c. Absence of abnormal fluid retention, such as peripheral edema or ascites
   d. Normal renal, thyroid, and adrenal function
   e. Serum hypotonicity along with urine that is not maximally dilute. A normal adult should be able to dilute urine to an osmolality of 50 to 75 mOsm/kg in the presence of decreased plasma osmolality; higher values are presumptive evidence for ADH activity at the renal tubules. Urine must be less than maximally dilute but need not be hypertonic relative to serum. Urine osmolality >75 to 100 mOsm/kg (or urine specific gravity >1.003) with plasma osmolality <260 mOsm/kg is suggestive of SIADH.
C. Management. Control of the responsible cancer usually corrects the problems associated with ectopic SIADH.
   1. Severe, symptomatic hyponatremia (serum sodium <110 mEq/L, or <120 mEq/L with severe symptoms such as seizure). Comatose or seizing patients with severe hyponatremia must receive aggressive management, preferably in an intensive care unit. Urgent treatment with hypertonic (3%) saline, 100 mL bolus should be given, with repeat dose once or twice more (total of three doses) every 10 minutes for persistent neurologic symptoms. Slow infusion of hypertonic saline (10 to 30 mL/hr) may then be continued, if necessary, with close monitoring of serum sodium concentration. The goal rate of correction depends upon the acuity of the hyponatremia: an increase of 4 to 6 mmol/L in the first 6 hours is appropriate for hyponatremia of <48 hour duration, whereas chronic hyponatremia goal correction rate is 6 to 8 mmol/L in the first 24 hours.
   2. Moderately severe hyponatremia (serum sodium >110 mEq/L, mild symptoms such as lethargy without seizure or coma).
      a. Fluid restriction is of paramount importance in treatment of all patients with SIADH and should result in correction of hyponatremia within 3 to 5 days. Patients with serum sodium levels <125 mEq/L should be restricted to 500 to 700 mL/d. Patients with higher serum sodium levels can be restricted to 1,000 mL/d.
      b. Salt tablets, 3 g three times daily, are used to increase serum sodium concentration. This effect may be enhanced with the coadministration of a loop diuretic to increase water excretion.
      c. Vasopressin receptor antagonists (conivaptan, tolvaptan) are effective at inducing free water diuresis and raising serum sodium level in SIADH. High cost and potential for significant liver toxicity are factors that limit widespread and prolonged use of these agents.
      d. Demeclocycline 300 to 600 mg PO twice daily induces renal resistance to ADH and facilitates free water excretion. Although its effects are variable, the drug may be useful in patients who cannot tolerate chronic fluid restriction or who have insufficient improvement of hyponatremia with fluid restriction. The drug is nephrotoxic and has the potential to cause nausea and vomiting.

VII. HYPERKALEMIA

A. Mechanisms

1. Hyperkalemia in patients with or without cancer often develops as a consequence of renal failure.

2. Hyperkalemia may result from rapid tumor lysis after therapy.

3. Mineralocorticoid deficiency results in hyperkalemia.

4. Pseudohyperkalemia occurs in patients with persistent leukocytosis or thrombocytosis, especially in the myeloproliferative disorders.

5. Drugs associated with hyperkalemia:

   a. Potassium-sparing diuretics (spironolactone, eplerenone, amiloride, triamterene)

   b. Calcineurin inhibitors (cyclosporine, tacrolimus)

   c. Nonselective beta-blockers (propranolol, labetalol)

   d. Angiotensin-converting enzyme inhibitors and angiotensin receptor blockers

   e. Octreotide

   f. Diazoxide

   g. Minoxidil

B. Diagnosis

1. **Symptoms** mostly consist of weakness and other neuromuscular complaints.

2. **Laboratory studies**

   a. Serum potassium concentration

   b. The severity of the ECG abnormalities corresponds to the severity of hyperkalemia; as hyperkalemia gets worse, the ECG may show increased T-wave amplitude, decreased R-wave amplitude, and increased S-wave depth; prolongation of PR intervals and widening of the QRS complex; and then a sine wave pattern, eventuating in asystole or ventricular tachyarrhythmias.

3. **Differential diagnosis:** renal insufficiency, excessive potassium intake, especially with renal insufficiency, effect of drugs, adrenal insufficiency, acidosis, cell destruction (e.g., tumor lysis, rhabdomyolysis)

C. Management

1. In patients with significant ECG abnormalities, IV calcium gluconate (10 mL of 10% solution) is to be given to antagonize the effect of hyperkalemia on cardiac cell membranes. These patients must also be placed on continuous cardiac monitoring.

2. Immediate lowering of the potassium is achieved by IV administration of 10 units of regular insulin plus 50 to 100 mL of 50% dextrose solution. If the serum glucose is >250 mg/dL, insulin may be given without dextrose.

3. Beta-adrenergic agonists also shift potassium from serum into cells. Albuterol can be given by nebulizer in doses of 10 to 20 mg (these doses are much larger than those used for treating asthma). There is an additive effect when given with insulin.

4. Removal of potassium from the body can be achieved with cation exchange resins like Kayexalate, 15 to 30 g every 6 hours. Kayexalate should not be given to patients with ileus or other obstructive bowel disease.

5. If renal function is adequate and the patient is not dehydrated, a loop diuretic, such as furosemide 40 to 80 mg, may be given intravenously to increase urinary potassium excretion.

6. Hemodialysis is necessary for management of chronic or refractory hyperkalemia.

7. Hyperkalemia due to adrenal insufficiency may be corrected with the synthetic mineralocorticoid, fludrocortisone, 0.05 to 0.20 mg/d.

VIII. HYPOKALEMIA

A. Ectopic Secretion of ACTH

1. **Mechanism.** A variety of tumors, especially small cell lung cancer, malignant thymoma, pancreatic cancer, islet cell tumors, and bronchial carcinoids, may ectopically synthesize ACTH and produce Cushing syndrome. Hypokalemia may occur in Cushing syndrome due to any cause, but it is particularly common (>50%) in patients with Cushing syndrome due to ectopic ACTH secretion.

2. **Diagnosis**
   a. **Symptoms and signs.** The most common malignant causes of ectopic ACTH syndrome are rapidly fatal. The typical features of adrenal or pituitary Cushing syndrome are often absent. Presenting signs usually are cachexia, weakness, and hypertension. Slower-growing cancers and benign tumors give rise to the characteristic rounded facies, truncal obesity, purple striae in skin stretch areas, and overt diabetes mellitus.
   b. **Laboratory studies**
      (1) Cancer patients who complain of weakness should have serum electrolytes measured. Hypokalemia and metabolic alkalosis may be severe (serum potassium as low as 1 mEq/L, bicarbonate >30 mEq/L) in patients with ectopic ACTH syndrome.
      (2) The diagnosis of ectopic ACTH syndrome may be quickly made by demonstrating the failure of high-dose dexamethasone to suppress ACTH levels in most cases (see Chapter 16, Section V.C.2).

3. **Management of ectopic ACTH syndrome.** Control of the underlying tumor is the most effective method. Hypokalemia is often difficult to correct. Potassium replacement consists of PO or IV doses of 80 to 150 mEq/d. Severe symptoms may occasionally improve with the use of adrenal suppressant medications, such as various combinations of mitotane, metyrapone, ketoconazole, and aminoglutethimide. The toxicity of these drugs may be worse than the symptoms from the underlying disease. Spironolactone, 100 to 400 mg daily, may be useful. Adrenalectomy is a consideration in the rare patient with an indolent, unresectable tumor that causes the ectopic ACTH syndrome.

B. Other Causes of Hypokalemia

1. Gastrointestinal losses associated with alkalosis (vomiting, prolonged nasogastric suctioning, colonic neoplasms [villous adenoma], chronic laxative abuse)
2. Gastrointestinal losses associated with acidosis (chronic diarrhea, ureterosigmoidostomy, Zollinger-Ellison syndrome)
3. Hyperaldosteronism
4. Non–ACTH-dependent hypercortisolism
5. Licorice ingestion
6. Renal tubular acidosis
7. Hypercalcemia, hypomagnesemia
8. Hypophosphatemia in anabolic states (e.g., rapid tumor growth)
9. Respiratory therapy resulting in alkalosis in patients with chronic carbon dioxide retention
10. Drugs associated with hypokalemia:
    a. Potassium-wasting diuretics (loop, thiazide, carbonic anhydrase inhibitors)
    b. Amphotericin B
    c. Beta-agonists

    d. Corticosteroids
    e. Ephedrine and pseudoephedrine
    f. Cisplatin

IX. HYPERURICEMIA

A. Mechanisms. Hyperuricemia and hyperuricosuria pose a major problem for patients with myeloproliferative disorders, lymphomas, myeloma, or leukemias, but usually not for patients with solid tumors.

    1. Hyperuricosuria. Urinary uric acid excretion is increased in untreated patients who have myeloproliferative disorders, acute or chronic myelocytic leukemia, or acute lymphoblastic leukemia. Patients with lymphoma have normal or slightly increased uric acid excretion. During treatment with either cytotoxic agents or radiation, massive tumor lysis releases nucleic acids and results in excess production of uric acid, especially in patients with lymphoma or leukemia.

    2. Uric acid nephropathy results from the precipitation of uric acid crystals in the concentrated, acidic urine of the renal medulla, distal tubules, and collecting ducts. The resultant sludge leads to intrarenal obstructive nephropathy and distinct inflammatory interstitial changes.

    3. Xanthine stones, resulting from the inhibition of xanthine oxidase by allopurinol in the setting of purine hypermetabolism, rarely complicate malignancies.

    4. Oxypurinol stones have rarely developed after therapy with massive doses of allopurinol.

B. Diagnosis is established by measurement of serum and urine uric acid concentrations. The normal excretory rate for uric acid is 300 to 500 mg/d.

C. Management (see Chapter 32)

X. HYPOURICEMIA

A. Mechanisms. Hypouricemia is usually caused by defects in proximal renal tubular reabsorption of uric acid. It also occurs in severe liver disease due to loss of xanthine oxidase activity. Hypouricemia has also been reported to be associated with a variety of tumors, especially Hodgkin lymphoma and myeloma.

B. Diagnosis

    1. Symptoms. Patients do not generally have symptoms.

    2. Laboratory studies. Blood uric acid levels identify the abnormality; a concentration of <2 mg/dL is considered definitive of hypouricemia.

    3. Differential diagnosis

        a. Volume expansion of extracellular fluid in patients receiving high-volume intravenous fluids

        b. Proximal renal tubular disease: Fanconi syndrome (myeloma is a common cause in adults), Wilson disease, isolated defect in otherwise healthy patients

        c. Uricosuric agents: salicylates, radiographic contrast agents, atorvastatin, losartan, captopril, and enalapril, probenecid, fenofibrate, calcium channel blockers

        d. Treatment with xanthine oxidase inhibitors (allopurinol, febuxostat) or urate oxidase (rasburicase)

        e. Hereditary xanthinuria

        f. Neoplastic diseases, especially Hodgkin lymphoma

        g. Liver disease

        h. SIADH

        i. Total parental nutrition

C. **Complications**

1. **Acute kidney injury** has been reported in patients with mostly familial renal hypouricemia, following exercise.

2. **Uric acid** nephrolithiasis is reported at higher rates in patients with renal hypouricemia.

XI. HYPERGLYCEMIA

A. **Mechanisms**

1. **Diabetic glucose tolerance curves** with relative insulin deficiency are present in many patients with cancer, particularly those with poor nutrition or cachexia. Nutritional replenishment appears to improve these abnormalities.

2. **Tumors** that produce hormone, such as glucagonoma, somatostatinoma, pheochromocytoma, and ACTH-producing tumors with resulting hypercortisolism, cause hyperglycemia.

3. **Drugs**

   a. **Glucocorticoids.** Use of dexamethasone or other glucocorticoids as an antiemetic or as part of a chemotherapy regimen often causes hyperglycemia.

   b. Inhibitors of the PI3K/AKT/mTOR pathway, such as everolimus and temsirolimus, produce insulin resistance, with resulting hyperglycemia in 13% to 50% of patients taking these agents.

   c. Androgen deprivation therapy in prostate cancer increases insulin resistance.

4. **Pancreatic destruction** by carcinoma may also cause diabetes.

5. **Nonketotic hyperosmolar coma** can be a complication of treatment with cyclophosphamide, vincristine, asparaginase, or prednisone in patients with even mild diabetes mellitus.

B. **Diagnosis.** Random or 2-hour postprandial blood glucose determinations disclose the abnormality in most patients.

C. **Management**

1. **Nutritional** status should be improved in cancer patients with glucose intolerance, if feasible. Management of substantial hyperglycemia on account of tumor is effected by control of the neoplasm and by administration of insulin or oral hypoglycemics as needed.

2. **Hyperosmolar coma** must be vigorously treated with fluid replacement of volume losses with IV saline until the blood pressure is stable. Insulin infusion (1 to 4 units/h) usually controls the hyperglycemia.

3. **Avoidance of glucocorticoids** will prevent steroid-induced hyperglycemia.

XII. HYPOGLYCEMIA

A. **Mechanisms.** Insulin-like substances (most often proinsulin-like growth factor-2 [pro-IGF-2]) may be produced by some tumors, especially large, often retroperitoneal sarcomas, and occasionally other cancers. Hepatocellular carcinomas and extensive liver metastases from a variety of primary sites may deplete glycogen stores and impair gluconeogenesis. Insulinoma is discussed in Chapter 16, Section VI.C.

1. **Etiologies of hypoglycemia**

   a. **Malignant tumors**

      (1) Insulinoma

      (2) Large retroperitoneal tumor producing pro-IGF-2

      (3) Hepatocellular carcinoma

      (4) Extensive hepatic metastasis

b. Drugs

(1) Surreptitious or therapeutic insulin administration

(2) Oral hypoglycemic agents

(3) Alcohol

(4) Salicylates

(5) Pentamidine

(6) Jamaican vomiting sickness (ackee fruit)

(7) Quinine (in antimalarial doses)

c. Metabolic disorders

(1) Starvation

(2) Chronic hepatic or renal failure

(3) Hypoadrenalism

(4) Hypopituitarism

(5) Myxedema

(6) Glycogen storage diseases

(7) Reactive hypoglycemias (e.g., postgastrectomy or bariatric surgery)

(8) Sepsis

2. Pseudohypoglycemia. Falsely low glucose levels may occur in patients with marked granulocytosis, especially patients with myeloproliferative disorders, because of *in vitro* consumption of glucose.

B. Diagnosis

1. Symptoms and signs. Hypoglycemia produces mental status change, fatigue, convulsions, or coma. Some patients show features of fasting hypoglycemia, such as an altered morning personality that improves after breakfast. Tremors, sweating, tachycardia, and hunger pangs are suggestive of an acute decrease in blood sugar level.

2. Laboratory studies. A blood glucose concentration of <55 mg/dL establishes the presence of hypoglycemia. Patients who are thought to surreptitiously abuse insulin should have C-peptide and insulin serum levels measured during a hypoglycemic episode. Absent C-peptide with elevated insulin level suggests the diagnosis of exogenous insulin administration.

C. Management

1. Intravenous glucose. Any patient with unexplained hypoglycemia should have a blood sample drawn for glucose, insulin, and C-peptide determination, followed immediately by rapid IV infusion of 50 mL of 50% dextrose solution. Serum glucose may remain low even while concentrated glucose solutions are being administered. All patients with glucose levels of <40 mg/dL and symptomatic patients with glucose levels of <60 mg/dL should be treated by continuous infusion of 10% glucose at 50 to 150 mL/h; rates are adjusted to maintain glucose levels higher than 60 mg/dL. Blood glucose levels are measured every 3 to 4 hours until stabilization occurs.

2. Glucagon, 1 mg IM or IV, raises blood glucose by promoting glycogenolysis and gluconeogenesis. Long-term glucagon therapy has been given by infusion pump.

3. Octreotide, a somatostatin analog, can decrease insulin hypersecretion and has occasionally normalized serum glucose in patients with pro-IGF-2–secreting tumors but may sometimes worsen or provoke hypoglycemia by inhibiting glucagon and growth hormone secretion.

4. Other measures. If the blood glucose cannot be increased to safe levels with glucose infusions, prednisone or diazoxide should be administered.

ACKNOWLEDGMENT
The author would like to acknowledge Dr. Harold E. Carlson, who significantly contributed to earlier versions of this chapter.

Suggested Readings

Abu-Alfa AK, Younes A. Tumor lysis syndrome and acute kidney injury: evaluation, prevention and management. *Am J Kidney Dis* 2010;55(suppl. 3):S1.

Ariaans G, de Jong S, Gietema JA, et al. Cancer-drug induced insulin resistance: innocent bystander or unusual suspect. *Cancer Treat Rev* 2015;41:376.

Cooper MS, Gittoes NJL. Diagnosis and management of hypocalcaemia. *BMJ* 2008;336:1298.

Cryer PE, Axelrod L, Grossman AB, et al. Evaluation and management of adult hypoglycemic disorders: an Endocrine Society clinical practice guideline. *J Clin Endocrinol Metab* 2009;94:709.

Ellison DH, Berl T. The syndrome of inappropriate antidiuresis. *N Engl J Med* 2007;356:2064.

Gaasbeck A, Meinders AE. Hypophosphatemia: an update on its etiology and treatment. *Am J Med* 2005;118:1094.

Marinella MA. Refeeding syndrome in cancer patients. *Int J Clin Pract* 2008;62:460.

Reagan P, Pani A, Rosner MH. Approach to diagnosis and treatment of hypercalcemia in a patient with malignancy. *Am J Kidney Dis* 2014;63(1):141.

Ruggiero SL, Mehrotra B. Bisphosphonate-related osteonecrosis of the jaw: diagnosis, prevention and management. *Annu Rev Med* 2009;60:85.

Santarpia L, Koch CA, Sarlis NJ. Hypercalcemia in cancer patients: pathobiology and management. *Horm Metab Res* 2010;42:153.

Sood MM, Sood AR, Richardson R. Emergency management and commonly encountered outpatient scenarios in patients with hyperkalemia. *Mayo Clin Proc* 2007;82:1553.

Sterns RH. Disorders of plasma sodium – causes, consequences, and correction. *N Engl J Med* 2015;1372(1):55.

Tisdall M, Crocker M, Watkiss J, et al. Disturbances of sodium in critically ill adult neurologic patients. *J Neurosurg Anesthesiol* 2006;18:57.

Vaidya C, Ho W, Freda BJ. Management of hyponatremia: providing treatment and avoiding harm. *Cleve Clin J Med* 2010;77:715.

Wagner J, Arora S. Oncologic Metabolic Emergencies. *Emerg Med Clin North Am* 2014;32:509.

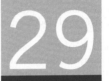

29 Cutaneous Complications

Bartosz Chmielowski and Richard F. Wagner Jr

I. METASTASES TO THE SKIN

A. **Incidence and pathology.** Skin is not an uncommon metastatic site of solid tumors. Of patients with metastatic disease, 2% to 10% develop skin metastases. In men, the most common internal malignancies leading to cutaneous metastases are lung cancer (24%), colon cancer (19%), melanoma (13%), squamous cell carcinoma of the oral cavity (12%), and renal cell carcinoma (6%). In women, these are breast cancer (69%), colon cancer (9%), melanoma (5%), lung cancer (4%), and ovarian cancer (4%). Cutaneous involvement by cancer can occur both as a metastatic process and as a direct extension of the tumor to the skin.

B. **Natural history.** Metastases to the skin may be delayed 10 to 15 years after the initial surgical treatment of primary melanoma, breast carcinoma, and renal cancer or may be the first indication of an internal malignancy. The mechanisms of spread include hematogenous and lymphatic spread, direct contiguous tissue invasion, and iatrogenic implantation.

1. **Breast cancer** represents almost 75% of female patients with cutaneous metastases. It shows eight distinct clinicopathologic types of cutaneous involvement:

   a. Inflammatory (erysipelas—resembling erythematous patch or plaque with active border, usually affecting the breast; but other skin sites can also be involved)

   b. En cuirasse (a diffuse morphea-like induration)

   c. Telangiectatic (papules with violaceous hue caused by accumulation of blood in vascular channels)

   d. Nodular (usually multiple firm papulonodules, sometimes ulcerated)

   e. Alopecia neoplastica (painless, well-demarcated, pinkish oval plaques of alopecia caused by hematogenous spread of breast carcinoma), which can occur with other neoplasms as well

   f. Paget disease (a sharply demarcated, scaling plaque on the nipple or areola representing cutaneous infiltration of cancer)

   g. Breast carcinoma of the inframammary crease (a cutaneous nodule that may resemble basal cell carcinoma)

   h. Histiocytoid nodule of the eyelid (presents as a painless eyelid swelling with induration)

2. **Lung cancer.** Cutaneous metastases from lung cancer may appear on any surface, but they are most common on the chest wall and the posterior abdomen; small cell lung cancer metastasizes most frequently to the skin of the back. Between 1.5% and 16% of patients with lung cancer develop skin metastases; in half of these patients, it is a presenting sign of the disease. Lung cancer also has a rare but peculiar tendency to metastasize to the anal area, fingertips, or toes.

3. **Gastrointestinal (GI) tract cancers.** Skin metastases from colon cancer and rectal cancer usually develop after malignancy has been recognized. Abdominal wall and the perineal area are the most common sites.

4. **Melanoma.** Both cutaneous and extracutaneous melanoma can produce skin metastasis. They usually present as multiple pigmented nodules, but they can also be erythematous or apigmented.

5. **Urologic malignancies.** Of all urologic malignancies, renal cell carcinoma metastasizes to the skin most frequently, but skin metastases from bladder, prostate, and testicular cancer have also been reported. These metastases are frequently the first sign of renal cell carcinoma, and they can appear very late, up to 10 years after diagnosis.

6. **Subungual metastases.** Malignant lesions in the nail unit can be classified into three groups: metastatic lesions from a distant primary, cutaneous involvement of a hematopoietic or lymphoproliferative malignancy, and primary cancer at this location. Lung cancer is the most common type of malignancy that can metastasize to the nail bed, followed by genitourinary, breast, and head and neck cancers and sarcomas. Subungual metastases typically present as erythematous enlargement, swelling of the distal digit, or a violaceous nodule. They are frequently painful, but they can also bleed or be hot, pulsatile, and fluctuant. These lesions can be mistaken for infection or trauma; in almost half of affected persons, they are a presenting sign of malignancy.

7. **Umbilical metastasis** (Sister Mary Joseph nodule) is encountered in 1% to 3% of patients with abdominopelvic malignancy. The term Sister Mary Joseph nodule was assigned to the Mayo brothers' surgical nurse who recognized that umbilical metastasis denoted incurable disease when the patient underwent laparotomy. The most common origins are GI (52%), gynecologic (28%), stomach (23%), and ovarian (16%) cancer.

C. **Prognosis.** Skin metastases usually indicate advanced disease and prognosis depends on the success of treatment of the primary malignancy.

D. **Diagnosis** is based on biopsy results.

E. **Management.** Most skin metastases are treated symptomatically, and they tend to regress when the primary tumor responds to systemic therapy. Occasionally, these lesions require treatment with local radiation therapy (RT), surgery, cryotherapy, or photodynamic therapy.

II. CUTANEOUS PARANEOPLASTIC SYNDROMES

Cutaneous paraneoplastic syndromes comprise a heterogeneous group of dermatologic syndromes describing skin lesions that do not contain malignant cells, but they appear in the presence of underlying malignancy.

A. **Acanthosis nigricans** is characterized by hyperpigmented, velvety plaques on the neck, in the axilla, groin, and antecubital fossa. In most cases, it reflects metabolic disturbances seen in patients with obesity, metabolic syndrome, or diabetes. If the lesions appear abruptly and progress rapidly, or they are associated with tripe palms or mucous membrane involvement, they can reflect underlying malignancy, mainly adenocarcinoma of the GI tract (in >50% of cases, gastric cancer). **Benign causes** of acanthosis nigricans are more common than are malignant.

B. **Amyloidosis** (primary systemic) secondary to nonmalignant disease rarely involves skin. Patients with multiple myeloma or, less commonly, Waldenström macroglobulinemia may develop "pinch purpura" (ecchymoses or purpuric patches occurring spontaneously or with minor trauma). The lesions are primarily in flexural areas, paranasal skin, anogenital regions, the neck, and around the eyes.

C. **Bazex syndrome** (acrokeratosis paraneoplastica) consists of psoriasiform lesions in the acral areas (ears, nose, nails, hands, feet, elbows, knees). In 18% of cases, lesions can be pruritic. This syndrome is universally associated with malignancy, mainly carcinoma of the upper aerodigestive tract, but also prostate carcinoma, hepatocellular carcinoma, lymphoma, and bladder carcinoma. In nearly two-thirds of cases, cutaneous lesions precede the diagnosis of malignancy.

D. **Dermatomyositis** and polymyositis belong to a group of idiopathic inflammatory myopathies. Between 15% and 25% of cases of dermatomyositis and about 10% of polymyositis are associated with malignancy. Almost any type of malignancy has been reported in patients with dermatomyositis, but ovarian carcinoma and lung and breast cancer are the most common. Dermatomyositis may precede development of the neoplasm for up to 5 years. Treatment of the malignancy results in symptom improvement, and worsening of symptoms may herald tumor recurrence.

These myopathies are typified by proximal muscle weakness with or without tenderness. Patients typically report that they are not able to brush their hair. Flat-topped erythematous papules over the phalangeal joints (Gottron papules) and pinkish-purple discoloration around the eyes (a heliotrope rash) are pathognomic signs of dermatomyositis. Other signs include periungual telangiectasias; patchy discoloration of the skin; red, scaly scalp rash; and photosensitivity. Laboratory work commonly reveals elevated creatinine kinase level, although the cases with normal level of creatinine kinase have been reported, and possibly they are more frequently associated with malignancy.

E. **Ectopic Cushing syndrome** is caused by the secretion of an adrenocorticotrophic hormone (ACTH) prohormone or ACTH, most commonly by small cell lung carcinoma and bronchial carcinoids, and occasionally by thymoma, islet cell tumor, non–small cell lung carcinoma, and pheochromocytoma. It presents as proximal muscle wasting, hypertension, hypokalemia, usually weight loss (not weight gain), and frequently with hyperpigmentation.

F. **Erythema gyratum repens** is characterized by an extensive eruption of erythematous, scaly, rapidly progressing, ring-forming, wood-grain–resembling lesions over most of the body, sparing the hands, feet, and face. It is frequently accompanied by severe pruritus. It is almost always a representation of underlying malignancy, and it precedes the detection of malignancy by 1 to 24 months. Lung cancer is most commonly reported, followed by esophageal and breast cancer.

G. **Exfoliative erythroderma syndrome** is a generalized erythema of the skin accompanied by a variable degree of scaling. It is frequently accompanied by severe pruritus and generalized lymphadenopathy. Malignancy accounts for 5% to 12% of cases, and it is most frequently associated with cutaneous T-cell lymphoma, rarely with solid tumors or acute myelogenous leukemia.

H. **Hypertrichosis lanuginosa acquisita** ("malignant down") refers to the development of fine, unpigmented hair predominantly localized to the head and neck. It has been associated with lung and colon cancer, but it can also occur in conjunction with shock, thyrotoxicosis, porphyria, and cyclosporine, minoxidil, phenytoin, and penicillin ingestion. Treatment should be directed toward the removal of malignancy.

I. **Ichthyosis.** Acquired ichthyosis is manifested by symmetric scaling ranging in severity from minor roughness and dryness to dramatic desquamation of white-to-brown scales. The diameter of the scales can range from <1 mm to >1 cm. It primarily affects the trunk and limbs. The lesions are usually more accentuated on extensor surfaces. It should be differentiated from the late-onset ichthyosis vulgaris, xerosis, and Refsum disease. Hodgkin lymphoma is the most common malignancy associated with acquired ichthyosis, but it can also occur in patients with a cutaneous T-cell lymphoma or carcinomas of the breast, lung, or bladder. It may be also a result of nonmalignant disease (e.g., autoimmune syndromes, endocrinologic disorders, nutritional abnormalities, infectious diseases, and finally a drug reaction).

J. **Multicentric reticulohistiocytosis** is characterized by pink, brown, gray papules appearing initially on the hands and then spreading to the face. The lesions can be also present on the knees, elbows, ankles, shoulders, feet, or hips, and they may have pathognomic coral-bead appearance. Approximately 20% to 25% of multicentric reticulohistiocytosis cases are associated with malignancy, including hematologic, breast, ovarian, gastric, and cervical neoplasms.

K. **Necrolytic migratory erythema (NME)** is an uncommon inflammatory dermatosis usually associated with *glucagonoma* and rarely with benign conditions, such as liver disease, inflammatory bowel disease, pancreatitis, and malabsorption disorders. The clinical features of NME include transient eruptions of irregular erythematous lesions in which a central bulla develops, subsequently erodes, and heals with hyperpigmentation. The lesions follow a periorificial distribution, or they are located in the areas subject to greater pressure and friction (i.e., the perineum, buttocks, groin, lower abdomen, and lower extremities).

L. **Necrotizing leukocytoclastic vasculitis** is a rare representation of malignancy. It appears as a palpable purpura, typically in dependent areas. This vasculitis is more common with hematologic malignancies than with solid tumors. Occasionally, it can also be a complication of antineoplastic therapy.

M. **Pachydermoperiostosis** exhibits thickening of skin and creation of new skin folds (leonine facies). The scalp, forehead, lids, ears, and lips are the typical sites. The tongue, thenar and hypothenar eminences, elbows, and knees may be enlarged. The fingers are clubbed. Biopsy shows thickening of the horny layer and hypertrophy of the sweat and sebaceous glands. The familial form of pachydermoperiostosis is not usually associated with malignant tumors.

N. **Paget disease.** *Extramammary* Paget disease is a nonhealing neoplasm occurring in the apocrine gland–bearing areas, mainly axilla and the perineum. It can be associated with either contiguous or a distant cancer. Surgical excision is the primary treatment for the skin lesions. It can also respond to topical 5-fluorouracil or imiquimod.

O. **Palmoplantar hyperkeratosis** is characterized by yellowish, symmetric thickening of palms and soles. It occurs in hereditary and nonhereditary forms. Acquired form can be associated with Hodgkin lymphoma, leukemia, breast cancer, and gastric cancer. Familial forms are strongly associated with squamous cell carcinoma of the esophagus, breast, and ovarian carcinoma. In familial forms, the development of malignancy is delayed >30 years after the appearance of hyperkeratosis. Arsenic exposure can predispose to punctuate palmar hyperkeratosis and higher cancer risk.

P. **Papillomatosis.** Florid cutaneous papillomatosis describes the sudden appearance of multiple acuminate *keratotic papules* that morphologically resemble viral warts. They initially develop on hands and wrists and later spread on the entire body and the face. This syndrome always reflects underlying malignancy, most commonly gastric adenocarcinoma.

Q. **Pemphigus.** Paraneoplastic pemphigus is a rare autoimmune bullous mucocutaneous disorder that presents typically with painful mucosal erosive lesions and pruritic papulosquamous eruptions that often progress to blisters. Immunofluorescence testing reveals IgG autoantibodies and C3 deposited intercellularly in the epidermis and in a linear fashion along the dermal–epidermal junction. The most common underlying neoplasms include non-Hodgkin lymphoma, chronic lymphocytic leukemia, and Castleman disease.

R. **Pityriasis rotunda** manifests as round, scaly hyperpigmented lesions on the trunk, buttocks, and thighs. It is very rarely diagnosed in whites. In 6% of cases, it develops in patients with malignancies, mainly hepatocellular carcinoma and gastric carcinoma.

S. **Pruritus.** Refractory pruritus, in patients without liver disease, can be associated with iron deficiency, thyroid disorders, renal insufficiency, and also with malignancy, most commonly lymphoma, myeloproliferative disorders, multiple myeloma, leukemia, and carcinoids.

T. **Pyoderma gangrenosum** is an idiopathic *neutrophilic dermatosis*. It presents classically as tender, fluctuant pustules or nodules, which expand peripherally to form ulcers with sharp, raised edges. Of cases, 50% to 70% are associated with underlying systemic disease, including ulcerative colitis, Crohn disease, diverticulitis, hematologic and rheumatologic conditions, hepatopathies, visceral carcinomas, and immunodeficiency states. The associated hematologic disorders include acute lymphoid and myeloid leukemia, myeloproliferative diseases, myeloma, Waldenström macroglobulinemia, and Hodgkin and non-Hodgkin lymphomas. It has been also reported in patients with colon, bladder, prostate, breast, bronchus, ovary, and adrenocortical carcinoma.

U. **Sweet syndrome** (acute febrile neutrophilic dermatosis) presents as an acute eruption of tender, erythematous plaques or nodules with irregular surfaces. The lesions can occur anywhere on the body but are most common on the face and the trunk. Histologic examination reveals dense neutrophilic infiltration. The rash is usually accompanied by fever, peripheral blood neutrophilia, arthritis, and conjunctivitis. Approximately 10% of patients have underlying malignancy, and acute myelogenous leukemia has been reported most frequently. Therapy with prednisone appears to be most effective.

V. **The sign of Leser-Trélat** is ominous of internal malignancy, and it is described as the sudden eruption of multiple pruritic seborrheic keratoses. These lesions have, frequently, an inflammatory base. The sign of Leser-Trélat has to be differentiated from the presence of multiple benign seborrheic keratoses. The predominant types of malignancy are GI adenocarcinomas, lymphoproliferative disorders, and cancers of the lung or breast.

W. **Urticaria pigmentosa** is a presenting feature in 55% to 100% of patients with systemic mastocytosis. The primary lesion is a hyperpigmented macule or papule that transforms into a wheal when irritated mechanically (Darier sign). In some cases, lesions can be pigmentless, telangiectatic, and nodular.

X. **Vitiligo** is the hypopigmentation of skin caused by the loss of melanocytes, and it frequently occurs in individuals with malignant melanoma. Vitiligo is the consequence of the immune-mediated response against antigens shared by normal melanocytes and melanoma cells. The appearance of vitiligo in patients with melanoma is associated with better prognosis. It is a common side effect of successful immunotherapy in patients with melanoma.

Y. **Miscellaneous cutaneous paraneoplastic disorders**

1. **Alopecia mucinosa** can develop during the course of lymphoreticular neoplasms as a consequence of mucinous degeneration of collagen around hair follicles and sebaceous glands. The resultant alopecia is unrelated to therapy.

2. **Circinate erythemas.** Erythema figuratum perstans is a circular elevation of the skin that remains stable for weeks to months. Erythema annulare centrifugum initially is a small erythematous area that slowly enlarges, leaving a central circle of normal-appearing skin. Lesions may be pruritic.

Circinate erythemas are associated most commonly with nonmalignant diseases (especially collagen vascular syndromes, angiitides, and infections). Many cases are idiopathic. Less commonly, they are associated tumors that include lymphoma and, occasionally, visceral cancer.

3. **Erythromelalgia** presents as painful, warm extremities (particularly the digits) that appear erythematous. Myeloproliferative diseases are the most common associated malignancies. Aspirin provides relief.

4. **Pigmentation of the skin.** Gray discoloration of the skin because of melanosis may develop in patients with extensive malignant melanoma. Periorbital purplish discoloration can develop in patients who have amyloid deposition in the eyelids from infiltration and purpura. The syndrome of postproctoscopic palpebral purpura is well described in these patients.

5. **Porphyria cutanea tarda** (PCT) is a blistering disease that appears in skin exposed to sunlight. Hepatocellular carcinoma and metastatic liver tumors are occasionally associated with paraneoplastic PCT.

6. **Tripe palms** resemble bovine foregut and appear as thickened palmar skin with exaggerated dermatoglyphics. More than 90% of patients with tripe palms have associated malignancy, most frequently of the lung, stomach, and genitourinary tract.

III. INHERITED MALIGNANCY-ASSOCIATED SYNDROMES

Several genetic syndromes involving the skin predispose to internal malignancy without having a paraneoplastic association.

A. **Ataxia telangiectasia** is an autosomal-recessive disorder caused by mutations in the *ATM* gene, which has a crucial role in the cellular response to DNA damage. The syndrome is characterized by progressive neurodegeneration, ocular and cutaneous telangiectasias, immunodeficiency, and premature aging. These individuals are at high risk for development of hematologic malignancies, including Hodgkin and non-Hodgkin lymphoma and leukemia.

B. **Basal cell nevus syndrome** (Gorlin syndrome) (see Chapter 17).

C. **Cowden disease** (multiple hamartoma–neoplasia syndrome) is an autosomal-dominant genodermatosis with incomplete penetrance characterized by multiple trichilemmomas (adnexal tumors), mucocutaneous papules, and high risk for malignancy. It is caused by an inactivation of PTEN (phosphatase and tensin homolog deleted on chromosome 10), a dual-phosphatase tumor suppressor gene. Patients with loss of wild-type PTEN expression from one allele carry an increased risk of malignant breast, thyroid, endometrial, and brain tumors.

D. **Cronkhite-Canada syndrome** is a rare, acquired, nonfamilial GI polyposis syndrome associated with protein-losing gastroenteropathy, alopecia, nail dystrophy, and hyperpigmentation. Patients are at high risk for the development of gastric, colon, and rectal carcinomas.

E. **Gardner syndrome** is a variant of familial adenomatous polyposis (FAP) with extracolonic symptoms; it is caused by mutations in the tumor suppressor gene adenomatous polyposis coli (APC). It is an autosomal-dominant disease characterized by the presence of colonic polyposis, osteomas, and mesenchymal tumors of the skin and soft tissues. In most patients, cutaneous and bone abnormalities develop approximately 10 years before polyposis. The most common skin manifestations of Gardner syndrome are epidermoid or sebaceous cysts (66%), which are found on the face, scalp, and extremities. Other skin manifestations are fibromas, neurofibromas, lipomas, leiomyomas, and pigmented skin lesions. The patients are at high risk for development of colon cancer and desmoid tumors.

F. **Howel-Evans syndrome** is a rare familial syndrome that links focal nonepidermolytic palmoplantar keratoderma (tylosis) with the early onset of esophageal squamous cell carcinoma. The locus has been located on chromosome 17q25 (*TOC* gene).

G. **Muir-Torre syndrome** is a rare genodermatosis associated with mutations in mismatch repair proteins, hMSH-2 and hMLH-1. It is most often diagnosed by the synchronous or metachronous occurrence of at least one sebaceous gland neoplasm and at least one internal malignancy. The syndrome is characterized by an autosomal-dominant inheritance pattern with variable penetrance and expression. The visceral malignancies include colorectal carcinoma or carcinoma of the urogenital system.

H. **Peutz-Jeghers syndrome** is an autosomal dominant disorder caused by germline mutations or epigenetic silencing of the serine/threonine kinase LKB1 (also known as STK11). It is characterized by skin and mucosal hyperpigmentation (perioral blue-black freckling) and development of multiple intestinal polyps that can transform into GI adenocarcinoma.

I. **Von Recklinghausen disease (neurofibromatosis type 1)** is inherited as an autosomal-dominant condition caused by mutations in the tumor suppressor gene *NF1*. About one-half of affected individuals inherit the gene from an affected parent with the remainder of cases caused by spontaneous mutation. Hyperpigmented, oval-shaped macules with smooth borders (café au lait spots) are seen in the early childhood. Other skin lesions include freckling in non–sun-exposed areas, iris hamartomas, and cutaneous neurofibromas. Individuals with von Recklinghausen disease have an increased risk of malignancy compared with the general population. A 10% lifetime risk exists of malignant peripheral nerve sheath tumors. Other malignancies (pheochromocytoma, urogenital rhabdomyosarcoma, astrocytoma, brainstem glioma, and juvenile chronic myelogenous leukemia) are seen less frequently.

J. **Werner syndrome** is an autosomal recessive disorder caused by mutations in the *WRN* gene, which is involved in abnormal telomere maintenance. It is characterized by premature aging and by early onset of age-related pathologies (alopecia, ischemic heart disease, osteoporosis, cataracts, diabetes mellitus, hypogonadism) and cancer (especially sarcomas).

K. **Wiskott-Aldrich syndrome** is an X-linked immunodeficiency disease caused by mutations in the *WAS* gene, which has a key role in actin polymerization. Its clinical phenotype includes thrombocytopenia with small platelets, typical in appearance and distribution eczema, recurrent infections caused by immunodeficiency, and an increased incidence of autoimmune manifestations and malignancies. The most frequent malignancy reported is B-cell lymphoma, often positive for Epstein-Barr virus.

IV. ADVERSE CUTANEOUS EFFECTS OF RADIATION THERAPY

The severity of skin reactions is influenced by both treatment-related and patient-related factors. Treatment-related factors include a larger treatment volume per field, a larger total dose, a large fraction size, longer duration of treatment, and type of energy used. Patient risk factors include radiation to skin areas of increased moisture and friction (axilla, breast, perineum), poor skin hygiene, concurrent chemotherapy, older age, comorbid conditions, compromised nutritional status, smoking, and chronic sun exposure.

A. **Early effects** are usually defined as side effects occurring within 90 days from the initiation of therapy. Erythema, dryness, epilation, and pigmentation changes occur between the second and the fourth week. Dry desquamation can develop between weeks 3 and 6 of treatment. It can also be followed by moist desquamation, which usually occurs after week 5. Finally, skin damage may progress to dermal necrosis and secondary ulceration.

B. Late effects are associated with injury to the dermis. The list includes dermal atrophy, telangiectasias, and invasive fibrosis. There may be permanent loss of nails and skin appendages, alopecia, and decreased or absent sweating. Patients treated with RT are at higher risk for development of secondary cutaneous malignancy, especially squamous cell carcinoma.

C. Prophylaxis of skin damage. To decrease the risk of skin damage, patients should wash the skin gently with lukewarm water and mild soap to keep the irradiated area clean and to decrease the risk of superimposed bacterial infection. Moreover, they should avoid rubbing the skin, should not use skin irritants or metallic-based topical agents (zinc oxide–based creams, aluminum-containing deodorants), should wear loose cotton clothing, and avoid extreme temperatures.

D. Management of skin reactions. Patients with erythema and dry desquamation benefit from use of nonscented, lanolin-free hydrophilic or moisturizing creams. These creams should not be applied to skin breakdowns. Petroleum jelly–based products containing skin irritants such as alcohol, perfume, other additives, and alpha hydroxyl acids should be avoided, but Vaseline or white petrolatum is generally well tolerated. Patients should also avoid swimming in chlorinated pools, hot tubs, and lakes and exposure to extremes of hot and cold. Low-dose steroids (1% hydrocortisone, 0.1% mometasone furoate, 0.1% betamethasone) decrease the degree of inflammation and pruritus.

If moist desquamation develops, it is the general principle that wounds heal more rapidly in moist environment. The affected area should be cleaned with room temperature normal saline; moisture retentive protective barrier ointment can be applied. Hydrocolloid dressings and hydrogels in a form of sheets or amorphous gel are frequently utilized.

Atrophic skin has a high predisposition for ulcers and skin breakdowns; it is mainly treated with use of ointments and avoidance of trauma. The goal of treatment of chronic ulcers is to control the amount of secretions and prevent superimposed bacterial infections. These patients may require surgical intervention. Chronic fibrosis is the most difficult complication to treat, but a decreased frequency was seen with a prophylactic use of pentoxifylline and tocopherol (vitamin E 1,000 units/d).

V. ADVERSE CUTANEOUS EFFECTS OF CHEMOTHERAPY

A. Alopecia induced by chemotherapy usually begins 1 to 2 weeks after the initial treatment, and it becomes most prominent in 1 to 2 months. The severity of alopecia may be reduced with a use of scalp tourniquets and scalp cooling. In most cases, it is reversible and hair frequently regrows with a change of color and structure. The use of cranial prostheses (wigs) and scarves should be encouraged.

B. Hypersensitivity reactions have been documented with almost all chemotherapeutic agents. The types of reaction can range from urticaria, pruritus, and angioedema, through erythema multiforme, up to toxic epidermal necrolysis. Anaphylaxis may be associated with the use of platinum drugs and taxanes. Taxanes are routinely administered together with steroids and H1 and H2 blockers. Asparaginase can cause reactions ranging from urticaria to anaphylactic shock in 25% of patients, and an intradermal skin testing with two units of the drug before the initial administration is generally recommended.

Chimeric and humanized monoclonal antibodies, such as obinutuzumab, rituximab, cetuximab, alemtuzumab, and trastuzumab, are given together with diphenhydramine and acetaminophen to reduce the incidence of infusion-related reactions. Infusion reactions are very common (up to 45%) in patients treated with ofatumumab.

C. **Hyperpigmentation** can occur locally in the infusion site or diffusely throughout the skin; it can also affect nails and mucous membranes. Busulfan is known to cause "busulfan tan," a dusky diffuse hyperpigmentation that may resemble Addison disease. Bleomycin is a cause of flagellate hyperpigmentation, linear, band-like streaks of discoloration in areas of trauma predominantly on the trunk and the proximal extremities. Repetitive administration of fluorouracil results in serpentine supravenous hyperpigmentation of the skin overlying veins. Methotrexate given weekly can cause the "flag sign," the hyperpigmented bands alternating with the normal color of the patient's hair. Other drugs that can result in hyperpigmentation include cisplatin, cyclophosphamide, dactinomycin, daunorubicin, doxorubicin, etoposide, hydroxyurea, ifosfamide, nitrosoureas, paclitaxel, plicamycin, procarbazine, thiotepa, and vinca alkaloids.

D. **Hand–foot syndrome** (acral erythema, palmar–plantar erythrodysesthesia) is traditionally associated with use of high-dose cytarabine, fluorouracil, capecitabine and liposomal doxorubicin (see Section VI). Application of cold during infusion of chemotherapy may prevent acral erythema. In patients treated with liposomal doxorubicin, oral dexamethasone and topical 99% dimethyl sulfoxide (DMSO) applied four times daily for 14 days attenuated the symptoms of hand–foot syndrome.

E. **Extravasation of chemotherapeutic agents** describes the process of leakage or direct infiltration of a chemotherapeutic drug into tissue. The agents are divided into three groups, based on their potential to cause local tissue injury: **vesicant drugs** (they induce the formation of blisters and ulcers and cause tissue destruction); **irritant drugs** (they cause pain at the extravasation site or along the vein, with or without inflammatory response); and **nonvesicant drugs** (they rarely produce reactions). The group of vesicant agents includes drugs with a high vesicant potential including actinomycin D, amsacrine, daunorubicin, doxorubicin, epirubicin, idarubicin, mechlorethamine, mitomycin C, mitoxantrone, trabectedin, vinblastine, vincristine, vindesine, vinorelbine. Irritant drugs include bendamustine, bleomycin, bortezomib, busulfan, carboplatin, carmustine, cisplatin, cladribine, cyclophosphamide, cytarabine, dacarbazine, docetaxel, etoposide, fluorouracil, gemcitabine, ifosfamide, irinotecan, ixabepilone, melphalan, oxaliplatin, paclitaxel, streptozocin, teniposide, topotecan, and trastuzumab emtansine.

1. **Prevention.** All vesicant chemotherapeutics should be administered through the central line whenever possible. Central lines significantly reduce, but do not eliminate, the chance of drug extravasation. If peripheral lines have to be used, they should be used only for short infusions under direct monitoring of nursing staff. The dorsum of the hand and the areas near joints should be avoided because extravasation can cause significant functional damage. When an IV line is placed, the vein should be accessed using a single approach and the entry site should not be covered by tape. Line patency is checked by gently withdrawing blood and administering IV fluids before a cytotoxic agent is started. Patients are asked to report any discomfort promptly.

2. **Clinical presentation.** Extravasation usually causes immediate pain, which is followed by erythema and edema within a few hours and increasing

induration over a period of several days. Skin ulceration and necrosis can occur within the next 1 to 3 weeks. Necrosis can involve underlying tendon, fascia, and periosteum. Occasionally, extravasation is painless, and it may be detected late, resulting in worsening of tissue damage.

   3. **Management.** As soon as extravasation is noted, the drug infusion must be stopped and the affected extremity elevated. The IV catheter should not be removed immediately; it should be used for aspiration of the fluid from the site and administration of a possible antidote. If no antidote is available, the catheter can be removed.

   Never flush the line and avoid applying pressure to the area. Intermittent cooling for 24 to 48 hours with ice or cold packs is recommended in all cases of extravasation, except the vinca alkaloids and epipodophyllotoxins (etoposide). Warm compresses are used for drugs from these two groups. Most clinicians also use warm compresses for paclitaxel and docetaxel extravasation.

   Patients who develop nonhealing ulcers and tissue necrosis are treated surgically. A limited number of specific antidotes are available.

   a. **Sodium thiosulfate** is used as antidote for mechlorethamine, cisplatin, and dacarbazine: 4 mL of 10% sodium thiosulfate solution is mixed with 6 mL sterile water, and 2 mL for 100 mg of cisplatin is injected through the existing IV line, followed by SC injection of 1 mL around the area of extravasation.

   b. **Hyaluronidase** (150 to 900 U through the IV line and around the site) is used for treatment of extravasation of vinca alkaloids, paclitaxel, ifosfamide, and epipodophyllotoxins.

   c. **Dexrazoxane** is used in anthracycline extravasation. It is given intravenously through a different IV access daily for 3 days starting within 6 hours of extravasation at the doses 1,000 mg/m², 1,000 mg/m², and 500 mg/m².

   d. **Dimethyl sulfoxide:** 1 to 2 mL of 50% DMSO is applied topically and allowed to air-dry in patients with extravasation of anthracyclines (dexrazoxane is preferred) or mitomycin C.

   e. **Corticosteroids** may be helpful in cases of oxaliplatin extravasation.

F. **Radiation reactions**

   1. **Photosensitivity** can be observed in patients receiving dacarbazine, dactinomycin, fluorouracil, hydroxyurea, methotrexate, mitomycin, procarbazine, and vinblastine.

   2. **Enhancement of skin toxicity caused by RT** has been associated with bleomycin, dactinomycin, doxorubicin, fluorouracil, gemcitabine, hydroxyurea, methotrexate, and paclitaxel.

   3. **Radiation recall** (i.e., inflammatory reaction of a previously radiated area after exposure to a chemotherapeutic agent) has been described with bleomycin, capecitabine, cyclophosphamide, cytarabine, dactinomycin, daunorubicin, docetaxel, doxorubicin, etoposide, fluorouracil, gemcitabine, hydroxyurea, lomustine, methotrexate, melphalan, paclitaxel, tamoxifen, and vinblastine.

   4. **Reactivation of UV light–induced erythema** has been associated with methotrexate, gemcitabine, and taxanes.

G. **Nail dystrophies.** Nails are commonly affected by chemotherapy. Bleomycin, cyclophosphamide, and doxorubicin can be responsible for development of Beau lines, transverse ridgings that move distally and disappear in the treatment-free intervals. Mees lines, multiple white lines whose number correlates with the number of cycles of chemotherapy, are associated with daunorubicin.

Onycholysis can result from therapy with docetaxel, doxorubicin, fluorouracil, and mitoxantrone.

H. Neutrophilic eccrine hidradenitis has a distinct histopathology consisting of neutrophilic infiltrates in eccrine glands with areas of necrosis. It appears as an erythematous eruption of hemorrhagic nodules, pustules, and plaques typically confined to the head, neck, trunk, or extremities. The rash usually presents 2 to 3 weeks after chemotherapy, and it was most frequently described with use of cytarabine but also bleomycin, chlorambucil, daunorubicin, doxorubicin, and mitoxantrone. The eruption clears spontaneously without scar formation.

VI. ADVERSE CUTANEOUS EFFECTS OF MOLECULARLY TARGETED THERAPY AND IMMUNOTHERAPY

A. Acneiform rash. Both small molecules (afatinib, erlotinib, gefitinib, lapatinib, osimertinib) and monoclonal antibodies (cetuximab, necitumumab, panitumumab) that target epidermal growth factor receptor (EGFR) are associated with the development of a unique acneiform rash in up to 70% of patients. Typical lesions surround hair follicles and consist of pruritic maculopapular eruptions that may evolve into pustules. The rash has predilection to the seborrheic areas (upper trunk, face, scalp, neck). The rash may be complicated by secondary infections caused most frequently by *Staphylococcus aureus*.

As acneiform rash prophylaxis, minocycline (100 mg daily) or doxycycline (100 mg twice daily) can be used. These should be combined with application of emollients and the use of the broad-spectrum sunscreen creams. In patients who develop the rash, avoidance of sun exposure and use of moisturizing or colloidal oatmeal lotions are recommended. Topical 1% clindamycin and low-potency steroids (2.5% hydrocortisone or 0.05% alclometasone) are helpful. If rash worsens, topical 0.05% fluocinonide or oral prednisone 0.5 mg/kg can be used, and the EGFR-blocking agent should be temporarily withheld.

Similar rash can also be seen with imatinib, ponatinib, trametinib, vandetanib, and the new mTOR inhibitors, such as temsirolimus and everolimus.

B. Paronychia is also associated with the use of EGFR-blocking agents; it has been also described in patients treated with vandetanib.

C. Exanthematous papular rash can be seen with the use of axitinib, bosutinib, imatinib, dasatinib, pazopanib, and regorafenib. It is frequently mild and self-limiting.

D. Hand–foot syndrome (acral erythema, palmar–plantar erythrodysesthesia) presents initially with tingling and burning of the palms and soles that progress to severe pain, tenderness, edema, and development of well-demarcated, symmetric erythematous plaques. The lesions can spread to the dorsum of the hands and feet. Areas of pallor progress into formation of vesicles and bullae that desquamate. It is most commonly associated with the use of axitinib (29%), cabozantinib (50%), regorafenib (47%), pazopanib (6%), sorafenib (30% to 60%), sunitinib (10% to 20%), and vandetanib.

Hand–foot syndrome is generally treated by cessation of the chemotherapeutic agent or a decrease in the dose. Patients are recommended to wear cotton socks or gel inserts and to avoid pressure points, to soak the affected skin in lukewarm water mixed with Epsom salts, to use 20% to 40% topical urea or 6% to 10% salicylic acid to remove callus buildup (prophylactic callus removal may decrease the risk of the development of hand–foot syndrome), and to apply moisturizing creams to prevent skin hardening. Erythematous areas are treated with topical steroids, and 2% lidocaine can be used to relieve pain.

Plantar hyperkeratosis (increased callus formation without erythematous changes) is seen in patients treated with vemurafenib and dabrafenib.

E. **Squamoproliferative lesions.** The development of keratoacanthomas and cutaneous squamous cell carcinomas has been described in about 5% of patients treated with sorafenib. The frequency of these lesions increased significantly upon introduction of the specific BRAF inhibitors, such as vemurafenib (18% to 26%) and dabrafenib (6% to 26%). The frequency of SCCs is significantly reduced when BRAF inhibitors are used in combination with MEK inhibitors (vemurafenib/cobimetinib, dabrafenib/trametinib). In addition, verrucal keratotic lesions are commonly induced by BRAF inhibitors. Patients treated with these agents should be under a regular dermatologic surveillance.

F. **Hypopigmentation/hyperpigmentation.** Hair depigmentation is seen in 38% of patients treated with pazopanib, and less frequently with sorafenib and sunitinib, and rarely with imatinib. These agents can also cause skin hypopigmentation. Imatinib can also cause skin hyperpigmentation.

G. **Alopecia.** Complete hair loss is seen in patients treated with sonidegib and vismodegib and partial hair loss, with dabrafenib and vemurafenib.

H. **Cutaneous complications of immunotherapy.** The treatment with CTLA-4–blocking antibodies (ipilimumab) and PD1-blocking antibodies (nivolumab, pembrolizumab) can be complicated by the development of immune-related adverse events. Pruritus (managed with oral diphenhydramine, hydroxyzine, topical steroids) and maculopapular rash are seen commonly (20% to 68%), but occasionally, Stevens-Johnson syndrome, toxic epidermal necrolysis, or rash complicated by full-thickness dermal ulceration or necrotic, bullous, or hemorrhagic manifestations occurred. These patients must be treated with high-dose IV methylprednisolone or oral prednisone at 1 to 2 mg/kg/d and the therapy must be permanently discontinued.

Suggested Readings

Alcaraz I, Cerroni L, Rütten A, et al. Cutaneous metastases from internal malignancies: a clinico-pathologic and immunohistochemical review. *Am J Dermatopathol* 2012;34(4):3.

Bentzen SM. Preventing or reducing late side effects of radiation therapy: radiobiology meets molecular pathology. *Nat Rev Cancer* 2006;6(9):702.

Hymes SR, Strom EA, Fife C. Radiation dermatitis: clinical presentation, pathophysiology, and treatment 2006. *J Am Acad Dermatol* 2006;54:28.

Melosky B, Anderson H, Burkes RL, et al. Pan Canadian Rash Trial: a randomized phase III trial evaluating the impact of a prophylactic skin treatment regimen on epidermal growth factor receptor-tyrosine kinase inhibitor-induced skin toxicities in patients with metastatic lung cancer. *J Clin Oncol* 2016;34(8):810.

Pérez Fidalgo JA, García Fabregat L, Cervantes A, et al. Management of chemotherapy extravasation: ESMO–EONS clinical practice guidelines. *Eur J Oncol Nurs* 2012;16(5):528.

Reyes-Habito CM, Roh EK. Cutaneous reactions to chemotherapeutic drugs and targeted therapies for cancer: Part I. Conventional chemotherapeutic drugs. *J Am Acad Dermatol* 2014;71:203.

Reyes-Habito CM, Roh EK. Cutaneous reactions to chemotherapeutic drugs and targeted therapy for cancer: Part II. Targeted therapy. *J Am Acad Dermatol* 2014;71:217.

30 Thoracic Complications
Bartosz Chmielowski

I. SUPERIOR VENA CAVA (SVC) OBSTRUCTION
A. Epidemiology and etiology
1. **Malignant etiologies** (60% to 85% of cases)
   a. **Lung cancer** accounts for 75% of malignancy causing SVC obstruction. Non–small cell lung cancer (NSCLC) accounts for 50% and small cell lung cancer (SCLC) 25% of all cases. SVC syndrome develops in about 3% of patients with lung cancer.
   b. **Non-Hodgkin lymphoma** (NHL) accounts for 10% to 15% of cases of malignant SVC obstruction. Nearly all cases have intermediate-/high-grade histology. Hodgkin lymphoma or low-grade lymphomas rarely cause SVC obstruction.
   c. **Other malignant etiologies.** Other malignant tumors that are less commonly associated with the SVC syndrome include thymoma, primary mediastinal germ cell neoplasms, mesothelioma, and solid tumors with mediastinal lymph node metastases.
2. **Benign etiologies** (approximately 30% of cases)
   a. **Mediastinal fibrosis and chronic infections**
      (1) Currently, as many as 50% of cases of SVC syndrome not due to malignancy are attributable to fibrosing mediastinitis, of which the most common cause is an excessive host response to *a prior* infection with *Histoplasma capsulatum*. Other infections associated with fibrosing mediastinitis include tuberculosis, actinomycosis, aspergillosis, blastomycosis, and lymphatic filariasis.
      (2) Idiopathic fibrosing mediastinitis
      (3) Associated with Riedel thyroiditis, retroperitoneal fibrosis, sclerosing cholangitis, and Peyronie disease
      (4) After radiation therapy (RT) to the mediastinum
   b. **Thrombosis of vena cava** is usually related to the presence of indwelling intravascular devices. However, considering the frequency of use of central venous access catheters, the incidence of catheter-related SVC thrombosis appears to be low.
      (1) Long-term central venous catheterization, transvenous pacemakers, balloon-tipped pulmonary artery catheters, peritoneal venous shunting
      (2) Polycythemia vera, paroxysmal nocturnal hemoglobinuria
      (3) Behçet syndrome
      (4) Idiopathic
   c. **Benign mediastinal tumors**
      (1) Aneurysm of the aorta or right subclavian artery
      (2) Dermoid tumors, teratomas, thymoma
      (3) Goiter
      (4) Sarcoidosis

B. Pathogenesis

1. **Obstruction and thrombosis.** Tumors growing in the mediastinum compress the thin-walled vena cava, leading to its collapse. Venous thrombosis, because of stasis or vascular tumor invasion, often appears to be responsible for acute-onset SVC syndrome.

2. **Collateral circulation.** The rapidity of onset of symptoms and signs from SVC obstruction depends upon the rate at which complete obstruction of the SVC occurs in relation to the recruitment of venous collaterals. Vena cava obstruction caused by malignancy often progresses too rapidly to develop sufficient collateral circulation, which might alleviate the syndrome. If the obstruction occurs above the azygos vein, the obstructed SVC could then drain into the azygos system. The azygos vein, however, is frequently obstructed by malignancy below its origin.

3. **Incompetent internal jugular vein valves,** a rare occurrence, cause a dire emergency that is manifested by the filling of these veins. Approximately 10% of patients can experience a rapid demise due to cerebral edema.

C. Diagnosis. The diagnosis of SVC syndrome is usually based on the clinical findings and the presence of a mediastinal mass. CT scan evidence of collateral flow due to a mass is also supportive evidence for the diagnosis. *SVC syndrome rarely has to be treated before a histologic diagnosis is made.*

1. **Symptoms.** Patients with malignant disease may develop symptoms of SVC syndrome within weeks to months because rapid tumor growth does not allow adequate time to develop collateral flow.

   a. The most common presenting symptoms are shortness of breath (50% of patients), neck and facial swelling (40%), and swelling of trunk and upper extremities (40%). Sensations of choking, fullness in the head, and headache are also frequent symptoms.

   b. SVC obstruction may occasionally be accompanied by spinal cord compression, usually involving the lower cervical and upper thoracic vertebrae. The SVC syndrome consistently precedes spinal cord compression in these cases. The coexistence of these two complications should be seriously suspected in patients with upper back pain.

2. **Physical findings.** The most common physical findings are thoracic vein distention (65%), neck vein distention and edema of face (55%), tachypnea (40%), plethora of the face and cyanosis (15%), edema of upper extremities (10%), and paralysis of vocal cords or Horner syndrome (3%). Veins in the antecubital fossae are distended and do not collapse when elevated above the level of the heart. Retinal veins may be dilated on funduscopic examination. Dullness to percussion over the sternum may be present. Laryngeal stridor and coma are grave signs.

3. **Radiographs**

   a. **Chest radiograph** demonstrates a mass in >90% of patients.

   b. **Chest CT scan.** Contrast-enhanced CT can pinpoint the area of obstruction, the degree of occlusion, and the presence of collateral veins. CT scans show absence of contrast in central venous structures with opacification of collateral routes. It can guide fine needle aspiration.

   c. **Superior venocavogram.** Contrast-enhanced CT with multidetector technology demonstrates the exact site of obstruction and is the procedure of choice in planning stenting procedures.

      (1) **Bilateral upper extremity venography** is infrequently used currently.

      (2) **MR venography** is an alternative approach that may be useful for patients with contrast dye allergy or those for whom venous access cannot be obtained for contrast-enhanced studies.

   d. MRI scans of the cervical and upper thoracic vertebrae should be planned in patients with SVC syndrome and back pain, particularly in the presence of Horner syndrome or vertebral destruction on plain films.
4. **Histologic diagnosis** is important for identifying malignancies that must be treated with cytotoxic agents to improve survival. After RT is started, tissue diagnosis is difficult to interpret due to necrosis from radiation. Likewise, steroids can affect histology if the underlying diagnosis is lymphoma.
   a. Cytology of sputum and of pleural effusion fluid is positive in nearly all patients with SVC syndrome due to lung cancer.
   b. Bronchoscopy and bronchial brushings are positive in 60% of patients. Bronchoscopy and bronchial biopsy in patients with SVC syndrome are rarely associated with serious complications when performed by experienced endoscopists.
   c. Lymph node biopsy of palpable nodes can be helpful.
   d. Imaging-guided transthoracic biopsy can be attempted for peripheral lesions that cannot easily be approached by bronchoscopy or in whom bronchoscopy results are nondiagnostic.
   e. Video-assisted thoracoscopic surgery (VATS) nearly always results in a definitive histologic diagnosis. Bleeding points are usually visualized and controllable.
   f. Mediastinoscopy with biopsy risks hemorrhage and other complications. However, when mediastinoscopy is performed on a highly selected group of patients, positive results are obtained in 80% of cases.
   g. Bone marrow biopsy can be helpful in patients suspected of having SCLC or lymphoma.
D. Management. There is little clinical or experimental evidence that unrelieved SVC syndrome is life threatening. Current management guidelines stress the importance of accurate histologic diagnosis prior to starting therapy. Emergency treatment is indicated only in the presence of cerebral dysfunction, decreased cardiac output, or upper airway obstruction.
1. **Endovascular stents.** Percutaneous placement of self-expanding metal endoprostheses gives rapid symptomatic relief in 90% to 100% of patients. The stent is placed via a guidewire percutaneously via the internal jugular, subclavian, or femoral vein, under local anesthesia. One stent may not be sufficient to bridge the entire extent of the stenotic area; sometimes two or even three stents in series are needed. Balloon angioplasty or catheter-directed thrombolysis or mechanical thrombectomy may be necessary in some cases prior to stent placement.
   a. Clear indications for placement of endovascular stents for SVC syndrome are patients with severe symptoms, especially when tissue diagnosis is not known yet.
   b. Short-term anticoagulation is often recommended after stent placement. Reasonable approaches include dual antiplatelet therapy (e.g., clopidogrel 75 mg daily plus aspirin) for 3 months after stent placement or warfarin (with the goal of maintaining an INR of 1.5 to 2.0).
2. **RT** is indicated alone in patients with symptomatic SVC syndrome caused by radiosensitive tumors. The total dose of RT varies between 3,000 and 5,000 cGy, depending on the general condition of the patient, severity of the symptoms, anatomic site, and histologic type of underlying malignant tumor. Symptoms may resolve dramatically even without establishment of patency of the SVC.

RT is associated with complete relief of symptoms of SVC obstruction within 2 weeks in about 70% of patients with lung cancer. Relief of symptoms, however, may not be achieved for up to 4 weeks, and approximately 20% of patients achieve no relief from RT. Furthermore, the benefits of RT are often temporary, with many patients developing recurrent symptoms before dying of the underlying disease.

3. **Chemotherapy** is indicated as initial treatment in patients with NHL, SCLC, germ cell cancer, and (possibly) breast cancer with symptomatic SVC syndrome. In these settings, the clinical response to chemotherapy alone is usually rapid. Furthermore, these patients can often achieve long-term remission and durable palliation with standard treatment regimens. In certain situations (e.g., limited-stage SCLC, some subtypes of NHL), the addition of RT to systemic chemotherapy may decrease local recurrence rates and improve overall survival.

4. **Emergency treatment.** For patients with clinical SVC syndrome who present with stridor, respiratory compromise, or depressed central nervous system function, emergent treatment with endovascular stenting followed by RT is recommended.

5. **Supportive therapy.** Airway obstruction should be corrected and hypoxia treated by oxygen administration. The head should be raised to decrease hydrostatic pressure and head and neck edema. Corticosteroids reduce brain edema and improve the obstruction by decreasing the inflammatory reaction associated with the tumor and RT. Diuretics may be helpful.

6. **Anticoagulants and antifibrinolytic agents** may be helpful if the underlying cause of the SVC thrombosis is an indwelling catheter. Removal of the catheter is indicated, in conjunction with systemic anticoagulation. These agents rarely result in disappearance of caval thrombosis but may be used in conjunction with stent placement. When extensive thrombosis occurs as a complication of SVC stenosis, local catheter-directed thrombolytic therapy may be of value to reduce the length of the obstruction and the number and length of stents required and also reduce the risk of embolization. The thrombus may also be removed by mechanical thrombectomy, although this is used less often than thrombolysis.

7. **Surgical decompression** of acute SVC obstruction and incompetence of jugulosubclavian valves consists of reconstructing or bypassing the SVC using a spiral saphenous vein graft or left saphenoaxillary vein bypass, which can be done under local anesthesia. The experience with this procedure has been mainly in SVC associated with nonmalignant causes.

II. PULMONARY METASTASES

A. **General aspects**

1. **Occurrence.** The lungs are the most frequent site of distant metastases for nearly all malignant tumors except those arising in the gastrointestinal tract.

2. **Dissemination to the lungs.** Malignant melanoma, bone and soft tissue sarcomas, trophoblastic tumors, and renal cell, colonic, and thyroid carcinomas tend to spread to vascular routes and usually produce discrete metastatic lung nodules. Malignant tumors of the breast, pancreas, stomach, and liver may spread directly through lymphatic channels, involve mediastinal lymph nodes, and produce diffuse interstitial or lymphangitic infiltration, focal or segmental atelectasis, and pleural metastasis or effusion. Germ cell tumors and sarcomas may also involve the mediastinum.

3. **Types of metastases**
   a. **Endobronchial metastasis** is not uncommon in Hodgkin lymphoma, hypernephroma, and breast carcinoma.
   b. **Solitary pulmonary metastasis** is relatively uncommon but can occur in patients with malignant melanoma or carcinoma of the breast, uterus, testis, kidney, or urinary bladder.
   c. **Isolated pulmonary metastasis.** Osteogenic sarcoma, soft tissue sarcoma, and testicular carcinoma are the tumors that are most likely to have lung metastases without involvement of other organs. Renal and uterine carcinomas may also produce isolated lung metastases. Malignant melanoma rarely has pulmonary metastases without other organ involvement as well.
   d. **Lymphangitic pulmonary metastases** are rapidly lethal. Median survival is <2 to 3 months for patients without effective treatment.
   e. **Central pulmonary metastases.** Malignant tumors that invade hilar or mediastinal structures may result in SVC obstruction, major airway obstruction, postobstructive pneumonia, and invasion of the pericardium, myocardium, or esophagus.

B. **Diagnosis.** A new pulmonary lesion in a patient with a known malignancy may represent a metastasis, a second primary lung cancer (particularly if the patient is a smoker), or a benign lesion.

1. **Symptoms and signs.** Most patients with solitary or multiple pulmonary metastases do not have symptoms. The patients who are most likely to be symptomatic with cough, chest pain, hemoptysis, or progressive dyspnea have central, hilar, mediastinal, or lymphangitic metastatic involvement. Dyspnea out of proportion to the radiographic findings in the absence of radiologic findings should raise suspicion of lymphangitic spread. Physical examination may also be absolutely normal.

2. **Radiographic studies.** No current imaging modality can distinguish a benign tumor from a malignant tumor or a primary tumor from a metastasis. Plain films do not detect lesions smaller than 1 cm in diameter. High-resolution helical CT detects approximately 25% more nodules than conventional CT and nodules as small as 2 to 3 mm; however, this improved sensitivity is at the expense of specificity.
   a. Metastatic nodules are typically well-circumscribed, round deposits with smooth margins and are predominantly subpleural or located in the outer third of the lung fields. In contrast, primary lung cancers are usually single, often have irregular borders and associated linear densities, and are more often located centrally.
   b. When multiple nodules are present, the probability of metastatic disease increases significantly. However, multifocal abnormalities may be seen with primary bronchioloalveolar carcinomas, which may present with multiple pulmonary nodules and ground-glass opacification, and with severe acute and chronic nonmalignant pulmonary disease.
   c. About half of patients with lymphangitic lung metastases have normal chest radiographs; the remainder of patients have nonspecific interstitial changes.

3. **Positron emission tomography (PET).** The main value of PET is for detecting extrathoracic disease.

4. **Sputum cytology** is positive in only 5% to 20% of patients with nodular metastases.

5. **Pulmonary function studies** with lymphangitic metastases characteristically produce a restrictive defect with hypocapnia but without hypoxemia.

Restrictive lung disease can be confirmed by finding impaired diffusion capacity of the lung for carbon monoxide (DLCO) and low residual and total lung volumes.

6. **Bronchoscopy** (with or without endobronchial ultrasound) is indicated as part of the evaluation in cases of centrally located lesions identified on CT, in patients with symptoms of airway involvement, and for cell types that are prone to endobronchial involvement, such as breast, colon, and renal cell cancer.

C. **Resection (metastasectomy) of pulmonary metastases.** Aggressive surgical resection of lung metastases in appropriately selected patients offers a chance for extended disease-free survival that would not be possible with systemic therapy.

1. **Considerations for surgical resection of metastases with specific primary cancers**

a. **Head and neck cancers.** Patients with a history of head and neck carcinoma (especially laryngeal carcinoma) and who develop a lung nodule should be approached as if they have developed a new primary lung cancer. There is no way to differentiate a solitary metastasis from a second primary cancer in these patients.

b. **Testicular carcinoma.** Solitary lung nodules in the treated patient may develop into malignant teratomas or be lesions harboring active cancer. These have to be considered for resection.

c. **Sarcomas.** Patients with sarcomas are routinely followed with CT scans of the chest, monitoring for the development of pulmonary metastases amenable to resection, because the lungs are frequently the only site of metastasis. Osteogenic sarcomas are best treated with preoperative chemotherapy if the tumors are multiple.

d. **Breast cancer.** Resection of pulmonary metastases that are solitary in patients with a previous history of breast cancer is appropriate as 50% of these patients may have a benign lesion or a new primary lung cancer.

2. **Factors associated with a better outcome**

a. **Completeness of resection.** Nearly all reports indicate that complete resection of metastatic disease is associated with the best outcomes.

b. **Disease-free interval (DFI)** between the diagnosis of the primary tumor and metastasis. Higher 5-year survival rates are observed for patients with a DFI of >36 months compared to patients with a DFI of <1 year.

c. **Number of metastases.** A single or few and unilateral metastases have a better prognosis than many or bilateral metastases.

d. **Delaying intervention** after a pulmonary metastasis is first identified may allow initially occult metastases to become clinically apparent; if in the lungs, a more complete resection would be permitted; if at other sites, unhelpful surgery would be avoided. On multivariate analysis, waiting more than 3 months from the detection of pulmonary metastases to resection was an independently significant prognostic factor for improved survival.

3. **Studies to be performed prior to metastasectomy**

a. Thin-section, high-resolution helical CT is preferred over conventional CT in order to maximize detection of all sites of intrathoracic disease.

b. Imaging (CT or PET–CT) to exclude extrapulmonary metastases.

c. Brain imaging for patients who have tumors that frequently metastasize to the brain (e.g., lung cancer, breast cancer, melanoma).

d. Evaluation of the mediastinal lymph nodes as would be done for a patient with a primary lung cancer. Surgical staging of the mediastinal and hilar lymph nodes prior to pulmonary metastasectomy appears to provide diagnostic and prognostic information.

4. **Criteria for resection.** VATS can be used for patients with one or a limited number of small metastases in the periphery of one lung. The type of histology, number of lesions, and whether they are bilateral do not appear to contraindicate resection or adversely influence the survival if the selection criteria discussed below are adhered to. Wedge resection is the recommended treatment of pulmonary metastases in patients who meet all of the following criteria:

   a. The patient's general medical condition and pulmonary function status are suitable for surgery.

   b. The primary tumor is under control (no evidence of local recurrence) or controllable.

   c. Metastases are limited to the lung (no uncontrollable extrapulmonary tumor exists), and all metastases appear to be completely resectable.

   d. Resection of one or more lung lesions may also be indicated in a patient with a known malignancy when a new primary lung cancer cannot be excluded.

   e. No better method of treatment exists.

5. **Timing for metastasectomy** depends upon the anticipated surgical approach (open thoracotomy vs. VATS). VATS metastasectomy may be selected for an isolated peripheral nodule in a favorable location because recovery time and surgical risk are minimal. However, open thoracotomy would be required for a deep nodule or numerous nodules of varying sizes. Delaying open surgery and performing repeat CT scanning for 2 to 3 months allow the full extent of disease to be revealed and prevent unnecessary surgery without affecting prognosis.

D. **Management of nonresectable pulmonary metastasis**

1. **Systemic therapy** (chemotherapy, targeted therapy, hormonal therapy, immunotherapy) can be applied in responsive tumors. Germ cell and trophoblastic tumors can be cured despite the presence of pulmonary metastasis.

2. **Local control.** RT is useful for palliation of local complications of metastatic tumors, such as bronchial obstruction, vena cava obstruction, hemoptysis, or pain caused by tumor invasion of the chest wall. Stereotactic RT, radiofrequency ablation, or cryotherapy may offer alternative options.

3. **Lymphangitic lung metastases** represent an emergent problem in diagnosis and management. Symptomatic relief of dyspnea can often be rapidly achieved with prednisone, 60 mg PO daily. Chemotherapy is effective in responsive tumors. Hormonal manipulation is usually ineffective or achieves a response too slowly to be helpful. Symptoms from refractory lymphangitic lung metastases may be palliated by low-dose lung irradiation.

III. MALIGNANT PLEURAL EFFUSIONS

A. **Pathogenesis**

1. **Etiology.** Malignant tumors causing pleural effusions are as follows: lung cancer (especially adenocarcinoma), breast carcinoma, lymphoma, unknown primary, gastric carcinoma, ovarian carcinoma, melanoma, and sarcoma.

2. **Types of pleural effusions.** Malignant pleural effusion is caused by a direct infiltration of the pleura by cancer (cytology/pleural biopsy is positive for malignancy). Paramalignant pleural effusions result from bronchial, lymphatic, or venous obstruction. Atelectasis, pneumonia, and severe hypoalbuminemia that complicate malignancy may also cause pleural effusion.

B. Natural history. Malignant pleural effusion is a sign of advanced disease. The pleural space is progressively obliterated by fibrosis and serosal tumor. Patients with carcinomatous pleural effusions have a median survival of 4 months from the time of diagnosis, but this varies with the responsiveness of the underlying tumor to systemic therapy.

C. Differential diagnosis. The differentiation of pleural fluid from pleural fibrosis or pulmonary consolidation may not be possible by physical examination or chest radiographs. Aspiration of fluid may be difficult because of loculation. Ultrasonography is helpful for identifying and sampling small pockets of effusion.

1. **Symptoms and signs.** Cough and dyspnea are the most common symptoms of pleural effusion. Dullness to percussion, decreased breath and voice sounds, decreased vocal fremitus, and egophony are the classic physical findings. The trachea may be shifted to the side opposite the effusion. Thickened pleura from fibrosis or neoplastic involvement also produces dullness and decreased vibration.

2. **Thoracentesis** should be performed in any patient with a suspected malignant, infectious, or empyemic pleural effusion. Pleural fluid should be assayed for protein, lactate dehydrogenase (LDH) level, pH, glucose, cell count, and cytology and stained and cultured for bacteria (especially mycobacteria) and fungi. If the effusion appears chylous, triglyceride and cholesterol concentrations should be measured. Malignant effusions are usually exudative but may be transudative. Results of fluid examination frequently are nonspecific.

   a. **Discrimination between transudates and exudates** is facilitated by relating the concentration of key parameters in the pleural fluid to those values in the serum or to the laboratory's upper limit of normal (ULN). Diagnostic rules vary among systems of classification. **Characteristics for exudates** in various systems are
   - Pleural fluid/serum ratio for protein >0.5
   - Pleural fluid protein >2.9 g/dL (29 g/L)
   - Pleural fluid/serum LDH ratio >0.6
   - Pleural fluid LDH >0.45× or >0.67× ULN for serum LDH
   - Pleural fluid cholesterol >45 mg/dL (1.165 mmol/L)

   b. **Cytology** is positive in half of malignant pleural effusions. Repeated cytologic analysis increases the yield if the first thoracentesis is negative.

   c. **Leukocyte counts** in malignant pleural fluid may be low or high; the predominant cells may be neutrophils, lymphocytes, or eosinophils.

   (1) **Lymphocytosis.** Pleural fluid lymphocytosis, particularly with lymphocyte counts representing about 95% of the total nucleated cells, suggests tuberculous pleurisy (it can be confirmed by measurement of adenosine deaminase level), lymphoma, sarcoidosis, chronic rheumatoid pleurisy, yellow nail syndrome, or chylothorax. Carcinomatous pleural effusions will be lymphocyte predominant in over one-half of cases.

   (2) **Eosinophilia** (pleural fluid eosinophils representing more than 10% of the total nucleated cells) is usually seen in patients with a benign etiology of pleural effusion such as drugs, infection (fungal or parasitic), pneumothorax, hemothorax, pulmonary infarction, benign asbestos pleural effusion, and even prior thoracentesis. Malignancy rarely causes eosinophilia.

d. pH. In patients with bronchopneumonia, a pH <7.2 at the initial thoracentesis may be predictive for the development of an empyema that has to be drained by tube. Values of <7.2, however, may also be found in patients with malignancy or collagen vascular disease.

3. Pleural biopsy

    a. Pleural needle biopsy is a blind procedure and is less sensitive than cytology. Among patients with a cytology-negative malignant effusion, the yield of this procedure is only about 7%.

    b. VATS is more commonly used in the United States. The entire costal pleura and a good portion of the diaphragmatic and mediastinal pleura can be visualized, thus allowing direct biopsy of any pleural lesion. Although VATS is well tolerated, it does have some risks and carries with it a significant expense.

D. Management. Respiratory insufficiency caused by malignant effusion may be relieved by removing up to 1,500 mL of fluid by needle aspiration. Removal of excessive amounts of pleural fluid can be associated with reactive pulmonary edema. In a small percentage of patients, no recurrence of the effusion develops after a single evacuation. In most cases, the effusion recurs, and more definitive methods of therapy are required.

1. Chemotherapy. Pleural effusion secondary to metastatic tumors that are sensitive to systemic therapy (lymphoma, breast, ovarian, testicular carcinoma, cancers with molecular targets and available molecular agents, cancers responsive to immunotherapy) should be treated with appropriate combinations of agents. The results may be dramatic if the effusion presents early in the disease before resistance to the chemotherapeutic drugs develops. Pleural effusions that occur in the late or terminal stages are usually resistant to systemic therapy.

2. RT. Pleural effusions caused by mediastinal lymphadenopathy may be best treated with RT.

3. Indwelling pleural catheter. A more aggressive intervention may be required if the malignant pleural effusion recurs rapidly (e.g., <1 month), such that the frequency of repeat therapeutic thoracentesis would be troublesome. Placement of an indwelling pleural catheter with intermittent drainage by the patient is the preferred initial step for patients with recurrent malignant effusions according to some authorities. This procedure is the least invasive option and requires little if any time in the hospital. Additionally, indwelling pleural catheter drainage is indicated when there is permanent lung entrapment or endobronchial obstruction by tumor; chemical pleurodesis is contraindicated in these patients due to high failure rates when the lung is unable to expand against the chest wall. Pleurodesis may develop spontaneously or may be attempted later with a sclerosing agent if the indwelling catheter fails.

4. Pleurodesis (visceroparietal pleural symphysis) is accomplished with tube thoracostomy. The decision to undergo chemical pleurodesis is often based on a relatively longer anticipated survival (e.g., longer than 3 months) and a desire for a single definitive procedure.

    a. Patient selection. Pleurodesis should be performed in patients who meet the following conditions:

        (1) The patient's symptoms (shortness of breath) are caused by the pleural effusion and not by lymphangitic or intrapulmonary metastasis (i.e., symptoms improve after aspiration of fluid).

        (2) The pleural effusion recurs after repeated needle aspirations or rapidly reaccumulates (within a few days).

        (3) The patient's life expectancy is estimated to be longer than 1 month.

b. Drainage procedure

 (1) The chest tube is inserted in the most dependent location, preferably at the anterior axillary line. The pleural fluid is first allowed to drain through a water seal gravity drainage system. Negative suction may be later applied to ensure completeness of drainage.

 (2) When <100 mL drains in 24 hours, a chest radiograph is obtained to assess the amount of residual fluid and the extent of reexpansion of the underlying lung.

 (3) The evacuation of pleural fluid may take a few days. The expansion of the underlying lung is necessary to bring the visceral and parietal pleural surfaces in close proximity in preparation for symphysis. Injecting sclerosing agents without apposition of the pleural surfaces is ineffective and may result in loculation.

c. Instilling sclerosing agents

 (1) The chest tube is first cross-clamped and is cleaned with antiseptic solution. A narcotic is given to prevent pain.

 (2) The sclerosing agent in 30 mL of normal saline is injected into the chest tube, which is then flushed with 50 mL of saline. Changing the patient's position to distribute the agent throughout the pleural space usually is not necessary.

 (3) The chest tube should remain clamped for 6 hours. The pleural fluid is then allowed to drain, preferably with negative suction, until <100 mL drains in 24 hours.

 (4) After a drug has been instilled, there may be a great deal of drainage because of pleural weeping from drug irritation. A nonfunctioning or blocked tube may produce complications (pain, atelectasis, and infection) and should be removed.

d. Choice of sclerosing agents

 (1) Talc is a preferred sclerosing agent. Asbestos-free, sterilized talc may be used as a powder at thoracotomy (poudrage) or thoracoscopy (insufflation) or as slurry through a chest tube. The last example is associated with efficacy rates of 90% to 100% in control of malignant pleural effusions. A meta-analysis of 10 randomized trials found that nonrecurrence of effusion was more likely with talc than other sclerosants (i.e., bleomycin, tetracycline) or tube drainage alone. It is unclear whether talc insufflation during VATS or talc slurry instillation via chest tube is preferable.

 (2) Doxycycline. The tetracycline derivative doxycycline is an alternative sclerosant with reported success rates of about 80%. Doxycycline may require repeat installations.

 (3) Bleomycin is used rarely. This agent is nearly 50% systemically absorbed, but it can cause systemic side effects.

e. Complications of pleural sclerosis

 (1) Pneumothorax. Suction may be applied to reexpand the lung if the chest tube is not blocked. If the chest tube is obliterated (no fluid oscillation), insertion of a new chest tube is indicated.

 (2) Cough may result from reexpansion of an atelectatic lung after the compressing pleural fluid is removed. This symptom is self-limited and may be advantageous because it further clears atelectasis.

 (3) Chest pain may be secondary to the chest tube insertion or the instillation of drugs. Pain usually dissipates within 5 days but may require opioids.

     (4) **Fever** may be caused by atelectasis or pneumonitis or by the sclerosing agent.

     (5) **Loculation of fluid** may be caused by inadequate drainage or the instillation of sclerosing agents before the lung has completely reexpanded. Injection of radiopaque material into the pleural space followed by upright and lateral decubitus chest radiographs may confirm this problem. Trying to break the loculation by tube manipulation is not recommended.

     (6) **Empyema and pleurocutaneous draining sinus** may occur when tumor seeds the chest tube site. Empyema may be the result of either contamination or bronchopleural communication.

  5. Pleurectomy. Total or subtotal pleurectomy (resection of visceral and parietal pleura) and decortication (removal of fibrous pleural rind) can control malignant pleural effusions in patients who have failed chemical pleurodesis. The procedure carries high morbidity and mortality and is considered only for otherwise healthy patients in whom all of the more conservative measures have failed.

  6. Pleuroperitoneal shunting is a rarely used option for patients who have lung entrapment, malignant chylothorax, or have failed pleurodesis.

IV. PULMONARY COMPLICATIONS OF SYSTEMIC THERAPY

  A. Etiology

    1. Mechanisms of lung injury. The pathogenesis of antineoplastic agent–induced lung injury is poorly understood. Most toxic effects are thought to result from direct cytotoxicity.

    2. Types of pulmonary reactions to chemotherapeutic agents include bronchospasm, acute interstitial pneumonitis, hypersensitivity pneumonitis, bronchiolitis obliterans with organizing pneumonia (BOOP), noncardiogenic pulmonary edema, chronic interstitial pneumonitis with the insidious development of diffuse parenchymal fibrosis, and/or pleural disease. Pulmonary embolism may be seen with thalidomide or lenalidomide. Acute lung injury owing to hemolytic uremic syndrome may be seen with mitomycin C.

    3. Associated drugs.

      a. Chemotherapy: bleomycin (1% to 10%), carmustine (BCNU) (2% to 30%), busulfan (5%), cytarabine (20%), mitomycin C (3% to 10%), fludarabine (10%), gemcitabine (2% to 13%), and methotrexate (2% to 8%) have been associated with pulmonary toxicity with significant frequency. Other drugs (chlorambucil, cyclophosphamide, etoposide, irinotecan, paclitaxel, docetaxel, procarbazine) have been associated with pulmonary toxicity rarely. Other agents can cause lung injury sporadically.

      b. Molecularly targeted drugs. Interstitial lung disease/pneumonitis has been described in 1% to 8% of patients treated with:

        – EGFR inhibitors (gefitinib, erlotinib, osimertinib). It can be fatal in 15% to 30% of cases. The risk is also increased in patients treated with panitumumab, but not cetuximab.

        – ALK inhibitors (crizotinib, ceritinib, alectinib).

        – Imatinib—It more commonly causes fluid edema.

        – Dasatinib—Pleural effusions are more common, and pulmonary artery hypertension has also been described.

        – Trametinib.

   – Idelalisib.
   – Rituximab.
   – Ado-trastuzumab emtansine.
   – mTOR inhibitors: everolimus (8% to 14%), temsirolimus (1% to 5%). Pulmonary hemorrhage was seen in patients treated with VEGF inhibitors (bevacizumab, sorafenib, sunitinib)

  4. Risk factors that promote chemotherapy-induced lung damage include
   a. Advanced age, history of smoking, prior chronic lung disease, and renal dysfunction for some drugs.
   b. Thoracic RT administered concomitantly or sequentially, particularly with radiosensitizing drugs such as gemcitabine, doxorubicin, or bleomycin.
   c. Other chemotherapeutic agents, such as concomitant bleomycin with cisplatin, gemcitabine with a taxane, or mitomycin C with vinblastine.
   d. Exposure to high inspired oxygen therapy.
   e. Granulocyte-colony stimulating factor (G-CSF, filgrastim) was identified as a possible risk factor for the development of bleomycin-induced lung injury in animal studies.

B. Differential diagnosis. Pneumonitis has no characteristic radiographic pattern and may be associated with a normal chest radiograph or diffuse infiltrates. Establishing the diagnosis of drug pulmonary toxicity is often difficult because cancer patients may also have other concomitant pulmonary abnormalities.

C. Diagnosis. Drug-induced pulmonary toxicity may be insidious or acute in onset, and it rarely develops after the drugs have been discontinued. Except for rare cases of delayed fibrosis seen with nitrosoureas and bleomycin, lung toxicity typically occurs within weeks to a few months after initiation of therapy. Clinical features are similar regardless of the specific drug involved.

  1. Symptoms. Dry cough and dyspnea are prominent.
  2. Signs. Fever, tachypnea, and rales are common in the acute varieties. Incomplete or asymmetric chest expansion (respiratory lag) may be an early finding. Skin eruptions are common with methotrexate pulmonary toxicity.
  3. Eosinophilia is occasionally an associated finding, especially if methotrexate, procarbazine, or tretinoin has been used.
  4. Chest radiographs may be normal. The most typical abnormalities are bibasilar linear densities. Nodular, interstitial, alveolar, and mixed patterns also occur. Hilar lymphadenopathy is uncommon, except in the case of methotrexate-induced lung disease.
  5. CT. The most common abnormalities on high-resolution CT are ground-glass opacities, consolidation, interlobular septal thickening, and centrilobular nodules. The pattern, distribution, and extent of abnormalities are of limited diagnostic and prognostic value.
  6. Pulmonary function tests (PFTs) usually show hypoxemia, a decreased DLCO, and a restrictive ventilatory defect (decreased vital and total lung capacities). The routine monitoring of DLCO during drug treatment with agents known to cause pulmonary toxicity is controversial at best. PFTs, including DLCO, are neither sensitive nor specific for drug-induced lung toxicity, and many have questioned the clinical significance of changes in their results.
  7. Bronchoscopy and bronchoalveolar lavage. There are no specific findings for drug-induced lung toxicity on bronchoscopy or bronchoalveolar lavage.
  8. Lung biopsy via VATS may be considered when the etiology remains unclear, although histopathologic findings of drug-induced lung toxicity are nonspecific.

D. **Management** includes careful patient selection before administering potentially pulmonary toxic drugs or using drugs that potentiate the effect of radiation.
   1. Drugs should be discontinued in patients who get symptoms and signs of toxicity.
   2. Glucocorticoids, such as prednisone, are advocated to minimize lung injury in the symptomatic patient who does not improve with drug withdrawal. Dosage schemes for corticosteroids and their effectiveness are anecdotal and inconsistent.
   3. Reinitiation of offending drugs is possible and tricky, although this maneuver has been successful at times. The critical need for a specific drug for a specific malignancy weighs heavily in this important decision. However, reinitiation is generally not recommended and is contraindicated in patients with pulmonary fibrosis.

E. **Pulmonary complications associated with immunotherapy.** PD1-blocking antibodies (pembrolizumab and nivolumab) have been associated with immune-mediated pneumonitis in 1% to 3% of treated patients. Most cases are mild, but some cases were fatal. The treatment with ipilimumab (CTLA4-blocking antibody) exacerbated sarcoidosis and induced organizing pneumonia. Lung toxicities are very rare with ipilimumab.

V. OTHER PULMONARY COMPLICATIONS
A. **Radiation-induced lung disease (RILD)**
   1. **Patients who undergo RT to the thorax or neck for malignancy** are at risk for RILD (acute or subacute pneumonitis or fibrosis). Many factors affect the risk for RILD, including the method of irradiation, the volume of irradiated lung, the total dosage and frequency of irradiation, preexisting pulmonary disease, smoking history, performance status, associated chemotherapy, and perhaps genetic factors.
   2. **Radiosensitizing drugs.** Several chemotherapeutic agents are known sensitizers to RT, including doxorubicin, taxanes, dactinomycin, bleomycin, mitomycin, cyclophosphamide, vincristine, and gemcitabine. Patients receiving these drugs are at a higher risk of developing RILD.
      a. **Gemcitabine** is included in many lung cancer treatment protocols and is a potent radiation sensitizer; when given as concurrent therapy, pulmonary toxicity is prohibitive, even with reduced doses.
      b. **Glucocorticoid withdrawal** during RT has been reported to increase the risk for radiation pneumonitis.
      c. The frequency of radiation-induced pneumonia appears to be increased by **concurrent endocrine therapy** for breast cancer. Many RT oncologists prefer to start endocrine therapy for these patients after RT is completed.
   3. **Radiation recall pneumonitis** can occur when certain antineoplastic agents (e.g., doxorubicin, etoposide, gemcitabine, paclitaxel, carmustine, gefitinib, and trastuzumab) are administered to a patient who has received prior RT to the lung.
   4. **Acute radiation pneumonitis.** An acute alveolar infiltrate can develop 3 to 10 weeks after the completion of RT. Pneumonitis is proportionately more frequent with increasing radiation doses and portal sizes.
      a. **Manifestations.** The patient usually does not have symptoms, although a dry cough, dyspnea, fever, and leukocytosis may be present. Symptoms caused by subacute radiation pneumonitis usually develop approximately 4 to 12 weeks following irradiation and usually subside within 2 weeks.

On chest radiograph, a sharply outlined abnormality, which conforms to the confines of the radiation port, is often seen and is virtually diagnostic of RILD. However, conformal and stereotactic treatment strategies do not cause this "straight line" finding due to the complex distribution of the RT. CT may show patchy alveolar ground-glass or consolidative opacities. Pulmonary function testing generally demonstrates a reduction in lung volumes, diffusing capacity, and lung compliance.

  b. **Management.** Glucocorticoids are useful in relief of symptoms of pneumonitis caused by drugs and radiation. The usual dose is at least 60 mg of prednisone per day for 2 to 3 weeks with a slow taper for 3 to 12 weeks. Immunosuppressive agents may be considered if glucocorticoids fail. Antibiotics are generally not helpful unless infection is present. Pentoxifylline (400 mg three times a day) has immunomodulating and anti-inflammatory properties and has possibly a modest preventive benefit.

  5. **Pulmonary interstitial fibrosis** may appear as early as 4 months after RT. Patients may develop restrictive lung disease, alveolar–capillary block, or cor pulmonale. Corticosteroids have a doubtful role in preventing or treating progression of fibrosis.

B. **Pulmonary tumor thrombotic microangiopathy with pulmonary hypertension** is characterized by fibrocellular intimal proliferation of small pulmonary arteries and arterioles in patients with metastatic carcinoma, particularly adenocarcinoma. This condition develops when microscopic tumor cell embolism induces both local activation of coagulation and fibrocellular proliferation of intima but does not occlude the affected vessels. The increased vascular resistance results in pulmonary hypertension. This complication should be considered in the differential diagnosis in patients with known carcinoma who develop acute or subacute cor pulmonale.

C. **Pulmonary infections** are discussed in Chapter 36.

VI. PERICARDIAL AND MYOCARDIAL METASTASES

A. **Epidemiology and etiology.** Metastatic involvement of the heart is relatively common; 8% of patients have metastatic disease involving the heart. Cardiac involvement may arise from hematogenous metastases, direct invasion from the mediastinum, or tumor growth into the vena cava and extension into the right atrium.

  1. Malignant pericardial effusion is usually a preterminal event. The epicardium is involved in 75% of metastatic lesions, and pericardial effusions are associated with 35% of epicardial metastases.

  2. Carcinomas of the lung and breast constitute about 75% of all cases of malignant pericardial effusion. Melanoma, leukemia, lymphoma, soft tissue sarcomas, renal carcinoma, esophageal carcinoma, hepatocellular carcinoma, and thyroid cancer also commonly affect the heart. Pericardial effusion, which is usually insignificant, occurs in 20% of patients with NHL at the time of presentation.

B. **Natural history**

  1. Most myocardial and pericardial metastases are clinically silent; about two-thirds are not diagnosed antemortem. Prognosis appears to be related to tumor type. Pericardial metastases produce symptoms by causing pericardial effusion with tamponade, constrictive pericarditis, or arrhythmias.

  2. Myocardial metastases produce symptoms by causing conduction blocks and arrhythmias. Metastases infrequently cause myocardial rupture, valvular disease, or emboli to other organs.

C. **Diagnosis of pericardial effusion.** Clinical manifestations arise from decreased cardiac output and venous congestion. Frequently, pericardial tamponade develops slowly, and symptoms resemble those of congestive heart failure.

1. **Signs of pericardial tamponade**
   a. Neck vein distention that increases on inspiration (Kussmaul sign).
   b. A fall in systolic pressure of >10 mm Hg at the end of inspiration (pulsus paradoxus).
   c. Distant heart sounds with decreased cardiac impulse; possible pericardial friction rub.
   d. Pulmonary rales, hepatosplenomegaly, or ascites may be seen.

2. **Diagnostic studies**
   a. **Chest radiographs** may show enlargement of the cardiac silhouette or a "water bottle" configuration.
   b. **Electrocardiogram (ECG) abnormalities** are generally not specific. Total electrical alternans involving both the P wave and QRS complex is almost pathognomic of pericardial tamponade. Alternans of only the QRS complex is suggestive of but not specific for cardiac tamponade.
   c. **Echocardiography** can detect as little as 15 mL of fluid. The findings on echocardiogram of right atrial and ventricular collapse in diastole strongly suggest tamponade.
   d. **Cardiac catheterization** is the gold standard for diagnosis and monitoring. Equalization of pressures across the chambers defines tamponade.
   e. **Cardiac MRI** provides more detailed information.
   f. **Pericardiocentesis.** A small catheter should be introduced through the needle into the pericardial sac and attached to water seal gravity drainage to prevent the recurrence of effusion until the final diagnosis is made.
   g. **Fluid analysis.** Malignant pericardial fluids are usually exudative and often hemorrhagic. Fluid analysis and interpretation are the same as for pleural effusions (see Section III.C.2). Cytologic findings may be difficult to interpret in patients who have received RT. Negative cytologic results do not exclude the diagnosis of malignant effusion.

D. **Management**

1. **Pericardiocentesis and catheter drainage.** Conservative treatment of malignant pericardial effusion using pericardiocentesis or short-term catheter drainage as needed (with or without instillation of intrapericardial chemotherapeutic drugs) may be effective treatment for some patients. Serious complications of pericardial aspiration through a left parasternal or xiphisternal approach are rare, but they include laceration of the heart or coronary arteries, other vessels, liver, or stomach and (very rarely) a dramatic shock-like reaction. Pneumothorax and arrhythmia occur rarely. Emergency subxiphoid pericardial decompression under local anesthesia, however, is reported to be associated with no operative mortality. The drainage catheter can be left in place for several days if necessary without increased risk of infection. The catheter can be removed when drainage is <75 to 100 mL/h. Systemic therapy should always be considered and used whenever possible.

2. **RT** may be used in radiosensitive tumor types. Overall response rates are reported to be 60% with a dose of 3,500 cGy given over 3 to 4 weeks.

3. **Sclerosing agents.** Chemotherapeutic drugs or doxycycline may be instilled intrapericardially to induce pericardial sclerosis and obliterate the pericardial space. Pericardial sclerosis results in decreased pericardial fluid reaccumulation in 50% to 75% of patients. Drug instillation should be performed with ECG monitoring and an intravenous line in place in case arrhythmia

develops. The development of constrictive pericarditis and refractory heart failure has been reported.

4. **Pericardiectomy.** Surgery should be reserved for patients with (1) rapidly accumulating pericardial effusions that cannot be controlled conservatively, (2) radiation-induced constrictive pericarditis, and (3) a life expectancy of 6 months or more.

   a. **Subtotal pericardiectomy** (resection of entire pericardium anterior to the phrenic nerves) is the surgical procedure of choice in patients whose expected survival is reasonably long. Subtotal pericardiectomy is superior to the pericardiopleural window, which may seal off shortly after surgery. Success rates range from 90% to 95%.

   b. **Alternative surgical interventions for pericardial tamponade**

      (1) **Percutaneous balloon pericardiotomy** proved successful in relieving the cardiac tamponade in >90% of cases with few complications.

      (2) **Subxiphoid pericardiotomy** was safe and efficacious in 85% of patients at 6 months.

      (3) **VATS** offers a minimally invasive technique for treatment of pericardial effusions but still requires general anesthesia and the ability to tolerate single-lung ventilation. VATS offers little advantage over subxiphoid pericardiostomy and should be applied in situations for which the subxiphoid approach failed.

5. **Myocardial metastases.** Patients with disseminated malignancy and new, unexplained cardiac arrhythmias that are refractory to treatment should be considered for cardiac irradiation, particularly if there is known mediastinal or pericardial involvement.

VII. OTHER CARDIAC COMPLICATIONS

A. **Nonbacterial thrombotic ("marantic") endocarditis** is rare, but if it occurs, it is most common in patients with mucinous adenocarcinoma of the lung, stomach, or ovary. Noninfected fibrin vegetations appear on heart valves that are otherwise normal. Treatment with anticoagulants or antiplatelet drugs may be reasonable in some cases, but the results of such treatment are not encouraging.

B. **Bacterial endocarditis** is not more frequent in cancer patients than in the general population.

C. **Radiation pericarditis and pancarditis**

1. **Acute pancarditis or pericarditis** is seen rarely because much lower doses of radiation are used in the management of mediastinal tumors.

   a. **Manifestations.** Symptoms and signs resemble acute or chronic pericarditis of other etiologies: pleuritic chest pain, pericardial friction rub, ECG abnormalities, and enlargement of the cardiac silhouette on radiographs. Most patients, however, do not have symptoms.

   b. **Management.** Treatment in the acute phase includes giving corticosteroids and antipyretics and doing pericardiocentesis.

2. **Myocardiopathy** is a rare sequel of large doses of irradiation to the heart, particularly with concomitant or prior use of doxorubicin. Refractory heart failure may result.

D. **Anthracycline-induced cardiomyopathy.** A major dose-limiting toxicity of the anthracyclines (doxorubicin, liposomal doxorubicin, daunorubicin, epirubicin, and idarubicin) is cardiomyopathy. Mitoxantrone appears to be less cardiotoxic. The mechanisms of cardiac toxicity are not well understood. Topoisomerase II (Top2) is the main target for anthracyclines. Tumor tissues contain an increased amount of Top2-alpha, and cardiac tissue contains mainly Top2-beta. It is postulated that binding of doxorubicin to Top2-beta is responsible for cardiac damage.

1. **Types of cardiac toxicity**
   a. **Acute cardiotoxicity** is a relatively uncommon event and is not related to total dose. Manifestations include the following: arrhythmias, especially sinus tachycardia and atrial fibrillation, which do not correlate with subsequent development of chronic cardiomyopathy; heart block; nonspecific ST–T-wave changes; pericardial and pleural effusions (after 1 to 2 days); and clinically unapparent decreases in left ventricular ejection fraction (LVEF) (reversible congestive heart failure may develop after the first dose). These events usually resolve within a week.
   b. **Chronic cardiomyopathy** is related to the total dose and method of administration. Microscopy is nonspecific and reveals interstitial edema, cytoplasmic vacuolization, muscle fiber degeneration, and deformed mitochondria. The heart becomes dilated and may contain mural thrombi.

      Subclinical left ventricular dysfunction occurs commonly. Overt congestive heart failure usually develops within 3 months of the last anthracycline dose but can occur even 10 years later. In adults, late/delayed toxicity is primarily of concern in clinical situations where anthracyclines are used as part of a curative or adjuvant regimen. Since the introduction of angiotensin-converting enzyme (ACE) inhibitors and beta-blockers in the management of heart failure, the outcome improved significantly.
   c. **Risk factors. Cumulative dose is the strongest predictor.** The overall incidence of congestive heart failure related to doxorubicin use is about 3% to 4%. The incidence is 1% to 2% for total doses of 300 mg/m^2, 3% to 5% for 400 mg/m^2, 5% to 8% for 450 mg/m^2, and 6% to 20% for 500 mg/m^2 and 25% for >550 mg/m^2. Other risk factors are as follows:
      (1) Age. Patients older than 65 and children are at higher risk. Among children, cardiotoxicity can be seen with lower cumulative doses.
      (2) Preexisting heart disease, peripheral vascular disease, hypertension, or diabetes mellitus.
      (3) Concurrent or prior chest RT (especially if >4,000 cGy); this factor is particularly important in women who received prior chest wall irradiation for left-sided breast cancer.
      (4) Concurrent treatment with other cardiotoxic chemotherapeutic drugs (especially trastuzumab, paclitaxel, docetaxel, or cyclophosphamide).
2. **Evaluation of cardiac injury.** Symptoms, physical findings, and ECG abnormalities (reduction of QRS voltage by 30%) occur too late to be helpful.
   a. **Endomyocardial biopsy** is the most specific method for determining anthracycline cardiotoxicity, although it is invasive and can be associated with complications.
   b. **Echocardiography and multigated radionuclide angiography** (MUGA) are noninvasive methods for determining LVEF. They should be obtained at baseline (although this is controversial), especially in patients with risk factors. Suggested intervals to repeat echocardiography are at 300 mg/m^2, 450 mg/m^2, and each 100 mg/m^2 thereafter. MUGA is preferred for patients with poor windows on echocardiography (e.g., obesity).
   c. **Cardiac MRI** may be useful in selected patients when the results of echocardiography and MUGA are suboptimal or conflicting.
   d. **Biomarkers,** such as troponins and brain natriuretic peptide (BNP), are of interest but have not been established as having a role in monitoring potential cardiotoxicity of anthracyclines.

3. Prevention

   a. Cumulative lifetime doses should be ≤450 to 500 mg/m^2 for doxorubicin and daunorubicin and <800 to 900 mg/m^2 for epirubicin. Some patients can tolerate higher cumulative doses.

   b. Results of surveillance during therapy. Baseline echocardiogram or MUGA should be obtained for all patients who are expected to receive ≥300 mg/m^2 of doxorubicin or daunorubicin or ≥240 mg/m^2 of epirubicin. Studies should be performed serially during (most commonly, it is done after cycle 4) and after treatment for an unspecified period of time; the patient should be considered at risk for the development of cardiomyopathy for years after treatment.

   The anthracycline should be discontinued if the patient develops clinical evidence of congestive heart failure or **if the LVEF decreases**

   (1) below 45% in adults and below 55% in children

   (2) by ≥10% to below the lower limit of normal

   (3) by 20% from any level

   c. Infusion rates. The development of cardiac toxicity is related to peak serum levels of doxorubicin. Weekly administration (20 mg/m^2) is associated with a lower incidence of cardiotoxicity when compared with monthly administration (60 mg/m^2). Continuous infusion over 24 to 96 hours through a central venous catheter also is less cardiotoxic than bolus administration.

   d. Liposomal anthracyclines (doxorubicin, daunorubicin) have efficacy in various malignancies (such as ovarian cancer, breast cancer, myeloma, and Kaposi sarcoma) and are associated with decreased risks of clinical and subclinical cardiac toxicity.

   e. Angiotensin-converting enzyme inhibitors, angiotensin II receptor blockers (ARBs), and beta-blockers (e.g., carvedilol) have been shown to protect against cardiotoxicity of anthracyclines in limited studies.

   f. Dexrazoxane is a cardioprotectant that can decrease the incidence and severity of cardiomyopathy, but some studies suggested that it can also decrease the response rate. Because of this observation, it should not be used in adults in the adjuvant setting. It can be used in patients with metastatic disease whose cumulative dose reached more than 300 mg/m^2.

E. Nonanthracycline chemotherapy–induced cardiotoxicity. Many chemotherapy agents have been associated with cardiotoxicity. The serious complications include vasospasm or vasoocclusion resulting in angina or myocardial infarction, arrhythmias, myocardial necrosis causing a dilated cardiomyopathy, and pericarditis.

1. Ischemic cardiotoxicity

   a. 5-Fluorouracil can cause cardiac ischemia with angina, hypotension, or congestive heart failure. The mechanism appears to be coronary artery vasospasm. The incidence of such toxicity is uncertain but has been reported to occur in 2% to 8% of patients, particularly when the drug is given by continuous intravenous infusion and when the patients have *a prior* history of cardiac disease. These manifestations are reversible when the drug is stopped; patients respond well to conventional cardiac treatments. However, the mortality rate is 2% to 15% in affected patients.

   b. Capecitabine therapy has been associated with observations similar to those with 5-fluorouracil; cardiac ischemia develops in 3% to 9% of patients.

2. **Mitoxantrone** has a similar structure to anthracyclines and it can cause a decrease in LVEF in 3% to 6% of patients and overt congestive heart failure in 1% to 3% of patients. This toxicity is related to cumulative dose and occurs in >10% of patients who receive >120 mg/m^2 or who have received prior doxorubicin. Mitoxantrone is also associated with a myocarditis–pericarditis syndrome.

3. **Monoclonal antibodies**

   a. **Trastuzumab** can cause decreased LVEF and, less commonly, congestive heart failure, particularly when used with anthracyclines. Cardiomyopathy develops in about 3% of patients with breast cancer treated with doxorubicin and cyclophosphamide followed by a taxane and trastuzumab. Trastuzumab-related cardiotoxicity is largely reversible in the majority of cases. Resumption of trastuzumab after resolution of cardiac abnormalities may be safe in some women.

      In the adjuvant setting, a baseline assessment prior to starting trastuzumab and serial LVEF monitoring are appropriate to screen for cardiac dysfunction. In the metastatic setting, the decision is more complex, given the clinical benefit provided by trastuzumab.

   b. **Bevacizumab.** Cardiovascular toxicity includes angina, myocardial infarction, heart failure, hypertension, stroke, and arterial thromboembolic events. When given as a single agent, left ventricular dysfunction can occur in 2% of patients. The risk of heart failure in those who receive concurrent anthracyclines may be as high as 14%, while those who had previously been treated with an anthracycline have an intermediate level of risk. Other antiangiogenic drugs (**aflibercept, ramucirumab**) are associated with an increased risk of thrombotic events.

   c. **Rituximab** is associated with arrhythmias or angina in <1% of infusions.

   d. **Alemtuzumab** is associated with a significant risk of heart failure and/ or arrhythmias.

4. **Tyrosine kinase inhibitors**

   a. **Imatinib.** Despite a theoretical causative factor via *bcr-abl*, significant heart failure occurs in <2% of patients with chronic myelogenous leukemia treated with imatinib. Left ventricular dysfunction has not been observed in patients receiving imatinib for the treatment of gastrointestinal stromal tumor.

   b. **Lapatinib.** Less than 2% of treated patients have experienced declines in LVEF, and these were usually asymptomatic.

   c. **Sunitinib and sorafenib** have been associated with a definite risk of cardiotoxicity. Sunitinib has been associated with a decline in LVEF in about 20% and clinical CHF in up to 10% of treated patients; cardiotoxicity was reversible and not associated with an adverse clinical outcome. Less data are available with sorafenib.

   d. **Nilotinib, dasatinib, and bosutinib** have been associated with QT prolongation and sudden death. Abnormalities in serum potassium and magnesium levels must be corrected prior to drug initiation. Other drugs that may affect the QT interval should be avoided. ECGs should be followed serially.

   e. **Vandetanib** is used mainly for treatment of medullary thyroid cancer. It has been associated with prolongation of the QT interval, torsades de pointes, and sudden death. Largely because of the cardiovascular risk, vandetanib is only available through a restricted distribution program.

   f. **Cobimetinib and trametinib** (MEK inhibitors) have been associated with a decreased LVEF and routine monitoring while on therapy is recommended.

    g. Axitinib, lenvatinib, pazopanib, and regorafenib (multikinase inhibitors, including VEGFR) can cause hypertension and increase the risk of thrombotic events.

    h. Ponatinib: 20% of patients developed severe thrombotic events, and 4% had serious decrease in LVEF.

    i. Ceritinib, crizotinib, osimertinib, and vemurafenib can cause QTc prolongation.

5. Alkylating agents

    a. Cyclophosphamide can potentiate doxorubicin-induced cardiotoxicity. When given in high doses, cyclophosphamide can cause myocardial necrosis and hemorrhagic myocarditis.

    b. Ifosfamide is associated with arrhythmias, ST–T-wave changes, and dose-related heart failure.

    c. Cisplatin has occasionally caused bradycardia, supraventricular tachycardia, bundle branch block, hypertension, ischemic cardiomyopathy, and congestive heart failure.

    d. Busulfan can cause endocardial fibrosis.

6. Taxanes may potentiate anthracycline-induced cardiomyopathy.

    a. Paclitaxel commonly results in asymptomatic bradycardia but can also occasionally cause conduction defects, cardiac ischemia, and ventricular tachycardia.

    b. Docetaxel occasionally causes pericardial effusion, but other cardiac events are rare.

7. Miscellaneous agents

    a. Cytarabine has caused pericarditis rarely.

    b. Bleomycin. Pericarditis is an uncommon but potentially serious complication associated with bleomycin. Coronary artery disease, myocardial ischemia, and myocardial infarction have been observed in young patients.

    c. Mitomycin C at cumulative doses >30 mg/m^2 has been associated with the development of heart failure. Cardiotoxicity may be additive if given with anthracyclines.

    d. Tretinoin (ATRA) can cause pericardial effusions, myocarditis, pericarditis, and, rarely, cardiac ischemia as part of the "retinoic acid syndrome." Similar events occur with **arsenic trioxide** when used to treat relapsed acute promyelocytic leukemia. Arsenic trioxide can also cause QT prolongation and arrhythmias and requires careful attention to potassium and magnesium levels when using.

8. Immunotherapy

    a. Interferon α has been associated with reversible cardiac dysfunction.

    b. Interleukin-2 causes capillary leak syndrome with hypotension and peripheral edema, but it can cause direct myocardiotoxicity.

    c. Ipilimumab. Rare cases of pericarditis have been described.

ACKNOWLEDGMENT

The author would like to acknowledge Dr. Dennis A. Casciato, who significantly contributed to earlier versions of this chapter.

Suggested Readings

Fagedet D, Thony F, Timsit JF, et al. Endovascular treatment of malignant superior vena cava syndrome: results and predictive factors of clinical efficacy. *Cardiovasc Intervent Radiol* 2013;36:140.

Heffner JE, Klein JS. Recent advances in the diagnosis and management of malignant pleural effusions. *Mayo Clin Proc* 2008;83:235.

McCurdy MT, Shanholtz CB. Oncologic emergencies. *Crit Care Med* 2012;40:2212.

Meadors M, Floyd J, Perry MC. Pulmonary toxicity of chemotherapy. *Semin Oncol* 2006;33:98.

Monsuez JJ, et al. Cardiac side-effects of cancer chemotherapy. *Int J Cardiol* 2010;144:3.

Movsas B, et al. Pulmonary radiation injury. *Chest* 1997;111:1061.

Quiros RM, Scott WJ. Surgical treatment of metastatic disease to the lung. *Semin Oncol* 2008;35:134.

Rice TW, Rodriguez RM, Light RW. The superior vena cava syndrome: clinical characteristics and evolving etiology. *Medicine (Baltimore)* 2006;85:37.

Silvestri F, et al. Metastases of the heart and pericardium. *G Ital Cardiol* 1997;27:1252.

Swain SM, Whaley FS, Ewer MS. Congestive heart failure in patients treated with doxorubicin: a retrospective analysis of three trials. *Cancer* 2003;97:2869.

Tan C, Sedrakyan A, Browne J, et al. The evidence on the effectiveness of management for malignant pleural effusion: a systematic review. *Eur J Cardiothorac Surg* 2006;29:829.

Torrisi JM, Schwartz LH, Gollub MJ, et al. CT findings of chemotherapy-induced toxicity: what radiologists need to know about the clinical and radiologic manifestations of chemotherapy toxicity. *Radiology* 2011;258:41.

Treasure T, Milošević M, Fiorentino F, et al. Pulmonary metastasectomy: what is the practice and where is the evidence for effectiveness? *Thorax* 2014;69:946.

Wilson LD, Detterbeck FC, Yahalom J. Clinical practice. Superior vena cava syndrome with malignant causes. *N Engl J Med* 2007;356:1862.

Zhang S, Liu X, Bawa-Khalfe T, et al. Identification of the molecular basis of doxorubicin-induced cardiotoxicity. *Nat Med* 2012;18:1639.

31 Abdominal Complications

Bartosz Chmielowski

I. GASTROINTESTINAL BLEEDING

A. Etiology

1. **Benign causes.** Gastrointestinal (GI) bleeding in patients with active cancer is usually caused by acute gastritis, peptic ulcer disease, esophagitis, Mallory-Weiss tears, esophageal varices, ischemic colitis, diverticular disease, or angiodysplasia; only 10% to 15% is caused by direct tumor bleeding.

2. **Malignant causes.** The most common malignant causes of upper GI bleeding are esophageal cancer, gastric cancer, gastric lymphoma, gastrointestinal stromal tumors (GISTs), and metastatic tumors involving the stomach. Lower GI bleeding is usually caused by colorectal cancer or metastatic cancer to the bowel (i.e., melanoma). In order to diagnose bleeding from the small bowel, patients may require enteroscopy or capsule endoscopy.

3. **Secondary to cancer treatments.** Bleeding is a common complication of radiation therapy (RT), that is, radiation esophagitis, enteritis, or proctitis. Chemotherapy can induce enteric mucositis. In addition, patients may suffer from superimposed infections (*Candida* or cytomegalovirus [CMV] esophagitis; *Clostridium difficile*, or gram-negative bacillus enteritis; or typhlitis). Antiangiogenic cancer medications (bevacizumab, sunitinib, sorafenib, pazopanib) increase the risk of bleeding and the risk of hemorrhagic complications during surgery.

4. **Secondary to supportive therapy in cancer patients.** Cancer patients may bleed from erosive esophagitis secondary to oral bisphosphonate or potassium chloride or erosive gastritis secondary to steroids or nonsteroidal anti-inflammatory drugs (NSAIDs).

B. Management.
The status of malignancy may influence the aggressiveness of the management. The bleeding is most commonly caused by benign causes, and it is frequently reversible. Therefore, aggressive management should be applied in all patients with good performance status.

Initially, patients are resuscitated with intravenous fluids and blood products, and then diagnostic efforts are concentrated on establishing the etiology. Surgical intervention is frequently required in cases of tumor bleeding; patients with persistent GI bleeding from unresectable tumors may be managed with RT. Long-term, successful systemic therapy against cancer is most helpful in the management of bleeding from the tumor.

II. BOWEL OBSTRUCTION

A. Etiology.
Bowel obstruction is defined by the inability of intestinal contents to traverse through the bowel and can be classified as complete or partial, and mechanical, or functional. In patients with a history of cancer, it is due to the original tumor or its metastases in 60% to 70% of cases. About 20% to 30% of patients have a benign cause of obstruction, and 10% to 20% have a new primary lesion. Duodenal obstruction is most commonly caused by cholangiocarcinoma, pancreatic carcinoma, and gallbladder carcinoma; distal bowel obstruction is secondary mainly to colon and ovarian cancer.

1. **Mechanisms** of bowel obstruction in malignancy include the following:
   a. External pressure on the intestine caused by mesenteric or omental masses.
   b. Obstructing masses in the bowel lumen.
   c. Intraluminal masses invading mucosa and impairing peristalsis (pseudo-obstruction).
   d. Invasion of the intestine's neural plexus, causing localized or diffuse ileus clinically indistinguishable from mechanical obstruction.
   e. Intussusception with certain tumors, notably melanoma.
   f. Pseudo-obstruction occurs in patients with peritoneal carcinomatosis in the absence of mechanical obstruction.
   g. Adhesions secondary to previous surgeries.
   h. Complications of RT or intraperitoneal chemotherapy.
   i. Use of cholinergic or sympathomimetic drugs (ileus, pseudo-obstruction).

2. **Differential diagnosis.** Diagnostic considerations in cancer patients include the following:
   a. **Vinca alkaloid neurotoxicity** may produce constipation. Particularly in elderly patients, paralytic ileus or decreased bowel tone may lead to high fecal impaction with bowel obstruction. Impaction is better prevented than treated.
   b. **Radiation injury of small bowel** (see Section VI.D) may be seen on small bowel radiographs or CT scan as mucosal effacement, ulcers, rigidity, narrowing, adhesions, bowel wall thickening, and bowel dilation.
   c. **Diverticulitis** may produce tightly narrowed areas in the distal colon that are often radiologically indistinguishable from constricting carcinoma. In the absence of metastatic disease elsewhere, these lesions must be resected regardless of coexistent tumor.
   d. **Other nonmalignant causes of ileus and obstruction** include adhesions, hernia, inflammatory bowel disease, volvulus, spontaneous intussusception, acute pancreatitis, and bowel infarction.

B. **Management of bowel obstruction caused by cancer.** The status of a patient's cancer should be always included in decision-making on the aggressive management of GI obstruction. Patients with terminal cancer benefit from the aggressive symptom management, but not from surgical intervention, parenteral nutrition, or long-term nasogastric (NG) tube placement.
   1. **Fluid resuscitation.** Intraluminal volume sequestration results in fluid depletion. In terminal patients, excessive hydration may worsen patient symptoms since it can increase intraluminal fluid secretion or lead to volume overload.
   2. **Decompression.** Patients with evidence of intestinal obstruction should have decompression by placement of an NG tube and intermittent suction. Complications of prolonged NG tube use include nasal erosion and sinusitis. The goal is to use decompression with other modalities listed later to minimize time with the NG tube. In refractory cases, venting gastrostomy/percutaneous endoscopic gastrostomy tube decompression is often the only palliative modality available when other measures fail.
   3. **Stents.** Expandable metallic stents have been used to treat obstruction in nearly all portions of the GI tract, including the esophagus, gastric outlet, duodenum, proximal jejunum, terminal ileum, colon, and rectum. Although stent placement requires a trained endoscopist or interventional radiologist, this procedure palliates obstruction in >80% of patients

and may obviate the need for surgery in patients who cannot be cured. Complication rates are low but include bleeding, stent migration, and tumor growth into stent.

4. **Surgical intervention.** A history of cancer or even the presence of active tumor is not necessarily a contraindication to surgery. About 75% of patients with a bowel obstruction resume normal bowel function after surgery. Function is maintained until death in 45% of patients. About 25% of these patients do not experience improvement of symptoms with surgery. Surgical intervention should be considered if the obstruction does not improve after 4 to 5 days of decompression.

5. **Other modalities of management**
   a. **Chemotherapy** may be tried in patients with obstruction caused by carcinomatosis. In some tumors, such as lymphomas treated with chemotherapy or GIST and melanomas treated with targeted therapy, symptomatic improvement is seen within days after starting the therapy.
   b. **RT** to relieve bowel obstruction may be beneficial in patients who have peritoneal carcinomatosis from ovarian carcinoma or extensive abdominal lymphoma that is resistant to chemotherapy. Targeted RT to a single obstructing lesion may also be helpful.
   c. **Treatment of preterminal patients with refractory obstruction caused by cancer**
      (1) **NG suction** is used to alleviate abdominal pain. Intravenous fluids are given to maintain hydration.
      (2) **Opioids** are given SC or IV for pain control; they are appropriate for continuous abdominal pain but can aggravate colic.
      (3) **Anticholinergic agents,** such as hyoscine butylbromide, 60 to 380 mg/d, or glycopyrrolate, may alleviate pain, especially colic, and can also reduce nausea and vomiting. Nausea and vomiting can be treated with various drugs.
      (4) **Phenothiazines** (prochlorperazine, promethazine, chlorpromazine) reduce nausea and vomiting.
      (5) **Metoclopramide** can have its place in patients with functional or partial bowel obstruction; it should not be used with anticholinergics or in patients with colic or complete bowel obstruction.
      (6) **Haloperidol,** 1 to 5 mg SC three times daily, is helpful in patients with nausea and delirium.
      (7) **Dexamethasone,** 6 to 16 mg/d parenterally, can help decrease edema and possibly help decrease obstructive symptoms.
      (8) **Octreotide,** 100 to 300 mg every 8 hours SC, is an effective drug that decreases GI secretions, decreases distention, and in many cases allows the NG tube to be taken out.
      (9) **Olanzapine,** in doses of 2.5 to 20 mg/d, can reduce vomiting in patients who failed other medications.

III. METASTASES TO THE LIVER AND BILIARY TRACT

A. **Incidence and pathology**
   1. **Liver.** The liver is a common site of metastases. Liver metastases account for more than half of the deaths in certain malignancies, such as colorectal cancer.
      a. **Liver commonly involved:** GI tract cancers (including carcinoids, pancreatic adenocarcinoma, and islet cell tumors), lung cancer, breast cancer, choriocarcinoma, melanoma, lymphomas, and leukemias

    b. Liver occasionally involved: carcinoma of the distal esophagus, kidney, prostate, endometrium, adrenal gland, and thyroid; testicular cancers, thymoma; angiosarcoma

    c. Liver rarely involved: carcinoma of the proximal esophagus, ovary, and skin; plasma cell myeloma; most sarcomas

  2. Extrahepatic biliary obstruction can occur from lymph node metastases in the porta hepatis, particularly from GI cancers and lung cancers (especially the small cell type).

B. Natural history. The clinical course of liver metastases depends on the tumor's behavior and responsiveness to chemotherapy. A liver that appreciably increases in size in <8 weeks is typical in small cell lung cancer and high-grade lymphoma; both of these tumors respond well to treatment. Rapid liver enlargement in patients with other tumor types is less common.

C. Diagnosis

  1. Symptoms and signs. Any combination of pain or discomfort in the right upper quadrant, weight loss, fatigue, anorexia, jaundice, or fever should raise the possibility of liver metastases, particularly in patients with a history of cancer. Symptoms are present in 65% of patients and hepatomegaly in 50% when liver metastases are discovered.

  2. Laboratory studies

    a. LFTs should be obtained in all patients suspected of having liver metastases. An elevation of the alkaline phosphatase level that is out of proportion to that of the transaminases suggests either a mass lesion or a biliary obstruction.

    b. Liver imaging is obtained in all patients with history, physical findings, or laboratory values suggestive of hepatic metastases. Hepatic CT or MRI scans are the most sensitive techniques. Ultrasound may be useful in determining whether a lesion is solid or fluid.

  3. Liver biopsy should be performed to confirm the presence and type of tumor in the following circumstances:

    a. There is no primary history of cancer, and the liver is the only obvious site of disease.

    b. There has been a long disease-free interval (>2 years) since the removal of the primary tumor.

    c. The liver abnormality is *not typical* of the natural history of the primary cancer and in any case when the results are likely to affect therapeutic decisions.

  4. Extrahepatic biliary obstruction. These patients must have special studies to exclude benign causes of obstruction, such as gallstones or bile duct strictures.

    a. CT scan of the liver is performed to look for parenchymal or porta hepatis masses and obstruction of the biliary tree.

    b. Percutaneous transhepatic cholangiogram or retrograde contrast study of the biliary tree is performed, depending on the availability of experienced radiologists and gastroenterologists.

    c. Magnetic resonance cholangiopancreatography (MRSCP) is a noninvasive method to evaluate the biliary treat and pancreatic ducts, and it is accurate in 95% of cases provided the patient complies with the exam.

    d. Laparotomy is indicated for both definitive diagnosis and treatment if the other studies suggest extrahepatic obstruction and if other sites of tumor are well controlled or not evident.

D. Management

1. **Surgery**

   a. **Resection of hepatic metastases** has been used in highly selected patients and should be considered, especially in patients with colon cancer and metastasis only to the liver. Modern anatomic techniques have decreased surgical mortality to <6%. Overall, in properly selected patients (those with four or fewer metastases, absence of disease outside the liver, and good performance status), 20% to 40% of patients survive 5 years. Success is greater in patients with slow-growing tumors and with a disease-free interval of >1 year.

   b. **Extrahepatic biliary tract obstruction** may be decompressed surgically if pruritus is severe. Jaundice *per se* is generally not an indication for surgery unless the patient must have a laparotomy for diagnosis.

      (1) **Percutaneous drainage** through internal or external catheter placement offers reasonable palliation. Drainage is achieved in 60% to 85% of cases. The most frequent complication is cholangitis, which appears to relate to multiple sites of obstruction or inadequate drainage. Further intervention with tube manipulation, tube replacement, or surgery is required in 20% to 75% of patients. The success rate for palliation is about 80%, similar to that achieved with cholecystojejunostomy.

      (2) **Endoscopic placement of prostheses** is another option that is successful in about 80% of patients. Cholangitis from inadequate drainage results in a 2% to 5% mortality rate. Morbidity rates are similar to those associated with percutaneous procedures. Drainage is internal and more convenient for patients.

2. **RT** in low doses (<2,400 cGy) is useful to palliate refractory pain from liver metastases. RT to portal masses may relieve biliary tract obstruction. External-beam therapy is best suited for patients with a good performance status, bilirubin <1.5 mg/dL, and no extrahepatic metastasis. Stereotactic radiosurgery is effective when a limited number of metastases are present.

3. **Chemotherapy**

   a. **Oral and IV chemotherapy** is useful for treating responsive tumors. The primary tumor determines the selection of drugs. Dexamethasone (4 mg PO, IV, or SC twice daily) can reduce pain due to distention and inflammation of the hepatic capsule.

   b. **Direct perfusion of chemotherapy** into the liver through hepatic artery cannulation is used by some physicians to treat isolated liver metastases. The benefit remains unclear, and since systemic therapies improved significantly, it is used rarely.

4. **Transarterial chemoembolization (TACE)** is a treatment method in which a chemotherapeutic agent is injected into the hepatic artery (or its branch) followed by embolization with a procoagulant. The method relies on the observation that the tumor gets blood supply through the hepatic artery, and the liver uses both the hepatic artery and the portal vein. It is used commonly in patients with hepatocellular carcinoma, but it can be used in other tumors with a small number of liver metastases, for example, uveal melanoma.

5. **Other options** for hepatic metastases include radiofrequency ablation, cryoablation, and alcohol instillation.

IV. CANCER-ASSOCIATED ASCITES

A. Pathogenesis

1. **Peritoneal carcinomatosis** with malignant ascites but without liver metastasis is most often caused by ovarian and bladder cancer and mesothelioma. Malignant ascites in colon, gastric, and biliary tract carcinomas is usually accompanied by liver metastasis. The most common extra-abdominal malignancies to produce peritoneal carcinomatosis include breast and lung carcinomas. Malignant ascites is caused by increased production of fluid induced by the tumor, increased vessel permeability, and marked neovascularization of the peritoneum.

2. **Massive liver metastasis**

3. **Hepatocellular carcinoma in a patient with cirrhosis** is seen in patients with chronic hepatitis B, chronic hepatitis C, and alcoholic cirrhosis.

4. **Chylous ascites** may result from obstruction or rupture of the major abdominal lymphatic passages. It is usually caused by lymphoma.

5. **Occlusion of the hepatic veins (Budd-Chiari syndrome)** is seen in patients with hyperviscosity states, particularly polycythemia vera. Patients with hepatic venous obstruction have large, tender livers, and rapidly evolving ascites.

6. **Peritonitis** caused by *Streptococcus bovis* may be a presenting feature for right-sided colon carcinoma. Ascites from any cause may become infected.

B. Diagnosis

1. **Differential diagnosis of ascites.** Neoplastic diseases that cause ascites include liver metastases, peritoneal metastases, pseudomyxoma peritonei, and primary mesothelioma. The etiologies of ascites can be best classified by the serum–ascites albumin gradient, which is the difference between serum and ascitic fluid albumin concentration (Table 31-1). This gradient predicts the presence or absence of portal hypertension and, in parallel, the responsiveness to treatment with diuretics.

2. **Paracentesis** should be done in all patients with presumed malignant ascites for diagnosis and to rule out complicating infections. Ascites from carcinomatosis is usually exudative and often bloody. Ascitic fluid should be studied for the following:

   a. **Appearance.** Clear fluid is seen in patients with cirrhosis and liver metastasis; turbid/cloudy fluid is caused by the increased number of cells secondary to peritoneal carcinomatosis; milky fluid is typical for chylous ascites; pink/bloody ascites is secondary to the increased number of red blood cells in the fluid.

   b. **Culture** for bacteria (including acid-fast bacilli) and fungi.

   c. **Albumin** should be measured to calculate the gradient.

TABLE 31-1	Serum–Ascites Albumin Gradient
High Albumin Gradient (≥1.1 g/dL; Portal Hypertension Likely)	**Low Albumin Gradient (<1.1 g/dL; Portal Hypertension Unlikely)**
Massive hepatic metastases	Peritoneal carcinoma
Chronic liver disease	Peritoneal inflammation (fungal, tuberculous, vasculitic)
Hepatic vein obstruction (Budd-Chiari syndrome)	Oncotic ascites secondary to hypoalbuminemia
Hepatic sinusoidal obstruction syndrome	Pancreatitis
Cardiac failure	Idiopathic
Hemodialysis with fluid overload	

  d. Exudates are associated with total protein values >2.5 g/dL, white blood cell count >250/mL (lymphocytosis suggests tuberculous peritonitis), and a lactate dehydrogenase level >50% of serum values.

  e. Values in ascitic fluid significantly greater than in serum of **amylase or triglyceride** indicate a pancreatic etiology or chylous content, respectively.

  f. Glucose level is often <60 mg/dL in carcinomatosis.

  g. Cytology is positive in more than half of the cases of peritoneal carcinomatosis.

C. Management. Treatment of the primary cancer with the effective therapy (cytoreductive surgery may be used in patients with ovarian cancer) is the most important. Otherwise, management of malignant ascites is principally directed toward the palliation of symptoms.

 1. Diuretics, such as furosemide and spironolactone, may be tried but are unlikely to be effective for ascites from peritoneal carcinomatosis. Diuretics may be beneficial for patients with a high albumin gradient.

 2. Large-volume paracentesis is reserved for patients with symptoms of shortness of breath, anorexia, early satiety, nausea, vomiting, or pain. A 14- to 16-gauge plastic catheter or a peritoneal dialysis catheter can be used; the latter is preferred for removing a large volume of fluid. A single suture should hold the catheter in place.

  a. Removal of large volumes of peritoneal fluid should not be done if a hepatic cause, such as cirrhosis or Budd-Chiari syndrome, is suspected.

  b. If cancer is suspected, as much fluid as possible should be removed. Removal of large volumes of ascites fluid that is a result of peritoneal carcinomatosis does not usually cause dangerous fluid shifts.

 3. Systemic chemotherapy is the treatment of choice for responsive tumors. The addition of bevacizumab, an antiangiogenic drug, may be especially important in women with ovarian cancer complicated by ascites.

 4. Intraperitoneal chemotherapy. Instillation of chemotherapy directly into the abdomen may control some malignant effusions. First, the maximum volume of ascites is removed, preferably using a peritoneal dialysis catheter. The chosen drug is dissolved in 100 mL of normal saline, injected into the catheter, and followed by another 100 mL of normal saline for flushing. The patient's position is shifted every few minutes for an hour to disperse the drug. If treatment is effective, the dose may be repeated at intervals. Fever or abdominal pain or tenderness may develop after the procedure, may persist for up to 1 week, and may require paracentesis to confirm that the peritonitis is sterile.

  a. Effective agents include cisplatin, paclitaxel, rituximab, mitomycin C, thiotepa, bleomycin, 5-fluorouracil, and bevacizumab. Hyperthermic intraperitoneal chemotherapy (HIPC) is sometimes used perioperatively in patients with peritoneal carcinomatosis.

 5. Peritoneovenous shunts (LeVeen and Denver) may be used to treat refractory cases if the patient has a life expectancy of >1 month and does not have significant cardiac or renal disease or disseminated intravascular coagulation (DIC). The ascitic fluid should not be hemorrhagic, infected, or loculated, and it should not contain large numbers of malignant cells. Complications of these shunts include primary fibrinolysis or clinically silent DIC (nearly 100%), sepsis (20%), pulmonary edema (15%), pulmonary emboli (10%), upper GI bleeding, fever without sepsis, superior vena cava thrombosis, pneumonia, shunt displacement, seromas around the catheter (10%), and neoplastic seeding to the superior vena cava on adjacent subcutaneous tissues. Thrombocytopenia is caused by both DIC and hemodilution. There is no evidence that shunts improve quality of life.

6. **Pseudomyxoma peritonei.** Mucinous adenocarcinomas, benign mucin-producing tumors, and appendiceal mucoceles can produce abundant gelatinous material that is impossible to remove by paracentesis. Recurrent bowel obstruction and progressive ascites develop. Laparotomy with removal of as much of the jellylike substance as possible is indicated. The procedure may be repeated if there is recurrence, depending on the changing anatomy and formation of adhesions.

V. PANCREATITIS AND METASTASES TO THE PANCREAS

A. **Etiology.** Pancreatitis in patients with cancer is most commonly caused by the same conditions as in the general population (namely, gallstones and alcohol consumption), but hypertriglyceridemia and hypercalcemia may also contribute. Less commonly, it can be caused by malignancy itself, drugs, or iatrogenic injury.

Acute pancreatitis occurs in up to 16% of patients treated with L-asparaginase. It has been described also in patients treated with cytarabine, cisplatin, methotrexate, cyclophosphamide, doxorubicin, ifosfamide, and steroids. Tyrosine kinase inhibitors (sorafenib, sunitinib, pazopanib, and others) can frequently cause asymptomatic elevation of lipase, but overt pancreatitis is seen in fewer than 1% of patients.

The list of procedures that can be complicated by pancreatitis includes ERCP and TACE of the liver. Small cell lung cancer metastasizes to the pancreas most commonly, but pancreatic metastasis of lymphoma, melanoma, and carcinomas of the breast, colon, and kidney also has been described.

Recently, chronic autoimmune pancreatitis has been identified that is associated with tissue infiltration by IgG4-positive plasma cells and increased levels of IgG4 in serum. This condition is treated with corticosteroids.

B. **Diagnosis** of pancreatitis depends on signs and laboratory findings. Blood work shows elevation of lipase and amylase, frequently accompanied by leukocytosis, hypo- or hyperglycemia, and hypocalcemia. CT scan of the abdomen is the best technique to demonstrate a mass in the pancreas.

C. **Management.** Pancreatitis complicating metastatic cancer should be treated with bowel rest, intravenous fluids, and analgesics. It is also important to remove the offending drug if possible. Severe pancreatitis can be complicated by systemic inflammatory response syndrome (SIRS), and patients may require support with vasopressors and mechanic ventilation.

VI. ADVERSE EFFECTS OF RADIATION TO THE LIVER AND ALIMENTARY CANAL

A. **Radiation-induced liver disease (RILD).** The liver is not able to tolerate high doses of radiation. About 5% of patients treated with the whole-liver doses of 30 to 35 cGy develop RILD. Therefore, RT has a limited function in the treatment of hepatic metastasis. Acute hepatitis from radiation can be mild to severe and may result in cirrhosis.

1. **Manifestations.** Signs and symptoms become evident 2 weeks to 3 months after irradiation. Patients present with anicteric hepatomegaly, ascites, and elevation of liver enzymes. Alkaline phosphatase is usually elevated more than transaminases. Liver biopsy demonstrates endophlebitis with thickening and obstruction of central veins and mild cellular necrosis or atrophy, findings similar to those seen with veno-occlusive disease (VOD) induced by chemotherapy (see Section VII below).

2. **Management** is symptomatic. Corticosteroids and diuretics may help.

B. **Radiation esophagitis**

1. **Acute esophagitis** usually occurs within 2 to 3 weeks from the initiation of RT and presents with dysphagia, odynophagia, and mediastinal discomfort. Concomitant administration of chemotherapy increases the risk of esophagitis. These patients are treated with viscous lidocaine solution, analgesics (opioids, NSAIDs), proton-pump inhibitors, and promotility agents (metoclopramide). When symptoms occur, patients are advised to eat small, frequent, bland meals; the food frequently must be pureed. Occasionally, nutritional supplementation may be required through a gastrostomy tube.

2. **Esophageal stricture** is a rare late complication that is more common when chemotherapy is given concomitantly. Dilation is performed in patients with symptoms. Antiacids and promotility agents are usually prescribed to decrease the risk of restenosis.

C. **Radiation gastritis**

1. **Acute radiation gastritis.** Symptoms can begin as early as 24 hours after starting the treatment. It usually presents with anorexia, nausea, vomiting, and abdominal pain. Occasionally, it can be complicated by development of a gastric ulcer.

2. **Late radiation gastritis** presents as chronic atrophic gastritis, dyspepsia, or ulcerative gastritis. These patients are treated with proton-pump inhibitors, H_2 blockers, or sucralfate.

D. **Radiation enteritis**

1. **Acute radiation enteritis**

   a. **Manifestations** are usually related to the volume of the bowel irradiated and to the daily dose. Most injuries involve the terminal ileum. Patients treated with concomitant chemotherapy (oxaliplatin, irinotecan) or EGFR-blocking antibodies (cetuximab, panitumumab) are at higher risk for radiation enteritis.

      (1) Nausea, vomiting, and anorexia usually do not persist >3 days after RT is stopped.

      (2) Diarrhea is more severe in patients who have had laparotomies and have developed adhesions. Symptoms can occur after the 2nd week of RT and usually disappear within 2 weeks after its completion.

   b. **Management**

      (1) **Antiemetics**, mainly 5-HT3 receptor antagonists, are given regularly throughout the day for patients with persistent vomiting. If symptoms are severe, parenteral hyperalimentation and reduction of the daily dose of radiation may be necessary.

      (2) **Diarrhea** is managed by eliminating alcoholic beverages, roughage, and milk products from the diet. Paregoric (tincture of opium), cholestyramine, or diphenoxylate–atropine may be useful.

2. **Chronic radiation enteritis.** Abdominal pain syndromes, malabsorption, bowel strictures, hemorrhage, perforations, and fistulas usually occur with doses to the abdomen of >4,500 cGy and are more frequent in the presence of postsurgical adhesions. Symptoms may develop months to many years after completion of therapy. Parenteral hyperalimentation may be necessary while the bowel abnormality is being corrected.

   a. **Abdominal pain syndromes** are treated with analgesics, bulk laxatives, and dietary modifications.

   b. **Perforations and fistulas** indicate a poorer prognosis than strictures and hemorrhage; malignancy recurs in 70% of these patients.

c. **Bowel obstruction.** Tube decompression may lead to resolution. Laparotomy should be avoided if possible. If the obstruction progresses, intestinal bypass (10% mortality rate) rather than bowel resection should be performed in the absence of gangrenous bowel (75% mortality rate).

d. **Chronic diarrhea** with malabsorption is rare and is treated symptomatically. Anorexia, nausea, and vomiting may occur. Medium-chain triglycerides may be of help to decrease stool fat loss and to relieve radiation-induced intestinal lymphangiectasia with protein loss. Steatorrhea may result from bacterial overgrowth; tetracycline, 250 mg given four times daily, may be tried for 10 to 14 days on an empiric basis. Prednisone and sulfasalazine may also be used.

E. **Radiation proctitis** is most commonly seen as a complication of the treatment of prostate cancer, but it can also occur in patients with anal, rectal, cervical, uterine, urinary bladder, and testicular cancers.

1. **Acute transient proctitis**

a. **Manifestations.** Tenesmus, diarrhea, and, occasionally, minor bleeding develop. Symptoms usually resolve soon after RT is completed.

b. **Management** is usually not indicated. If symptoms are prolonged or severe, steroid enemas and suppositories, stool softeners, mineral oil, low-residue diet, paregoric, diphenoxylate–atropine, rectal sucralfate, hyperbaric oxygen, and metronidazole may be helpful.

2. **Late radiation proctitis** usually occurs 6 months to 2 years after RT, but occasionally it can develop many years after treatment.

a. **Manifestations.** Symptoms include tenesmus, diarrhea, and hematochezia. Proctoscopic examination reveals hemorrhagic, edematous mucosa with decreased pliability, and, occasionally, ulcers.

b. **Management**

(1) **For severe inflammation,** treat as described for acute proctitis.

(2) **For rectal ulcers** refractory to conservative management, surgery is advised.

(3) **For late rectal narrowing,** treat with dilation and stool softeners.

VII. HEPATIC SINUSOIDAL OBSTRUCTION SYNDROME

Sinusoidal obstruction syndrome (SOS) was previously known as veno-occlusive disease. Hepatic SOS is a nonthrombotic obliterative process of the central or sublobular hepatic veins characterized by rapid onset of hyperbilirubinemia, ascites, and painful hepatomegaly and by varied clinical outcome.

A. **Causes**

1. The hepatotoxic pyrrolizidine alkaloids that occur naturally in plants (other implicated dietary contaminants include aflatoxin and nitrosamines) are the most common cause worldwide. Chemotherapy and irradiation, especially in patients who have had bone marrow, liver, or kidney transplantation and graft versus host disease, are important causes in the Western world.

2. Virtually any high-dose chemotherapeutic regimen can cause hepatic SOS. Azathioprine, 6-mercaptopurine, 6-thioguanine, and dacarbazine have been implicated as causes of hepatic vascular damage.

3. Other causes include postnecrotic cirrhosis, metastatic or primary hepatic malignancy, myeloproliferative disorders (particularly polycythemia vera), and a variety of other hypercoagulable states.

B. **Diagnosis.** The diagnosis of hepatic SOS is suggested by a typical clinical picture in a patient with risk factors. The reversal of flow in the portal vein by Doppler ultrasound is frequently seen. Liver biopsy can be helpful in establishing the diagnosis but is performed rarely. The transvenous approach is useful for patients with thrombocytopenia.

C. **Management**

1. **Supportive care** is indicated because most patients recover (70%). Management of fluid balance and diuretics is useful. In those with severe SOS, modalities such as dialysis and mechanical ventilation have little impact on outcome, and the continued use of these modalities will have to be discussed based on the overall prognosis of the patient.

2. **Defibrotide** is a polydeoxyribonucleotide characterized by antithrombotic, fibrinolytic, and angiogenic activity. The study of defibrotide in patients with severe SOS after hematopoietic stem cell transplantation showed responses in 36% to 55% of patients. Historically, resolution was seen only in 9% of patients. Defibrotide is approved for patients with hepatic SOS with renal or pulmonary dysfunction.

3. **Liver transplant** for severe SOS has been tried in patients where the underlying disease has a good chance of being cured with cytoreductive therapy.

4. **Other surgical procedures,** such as peritoneovenous or intrahepatic shunts, have had variable outcomes with SOS.

5. **Ursodeoxycholic acid** in divided doses of 600 to 900 mg a day is used in some transplant centers as SOS prophylaxis.

VIII. COMPLICATIONS OF IMMUNOTHERAPY

The treatment with CTLA4-blocking antibodies (ipilimumab) or PD-1-blocking antibodies (pembrolizumab, nivolumab) can be associated with the development of unique immune-mediated adverse events that can occasionally be life threatening or fatal.

A. **Diarrhea** with or without symptomatic **enterocolitis** (fever, cramps, abdominal tenderness). Severe diarrhea/colitis is seen in 5% to 7% of patients treated with ipilimumab, 2% to 4% treated with nivolumab or pembrolizumab, and 26% treated with combination of ipilimumab and nivolumab.

B. **Hepatitis** presenting as AST, ALT, bilirubin level elevation. It can be accompanied by nausea, vomiting, fatigue, and jaundice. Severe hepatitis is seen in 1% to 2% of patients treated with ipilimumab, 1% treated with nivolumab or pembrolizumab, and 13% treated with combination of ipilimumab and nivolumab.

C. **Autoimmune pancreatitis** presents with endocrine pancreatic insufficiency (insulin-dependent diabetes) and exocrine insufficiency (malabsorption, diarrhea). It is seen in fewer than 1% of patients. Asymptomatic lipase elevation can be seen in 9% to 20% of patients. These patients are treated with replacement insulin, pancreatic enzymes. It is unclear if high-dose steroids can reverse the process.

D. **Management.** When mild symptoms/signs are present, for example, fewer than four bowel movements a day, elevation of liver enzymes <2.5 times of the upper limit of normal, the therapy can be continued. As the side effects worsen, the therapy should be stopped and the treatment with steroids must be started at the dose of 0.5 to 2 mg/kg of prednisone or its equivalent. Patients who are acutely ill may require intravenous steroids. Other medications may be also helpful if there is no response to steroids such as infliximab 5 mg/kg once for colitis or mycophenolate mofetil 1 g twice a day for hepatitis. Antidiarrheals and hydration should be started early.

    The early initiation of steroids leads to a faster resolution of symptoms. After the side effects have resolved, steroids should be tapered slowly, generally over a period of 4 weeks. Antifungal and PCP prophylaxis should be considered while high-dose steroids are administered.

Suggested Readings

Adam RA, Adam YG. Malignant ascites: past, present and future. *J Am Coll Surg* 2004;198(6):999.

Barish MA, Yucel EK, Ferrucci JT. Magnetic resonance cholangiopancreatography. *N Engl J Med* 1999;341:258.

Clark K, Smith JM, Currow DC. The prevalence of bowel problems reported in a palliative care population. *J Pain Symptom Manage* 2012;43:993.

Dawson LA, Ten Haken RK. Partial volume tolerance of the liver to radiation. *Semin Radiat Oncol* 2005;15(4):279.

Imbesi JJ, Kurtz RC. A multidisciplinary approach to gastrointestinal bleeding in cancer patients. *J Support Oncol* 2005;3(2):101.

Lawrence TS, Robertson JM, Anscher MS, et al. Hepatic toxicity resulting from cancer treatment. *Int J Radiat Oncol Biol Phys* 1995;31:1237.

Parikh AA, et al. Radiofrequency ablation of hepatic metastasis. *Semin Oncol* 2002;29:168.

Rubbia-Brandt L. Sinusoidal obstruction syndrome. *Clin Liver Dis* 2010;14(4):651.

Sasson AR, Sigurdson FR. Surgical treatment of metastasis. *Semin Oncol* 2002;29:107.

Shadad AK, Sullivan FJ, Martin JD, et al. Gastrointestinal radiation injury: symptoms, risk factors and mechanisms. *World J Gastroenterol* 2013;19:185.

Soriano A, Davis MP. Malignant bowel obstruction: individualized treatment near the end of life. *Cleve Clin J Med* 2011;78(3):197.

Sussman-Schnoll F, Kurtz RC. Gastrointestinal emergencies in the critically ill cancer patient. *Semin Oncol* 2000;27:270.

32 Renal Complications

Sandy T. Liu and Alexandra Drakaki

I. OVERVIEW

Acute kidney injury (AKI) syndrome is a constellation of worsening renal function, electrolyte, acid–base changes, and changes in fluid and volume status. The three categories of AKI syndrome are **prerenal failure, direct renal tubular damage** (acute tubular necrosis [ATN], tubulointerstitial nephritis, acute glomerulonephritis), and **postrenal failure** (obstruction of the renal and urinary collecting system).

The renal failure may be due to direct or indirect consequences of the tumor, anticancer therapy, immunosuppression, infectious complications, and antibiotic use, as well as contrast use in diagnostic tests. A careful and thorough history, physical examination, and appropriate diagnostic tests including kidney ultrasound, urinalysis, and 24-hour urine collection are the first steps for the initial workup.

II. PRERENAL FAILURE

A. **Pathogenesis.** Decreased effective circulating volume (ECV, i.e., from vomiting, diarrhea, blood loss) provides a physiologic stimulus for metabolic and biochemical changes, which lead to reduced renal blood flow and glomerular filtration rate (GFR). Furthermore, patients with decreased ECV have a baroreceptor-mediated stimulus for increased secretion of antidiuretic hormone (ADH), diminished renal blood flow, and physiologically increased circulating levels of renin, angiotensin II, and aldosterone. The combined effects of decreased renal blood flow and increased levels of ADH, angiotensin II, and aldosterone result in excretion of a low urine volume that is highly concentrated (elevated urine specific gravity and osmolality), contains little sodium, and often contains large amounts of potassium (the potassium can be variable and is typically not used as a diagnostic test). The body is trying to maintain blood pressure and hemodynamic stability at the expense of renal function. Table 32-1 shows laboratory values that distinguish prerenal failure from renal failure in oliguric patients.

1. **Decreased GFR** leads to retention of urea (along with sodium) and creatinine.

2. **The serum creatinine level** is primarily reflective of muscle mass and GFR, when in a "stable state." Elderly patients and poorly nourished patients with less muscle mass have a relatively low serum creatinine. Because of this, an important clinical pearl/caveat is that serum creatinine levels may still be in the "normal lab range," yet GFR may have dropped significantly.

3. **BUN** is a metabolic waste product of protein intake, produced within the liver and excreted by the kidney. Although AKI will lead to increases in creatinine and BUN, a lower protein intake and/or diminished liver function, and cachexia with muscle wasting may result in BUN levels that may not be as elevated. Conversely, high protein intake, significant catabolic states, blood in the gastrointestinal tract, and severe prerenal states may result in BUN levels that are dramatically elevated in relation to the serum creatinine.

TABLE 32-1	Distinguishing Prerenal from Renal Causes of Azotemia	
Characteristic	**Prerenal**	**Renal**
Fractional excretion of sodium: $FE_{Na} = [(U_{Na} \times S_{creat}) \div (S_{Na} \times U_{creat})] \times 100$	≤1%	≥2%
U_{Na}	<15 mEq/L	>30 mEq/L
U_{creat}: S_{creat} ratio	>40	<20
BUN: S_{creat} ratio	>20	<20
Response to fluid or loop diuretics	Positive	Negative

FE, fractional excretion; U, concentration in urine; S, concentration in serum; Na, sodium; creat, creatinine; BUN, blood urea nitrogen.

B. Causes of prerenal failure. Table 32-2 shows general causes of prerenal failure with specific factors that may predispose patients with malignancies to prerenal failure.

C. Diagnosis. The medical history could guide identifying the possible causes of increased fluid loss (e.g., diarrhea, vomiting, bleeding) or of sequestration (e.g., pleural effusions, ascites, edema, "third spacing," retroperitoneal hemorrhage, congestive heart failure). The physical examination is of paramount importance in assessing volume status and finding clues to the pathogenesis of aberrations, as follows:

    1. Hypotension is recognized with a supine systolic blood pressure (BP) of <90 mm Hg. Changes in hemodynamic parameters (orthostatic changes) are recognized by a drop in systolic BP of 20 mm Hg or in diastolic BP of

TABLE 32-2	Cause of Decreased Effective Circulating Volume and Prerenal Failure in Patients with Malignancies
General Cause	**Predisposing Factors in Patients with Malignancies**
Hypovolemia	
Decreased intake	Anorexia from malignancy or chemotherapy, intercurrent illness, obtundation, neglect
Increased loss	
Vomiting	Intestinal obstruction, chemotherapy
Diarrhea	Enteral hyperalimentation, carcinoid, VIPoma, chemotherapy, antibiotic-associated
Blood loss	Tumor- or chemotherapy-related
Renal	
Diabetes insipidus (DI)	Primary pineal tumor, craniopharyngioma, metastasis (breast cancer)
Nephrogenic DI	Chronic renal insufficiency, myeloma kidney, lithium, demeclocycline, nephrocalcinosis
Osmotic diuresis	Hypercalcemia, hyperglycemia
Hypoalbuminemia	Poor nutrition, severe liver disease, nephrotic syndrome
Intra- and Extravascular Shifts	
Congestive heart failure, low cardiac output	Malignant pericardial effusion, radiation-induced pericarditis or myocarditis
Sepsis, shock	Lymphoma, leukemia, myeloma, neutropenia due to chemotherapy
Decreased Renal Blood Flow per se	
Renal artery obstruction	
Intrinsic	Renal artery stenosis, atheroemboli
Extrinsic	Tumor (rare)
Hepatorenal syndrome	Hepatic metastases
Drugs	ACE inhibitors, angiotensin receptor blockers, cyclosporine, tacrolimus, NSAIDs

10 mm Hg and increased heart rate (10 to 20 beats/min) when moving the patient from the supine to sitting or standing positions. These findings are suggestive of intravascular volume depletion and thus low ECV. Medications that affect blood pressure (antihypertensives) and heart rate (beta-blockers and calcium channel blockers) should be taken into account and be associated with more modest changes in these hemodynamic parameters.

2. **Flat neck veins** in the supine position suggest volume depletion.

3. **Obstruction: In patients without obvious volume depletion,** careful palpation and percussion of the bladder, rectal examination of the prostate of male patients, and pelvic examination in female patients may divert attention to an obstructive cause.

D. **Management of prerenal failure** is to correct the underlying cause and, when possible, to restore ECV to normal.

1. **Hypovolemic patients** usually require large volumes of crystalloids (i.e., 0.9% sodium chloride with or without glucose) or colloidal solutions (i.e., albumin). Although albumin solutions specifically increase intravascular volume, they are expensive, and the effect is often transient.

2. **Reversible renal failure** is diagnostic of prerenal failure and often not known until after a therapeutic trial and repeat blood and urine testing. If not treated effectively or completely, prerenal failure can lead to more significant kidney damage and ATN.

III. POSTRENAL FAILURE: OBSTRUCTIVE UROPATHY

A. **Pathogenesis**

1. **Ureteral obstruction.** Uremia may be caused by bilateral obstruction (or unilateral obstruction in the case of a single functioning kidney) as a result of the following:

   a. Bladder tumors and tumors of the collecting systems.

   b. Uterine tumors, especially carcinoma of the cervix.

   c. Retroperitoneal tumors (rare), including lymphoma, sarcomas, and metastatic tumors.

   d. Intrinsic renal tumors (rare).

   e. Retroperitoneal fibrosis, including that induced by irradiation, drugs (busulfan), carcinoid tumors (especially rectal), Gardner syndrome (familial colorectal polyposis), or desmoplastic reactions to metastases.

   f. Blood clots within the collecting system or bladder from bleeding.

   g. Renal papillary necrosis (RPN).

   h. Nephrolithiasis.

   i. Stone and/or crystal accumulations from high production or excretion of uric acid.

   j. Some medications could crystallize from supersaturation of the agent and become the primary component of stones. Drugs that induce calculi include magnesium trisilicate, ciprofloxacin, sulfa medications, triamterene, indinavir, and ephedrine.

2. **Outlet obstruction of the urethra.** Causes include primary cancer of the prostate, urethra, cervix, ovary, bladder, or endometrium. Metastases from the lung, gastrointestinal tract, breast, and melanoma to the pelvic organs, prostate, or urethra are rare causes of this complication.

B. **Diagnosis**

1. **Symptoms** are often absent or insidious in onset. Anuria is highly suggestive, but partial high-grade obstruction of ureters can occasionally cause renal failure with a normal urine volume. A variable urine output or overflow incontinence causing dribbling suggests bladder outlet obstruction.

2. **Physical findings** are those of the underlying disease. Dullness to percussion in the suprapubic region suggests a mass or distended bladder.

3. **Ultrasonography** may show hydronephrosis. However, acute obstruction or chronic obstruction wherein the collecting system is encased in tumor may show minimal abnormalities. A normal-appearing but full collecting system in an oliguric patient suggests obstruction. Blockage of only one kidney may be less severe. In some cases, ultrasound may miss obstruction, especially when ECV and urine volume are low.

4. **Postvoid residual urine** determination is often useful in evaluating for outlet obstruction from urethral swelling, stenosis, or scarring; benign prostatic hypertrophy in the male; or an ovarian mass in the female patient. In such patients, insertion of a Foley catheter should be performed along with ultrasonography. Computed tomography (CT) scan of the pelvis may also be useful diagnostically, although intravenous dye should be avoided as it can be nephrotoxic, especially in the patient with a low ECV.

5. **Cystoscopy** could demonstrate bladder outlet obstruction, show the extent of bladder tumors, and permit retrograde ureterography, which may demonstrate ureteral stenosis or blockage of the ureterovesicular junction.

C. **Management**

1. **Obstruction of the urinary tract** could be accompanied by infection and in some cases renal calculi. Obstruction is a medical emergency requiring immediate diagnosis, treatment, and management. As in prerenal failure, postrenal obstruction, if not corrected, can lead to ARF syndrome and is also a cause of CKD.

2. **Stones** may pass spontaneously or can be removed by shock lithotripsy or by one of several available urologic procedures.

3. **Blood clots** in the collecting system will lyse spontaneously; larger clots in the bladder should be removed by continuous bladder irrigation and/or cystoscopy.

4. **Retroperitoneal fibrosis** may be treated by percutaneous nephrostomies or by surgical release of the involved ureters.

5. **Obstructing lymphomas** are usually successfully managed with chemotherapy, with or without focal radiation therapy.

6. **Solid tumors**. Most patients with pelvic tumors causing obstruction are at an advanced stage of disease; therapy, including percutaneous drainage of the renal pelvis, must be carefully considered in light of the potential for palliation, the extent of disease, and the overall prognosis.

IV. DIRECT RENAL TUBULAR DAMAGE CAUSING RENAL FAILURE

A. **Acute kidney injury** may have an abrupt onset immediately after renal insult (e.g., radiocontrast administration, hyperuricemia after tumor lysis, cholesterol embolization after intravascular procedures). AKI may also arise more insidiously over days to weeks as an indirect consequence of malignancy (e.g., hypercalcemia, myeloma kidney resulting from deposits of Bence Jones proteins) or therapy (e.g., interstitial nephritis after administration of certain therapeutic agents).

1. **Oliguria** is often present in more severe and dramatic episodes of AKI. Most causes of AKI, however, present with normal or nearly normal urine volumes.

2. **Oliguria** is defined as >400 to 500 mL/24 hours. Since 600 mOsm of solute need to be excreted each day, and the maximal concentrating ability of the kidney is 1,200 mOsm, a minimum of 400 to 500 mL of urine needs to be excreted each day to excrete these solutes. Also called "nonoliguric" renal failure, a normal or higher urinary output in AKI is typically related to less

severe renal failure. Despite the reduction in GFR and inability to remove adequate metabolic waste products, kidney tubular cells increase fractional excretion of water and maintain what appears to be a normal urine volume, often fooling the patient and clinical staff into complacency despite a marked reduction in GFR and highly abnormal laboratory markers of renal function.

3. The finding of complete anuria is typically only seen in extreme cases of severe renal failure (renal cortical necrosis, profound ATN, and acute glomerulonephritis) or complete obstruction that affects both kidneys or, in some cases, one anatomic or functional kidney. Anuria leads to more dramatic and quicker changes in electrolyte and fluid complications and requires more immediate management.

4. Although AKI is often transient and reversible, certain causes can result in permanent renal failure (e.g., cisplatin toxicity, mitomycin-induced hemolytic–uremic syndrome). Drugs may cause injury to the kidney by a variety of mechanisms (Table 32-3). Although AKI may resolve, patients are often left with residual renal dysfunction and CKD.

B. **Acute tubular necrosis (ATN)** usually has an abrupt onset, but there may often be an overlap between "prerenal," acute renal damage, and postrenal disease.

1. **Urinalysis in ATN**
   a. **Urine specific gravity** is usually near isosthenuria (1.010).
   b. **Mild proteinuria** is typical (nephritic, usually 1+ to 2+ on a urine dipstick exam) as opposed to nephrotic range proteinuria (which is often 3+ or 4+ on the dipstick).

TABLE 32-3	Drugs That Affect the Kidneys of Cancer Patients
Acute tubular necrosis	
Antibiotics	Aminoglycosides, amphotericin, pentamidine, cephalosporin (rare), vancomycin (rare, but especially with aminoglycosides)
Chemotherapeutics	Methotrexate, cisplatin (often irreversible damage), carboplatin (especially in high doses), streptozocin and other nitrosoureas, cyclosporine (acute: hemodynamic changes; chronic: interstitial fibrosis), tacrolimus, ifosfamide (especially when combined with cyclophosphamide), interferon-α (mainly by intravascular volume depletion), suramin, and pentostatin
Tyrosine kinase inhibitors	Sorafenib, sunitinib, imatinib, and dasatinib
Tubular obstruction	Acyclovir, methotrexate, and sulfa drugs (crystal-induced acute renal failure)
Acute interstitial nephritis	Penicillins, cephalosporins, ciprofloxacin (possibly with other fluoroquinolones as well), sulfa drugs, thiazide, furosemide, bumetanide (but not ethacrynic acid), antituberculous drugs, nonsteroidal anti-inflammatory drugs (NSAIDs, usually after 3–6 mo of use), and allopurinol, sorafenib, sunitinib, ipilimumab, nivolumab, pembrolizumab, avelumab, atezolizumab, durvalumab
Chronic irreversible renal failure (mild to severe)	
Acute hemolytic–uremic syndrome	Mitomycin (most often reported cytotoxic agent; potentiated by tamoxifen), cisplatin, cyclosporine, gemcitabine, streptozocin, and interferon-α (rare)
Tubular interstitial fibrosis	Cisplatin, cyclosporine, tacrolimus, ifosfamide, carmustine, streptozocin,
Fanconi syndrome (partial or complete)	Ifosfamide, azacitidine

   c. Sediment. Early on, the sediment may be remarkably bland. ATN can often be suspected by the presence of many "dirty brown" granular casts in the urine. Usually, only small numbers of white and red blood cells are seen, except in cases of acute glomerulonephritis. Red blood cell casts are rare. The finding of renal tubular epithelial cells (larger cells with larger nuclei) is diagnostic of renal tubular damage.

2. **Several pathogenetic mechanisms** are recognized (see Table 32-3). A careful review of inpatient and outpatient medications is necessary, especially with the increasing use of medications purchased "over the counter" that could be potentially nephrotoxic.

3. **The major histologic finding** is sloughing of tubular epithelial cells with preservation of tubular basement membranes and evidence of epithelial regeneration (mitotic figures). Proteinaceous casts and inflammatory cells may be present. Glomeruli are generally preserved. The lesion may be spotty with some nephrons appearing nearly normal. Disruption of tubular basement membranes (tubulorrhexis) and disrupted glomeruli suggest cortical necrosis, which carries a poor renal prognosis. Management includes avoidance of fluid imbalance and other supportive measures until function returns. Dialysis may be needed in some cases.

4. **Radiocontrast** is a particularly important cause of ARF in patients with malignancies because of the frequency with which these patients undergo radiocontrast studies. Predisposing factors include age older than 60 years, diabetes mellitus, volume depletion, other recent radiocontrast studies, high dose of contrast, concomitant nephrotoxic drug therapy, and, possibly, hyperuricemia.

   a. Iodinated contrast media are strongly linked to the development of ATN and ARF syndromes, especially in patients with preexisting renal disease. Hyperosmolar contrast agents appear to be more toxic. With the increasing clinical use of isotonic and hypotonic contrast agents, the risk of ARF can be lessened. Intravenous (not oral) hydration using isotonic (normal) saline is superior to 0.45% saline and is the most proven method to prevent or limit consequences of renal tubular damage. *N*-acetylcysteine has also been used in high-risk patients to prevent contrast-induced nephropathy. The mechanism is via a decrease of vasoconstriction and oxygen free radical generation.

   b. Nephrogenic systemic fibrosis (NSF) is a relatively recently recognized syndrome that occurs exclusively in patients with kidney disease. Greater than 95% of cases of NSF are associated with intravenous **gadolinium used as a "contrast agent" for MRI studies.** Different gadolinium contrast agents may be associated with a lesser risk of NSF, which may be irreversible. Gadolinium is relatively contraindicated in patients with renal insufficiency, especially those on dialysis.

5. **Prevention of ATN** is often difficult in complicated patients who may be septic or hypotensive and who may have received or required nephrotoxic drugs and/or participated in studies using radiocontrast materials. The following measures are reasonable:

   a. Avoid nephrotoxic agents and monitor drug levels when such drugs are needed.

   b. Keep patients optimally hydrated with attention to intravascular volume and frequent monitoring of vital signs including BP, pulse rate, cardiac output, urine volume, and oxygen saturation.

    c. Maintain high urine flow rate in patients at risk of crystal deposition in tubules, with fluids and loop diuretics, and alkalinize the urine for patients with rhabdomyolysis, hyperuricemia, or high-dose methotrexate therapy.

    d. Prevention of radiocontrast-induced ATN is best managed by hydrating patients and avoiding serial studies in a short period of time. *N*-acetylcysteine 600 mg PO twice daily periprocedure could be used.

C. Tubulointerstitial nephritis occurs acutely after the administration of a growing list of drugs but can occur more insidiously after 6 to 12 months of therapy with nonsteroidal anti-inflammatory drugs (NSAIDs; see Table 32-3). The acute presentation is that of nonoliguric acute renal failure with variable systemic findings of allergic skin rash, fever, or arthralgias. Leukocytosis with eosinophilia may be seen, but pyuria with eosinophiluria is probably more common. Microscopic hematuria is a remarkably frequent finding in acute allergic tubulointerstitial nephritis.

    1. Histologically, there is a diffuse inflammatory reaction in the interstitium, sometimes with invasion of tubules by white blood cells. Eosinophils may dominate or may be only minimally present.

    2. The renal prognosis is good if the offending agent is discontinued. Anecdotal evidence favors the use of a short course of corticosteroids (40 to 60 mg/d of prednisone) if renal failure is severe or persists. Dialysis is only rarely required.

D. Tumor invasion

    1. Primary renal tumors commonly invade renal parenchyma, of course, but renal failure requires extensive bilateral renal involvement and is a rare event. The more common cause of renal failure in patients with primary renal tumors is surgical ablation of renal tissue, the consequence of attempts to extirpate the tumor.

    2. Solid tumor metastasis to kidneys is a rare cause of renal failure or death.

    3. Lymphoproliferative tumors. Renal involvement is common in acute lymphoblastic leukemia (about half of the cases) and lymphoma. Renal failure is less common but does occur. Urinary findings include mild proteinuria, hematuria, and often tumor cells that, when present, are highly suggestive of renal invasion. Imaging studies show large, poorly functioning kidneys without hydronephrosis. Treatment with local irradiation or chemotherapy is associated with resolution of renal failure and diminution of renal size to or toward normal; both abnormalities may recur with recurrence of the tumor.

E. Acute glomerulonephritis causing renal failure is as rare in patients with underlying malignancies as it is in the general population. Certain lymphoproliferative disorders may result in mixed cryoglobulinemia that can cause rapidly progressive (crescentic) glomerulonephritis.

F. Renal cortical necrosis is a rare cause of AKI secondary to ischemic necrosis of the renal cortex. The lesions are usually caused by significantly diminished renal arterial perfusion secondary to vascular spasm, microvascular injury, or intravascular coagulation. Cases of renal cortical necrosis are usually bilateral. Although the pathogenesis of the disease remains unclear, the presumed initiating factor is intense vasospasm of the small vessels. If this vasospasm is brief and vascular flow is reestablished, ATN results. More prolonged vasospasm can cause necrosis and thrombosis of the distal arterioles and glomeruli, and renal cortical necrosis ensues. In hemolytic–uremic syndrome, an additional mechanism involves endotoxin-mediated endothelial damage that leads to vascular thrombosis.

G. **Renal papillary necrosis (RPN)** is characterized by coagulative necrosis of the renal medullary pyramids and papillae brought on by several associated conditions and toxins that exhibit synergism toward the development of ischemia. The clinical course of RPN varies, depending on the degree of vascular impairment, the presence of associated causal factors, the overall health of the patient, the presence of bilateral involvement, and, specifically, the number of affected papillae.

1. RPN can lead to secondary infection of desquamated necrotic foci, deposition of calculi, and/or separation and eventual sloughing of papillae, with impending acute urinary tract obstruction.

2. RPN is potentially disastrous and, in the presence of bilateral involvement or an obstructed solitary kidney, may lead to renal failure. The infectious sequelae of RPN are more serious if the patient has multiple medical problems, particularly diabetes mellitus.

V. CHRONIC KIDNEY DISEASE IN PATIENTS WITH CANCER

The successful development of advanced medical therapies has led to a dramatic increase in the number of patients living with chronic kidney disease (CKD), those living with successfully treated cancer, and those living with both conditions and other illnesses as well. Many countries will allow the patient with progressive and advanced kidney disease artificial kidney treatments (dialysis) or kidney transplantation. In the United States, there are estimated to be nearly 30 million individuals with or at risk of CKD, with around 600,000 receiving regular dialysis therapy.

A. **Classification of CKD.**

Stage 0: GFR $\geq$90 mL/min/1.73 m^2. The patient is at increased risk of CKD (e.g., diabetes, hypertension, family history of kidney disease). Management involves reduction of CKD risk.

Stage 1: GFR $\geq$90 mL/min/1.73 m^2. The patient has urinary abnormalities (e.g., hematuria, proteinuria). Management involves treatment of comorbid conditions and slowing progression.

Stage 2: GFR 60 to 89 mL/min/1.73 m^2. Management involves estimating progression.

Stage 3: GFR 30 to 59 mL/min/1.73 m^2. Management involves evaluating and treating complications (e.g., treatment for anemia owing to erythropoietin deficiency, vitamin D deficiency, and secondary hyperparathyroidism).

Stage 4: GFR 15 to 29 mL/min/1.73 m^2. Management involves preparation for kidney replacement therapy (e.g., treatment for hyperkalemia, hyponatremia, and significant acid–base changes).

Stage 5: GFR $\leq$15 mL/min/1.73 m^2; previously termed end-stage renal disease ("ESRD"). Management nearly always requires some form of dialysis or "renal replacement therapies," including kidney transplantation.

B. **CKD in cancer patients.** The survival rate at 2 years is significantly lower for cancer patients with kidney disease than those without CKD. This reduced survival has been hypothesized to be related to the cardiovascular complications of CKD and drug dose adjustment. With increasingly successful anticancer treatment, patients may develop CKD after recovery from AKI or as a long-term consequence of therapies.

VI. NEPHROTIC SYNDROME

The nephrotic syndrome is an unusual but recognized complication of neoplasms. The syndrome may be caused by glomerular deposits of amyloid, by the deposition of immune complexes, or by less well-defined immunologic mechanisms.

A. **Incidence.** The incidence of nephrotic syndrome as a consequence of malignancies is unknown. From 6% to 10% of patients with nephrotic syndrome eventually manifest a malignancy. Patients with nephrotic syndrome should be evaluated with a careful history and physical examination, coupled with a complete blood count, chest radiograph, and stool for occult blood unless symptoms or findings suggest the need for further workup. Colonoscopy should be done in patients over age 50 years or with a family history of colon cancer. Women should undergo mammography and pelvic examination with Papanicolaou smear as part of their routine examination.

The 24-hour urine measurement of protein is a gold standard. The measurement of the urine protein/creatinine ratio on a "spot urine" is a faster test; a ratio of 3.5 or greater or 4+ protein on a dipstick in a well-hydrated patient is typically seen and diagnostic of nephrotic range proteinuria.

B. **Associations of nephrotic syndrome** exist with many malignancies, including Hodgkin lymphoma (most common); many other lymphoproliferative disorders (including cutaneous T-cell lymphoma); thymoma; squamous cell carcinoma; adenocarcinomas of the lung, breast, kidney, thyroid, cervix, prostate, and gastrointestinal tract (including esophagus, stomach, pancreas, and colon); mesothelioma; and multiple melanoma. Membranous nephropathy has been frequently reported in patients undergoing graft versus host disease following bone marrow transplantation.

The nephrotic syndrome may occur simultaneously with the clinical manifestation of malignancy. More often, what appear to be true associations of nephrotic syndrome occur months before or after manifestations of the tumor. Recurrence of previously treated tumor may be heralded by the return of the nephrotic syndrome by weeks or months.

C. **Management.** Remission of nephrotic syndrome may occur with partial or complete elimination of the tumor, especially in Hodgkin lymphoma. Corticosteroid therapy for tumor-associated nephrotic syndrome is usually ineffective if the tumor cannot be controlled.

VII. RENAL EFFECTS OF ANTICANCER THERAPIES

Chemotherapy can cause nephrotoxicity by a variety of mechanisms. Factors that can potentiate renal dysfunction and contribute to the nephrotoxic potential of antineoplastic drugs include intravascular volume depletion, the concomitant use of other nephrotoxic drugs or radiographic ionic contrast media in patients with or without preexisting renal dysfunction, tumor-related urinary tract obstruction, and intrinsic renal disease that is idiopathic and related to other comorbidities or to the cancer itself.

A. **Tumor lysis syndrome (TLS)**

1. **Mechanism.** TLS is an oncologic emergency that is caused by massive tumor cell lysis with the release of large amounts of potassium, phosphate, and nucleic acids into the systemic circulation. Hyperuricemia is a consequence of the catabolism of purine nucleic acids to hypoxanthine and xanthine and then to uric acid via the enzyme xanthine oxidase. Uric acid is poorly soluble in water, particularly in the usually acidic environment in the distal tubules and collecting system of the kidney. Overproduction and overexcretion of uric acid in TLS can lead to crystal precipitation and deposition in the renal tubules, and acute uric acid nephropathy with AKI. Hyperphosphatemia with calcium phosphate deposition in the renal tubules can also cause renal failure.

TLS most often occurs after the initiation of cytotoxic therapy in patients with tumors that have a high proliferative rate, large tumor burden, and high sensitivity to cytotoxic therapy (e.g., particularly with high-grade lymphomas and acute lymphoblastic leukemia).

2. **Manifestations.** The symptoms associated with TLS largely reflect the associated metabolic abnormalities (hyperkalemia, hyperphosphatemia, and hypocalcemia). They include nausea, vomiting, diarrhea, anorexia, lethargy, hematuria, heart failure, cardiac dysrhythmias, seizures, muscle cramps, tetany, syncope, and possible sudden death.

3. **Prevention.** The best management of TLS is prevention. The preventive regimen consists of aggressive IV hydration and the administration of hypouricemic agents (allopurinol, rasburicase, or febuxostat). Febuxostat can be given in full dosages in kidney or liver disease.

   a. **IV hydration** is recommended prior to therapy in all patients at intermediate or high risk for TLS. The goal is induction of a high urine output of 80 to 100 mL/m^2/hr, which will minimize the likelihood of uric acid precipitation in the tubules. The recommended hydration fluids are 5% dextrose/0.45% sodium chloride and in hyponatremic patients 0.9% sodium chloride. Furosemide can be used to maintain urinary output.

   b. **Urinary alkalinization.** The role of urinary alkalinization (to keep the urine pH as high as 7 since uric acid crystals are more likely to form in an acid urinary environment) with sodium bicarbonate is controversial. Use of sodium bicarbonate is only clearly indicated in patients with metabolic acidosis.

   c. **Hypouricemic agents**
      (1) **Allopurinol** is a hypoxanthine analog that competitively inhibits xanthine oxidase, blocking the metabolism of hypoxanthine and xanthine to uric acid. The usual allopurinol dose in adults is 100 mg/m^2 every 8 hours (maximum 800 mg/d), is generally initiated 24 to 48 hours before the start of induction chemotherapy, and is continued until there is normalization of serum uric acid and other laboratory evidence of tumor lysis (e.g., elevated serum LDH levels).

      (2) **Rasburicase** (recombinant urate oxidase) is well tolerated, rapidly lowers serum uric acid, and is effective in preventing and treating hyperuricemia in TLS. The rapid reduction in serum uric acid is in contrast to the effect of allopurinol, which decreases uric acid formation and therefore does not acutely reduce the serum uric acid concentration. The recommended rasburicase dose is 0.15 to 0.2 mg/kg once daily for 5 days. However, lower doses (3 to 6 mg) or a shorter duration of therapy (or even as a single dose) may be effective in selected patients, based upon whether the indication is for prevention of TLS or for treatment of established TLS. Rasburicase rather than allopurinol is recommended if pretreatment uric acid levels are ≥7.5 mg/dL and for high-risk patients. Rasburicase is **contraindicated** in pregnant or lactating women and in patients with glucose-6-phosphate dehydrogenase (G6PD) deficiency because hydrogen peroxide, a by-product of uric acid breakdown, can cause anaphylaxis, severe hemolysis, and methemoglobinemia in patients with G6PD deficiency.

      (3) **Febuxostat** is a more potent xanthine oxidase inhibitor, which can be given in renal failure. The data are unclear if it is superior to

allopurinol. Febuxostat is 500 times more potent than allopurinol. Flat dosing is given in renal and liver disease. However, in some cases, colchicine may need to be given to prevent acute gout since the drug lowers uric acid quickly.

4. **Treatment of electrolyte disturbances** is discussed in Chapter 28.

B. **Radiation nephritis** can occur 6 to 12 months to years after doses to the kidneys exceeding 2,000 cGy as a function of dose and proportion of kidney tissue irradiated. Cases with earlier onset may manifest as severe or malignant hypertension, proteinuria of <2 g/d, and an active urinary sediment with microscopic hematuria and granular casts. Cases occurring later mimic chronic interstitial nephritis with a bland urinary sediment, possible salt wasting, or hyporeninemic hypoaldosteronism. Treatment of either presentation involves controlling the blood pressure when elevated.

C. **Drug-induced thrombotic thrombocytopenic purpura/hemolytic–uremic syndrome (TTP–HUS)** is discussed in Chapter 35. The mechanism based on which drugs are triggering the development of TTP–HUS is either due to systemic cytotoxic effects or via immune-mediated reactions.

1. **Systemic toxicity** (appears to be related to cumulative dose of the drug): mitomycin C, gemcitabine, cisplatin with or without bleomycin, cyclosporine, tacrolimus, the newer targeted therapies (pazopanib, bevacizumab and sunitinib), and use of radiation and high-dose chemotherapy prior to hematopoietic stem cell transplantation

2. **Immune mediated:** quinine, ticlopidine, and, less often, clopidogrel

D. **Retinoic acid syndrome.** Leukocytes may infiltrate the kidney and cause AKI as part of the retinoic acid syndrome, which is caused by the treatment of acute promyelocytic leukemia with all-*trans*-retinoic acid (see Chapter 26). The syndrome responds to corticosteroids.

E. **Cisplatin nephrotoxicity**

1. **Mechanisms** include tubular epithelial cell toxicity, vasoconstriction in the renal microvasculature, and proinflammatory effects. Cisplatin nephrotoxicity also appears to be mediated by the organic cation transporter (hOCT2). High peak plasma-free platinum concentrations are associated with an increased risk of AKI. The incidence and severity of renal failure increases with subsequent courses and can eventually become irreversible. Cisplatin may also be associated with a thrombotic microangiopathy with features of TTP–HUS when given with bleomycin.

2. **Manifestations.** The most important manifestation of cisplatin nephrotoxicity is renal impairment, which can be progressive. Other renal manifestations include urinary magnesium and salt wasting, glucosuria, and aminoaciduria (a Fanconi-like syndrome).

3. **Prevention.** The standard approach to prevent cisplatin-induced nephrotoxicity is the administration of IV isotonic saline to establish a urine flow of at least 100 mL/hr for 2 hours prior to and 2 hours after chemotherapy administration.

   a. The optimal hydration regimen to prevent nephrotoxicity associated with cisplatin administration is unclear. Mannitol is frequently used to induce diuresis, although there is no evidence that this is required. The addition of furosemide is generally not required, unless there is evidence of fluid overload.

   b. Patients with intraperitoneal tumors may be treated with intraperitoneal cisplatin or carboplatin to achieve high local drug levels and relatively low plasma concentrations. In this setting, IV **sodium thiosulfate** can be given concurrently to bind covalently with the platinum that enters the systemic circulation. The resulting complex has no systemic or renal toxicity and also has no antitumor effect.

   c. Avoid the coadministration of other potentially nephrotoxic agents, such as aminoglycosides, nonsteroidal anti-inflammatory agents, or iodinated contrast media.

   d. Generally, avoid using cisplatin among patients with a serum creatinine concentration >1.5 mg/dL or an estimated GFR of <50 mL/min. Possible exceptions are when cisplatin has a proven curative role, such as in patients with testicular cancer.

F. Ifosfamide nephrotoxicity

  1. Mechanisms. In vitro studies suggest that the metabolite chloracetaldehyde is toxic to the tubular cells, rather than the parent drug or another metabolite acrolein. Another possible mechanism of toxicity may be energy depletion via mitochondrial damage.

  2. Manifestations. Although ifosfamide can lead to a mild reduction in GFR, renal injury is primarily manifested by one or more of the following signs of tubular dysfunction:

    a. Impairment in proximal tubular function as manifested by renal glucosuria, aminoaciduria, tubular proteinuria (i.e., low molecular weight proteins but not albumin), and a marked increase in beta-2-microglobulin excretion.

    b. Hypophosphatemia induced by decreased proximal tubular phosphate reabsorption.

    c. Renal potassium wasting.

    d. Metabolic acidosis with a normal anion gap (hyperchloremic) acidosis due to distal (type 1) or proximal (type 2) renal tubular acidosis.

    e. Polyuria due to nephrogenic diabetes insipidus (i.e., resistance to ADH) causes a dilute urine and is relatively rare. When polyuria does occur, it is more often an appropriate response to isotonic saline therapy that causes sodium diuresis.

  3. Prevention. The cornerstone of prevention of ifosfamide nephrotoxicity is to limit the cumulative dose of the drug. The risk of nephrotoxicity is low at cumulative ifosfamide doses of 60 g/m^2 or less, and when toxicity does occur, it is usually mild to moderate. Mesna reduces the risk of hemorrhagic cystitis, but it is unclear if it reduces the risk of nephrotoxicity.

G. Methotrexate (MTX) nephrotoxicity

  1. Mechanisms. MTX is primarily cleared via the kidneys, with about 90% being excreted unchanged in the urine. Thus, any impairment of GFR will result in sustained serum levels of the drug that may induce bone marrow or other toxicities. At low doses, MTX is not nephrotoxic. However, when given in high doses, MTX can precipitate in the tubules and directly induce tubular injury, and it also causes a transient decline in GFR after each dose, with complete recovery within 6 to 8 hours.

  2. Manifestations. MTX-induced ARF is typically nonoliguric and is reversible in almost all cases within 1 to 3 weeks. The major risk with MTX-induced renal dysfunction is that MTX clearance is severely compromised, resulting in delayed excretion of the drug, higher-than-expected plasma concentrations, and increased systemic toxicity.

  3. Prevention. The likelihood of HDMTX-induced renal dysfunction can be minimized (but not eliminated) by hydration both to maintain a high urine flow and to lower the concentration of MTX in the tubular fluid and by alkalinization of the urine to a pH above 7.0.

H. Bisphosphonate nephrotoxicity

1. **Mechanisms**

   a. **Pamidronate** has been associated with the development of nephrotic syndrome due to a number of different mechanisms, including collapsing focal segmental glomerulosclerosis. Most cases are reported in patients with multiple myeloma.

   b. **Zoledronic acid.** Significant renal impairment attributable to zoledronic acid is uncommon and appears to be predominantly associated with higher doses and with infusion durations <15 minutes. The mechanism of nephrotoxicity appears to be different from that in patients receiving pamidronate.

2. **Management and prevention.** Serum creatinine should be monitored prior to each dose of pamidronate or zoledronic acid. Otherwise, unexplained azotemia (an increase of ≥0.5 mg/dL in serum creatinine or an absolute level of >1.4 mg/dL among patients with normal baseline values) should prompt temporary discontinuation of the bisphosphonate.

   a. **Restarting bisphosphonates**. One can consider increasing the infusion time of pamidronate to more than 2 hours and of zoledronic acid to 30 to 60 minutes every 4 weeks if renal function returns to within 10% of baseline.

   b. **Hypocalcemia**. Most patients receiving high-potency bisphosphonates do not become hypocalcemic because of compensatory mechanisms. However, in some cases, these compensatory mechanisms may be blocked (e.g., prior parathyroidectomy, low vitamin D levels, hypomagnesemic hypoparathyroidism, renal failure) and result in hypocalcemia.

I. Other potentially nephrotoxic chemotherapeutic agents

1. **Carboplatin** may cause reversible tubular injury manifested by hypomagnesemia and recurrent salt wasting but rarely causes ARF.

2. **Vinca alkaloids** can result in hyponatremia by inducing the syndrome of inappropriate antidiuretic hormone (SIADH) secretion.

3. **Nitrosoureas** may cause interstitial nephritis with progressive renal failure via glomerular sclerosis and tubular fibrosis. Streptozocin causes proteinuria commonly, as well as other tubular syndromes, via proximal tubular damage.

J. Monoclonal antibodies

1. **VEGF pathway inhibitors. Bevacizumab, aflibercept** and **ramucirumab** may cause hypertension, proteinuria, or nephrotic syndrome. The mechanism appears to be a renal thrombotic microangiopathy. Studies have shown that preexisting hypertension was a significant risk factor for the development of hypertension with VEGF-targeted therapy.

   Patients should be screened for hypertension before administration of any anti-VEGF agents, and blood pressure should be monitored regularly after starting therapy and then every 2 to 3 weeks as long as the blood pressure remains stable. The target blood pressure in patients receiving angiogenesis inhibitors is 140/90 mm Hg. The hypertension caused by antiangiogenic agents is often easily managed with routine antihypertensive agents. Angiotensin-converting enzyme (ACE) inhibitors are preferred since they have the added benefit of decreasing proteinuria. Other antihypertensive agents may also be needed to control the blood pressure. Nitrates can increase production of nitric oxide and cause vasodilation, thereby facilitating blood pressure control. It is recommended that therapy be discontinued in patients who develop a hypertensive emergency or encephalopathy.

Patients should undergo a screening urine analysis for proteinuria prior to receiving antiangiogenic therapy. If proteinuria of grade 1+ is present on screening urine analysis, then urine protein excretion should be quantified using a spot urine albumin/creatinine ratio. Referral to a nephrologist is recommended for additional evaluation and for the treatment of CKD. In case proteinuria develops while on therapy, if the level of proteinuria is ≥2 g/24 hours, current guidelines recommend that the antiangiogenic agent be suspended until the return of urine protein level to baseline. Nephrotic range proteinuria and thrombotic microangiopathy are generally considered reasons to discontinue therapy.

2. **EGFR pathway inhibitors. Panitumumab, cetuximab and necitumumab** may cause hypomagnesemia and hypokalemia. The mechanism of hypomagnesemia appears to be through renal wasting. Careful management of hypomagnesemia is indicated in patients receiving EGFR antibodies because of the potential serious cardiac arrhythmias. Serum magnesium levels should be monitored regularly, and the frequency should be determined by the severity of the deficit. Intravenous replacement is the most effective. Amiloride is a potassium-sparing diuretic that has been shown to increase serum magnesium and may be an option for patients who are normovolemic and normotensive on cetuximab. Hypomagnesemia usually resolves within 4 to 6 weeks after cessation of treatment. The mechanism of hypokalemia may be due to a direct toxic effect on the kidney. Another contributing factor may be concomitant hypomagnesemia.

K. **Molecularly targeted therapies**
   1. **Tyrosine kinase inhibitors.** Renal dysfunction, including proteinuria, hyponatremia, hypophosphatemia, and elevated creatinine, has been observed with all tyrosine kinase inhibitors. The pathology of renal toxicity can be due to thrombotic microangiopathy, acute interstitial nephritis, ATN, glomerulonephritis, and focal segmental glomerulosclerosis.
      a. **Sorafenib and sunitinib** may cause proteinuria or nephrotic syndrome. The mechanism appears to be a renal thrombotic microangiopathy. There have been case reports of biopsy-confirmed occurrence of acute interstitial nephritis causing AKI. Patients require regular monitoring, and if laboratory values show proteinuria, especially in the nephrotic range, then the dose should be decreased or medication should be discontinued. Other antiangiogenic TKIs such as **pazopanib**, **lenvatinib**, and **axitinib** were associated with asymptomatic proteinuria.
      b. **Imatinib and dasatinib** can cause AKI through development of TLS that leads to the deposition of uric acid in the collecting tubules. Another postulated mechanism appears to be the development of tubular damage in the form of ATN tubular vacuolization and partial Fanconi syndrome with apical vacuoles in some tubular cell. Imatinib can inhibit PDGF-dependent renal mesangial cell proliferation in a dose-dependent fashion and may hamper tubular repair, resulting in the development of ATN. In patients who are at higher risk of developing AKI, close monitoring is necessary. The lowest possible dose of imatinib should be used, as some of the effects may be dose dependent. Prevention of nephrotoxicity also entails the avoidance of administration of concomitant nephrotoxic drugs, prevention of dehydration, and avoidance of loop diuretics. Hypophosphatemia can also occur secondary to inhibition of renal tubular reabsorption of phosphorus. Hypophosphatemia should be managed aggressively because of its possible effects on bone metabolism.

Vitamin D replacement may attenuate the effects of hypoparathyroidism and hypophosphatemia and should be considered in patients with low vitamin D levels. Calcitriol may be a better option for patients with severe phosphate deficiency as oral phosphate supplements could potentially bind to dietary calcium. A decline if GFR was also seen in patients treated with **bosutinib.**

   c. **Ibrutinib.** The treatment with ibrutinib was associated with cases of severe renal failure and creatinine should be monitored periodically.

2. **mTOR inhibitors.**

   a. **Everolimus** can cause proteinuria although the mechanisms are unclear, and a possibility can be due to the decreased production of VEGF seen in podocytes, which leads to podocyte damage. Several other proposed mechanisms include decreased expression of cubilin and megalin, which mediate the endocytosis of proteins such as albumin, into the proximal tubules, which leads to decreased albumin reuptake and subsequent proteinuria. Patients who receive mTOR therapy should be monitored regularly for the development of proteinuria. Mild proteinuria can be managed with an ACE inhibitor or angiotensin receptor blocker in conjunction with diet and lifestyle modifications aimed at controlling blood pressure. Proteinuria resolves after discontinuation of the offending agent without any long-term effects on the kidney. Patients who develop focal segmental glomerulosclerosis and membranoproliferative glomerulonephritis may benefit from plasmapheresis.

L. **Checkpoint inhibitors: ipilimumab (anti–CTLA-4 antibody), nivolumab and pembrolizumab (anti–PD-1 antibodies), avelumab, atezolizumab, durvalumab** (anti–PD-L1 antibodies).

   This class of medications augments the immune response and leads to immune-related adverse events (irAEs) through either cell-mediated immunity or autoimmunity. Although rare, treatment-related renal injury is seen in 0% to 4% and includes elevated creatinine, autoimmune, interstitial nephritis, and nephrotic syndrome. Steroids are administered when the severity of an irAE warrants reversal.

   Renal injury with ipilimumab is usually associated with hypersensitivity, such as rash, fever, and eosinophilia. Kidney injury is most often seen within 3 weeks after starting therapy and presents as sudden worsening of renal function associated with mild proteinuria and abnormal urinalysis in the setting of a normal blood pressure and a lack of edema.

   An indirect mechanism by which those checkpoint inhibitors could cause renal failure is via immune-mediated rhabdomyolysis as the muscle breakdown products could precipitate in the kidneys and lead to renal function impairment. It is a rare complication but definitely well described and seen in clinical practice. In such cases, measurement of serum CK, aldolase, troponin, and urine myoglobin is needed.

ACKNOWLEDGMENTS

The authors would like to acknowledge Drs. Kenneth S. Kleinman and Dennis A. Casciato, who significantly contributed to earlier versions of this chapter.

Suggested Readings

Abbas A, et al. Renal toxicities of targeted therapies. *Target Oncol* 2015;10:487.

Aspelin P, et al. Nephrotoxic effects in high-risk patients undergoing angiography. *N Engl J Med* 2003;348:491.

Cairo MS, et al. Recommendations for the evaluation of risk and prophylaxis of tumour lysis syndrome (TLS) in adults and children with malignant diseases: an expert TLS panel consensus. *Br J Haematol* 2010;149:578.

Coresh J, Selvin E, Stevens LA, et al. Prevalence of chronic kidney disease in the United States. *JAMA* 2007;298:2038.

Cortes J, Moore JO, Maziarz RT, et al. Control of plasma uric acid in adults at risk for tumor lysis syndrome: efficacy and safety of rasburicase alone and rasburicase followed by allopurinol compared with allopurinol alone—results of a multicenter phase III study. *J Clin Oncol* 2010;28:4207.

Giraldez M, Puto K. A single, fixed dose of rasburicase (6 mg maximum) for treatment of tumor lysis syndrome in adults. *Eur J Haematol* 2010;85:177.

Janus N, et al. Proposal for dosage adjustment and timing of chemotherapy in hemodialyzed patients. *Ann Oncol* 2010;21:1395.

Kapoor M, Chan G. Malignancy and renal disease. *Crit Care Clin* 2001;17:571.

Kini A, et al. A protocol for prevention of radiographic contrast nephropathy during percutaneous coronary intervention: effect of selective dopamine receptor agonist fenoldopam. *Catheter Cardiovasc Interv* 2002;55(2):169.

Kintzel PE. Anticancer drug-induced kidney disorders. *Drug Saf* 2001;24:19.

Kintzel PE, et al. Anti-cancer drug renal toxicity and elimination: dosing guidelines for altered renal function. *Cancer Treat Rev* 1995;21:33.

Klag MJ, Whelton PK, Randall BL, et al. Blood pressure and end-stage renal disease in men. *N Engl J Med* 1996;334:13–18.

Launay-Vacher V. Epidemiology of chronic kidney disease in cancer patients: lessons from the IRMA study group. *Semin Nephrol* 2010;30:548.

National Kidney Foundation. K/DOQI clinical practice guidelines for chronic kidney disease: evaluation, classification, and stratification. *Am J Kidney Dis* 2002;39:S1.

Spain L, et al. Management of toxicities of immune checkpoint inhibitors. *Cancer Treat Rev* 2016;44:51.

Tepel M, et al. Prevention of radiographic-contrast-agent-induced reductions in renal function by acetylcysteine. *N Engl J Med* 2000;343:180.

Weber JS, et al. Toxicities of Immunotherapy for the practitioner. *J Clin Oncol* 2015;33:2092.

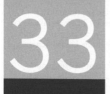

Neuromuscular Complications

Yoshie Umemura and Lisa M. DeAngelis

I. METASTASES TO THE BRAIN

A. **Pathogenesis**

1. **Incidence.** Autopsy series show that 25% of patients who die of cancer have intracranial metastases; 15% have brain and 10% have dural or leptomeningeal metastases.

2. **Tumor of origin.** The tumor that most commonly metastasizes to the brain is lung cancer, which is responsible for almost one-half of all brain metastases. Brain metastases from pulmonary tumors can occur early in the course of malignancy, and their diagnosis is synchronous (i.e., before or at the same time as the primary tumor) in about one-third of cases. Other types of tumors that commonly metastasize to the brain include breast and renal cancers and melanoma (each comprising 20%, 5%, and 10% of cases, respectively), along with metastases from tumors of unknown primary sites (5%). Carcinomas of the gastrointestinal tract, ovary, and uterus rarely produce intracerebral metastases.

3. **Mechanism.** Tumor dissemination to the central nervous system (CNS) is usually by the hematogenous route, and the distribution of lesions parallels the distribution of arterial blood flow. Of brain metastases, 80% are supratentorial, 15% are cerebellar, and 5% are in the brainstem. However, metastases from certain primaries have a predilection for particular regions in the brain. For example, colon cancer and pelvic primaries have a propensity to metastasize to the posterior fossa, whereas lung cancer tends to metastasize to the supratentorial compartment. About one-half of the metastases are single, especially those from lung, renal, and colon cancers; metastases from melanoma and breast cancer are more likely to be multiple. Metastases can be solid, cystic, or hemorrhagic (especially lung, choriocarcinoma, melanoma, and thyroid carcinoma).

B. **Natural history.** Left untreated, metastatic brain tumors cause progressive neurologic deterioration leading to coma and death; the median survival time is only 1 month. About one-half of patients with brain metastases die of their neurologic disease, and the remainder die of systemic causes. Among treated patients, the overall median survival is broad at 3 to 25 months depending upon number of metastases, presence of active systemic disease, and range of therapeutic options.

C. **Clinical presentation.** Metastases can cause focal or global cerebral dysfunction at presentation. Symptoms usually develop insidiously and progress over a few weeks. Occasionally, the onset is sudden when there is an acute hemorrhage into the metastasis.

1. **Global signs and symptoms.** Headache and mental status changes are each seen in 50% of patients. Other nonlocalizing findings include symptoms of increased intracranial pressure, such as papilledema, nausea, and vomiting.

2. **Focal signs and symptoms,** including hemiparesis, visual field defect, and aphasia, depend on the site of metastasis.

3. **Seizures** are the presenting manifestation in about 20% of patients.
4. **Differential diagnosis.**
   a. **Metabolic encephalopathy,** including hyponatremia, hypercalcemia, hypoxemia, uremia, hepatic encephalopathy, and hypothyroidism
   b. **Drug-induced encephalopathy** from analgesics, sedatives, glucocorticoids, chemotherapeutic agents, and other drugs
   c. **CNS infections,** including bacterial and fungal meningitis, herpes encephalitis, progressive multifocal leukoencephalopathy, and cerebral abscess (see Chapter 36)
   d. **Nutritional deficiency,** such as Wernicke encephalopathy
   e. **Cerebrovascular disease (CVD),** owing to thrombotic disorders and disseminated intravascular coagulation (DIC)
   f. **Paraneoplastic disorders.** See Section V.

D. **Evaluation.** An MRI is the optimal test to detect brain metastases. A CT scan should only be used if MRI is not feasible (e.g., pacemaker). Most metastatic tumors are contrast enhancing, and both a noncontrast and contrast study should be performed in every patient. Lesions detectable by CT or MRI that may resemble brain metastases include cerebral abscesses, parasitic disease, and occasionally stroke. Lumbar puncture is not useful in diagnosing brain metastases and is often contraindicated.

E. **Management.** The aims of therapy for patients with brain metastases are to relieve neurologic symptoms and prolong survival. Exact treatment recommendations depend on the tumor histology, the degree of systemic dissemination, and clinical condition.

   1. **Dexamethasone,** usually 10 mg IV followed by 2 to 4 mg PO or IV twice a day, results in a dramatic reversal of neurologic deficits and alleviates headache. Dexamethasone is unnecessary for asymptomatic patients. In most patients, steroids can be tapered off once definitive therapy has been administered.

   2. **Anticonvulsant therapy** should be administered only to patients who have had a seizure. Antiepileptics that do not induce the hepatic microsomal system, such as levetiracetam, lacosamide, or lamotrigine, are the best options. There is no role for prophylactic anticonvulsants in patients with brain metastases. They do not protect against future seizures, are associated with frequent side effects, and can enhance the metabolism and thus reduce the efficacy of many chemotherapeutic agents.

   3. **Radiation therapy (RT)** is the standard treatment for multiple or unresectable metastases, and for lesions too large for radiosurgery. It is palliative and can be useful when both CNS and systemic disease are progressing. The field usually encompasses the whole brain, with a recommended dose of 3,000 cGy in 10 daily fractions.

   4. **Surgery** provides a significant survival advantage for patients with a single brain metastasis. Median survival for surgically treated patients is 9 to 16 months, and 12% of patients live 5 years or longer. Candidates for surgical resection should have a single or possibly two brain metastases and limited or controlled systemic disease. Surgical resection is considered in other cases on an individual basis and may be influenced by the need for a tissue diagnosis. Whole-brain RT and radiosurgery after surgical resection improves control of CNS disease but does not prolong survival.

   5. **Radiosurgery** delivers a single large dose of radiation to a well-defined target; the steep dose curve of this technique ensures that little radiation is delivered to surrounding tissues. Radiosurgery can be delivered with

equal efficacy by a gamma knife, cyberknife, or linear accelerator. It is an effective, minimally invasive outpatient procedure that is a treatment option for patients with one to three or possibly more intracranial metastases. Radiosurgery may be used in place of surgical resection or whole-brain RT or as an adjunct to either treatment. Local control rates appear to be equal for surgery and radiosurgery. Radiosurgery offers an advantage for metastases that are not surgically accessible, for multiple metastases, or for tumor types that are resistant to standard RT (e.g., renal cell carcinoma, melanoma) where control by radiosurgery appears to be superior. Radiosurgery must be limited to lesions ≤3 cm in diameter and can occasionally produce symptomatic radionecrosis or a prolonged dependence on corticosteroids.

6. **Chemotherapy.** Cytotoxic agents are primarily used to treat brain metastases at relapse or occasionally asymptomatic lesions found on screening MRI. Responses have been documented in patients with metastatic breast cancer, small cell lung cancer (SCLC), and lymphoma. Effective regimens are selected on the basis of the underlying primary and the patient's prior therapies.

Targeted therapy has proven effective against CNS metastases that harbor sensitizing mutations such as erlotinib in EGFR mutant non–small cell lung cancer (NSCLC), lapatinib and capecitabine in HER2-positive breast cancer, or BRAF inhibitors in BRAF mutant melanomas. Immunotherapy such as ipilimumab and nivolumab are additional therapeutic options for patients with brain metastases from melanoma or lung cancer.

II. METASTASES TO THE MENINGES
A. Pathogenesis
1. **Incidence.** Leptomeningeal metastases have been demonstrated at autopsy in 8% of patients with systemic malignancy.
2. **Associated tumors.** Although any systemic tumor can metastasize to the leptomeninges, those that do so most commonly are lymphoma, leukemia (especially acute), lung carcinoma (especially small cell), breast carcinoma, and melanoma.
3. **Mechanism.** Metastasis to the leptomeninges occurs by hematogenous spread through arachnoid vessels or the choroid plexus, by infiltration along nerve roots, and by extension from brain or dural metastases. The sites of heaviest infiltration are usually at the base of the brain, the major brain fissures, and the cauda equina.

B. Natural history.
Leptomeningeal metastasis can involve any area of the CNS in direct contact with the cerebrospinal fluid (CSF). Tumor can grow as a sheet along the surface of the brain, spinal cord, cranial nerves, or nerve roots and can also invade these structures causing focal dysfunction. Tumor cells can obstruct the arachnoid villi and impair CSF reabsorption causing hydrocephalus.

C. Clinical presentation.
The hallmarks of leptomeningeal metastasis are evidence of multilevel, noncontiguous neurologic signs and more neurologic findings identified on examination than the patient has symptoms. There are four basic clinical presentations that may be seen alone or in combination; meningismus is rarely present.
1. **Spinal.** At least 50% of patients with leptomeningeal metastasis have spinal symptoms. Symptoms and signs include back pain, radicular pain, weakness, numbness (leg more often than arm), and loss of bowel and bladder control.
2. **Cerebral.** About one-half of the patients present with cerebral symptoms and signs including headache, lethargy, change in mental status, ataxia, and seizures (partial and generalized).

3. **Cranial nerve.** Symptoms and signs include visual loss, diplopia, facial numbness, facial weakness, dysphagia, and hearing loss.

4. **Hydrocephalus.** Symptoms and signs of increased intracranial pressure include headache, decreased level of consciousness, gait apraxia, and urinary incontinence.

D. **Evaluation.** The diagnosis of leptomeningeal metastasis is often strongly suspected on clinical grounds, but it can sometimes be difficult to make a definitive diagnosis. The diagnosis may be confirmed by characteristic findings on MRI or by the demonstration of tumor cells in the CSF.

1. **Imaging studies.** Contrast-enhanced MRI of the brain and complete spine should be obtained in all patients to evaluate the full extent of disease. If the patient cannot have an MRI, CT scan of the head and CT myelography of the spine can be performed. Definitive neuroimaging findings include nodules on the cauda equina, enhancement of the cranial nerves, enhancement within sulci or the cisterns, or enhancement along the surface of the spinal cord. In a patient with known cancer, these findings suffice to establish the diagnosis and do not require CSF confirmation of tumor cells. Radiographic evidence of communicating hydrocephalus or brain metastases adjacent to a ventricular surface, or deep within sulci, are suggestive of leptomeningeal disease but require definitive spinal imaging or the demonstration of tumor cells in the CSF to confirm the diagnosis.

2. **CSF examination.** CSF is examined for protein and glucose concentrations, cell count, and cytology. Routine cultures should be performed because the differential diagnosis includes chronic infectious meningitis. CSF may be obtained by lumbar puncture or, in cases of suspected spinal block, by cervical puncture under radiographic guidance.

   a. **Opening pressure.** The opening pressure should always be measured to assess the intracranial pressure (ICP). Patients can have marked elevation of ICP even in the absence of hydrocephalus.

   b. **Routine studies.** Elevated protein and pleocytosis (usually lymphocytic) are nonspecific findings that occur in about 75% of patients with leptomeningeal metastases. A low glucose concentration occurs in <25% but is strongly suggestive when present.

   c. **Cytologic examination** confirms the diagnosis in about one-half of patients on the first lumbar puncture. The diagnostic yield increases to about 90% by the third tap, but 10% of patients remain undiagnosed. The use of molecular diagnostic techniques, particularly for hematopoietic neoplasms, may be useful. Immunohistochemical staining and fluorescence *in situ* hybridization (FISH) (i.e., in hematologic malignancies, or to detect aneusomy of chromosome 1 in breast or other solid tumors) may enhance the diagnostic yield. Flow cytometry studies, which evaluate DNA abnormalities and estimate the degree of aneuploidy, may also be useful in cases of suspected leptomeningeal metastasis (especially from leukemia or lymphoma) with a nondiagnostic CSF cytology.

   d. **Tumor markers** may serve as additional diagnostic tests and are useful in following response to therapy. Tumor-specific biochemical markers include β_2-microglobulin (leukemia and lymphoma), carcinoembryonic antigen (lung, colon, and breast cancer), cancer antigen 15-3 (breast cancer), human chorionic gonadotropin and α-fetoprotein (germ cell tumors), and lymphocyte markers (especially B-cell markers) to differentiate leukemic or lymphomatous cells from normal reactive T lymphocytes. Nonspecific markers that may be elevated in a variety of tumor types include β-glucuronidase and lactate dehydrogenase isoenzyme 5; newer markers also include telomerase and vascular endothelial growth factor (VEGF). All tumor markers should be measured in the serum, and if the serum to CSF ratio is <60:1, the marker is being produced inside the CNS. Brain metastases do not increase CSF tumor marker concentration.

E. **Management.** The optimal therapy for neoplastic meningitis has not been established. The basic premise has been to treat clinically active or bulky disease with RT and to treat the remainder of the neuraxis with intrathecal chemotherapy. Systemic chemotherapy appears, however, to have an important role and may be associated with improved outcome. A response can be achieved in about one-half of patients, but the median survival is <6 months. Patients with breast cancer, leukemia, and lymphoma have the best prognosis.

1. **Dexamethasone** is of limited benefit in patients with leptomeningeal disease, except in patients with lymphoma where it acts as a chemotherapeutic agent. It should be avoided unless the patient has elevated ICP.

2. **RT** is limited to areas of clinical involvement even if disease is not evident at that location radiographically. The typical dose is 3,000 cGy delivered in 10 fractions. This frequently relieves pain and may stabilize the patient neurologically. Fixed neurologic deficits do not usually improve. Complete neuraxis RT is avoided because it is associated with a high morbidity, causes myelosuppression, and does not improve outcome.

3. **Intrathecal chemotherapy** may be used to treat the entire subarachnoid space, although intrathecal drug does not penetrate into nodules of subarachnoid disease. The drug can be administered by lumbar puncture or preferably through an intraventricular reservoir (an Ommaya reservoir). The drug is usually given twice weekly until abnormal cells are no longer found in the CSF, and it is then given at progressively longer intervals. Preservative-free agents should be used. The dose is fixed and not calculated on a meter-squared basis because the volume of CSF is identical in all adults regardless of size. There must be normal CSF flow dynamics for intrathecal chemotherapy to be effective. Patients with large bulky lesions or hydrocephalus always have impaired CSF flow, and intrathecal drug should not be administered to these patients until normal CSF flow is documented by an intrathecal indium radionuclide study. Intrathecal chemotherapy can be complicated by an acute chemical meningitis or arachnoiditis. This can cause headache, nausea, fever, and neck stiffness mimicking infectious meningitis. Arachnoiditis may be seen with any agent but is pronounced with liposomal cytarabine (DepoCyt), and patients must be treated with corticosteroids for several days before and after each DepoCyt injection to minimize this toxicity.
   a. Methotrexate, 12 mg twice weekly followed by leucovorin rescue
   b. Cytarabine, 30 to 60 mg twice weekly
   c. Thiotepa, 10 mg twice weekly
   d. DepoCyt (liposomal cytarabine), 50 mg every other week
   e. Rituximab, 25 mg twice weekly

4. **Systemic chemotherapy** has the advantage of reaching all areas of disease, penetrating into bulky lesions that intrathecal drug cannot reach, and being independent of CSF flow to reach the whole subarachnoid space. The choice of drug is based on its ability to penetrate into the CSF and on the chemosensitivity spectrum of the underlying primary. The most widely used agents are high-dose methotrexate (≥ 3 g/m^2), high-dose cytarabine (3 g/m^2), and

thiotepa. A wide variety of other drugs, however, have been used effectively, such as capecitabine for breast cancer. There are isolated reports that bevacizumab has been beneficial.

III. EPIDURAL SPINAL CORD COMPRESSION

Epidural spinal cord compression is a neuro-oncologic emergency. Any cancer patient with back pain should receive a prompt and thorough evaluation, and those with neurologic dysfunction localizing to the spinal cord or cauda equina require emergency evaluation and treatment.

A. Pathogenesis

1. **Incidence.** About 5% of patients with cancer develop clinical evidence of spinal cord compression.

2. **Distribution.** About 10% of epidural metastases occur in the cervical spine, 70% in the thoracic spine, and 20% in the lumbosacral spine. About 10% to 40% of patients have multifocal epidural tumor.

3. **Responsible tumors.** Any tumor can cause spinal cord compression, but lung cancer accounts for 15% of cases; breast, prostate, carcinoma of unknown primary site, lymphoma, and myeloma each account for about 10% of cases.

4. **Mechanisms.** A tumor reaches the epidural space by either (1) direct extension from a metastasis to the vertebral body growing into the epidural space or (2) tumor such as lymphoma can grow into the spinal canal through the intervertebral foramina without destroying bone. Secondary vascular compromise may cause venous infarction resulting in the sudden, irreversible deterioration seen in some patients. Direct metastasis to the spinal cord parenchyma is a rare cause of spinal cord dysfunction in cancer patients.

B. Diagnosis

1. **Natural history.** The progression of disease from the spinal column to the epidural space with neural encroachment is manifested clinically as local back pain followed by radicular symptoms and eventually myelopathy.

   a. The initial stage of localized pain can last for several weeks or, in tumors such as breast or prostate cancer and lymphoma, for several months.

   b. Radicular symptoms, such as pain radiating in a root distribution, heralds further tumor progression but is still a relatively early symptom.

   c. Once paraparesis or ascending numbness of the legs occurs, the progression may be extremely rapid and a complete myelopathy may develop within hours.

2. **Clinical presentation** depends on the level of spinal involvement.

   a. Back pain is the initial symptom in >95% of patients with spinal cord compression caused by malignancy. The pain is dull, aching, and often localized to the upper back; it typically worsens with recumbency, unlike back pain from spinal degenerative disease. Tenderness over the appropriate spinal level may be readily elicited.

   b. Radiculopathy is usually manifested by pain in a dermatomal distribution but can also include sensory or motor loss in the distribution of the involved roots. Cervical and lumbar diseases usually cause unilateral radiculopathy, whereas thoracic disease causes bilateral radiculopathy, resulting in a band-like distribution of pain around the torso. The pain from thoracic radiculopathies can sometimes be similar to pain from pleurisy, cholecystitis, or pancreatitis. The pain from cervical or lumbar radiculopathies can simulate disk herniation.

c. **Myelopathy** can occur rapidly, and the signs include bilateral leg weakness and numbness and loss of bowel and bladder function depending on the level of spinal involvement. Associated neurologic findings include hyperactive deep tendon reflexes, Babinski responses, and decreased anal sphincter tone. Disease at the level of the cauda equina usually causes urinary retention and saddle anesthesia. Unusual presentations of spinal cord compression include ataxia without motor, sensory, or autonomic dysfunction. Metastasis to the spinal cord parenchyma can cause a myelopathy without back pain.

3. **Evaluation.** Because the prognosis worsens when myelopathy develops, the diagnosis of epidural metastasis should be established before the onset of spinal cord injury.

   a. **MRI** is the procedure of choice for evaluating patients with suspected cord compression. MRI defines the degree of neural impingement and the extent of bone involvement; it is noninvasive and accurately detects other entities in the differential diagnosis of myelopathy. In addition, the entire spine can be imaged, which is essential in any patient with an epidural metastasis. Epidural tumor is best visualized without gadolinium. Contrast will identify leptomeningeal metastasis or a spinal cord metastasis if they are diagnostic considerations.

   b. **CT myelography** can be used if the patient cannot undergo an MRI. If myelography shows a complete block, contrast material needs to be administered at both the lumbar and the high cervical levels to establish the extent of disease. If myelography is performed, CSF should always be sent for routine studies and cytologic examination. Myelography is contraindicated in patients with coagulopathy and may worsen a neurologic deficit below the level of a complete spinal block.

4. **Differential diagnosis**

   a. **Structural lesions.** Epidural hematoma (may occur spontaneously or after invasive procedures, especially in patients with a coagulopathy), epidural abscess, herniated disk, or osteoporotic vertebral collapse.

   b. **Nonstructural lesions.** Paraneoplastic syndromes (see Section V), radiation myelopathy (see Section VI.B.3), or Guillain-Barré syndrome.

   c. **Back pain** in the absence of neurologic findings in patients with normal imaging studies of the spine may be caused by leptomeningeal, lumbosacral, or brachial plexus or retroperitoneal metastases, which can be diagnosed by enhanced MRI, CSF studies, or body MRI or CT scans.

C. **Prognosis.** The outcome is greatly improved if treatment is initiated before spinal cord symptoms appear. In general, if the patient is walking at diagnosis, he or she will remain ambulatory after treatment, but if the patient is not walking at diagnosis, restoration of ambulation is less likely. Other prognostic factors include the level of spinal cord involvement and the rate of neurologic progression. Patients with breast cancer and lymphoma tend to do better because their tumors respond to therapy. Patients with lung or prostate cancer that is refractory to treatment, and who have cord compression that has progressed rapidly, tend to do poorly.

D. **Management.** Once the diagnosis of epidural tumor has been established, rapid therapeutic intervention is essential.

1. **Dexamethasone** is useful for alleviating neurologic symptoms and helps to control pain associated with epidural cord compression. Treatment should

begin immediately, even before diagnostic studies are performed, unless the patient has lymphoma in which case corticosteroids can cause tumor regression and a false-negative finding on MRI. Dosing depends on the degree of neurologic involvement. For radiculopathy only, doses are usually 10 mg IV followed by 4 to 8 mg IV or PO twice a day. For rapidly evolving disease, or with evidence of myelopathy, treat with 100 mg IV followed by 24 mg IV twice a day; a rapid taper is essential for these high-dose regimens and should start within 48 hours.

2. **RT** is effective for spinal cord compression. It not only retards tumor growth but also alleviates pain. RT is especially useful for tumors that are sensitive to radiation (e.g., lymphoma, breast), early and slowly progressive lesions, and metastases below the conus medullaris. The usual dose is 3,000 cGy divided in 10 fractions, but recent data suggest a shorter course with 2,000 cGy divided in 5 fractions is equally effective.

3. **Surgery** is used in the treatment of some patients with tumor metastatic to the spine. A randomized, prospective trial demonstrated that surgery followed by RT is superior to RT alone, giving significantly longer survival and better neurologic outcome, including restoration of ambulation in paraplegic patients. These operations involve resection of the vertebral body through an anterior approach; the body is reconstructed and the spine stabilized with hardware. Patients must be in reasonable condition with controlled systemic disease to qualify for this approach. RT may be performed after surgery, depending upon the primary cancer. Laminectomy has limited value in the management of metastatic spinal disease because the tumor usually originates anteriorly and posterior decompression does not relieve pressure on the spinal cord. Other specific indications for surgery include the following:

   a. Need for a pathologic diagnosis.

   b. Progression of neurologic abnormalities during RT; surgery rarely restores lost neurologic function in this situation.

   c. Recurrent spinal cord compression in a previously irradiated area.

   d. Spinal instability.

4. **Chemotherapy** is used in highly responsive tumors, such as lymphoma or germ cell tumors, if neurologic involvement is limited.

IV. METASTASES TO THE PERIPHERAL NERVOUS SYSTEM

A. Brachial plexus

1. **Anatomy.** The brachial plexus is composed of the C5 through T1 nerve roots. The upper portion of the plexus innervates the proximal arm musculature and sensation to the forearm and thumb. The lower portion innervates the hand musculature and sensation to the fifth digit. The lower portion of the plexus is in close proximity to the lymphatic system in the axilla.

2. **Mechanism.** Tumor is most likely to involve the brachial plexus by contiguous growth from the upper lobe of the lung or the axillary or paraspinal lymph nodes. Lung cancer, breast cancer, and lymphoma are the most common tumors to cause a metastatic brachial plexopathy.

3. **Clinical presentation.** The most common presenting symptom is pain, which tends to radiate from the shoulder to the digits and is exacerbated by shoulder movement. Paresthesias and weakness, with loss of deep tendon reflexes and evidence of muscle atrophy, occur in relation to the extent of involvement of the brachial plexus. Associated findings may include a palpable axillary or supraclavicular mass or Horner syndrome.

4. **Differential diagnosis.** The primary differential diagnosis is radiation plexopathy in patients who have been irradiated as treatment for their primary disease (e.g., breast cancer). Metastatic tumors tend to involve the lower trunk of the plexus because of its close proximity to lymphatic vessels, whereas RT plexopathy is more likely to involve the upper trunk. Features of both upper and lower plexus involvement are usually found, however, so this distinction is not diagnostic. Other causes of plexopathy include surgical trauma, trauma secondary to poor limb placement during anesthesia, brachial neuritis, and radiation-induced tumors of the plexus.

   a. **Metastatic plexopathy** is suggested by early severe pain, hand weakness, and Horner syndrome.

   b. **Radiation plexopathy** is suggested by absent or mild pain, weakness of the shoulder girdle, and progressive lymphedema. Often, cutaneous radiation changes, such as telangiectasias, can be identified within the previous RT port.

5. **Evaluation.** Imaging with CT, MRI, or positron emission tomography (PET) will demonstrate a tumor mass in the plexus in most patients with metastatic plexopathy. Surgical exploration and biopsy are rarely required to confirm the diagnosis but are necessary in patients who have diffusely infiltrative disease that does not form a discrete mass. Epidural disease of the cervical or upper thoracic spine may accompany metastatic plexopathy in some patients, particularly those with Horner syndrome, necessitating imaging of the spine in these patients.

6. **Management.** The tumor is usually treated with RT if not previously administered; otherwise, chemotherapy may be helpful. The primary management problem is often pain control; neurologic function may not return even with effective treatment of the metastatic lesion. No treatment exists for radiation plexopathy. Physical therapy can help maintain residual arm and hand function after both types of plexus injury.

B. **Lumbosacral plexus**

1. **Mechanism.** Malignant lumbosacral plexopathy is caused primarily from direct extension of intra-abdominal tumors, but 25% of cases are from metastases of extra-abdominal tumors. Nearly one-half of the patients with metastatic plexopathy also have spinal epidural disease. Radiation plexopathy can result from pelvic irradiation and present in a similar fashion.

2. **Clinical presentation.** The most common presenting symptom is pain; severe, unremitting low back or pelvic pain usually radiates into one leg. Pain is followed by paresthesias, weakness, and loss of reflexes. Bladder function is usually preserved. Lymphedema, painless weakness, and paresthesias are more commonly seen with radiation plexopathy.

3. **Evaluation.** CT or MRI scans will detect tumor involving the plexus or presacral areas. MRI of the spine may also be required.

4. **Management.** RT and chemotherapy are used to treat the malignancy as indicated. Pain control and physical therapy are often required.

C. **Peripheral nerves.** Spread of systemic tumors to peripheral nerves is a rare neurologic complication of malignancy. It occurs primarily in two settings:

1. **Infiltrative polyneuropathy** results from invasion of the endoneurium by lymphoma or leukemia, causing neurolymphomatosis. Over weeks to months, it causes a widespread, asymmetric, often painful, multifocal neuropathy, which may be fulminant in some cases leading to death. Secondary

seeding of the CSF may develop with subsequent leptomeningeal metastasis. The diagnosis may be made by biopsy of an involved sensory nerve or more frequently by hypermetabolism seen on body PET as tumor tracks along the roots and peripheral nerves.

2. **Perineural spread of tumors** is seen with cutaneous and primary cancers of the head and neck (i.e., cancers of the skin, larynx, pharynx, and tongue). Tumor invades the perineural space, spreads proximally along the nerve, and may enter the intracranial cavity and extend into the brainstem. The trigeminal and facial nerves are most commonly involved, often together, probably because of their rich coinnervation of the face. Orbital nerves may also be involved. The diagnosis is based on clinical suspicion and is confirmed by biopsy of a cutaneous nerve. MRI rarely shows thickened, enhancing cranial nerves.

V. PARANEOPLASTIC SYNDROMES

Neurologic paraneoplastic syndromes are rare and frequently present before the cancer is diagnosed. Patients with paraneoplastic syndromes tend to present with less extensive tumor and have a prolonged survival time compared with the standard population with the same cancer. An autoimmune pathogenesis has been demonstrated for some of these disorders, and specific antibodies are associated with many of the paraneoplastic disorders. These antibodies are generated as an antitumor response and are directed against the patient's tumor; they are thought to cross-react with specific neuronal subgroups, producing neurologic dysfunction and the clinical syndrome. It is important to realize that clinically identical disorders can occur in patients without cancer, but such patients do not demonstrate these autoantibodies.

A. **Paraneoplastic cerebellar degeneration (PCD)** is a syndrome of pancerebellar dysfunction of subacute onset. Manifestations include truncal and appendicular ataxia, dysarthria, and nystagmus; patients are usually so severely affected that they are bedridden, have unintelligible speech, and are unable to care for themselves. Associated neurologic symptoms, such as dementia or neuropathy, may be present, but they tend to be much less severe.

1. **Pathogenesis.** The tumors in patients with PCD express antigens normally present only in the cerebellum, and the paraneoplastic syndrome is believed to result as a consequence of circulating antibodies that bind to both tumor and Purkinje cells in the cerebellum. About 50% of the affected patients have antitumor antibodies. The most common antibody in PCD is anti-Yo, seen primarily in women with breast and gynecologic malignancies. Other associated antibodies include anti-Hu (mostly with SCLC), anti-Ri (breast cancer), and anti-Tr (mostly in men with Hodgkin lymphoma).

2. **Diagnosis.** The neurologic presentation may suggest PCD, and a definitive diagnosis is possible when anti-Yo, anti-Hu, or anti-Ri antibodies are detected in the serum or CSF. Other diagnostic features include inflammatory cells in the CSF, isolated cerebellar atrophy on imaging, and the absence of other causes of cerebellar dysfunction. If there is no known malignancy, a thorough search for cancer must be undertaken. Occasionally, exploratory surgery with hysterectomy and oophorectomy are performed in the absence of an obvious mass and microscopic tumors are identified. An occult malignancy may be seen at autopsy along with loss of cerebellar Purkinje cells.

3. **Therapy.** Patients with PCD do not respond to plasmapheresis, immunosuppressive treatment with steroids or cytotoxic agents, or treatment of the underlying malignancy. The patient's condition usually stabilizes at a level of severe disability.

B. **Paraneoplastic sensory neuronopathy (PSN)**, also referred to as *dorsal root ganglionitis*, is a syndrome of subacute progressive loss of proprioception and vibratory sense, resulting in a severe sensory ataxia that leaves patients unable to walk. Pain, temperature, and touch modalities of sensation are affected at a lesser degree. Painful dysesthesias and paresthesias are usually present. The neuropathy may affect the autonomic system, causing urinary retention, hypotension, pupillary changes, impotence, and hyperhidrosis. Sparing of the motor system is a hallmark of the syndrome, although patients may have mild weakness from disuse atrophy. In patients with more widespread neurologic disease, such as dementia, myelopathy, or cerebellar dysfunction, the disorder is referred to as *paraneoplastic encephalomyelitis* (PEM).

1. **Pathogenesis.** A circulating antibody, anti-Hu (also called ANNA-1 for antineuronal nuclear antibody type 1), has been demonstrated in patients with PSN or PEM; it is primarily associated with SCLC. Clinically, the antibody mainly targets the dorsal root ganglia, causing inflammation and loss of neurons. Despite the presence of antigen in all small cell cancers, only about 15% of patients develop the antibody, and few of these patients develop the neurologic syndrome that is associated with very high titers of anti-Hu. Rarely, an isolated brainstem syndrome has been described.

2. **Diagnosis.** PSN is often suspected clinically because the neurologic syndrome is highly specific. Electromyographic (EMG) studies in patients with PSN usually show a total absence of sensory action potentials and normal or nearly normal compound muscle action potentials. A definitive diagnosis can be made by detecting the anti-Hu antibody in serum and CSF. CSF studies show increased protein, a mild pleocytosis, and oligoclonal bands.

3. **Therapy.** Plasmapheresis, immunosuppressive therapy, or treatment of the underlying malignancy does not reverse neurologic deficits, although it may arrest progression.

C. **Opsoclonus–myoclonus.** Opsoclonus is an ocular motility disorder consisting of irregular, involuntary, multidirectional eye movements that persist with eye closure and sleep. It may be associated with myoclonus (brief, jerking contractions of flexor muscles). Opsoclonus–myoclonus is classically associated with neuroblastoma in children, in whom it heralds a good prognosis. Less commonly, it is associated with the anti-Ri antibody (or ANNA-2) in patients with breast cancer, causing ataxia and encephalopathy. Opsoclonus–myoclonus can be relapsing and remitting and may resolve spontaneously.

D. **Cancer-associated retinopathy** is a syndrome of visual loss that begins with obscurations and night blindness and proceeds to total blindness. It is most commonly associated with small cell lung carcinoma and melanoma. This disorder is associated with an antibody that recognizes the protein *recoverin* in the photoreceptor cells of the retina. It can be diagnosed by detection of this antibody in serum and by electroretinography.

E. **Limbic encephalitis.** Early manifestations include personality changes (depression and anxiety), followed by a profound loss of short-term memory. Seizures, hallucinations, and hypersomnia may also be present. Paraneoplastic limbic encephalitis is most commonly associated with antibodies against intracellular antigens seen in SCLC (anti-Hu antibody) or in germ cell tumors (anti-Ma2 antibody). It can also result from antibodies against cell surface antigens such as the AMPA and GABA-B receptors seen in lung, breast, and thymus cancers. Autoimmune and not paraneoplastic limbic encephalitis is associated with an antibody directed against LGI1, a component of the voltage-gated potassium channel.

F. **Anti-NMDAR encephalitis** occurs predominantly in young women and is associated with ovarian teratomas when it is paraneoplastic (about 50% of cases). Patients develop a multistage illness characterized by psychosis, memory deficits, and seizures that progresses to unresponsiveness, abnormal movements, and autonomic instability. The diagnosis is established by the presence of antibodies against the N-methyl-D-aspartate receptor (NMDAR). Patients improve with tumor resection and immunosuppressive therapy.

G. **Motor neuronopathy, or motor neuron disease,** is a spectrum of disorders for which the association with malignancy is poorly characterized. This syndrome can arise late in the course of the malignancy, even during remission. It is most commonly seen in both non-Hodgkin and Hodgkin lymphoma and is frequently associated with a paraproteinemia. A similar condition can be seen as part of the spectrum of disease associated with the anti-Hu antibody and SCLC. These disorders are characterized by a progressive loss of motor function that may resolve spontaneously; the sensory system is spared. Loss of anterior horn cells is seen pathologically. EMG studies can help establish the diagnosis.

H. **Neuropathies associated with plasma cell dyscrasias.** A symmetric, distal sensorimotor polyneuropathy may be associated with plasma cell dyscrasias, including monoclonal gammopathy of undetermined significance (MGUS), multiple myeloma with or without amyloidosis, osteosclerotic myeloma, and Waldenström macroglobulinemia. The polyneuropathy can occur as part of the POEMS (**p**olyneuropathy, **o**rganomegaly, **e**ndocrinopathy, **m**onoclonal gammopathy, and **s**kin changes) syndrome. It is often associated with a monoclonal paraprotein resulting in a demyelinating neuropathy. The neuropathy is progressive, but usually no pain or autonomic involvement occurs. Treatment of the underlying disease or with plasmapheresis is beneficial in some patients.

I. **Polymyositis and dermatomyositis.** These disorders cause painful symmetric, proximal muscle weakness manifested as difficulty rising from a chair or combing hair. Only a small minority of patients with these disorders have an associated malignancy.

J. **Myasthenia gravis** causes progressive fatigue with exercise. It occurs in 30% of patients with a thymoma, and 10% of patients with myasthenia gravis have a thymoma. The syndrome is caused by anti–acetylcholine receptor antibodies that block function at the postsynaptic membrane of the neuromuscular junction or anti–muscle-specific kinase (MuSK) antibodies that have both pre- and postsynaptic effects. The diagnosis is made by detecting an antibody in the serum, by the response to edrophonium (Tensilon), and by the characteristic EMG response to repetitive stimulation. Treatments include pyridostigmine bromide, steroids, plasmapheresis, and resection of an associated thymoma or the thymus.

K. **Lambert-Eaton myasthenic syndrome (LEMS)** is characterized by proximal muscle weakness, especially of the pelvic girdle. In contrast to myasthenia gravis, the weakness improves with exercise. Hyporeflexia, muscle tenderness, and autonomic dysfunction (orthostatic hypotension, impotence, dry mouth) may be associated with the condition. LEMS results from an autoantibody that reacts with voltage-gated calcium channels (VGCC) of peripheral cholinergic nerve terminals, mostly associated with SCLC but also seen with lymphoma and thymoma. One-third of patients have no malignancy.

1. **Diagnosis.** The diagnosis of LEMS is established by detection of the antibody against P/Q-type VGCC and by EMG with small compound muscle action potentials that increase after brief exercise or repetitive stimulation at high frequencies (20 to 50 Hz).

2. **Therapy.** Effective therapies include treatment of the underlying malignancy and 3,4-diaminopyridine (10 to 20 mg PO two or four times daily) for symptomatic treatment. When 3,4-diaminopyridine is ineffective or unavailable, guanidine hydrochloride, pyridostigmine, steroids, IV immune globulin, and plasmapheresis may be utilized.

VI. ADVERSE EFFECTS OF RADIATION TO THE NERVOUS SYSTEM

A. **Mechanism.** The CNS is highly susceptible to damage from radiation. The degree of neural dysfunction depends on the total radiation dose and fraction size, the volume of irradiated brain or spinal cord, and the time elapsed since RT. Reactions are classified as acute, early delayed, and late delayed. Acute reactions during RT are believed to be caused by a transient breakdown in the blood–brain barrier, leading to increased ICP. The risk for acute reactions increases with fraction sizes >200 cGy. Early delayed reactions, occurring weeks to months after irradiation, are usually self-resolving and are thought to be caused by demyelination. Late delayed reactions, occurring months to years after irradiation, result in permanent CNS damage. Tissue destruction with coagulative necrosis of the involved white matter is seen pathologically. Hyalinization of blood vessels leading to vascular thrombosis is a specific feature of radionecrosis.

B. **Radiation syndromes.** Specific neurologic syndromes occur in response to RT, depending on the site of irradiation.

1. **Radiation encephalopathy.** Acute radiation encephalopathy manifests as headache, nausea, and vomiting. Early delayed encephalopathy often mimics tumor recurrence, both clinically and radiographically, and consists of headache, lethargy, and worsening or reappearance of lateralizing neurologic symptoms. Chronic radiation encephalopathy is associated with atrophy of the brain and is more likely to occur after whole-brain RT than after focal RT. Clinical findings include memory loss, cognitive dysfunction (learning disabilities in children), gait abnormalities, and urinary incontinence. This chronic disorder sometimes responds to CSF shunting.

2. **Radiation necrosis** is a late delayed reaction to RT that mimics tumor recurrence. It causes worsening focal neurologic deficits and progressive enhancing lesions on imaging studies. PET or perfusion MRI may be useful in differentiating radiation necrosis from tumor recurrence, but these tests can also give false-negative and false-positive results. Glucocorticoids are beneficial, and because the necrotic lesion has mass effect, surgical extirpation is often useful. Bevacizumab has been reported to improve radiation necrosis and may help reduce corticosteroid requirements. However, clinical deterioration with continued bevacizumab can develop after an initial improvement.

3. **Radiation myelopathy.** No acute reactions to irradiation of the spine occur. Early delayed reactions occur as electric shock-like sensations in the arms or legs that last for several seconds and are precipitated by flexion of the neck (Lhermitte symptom). The condition is usually self-limited. Late delayed damage to the spinal cord results in a progressive myelopathy that may be asymmetric in onset; typically, numbness and weakness ascend and progress to symmetric paraplegia. This disorder is secondary to necrosis of the white

matter and usually occurs with doses ≥5,000 cGy given by conventional fractionation.

4. **Radiation plexopathy.** Brachial and lumbosacral plexopathy, a late delayed reaction to RT, is discussed in Section IV.A.4.

5. **Loss of special senses.** Loss of vision and hearing is a relatively common sequelae of cranial irradiation. Visual loss can result from radiation-induced optic neuropathy, retinopathy, glaucoma, cataract formation, and dry-eye syndrome. Hearing loss is caused by otitis media (acute or early delayed effect) or by sensorineural damage (late delayed effect).

6. **Hormonal deficiencies** occur as a result of hypothalamic and pituitary dysfunction after cranial irradiation. The most common deficiency involves growth hormone, but thyroid, adrenal, and gonadal dysfunctions also occur.

C. **Management.** Acute and early delayed reactions are self-limited but often respond to treatment with steroids. Acute reactions and some early delayed reactions may be prevented by premedicating patients with steroids before the start of cranial RT. Patients with large CNS tumor(s) and surrounding edema should always receive steroids for at least 48 hours before RT is started. Late delayed reactions, which are usually caused by neuronal and glial injury, do not recover with treatment; however, steroids can reduce swelling and symptoms in patients with radionecrosis. If small, the radionecrosis will eventually resolve on its own, but if the involved region is large, resection of the dead tissue may be necessary.

D. **Radiation-induced** tumors tend to occur decades after irradiation and include meningiomas, nerve sheath tumors, astrocytomas, and sarcomas; these tumors are usually malignant.

E. **Radiation-induced CVD disease** is caused by accelerated atherosclerosis that becomes manifest years after irradiation. It is thought to result from occlusion of the vasa vasorum. Patients are at high risk for transient ischemic attacks and strokes.

VII. NEUROLOGIC COMPLICATIONS OF CHEMOTHERAPY

Neurologic complications of chemotherapy are common and depend on the dose of the chemotherapeutic agent, whether the drug is given as part of a multidrug regimen and whether it is given in conjunction with RT. Chemotherapeutic agents may be toxic to the entire nervous system or cause more limited neurotoxicity, affecting only the central or peripheral nervous system. A variety of clinical syndromes are seen, many of which are drug specific.

A. **Encephalopathy** (insomnia, agitation, drowsiness, depression, confusion, headache) usually develops acutely after administration of the offending agent. Responsible agents include methotrexate, cytarabine, procarbazine, mitotane, L-asparaginase, ifosfamide, cisplatin, vincristine, 5-fluorouracil, tamoxifen, nitrosourea, etoposide, interferon-alpha, blinatumomab, brentuximab and, rarely, fludarabine, and 5-azacitidine. Although not a chemotherapy, chimeric antigen receptor (CAR) T cells can produce encephalopathy days after infusion characterized by seizures, obtundation, and decreased verbal output.

B. **Cerebellar syndrome** (ataxia, nausea and vomiting, nystagmus) can be seen after the use of cytarabine, procarbazine, fluorouracil, and the nitrosoureas.

C. **Seizures** may occur after cisplatin, hydroxyurea, L-asparaginase, ifosfamide, procarbazine, and, rarely, vincristine.

D. **Peripheral neuropathy** (paresthesias, loss of deep tendon reflexes, distal extremity weakness) is a common neurologic complication of chemotherapy. It is cumulative and at least partially (if not completely) reversible with discontinuation of the offending agent. Vincristine, paclitaxel, and cisplatin cause some degree of peripheral neuropathy in almost all patients. Other drugs that can cause neuropathy include bortezomib, docetaxel, oxaliplatin, thalidomide, vindesine, vinblastine, procarbazine, etoposide, and teniposide.

E. **Cranial neuropathy** (loss of hearing, vision, taste) may develop from the use of cisplatin, vincristine, and the nitrosoureas.

F. **Myelopathy** (quadriparesis, paraparesis, bowel and bladder dysfunction) is a rare complication of intrathecal chemotherapy, including methotrexate and cytarabine. Myelopathy has been reported only after drug administration via lumbar puncture, not through an intraventricular (Ommaya) reservoir.

G. **Combined radiation and chemotherapy-induced neurotoxicity.** The combination of cranial irradiation and chemotherapy, particularly with methotrexate, nitrosoureas, or cytarabine, can have a synergistic toxic effect on normal brain structures. This can lead to permanent damage, often affecting the white matter and causing a leukoencephalopathy that produces a progressive dementing process. No known treatment exists, but some patients temporarily benefit from a ventriculoperitoneal shunt.

VIII. OTHER COMPLICATIONS OF CANCER

A. **Cerebrovascular disease (CVD).** Strokes and hemorrhages are the second most common cause of CNS lesions in cancer patients after metastases. Autopsy series show that 15% of cancer patients have CVD, of whom one-half have symptoms during their lifetime. In addition to standard risk factors that apply to the general population, patients with cancer have additional conditions that predispose to CVD.

1. **Cerebral embolism** can result from the following:
   a. Nonbacterial thrombotic endocarditis, seen especially with adenocarcinoma of the lung and gastrointestinal tract, is probably the most common cause of cerebral infarction in patients with carcinoma, although it is difficult to diagnose. Diagnosis of the valvular lesions is best established by transesophageal echocardiogram.
   b. Septic emboli from systemic fungal infections, most commonly *Aspergillus* species.
   c. Tumor emboli (uncommon).

2. **Thrombosis** can cause strokes (arterial) as well as occlusion of the superior sagittal sinus (venous). The latter syndrome presents with headache, obtundation, and sometimes bilateral venous infarcts that may be hemorrhagic. Thrombotic disorders in cancer are caused by the following:
   a. DIC
   b. Hyperviscosity syndrome
   c. Chemotherapy, especially L-asparaginase, which causes venous sinus thrombosis
   d. Vasculitis, usually as a complication of herpes zoster infection or seen in patients with Hodgkin disease.

3. **Hemorrhages** are more common in patients with leukemia but can occur in those with solid tumors as well. Specific causes include:
   a. Thrombocytopenia
   b. DIC
   c. Hyperleukocytosis (acute myelogenous leukemia)
   d. Tumor invasion of blood vessels
   e. Bleeding diatheses/coagulopathy (e.g., in hepatic failure)
   f. Brain metastasis

4. **Subdural hematomas** can result from:
   a. Metastases
   b. Lumbar puncture producing intracranial hypotension
   c. Thrombocytopenia
   d. Head trauma (minor or postoperative)
B. **CNS infections** are discussed in Chapter 36
C. **Ocular complications in cancer**
   1. **Metastases to the eye and orbit**
      a. **Etiology.** Ocular and orbital metastases occur most frequently in breast cancer. Hematogenous dissemination to the eye or globe also complicates acute leukemia, lymphoma, melanoma, sarcoma, and carcinomas of the lung, bladder, and prostate. Head and neck cancers can erode directly into the orbit.
      b. **Diagnosis.** Patients develop eye pain, diplopia, loss of vision, and exophthalmos. Fundal hemorrhages, leukemic infiltrates, or masses may be evident on ophthalmoscopy. MRI brain or CT scans of the orbits, brain, and surrounding tissues may be diagnostic. Biopsy is performed if the retro-orbital mass is the sole site of disease.
      c. **Management.** Prednisone, 40 mg/m² PO daily, decreases pain. RT to the orbit can improve vision. Emergency treatment of the eye with small doses of RT may prevent blindness in patients with ocular involvement from acute leukemia. Ocular or orbital RT can produce subsequent cataracts but rarely causes permanent visual loss.
   2. **Central retinal vein thrombosis**
      a. **Etiology.** Central retinal vein thrombosis occurs in hyperviscosity syndromes associated with Waldenström macroglobulinemia and occasionally with plasma cell myeloma and with marked erythrocytosis from polycythemia vera.
      b. **Diagnosis.** Patients develop a sudden, painless loss of vision. "Sausage-link" widening of conjunctival and fundal veins may be present. The fundus may also have hemorrhages, hard and soft exudates, and microaneurysms.
      c. **Management.** Plasmapheresis is used for malignant paraproteinemias (see Chapter 23) and phlebotomy for polycythemia vera (see "Polycythemia Vera" in Chapter 25).
   3. **Retinal artery occlusion**
      a. **Etiology.** Embolic retinal artery occlusion is most commonly caused by atherosclerosis but may rarely occur with atrial myxoma, nonbacterial thrombotic endocarditis, and cryoglobulinemia.
      b. **Diagnosis.** Patients develop sudden, painless loss of vision and a pale fundus with a bright red spot over the fovea.
      c. **Management.** Ophthalmologic consultation should be obtained immediately, and in appropriate candidates, intra-arterial thrombolytic therapy is considered if symptoms are only of a few hours duration. Conservative measures include vigorous massage of the eye, administration of a vasodilator, and aspiration of aqueous humor.
   4. **Amaurosis fugax** can occur in patients with marked thrombocytosis (platelet count >800,000/μL) caused by myeloproliferative diseases, especially essential thrombocythemia or polycythemia vera. Treatment consists of antiplatelet drugs (e.g., aspirin, 81 to 325 mg/d) and chemotherapy. Plateletpheresis may also be used in severe cases.

Suggested Readings

Chamberlain M, Soffietti R, Raizer J, et al. Leptomeningeal metastasis: a response assessment in neuro-oncology critical review of endpoints and response criteria of published randomized clinical trials. *Neuro Oncol* 2014;16:1176.

DeAngelis LM, Posner JB. *Neurologic Complications of Cancer.* 2nd ed. New York: Oxford University Press, 2009.

Lin X, DeAngelis LM. Treatment of brain metastases. *J Clin Oncol* 2015;33:3475.

Magge RS, DeAngelis LM. The double-edged sword: neurotoxicity of chemotherapy. *Blood Rev* 2015;29:93.

Navi BB, Reiner AS, Kamel H, et al. Association between incident cancer and subsequent stroke. *Ann Neurol* 2015;77:291.

Rades D, Šegedin B, Conde-Moreno AJ, et al. Radiotherapy with 4 Gy × 5 versus 3 Gy × 10 for metastatic epidural spinal cord compression: final results of the SCORE-2 trial (ARO 2009/01). *J Clin Oncol* 2016;20:597.

Rosenfeld MR, Titulaer MJ, Dalmau J. Paraneoplastic syndromes and autoimmune encephalitis: five new things. *Neurol Clin Pract* 2012;2:215.

Stone JB, DeAngelis LM. Cancer-treatment induced neurotoxicity-focus on newer treatments. *Nat Rev Clin Oncol* 2016;13:92.

34 Bone and Joint Complications

Rodolfo Zamora, Darin J. Davidson, and
Howard A. Chansky

I. METASTASES TO CORTICAL BONE

A. Pathogenesis. Metastases from carcinoma are the most frequent malignant tumor involving the skeleton with the most frequently affected sites being the spine, pelvis, ribs, and femur. Tumor cells may metastasize to vertebral bodies or the skull without entering the systemic circulation by seeding through Batson vertebral venous plexus (a valveless system of veins along the entire vertebral column that communicates with other venous systems, from the pelvis to the brain).

1. **Mechanisms.** Osteoclast-mediated destruction and direct tumor cell–mediated destruction are the two mechanisms by which skeletal metastases destroy bone. Stimulation or inhibition of osteoblastic activity also occurs. The relative balance of osteoclastic and osteoblastic activity determines whether a lesion is osteolytic or osteoblastic. Malignant cells secrete many factors known to both stimulate the proliferation and activity of osteoclasts and produce osteolysis, possibly indirectly through the osteoblasts. These factors include the following:

   a. Transforming and fibroblastic growth factors; tumor necrosis factors

   b. Prostaglandins; interleukin-1 (IL-1), IL-6, and IL-11

   c. Parathyroid hormone–related protein

   d. Bone morphogenic proteins

   e. Matrix-degrading proteins, such as specific metalloproteinases

   f. Receptor activator of nuclear factor kappa B ligand (RANKL), the essential osteoclast differentiation factor

   g. Chemokines and chemokine receptors

   h. Osteoblast inhibitory proteins: Dickkopf-1 and secreted frizzled protein 2

2. **Frequency.** A relatively small number of different malignancies account for most tumors that spread to bone.

   a. Tumors that commonly metastasize to bone. Carcinomas of unknown primary site, lung, breast, kidney, prostate, and thyroid; lymphoma; melanoma; and occasionally primary sarcomas of bone.

   b. Tumors that rarely metastasize to bone. Ovarian carcinoma and most soft tissue sarcomas.

   c. Certain carcinomas have a predilection for metastasizing to particular skeletal sites. For example, skeletal metastases to the hands are unusual, but about 50% of these metastases arise from a lung primary, whereas foot metastases are most commonly caused by gastrointestinal and genitourinary tract tumors. Renal cell carcinomas often metastasize to the bones of the shoulder girdle.

3. **Types of bone metastases** and their occurrence in various tumors are shown in Table 34-1. Osteolytic lesions are the most common presentation, followed by mixed and osteoblastic lesions.

TABLE 34-1	Radiologic Characteristics of Bone Metastases		
Predominantly Osteolytic Tumors	**Mixed Osteolytic and Osteoblastic Tumors**	**Predominantly Osteoblastic Tumors**	**Other Causes of Osteoblastic Bone Lesions**
Non–small cell lung cancer	Breast cancer	Small cell lung cancer	Tuberculosis
Renal cancer	Squamous cell cancers (most primary sites)	Prostate cancer Carcinoids	Fluorosis Osteoarthritis
Multiple myeloma	Gastrointestinal cancers (most)	Gastrinoma	Osteopetrosis
Melanoma	Thyroid cancer	Gastric cancers Mastocytosis Lymphomas	Paget disease Tuberous sclerosis

    a. Osteolytic lesions are characterized by specific radiolucent areas: commonly in renal cell and breast carcinomas.

    b. Osteoblastic lesions are characterized by radiopaque areas: commonly in prostate cancer.

    c. Mixed lesions: commonly in breast carcinoma and most tumors.

B. Natural history. Bone metastases are usually confined within the bony substance and generally do not cross joint spaces. They lead to pain, pathologic fracture, neurologic compromise, progressive immobility, and resulting loss of quality of life. Crippling bone disease can make bedridden patients susceptible to decubitus ulcers, hypercalcemia, and infections.

    1. Spine metastases commonly result in pain. Cervical spine metastases compressing the cord may result in myelopathy and weakness of the muscles of respiration, resulting in paralysis, pneumonia, and possibly death. Thoracic spine metastases compressing the cord can result in paraplegia.

    2. Osteoblastic metastases (e.g., with prostate cancer) or extensive involvement of bone marrow spaces can result in refractory pancytopenia. Pathologic fracture is less likely in the osteoblastic variant.

C. Prognosis. The expected survival of patients with skeletal metastasis varies, but in general, the presence of skeletal metastasis marks the lethality of the disease.

D. Diagnosis

    1. Symptoms and signs

        a. Dull, aching, or boring pain that is worse at night than with physical activity is characteristic of pain from bone metastases. As disease progresses, weight-bearing pain becomes more prominent meaning involvement of the cortex and increased risk of pathologic fracture. These characteristics are directly opposite to the typical pain of degenerative diseases, in which pain related to activity is present earlier and worse than pain at rest. Direct compression of the affected bone may reproduce the pain.

        b. Bone pain intensified by activity is often the first symptom of imminent fracture. On the other hand, pathologic fractures, particularly in non–weight-bearing bones, can also be painless. Patients often report falling down, but it is often not clear whether the fracture was the cause or the effect of the fall.

        c. Spinal instability secondary to bone loss can cause excruciating mechanical pain. The patient is comfortable only when lying absolutely still.

d. C-7 to T-1 vertebral pain is usually referred to the interscapular region; radiography of both cervical and thoracic spines is essential in these patients.

e. T-12 to L-1 vertebral pain is usually referred to the iliac crest or sacro-iliac joint.

f. Sacral pain is usually referred to the buttocks, perineum, and posterior thighs. The pain typically is exacerbated by sitting or lying down and relieved by standing.

2. **Serum alkaline phosphatase levels** are usually elevated in patients with bone metastases. Elevations appear to reflect an osteoblastic (or healing) response to tumor destruction. In pure osteolytic tumors, the serum alkaline phosphatase level is normal.

3. **Radionuclide bone scan,** using ^{99m}Tc-methylene bisphosphonate, is the most effective screening test for skeletal metastases. The scan often detects metastases several months before radiologic changes are evident. Radionuclide bone scans reflect osteoblastic activity; thus, purely osteolytic lesions may not be apparent on a bone scan.

   a. Specificity. Patients with a known cancer and bone pain have positive bone scans in 60% to 70% of cases; patients without bone pain have positive scans in 10% to 15% of cases. Multiple "hot spots" are more specific than one or two.

   (1) Retroperitoneal tumors often cause a bony response, characterized by diffuse isotope uptake over the anterior aspect of the spine.

   (2) Patients with metastases from breast or prostate cancer, when clinically responding to endocrine therapy, may develop new abnormal areas on scans because of bone healing and increased osteoblastic activity.

   (3) Multiple myeloma, a predominantly osteolytic process except in the presence of pathologic fracture, is the most frequent cause of false-negative bone scans.

   (4) Decreased uptake of radioisotope is seen in irradiated bone and thus cannot be interpreted as a sign of absence of metastases or of reduced tumor burden.

   b. Benign conditions that can cause a positive bone scan: bone healing after fracture, radiation osteitis, arthritis and spondylitis, osteomyelitis, osteonecrosis, regional osteoporosis, Paget disease of bone, hyperostosis frontalis interna, Albers-Schönberg disease, osteogenesis imperfecta.

4. **Plain radiographs** remain essential for the diagnosis and characterization of bone metastases. Metastatic lesions must involve 30% to 50% of bone matrix to be visualized on plain radiographs. *Skeletal infections* with pyogenic bacteria are frequently associated with sclerotic reactions; chronic granulomatous infections, however, may result in purely osteolytic lesions. Blown-out lytic metastases are seen in renal cell and thyroid carcinoma and express the presence of soft tissue component.

   a. Indications. Radiographs should be obtained and compared with previous films of the involved areas in patients with bone pain, abnormalities on physical examination suggestive of fracture, or asymptomatic abnormalities in bone scans.

   b. Vertebral involvement from metastatic cancer is manifested by loss of the pedicles or lateral spinous processes and vertebral collapse with sparing of the intervertebral space. Infections that involve the intervertebral disk space destroy it. Some chronic infections (e.g., tuberculosis or

brucellosis), however, may involve the vertebrae and not the intervertebral spaces, result in vertebral collapse, and thereby mimic malignancy.

c. **Postirradiation osteitis** produces irregular, diffuse (rather than localized) osteolytic or mixed lesions confined to the radiation portal.

5. **Positron emission tomography (PET)** scans cannot provide as detailed
anatomic information as standard radionuclide bone scans, but this limitation can be overcome by performing a combined PET/CT scan. PET scans
have greater specificity for detecting skeletal metastases, but radionuclide
bone scans retain improved sensitivity and are much less expensive than PET
scans. Radiation exposure of PET scans and cost should also be considered.

6. **CT scans** are useful to characterize metastases of bone, particularly in the
spine and pelvis, when hot spots are detected on the radionuclide scan. CT
scans elucidate cortical erosion, subtle fractures, and matrix calcification
or ossification. Skeletal metastases around the spine and pelvis are better
described with CT scans, and in some cases, 3D reconstruction is somewhat
useful to plan surgery.

7. **MRI** scanning is best at delineating the extraosseous extension of a soft tissue
mass through the bone cortex (e.g., epidural compression). This technique
demonstrates in detail the intraosseous extension. MRI may also be used to
reveal subtle insufficiency or pathologic fractures about the hip and pelvis or
to evaluate specific sites associated with pain. MRI may overestimate the size
of lesions and presence of fractures.

8. **Biopsy.** Specific expertise in bone histopathology must be available. If only a
single bone is involved, the biopsy must be approached as if the lesion were
resectable for cure. Likewise, primary bone sarcomas may imitate a single
metastatic lesion.

a. **Indications.** If other sites associated with a lower risk for morbidity are
not available, bone biopsy for the differential diagnosis of cancer is indicated in patients with the following conditions:

(1) An isolated bone lesion that the radiologist interprets as being compatible with a primary bone tumor

(2) An osteolytic bone lesion in a crucial area (e.g., cervical spine or
femoral neck) and no history of cancer

(3) A history of a cancer that metastasizes to bone, localized bone pain,
normal radiographs of the area, equivocal bone scan and alkaline
phosphatase results, and no evidence of disease elsewhere

(4) Isolated bone pain in a region that was previously irradiated and
radiographic findings that are not typical of postirradiation osteitis

b. **Contraindications.** Bone biopsy should not be done in asymptomatic
patients known to have cancer but with isolated, osteolytic lesions in
noncrucial areas that are suspected to be benign lesions or metastatic
disease.

E. **Medical management** is necessary in patients with multiple painful metastatic
sites.

1. **Systemic therapy** is a critical part of the treatment of patients with bone
metastasis. If a tumor responds to systemic therapy, it may lead to a rapid
improvement in the patient's symptoms.

2. **Denosumab** is a monoclonal antibody with affinity for nuclear factor kappa
ligand (RANKL). It is currently the preferred agent for treatment of bone
metastasis.

a. **Mechanisms.** Osteoblasts secrete RANKL; RANKL activates osteoclast
precursors and subsequent osteolysis. Denosumab binds to RANKL,

blocks the interaction between RANKL and RANK (a receptor located on osteoclast surfaces), and prevents osteoclast formation.

b. Use. Denosumab is approved by the FDA for reduction of skeletal-related events (SREs) in patients with bone metastases from solid tumors (120 mg SQ every 4 weeks). Dosage adjustment is not needed for renal impairment. The prevention against SRE is superior to the prevention obtained with zoledronic acid.

c. Adverse reactions include limb pain, rash, and osteonecrosis of the jaw (ONJ). At 120 mg monthly dosing, hypocalcemia, hypophosphatemia, fatigue, headache, nausea, diarrhea, and dyspnea can also occur. Prophylactic vitamin D and calcium should be administered to prevent hypocalcemia.

3. **Bisphosphonates** are potent inhibitors of osteoclast-mediated bone resorption, and they are analogs of the endogenous pyrophosphonate with a carbon replacing the oxygen atom. The wide variety of alternative carbon substitutions results in marked differences in antiresorptive properties and side effects.

   They are highly concentrated in bone and become biologically inactive once the drug becomes a part of bone that is not remodeling. As a result, continued administration of bisphosphonates is required to achieve the desired lasting inhibition of bone resorption. After the absorption of bisphosphonates into bones, this drug has a very long terminal elimination half-life, approximately 10 years.

   a. Intravenous bisphosphonates. Zoledronic acid (4 mg IV over 15 minutes) or pamidronate (90 mg IV over 2 hours) every 3 to 4 weeks reduces morbidity and subsequent skeletal events for patients with myeloma and metastatic bone disease. Although both pamidronate and zoledronic acid have shown efficacy for patients with osteolytic bone disease caused by breast cancer or myeloma, only zoledronic acid has reduced skeletal events among patients with other cancers, regardless of whether the disease results from osteolytic, osteoblastic, or mixed metastatic bone lesions. Pain is improved in about half of the patients given pamidronate even without anticancer treatments. Recent trials show that after 9 to 12 months of the therapy, dosing can be switched to every 12 weeks without an impact on the frequency of skeletal events.

   Glucocorticosteroids and gonadal ablation with drugs such as GnRH agonists or aromatase inhibitors lead to enhanced loss of bone and induce fractures. Several studies have shown the ability of IV bisphosphonates administered less frequently to prevent bone loss and actually increase bone density. However, more studies are needed to establish the long-term safety and efficacy of this approach for this at-risk cancer population.

   Bisphosphonates may also have a bone metastasis antitumor effect. Some randomized trials have shown a reduction in both skeletal and visceral metastases in patients with myeloma or breast cancer.

   b. Adverse effects of bisphosphonates.

   (1) Renal dysfunction. The type of renal lesion is different between the two bisphosphonates. Pamidronate more often will cause a glomerular lesion initially associated with proteinuria. By contrast, zoledronic acid more often causes tubular dysfunction and thus is not often associated with albuminuria.

The nephrotoxicity is both dose- and infusion time dependent. After the bisphosphonate is temporarily discontinued and renal function returns to baseline, the drug may be cautiously reinstituted using longer infusion times (e.g., 30 to 60 minutes for zoledronic acid).

(2) **Hypocalcemia.** Most patients receiving high-potency bisphosphonates do not become hypocalcemic because of compensatory mechanisms, most importantly, increased secretion of parathyroid hormone. Hypomagnesemia and/or reduced creatinine clearance frequently are simultaneous factors. Thus, serum creatinine, magnesium, calcium, and phosphate should be monitored during bisphosphonate therapy.

(3) **Osteonecrosis of the jaw** is defined as the presence of exposed bone in the maxillofacial region that does not heal within 8 weeks of treatment. IV bisphosphonates are associated with an increased risk of ONJ (3% to 8% of patients). The concomitant use of angiogenesis inhibitors (e.g., bevacizumab, sunitinib) may be additive risk factors for the development of ONJ in patients receiving bisphosphonates.

This complication occurs more frequently among patients who have had recent dental surgery (especially dental extraction or implant) or trauma or who abuse alcohol, use tobacco, or have poor dental hygiene. Before initiating bisphosphonate treatment, patients should have a complete dental exam, and any dental extractions or removal of jawbone(s) should be completed several months before initiating these drugs to reduce the risk of ONJ. Conservative management of ONJ with limited debridement, antibiotic therapy, and topical mouth rinses may result in healing. Surgical intervention to treat this problem should be minimized and only undertaken by dental professionals experienced with this problem.

(4) **Other adverse effects of IV bisphosphonates**

(a) In about 15% to 30% of naive patients to these drugs, the intravenous agents may cause transient fever and an influenzalike syndrome.

(b) Severe and rarely incapacitating bone, joint, or muscle pain can occur within days, months, or years after starting a bisphosphonate and does not always resolve completely with discontinuation of therapy.

(c) Conjunctivitis, uveitis, scleritis, and orbital inflammation may rarely occur, but these manifestations require a prompt ophthalmologic evaluation; further treatment with the offending bisphosphonate is not recommended.

(d) A modest association between the use of oral and intravenous bisphosphonates and atrial fibrillation and stroke has been suggested.

4. **Criteria for response of bone metastases to therapy.** The appearance of new osteoblastic lesions on radiographs or bone scans or increasing size of sclerotic lesions does not necessarily indicate progression of metastases. Indeed, these findings may represent clinical improvement. Although the response of bone metastases to treatment is difficult to quantitate, it may be evaluated by assessing pain relief and quality of life, serum tumor markers, biochemical markers of bone resorption (e.g., urinary hydroxyproline excretion), and CT scans. PET is a promising but not validated technique to assess response of metastases to therapy.

5. **Bracing of the vertebral column** may help relieve pain and protect neurovascular structures while the lesions are resolving with radiation therapy (RT) or systemic treatments. Bony strength to resist gravitational forces must be adequate. Bracing of the lower extremities is seldom helpful.

F. **Management with radiation**

1. **External beam RT** ameliorates pain and may produce bone union and prevent fracture. The optimal dose of RT has not been defined. Smaller doses (e.g., 800 cGy given once) may be as effective as 2,500 to 4,000 cGy given over 2 to 4 weeks. This undoubtedly convenient, single, or very short dose schedule, however, may not be adequate for patients with a relatively good prognosis.

   a. **Pathologic fractures.** The administration of RT after orthopedic fixation of pathologic fractures is considered standard therapy. After orthopedic fixation, the bone encompassing the entire prosthesis is typically included in the radiation portal. RT may begin as soon as possible, especially if the incision can be spared; otherwise, treatment is delayed until the skin has healed.

   b. **Isolated sites of bone pain.** RT controls local pain from bony metastases in more than 80% of patients within 2 weeks to 3 months. Irradiating a few severely painful sites may reduce the analgesic dose needed to manage patients with multiple sites of pain.

   c. **Asymptomatic osteolytic lesions** of the cervical spine are irradiated when they are not at risk of fracture, to prevent complications.

2. **Radiopharmaceuticals,** strontium-89 (^{89}Sr), samarium-153 (^{153}Sm), and radium-223 (^{223}Ra), can decrease pain for several months in about 75% of patients with skeletal metastases from breast or prostate cancer.

   a. ^{223}Ra emits alpha particle. The drug resembles calcium and gets incorporated into bone in the areas of increased turnover. It is approved for the treatment of patients with symptomatic bone metastasis of prostate cancer. The treatment resulted in improvement not only of symptoms but also of overall survival.

   b. ^{89}Sr and ^{153}Sm are beta particle–emitting radiopharmaceuticals, and they are preferentially taken up and retained at sites of increased bone mineral turnover; uptake in bone adjacent to metastases is up to five times greater than for normal bone. These therapies have the potential to provide significant palliation of bone pain, with no survival benefit and with significant myelosuppression, which has limited their use.

G. **Surgical management.** Surgery plays a crucial role in managing bony metastases that endanger neurologic function; ambulation or pain is not well controlled with medical treatments as RT or systemic therapy.

   Orthopedic consultation should be obtained in all patients with metastatic lesions deemed to be at risk for impending or actual pathologic limb fracture. Pathological fracture is a real and severe emergency that needs to be avoided. The median survival of patients with pathological fracture is shorter than that of patients without fracture, underlying the importance of prophylactic fixation in patients with impending fracture. When considering operative treatment, the major factors include the patient's general medical condition, functional goals, and comfort and quality of life; the anticipated responsiveness of the tumor to RT alone; the ease of delivering nursing care; and the morbidity of the contemplated procedure.

1. **Methyl methacrylate,** an acrylic bone cement. It is frequently included in orthopedic procedures treating metastatic disease. It increases compressive

strength and torque capacity, promotes hemostasis, and should be used with fixation devices whenever bone stock is inadequate to permit rigid fixation or implantation. The circulating monomer may be associated with intraoperative cardiac complications, although this is uncommon.

2. **Complications.** The risk for infection increases in previously irradiated sites and in immunocompromised patients. Common reasons for failure of internal fixation include poor initial fixation, improper implant selection, and progression of disease within the operative field.

3. **Embolization.** Blood loss during surgical stabilization or biopsy of a metastatic lesion may be life threatening. Preoperative angiography and occlusion of feeding vessels, particularly for lesions of the acetabulum or spine, may be indicated.

4. **Rehabilitation.** Patients treated surgically for pathologic fractures caused by metastases are good candidates for intensive rehabilitation programs unless they have hypercalcemia or require parenteral narcotics, which are associated with very short survival times.

5. **Prognosis.** In general, median survival is <1 year after surgical treatment of an impending or actual pathologic fracture.

H. **Surgical management of the appendicular skeleton.** The threshold to treat lower extremity lesions is lower than that for upper extremity disease due to the weight-bearing function of the legs and the increased mechanical load on the involved bone, carrying higher risk of fracture. However, lifting and pulling with the arms generate high distractive and rotational forces. In addition, patients with metastases to the lower extremities often require crutches or a walker, which generate high compressive loads in the bones of the arms.

1. **Surgical methods** for metastases to long bones of the limbs include the following:

   a. **Reinforcement of the involved bone** with internal splints (bone plates, compression hip screws and side plates, intramedullary rods). Whenever possible, intramedullary fixation (nails or endoprostheses) is preferred, particularly in the femur and around the hip, because of the smaller dissection, more durable fixation, and more rapid return to weight bearing. Exceptions are humerus fixation for extensile metastatic disease and forearm, in which, plates and bones filled with cement allow patients to return to weight-bearing activities sooner.

   b. **Removal of the metastatic tumor** from the bone (either by surgical resection or by curettage), insertion of an internal fixation device or prosthesis, and supplemental fixation with bone cement.

   c. **Reconstruction of the articular surfaces** of the proximal humerus, hip, or knee after *en bloc* excision of involved segments of periarticular bone with either total joint arthroplasty or hemiarthroplasty. Prosthetic arthroplasty is useful in reconstruction of large destructive periarticular lesions, salvage of failed internal fixation devices, and salvage of lesions in which there are no RT options to prevent disease progression.

   d. **Amputation of dysfunctional extremities** riddled with tumor in patients with intractable pain, reasonable life expectancy, and an absence of limb-sparing treatment.

2. **Upper extremities.** Lesions that are larger and in patients using walkers or crutches may be best treated with surgical treatment followed by RT. The preferred surgical options are stabilization for nonarticular lesions and prosthetic replacement when the lesion affects the adjacent joint.

3. **Lower extremities: prophylactic orthopedic surgery.** Prophylactic internal fixation, followed by RT to inhibit further tumor growth, is always considered in patients with osteolytic lesions in the femoral neck or shaft that are at risk for pathologic fracture. Sometimes the prophylactic fixation includes the resection of the lesion and the replacement with an oncologic prosthesis. Prophylactic surgery should be considered in the following circumstances:
   a. The patient is in good general medical condition.
   b. The osteolytic lesion of the femur or tibia is >2.5 cm in diameter or involves more than half of the total cortical width (implies a 50% likelihood of fracture if untreated).
   c. Spontaneous avulsion of the lesser trochanter has occurred.
   d. Painful peritrochanteric lytic lesion.
   e. Pain from osteolytic lesions persists despite RT.
4. **Lower extremities: pathologic fractures.** Untreated pathologic fractures rarely heal, and although RT may achieve local control, bony union remains unlikely. Internal fixation is indicated for pathologic fractures of the femur or tibia to decrease pain and to permit early ambulation.
   a. **Femoral head and neck fractures.** Internal fixation may be considered but is usually inadequate. A cemented femoral hemiarthroplasty is safe, provides long-lasting relief from pain, permits early ambulation, and is preferred. Prosthetic replacement is particularly required if extensive cortical destruction would not allow a stable construction even with bone cement augmentation. The complication rate is 20%. Protecting the entire femur with long-stem replacements is not necessary when distal lesions are not present. Cemented implants are preferred as the patient can progress sooner to full weight bearing.
   b. **Intertrochanteric fractures.** Intramedullary devices are usually preferred so that the entire femur is reinforced with a load-sharing device. Prosthetic replacement is considered if there is extensive bony loss, making structural stability difficult. It is important to preserve the abductor mechanism, improving the function of the extremity. At 5 and 10 years, the implant survival rate is 84% and 70%, respectively. The complication rate, however, is substantial.
   c. **Subtrochanteric fractures** often extend into the intertrochanteric area or femoral shaft. The fractures are usually stabilized with a reconstruction nail with cementation as needed. Sliding hip screws are associated with a high frequency of implant failure. Extensive destruction may require the use of a modular oncologic or calcar-replacing prosthesis.
   d. **Femoral shaft fractures** require intramedullary fixation supplemented with interlocking screws and bone cement if there has been extensive cortical loss.
   e. **Lesions of the acetabulum.** Reconstructive surgery with total hip replacement is often beneficial in patients with reasonable life expectancy. Harrington procedure is described for reconstruction of the supra-acetabular area including the use of Steinmann pins running from the ilium to the superior pubic ramus and to the posterior column filling the cavity with bone cement. This procedure is generally followed by a hip replacement. A protrusio acetabulum often needs to provide additional structural support to the medial wall of the acetabulum (e.g., as cage reconstruction or composite with cement and wires). Custom oncologic prostheses can also be considered for managing these lesions.

I. **Surgical management of the axial skeleton.** Most cancer patients with mild mechanical instability of the spine and neck or back pain can be successfully treated with supportive medical care (e.g., chemotherapy, corticosteroids), bracing, and RT. Surgery is associated with a significant rate of complications (about 20%) but becomes important when the spine is unstable. Segmental spinal fixation systems use pedicle screws to attach rods to the posterior spine at multiple vertebral levels. Newer techniques use combinations of bone cement, allograft bone, and metallic implants (cages) to replace or supplement diseased vertebral bodies. Patients may get out of bed on the first postoperative day and typically require a custom-fitted, low-profile plastic orthosis.

As a generalization in the appropriate patient, surgical decompression and stabilization combined with RT are more efficacious than RT alone.

1. **Surgery for spinal metastases** may be indicated in the following circumstances:
   a. The diagnosis of metastatic cancer has escaped diagnosis at other sites.
   b. Mechanical instability from fracture causes pain and progressive deformity.
   c. Pathologic fracture or tumor extension causes compression of the spinal cord or nerve roots.
   d. A symptomatic tumor is known to be resistant to RT (e.g., renal cell carcinoma) or continues to progress despite adequate RT.

2. **Stabilization of the spine may not be indicated** in the following circumstances:
   a. Multiple osseous and soft tissue metastases exist.
   b. More than two or three contiguous vertebrae are destroyed and need replacement.
   c. The patient has poor nutritional, immunologic, or pulmonary status or severe disease not related to the malignancy.
   d. Life expectancy is very limited (typically <3 months).

3. **Stability of the spine** is commonly evaluated with the spinal instability neoplastic score (SINS). This score includes the location of the lesion, the presence of mechanical pain, the type of lesion (blastic, lytic or mixed), the alignment of the spine, the severity of vertebral collapse, and the involvement of facets, pedicle, or costovertebral junction by tumor or fracture. Scores equal or over 13 suggest spine instability and require surgical stabilization (Table 34-2).

4. **Cervical spinal metastases** often require RT regardless of symptoms. A soft cervical collar should be used only in patients with minimal disease. A rigid collar-like brace is adequate support if there is some intrinsic stability.

   Metal implants to replace vertebral bodies anteriorly, and screws into the pedicles or lateral masses posteriorly, can restore spine and spinal cord integrity. In patients with severely limited life expectancy, in lieu of major surgery, the head can be immobilized permanently with a special halo device and placement of screws into the skull.

5. **Thoracolumbar spinal metastases**
   a. **Painful lesions** may require RT. MRI should be done first to search for potential sites of epidural compression and to map out radiation fields. Many patients have a soft tissue mass extending around the involved vertebrae. These masses compress nerves, contribute to pain, and should be included in the radiation port. Fiberglass braces and corsets may reduce back pain and help stabilize the spine.
   b. **Rapidly progressive metastases** that are refractory to RT may be treated with an open decompression of the spinal cord and internal fixation to permit early mobility (1 to 3 weeks), but the outlook for these patients is poor.

TABLE 34-2	Spine System for Spine Instability Neoplastic Score (SINS)

Spine Location

Junctional (occiput-C2, C7-T2, T11-L1, L5-S1)	3
Mobile spine (C3-C6, L2-L4)	2
Semirigid (T3-T10)	1
Rigid (S2-S5)	0

Pain with Movement/Loading of the Spine

Yes	3
No or not mechanical	1
Pain-free	0

Bone Lesion Quality

Lytic	2
Mixed lytic/blastic	1
Blastic	0

Radiographic Spinal Alignment

Subluxation/translation present	4
Recent deformity (kyphosis/scoliosis)	2
Normal alignment	0

Vertebral Body Collapse

>50% collapse	3
<50% collapse	2
50% body involved but no collapse	1
None of the above	0

Posterolateral Involvement of the Spinal Elements

Bilateral	3
Unilateral	1
No involvement	0

Score	Classification	Management
0–6	Stable Spine	Medical management
7–12	Impending instability	Surgical consultation
13–18	Instability	Warrant surgical consultation and possible surgery

6. **Spinal decompression**
   a. **Laminectomy** provides direct access to posterior and posterolateral tumors but compromises the stability of the spine. Spinal cord compression is usually a result of tumors of the vertebral body (i.e., anterior to the spinal cord); thus, laminectomy does not reliably relieve symptoms. Below the level of the third cervical vertebra, laminectomy should only be used for lesions in the dorsal elements, laminae, and pedicles.
   b. **Anterior surgical decompression** of the spinal cord is performed using thoracotomy or laparotomy. Anterior decompression involves the removal of the vertebral body and all tumors anterior to the spinal cord (vertebrectomy). The spinal column is reconstructed with a graft or cage, and posterior stabilization with rods and pedicle screws is also usually needed. The anterior route provides immediate mechanical stability and the best chance for neurologic improvement. The associated success rate is reported to be 75% to 90%, with less blood loss and fewer complications than with laminectomy.

c. **Posterolateral surgical decompression** is an alternative for the technically difficult lesions above the sixth thoracic vertebra and is useful in more debilitated patients.

(1) Posterolateral decompression removes a part of the rib and lamina to gain access to the vertebral body and decompress the anterior aspect of the spinal cord from the side. After completing vertebrectomy and removing the disks, the surgeon inserts a vertical strut (graft or cage) between the end plates of the healthy vertebrae above and below the tumor site. Posterior fixation rods, which can be placed through the same incisions, provide immediate stability.

(2) The advantage of this approach is that it does not require thoracotomy. Posterior spinal instrumentation can be carried out at the same time as tumor removal, often with video-assisted endoscopic techniques. This procedure may reduce patient morbidity, days in intensive care, and days of hospitalization. Access to the tumor, however, is usually limited because the surgeon is working around the spinal cord.

7. **Percutaneous vertebroplasty and balloon kyphoplasty** are minimally invasive procedures consisting of the percutaneous injection, under fluoroscopic guidance, of methyl methacrylate into a diseased vertebral body. The kyphoplasty procedure uses a balloon to restore vertebral height and compress both cancellous bone and tumor before injecting the cement. Both procedures can be done quickly, have been shown to lead to very rapid and sustained reduction in back pain for patients with metastases, and are associated with low surgical risk and minimal morbidity. Cement extrusion is the most frequent complication, generally asymptomatic.

a. **Contraindications.** Vertebroplasty and kyphoplasty are contraindicated in presence of epidural compression or severe involvement of the posterior vertebral body adjacent to the spinal canal.

b. **Methyl methacrylate pulmonary emboli**, one of the most serious potential complications, are estimated to occur in 3% to 23% of patients depending on whether patients are evaluated with a plain chest radiograph or CT. This risk appears to be higher with vertebroplasty than with kyphoplasty. Asymptomatic peripheral embolisms predominate and require no therapy. Symptomatic emboli to the pulmonary arteries are treated with warfarin for 6 months, which appears to stop the progression of the foreign body–induced thrombotic occlusion while the cement theoretically becomes endothelialized. Open thoracic thrombectomy and percutaneous vascular retrieval have been used in cases of acute life-threatening cardiopulmonary compromise.

II. PARANEOPLASTIC, INFILTRATIVE, AND TREATMENT-RELATED BONE AND JOINT CONDITIONS

A. **Hypertrophic osteoarthropathy** (HOA) is manifested by clubbing of the fingers, pain and effusion in large joints, and periostosis of tubular bones. The ankles, knees, elbows, and wrists are the most frequently involved joints. The extremely painful periosteal reaction usually involves the extensor surfaces of the legs and forearms. The change in the overlying skin resembles cellulitis with induration, erythema, and *peau d'orange.*

1. **Associated tumors.** HOA develops most frequently with lung adenocarcinoma and occasionally with gastrointestinal adenocarcinomas and intrathoracic sarcomas. Benign causes need to be ruled out.

2. **Diagnosis.** Clubbing should be self-evident; patients should be questioned about the duration of the abnormality. Sponginess, by palpation, of the proximal nail beds may indicate early clubbing. Radiographs of painful joints or long bones often show periosteal reactions.

3. **Therapy.** Control of the associated tumor usually alleviates symptoms of HOA. The pain can be relieved by a variety of nonsteroidal anti-inflammatory drugs (NSAIDs). Pamidronate and zoledronic acid have been reported to be effective.

B. **Other paraneoplastic rheumatic syndromes**

1. **Pachydermoperiostosis** associated with lung cancer consists of a dense over-growth of periosteum resulting in clubbing and leonine facies (see Chapter 29, Section II.M).

2. **Joint pain, subcutaneous fat necrosis (panniculitis), and eosinophilia** occasionally constitute the presenting features of pancreatic cancer.

3. **Hypercalcemia and hypocalcemia** (see Chapter 28).

4. **Myelodysplastic syndromes** are associated with a variety of phenomena of suspected autoimmune pathogenesis. Among the rheumatic manifestations are monoarticular arthritis, relapsing polychondritis, Raynaud phenomenon, Sjögren syndrome, and vasculitis.

C. **Rheumatic manifestations that suggest an occult malignancy.** No distinguishing features of rheumatic syndromes define the coexistence of cancer. Manifestations may improve or disappear with therapy directed at the malignancy. The following syndromes should strongly suggest a thoughtful search for malignancy, *particularly if they first occur at ≥50 years of age.*

1. Explosive seronegative polyarthritis presenting with swollen and tender joints, with a predilection for the lower extremities sparing the small joints and wrists, and with mild nonspecific synovitis identified by synovial biopsy

2. Monoclonal gammopathy in a patient with typical rheumatoid arthritis

3. Palmar fasciitis and polyarthritis

4. Eosinophilic fasciitis unresponsive to steroidal therapy

5. Raynaud phenomenon (often with asymmetric involvement of the fingers and progression to necrosis)

6. Cutaneous leukocytoclastic vasculitis

D. **Direct infiltration of malignancy into articular tissues**

1. **Sarcomas** rarely present as primary malignancies of any joint. Intra-articular involvement of a sarcoma is typically the result of direct seeding into the joint.

2. **Metastases** can affect any joint and mimic inflammatory arthritis.

3. **Acute leukemic arthritis** is caused by leukemic infiltration of synovium. It is usually symmetric and may resemble rheumatic fever or juvenile rheumatoid arthritis. In 25% of cases, adjacent bone may develop osteolytic lesions, osteoporosis, or osteoblastic changes. Treatment of the underlying leukemia resolves with arthritis.

4. **Chronic leukemic arthritis** is uncommon; it is usually symmetric but is otherwise similar to the acute type both in radiographic patterns and in response to therapy.

III. ADVERSE EFFECTS OF RADIATION TO BONE

A. **Radio-osteonecrosis of the mandible** may complicate RT of head and neck cancers. The problem occurs more often in patients with large tumors, bone invasion, history of large alcohol intake and heavy smoking, poor dentition, poor oral hygiene, and poor nutritional status. The mandible becomes brittle and superinfected, resulting in pain, fractures, and draining fistulas.

1. **Diagnostic criteria** includes localized pain and tenderness, mucosal ulceration or necrosis (occasionally, a fistula) with exposure of bone, loose teeth in the suspected area and radiographs showing a osteolytic lesion of the mandible, sometimes with a radiodense sequestrum or involucrum. Manifestations should not be clinically evident for at least 4 months after completion of treatment.

2. **Prevention** of radio-osteonecrosis involves proper dental extractions before RT and oral hygiene and fluoride treatment regimen during and after RT. If possible, the patient should not have any dental extractions for 2 years after RT. Even with these precautions, osteonecrosis develops in 5% to 10% of patients when a high-dose RT portal overlies the mandible.

3. **Treatment**
   a. **Conservative management involves** frequent mouthwashes with dilute hydrogen peroxide or a baking soda and salt solution, systemic antibiotics, usually penicillin; topical nystatin or bacitracin ointment and gentle debridement.
   b. **Aggressive management includes** hyperbaric oxygen treatments and surgical resection of the nonviable portion of the mandible.

B. **Radiation osteitis** may mimic bony metastases. Differentiation of these disorders is discussed in Section I.D.

C. **Radiation-induced bone sarcomas** have been reported after high-dose irradiation of both benign and malignant lesions. The incidence is <0.1% of all 5-year survivors; the latent period is >5 years. Sarcomas induced by radiation are generally high grade, and most patients present with a locally advanced tumor. The prognosis is poorer than for comparable de novo sarcomas.

D. **Premature closure of bone epiphyses and apophyses** can result in shortening, kyphosis, and asymmetry of osseous structures in children who have received RT.

E. **Soft tissue radiation injury** depends on dose and those structures that are encompassed by the radiation fields directed to the bony site.

F. **Hypothyroid myopathy.** Myalgia, stiffness, and elevation of serum creatine kinase following external neck irradiation may be the result of radiation-induced hypothyroidism. These symptoms may follow RT by months or even years.

IV. RHEUMATIC DISORDERS RELATED TO SYSTEMIC THERAPY FOR MALIGNANT DISEASE

A. **Aseptic necrosis of the hip** is a complication of high doses of glucocorticoids. The risk is proportional to the dose of drug and not to the duration of therapy. Increased pressure in the intramedullary space causes the sudden onset of hip pain. Early diagnosis is best established by MRI. Removal of bony cores from the necrotic areas predictably, if incompletely, relieves pain and may favorably alter the natural history of osteonecrosis. Hip replacement is preferred at post-collapse symptomatic stages.

B. **Postchemotherapy rheumatism** is a syndrome of myalgias and arthralgias that usually develops within 1 to 3 months after completing adjuvant chemotherapy for breast cancer. Mild periarticular swelling occurs in some cases. NSAIDs are not effective. Symptoms are self-limiting and generally resolve over several months.

1. **Arthralgias associated with taxanes** (paclitaxel and docetaxel) usually begin 2 to 3 days after treatment and resolve within 5 days.

2. **Arthralgias associated with hormonal therapy** occur frequently in patients being treated with aryl aromatase inhibitors (anastrozole, letrozole,

exemestane) for breast cancer. Arthralgia and subjective joint stiffness are common complaints, occurring in up to 40% of women who are being treated with one of these agents. The problem often is not solved by changing agents within that class of drugs and may lead to discontinuance of such therapy. Arthralgias have also been reported in patients treated with tamoxifen but to a lesser extent and severity. These occurrences remain significant because long-term treatment is affected by their development.

3. The use of bleomycin has been associated with cases of scleroderma.

C. **Raynaud phenomenon** is a common toxicity of treatment with cisplatin, oxaliplatin, vinblastine, or bleomycin.

D. **Osteoporosis.** Many therapeutic regimens in cancer treatment carry the risk of promoting osteoporosis. Therapies involving corticosteroids or causing hypogonadism, including androgen-deprivation therapy and aromatase inhibitors, are the most common causes. Cytotoxic drugs that have been implicated in the development of osteoporosis include methotrexate and ifosfamide. The risk of osteoporosis should be assessed with osteodensitometry when indicated. Treatment with hormone replacement, calcium with vitamin D, bisphosphonates, and/or denosumab can be considered when appropriate.

E. **Immunotherapy with checkpoint inhibitors** (ipilimumab, pembrolizumab, nivolumab). Checkpoint inhibitors are a new group of antineoplastic medications working through unleashing immune responses. The treatment can be associated with immune-related adverse events: preexisting autoimmune disorders (e.g., rheumatoid arthritis, psoriatic arthritis) may get exacerbated or new polyarthritis may develop that resembles rheumatologic entities, but it is almost always negative for rheumatoid factor and other antibodies.

ACKNOWLEDGMENTS

The authors would like to acknowledge Drs. Dennis A. Casciato and James R. Berenson, who significantly contributed to earlier versions of this chapter.

Suggested Readings

Bauer HCF. Controversies in the surgical management of skeletal metastases. *J Bone Joint Surg Br* 2005;87:608.

Berenson J, et al. Long-term pamidronate treatment of advanced multiple myeloma patients reduces skeletal events. *J Clin Oncol* 1998;16:593.

Berenson J, et al. Balloon kyphoplasty versus non-surgical fracture management for treatment of painful vertebral body compression fractures in patients with cancer: a multicenter, randomized controlled trial. *Lancet Oncol* 2011;12:225.

Blacksburg SR, Witten MR, Haas JA. Integrating bone targeting radiopharmaceuticals into the management of patients with castrate-resistant prostate cancer with symptomatic bone metastases. *Curr Treat Options Oncol* 2015;16:325.

Dougall WC, Chaisson M. The RANK/RANKL/OPG triad in cancer-induced bone diseases. *Cancer Metastasis Rev* 2006;25:541.

Filleul O, Crompot E, Saussez S. Bisphosphonate-induced osteonecrosis of the jaw: a review of 2,400 patient cases. *J Cancer Res Clin Oncol* 2010;136:1117

Fisher CG, et al. A novel classification system for spinal instability in neoplastic disease: an evidence-based approach and expert consensus from the Spine Oncology Study Group. *Spine* 2010;35(22):E1221–E1229.

Fizazi K, et al. A randomized phase III trial of denosumab versus zoledronic acid in patients with bone metastases from castration-resistant prostate cancer. *J Clin Oncol* 2010;28:951s.

Johnson DB, Sullivan RJ, Ott PA, et al. Ipilimumab therapy in patients with advanced melanoma and preexisting autoimmune disorders. *JAMA Oncol* 2016;2:234.

Krueger A, et al. Management of pulmonary cement embolism after percutaneous vertebroplasty and kyphoplasty: a systematic review. *Eur Spine J* 2009;18(9):1257.

Lipton A. Treatment of bone metastases and bone pain with bisphosphonates. *Support Cancer Ther* 2007;4:92.

Lipton A, et al. Effect of denosumab versus zoledronic acid in preventing skeletal-related events in patients with bone metastases by baseline characteristics. *Eur J Cancer* 2015;53:75–83.

Loprinzi CL, Duffy J, Ingle JN. Postchemotherapy rheumatism. *J Clin Oncol* 1993;11:768.

Naschitz JE, Rosner I. Musculoskeletal syndromes associated with malignancy (excluding hypertrophic osteoarthropathy). *Curr Opin Rheumatol* 2008;20:100.

Patchell RA, et al. Direct decompressive surgical resection in the treatment of spinal cord compression caused by metastatic cancer: a randomised trial. *Lancet* 2005;366:643.

Pelton WM, et al. Methylmethacrylate pulmonary emboli: radiographic and computed tomographic findings. *J Thorac Imaging* 2009;24:241.

Piccioli A, Spinelli MS, Maccauro G. Impending fracture: a difficult diagnosis. *Injury* 2014; 45(suppl 6):S138–S141.

Saad F, Lipton A, Cook R, Chen YM, et al. Pathologic fractures correlate with reduced survival in patients with malignant bone disease. *Cancer* 2007;110:1860–1867.

Schneiderbauer MM, et al. Patient survival after hip arthroplasty for metastatic disease of the hip. *J Bone Joint Surg Am* 2004;86-A(8):1684.

Smith MR, et al. Denosumab in men receiving androgen-deprivation therapy for prostate cancer. *N Engl J Med* 2009;361:745.

Thambapillary S, et al. Implant longevity, complications and functional outcome following proximal femoral arthroplasty for musculoskeletal tumors: a systematic review. *J Arthroplasty* 2013;28(8):1381–1385.

Hematologic Complications

Mary Territo

I. ERYTHROCYTOSIS (POLYCYTHEMIA)

Erythrocytosis is defined as an elevation of the hematocrit and red blood cell (RBC) count above the upper limits of normal. Levels vary depending on the laboratory, but in general, males with hematocrit >52% and hemoglobin >18 and females with hematocrit >48 and hemoglobin >16 are considered to have erythrocytosis.

A. **Relative erythrocytosis** is characterized by normal RBC mass and decreased plasma volume. Causes of relative erythrocytosis include dehydration, diuretics, burns, capillary leak, decreased oncotic pressure ("third spacing"), hypertension, and stress ("Gaisböck syndrome").

B. **Primary erythrocytosis** is caused by intrinsic defects of erythroid progenitors.

1. **Acquired primary erythrocytosis** (polycythemia vera [PV]) is a clonal disorder. The majority of patients with PV have a somatic mutation in a gene on chromosome 9p (the *JAK2* gene). Erythrocytosis develops independently of serum erythropoietin (EPO) concentration. Uncontrolled proliferation of marrow elements results in an increased RBC mass and is discussed in Chapter 25, "Polycythemia Vera."

2. **Primary familial and congenital polycythemias** result from germ line rather than somatic mutations. Can involve abnormal oxygen-sensing (von Hippel-Lindau gene mutations) or mutations of the EPO receptor.

C. **Secondary erythrocytosis** is associated with increased RBC mass due to extrinsic stimulation of progenitors by circulating substances such as EPO.

1. **Appropriate erythrocytosis:** the bone marrow is responding to appropriate EPO.

a. **Congenital disorders** include hemoglobinopathies with high oxygen affinity, overproduction of EPO, and familial deficiency of 2,3-diphosphoglycerate.

b. **Chronic hypoxemia** is a potent stimulus for EPO production. Causes of hypoxemia include pulmonary diseases, right-to-left intracardiac shunts, low atmospheric pressure (high altitudes), alveolar hypoventilation (brain disease or pickwickian syndrome), and portal hypertension. Intermittent arterial desaturation and erythrocytosis may be caused by sleep apnea or by supine posture, particularly in obese patients with pulmonary disease.

c. **Heavy smoking.** Excessive and sustained exposure to carbon monoxide from cigarettes or cigars, which produces an increased affinity between the remaining oxygen and the hemoglobin molecule, is a common cause of erythrocytosis.

d. **Androgen therapy** stimulates erythropoiesis.

e. **Cobalt chloride** induces tissue hypoxia and consequent increased EPO production.

2. **Inappropriate erythrocytosis** occurs with elevated EPO levels in the absence of generalized tissue hypoxia. This can be seen in a variety of diseases and may be a presenting symptom or associated with ectopic EPO production of some tumors.

a. **Renal diseases** account for about 60% of all cases of inappropriate erythrocytosis, and renal adenocarcinomas account for half of those cases. Cysts, other tumors, hydronephrosis, and transplantation make up the remaining renal causes of erythrocytosis.

(1) **Renal cell carcinomas** synthesize EPO in association with erythrocytosis in 1% to 5% of cases.

(2) **Renal transplantation** is associated with erythrocytosis in 10% of patients. The erythrocytosis has been attributed to transplanted artery stenosis, graft rejection, hypertension, hydronephrosis, diuretic use, and EPO overproduction from residual renal tissue, especially in polycystic disease.

b. **Hepatocellular carcinoma and cerebellar hemangioblastoma** each account for 10% to 20% of the cases of inappropriate erythrocytosis in the literature.

c. **Other causes** of inappropriate erythrocytosis are rare. Huge uterine leiomyomas and ovarian carcinoma can cause renal hypoxia or ectopic EPO production. Pheochromocytomas and aldosteronomas can cause erythrocytosis through multiple mechanisms.

D. **Evaluation of patients with erythrocytosis**

1. **Initial evaluation.** The following studies are obtained in all patients with persistent erythrocytosis:

a. **Perform a complete history and physical examination** to search for known causes of elevated hematocrits. Search for treatments that are associated with absolute or relative erythrocytosis (androgen therapy, diuretics) and for splenomegaly, which would suggest PV. If intravascular volume depletion is suspected, replete the volume and then reassess.

b. **Analyze the hemogram.** The presence of granulocytosis, eosinophilia, basophilia, or thrombocytosis suggests PV.

c. **Measure arterial oxygen saturation.** The RBC mass is roughly proportional to the degree of arterial desaturation. Arterial oxygen saturation <90% and a PaO_2 < 60 to 65 mm Hg may result in erythrocytosis and suggest pulmonary or cardiac causes.

d. **If the patient smokes tobacco, measure the carboxyhemoglobin concentration;** values >5% are associated with erythrocytosis. Smoking may also cause granulocytosis. Pulmonary complications of smoking should also be evaluated.

e. **Serum EPO level** is decreased in PV and abnormalities of the EPO receptor. The concentration is normal or increased in the other disorders associated with erythrocytosis.

2. **Special diagnostic studies**

a. **RBC mass** determination previously was paramount for distinguishing absolute erythrocytosis from relative erythrocytosis. RBC mass is measured with ^{51}Cr-labeled erythrocytes, and plasma volume is measured concomitantly with ^{125}I-labeled albumin to assess for intravascular volume reduction. However, this useful test is becoming increasingly unavailable, and measurement of EPO levels is substituted.

b. **Abdominal radiography** (ultrasonography or CT scanning) is indicated in all patients with absolute erythrocytosis that is not explained by either PV or hypoxemia because the frequency of renal causes is high.

    c. *JAK2* **gene mutation** should be obtained if PV is suspected.

    d. Oxyhemoglobin dissociation curve is indicated in patients with a family history of unexplained erythrocytosis.

    e. Other diagnostic studies for inappropriate erythrocytosis are obtained *if* the screening evaluation exposes abnormalities that could indicate pathology of a specific organ.

    f. Bone marrow examination is not diagnostic of any disorder associated with erythrocytosis but in PV may show reduced iron stores, hyperplasia of other cell lines, or fibrosis.

II. NEUTROPHILIA

A. Definitions

1. **Neutrophilia.** Is an increase in the number of neutrophils (upper limit of normal is 8,000/µL). Granulocytosis is frequently used synonymously since neutrophils are usually the main cell line involved but can also refer to increases in eosinophils or basophils.

2. **Leukemoid reactions.** The term *leukemoid reaction* should be restricted to significant neutrophilia with some immature cells in the circulation (left shifting).

3. **Leukoerythroblastic reactions** are characterized by some immature neutrophils in association with nucleated erythrocytes in the peripheral blood. Platelet counts may be normal, increased, or decreased. This picture can be seen with (**a**) metastatic tumor in the marrow, (**b**) marrow fibrosis with extramedullary hematopoiesis, (**c**) marrow recovery after severe hematosuppression, (**d**) shock or hemorrhage, and (**e**) brisk hemolysis or hereditary anemias.

B. Mechanisms of neutrophilia

1. **Increased proliferation in the marrow** is seen in myeloproliferative neoplasms (MPNs, see Chapter 25), in marrow rebound after suppression by drug or virus, and as a response to infection, inflammation, or tumor. The mechanism of tumor-induced granulocytosis most often involves increased production of granulocyte and granulocyte-macrophage colony-stimulating factors (G-CSF, GM-CSF), interleukin (IL)-1, and IL-3.

2. **Increased marrow proliferation and increased granulocyte survival** are seen in chronic myelogenous leukemia (CML, Chapter 24).

3. **Shift from the marrow storage pool into the circulation** is seen in response to corticosteroids, stress, endotoxin, etiocholanolone, infection, and exercise.

4. **Decreased egress into the tissues** is seen after chronic treatment with corticosteroids.

C. Differentiation of leukemoid reactions from MPNs and CML involves complete clinical evaluation for signs of infections or other underlying disorders and presence of splenomegaly. The leukocyte differential count, neutrophil alkaline phosphatase score (low in CML, normal or increased in MPNs and reactive granulocytosis), cytogenetics and determination of BCR/ABL, JAK-2, or other mutations (see Chapters 24 and 25) are usually diagnostic. Bone marrow evaluation may be necessary.

III. EOSINOPHILIA

A. Definition.
The upper limit of normal in absolute eosinophil count in the peripheral blood is 550/µL. An increase in eosinophils can be seen in a variety of malignant and nonmalignant disorders. Persistent eosinophil counts >1,500/µL for at least 6 months without a known secondary cause is characteristic of

the hypereosinophilic syndrome (HES) and is usually accompanied by organ dysfunction. Specific clonal genetic abnormalities can now be identified for most HES patients and is discussed in Chapter 25.

B. **Causes of Eosinophilia:**

1. **Nonmalignant:** There are a number of nonmalignant causes of eosinophilia, which need to be excluded prior to attributing the findings to the neoplastic disorder. These include allergies, drug hypersensitivities, skin diseases (many types), infections (fungal, protozoan, metazoan), autoimmune disorders, eosinophilic pulmonary syndromes, chronic active hepatitis, and immunodeficiency syndromes.

2. **Solid Tumors:** Eosinophilia can be seen in association with many different solid tumors and tends to indicate advanced disease. This association can be related to tumor necrosis or to release of cytokines (CKs) by the tumors (G-CSF, IL-3, IL-5). The eosinophilia may resolve after surgical removal of the tumor but reappear with recurrence.

3. **Lymphoid Tumors:** Eosinophilia is seen in up to 20% of patients with Hodgkin lymphoma and is frequently associated with T-cell lymphomas. Bone marrow and tissue eosinophilia are also common in these disorders. The eosinophilia results from IL-5 and other CKs released by the tumor cells. A subset of B-cell leukemias is associated with a t(5;14) cytogenetic abnormality, which juxtaposes the IL-3 gene on chromosome 5 to the immunoglobulin heavy chain locus (IgH) on chromosome 14 frequently leading to eosinophilia.

4. **Myeloid Tumors:** Eosinophilia can be seen in association with the MPNs and with CML as part of the malignant clone and if extensive can be associated with eosinophil-induced tissue damage. Acute myelogenous leukemia (AML) patients with inversion or translocation of chromosome 16 have an associate eosinophilia and have a relatively favorable prognosis. Eosinophilia can also be seen in about 30% of AML patients with translocation 8:21. In these cases, the eosinophils are part of the malignant clone.

IV. BASOPHILIA

A. **Definition.** Basophils are the least common blood cell (<1%) in the normal peripheral blood. The upper limit of normal is 50 basophils/μL.

B. **Causes of basophilia**

1. **Nonmalignant:** Basophilia can be seen in association with hemolysis, infections, hypersensitivity reactions, chronic inflammatory disorders, and hypothyroidism, and in asplenic conditions.

2. **Malignant:** Basophilia is commonly seen in MPNs and may contribute to the pruritus accompanying PV in some patients. An increased basophil count can also be seen in association with Hodgkin disease.

V. MONOCYTOSIS

A. **Definition.** The upper limit of normal is 500 to 800/μL of peripheral blood.

B. **Causes of monocytosis**

1. **Nonmalignant:** Monocytosis can be seen with inflammatory bowel disease, sprue, alcoholic liver disease, collagen vascular disease (including rheumatoid arthritis, systemic lupus erythematosus, polyarteritis nodosa, and temporal arteritis), sarcoidosis, hyposplenism, and a variety of infections including mycobacteria, *Listeria*, subacute bacterial endocarditis, syphilis, varicella–zoster virus, and cytomegalovirus (CMV).

2. **Malignant:** Monocytosis can accompany leukemias, lymphomas, myeloma, and myelodysplastic syndromes. It is a hallmark of chronic myelomonocytic leukemia. Monocytosis can also be seen in a number of solid tumors with and without metastases.

VI. LYMPHOCYTOSIS

The differential diagnosis of lymphocytosis is discussed in Chapter 24, Section III.D in "Chronic Lymphocytic Leukemia."

VII. THROMBOCYTOSIS

A. **Thrombocytosis** (platelet count >450,000/µL) is often associated with solid tumors and can be a presenting finding or precede the diagnosis of an underlying cancer. Tumor cells can produce IL-6 or other CKs, which induce thrombopoietin and lead to an increased platelet count. Thrombocytosis can also be a consequence of tumor-associated bleeding or bone marrow metastases. Generally, thrombocytosis associated with solid tumors is mild, but values may occasionally exceed 1,000,000/µL.

In addition to contributing to the thrombotic risks of cancer, increased platelet counts can be associated with an increased likelihood of metastatic disease and poor outcomes in patients with solid tumors. Platelets can coat circulating tumor cells protecting them from immune surveillance, they can secrete CKs and growth factors that facilitate tumor metastases and growth, and they can produce angiogenic factors to help establish metastatic tumor blood supply.

B. **Causes.** Thrombocytosis can also be secondary to iron deficiency, infections or inflammation, acute hemorrhage, recovery from myelosuppression (viruses, ethanol, cytotoxic agents), hemolysis, hyposplenic states (postsplenectomy, splenic infarcts, and atrophy), and certain drugs (vinca alkaloids, epinephrine). Primary thrombocytosis is seen in myeloproliferative neoplasms (Essential Thrombocythemia, see Chapter 25).

CYTOPENIAS

Decreased cellular elements in the circulating blood can result from decreased or ineffective production within the bone marrow, increased destruction or utilization of cells, or sequestration in the spleen. Patients with cancer often have a combination of these factors. The type and duration of cytopenia can depend on multiple factors.

I. PANCYTOPENIA DUE TO BONE MARROW FAILURE

A. **Metastases to the marrow**

1. **Occurrence.** Carcinomas of the breast, prostate, and lung are the solid tumors most likely to be associated with extensive marrow metastases. Melanoma, neuroblastoma, and carcinomas of the kidney, adrenal gland, and thyroid also frequently have marrow metastases.

2. **Findings.** Tumor volume in the marrow does not correlate directly with the degree of hematosuppression. Marrow metastases are often found in patients without any hematologic abnormality. Patients occasionally have bone pain, bone tenderness, radiographic evidence of cortical bone involvement, or elevated serum alkaline phosphatase levels.

   a. **Bone marrow paraneoplastic alterations** can result in qualitative and quantitative abnormalities in hematopoiesis. In the absence of marrow metastases, changes can develop that are comparable to those seen in the primary myelodysplastic syndromes, including myelodysplasia in all cell lines, marked reactive changes, stromal modifications, and bone marrow remodeling.

   b. **Bone marrow biopsy** is superior to aspiration (with examination of the clot specimen) for detection of metastases, though both techniques are complementary. Cytologic preparations of bone marrow aspirates must be inspected at the edges of the smears for clumps of tumor cells. Immunohistochemical staining for epithelial markers and flow cytometry may be helpful in identifying carcinomas.

   c. **Peripheral blood abnormalities.** Nearly all patients with solid tumors having a leukoerythroblastic blood smear have demonstrable marrow metastases. Thrombocytopenia (in the absence of RT or chemotherapy) is the next best indicator. Leukocytosis, eosinophilia, monocytosis, and thrombocytosis each is associated with positive marrow biopsies in about 20% of cases.

B. Marrow fibrosis

1. **Occurrence.** Extensive marrow fibrosis is characteristic of primary myelofibrosis (MF) and late-stage PV (Chapter 25). Marrow fibrosis may also be secondary to neoplastic infiltration with leukemia or metastatic carcinoma or as a distant effect of some tumors without demonstrable tumor cells in the marrow.

   Secondary fibrosis in the marrow may also be seen in reaction to toxic agents (benzene, radiation, cytotoxic agents), infectious agents (especially tuberculosis and syphilis), hematologic diseases (myelodysplasia, pernicious anemia, hemolytic anemia), collagen vascular disorders, and in other disorders (osteopetrosis, mastocytosis, renal osteodystrophy, Gaucher disease, angioimmunoblastic lymphadenopathy).

2. **Findings.** A leukoerythroblastic blood smear is characteristic of marrow fibrosis of any cause, and splenomegaly may be seen.

C. Bone marrow abnormalities secondary to treatment.

1. **Bone marrow failure:** Ionizing radiation and most chemotherapeutic agents cause suppression of bone marrow function. Although recovery is usual after standard doses of chemotherapy, recovery after irradiation is inversely proportional to dose and volume treated and may never be complete. After doses in excess of 3,000 cGy, the bone marrow may be replaced by fatty and fibrous tissue.

2. **Therapy-related myelodysplasia and leukemia.** The occurrence of therapy-related myelodysplasia and AML should always be considered when developing treatment strategies. It should be remembered, however, that to develop this complication, the patient must have been effectively treated and then live long enough to manifest this toxicity so that effectiveness of the treatment is the prime consideration.

   a. **Occurrence.** Therapy-related myeloid neoplasms (tMN) account for 10% to 20% of AML patients. This incidence has been increasing as patients are living longer with possibly more aggressive therapies. Cases of tMN are seen in both solid tumor (especially breast, but also ovarian cancer, germ cell tumors, small cell lung cancer) and hematologic tumor (Hodgkin lymphoma, non-Hodgkin lymphoma, myeloma, and childhood acute lymphoblastic leukemia [ALL]). For children with ALL who achieve complete remission, the risk for therapy-related AML is greater than the risk for developing relapsed ALL. Modification of treatment strategies has shown a reduction in the risk of tMN for Hodgkin lymphoma from about 7% using older therapies, to 0.3% with current treatments.

   b. **Leukemogenic agents.** The risk of inducing AML is related to total cumulative dose and probably to dose intensity. The risk may also depend on the schedule of administration.

(1) Alkylating agents (i.e., melphalan, cyclophosphamide, cisplatin, dacarbazine) are most frequently associated with leukemogenic potential. There is a long latency period of 3 to 10 years after exposure, frequently with a preceding myelodysplastic phase.

(2) Topoisomerase II inhibitors (etoposide, teniposide, mitoxantrone) tend to have a shorter latency period (1 to 3 years) and do not usually have a preceding myelodysplastic phase. Other drugs nitrosoureas, procarbazine, and cisplatin are also concerning.

(3) Radiation therapy is associated with a minimally increased risk for AML when given alone but with a synergistically increased risk when combined with other leukemogenic drugs.

c. Chromosome abnormalities. Deletions involving chromosomes 5q and/or 7q are found in 70% of therapy-linked AML associated with alkylating agents, frequently in association with complex karyotypes. These same aberrations are seen in patients developing AML after exposure to leukemogenic solvents and pesticides. In contrast, certain balanced translocations involving 11q23 or 21q22 appear to be characteristic of AML occurring after treatment with topoisomerase II inhibitors, such as etoposide. Patients with these therapy-related leukemias tend to respond poorly to standard chemotherapy and overall have a poor prognosis. High-dose therapy with hematopoietic stem cell transplant can be considered for appropriate patients.

II. PANCYTOPENIA BECAUSE OF HYPERSPLENISM

A. Pathogenesis. Splenic enlargement from any cause (including carcinomatous metastases) may result in pooling and phagocytosis of the circulating blood cells in the spleen and lead to the development of cytopenias. Hypersplenism with severity sufficient to beg the question of splenectomy develops most often in lymphoproliferative disorders and myelofibrosis.

B. Diagnosis. The diagnosis of hypersplenism is based on clinical judgment. The only true diagnostic test for hypersplenism is improvement in the cytopenias after splenectomy.

C. Treatment

1. Indications for splenectomy for hypersplenism are all of the following present:

a. The patient has a significantly enlarged palpable spleen.

b. The cytopenia is severe (e.g., anemia requiring frequent transfusions; severe neutropenia associated with recurrent, serious bacterial infections; or thrombocytopenia with hemorrhagic manifestations).

c. Other causes of cytopenia have been ruled out (e.g., disseminated intravascular coagulation [DIC]).

d. A reasonable survival time after splenectomy is expected.

e. The patient's general medical condition is satisfactory enough to make the operative mortality risk acceptable.

f. Surgeons experienced in performing splenectomy under adverse conditions are available. Laparoscopic approach should be considered when appropriate.

2. Consequences of splenectomy

a. Postsplenectomy blood picture is characterized by Howell-Jolly bodies in the circulating red cells, neutrophilia, eosinophilia, basophilia, lymphocytosis, monocytosis, and thrombocytosis.

    b. Postsplenectomy sepsis is a potentially fatal complication, especially in children younger than 6 years of age. The most common infecting organisms are *Streptococcus pneumoniae* and *Haemophilus influenzae*. The incidence of sepsis in patients with Hodgkin lymphoma who undergo splenectomy has been reported to be 1% to 3%. Immunization prior to splenectomy should be undertaken. Febrile episodes must be treated immediately and aggressively in asplenic patients.

III. PANCYTOPENIA DUE TO HISTIOCYTOSIS

A. Hemophagocytic lymphohistiocytosis/macrophage activation syndrome (HLH/MAS) is an acquired syndrome of exaggerated histiocytic proliferation and activation. The acquired form is frequently associated with systemic viral infection (especially with Epstein-Barr virus [EBV]), although other microorganisms have also occasionally been implicated. HLH/MAS can develop on the background of another primary disease, such as autoimmunity, immunodeficiencies, or neoplasms. Lymphomas are the most commonly associated neoplasia (especially T-cell disorders, but also NK cell and Hodgkin disease) and should be searched for in all presenting patients. Abnormalities in genes involved in immune response pathways (i.e., PRF1, STX11, and MUNC13-4) are evident in children with the genetic form of the disease and are being identified in patients with the acquired forms of the disease with increased frequency, so that patients who do develop the disease may have an underlying genetic predilection.

    1. Pathogenesis. This is a systemic hyperinflammatory syndrome in which excessive stimulation of T cells and proliferation of these cells lead to disruption of immune regulation, CK storm, and systemic macrophage activation. This can lead to major organ failure of the liver, kidneys, brain, or lung. The severity of the syndrome varies from mild to lethal.

    2. Clinical findings include fever, severe malaise, myalgias, and often hepatosplenomegaly (which is less prevalent in adults than in children). At least two cytopenias are seen in nearly all cases. Neurologic symptoms and multiorgan failure may predominate and can be prominent.

        a. Bone marrow biopsy is often hypocellular with an increase in marrow macrophages. The macrophages are vacuolated and contain ingested RBCs and erythroblasts (and occasionally other hematopoietic elements).

        b. Lymph node biopsy may show evidence of lymphoma or can show normal nodal architecture with hemophagocytic histiocytes. These cells can also be seen on liver biopsies and may be evident in other effected organs.

        c. Blood studies

            (1) Acute phase reactants and proinflammatory CKs are elevated.

            (2) Triglycerides, ferritin, and LDH are frequently elevated. Fibrinogen and sodium are frequently decreased.

            (3) Increased soluble CD25, decreased or absent NK cell activity.

            (4) Parameters indicating DIC are frequently present (see Coagulopathy section).

    3. Treatment

        a. Patients with mild to moderately severe disease may recover in weeks if the infectious agent is treatable, or the disease may resolve naturally if the patient's immune system is intact.

        b. Patients receiving immunosuppressive therapy may require drug dosage reduction.

        c. Patients with the severe syndrome (EBV induced and others) may require 10 months or more of treatment with dexamethasone, etoposide, and cyclosporine A to suppress the CK release and reverse proliferation of

T cells. Alemtuzumab or allogeneic stem cell transplantation can be considered for aggressive disease. Etoposide alone, antithymocyte globulin, and γ-globulin have been used for less severe manifestations.

IV. ANEMIA IN PATIENTS WITH CANCER

A. **Anemia because of blood loss or iron deficiency**

1. **Pathogenesis** includes blood loss from ulcerating tumors, extensive surgery, benign gastrointestinal (GI) tract diseases, and hemosiderinuria from chronic intravascular hemolysis.

2. **Diagnosis.** Patients with known GI tract malignancies must not be presumed to be bleeding from an ulcerating tumor. Stools should be tested for occult blood.

   a. **Blood studies** may demonstrate microcytosis and hypochromia (although this may be modified by the tendency toward macrocytosis induced by some chemotherapeutic agents). Important clues that may signify a recent hemorrhage are polychromasia (often prominent 5 to 10 days after acute hemorrhage) or thrombocytosis (as a reaction to bleeding). Hypoferremia and hypertransferrinemia are often obfuscated in cancer patients by the presence of concomitant anemia of chronic disease (ACD); reduced serum ferritin levels are usually more helpful. Assays of soluble transferrin receptor (which is elevated in iron deficiency but not in ACDs) may be helpful.

   b. **Bone marrow examination** demonstrating the absence of stainable iron is unreliable in patients with cancer. The presence of stainable iron eliminates iron deficiency but could be compatible with ACD.

   c. **Therapeutic trials.** Ferrous sulfate, 325 mg PO given three times daily for 30 days, should elevate the hemoglobin concentration in patients with iron deficiency and otherwise intact hematopoiesis if ongoing bleeding is not present and marrow suppressing agents are not being used.

B. **Anemia because of nutritional deficiencies** results in megaloblastic anemia, with macro-ovalocytosis of erythrocytes, neutrophil hypersegmentation, and in severe cases, pancytopenia.

1. **Folic acid deficiency** is the most common cause of megaloblastic anemia in cancer patients. Decreased intake of folate is common with any advanced cancer. Increased requirements for folate develop with autoimmune hemolytic anemia, the postoperative state, prolonged IV therapy, and competition for use of folate by rapidly proliferating tumor cells. Folate deficiency may also develop after the use of folate antagonist drugs (e.g., methotrexate). Folinic acid (leucovorin) can bypass the folate inhibition of methotrexate.

2. **Vitamin B$_{12}$ deficiency** can be seen in cancer patients who have undergone gastrectomy or have extensive lymphoma involvement of the stomach (the site of intrinsic factor production). It can also occur secondary to lymphoma or resection of the terminal ileum (the site of vitamin B$_{12}$ absorption). Systemic B$_{12}$ replacement should be given to all patients who undergo gastrectomy or terminal ileectomy to avoid this complication.

C. **Anemia of chronic diseases (ACD)**

1. **Pathogenesis.** ACD is a multifactorial process in which CKs produced by the tumor and inflammation lead to restriction of iron availability, transient suppression of erythropoiesis, and mildly shortened erythrocyte lifespan. Inflammatory CKs (mainly IL-6) induce hepcidin release from the liver leading to a trapping of iron in macrophages, hepatocytes, and intestinal enterocytes. This results in less iron delivered to plasma

transferrin making iron unavailable for red cell production. This results in the characteristic low serum iron despite adequate tissue iron stores. Inflammatory CKs including TNF-α, IL-1, and interferon-γ can blunt the normal release and activity of EPO, leading to reduced erythropoiesis. These CKs can also lead to macrophage activation, which can result in premature RBC ingestion and destruction with decreased RBC survival. ACD is more severe with widespread metastases but may be observed in patients with localized tumors.

2. **Diagnosis**

   a. **Hemogram.** The erythrocytes in ACD are usually normocytic and normochromic. Some patients have microcytosis and hypochromia. The reticulocyte count is usually normal.

   b. **Serum iron studies.** Both serum iron and transferrin (total iron-binding capacity) are reduced, serum ferritin is normal or increased, and soluble transferrin receptor levels are normal (as opposed to iron deficiency anemia where you usually find elevated transferrin, decreased serum ferritin, and increased soluble transferrin receptors). Bone marrow iron stores are normal to increased.

3. **Treatment.** ACD is rarely severe enough to necessitate RBC transfusions. However, recombinant human EPO can correct ACD in many cases. Systemic iron replacement can also be considered if severe.

D. **Anemia caused by parvovirus B19.** Parvovirus B19 is the etiologic agent of transient acute aplastic crises in patients with underlying hemolytic anemias. This complication can be also seen in patients receiving chemotherapy, particularly as treatment of leukemia. An acute infection is manifested by worsening anemia, exanthema, and polyarthralgia. In immunocompromised hosts, antibody response against the virus may be blunted; an infection can persist and cause chronic bone marrow failure, primarily manifested by anemia. The viral target is an erythroid progenitor cell. The bone marrow shows erythroid hypoplasia. Treatment with commercial hyperimmune γ-globulins may be helpful.

E. **Pure red cell aplasia** (PRCA) is the isolated severe hypoplasia of erythroid elements in the marrow.

   1. **Pathogenesis.** Most commonly PRCA is idiopathic. Approximately 10% of cases are associated with thymoma. Lymphoproliferative disorders and various carcinomas have also been associated with PRCA.

   2. **Diagnosis.** A normocytic, normochromic anemia and reticulocytopenia are present. Bone marrow biopsy demonstrates markedly decreased-to-absent erythroid precursors and normal megakaryocytes and myeloid elements. Chest radiographs demonstrate a mediastinal mass if associated with thymoma.

   3. **Treatment.** Removal of a thymoma results in remission of PRCA in about 20% of these cases. Patients with and without thymoma have responded to therapy with cyclophosphamide, cyclosporine, or antithymocyte globulin.

F. **Warm antibody (IgG) immune hemolysis**

   1. **Pathogenesis.** Autoimmune hemolysis due to IgG antibodies most commonly occurs in patients with lymphoproliferative neoplasms. More than half of the patients in some series have an associated malignancy (usually lymphoid); only 2% of cases are associated with solid tumors. This complication has also been reported after treatment with various cytostatic drugs (e.g., fludarabine). The IgG-coated erythrocytes are removed from the circulation by the reticuloendothelial system, predominantly by the spleen (extravascular hemolysis).

2. **Diagnosis.** Patients with warm antibody autoimmune hemolysis usually have an insidious onset of severe anemia, mild jaundice, and splenomegaly. The blood smear shows polychromasia, a significant degree of spherocytosis, and, often, nucleated RBCs. Reticulocytes are typically increased but may be normal if any other cause of anemia is also present. The direct antiglobulin test (DAT, or direct Coombs test) is positive with anti-IgG or anticomplement antisera, frequently with specificity for the Rh blood group system. Other causes (i.e., viral, autoimmune, drugs) need to be ruled out.

3. **Treatment.** Prednisone +/– rituximab is usually successful. Patients with solid tumors associated with immune hemolysis respond to prednisone infrequently. Other treatments include cyclosporine, mycophenolate, azathioprine, or cyclophosphamide. Patients who have an unsatisfactory response or need chronic corticosteroid therapy may require splenectomy if their general condition permits.

G. **Cold antibody (IgM) immune hemolysis**

1. **Pathogenesis.** Cold agglutinins are IgM molecules that attach to RBC membranes at cold temperatures and fix complement. At 37°C, the IgM molecules dissociate from the cell, but the complement remains fixed. Cold agglutinins are most common in lymphoma and are rare in other malignancies. Antibodies are most commonly directed against the I/i system, but antibodies to the M, P, and precursors of ABH or Lewis systems are also seen. Overt hemolysis (often intravascular) is unusual except in patients with very high titers (>1:10,000) of cold agglutinins.

2. **Diagnosis.** Patients with high titers of cold agglutinins may have acrocyanosis or Raynaud phenomenon. RBC agglutination may be observed on blood smears, but spherocytes are not prominent. The DAT is strongly positive when performed at 4°C but is positive only with anticomplement antisera at 37°C.

3. **Treatment.** Rituximab, 375 mg/m^2 weekly for 4 weeks, is often effective. Chlorambucil or cyclophosphamide may be helpful for patients with symptomatic chronic cold agglutinin disease. Other drugs that may be useful include fludarabine, eculizumab, and bortezomib. Blood products and IV solutions should be warmed prior to infusion.

H. **Microangiopathic hemolytic anemia (MAHA)** with erythrocyte fragmentation has been described in patients with adenocarcinomas (particularly gastric cancer) and vascular sarcomas (i.e., hemangioendothelioma or angiosarcoma). The pathophysiology of MAHA involves fibrin strands of DIC, pulmonary intraluminal tumor emboli, narrowing of pulmonary arterioles by intimal proliferations, or a side effect of chemotherapy. Most patients with MAHA are in the spectrum with DIC and chemotherapy-associated thrombotic thrombocytopenia (see Section V. C below).

V. THROMBOCYTOPENIA BECAUSE OF INCREASED PLATELET DESTRUCTION

Increased destruction of platelets is usually associated with normal to increased megakaryocytes in the bone marrow and decreased platelet life spans.

A. **DIC** is a frequent cause of increased destruction of platelets in cancer patients and is discussed in Section III "Coagulopathy."

B. **Immune thrombocytopenic purpura (ITP)** can be seen as a complication of lymphoproliferative diseases and is rarely associated with carcinoma. Thrombocytopenia in ITP is due to reticuloendothelial system destruction of IgG-coated platelets.

1. **Diagnosis** of ITP is made presumptively in the absence of evidence of DIC or of drug-induced thrombocytopenia and with the finding of a

nondiagnostic bone marrow containing normal or increased numbers of megakaryocytes. Other causes of immune thrombocytopenia (viral, autoimmune, drugs) need to be ruled out.

2. **Treatment.** Control of the underlying disease is essential for satisfactory control of ITP.

   a. Treatment with glucocorticoids (e.g., prednisone 60 to 80 mg/d PO), intravenous immunoglobulins, anti-D immune globulin (only if RBCs are Rh(D)+ and patients did not have splenectomy), rituximab, single alkylating agents, or vinca alkaloids can successfully yield remission in some patients. Splenectomy may be indicated in patients who fail these measures and have symptomatic thrombocytopenia or require relatively high doses of prednisone chronically. Thrombopoietin receptor agonists (eltrombopag, romiplostim) may be effective for maintenance therapy.

   b. Many cases of ITP are chronic; platelet counts are 50,000 to 80,000/μL and don't usually result in bleeding problems. In the absence of symptoms, it is best to observe these patients without giving long-term immunosuppressive therapy.

C. **Thrombotic microangiopathic diseases (TMA): Thrombotic thrombocytopenic purpura (TTP) and hemolytic–uremic syndrome (HUS)** are disorders with multiple causes and overlapping symptoms and together are part of the thrombotic microangiopathies (TMAs). MAHA is frequently associated. These disorders are characterized by hyalin-like material in arterioles and capillaries, occlusive microvascular thrombosis, thrombocytopenia, hemolysis with schistocytosis, and end organ damage (renal, CNS, and others). CKs such as TNF-α and IL-8 have been shown to cause secretion of von Willebrand factor (VWF), while IL-6 inhibits cleavage of VWF multimers in vitro and may contribute to the pathologic thrombus formation in HUS. Endothelial activation and abnormalities of complement can also play a role. Primary TTP is associated with very low serum levels of the metalloprotease ADAMTS13 (either due to decreased production or to autoantibodies to the ADAMTS13). ADAMTS13 is responsible for cleaving multimeric VWF and regulating thrombus formation, so with very low levels, there is pathologic thrombus formation as seen in TTP. Plasmapheresis and/or plasma replacement have shown responsiveness in many of these patients.

   TMA can be seen in association with a variety of malignancies (usually late stages) and post–bone marrow transplantation (BMT). More commonly, TMA is seen secondary to treatment of the malignancies with cytotoxic or immunologic agents.

   1. **Chemotherapy-induced TMA** can be seen with mitomycin and gemcitabine and is thought to relate to nonspecific endothelial injury by the drugs resulting in exposure of the subendothelium, platelet activation, and subsequent clotting within the microvasculature. Cyclosporin or tacrolimus can cause similar problems.

   2. **Immunotherapy-related TMA:** Immunotherapeutic agents (i.e., alemtuzumab) have occasionally been associated with TMA, likely related to CK release (TNF-α, IL-6) leading to pathologic thrombus formation. Immunotoxins have also been associated with TMA.

   3. **Anti-vascular endothelial growth factor (VEGF) therapy-induced TMA:** TMA has been seen with agents that inhibit VEGF (bevacizumab, sunitinib). Lack of VEGF signaling may lead to endothelium compromise and subsequent pathologic thrombosis. Schistocytosis may not be evident in these patients.

   4. **Diagnosis.** Diagnostic hallmarks of TTP/HUS are microangiopathic hemolysis and thrombocytopenia; other features often include markedly

elevated serum LDH levels, rapidly changing neurologic abnormalities, fever, and renal dysfunction. Coagulation abnormalities associated with DIC are absent.

5. **Treatments:** The offending agent should be stopped or reduced. Treatment with corticosteroids, plasma exchange treatments, or plasmapheresis is used because of the effectiveness in primary TTP, although it is unclear of their activity when the plasma ADAMT13 levels are normal. Treatment with staphylococcal protein A extracorporeal immunoabsorption of circulating IgG immune complexes can also give responses in some patients. Responses are usually observed within the first 3 weeks. Rituximab has demonstrated effectiveness in many patients. Other agents to consider include cyclophosphamide, vincristine, and eculizumab for patients who are unresponsive.

VI. GRANULOCYTOPENIA

Granulocytopenia in cancer patients is usually the result of chemotherapy, radiotherapy, other drugs, severe infection, or tumor marrow involvement. An immune or CK basis is involved in the granulocytopenia associated with T-cell large granular lymphocyte leukemia and rare cases of thymoma.

Granulocytopenia predisposes patients to infections (See Chapter 36). Infection in patients with severe neutropenia (<500 neutrophils/µL) can be a lethal complication and should be treated rapidly with antimicrobial agents. Cultures should be obtained, and broad spectrum antibiotics should be instituted at the first signs of fever or infection; these can be modified later if a specific organism is identified. Because fungal infections are also a risk with severe neutropenia, the addition of antifungal agents should be considered in patients who fail to respond to antibiotics if no other cause is identified.

VII. LYMPHOCYTOPENIA

Pretreatment lymphopenia is an independent prognostic factor in a variety of solid tumors, including rectal cancer, cervical cancer, and metastatic breast cancer. Lymphocytopenia can be seen secondary to CT/RT. Corticosteroids are directly lympholytic, and many therapeutic antibodies (i.e., rituximab, alemtuzumab, ATG) are directed against lymphocyte populations. Treatment-related lymphopenia can be associated with adverse outcomes. Opportunistic infections (i.e., pneumocystis, CMV, zoster) can develop, and early treatment or consideration of prophylaxis should be undertaken (see Chapter 36).

VIII. MONOCYTOPENIA

Monocytopenia as an isolated finding has no specific clinical findings. Monocytopenia can be seen with CT/RT, in aplastic anemia, and is a constant finding in hairy cell leukemia, for which it can represent an important diagnostic clue. Severe monocytopenia is seen in patients with the MonoMAC syndrome and is associated with mycobacterial infections. The monocytopenia is usually accompanied by decreased B cells, NK cells, and Dendritic cells; and frequently have GATA2 mutations. These patients have an increased risk of opportunistic infections and a tendency to develop hematologic malignancies.

IX. BLOOD COMPONENT THERAPY

A. **Transfusion of erythrocytes**

1. **Indications:** Packed RBCs (PRBCs) are used for increasing blood volume (with saline or colloid solutions when acute blood loss threatens the integrity of the cardiovascular system) and for increasing oxygen-carrying capacity

(when anemia causes or threatens tissue hypoxia). Most patients tolerate chronic, moderately severe anemia well. No specific hemoglobin value mandates transfusion, and the clinical status of the patient should primarily dictate when RBC transfusions are needed. PRBCs are given to increase the oxygen-carrying capacity of blood for actual or incipient congestive heart failure or to reverse cardiac or central nervous system ischemic symptoms. When the hemoglobin level that precipitated symptoms is determined, patients with chronic anemia are transfused prophylactically to exceed that level.

2. **Transfusion reactions**
   a. **Fever and chills.** Most febrile reactions are caused by antibodies in the recipient directed against granulocytic antigens and specific human leukocyte antigens (HLAs) on leukocytes in the donor blood. Febrile reactions occur in up to 80% of patients who receive multiple transfusions. The reaction usually starts shortly into the transfusion, continues for 2 to 6 hours, and may persist for 12 hours.

      Premedication with an antipyretic and an antihistamine (usually acetaminophen and diphenhydramine), prestorage leukoreduction of PRBC units, and reduced plasma from platelet units can diminish but do not eliminate febrile transfusion reactions.

   b. **Allergic reactions** involving urticaria develop in 5% of transfused patients. Some of these reactions are due to antibodies in the recipient directed against immunoglobulin components and other proteins in the plasma of the donor. These reactions are usually mild and respond to antihistamines.

      These kinds of reactions or anaphylaxis are particularly likely to occur in patients with congenital IgA deficiency who have formed anti-IgA antibody (1 per 800 people). Reactions can be prevented by using washed or frozen RBCs because these components are prepared by procedures that remove donor plasma.

   c. **Major acute intravascular hemolytic transfusion reactions** are most likely to occur as a result of human error during blood preparation or administration. Fever and chills usually develop within the first 30 minutes into the transfusion and are often accompanied by back pain, sensations of chest compression, tachycardia, hypotension, tachypnea, nausea, vomiting, oliguria, hemoglobinuria, and DIC. The risk for a fatal hemolytic transfusion reaction is about 1:100,000. Plasma is examined for confirmatory findings and compared with the pretransfusion specimen: increased free plasma hemoglobin (pink plasma) and methemalbumin (brown plasma). Detailed evaluation of antibodies evaluated in the cross-matching process should follow.

   d. **Delayed hemolytic transfusion reactions** occur 5 to 14 days after transfusion, particularly in association with alloantibodies to antigens of the Kidd, Duffy, Kell, or Rh blood group systems. Hemolysis is extravascular and is manifested by jaundice and the absence of an improvement of hemoglobin levels after transfusion. In these cases, patients have become alloimmunized by a previous transfusion or pregnancy, but the antibody concentration was too low to be detected at the time of transfusion; an anamnestic antibody response was generated by the subsequent transfusion.

   e. **Posttransfusion purpura** is manifested by severe thrombocytopenia developing 5 to 8 days after transfusion and occurs in the 2% of patients who lack the platelet antigen Pl^{A1}.

f. **Bacterial contamination** occurs rarely in PRBC units (usually with cryopathic gram-negative bacteria) but is more likely with platelet packs that are stored (at room temperature) for >4 days.

g. **Viral contamination.** Predonation screening interviews and postdonation serologic testing have significantly reduced the incidence of some transfusion-transmitted viral infections (hepatitis B, hepatitis C, and human immunodeficiency virus [HIV]). The risks (per unit for blood units that are negative in laboratory testing) of transmitting viruses through transfusion are 1:150,000 for hepatitis B virus, 1:1,200,000 to 1,900,000 for hepatitis C virus, 1:1,400,000 to 2,100,000 for HIV, and 1:640,000 for human T-cell lymphotropic virus types 1 and 2.

h. **Graft versus host disease** (GVHD; see Chapter 38) can occur after blood cell transfusion in patients who have undergone a conditioning regimen for BMT. Transfusional GVHD can occur following blood transfusion in patients who are heavily immunosuppressed following chemotherapy or who have congenital immunodeficiencies. GVHD can also occur in patients who are less immunocompromised if the blood donor is homozygous for one of the HLA haplotypes of the recipient and particularly if the donor is a first-degree relative. Transfusional GVHD is preventable by irradiation of blood products prior to transfusion (see Section IX.A.3.f).

i. **Other complications** include those associated with massive transfusion (blood volume overload, hypocalcemia, hyperkalemia, hypothermia), iron overload with chronic transfusions, alloimmunization, and transfusion-related acute lung injury (TRALI. See section IX.D.2.d).

3. **Uses for erythrocyte preparations**

a. **Fresh whole blood.** None

b. **PRBCs.** The mainstay of erythrocyte transfusion therapy

c. **Saline-washed PRBCs** are indicated in patients who have IgA deficiency (particularly those with high anti-IgA titers), prior urticarial reactions with transfusions, the need to avoid transfusion of complement, or the rare patient who is hypersensitive to plasma.

d. **Leukocyte-reduced PRBCs** are used for patients requiring chronic transfusion therapy and those with prior febrile nonhemolytic transfusion reactions and also for immunocompromised patients in whom reducing the risk for transfusion-transmitted CMV is sought (particularly when seronegative units for CMV are not available). Leukocytes can be removed by centrifugation, washing, or filtration (the latter technique is most frequently used). These products yield $<5 \times 10^8$ leukocytes per unit of blood.

e. **Frozen RBCs** are a source for rare blood types, a backup supply for the common blood types, a substitute for saline-washed or leukocyte-filtered PRBCs when those methods fail to prevent febrile or allergic transfusion reactions, and an additional method of autologous donation. The extensive washing required to remove the cryopreservatives in frozen RBCs renders the suspension totally free of all leukocytes, platelets, and plasma constituents. The major limitations are the cost and the time required to prepare and store cells.

f. **Gamma-irradiated PRBCs** are given to prevent viable T lymphocytes from causing transfusion-induced GVHD in the recipient. The blood unit is usually treated with a dose of 1,500 cGy.

    g. Directed or designated donors from among family members or friends, contrary to expectation, are no safer for viral transmission than screened volunteer blood donors (probably because of the sometimes unreliability of the history taken from these candidates in the screening process prior to donation). Furthermore, if not irradiated, these units are associated with an increased risk for transfusional GVHD when provided by first-degree relatives to immunocompromised patients.

B. Transfusion of granulocytes. Granulocytes collected by apheresis are rarely helpful in treating patients with granulocytopenia. The paramount factors in determining the outcome of sepsis are effectiveness of antimicrobial therapy and the recovery of marrow function. Transfusion of granulocytes can occasionally be helpful as a temporary adjunct to antimicrobials in severely neutropenic patients with active infections. Transfusion of leukocytes can result in transfusional GVHD and transmission of CMV. If granulocyte transfusion is used, the transfused cells should be irradiated, and donors who are seronegative for CMV should be used for seronegative recipients.

C. Transfusion of platelets

    1. Factors influencing the decision to transfuse platelets

        a. Platelet count. Spontaneous hemorrhage rarely occurs with platelet counts above 20,000/µL. Platelet counts of <10,000/µL are associated with an increased risk for spontaneous hemorrhage, especially when the thrombocytopenia results from decreased production rather than from increased platelet destruction. Progressively worsening thrombocytopenia is more likely to be associated with active hemorrhage than with stable or increasing platelet counts.

        b. Platelet age. Young platelets (i.e., produced after peripheral destruction) are larger and better able to provide hemostasis than old platelets. Usually, patients with immune or postinfectious severe thrombocytopenia have no serious hemorrhagic sequelae.

        c. Active bleeding, uncontrollable by local measures, or bleeding into vital or inaccessible organs, is an absolute indication for platelet transfusion in patients with thrombocytopenia of nearly any severity.

        d. Fever, infection, and corticosteroid therapy increase the risk for serious hemorrhage in patients with very low platelet counts.

        e. Drugs and diseases adversely affecting platelet function may necessitate platelet transfusions in times of hemorrhage or surgery despite adequate platelet counts (see Section IX.C.6).

        f. Immune thrombocytopenia usually makes platelet transfusions useless.

        g. Patients with thrombocytopenia that is refractory to platelet transfusion may be alloimmunized, but they also may have DIC, TTP/HUS, or ITP.

    2. Problems associated with platelet transfusion. The majority of platelets are now produced by plateletpheresis, wherein the platelet concentrate contains <5 × 10^6 white blood cells (WBCs); these products can be considered "leukocyte depleted."

        a. Alloimmunization. Compatibility between donor and recipient for both ABO and HLAs is important for achieving a successful platelet count increment after transfusion. Alloimmunization requires the presence of class I and class II HLAs. Platelets alone do not result in the development of antibodies because they carry only class I HLAs and platelet-specific antigens; the class II antigens necessary for the development of alloimmunization are provided by transfused monocytes, lymphocytes, and dendritic cells. Rh antigens play only a minor role in alloimmunization after platelet transfusions.

  b. Reactions to platelet transfusion. Infectious contamination occurs rarely but more commonly than with PRBCs because platelets are stored at room temperature for up to 5 days. TRALI can occur following platelet transfusions (See section IX.D.2.d). Hemolysis of the small numbers of contaminating donor RBCs in donor platelet concentrates is of minor consequence. **Febrile reactions,** however, occur often even in ABO-compatible platelet transfusions because:

   (1) Recipient antibodies to WBCs attack donor WBCs contained in transfused platelet packs. This reaction is prevented by effective leukodepletion of platelet packs.

   (2) Cytokines released by leukocytes during storage, particularly TNF-α and IL-1 (which are exceptional pyrogens), are passively transfused. This reaction is prevented by performing leukodepletion before storage of the platelet packs.

   (3) Recipient antibodies to cells and proteins in the donor unit form immune complexes that trigger the release of CKs. This reaction involving incompatible platelets is unaffected by leukodepletion and justifies further testing for HLA antibodies or platelet-specific antibodies, if available.

  c. Leukodepletion filters remove donor leukocytes by barrier retention of the filters' microfibers, by adherence to the filter material, and by platelet–leukocyte–mediated interactions.

 3. Selection of which platelet preparation to transfuse depends on expected future transfusions and the presence of alloimmunization.

  a. Random (ABO-compatible) units. One random unit is the platelet concentrate from 1 unit of whole blood. These platelet units can be pooled and may be used in patients with transient thrombocytopenia that is not expected to recur and when platelets are needed immediately.

  b. Single-donor platelets (plateletpheresis packs) are the main platelet product used. They are obtained by density centrifugation using an apheresis machine. One plateletpheresis pack is equivalent to about 6 to 8 random platelet units and may be obtained from one donor two or three times weekly. Single-donor platelet packs are the preferred blood product in conditions that require recurrent platelet transfusions because alloimmunization is decreased.

  c. Platelets cross-matched for ABO compatibility are available for potential use in alloimmunized patients.

  d. HLA-compatible platelets. HLA-matched platelets (HLA class I only) are required in alloimmunized patients but are not always available. The likelihood of an identical HLA match is 1 in 4 among siblings and 1 in 1,000 in the general population.

  e. Platelets from family members should be avoided in patients who are possible candidates for BMT, but can be utilized posttransplant. The marrow donor may be used as the source of HLA-identical platelets, after the transplantation conditioning program has begun.

 4. Prophylactic transfusions

  a. Acute leukemia. Although there is some debate as to whether prophylactic platelet transfusions are superior to therapeutic-only platelet transfusions, prophylactic platelet transfusions are usually used to keep platelets above 10,000/μL. Higher levels are needed if patients are febrile or having bleeding symptoms.

    b. In aplastic anemia, prophylactic transfusions are avoided if possible.

    c. Pregnancy. Pregnant patients with thrombocytopenia induced by myelosuppressive therapy or leukemia are given platelet transfusions empirically.

5. Effectiveness of platelet transfusions is determined by measuring platelet counts just before, 1 hour after, and 24 hours after transfusions. If the patient does not respond with an increase of about 20,000 in the platelet count after 1 hour, the transfusion should be considered a failure. The result at 24 hours can be further affected by concurrent hematologic complications.

6. Other measures

    a. Diseases affecting platelet function. Patients with uremia who are actively bleeding require dialysis, cryoprecipitate, or desmopressin acetate (DDAVP) with aminocaproic acid to improve platelet function. In patients with platelet dysfunction secondary to paraproteins, it is necessary to control the underlying disease or to perform plasmapheresis.

    b. DDAVP may be useful in patients with aspirin-induced platelet dysfunction at a dose of 0.3 µg/kg given over 20 minutes.

    c. Alloimmunized patients who are refractory to transfused platelets. High-dose intravenous γ-globulin (400 mg/kg/d for 5 days) occasionally permits better platelet increments in patients who are refractory to platelet transfusion. Cross-matched or HLA-matched platelets may be helpful. Plasmapheresis may be tried empirically in difficult situations but is rarely helpful.

    d. Menorrhagia in patients with thrombocytopenia should be treated with medroxyprogesterone, 20 mg PO daily, to induce amenorrhea. Alternatively, leuprolide, 3.75 mg IM monthly, can be used if the platelet count is high enough to permit IM administration. Patients who will be treated with drugs causing an expected significant drop in platelet counts (i.e., acute leukemia treatment or stem cell transplant) should have anovulatory treatment started prior to the chemotherapy and continued until the platelet count recovers to >50,000/µL.

D. Transfusion of plasma proteins

    1. Preparations

        a. Fresh frozen plasma (FFP) contains all coagulation factors and is useful in replacement of all acquired clotting factor deficiencies (e.g., DIC, massive transfusion, liver disease), but frequently requires large volume infusions. FFP can be used in the following situations:

            (1) Replacement of isolated coagulation factor deficiencies

            (2) Reversal of documented coagulation factor deficiencies after massive blood transfusions

            (3) Reversal of warfarin effect in patients requiring immediate surgery or having active bleeding

            (4) Treatment of antithrombin (AT) deficiency or TTP

        b. Cryoprecipitate contains VWF, fibrinogen (factor I), factor VIII, and factor XIII. Cryoprecipitate is useful in treating acquired deficiencies of fibrinogen and factor VIII (e.g., DIC) when volume overload from plasma treatment is to be avoided or for replacement of fibrinogen due to massive hemorrhage.

        c. Plasma protein fractionation has resulted in the following commercially available products, which are obtained by pooling plasma from thousands of donors and then fractionating into components. Viral inactivation processes have improved the safety of these products.

(1) **Fibrinogen.** Can be used for fibrinogen replacement with massive hemorrhage.

(2) **Prothrombin complexes** (factors II, VII, IX, X, protein C, and protein S) are used in congenital factor deficiencies of these factors and in cases of coumarin overdose with life-threatening hemorrhage. Early products carried the risk of inducing venous thrombosis and/or DIC because of activated factors in the product, but the risk has been reduced with modern unactivated preparations.

(3) **Albumin and purified protein fraction** have the same concentration of albumin and the same cost. They are useful for blood volume expansion, but their use in chronic hypoalbuminemia of malabsorption, nephrosis, or cirrhosis or as a nutritional supplement is futile.

(4) **Gamma globulin. Intravenous immunoglobulin** (IVIG) is made from the gamma globulin fraction of pooled serum. It is useful as replacement factor in patients with hypogammaglobulinemia as may be seen in lymphomas, myelomas, or post–bone marrow transplant. For immunoglobulin replacement, doses of 200 to 400 mg/kg body weight are given about every 3 weeks. IVIG can also be used as an immunomodulatory agent for a wide range of immunologic disorders including immune cytopenias. In these situations, higher doses (i.e., 2 g/kg/mo) are used.

2. Hazards

a. **Allergy.** All plasma preparations are associated with a small incidence of serum sickness reactions. Fever, urticaria, or erythema may also occur.

b. **Volume overload** is an important consideration when administering FFP. Citrate toxicity may occur with very rapid transfusion rates (100 mL/min).

c. **Infection** with hepatitis B, hepatitis C, delta agent hepatitis, HIV, CMV, and EBV is a potential risk for all plasma products, but careful donor screening and viral inactivation procedures have reduced the risk.

d. **Transfusion-related acute lung injury (TRALI)** is a rare, but occasionally lethal, transfusion complication. It can be seen with any blood transfusion containing plasma (RBC, WBC, platelets, FFP). Patients develop acute respiratory distress with dyspnea, hypoxia, fevers, and noncardiogenic pulmonary edema usually occurring during or within 6 hours of a transfusion and without other known causes. There are likely two steps involved in the pathogenesis. First is a priming step where an underlying condition of the patient (usually inflammatory) leads to neutrophil recruitment and activation in the pulmonary vasculature. The second is provided when the transfused plasma contains antibodies to HLAs or human neutrophil antigens (HNA) that react with and activate the recipient's granulocytes and endothelial cells and cause vascular leak. This activation can also be caused on a nonimmune basis by biologically active lipids, CKs, or platelet microparticles released by the cells over time when blood is stored.

Treatment is symptomatic and based on oxygen therapy (intubation and mechanical ventilation are required about 70% of the time). Low tidal volume and low plateau pressure are used. Transfusions should be stopped immediately. Attempts at prevention by blood donor and collection strategies may be decreasing the incidence of TRALI. Since HLA and HNA antibodies are usually obtained by prior transfusions or pregnancy, avoidance of these individuals for FFP donation has been helpful. Leukoreduction and plasma reduction of RBC and platelet products prior to storage can also help.

COAGULOPATHY

Cancer patients can have abnormalities in their coagulation system leading to both thrombosis and bleeding. These processes are interrelated and sometimes occur at the same time, leading to difficult therapeutic decisions.

I. THROMBOSIS IN PATIENTS WITH CANCER

The presence of cancer, particularly when disseminated, is recognized to be a "hypercoagulable" or "thrombophilic" state. Multiple or migratory venous thromboembolism (VTE) in cancer patients has been repeatedly documented since Trousseau's description in 1865. Fibrin–platelet vegetations may form on mitral or aortic valves and result in noninfectious ("marantic") endocarditis with paradoxical emboli to peripheral organs. An accelerated course of intermittent claudication and of ischemic heart disease has also been described in cancer patients and probably represents additional variants of Trousseau syndrome.

A. Incidence. The overall incidence of thrombotic episodes in cancer patients is 10% to 15%, especially during postoperative periods. The postoperative risk of VTE in cancer patients is about double that in patients without cancer (37% vs. 20%), and the risk of fatal pulmonary embolism is about fourfold higher in cancer patients.

About 5% to 10% of patients with idiopathic VTE ultimately are shown to have a malignancy, particularly during the first 6 months after diagnosis. Pulmonary emboli have been found at necropsy in about half of the patients with disseminated cancer and have antedated the diagnosis of cancer in 1% to 15% of patients. The malignancies most commonly associated with thrombosis are MPNs and carcinomas of the GI tract, lung, or ovary. About 7% of patients with pancreatic cancer develop classic Trousseau syndrome.

B. Mechanisms for hypercoagulability

1. Cancer is associated with the following thrombophilic factors:

a. The tumor's **disruption of blood vessels** exposes collagen and endothelial basement membrane, which may trigger clotting. Tumor neovascularization activates both factor XII and platelet reactions.

b. Cancers can directly produce various procoagulants. The best characterized is **tissue factor–like procoagulant (TF).** TF forms a complex with factor VIIa to activate factors IX and X, initiating the clotting cascade leading to thrombin and fibrin formation. TF is produced by many solid tumor cells and leukemic blasts. TF also appears to be an important promoter of tumor growth and of angiogenesis. TF up-regulates expression of VEGF by tumor cells. VEGF in turn up-regulates TF. The induction of angiogenesis by TF also involves its interaction with the protease-activated receptors (PARs).

c. Inflammatory cytokines (CKs), particularly TNF and IL-1, can be released by tumor cells and immune regulatory cells under pathologic conditions. These CKs can induce TF expression on tumor-associated macrophages and endothelial cells. The endothelial cells become procoagulant under the influence of these CKs. The CKs also up-regulate adhesion molecules, platelet-activating factor, and plasminogen activator inhibitor type-1 (PAI-1). The CKs down-regulate the expression of thrombomodulin and endothelial cell protein C receptor.

d. Thus, a **hypercoagulable state** is established in cancer patients through activation of the clotting cascade, activation of platelets, enhancement of endothelial cell adhesion, suppression of fibrinolysis, and inhibition of the anticoagulant protein C pathway.

2. **Comorbid factors,** such as advanced age, previous history of VTE, immobility, obesity, hospitalization, surgery, catheterization, major medical conditions (such as infection), concomitant chemotherapy, and hereditary thrombophilia, play contributory roles for blood hypercoagulability to become manifest clinically. Venous stasis as a result of bed rest or extrinsic vessel compression from tumor masses also contributes.

3. **Cancer therapies** associated with enhanced risk for thrombosis are
   a. **Selective estrogen receptor modulators:** tamoxifen, raloxifene
   b. **Progestins:** megestrol
   c. **Thalidomide analogs:** thalidomide, lenalidomide, pomalidomide
   d. **Cytotoxic agents:** 5-fluorouracil, capecitabine, asparaginase, bleomycin, carmustine, cisplatin, mitomycin C, vinca alkaloids, high-dose chemotherapy with BMT
   e. **Vascular endothelial growth factor (VEGF) inhibitors:** bevacizumab, sunitinib, sorafenib, ponatinib
   f. **Epidermal growth factor receptor (EGFR) inhibitors:** cetuximab, panitumumab

C. **Management of cancer-associated thrombosis.** In the acute phase, low molecular weight heparin (LMWH) (enoxaparin, dalteparin, tinzaparin) is the preferred anticoagulant over unfractionated heparin (UH). There are not enough data on the use of fondaparinux and direct thrombin inhibitors (dabigatran) and factor Xa inhibitors (rivaroxaban, apixaban, edoxaban) in this patient population. As the long-term treatment, LMWH is also preferred over warfarin or direct oral anticoagulants. The therapy is continued for 3 to 6 months. Patients who are at high risk for recurrent thrombosis, for example, patients who are immobilized, with active cancer, with a high clot burden or persistent clot after therapy, should be considered for extended anticoagulation beyond 6 months.

Heparin-induced thrombocytopenia is uncommon (1% to 5% of patients treated with UH and in <1% of patients receiving LMWH) but needs to be considered if thrombocytopenia develops in these patients while on heparin.

D. **Management of recurrent thrombosis in cancer patients** is difficult because it is often resistant to therapy and because patients often have worrisome sites for potential hemorrhage.

1. **Anticoagulant therapy.** The use of LMWH is supported by observational data.
   a. If recurrent thrombosis develops while on warfarin therapy, switch to LMWH. Increasing the warfarin dosage limit excessively increases the risk for hemorrhage.
   b. If recurrent thrombosis develops while on LMWH therapy, increase the dose by 20% to 25%. If clinical improvement does not occur within a week, measure the peak anti-Xa level (the target would be 1.6 to 2.0 U/mL for once daily dosing or 0.8 to 1.0 U/mL for twice daily dosing).

2. **Contraindications to anticoagulant therapy** include the following:
   a. Preexisting clotting defect or bleeding source
   b. Inaccessible ulceration (e.g., GI tract)
   c. Recent hemorrhage or surgery in the eye or central nervous system
   d. Severe hypertension or bacterial endocarditis
   e. Regional or lumbar anesthesia, tube drainage

3. **Pregnancy:** If anticoagulation is needed, use UH or LMWH because it crosses the placenta less readily than warfarin.

4. **Vena cava interruption:** In general, vena cava filters should be avoided in these patients for the treatment of thrombosis because of their invasiveness, cost, and the lack of proven efficacy. However, retrievable inferior vena cava filter can be considered when anticoagulants are *contraindicated*. The filter is effective for preventing pulmonary embolism but increases the risk for recurrent VTE.

5. **Graduated compression stockings** should be used, if practical, particularly in postoperative and bedridden patients.

6. **Removal of the tumor** may control thrombotic episodes but is often impossible.

7. **Special considerations for anticoagulation in cancer patients.** The objective in treating VTE (prevention of death due to and other complications of pulmonary embolism) is not necessarily applicable in the preterminal patient with cancer. The goal of anticoagulation in these patients is more likely to prevent pain in the extremities or chest. Therapy with warfarin in cancer patients is often chaotic and associated with unpredictable changes in dose response because of the presence of poor nutrition, impaired liver function, infection, and concomitant medications (especially antibiotics). Furthermore, temporary cessation of anticoagulation may be necessary because of thrombocytopenia induced by chemotherapy.

E. **Prophylaxis against venous thrombosis in cancer patients**

1. **Cancer surgery** is associated with a 35% risk of venous thrombosis without prophylaxis. The use of LMWH decreases the rate to 13%. The addition of mechanical prophylaxis to the anticoagulant program reduces the risk to 5%. Fondaparinux has also been shown to be effective in this setting. Consensus guidelines recommend extending prophylaxis for at least 1 month after surgery in patients with cancer, particularly in patients with other risk factors for VTE.

2. **Hospitalization.** Consensus recommendations support thromboprophylaxis in patients with cancer when they are admitted to the hospital.

3. **Central venous catheters.** Low doses of warfarin or LMWH seem to have no effect on reducing catheter-related thrombotic complications. Increased risk for thrombosis is seen in those patients with a poorly positioned catheter tip, insertion of the catheter in left-sided veins, age >60 years, or metastatic disease.

4. **Chemotherapy.** The risk of VTE in cancer patients undergoing chemotherapy is particularly high. LMWH reduces clinically important VTE, but the optimal dose, duration, and specific patient populations are poorly defined.

F. **Diagnostic tests in patients with idiopathic (unprovoked) VTE**

1. **The clinical diagnosis of venous thrombosis** is made by physical examination and venous ultrasonography or venography. Venography and the fibrinogen uptake test have higher rates of detection than ultrasonography. It is estimated that about 20% of idiopathic VTE have an underlying malignancy. The presence of venous thrombosis, a heart murmur, and arterial embolism suggests an underlying mucin-producing carcinoma.

2. **An occult malignancy** may be a cause of idiopathic venous thrombosis, but aggressive testing for cancer does not improve survival, and it is generally not recommended. Diagnostic pursuit is justified in patients with signs and symptoms suggestive of cancer.

3. **Laboratory tests of coagulation** can be obtained during the first idiopathic thromboembolic event in an otherwise healthy person to seek a possible biologic defect predisposing to thrombosis. Such assays would include the following:

   a. Assays for lupus anticoagulant and serologic tests for antiphospholipid antibodies

   b. Functional assays for protein C and antithrombin 3 (AT3)

   c. Functional assays for protein S (immunologic assays of total and free protein S)

   d. Clotting assay for resistance to activated protein C (and genetic test for factor V Leiden)

   e. Screening for dysfibrinogenemia (thrombin time [TT], immunologic and functional assays of fibrinogen)

   f. Total plasma homocysteine

   g. Genetic test for prothrombin gene mutation (prothrombin 20210A)

   h. Various laboratory findings that are *not predictive* of thromboembolic disease in cancer patients include increased levels of platelets, markers of platelet activation, markers of thrombin generation, fibrinogen, and factors V, VIII, IX, and XI; decreased plasma levels of AT3; and suppression of fibrinolytic activity.

II. DISSEMINATED INTRAVASCULAR COAGULATION

DIC is an acquired syndrome characterized by systemic intravascular activation of coagulation, leading to deposition of fibrin in the bloodstream. It can be provoked by numerous disorders including obstetrical complications, trauma, infections, and carcinomas. DIC is a frequent complication for patients with metastatic cancer, either as a consequence of the metastases themselves or complicating infections. Local or diffuse thrombosis or hemorrhage can occur in all combinations.

A. Pathogenesis of DIC. DIC involves complex interactions between the coagulation, fibrinolytic, and inflammatory systems that result in the clinical syndrome of DIC. With all inciting conditions, procoagulants are produced or introduced into the blood and overcome the anticoagulant mechanisms, leading to the generation of thrombin and DIC. **Tissue factor** (TF) and the cascade of CKs produced by the tumors and adjacent injured tissues can lead to thrombosis. Once TF is expressed, the coagulation cascade generates thrombin through factor VII leading to fibrin and platelet deposition. **Thrombin** then amplifies both clotting and inflammation by activating factors VIII, V, and XI (leading to further thrombin and fibrin generation), platelets (leading to platelet aggregation and activation), factor XIII, and thrombin-activatable fibrinolysis inhibitor (making clots resistant to fibrinolysis). The coagulation proteases (thrombin, Xa, VIIa-TF) up-regulate inflammation. Tumor injury or inflammation can compromise the endothelium leading to microvascular thrombosis and ensuing multiorgan dysfunction. **Antithrombin (AT),** a circulating serine protease inhibitor that normally neutralizes thrombin, factor Xa, and the other coagulation serine proteases, is consumed in DIC allowing more thrombin generation. Plasminogen is activated to **plasmin,** which lyses fibrin creating fibrin degradation products (including D-dimers). Fibrinolysis can be impaired from PAIs in DIC resulting in persistent microthrombosis. With the chronic coagulation activation, there is utilization and consumption of platelets and clotting factors and also active fibrinolysis resulting in the paradoxical **hemorrhagic tendency** in the face of ongoing thrombosis.

B. Diagnosis. The widespread generation of thrombin in DIC induces the deposition of fibrin, which results in the consumption of platelets, fibrinogen, factors V and VIII, protein C, AT, and components of the fibrinolytic system. The severity of DIC manifestations depends on the underlying diagnosis, the acuteness of the DIC, and the intensity of secondary fibrinolysis. Some patients hemorrhage profusely and have marked abnormalities in all of the tests for DIC; others mainly have microthrombi and organ dysfunction. On the other hand, DIC may be subclinical and manifested only by mild laboratory abnormalities and thrombocytopenia.

1. **Clinical features**
   a. **Type of bleeding.** Patients with severe DIC bleed from multiple sites simultaneously. Petechiae, ecchymoses, mucosal bleeding, and oozing from venipunctures, lines, and catheters are common. Patients with chronic DIC (the usual DIC seen with malignancies) may have minimal bleeding.
   b. **End organ damage.** Microangiopathic hemolysis, hypotension, oliguria, and renal failure are frequent complications of serious DIC. Renal cortical ischemia induced by microthrombosis of afferent glomerular arterioles and acute tubular necrosis due to hypotension are the major causes of renal dysfunction in DIC. Both the underlying diseases and DIC itself can cause shock. Microvascular thrombi and thromboembolism can result in dysfunction of any organ (e.g., acral necrosis, neurologic manifestations, and pulmonary dysfunction).

2. **Laboratory tests.** No single test is diagnostic for DIC, but combination of findings can help make the diagnosis.
   a. **Blood smear.** Decreased platelets and fragmented erythrocytes or microspherocytes may be seen.
   b. **Platelet count.** Thrombocytopenia occurs nearly always, but DIC alone rarely causes platelet counts of <50,000/μL. Concomitant causes of thrombocytopenia should be sought for severe thrombocytopenia in the presence of DIC.
   c. **Clotting tests.** Prothrombin time (PT) and activated partial thromboplastin time (aPTT) may be slightly shortened, normal, or prolonged. TT prolongation occurs with severe hypofibrinogenemia (<50 mg/dL) or clinically significant elevation of fibrin degradation products. The TT can also be prolonged with heparin therapy, dysfibrinogenemia, or malignant paraproteinemia.
   d. **Fibrinogen level** is usually decreased. Fibrinogen levels >50 mg/dL (normal range is 200 to 400 mg/dL) should not result in abnormalities of the TT. It is important to remember that fibrinogen is an acute-phase reactant protein and is normally elevated in pregnancy and inflammatory states; thus, a normal result may actually be abnormal.
   e. **D-Dimer test:** D-dimers are produced when cross-linked fibrin is degraded by plasmin-induced fibrinolytic activity. D-dimers are expected to be elevated in patients with DIC. The finding of D-dimers does not make the diagnosis of DIC since other disorders (i.e., other thrombotic states) can cause a positive D-dimer elevation. A negative D-dimer test result however has a strong negative predictive value.

C. Management. Few patients with DIC are helped if the underlying problem is not corrected. Treatment is not necessary for laboratory manifestations alone. The following sequence is recommended:

1. **Treat the underlying disease.** This may be futile for patients with disseminated cancer alone, but the possible advantages of antimicrobial therapy, further surgery, RT, or chemotherapy should be considered. Hypotension, tissue perfusion, acidosis, hypoxemia, and the triggering event (e.g., sepsis) must be addressed vigorously.

2. **Administration of blood components.** Patients with low levels of fibrinogen, thrombocytopenia, and/or prolonged PT, who are actively bleeding or at a high risk for bleeding, with no evidence of venous or arterial thromboembolism, can be considered for replacement therapy. Platelet transfusions can be given for significant thrombocytopenia. Fibrinogen, cryoprecipitate (for fibrinogen and factor VIII), and occasionally FFP can be given to correct the coagulopathy. The unactivated prothrombin factor concentrates can be used to correct the vitamin K–dependent clotting factors when patients are euvolemic or hypervolemic, rather than use large volumes required for FFP.

3. **Patient surveillance.** The platelet count, fibrinogen level, and clinical evaluation are the most useful factors to follow.

III. OTHER HEMOSTATIC DEFECTS ASSOCIATED WITH CANCER

A. **Platelet function abnormalities are common in malignancies.**

1. **Mechanisms:** These can be due to coating of platelet surfaces by fibrin degradation products (with DIC) or with paraproteins (with myeloma), concomitant azotemia, inherent platelet dysfunction associated with myelodysplastic disorders or MPN s, or drugs with antiplatelet activity (i.e., aspirin, nonsteroidal anti-inflammatories, clopidogrel, ticlopidine).

2. **Diagnosis: Signs** of platelet dysfunction include easy bruisability, gingival bleeding with toothbrushing, and other minor mucosal bleeding. **Laboratory studies:** A variety of *in vitro* platelet function tests have uncertain clinical validity. Thrombocytopenia, DIC, and azotemia should be ruled out by appropriate tests.

3. **Treatment.** Patients with bleeding and platelet dysfunction require treatment of the underlying disorder and may require platelet transfusions. DDAVP, 0.3 µg/kg IV over 20 minutes, may also be helpful temporarily.

B. **Paraproteinemia.** Hemostatic abnormalities associated with plasma cell myeloma are discussed in Chapter 23.

C. **Liver metastases,** when extensive, can result in the inability to synthesize clotting factors. Treatment with vitamin K is usually ineffective. Active bleeding may be controlled by the administration of prothrombin factor concentrates and fibrinogen. FFP can be used, but the large volumes needed may not be tolerated.

D. **Dysfibrinogenemia.** Dysfibrinogens are abnormal fibrinogen molecules, which may be inherited or acquired in association with hepatocellular carcinoma or liver metastases. The PT, aPTT, and TT are all markedly abnormal. Fibrinogen levels are low when measured by clotting methods but are normal when measured by immunologic or physical precipitation methods. Hemorrhage is not common with dysfibrinogenemia but may occur. Thrombotic complications are more common.

E. **Acquired circulating inhibitors of coagulation** occur in a wide variety of tumors (e.g., a heparin-like inhibitor in mastocytosis, antibodies to coagulation factors in lymphomas). It is doubtful that these inhibitors are responsible for hemorrhage in the absence of other causes, such as uremia or thrombocytopenia.

F. **Specific factor deficiencies**

1. **Factor XIII deficiency or dysfunction** is common in patients with cancer but usually does not cause clinical problems. The PT, aPTT, and TT are normal, but the assay for factor XIII is abnormal. Hemorrhagic episodes are treated with FFP, 5 mL/kg weekly.

2. **Factor X deficiency** may occasionally be an isolated coagulation abnormality in patients with amyloidosis, which can also be associated with systemic fibrinolysis. Hemorrhagic episodes are treated with FFP or prothrombin complexes.

3. **Factor XII and Fletcher factor (prekallikrein) deficiencies** have been described in patients with cancer but have little clinical significance.

4. **Acquired von Willebrand disease** has been reported in cancer patients, particularly in the MPNs in association with marked thrombocytosis.

G. **Hemostatic abnormalities associated with cytotoxic agents**

1. **Hypofibrinogenemia** or dysfibrinogenemia, and antithrombin deficiency, is common with L-asparaginase use. Thrombotic episodes are also common.

2. **Vitamin K antagonism** occurs with actinomycin D therapy.

3. **Platelet dysfunction** (of questionable significance) has been reported with cytarabine, daunorubicin, melphalan, vincristine, mitomycin C, L-asparaginase, and high-dose chemotherapy in preparation for BMT.

4. **Budd-Chiari syndrome** is associated with dacarbazine therapy.

Suggested Readings

Blake-Haskins JA, Lechleider RJ, Kreitman RJ. Thrombotic microangiopathy with targeted cancer agents. *Clin Cancer Res* 2011;17:5858.

Churpek JE, Larson RA. The evolving challenge of therapy-related myeloid neoplasms. *Best Pract Res Clin Haematol* 2013;26:309.

Dasararaju R, Marques MB. Adverse effects of transfusion. *Cancer Control* 2015;1:16.

Feinstein DI. Disseminated intravascular coagulation in patients with solid tumors. *Oncology* 2015;29:96.

Filipovich AH. Hemophagocytic lymphohistiocytosis (HLH) and related disorders. *Hematology Am Soc Hematol Educ Program* 2009;127.

Lee AYY. Thrombosis in cancer: an update on prevention, treatment and survival benefits of anticoagulants. *Hematology Am Soc Hematol Educ Program* 2010;2010:144.

Lin RJ, Afshar-Kharghan V, Schafer AI. Paraneoplastic thrombocytosis: the secrets of tumor self-promotion. *Blood* 2014;124:184.

Nemeth E, Ganz T. Anemia of inflammation. *Hematol Oncol Clin North Am* 2014;28:671.

Schram AM, Berliner N. How I treat hemophagocytic lymphohistiocytosis in the adult patient. *Blood* 2015;125:2908.

Watkins T, Surowiecka MK, McCullough J. Transfusion indications for patients with cancer. *Cancer Control* 2015;22:38.

Zhang L, Wang SA. A focused review of hematopoietic neoplasms occurring in the therapy-related setting. *Int J Clin Exp Pathol* 2014;7:3512.

Zhang L, Zhou J, Sokol L. Hereditary and acquired hemophagocytic lymphohistiocytosis. *Cancer Control* 2014;21:301.

Infectious Complications

Bhagyashri Navalkele and
Pranatharthi H. Chandrasekar

I. BACKGROUND

Infection is a major cause of morbidity and mortality in cancer patients. Prompt recognition of infection and initiation of appropriate antimicrobial therapy is important in the management of febrile neutropenic patients. The disruption of host defense mechanisms such as natural mechanical barriers to infection, reduction in number of functional neutrophils, and altered cell-mediated and/or humoral immunity are predisposing risk factors resulting in development of infection. These risk factors can occur due to the underlying malignancy or its therapy. This chapter provides an overview on various types of infections encountered in cancer patients and summarizes standard treatment recommendations including recent advances. The recommendations are applicable to a majority of the cancer patients with suspected/proven infection with some exceptions requiring individual case-by-case decision. Involvement of infectious disease physicians with expert knowledge in the field is advised. This chapter does not address infections in bone marrow transplant recipients.

II. NEUTROPENIA AND FEVER

A. Principles. Neutropenic patients with fever alone or with clinical signs and symptoms of infection even in the absence of fever should be evaluated as a medical emergency. A majority of febrile neutropenic patients do not have an identifiable site of infection. Nevertheless, these patients should be rapidly assessed for identification of underlying infectious etiology and promptly initiated on empiric antimicrobial therapy.

B. Definitions

1. **Fever.** A single oral temperature measurement of 101°F (38.3°C) or a temperature of 100.4°F (38.0°C) sustained over 1 hour constitutes fever. Measurement of axillary and rectal temperatures is not advised.

2. **Neutropenia.** An absolute neutrophil count (ANC) <500 cells/mm³ or anticipated decline in ANC to <500 cells/mm³ in next 2 days is regarded as neutropenia. "Profound neutropenia" is ANC <100 cells/mm³. A variant type of neutropenia associated with normal white blood cell count but high infection risk is called "functional neutropenia" due to impaired phagocytic function of neutrophils in patients with hematologic malignancies.

3. **Low-risk patient:** Patients with expected duration of neutropenia of <7 days, with no comorbid conditions, and with stable renal and hepatic function tests are considered low-risk patients.

4. **High-risk patient:** Cancer patients with certain risk factors are considered to be at high risk for serious infections and require immediate hospitalization and initiation of empiric antimicrobial therapy. High-risk patients include patients with any of the following risk factors: ANC <100 cells/mm³ expected to last longer than 7 days, hemodynamic instability, systemic infections like mucositis resulting in dysphagia/vomiting/diarrhea/abdominal

pain, acute change in mental status, suspected catheter-associated bloodstream infection (BSI), new lung infiltrate, or hypoxemia. Patients with any comorbid conditions like underlying chronic lung disease, advanced age, metastatic or advanced malignancy, or poor functional status or abnormal laboratory studies with presence of acute hepatic failure (aminotransferase levels greater than five times the normal) or renal failure (creatinine clearance <30 mL/min) are also considered to be high risk. Patients with acute leukemia or myelodysplastic syndrome (MDS) or on induction chemotherapy for acute leukemia are considered to be high risk.

C. **Prevention of infections in neutropenia**
  1. **General measures**
     a. Regular hand hygiene, before entry and after exit from a patient room, is the most important preventive measure to reduce infection transmission.
     b. Daily care of neutropenic nonhematopoietic stem cell transplant patients does not require special precautions or use of single-patient room.
     c. Daily bathing with good oral, dental, and perineal hygiene is advised in all immunocompromised patients. Daily inspection of skin with special attention to portal of entry for infection like vascular sites and perineal examination should be performed.
     d. Fresh flowers, dried flowers, and plants should not be present in the rooms of neutropenic patients because they may carry molds, such as *Aspergillus* and *Fusarium* species.
     e. Pet therapy, or household pets at the bedside, should be avoided.
     f. A diet consisting of well-cooked food and cleaned fresh fruits and vegetables is acceptable. Prepared luncheon meats are not allowed.
     g. In the absence of an outbreak, infection control personnel are discouraged from performing routine bacterial surveillance culture from environment or devices.
  2. **Isolation**
     a. Standard barrier precautions using gloves, gowns, and masks should be practiced when contact with patient's body fluids is expected.
     b. Reverse or neutropenic isolation (caps, masks, gloves, and gowns) has no established benefit. In addition, it deters good patient care by limiting patient contact with the health care workers (HCWs) and families.
     c. Isolation precautions per hospital infection control policy should be followed for certain infections (e.g., MRSA infection, *Clostridium difficile* infection, multidrug-resistant (MDR) gram-negative rod infections).
     d. Special ventilation rooms consisting of high-efficiency particulate air filters and rooms with >12 air exchanges/hour are only recommended for allogenic hematopoietic stem cell transplant (HSCT) recipients and have no proven benefit in other neutropenic patients.
  3. **Instructions for healthcare workers and visitors**
     a. Visitors and HCWs with infections known to be transmitted via direct, airborne, or droplet route should avoid contact with or use appropriate barrier precautions before visiting or caring for neutropenic patients.
     b. It is highly recommended for HCWs and visitors to be up-to-date with immunizations such as yearly influenza, measles–mumps–rubella, and varicella to avoid spread of vaccine-preventable diseases to cancer patients.
  4. **Antimicrobial prophylaxis:** The main rationale for prophylaxis with antibacterial, antiviral, or antifungal agents is to prevent infections and infection-related mortality during neutropenia or immunosuppression. Routine

antimicrobial prophylaxis in all neutropenic cancer patients increases risk for antimicrobial agent–related side effects such as disruption of normal gastrointestinal flora and development of bacterial/viral/fungal resistance. Based on good evidence, prophylaxis is recommended only for high-risk cancer patients.

a. Prophylaxis with fluoroquinolones (e.g., ciprofloxacin or levofloxacin) can be considered in patients who are at high risk for infection and are expected to have prolonged or profound neutropenia for more than 7 days. Prophylaxis with fluoroquinolone reduces the rate of febrile episodes, documented bacterial infections, and both gram-positive and gram-negative bacteremias. Recent evidence demonstrated reduction in all-cause and infection-related mortality especially with ciprofloxacin use in patients at high risk for infections.

b. It is advised to initiate antibiotic prophylaxis in high-risk patients, on initiation or after completion of cytotoxic therapy and discontinue with engraftment or with initiation of empiric therapy for febrile neutropenia.

c. The risk of emergence in fluoroquinolone-resistant bacterial infections and *C. difficile* infection due to prophylaxis is a serious concern. Cancer center-based routine monitoring for these infections is advised.

d. Patients expected to have short duration of neutropenia (<7 days) are not recommended to be on antibiotic prophylaxis.

e. The routine use of sulfamethoxazole–trimethoprim to prevent *Pneumocystis jirovecii* pneumonia (PJP) is commonly recommended in AIDS patients with CD4 lymphocyte count <200 cells/μL or <15%. In non-HIV setting, the risk for PJP infection is associated with cytotoxic therapy affecting cell-mediated immunity. Prophylaxis with sulfamethoxazole–trimethoprim is recommended in patients receiving steroids (prednisone dose equivalent ≥20 mg/d for ≥3 weeks) with chemotherapy but is not recommended for all neutropenic patients.

f. Intravenous vancomycin prophylaxis, sometimes combined with quinolones, has been used to prevent catheter-associated gram-positive bacterial infections. This practice can lead to resistant organisms and is *strongly discouraged*.

g. Antifungal agents: Invasive fungal infections are rare; however, they are associated with serious complications and high mortality. Antifungal prophylaxis (posaconazole) is recommended in high-risk patients (undergoing intensive chemotherapy for acute leukemia/MDS) against two most important invasive fungal pathogens *Candida* and *Aspergillus*.

h. Low-risk patients, such as patients with lymphoma and multiple myeloma, are not recommended to receive routine antifungal prophylaxis.

i. Recently, a broad-spectrum antifungal agent isavuconazonium sulfate has demonstrated safety, tolerability, and efficacy against aspergillosis and mucormycosis. This triazole agent is currently not recommended for prophylaxis.

j. Antiviral agents: Acyclovir prophylaxis is strongly recommended for those HSV-seropositive patients undergoing induction chemotherapy for leukemia. Antiviral prophylaxis should be continued till resolution of neutropenia or until resolution of mucositis occurs. Longer duration of prophylaxis can be provided in special circumstances such as recurrent HSV infections.

k. Prophylactic myeloid colony-stimulating factors can be considered in patients on chemotherapy treatment (excludes palliative chemotherapy) at high risk (≥20%) for developing febrile neutropenia.

5. **Vaccination**

Vaccination of immunocompromised patients is an effective way to prevent and reduce morbidity and mortality from vaccine-preventable diseases. Though immunocompromised patients may not mount an adequate response to active immunization due to impaired immunity, benefit exists by reducing morbidity and mortality associated with preventable infections. The indicated vaccines are given prior to initiation of chemotherapy, immunosuppressive drugs, splenectomy, or radiation therapy.

a. Live vaccines are contraindicated in immunosuppressed patients. These include the viral vaccines for rubeola (measles), varicella, rubella, mumps, polio, smallpox, yellow fever, and live, attenuated, intranasally administered influenza vaccine (FluMist). Live vaccines should be avoided for at least 3 months after high-dose chemo or radiation therapy for hematologic malignancies.

b. Inactivated vaccines are considered safe to be administered in immunosuppressed patients. Permissible vaccines include those against diphtheria, tetanus, pertussis, typhoid, cholera, plague, influenza, hepatitis A and B, and *S. pneumoniae*, and these may be administered in appropriate circumstances.

c. Patients should be given annual influenza immunization because immunity is short lived, and antigenic drift of the "epidemic" strain(s) occurs each year.

d. Pneumococcal vaccination is strongly indicated for all cancer patients. There are two types of pneumococcal vaccines: pneumococcal conjugate vaccine (PCV13) and pneumococcal polysaccharide vaccine (PPSV23), both of which should be administered. First-time recipients of pneumococcal vaccine should receive PCV13 initially, followed by PPSV23 vaccination 8 weeks later. If PPSV23 was administered initially, PCV13 can be given after an interval of 1 year. In patients <65 years of age, repeat vaccination with PPSV23 (1 or 2 doses) can be given after 5 years from most recent dose of PPSV23.

e. Vaccines should not be administered during cycles of intense chemotherapy due to lower immune response, except annual inactivated influenza vaccine. Influenza vaccine, if necessary, may be administered during chemotherapy-induced neutropenia as well.

D. **Predisposition to infection**

1. The degree and the duration of neutropenia are the most important and easily measured risk factors that predispose to the development of infection. Infection that develops in the setting of neutropenia of relatively brief duration (5 to 7 days) is most likely due to a bacterial infection, reflecting the important role of granulocytes in the prevention or control of bacterial infections. Defects in granulocyte function, humoral immunity, and cell-mediated immunity are likely contributing factors, particularly when neutropenia is of longer duration. In patients with profound neutropenia lasting longer than 7 days, fungal infections become a major concern.

2. Defects in the normal mechanical barriers of the host to infection are an important predisposition to infection.

a. Most common sites of such breaches are the skin, the paranasal sinuses, and the alimentary tract; breaches of these barriers allow for local and disseminated infection by the indigenous (normal) and colonizing (environmental) flora of the skin and alimentary tract. The loss of mucosal barrier integrity results in translocation of colonizing microbial flora into the bloodstream resulting in severe infection even at low bacterial load due to absence of defensive neutrophils. Mucositis increases the risk for both bacterial and candidal BSIs. Placement of vascular access devices creates a portal for infection of the surrounding soft tissues and bloodstream by microorganisms. Other invasive procedures such as bone marrow biopsy pose risks for infection that relate to the site of the procedure.

b. Other types of impairment of the host's normal barriers to infection include tumor invasion of mucosal surfaces and of the integument; loss of protective reflexes, such as cough; and obstruction to drainage of hollow organs, such as the urinary bladder and the gall bladder.

3. Hospitalization increases risk for colonization and infection with resistant pathogens.

4. Newer biologic agents: Monoclonal antibodies like rituximab and alemtuzumab are being used as targeted therapy for treatment of lymphomas and leukemias. The use of these biologic agents has been associated with higher prolonged immunosuppression increasing the risk for bacterial, viral, fungal, and mycobacterial infections.

E. Microorganisms

1. Early in the course of neutropenia, during the first week, bacteria predominate as the microbiologically documented pathogens. Previously, gram-positive bacteria were the most common cause of BSI. Currently, both gram-positive and gram-negative bacterial infections have similar rates for BSI. Among resistant bacterial infections, methicillin-resistant *Staphylococcus aureus* (MRSA), vancomycin-resistant *Enterococcus* (VRE), and gram-negative infections like extended-spectrum beta-lactamase (ESBL)-producing Enterobacteriaceae (see Section V.D.) are the common cause of BSI. Carbapenemase-producing Enterobacteriaceae are less common, but serious bacterial infections with limited treatment options can occur.

2. Later in the course of neutropenia, after the first week, fungi, particularly yeast (*Candida* species), are commonly associated with mucosal infections and other less common serious infections like candidemia, hepatosplenic, or disseminated candidiasis. Molds (particularly *Aspergillus* species) must be considered as potential pathogens typically after 2 weeks of neutropenia.

F. Diagnosis

1. History and physical examination. A careful history should be taken, with a focus on new symptoms, prior infections, prior antimicrobial exposures, sick contacts, and other possible noninfectious etiologies for fever. Classic signs of inflammation may not be present because of the absence of neutrophilic exudates in infected tissues, although the presence of localized pain may be an important clue. A detailed examination should be performed of the ocular fundus; oropharynx, including teeth and supporting structures; lungs; perineum and perianal areas; and the skin, including vascular access catheter sites and other breaks in the integument related to diagnostic procedures. Digital rectal examination and pelvic examination are usually not advised because trauma to the mucosa during the examination may cause bacteremia.

2. Laboratory evaluation. In addition to routine laboratory tests, at least two sets of blood cultures should be obtained promptly, one set from central venous catheter (if present) and another from a peripheral vein. Blood cultures (two sets) may be obtained over consecutive 2 days if fever persists. Serum levels of β-D-glucan and β-galactomannan can be used as a guide for diagnosis of fungal infection.

a. If a CVC is present, the skin exit site should be carefully inspected. If there is drainage from the CVC exit site, the exudate should be submitted to the laboratory for Gram stain, bacterial culture, and fungal culture.

b. Cutaneous lesions should be carefully looked for; if present, they need to be either aspirated or biopsied for bacterial and fungal cultures and histopathologic examination.

c. Patients with respiratory symptoms or infiltrate on chest imaging should have sputum cultures sent for Gram stain and bacterial cultures. During seasonal outbreaks, nasal swab or wash should be tested for respiratory virus infections like adenovirus, RSV, influenza A and B virus, and para-influenza virus. Respiratory viral panel for PCR may be utilized.

d. Urine culture is indicated in symptomatic patients with dysuria or urinary frequency or patients with sepsis with indwelling urinary catheter.

e. If diarrhea is present, then samples should be submitted for *C. difficile* toxin assay. In patients with hospital stay <3 days, routine stool culture may be considered for *Salmonella, Shigella, Campylobacter, and Norovirus* infection. If diarrhea has been present for >7 days, tests for *Giardia, Cryptosporidium, Cyclospora,* and *Isospora* should be considered.

f. Inflammatory markers like C-reactive protein, ESR, procalcitonin levels should not be followed in neutropenic patients due to inadequate evidence to support their use.

3. **Imaging studies.** A baseline chest radiograph (posteroanterior and lateral views) should always be done as part of the initial evaluation. In the case of persistent fever and neutropenia with localizing signs and symptoms, CT scan of lungs, abdomen/pelvis, head, or sinuses should be performed as indicated. CT scan of chest is appropriate for early detection of fungal infection (aspergillosis) in patients with persistent fever and prolonged neutropenia, despite lack of pulmonary symptoms and normal chest x-ray.

G. **Management**

1. **Febrile neutropenic patients** should be rapidly assessed for evidence of infection. Even if there is no evidence of infection other than fever, prompt institution of *empiric* antimicrobial therapy (within 2 hours of initial presentation) is always indicated.

   Low-risk patients, based on clinical status, may be safely treated with either oral or intravenous antimicrobial therapy as outpatients with mandatory close follow-up. High-risk patients warrant hospitalization and intravenous antibiotic treatment, regardless of the anticipated duration and severity of neutropenia.

   Useful antibacterial, antiviral, and antifungal agents for the treatment of neutropenic fever are shown in Table 36-1.

2. **Intravenous antimicrobial therapy:** Most patients will likely fall into the "high-risk" category and require initiation of empiric therapy.

   a. The goal of empiric therapy is to provide coverage against likely pathogens pending receipt of culture results. Information from the antibiogram can be used to tailor empiric treatment based on local resistance patterns.

   b. Empiric antibacterial therapy: Infection with gram-positive bacteria is more common; however, infection with gram-negative *bacteria is associated with* higher mortality. The main goal of initial empiric therapy is coverage of gram-negative bacilli of gastrointestinal origin, including *Pseudomonas aeruginosa*; this coverage can usually be accomplished by monotherapy with a beta-lactam agent. Agents appropriate for this goal include piperacillin–tazobactam, cefepime, and selected carbapenems (either meropenem or

TABLE 36-1	Antimicrobials in Neutropenic Fever (NF)

Antibiotic (Brand Name)	Standard Dose in NF	Comments
Oral Antibacterials		
Ciprofloxacin (Cipro)	750 mg PO q12h	For oral therapy in low-risk neutropenic patients
Amoxicillin/clavulanate (Augmentin)	Amoxicillin 875 mg/clavulanate potassium 125 mg PO q12h	
Carbapenems		
Imipenem–cilastatin (Primaxin)[a]	0.5 g IV q6h	1.0 g q6–8h may predispose to seizures particularly in renal impairment.
Meropenem	1.0 g IV q8h	Less likely than imipenem–cilastatin to induce seizures
Extended-Spectrum Penicillins		
Piperacillin–tazobactam (Zosyn)	3.375 g IV q6h	Nosocomial pneumonia/septic shock: 4.5 g IV q6h
Cephalosporins		
Cefepime (Maxipime)	2.0 g IV q8h	Frequently used as a first-line agent in febrile neutropenia
Aminoglycosides[b]		
Gentamicin (Garamycin)	1.7–2.0 mg/kg IV q8h, or 5–7 mg/kg q24h	Increased risk of nephrotoxicity is a concern.
Tobramycin (Nebcin)	1.5–2 mg/kg IV q8h, or 5–7 mg/kg q24h	
Amikacin (Amikin)	7.5 mg/kg IV q12h, or 15 mg/kg q24h	
ANTIFUNGAL AGENTS		
Echinocandins		
Caspofungin (Cancidas)	70 mg IV × 1 loading dose, followed by 50 mg IV q24h	Echinocandins are initial treatment of choice for candidemia.
Anidulafungin (Eraxis)	200 mg IV × 1 loading dose, followed by 100 mg IV q24h	
Micafungin (Mycamine)	100 mg IV q24h	
Triazoles		
Fluconazole (Diflucan)	800 mg (12 mg/kg) PO/IV × 1 loading dose, followed by 400 mg IV or PO q24h	Alternative treatment option for noncritically ill patients with no prior azole exposure as a step-down therapy after clearance of candidemia
Itraconazole	200 mg PO q24h	Generally not preferred because of poor activity against mold. Suspension form is preferred over tablet form.
Voriconazole	400 mg b.i.d. PO (6 mg/kg) q12h × 2 loading dose, followed by 200 mg PO (3 mg/kg) q12h	Good activity against *Candida* and *Aspergillus*; many drug–drug interactions; has FDA indication for treatment of invasive aspergillosis
Posaconazole	400 mg b.i.d. or extended release tablets 300 mg oral daily (IV preparation not available)	Prophylaxis against invasive aspergillosis and *Candida* infection. May be used as a step-down therapy for mucormycosis
Isavuconazonium sulfate (Cresemba)	372 mg PO/IV q8h × 6 doses (48 hr) followed by 372 mg PO/IV daily	Approved for treatment of invasive aspergillosis and mucormycosis. No renal adjustment required

(Continued)

TABLE 36-1	Antimicrobials in Neutropenic Fever (NF) (Continued)	
Antibiotic (Brand Name)	**Standard Dose in NF**	**Comments**
Amphotericin Preparations[c]		
Liposomal amphotericin B	3–5 mg/kg IV daily	Effective agent but less preferred due to nephrotoxicity
Amphotericin B deoxycholate (Fungizone, AmBD)	0.5–0.7 mg/kg IV q24h	Infusion-related toxicity and nephrotoxicity
Amphotericin B lipid complex (Abelcet, ABLC)	3–5 mg/kg IV q24h	Amphotericin B lipid complex has infusion-related side effects of shakes and rigors, which are not seen with Ambisome.
ANTIVIRAL AGENTS		
Neuraminidase Inhibitors		
Oseltamivir	75 mg oral twice daily	Treatment for 5 d or longer in severely ill patients with influenza A/B
Zanamivir	10 mg (5 mg inhalation × 2) twice daily	
Peramivir	600 mg IV × 1 dose	Alternate IV agent in patients with poor absorption of oseltamivir
DNA Polymerase Inhibitors		
Acyclovir	HSV-localized infection 5 mg/kg IV q8h HSV encephalitis 10 mg/kg IV q8h VZV systemic infection 10 mg/kg IV q8h HSV oral/genital infection 400 mg PO t.i.d.	Treatment of HSV and VZV infections IV formulation is preferred for serious infections. Poor oral absorption Higher dosage recommended for CNS infections
Valacyclovir	Herpes zoster: 1 g PO t.i.d. HSV: 1 g PO b.i.d.	Effective step-down therapy for nonsevere HSV/VZV infections in noncritically ill patients
RNA Polymerase Inhibitor		
Ribavirin	6 g aerosolized given via face mask over twice daily	Used for treatment of lower respiratory tract RSV infection

[a]1.0 g q8h to q6h may be given in life-threatening situations or for infections by organisms that are only *moderately* susceptible to imipenem–cilastatin (primarily some strains of *P. aeruginosa*) and resistant to most other agents.
[b]All aminoglycosides are dosed based on ideal body weight.
[c]Amphotericin B deoxycholate has considerable nephrotoxicity and should be avoided in cancer patients. However, lipid preparations are expensive and need to be used judiciously.

imipenem–cilastatin), which also provide moderate to excellent coverage for many (but not all) gram-positive organisms and anaerobic bacteria and are often used as monotherapy for fever in the setting of neutropenia. Recent evidence demonstrated good efficacy of monotherapy with antipseudomonal beta-lactam agent compared to dual coverage with an antipseudomonal beta-lactam plus an aminoglycoside. Generally, monotherapy is appropriate when the patient has not been exposed repeatedly to antimicrobial therapy, and the microbiology laboratory at the treatment facility has not recorded appreciable resistance to these agents. If the patient is critically ill or there is concern about infection with more resistant bacteria, addition of other agents to the regimen may be warranted; these agents may include vancomycin, fluoroquinolones (ciprofloxacin and levofloxacin), aminoglycosides (particularly amikacin), and colistin.

    c. Modification to the initial empiric antibiotic regimen is appropriate for patients who are at risk for infection with resistant organisms or who are bacteremic or are clinically unstable. Infection with resistant organisms includes MRSA, VRE, ESBL-producing *Enterobacteriaceae*, or carbapenemase-producing gram-negative bacteria (see Section V.D). A significant degree of expertise with regard to local hospital bacterial resistance patterns is often needed to address these issues; infectious diseases consultation should be considered.

    d. The initial empiric use of vancomycin is indicated in patients who are suspected of having CVC-related infection, bacterial pneumonia, and skin and soft tissue infection or who are hemodynamically unstable. Routine addition of vancomycin for empiric coverage in febrile neutropenic patients is not advised as it has failed to show any benefit in reduction in duration of fever or overall mortality.

    e. A history of uncomplicated penicillin-induced skin rash is not a contraindication to the use of these beta-lactam agents (penicillins, cephalosporins, and carbapenems). In most cases, a history of allergy is false. However, these drugs should be avoided in patients with a history of immediate hypersensitivity to penicillins (or other beta-lactam agents) or history of penicillin-associated Stevens-Johnson syndrome or toxic epidermal necrolysis. In the occasional situation in which a beta-lactam agent is clearly contraindicated because of risk of serious allergic reaction, alternative empiric regimens include ciprofloxacin–clindamycin or aztreonam–vancomycin; data regarding efficacy of these alternative regimens are limited.

3. Oral antimicrobial therapy: Oral antimicrobial therapy with ciprofloxacin plus amoxicillin/clavulanate has been shown to be safe and appropriate, when limited to adult patients who are at low risk for infectious complications of neutropenia. Such patients do not have an identifiable focus of infection and lack clinical findings of systemic infection other than fever and do not have other risk factors. Use of fluoroquinolones as empiric therapy in febrile neutropenic patients already on fluoroquinolone prophylaxis is not advised. Patients on oral therapy still require careful observation and immediate access to medical care. Admission to hospital and empiric IV antimicrobial therapy is indicated if fevers persist or new signs of infection develop. Other options are initial hospitalization for administration of intravenous antibiotics, followed by switch to oral therapy and discharge, or discharge home on IV antibiotic therapy.

4. Management of antimicrobial therapy

Response of fever to initiation of empiric antimicrobial therapy, if it is to occur, sometimes requires 3 to 5 days. After initiation of antimicrobial therapy, several possible outcomes exist: deterioration during the ensuing 1 to 3 days, resolution of fever during the first 3 to 5 days, or persistence of fever during the first 3 to 5 days. In the event of clinical instability, immediate reassessment of both patient and treatment regimen is essential.

In many studies, the median time to defervescence after initiation of therapy is approximately 5 days. Therefore, in a patient who is clinically stable, except for persistent fever, the physician should consider waiting approximately 5 days before entertaining changes in the antimicrobial regimen, unless initial cultures yield an organism resistant to the treatment regimen. Changes in antimicrobial therapy should generally be made for specific reasons; an unintended consequence of aggressive, unjustifiably escalating antimicrobial therapy is the promotion of subsequent infection by more highly resistant microorganisms.

a. In patients who become afebrile within 3 days, broad-spectrum therapy should be maintained throughout the period of neutropenia, with appropriate modifications to the regimen based on results of cultures and other diagnostic tests. Cessation of therapy is appropriate when cultures and clinical assessment indicate eradication of infection and the ANC is >500 cells/mm^3. A switch from IV to oral antibiotic therapy is reasonable if the patient is clinically stable and impaired absorption of antibiotics from the gastrointestinal tract is not a concern. Clinically documented infection should be treated in a manner that is appropriate for the type of infection, irrespective of the rapidity with which neutropenia resolves.

b. For patients whose fever persists during the first 4 to 7 days of empiric therapy and in whom a specific infectious process has not been identified, a number of possibilities exist. In the event of persistent fever of unknown cause for more than 4 days, the most appropriate actions are as follows:

(1) Continue treatment with the initial regimen.

(2) Change or add antibacterial agents to the original regimen.

(3) Add an antifungal agent to the regimen (with or without making changes to the antibacterial regimen).

c. Persistent fever after resolution of neutropenia: The persistence of fever after broad-spectrum antimicrobial therapy and recovery of ANC >500 cells/mm^3 suggests drug fever, deep-seated bacterial infection, or infection with a mycobacterium or fungus (e.g., aspergillosis or candidiasis).

Causes of persistent fever include slow response to the treatment regimen, bacterial infection resistant to the treatment regimen, development of a second infection, inadequate antibiotic levels owing to suboptimal dosing, inadequate source control or penetration of drugs into an infected site such as infected necrotic tissue or CVC site, nonbacterial infection, fever of noninfectious origin such as drug fever or tumor fever, or pulmonary emboli during engraftment or resolution of neutropenia.

d. In reevaluating the patient's status after 3 to 4 days of therapy, the physician should repeat the initial diagnostic evaluation, review results of culture, obtain additional cultures, and consider obtaining radiographic imaging studies, if new localizing symptoms or signs are present. Any changes in therapy should be dictated by findings on reevaluation.

If the patient has remained clinically stable and the reevaluation was unrevealing, continuation of the initial regimen is reasonable. If neutropenia is expected to resolve within 5 days, this approach is quite appropriate.

e. With evidence of progressive disease, consideration should be given to changes in the antimicrobial regimen. The nature of these changes should be dictated by findings during clinical reassessment and the components of the initial antimicrobial regimen. Examples of new findings include development of abdominal pain (suggesting neutropenic enterocolitis or other intra-abdominal processes), development of diarrhea (suggesting *C. difficile* disease), detection of pulmonary infiltrates, drainage or inflammation at catheter entry sites, worsening stomatitis, and radiographic detection of sinus opacities. Further imaging with CT abdomen/pelvis or CT chest or sinuses for detection of invasive fungal infections and empiric broadening of antimicrobial therapy, including empiric treatment for *C. difficile*–associated diarrhea till infection is ruled out, can be considered.

f. Addition of antifungal therapy to the treatment regimens of patients who are febrile after initial antimicrobial therapy has been controversial, particularly with regard to the timing of such therapy and the particular antifungal agent to be used. Most experts believe that a patient with persistent fever and profound neutropenia after 4 to 7 days of **empiric** antimicrobial therapy should be considered for antifungal therapy. In most cases, this would not apply to patients with solid tumors but only to those with hematologic cancers receiving intensive chemotherapy. A thorough evaluation to detect systemic fungal infection should be done; this should include consideration of biopsy of suspicious lesions, chest radiographs, sinus radiographs, and CT of the chest and abdomen. If a focus of bacterial infection is not found, fungal infection should strongly be considered. The fungi most likely to cause fever relatively early in the course of neutropenia are *Candida* species.

g. Influence of antifungal prophylaxis needs to be carefully considered before empiric antifungal therapy. Detailed discussion of treatment of fungal infections and use of antifungal agents is provided in Section VI.

5. Duration of therapy

a. Antibacterial therapy: The most important indicator in deciding to discontinue antibacterial therapy is the neutrophil count. If the ANC is >500 cells/mm³ and the patient has been afebrile for 2 consecutive days, therapy may be stopped unless more prolonged therapy is indicated for treatment of a specific, documented infection (e.g., pneumonia or bacteremia).

For the patient who becomes afebrile but is persistently neutropenic, after completion of full course of antimicrobial therapy, fluoroquinolone prophylaxis may be resumed until marrow recovers (ANC >500 cells/mm³).

b. Antifungal therapy: If a specific fungal infection has been documented, then the duration of antifungal therapy will be determined by the pathogen and the nature of the infection. Because of the differing activities of the three main groups of antifungal agents commonly given to patients with neutropenic fever (echinocandins, triazoles, and amphotericin B preparations), a greater need now exists for establishing an etiologic diagnosis. Knowledge of the infecting fungus should allow for selection of the most effective therapeutic agent and facilitate limitation of toxicity.

If a fungal infection is not documented but empiric antifungal therapy is given, it is not clear how long antifungal therapy should be given. Antifungal therapy can be discontinued if neutropenia and fever have resolved, the patient appears well, cultures are negative, and imaging studies do not reveal lesions suspicious for fungal infection.

c. Antiviral therapy

Empiric use of antiviral agents is not recommended. Localized lesions caused by herpes simplex or varicella-zoster virus (VZV) may provide a portal of entry for other pathogens and can be treated with oral acyclovir, valacyclovir, or famciclovir. Cytomegalovirus (CMV) infection/disease is rare in the absence of profound immunosuppression that occurs in patients with AIDS or stem cell transplantation. CMV disease is an uncommon occurrence in patients with cancer undergoing standard chemotherapy.

6. **Granulocyte transfusions**

Prolonged neutropenia in patients receiving high-dose induction chemotherapy for leukemia remains a major risk factor for bacterial and fungal infections. Transfusion of granulocytes to reduce the infection rate, hospitalization, and associated morbidity and mortality has been investigated for many decades. Recently performed small underpowered multicenter randomized controlled trial demonstrated no added benefit in patients receiving antimicrobial therapy with or without granulocyte transfusion. A high-dose of granulocyte transfusion ($\geq 0.6 \times 10^9$ granulocytes/kg) has been associated with better outcome. The use of granulocyte transfusion in neutropenic patients is still controversial and not routinely recommended.

III. SPECIFIC INFECTIONS IN THE COMPROMISED HOST

A. **Pulmonary infiltrates**

1. **Noninfectious causes**

About 25% to 30% of cases of fever with pulmonary infiltrates in cancer patients are owing to noninfectious causes, which include radiation pneumonitis, drug-induced pneumonitis, pulmonary emboli and hemorrhage, and leukoagglutinin transfusion reaction.

2. **Infectious causes**

a. Acute, severe symptoms that progress in 1 to 2 days suggest a common bacterial pathogen, a virus, or a noninfectious process (pulmonary emboli, pulmonary hemorrhage). A subacute course (5 to 14 days) suggests pneumocystosis or, occasionally, aspergillosis or nocardiosis. A chronic course (over several weeks) is more typical of mycobacterial or fungal infection, radiation fibrosis, or drug-induced pneumonitis. Despite the susceptibility of cancer patients to opportunistic pathogens, *S. pneumoniae* and influenza virus are the most likely causes of pulmonary infections in the outpatient setting. *Escherichia coli, Klebsiella pneumoniae, Serratia marcescens, Pseudomonas aeruginosa, Acinetobacter* sp., *Stenotrophomonas*, and *S. aureus* are the most frequently acquired nosocomial bacterial pathogens. *Aspergillus* sp. and *Legionella pneumophila* may be hospital acquired.

b. The association between lung carcinoma and pulmonary tuberculosis is related to the increased susceptibility to opportunistic infections and tuberculosis in cancer patients. Erosion of tumor into a quiescent tuberculous focus likely accounts for some cases. Diagnosis of tuberculosis requires pathologic evidence from biopsies or bacteriology samples. Surgical treatment of early-stage bronchopulmonary carcinoma may have to be postponed and may even be contraindicated in the presence of active tuberculosis. Chemotherapy and radiotherapy may result in extension of the tuberculosis.

3. **Diagnostic approaches**

a. **Sputum examination.** If the sputum contains many neutrophils or macrophages and <10 epithelial cells per low-power field, the sputum culture results are probably valid. Neutropenic patients usually have no neutrophils in the sputum; hence, diagnostic utility of sputum becomes uncertain.

Aspiration pneumonia is usually caused by mouth flora, which renders routine culture meaningless.

S. pneumoniae is a fastidious organism that is difficult to recover from sputum, although approximately 25% of pneumococcal pneumonias are associated with concomitant bacteremia.

Many opportunistic organisms that produce pneumonia are infrequently retrieved from sputum (e.g., *Nocardia asteroides*, *Aspergillus* species, and other molds).

Sputum cultures of hospitalized patients, particularly those receiving antibiotics, often yield *Candida* on culture. Although candidemia and disseminated candidiasis are frequent and serious complications of immunosuppression, pneumonia because of *Candida* is remarkably uncommon. Therefore, recovery of *Candida* from sputum should not be considered to be diagnostic of infection, but simply colonization.

b. Serology may be useful for identifying infection caused by *Coccidioides immitis*. Serology is less useful for diagnosis of infections caused by *Aspergillus* species, *L. pneumophila*, *Mycoplasma pneumoniae*, *Toxoplasma gondii*, and CMV. There is a delay associated with most serologic tests, and some are not very sensitive or specific.

c. Antigen tests: Blood antigen tests are useful for diagnosis of infections caused by *Cryptococcus neoformans*. Urinary antigen tests are valuable tools for diagnosis of infections caused by *S. pneumoniae*; *L. pneumophila*, serogroup 1; and *Histoplasma capsulatum*. The detection of cryptococcal antigen in any body fluid is considered diagnostic of infection.

The use of nonculture methods for diagnosis of other fungal infections is evolving. Detection of *Candida* species depends primarily on culture. The serum galactomannan test for diagnosis of aspergillosis has become an important diagnostic tool. A meta-analysis found the test sensitivity ranged from 61% to 71% and specificity from 89% to 93%. Galactomannan testing in serum and bronchoalveolar lavage fluid has become useful. The serum beta-D-glucan assay can detect a cell wall component (1,3-beta-D-glucan) of many fungi. This is most useful in ruling out systemic candidiasis as it has high negative predictive value.

Blood cultures should be obtained in all patients.

d. Imaging and procedures: A normal chest radiograph makes pneumonia unlikely, but plain radiographs of the lungs may be too insensitive to detect early disease. Neutropenic patients with persistent fever and normal chest radiographs should undergo high-resolution CT scanning to detect occult cavitary disease or inflammatory pulmonary disease. CT is of particular value for diagnosis of invasive pulmonary mycoses, such as aspergillosis identified with presence of "halo" sign on CT chest. Thoracentesis should be performed in patients with pleural effusion (generally uncommon in the neutropenic setting). Diagnosis is paramount in the immunocompromised host. The highest yield and best control of bleeding is by direct visualization with open-lung biopsy or video-assisted thoracoscopic surgery (VATS). This approach may be necessary when the patient is critically ill. If the pneumonic process is less rapid, then bronchoscopy with lavage appears to be the best initial approach. When a mass or consolidation is present in the peripheral field, a fine needle biopsy may be adequate with less chance of complications.

Invasive techniques are often not justified late in the course of malignancy because they often add morbidity with little hope of significant benefit. Empiric antibiotic therapy directed at the most likely pathogen(s) may be justified in these cases.

4. Therapy for acute pneumonia should be initiated immediately after cultures are obtained. Patients with acid-fast bacilli, *N. asteroides*, *Cryptococcus*, or *Aspergillus* species in sputum should not be regarded as colonized with such organisms and should be treated. Rapid molecular testing is useful to differentiate *Mycobacterium tuberculosis* from atypical mycobacteria.

B. **Central nervous system infections:** Infections of the CNS can present either with simple changes to mentation or motor skills or with seizures and coma. Meningismus is a hallmark of disease, but this condition may be absent. MRI is indicated when cerebral edema, abscess, or demyelinating encephalitis is suspected. This scan is particularly useful in defining viral encephalitis and areas where enhanced foci are seen, such as in toxoplasmosis.

1. Special considerations in cancer patients suspected or proven to have CNS infections are as follows:

   a. **Meningitis:** Cancer patients have an increased incidence of atypical pathogens. These can occur as a direct result of immune suppression, CNS involvement by the malignancy, or opportunistic infections after craniofacial surgery.

   Neutropenic patients rarely develop gram-negative meningitis despite a relatively high incidence of gram-negative bacteremia. However, when meningitis does develop, the pathogens usually are members of the family *Enterobacteriaceae* (e.g., *E. coli*, *Klebsiella*), *P. aeruginosa*, or *Listeria monocytogenes*. Meningitis caused by aspergillosis or zygomycosis, though rare, has been described.

   Patients with defects in cell-mediated immunity: *L. monocytogenes* and *C. neoformans* are relatively likely pathogens in these patients. Meningitis and meningoencephalitis from VZV, herpes simplex virus (HSV), JC virus (progressive multifocal leukoencephalopathy), human immunodeficiency virus (HIV), CMV, *T. gondii*, and *Strongyloides stercoralis* also occur.

   b. **Brain abscesses** are most likely caused by mixed aerobic and anaerobic bacteria. In the immunocompromised patient, brain abscesses are also caused by *Aspergillus* species, the agents of mucormycosis, *N. asteroides*, or *T. gondii*. *Toxoplasma* can produce meningitis, necrotizing encephalitis, or abscess. In atypical cases, brain tissue should be obtained for examination at the time of surgical drainage.

2. **Diagnosis**

   a. **Lumbar puncture (LP)**

   An emergency CT scan of the brain must be performed first. Patients with space-occupying lesions seen on CT scan should have LP or cisternal puncture performed by a qualified neurologist or neuroradiologist.

   Spinal subdural hematoma occasionally complicates LP in patients with severe thrombocytopenia. Clinical evidence of CNS infection, however, supersedes consideration of risks. The following guidelines are recommended.

   If the platelet count is <50,000/µL, transfuse platelets just before performing LP. Transfuse additional platelets if back pain or neurologic signs develop.

   Cerebrospinal fluid should be evaluated for the following:

   (1) Glucose and protein concentrations, cell counts, routine bacterial culture and sensitivity, Gram stain, and cytology. The WBC count in the cerebrospinal fluid is >100/µL in about 90% of patients with bacterial meningitis and >1,000/µL in 15% to 20%. Neutrophils constitute >80% of the WBC count in 80% to 90% of patients; occasionally, lymphocytes predominate in the cerebrospinal fluid, especially in neutropenic patients and in about 25% of patients with meningitis caused by *L. monocytogenes*.

(2) Acid-fast culture and stain, fungal stains of smears and fungal cultures, India ink preparation, cryptococcal antigen, and "screening" and complement fixation serology for *Coccidioides immitis* (depending on geography and predominant soil fungus) should be done.

(3) Polymerase chain reaction (PCR) assays for HIV, JC virus, herpesviruses, *Toxoplasma*, and *M. tuberculosis* should be performed only if clinical or laboratory findings suggest the likelihood of that specific infection.

C. Skin infections

1. Neoplasms invading the skin (e.g., mycosis fungoides) are associated with infections involving common pathogens such as *S. aureus* and *Streptococcus pyogenes*.

2. Cell-mediated immunity deficiencies are typically associated with skin infection by VZV or HSV.

3. Neutropenic patients may have skin infections with atypical or few physical findings. *S. aureus* and *S. pyogenes* are common. More serious manifestations represent systemic infections; these include bullae formation, raised ecchymotic plaques or nodules, black necrotic ulcers, or ecthyma gangrenosum. These more pronounced cutaneous manifestations of systemic infection are typically caused by *P. aeruginosa*; however, other pathogens including *Aeromonas hydrophila*, members of the family *Enterobacteriaceae*, and fungi, including *Candida* species, *Aspergillus* species, and members of the class *Zygomycetes* (the latter infections are often referred to as mucormycosis), may cause them as well.

D. Alimentary tract and intra-abdominal infections

1. Esophagitis may be caused by *Candida* or HSV and rarely CMV.

2. Colitis with ulceration is occasionally produced by CMV. *Aspergillus* and *Mucor* may also involve the GI tract. In most medical centers, colonic infection due to *Clostridium difficile* is the most common.

3. Cecitis or typhlitis and ileocolitis are processes that probably develop as a consequence of several factors that include mucosal injury, neutropenia, and the resident bowel flora. They can usually be appreciated on CT scan of the abdomen and may be confused with *Clostridium difficile*–induced colitis when colonic wall thickening is present. Right lower quadrant pain mimicking appendicitis may indicate typhlitis during chemotherapy-induced neutropenia.

4. Intra-abdominal abscesses develop when the bowel or genital tract becomes obstructed, necrotic, or perforated because of tumor. Mixed infections derived from colonic flora involve gram-negative enteric bacilli; various species of streptococci and members of the *Bacteroides fragilis* family are common. *Streptococcus bovis* abscess and sepsis may occur with colonic or pancreatic carcinoma.

5. Perirectal infections frequently develop in neutropenic patients, especially those with acute leukemia; usually, they are caused by a mixture of aerobic and anaerobic bacteria. The hallmark of perirectal infection in neutropenic patients is pain on defecation.

6. Liver infections: Multiple abscesses secondary to systemic bacterial or fungal infection may occur. Hepatosplenic candidiasis can be an extremely difficult infection to diagnose. It usually clinically manifests with right upper quadrant pain during recovery from neutropenia. Imaging is helpful in diagnosis. Even herpesviruses, such as VZV, HSV, CMV, and Epstein-Barr virus (EBV), can present as mass or necrotic lesions in the liver of immunocompromised patients.

E. **Urinary tract infections** are frequent in cancer patients because of obstructive uropathies, the use of urinary catheters, and prolonged and repeated hospitalizations. These infections are often caused by resistant gram-negative bacteria or *Candida* species. *Candida* species often colonize the urinary tract of patients who have indwelling catheters or diabetes mellitus, particularly in the setting of recent antibacterial therapy. Recovery of *Candida* from urine may occasionally represent significant infection of the urinary tract (rather than colonization that resolves with removal of the bladder catheter) but should always lead to consideration of occult fungemia.

F. **Bone marrow suppression (infection)** usually reflects systemic or disseminated disease, considerations include viral infections, *M. tuberculosis*, *Mycobacterium avium* complex, fungi, *Salmonella*, and *Listeria*. Bone marrow biopsy for culture can be a useful diagnostic tool. Bone marrow suppression mimicking aplastic anemia occurs with adenovirus, HHV6, HHV7, CMV, parvovirus B19, mycobacterial infection, histoplasmosis, and brucellosis.

G. **Central line–associated infections**

The incidence of infection of IV catheters, including nontunneled central lines, tunneled silicone catheters (e.g., Hickman, Broviac, or Groshong), or implantable devices (e.g., Portacath), is significant and often poses a major challenge for the clinician.

Most central line infections are caused by *S. aureus* (coagulase-positive *Staphylococcus*) or coagulase-negative *Staphylococcus* species. The neutropenic patient is also at risk for infection of venous catheters by a variety of gram-negative bacilli, including *P. aeruginosa* and by *Candida* species and other fungi.

In almost all instances, infected peripheral vascular catheters and nontunneled CVC should be removed and appropriate antimicrobial therapy administered. In addition, CVC in which there is a tunnel (pocket) infection or a periport abscess should always be removed. Attempts at salvage of the CVC can be made, if the organism is of low virulence (e.g., coagulase-negative staphylococci), by the use of appropriate IV antibiotics. Clinical guidelines have been developed to assist clinicians with this vexing problem. In the neutropenic settings, catheter removal is not always necessary; judgment needs to be exercised.

Vancomycin, with dosage adjustment for renal dysfunction, should be used for initial therapy of infection due to gram-positive organisms; alternatives include daptomycin and linezolid. If the organism is subsequently found to be "methicillin susceptible," then oxacillin/nafcillin should be used.

"Antibiotic lock therapy," in which the catheter is filled with a high concentration of an appropriate antibiotic and then capped for varying periods of time, has been advocated by some, but controlled clinical studies are insufficient to permit conclusions to the utility of this method in the setting of neutropenia.

Treatment with systemic antimicrobial therapy for at least 14 days for uncomplicated and 4 to 6 weeks for complicated central line infections is advised.

All nontunneled peripheral and central catheters (the latter are often referred to colloquially as "PICC lines") should be removed, if bacteremia has been documented or there is evidence of insertion site infection.

As a general guideline, venous catheters should be removed in the following circumstances:

1. All tunnel infections or periport abscesses

2. All catheter infections caused by fungi

3. Persistence of bacteremia/fungemia after 48 to 72 hours of treatment, regardless of the pathogen

4. Bacteremia caused by *S. aureus*, VRE, *Bacillus* species, *Corynebacterium jeikeium*, or gram-negative bacilli

5. Infections associated with thrombophlebitis, septic emboli, or hypotension

6. Nonpatent (i.e., plugged) catheter

Individual consideration should be exercised in neutropenic patients.

Once removed, the tip of the central catheter can be sent for culture and identification of infection in septic patients with unidentified bacteremia.

IV. VIRAL INFECTIONS

A. Respiratory viruses

Respiratory viral infections are a common cause of fever during neutropenia. Most common causes are influenza/parainfluenza viruses, respiratory syncytial virus, adenovirus, and metapneumovirus. Viral infections usually result in upper respiratory illness, but at times with ongoing immunosuppression can spread into the lower respiratory tract resulting in pneumonia with a high mortality rate. The treatment for most of the viral infections is usually symptomatic management. Deferral of chemotherapy is advised during viral respiratory tract illness.

1. Influenza: Influenza A and B infections are frequent causes of upper respiratory tract illness during the flu season. It results in significant morbidity and mortality among cancer patients. Patients should be monitored for development of complications post influenza with secondary bacterial infection with *Streptococcus pneumoniae* or *S. aureus*.

Diagnosis is based on rapid influenza antigen testing, confirmed with PCR testing. Initiation of empiric **therapy** with oral oseltamivir 75 mg twice daily in influenza-like illness is recommended. Other treatment options for influenza include zanamivir 2 oral inhalations (5 mg/inhalation) twice daily. Influenza-confirmed patients should be treated for 5 days or longer based on clinical status. Recently, the first IV antiviral medication peramivir was approved as a single 600-mg dose for 1 day for treatment of uncomplicated influenza only. Use of peramivir should be considered in critically ill patients with poor GI absorption of oral oseltamivir.

2. Respiratory syncytial virus (RSV): RSV infection is associated with higher risk for progression from the upper respiratory tract to the lower respiratory tract in immunocompromised population. Infection of the lower respiratory tract may be associated with poor prognosis and mortality rate as high as 80%. RSV may be suspected based on respiratory symptoms suggestive of upper or lower tract disease and confirmed with positive RSV PCR on nasal wash or bronchoalveolar lavage specimen. Treatment of upper respiratory tract disease with RSV is not indicated. Lower respiratory tract disease may be treated with aerosolized ribavirin or a combination of ribavirin with IVIG. Effective ribavirin dosage is not known; aerosolized dose of 2 g every 6 hours given via face mask has been conventionally used. Newer and better antivirals against RSV are under study.

B. Herpes simplex virus (HSV): HSV reactivation occurs in 60% of HSV-seropositive immunocompromised patients. A frequent cause of fever in neutropenic patients is oral mucositis or ulceration in GI tract or perianal ulceration caused by HSV. The incidence of reactivation is reduced due to routine use of antiviral prophylaxis (usually acyclovir) in HSV-seropositive patients undergoing induction therapy for leukemia. Patients with reticuloendothelial neoplasms or T-lymphocyte defects or those receiving cytotoxic chemotherapy treatment may develop HSV viremia. The viremia often produces alimentary tract ulceration and hemorrhage, hepatitis (occasionally manifested by abscess-like lesions), and respiratory tract infections. Patients with Sézary syndrome or atopic dermatitis can develop progressive fulminant mucocutaneous disease (eczema herpeticum), which can recur and disseminate to visceral organs.

1. **Diagnosis:** Diagnosis of HSV is based on clinical suspicion and confirmed with laboratory testing.

    a. **PCR:** HSV PCR testing is the gold standard for diagnosis of HSV infection. Swab collected from base of ulcerative lesion or biopsy of tissue can be tested for amplification and identification of HSV DNA by PCR.

    b. Cytology demonstrates the characteristic intranuclear mass surrounded by marginated chromatosis and often a peri-inclusion halo. Cytoplasmic inclusions are absent. Immunofluorescence for HSV antigen is also rapid and specific.

    c. HSV grows rapidly in tissue cultures (24 to 72 hours) and produces a unique cytopathologic picture.

2. **Management**

    Acyclovir is a safe, effective treatment for HSV infections in normal and immunocompromised patients. Acyclovir reduces the amount of viral shedding and symptom severity and facilitates healing. Famciclovir and valacyclovir supercede acyclovir because they have easier dosing regimens and better bioavailability. **Valacyclovir** 1,000 mg PO b.i.d. or **famciclovir** 250 mg PO t.i.d. is the preferred treatment for HSV infection. Acyclovir dose is 200 mg PO five times daily or 400 mg t.i.d. for 7 to 10 days for mild to moderate mucocutaneous disease. As an ointment, acyclovir is useful for primary local infections but does not appear to prevent recurrent disease. Serious infections (e.g., HSV encephalitis) requiring IV therapy should be treated with acyclovir 10 mg/kg IV q8h for 7 to 10 days.

    Vidarabine is effective topically for keratitis.

C. **Cytomegalovirus (CMV):** CMV often presents as EBV-negative mononucleosis. CMV infection occurs in severely immunocompromised patients such as AIDS, bone marrow or solid organ transplantation, recipients of high-dose steroids, or tumor necrosis factor antagonists. In cancer patients undergoing standard chemo-/radiation therapy, CMV infection/disease remains rare. Fever, interstitial pneumonia, and alimentary canal ulcerative disease are the most common manifestations of CMV. CMV, which is tropic for endothelial cells, also causes retinitis, encephalitis, and peripheral neuropathy. CMV can suppress cell-mediated immunity, reticuloendothelial cell function, and granulocyte reserves.

Primary CMV infection can occur perinatally or later in life and inevitably results in latent infection. Infection may occur after transfusions of infected blood that contains granulocytes. Latent CMV burden and risk for recurrence are related to the extent of virus multiplication during primary infection. The risk for CMV recurrence is relatively high in severely immunocompromised patients.

CMV infection of the GI tract can cause serious inflammatory or ulcerative disease in immunocompromised patients. Manifestations include pain, ulceration, bleeding, diarrhea, and perforation. All levels of the GI tract, particularly the stomach and colon, may be involved. Pathologic examination reveals diffuse ulcerations and necrosis with scattered CMV inclusions.

1. **Diagnosis**

    a. CMV is slow growing (up to 6 weeks), and culture is generally not practical. Early antibody detected by application of enzyme-linked immunosorbent assay (ELISA) in cultures may accelerate identification.

b. Histology shows the characteristic enlarged cells with dense nuclear inclusions and wide peri-inclusion halos. Cytoplasmic inclusions are frequent, but multinucleation is absent.

c. Seropositivity for antibodies against CMV is indicative of latent infection but is insufficient as a predictor for the risk for recurrence.

Anticomplementary immunofluorescence assay, ELISA, and indirect fluorescent antibody (FA) assays are sensitive indicators of infection. IgG antibody occurs during the acute phase of the illness and persists for life, whereas IgM antibodies occur early and often disappear after 4 to 8 weeks. Recurrent IgM spikes occur in certain patients, indicating either partial immunity to CMV or exposure to new variants of the virus.

d. PCR assay, both *in situ* and in DNA extracted from gross specimens, is the most useful tool to isolate and identify the presence and location of CMV in clinical disease. In recent years, CMV antigen detection assay has been replaced by serum CMV PCR test. CMV PCR methodology is standardized and is currently used widely.

2. Management

a. Ganciclovir: The efficacy of this drug for CMV retinitis and colitis is well documented, but is less effective for CMV pneumonia or meningoencephalitis. After stem cell transplantation, the prophylactic administration of ganciclovir abrogates CMV pneumonitis and considerably reduces the incidence of CMV infection.

b. Foscarnet and cidofovir are other agents that may be useful for treatment of CMV reactivation/disease. Foscarnet is the alternate agent in patients with severe bone marrow suppression. Ganciclovir-resistant CMV is not uncommon in those with prior exposure to the drug.

D. Varicella–Zoster virus (VZV)

Chickenpox is often associated with extensive visceral dissemination and appreciable mortality in immunocompromised patients, particularly stem cell transplant recipients. Dermatomal shingles usually due to reactivation of latent varicella virus is characterized by the development of vesicles in clusters on erythematous bases, usually distributed along one to three dermatomes. Presence of several lesions outside a dermatomal distribution does not necessarily indicate dissemination. Disseminated VZV infections may be manifested by encephalopathy, Guillain-Barré syndrome, transverse myelitis, myositis, pneumonia, thrombocytopenia, hepatitis, and arthritis.

1. Diagnosis. Based on dermatomal distribution, VZV can usually be diagnosed on physical examination. PCR test/culture of vesicular fluid may be confirmatory.

2. Management. VZV is very easily transmissible by airborne route. In presence of disseminated infection, patients should be isolated with airborne and contact precautions.

a. IV acyclovir is the treatment of choice for ophthalmic zoster and disseminated VZV infection in immunocompromised patients (10 mg/kg IV every 8 hours for 7 to 10 days; renal function should be monitored for evidence of nephrotoxicity). "Localized" or nondisseminated zoster can be treated with IV acyclovir initially and then with oral agents to complete 7 to 10 days of treatment: acyclovir (800 mg five times daily), valacyclovir (1,000 mg t.i.d.), or famciclovir (500 mg t.i.d.).

b. Ganciclovir has considerable activity for VZV, but not preferred in view of its myelosuppressive potential.

    c. VZV live vaccines available for primary immunization against chicken-pox and prevention of recurrent VZV infection (shingles) are contraindicated in the immunocompromised patient.

    d. VZV immune globulin may prevent or ameliorate the severity of infection in immunocompromised patients, if given soon after exposure.

V. BACTERIAL INFECTIONS

A. **_Clostridium difficile:_** _C. difficile_ is currently the most common health care–associated infection. This toxin-mediated diarrheal disease of the colon is almost invariably associated with recent or concurrent use of antimicrobial therapy. In cancer centers where antibiotic use (prophylactic and empiric) is usually very common, _C. difficile_ infection is a vexing problem. Horizontal spread of _C. difficile_ within health care facilities has become extremely common. An epidemic clonal strain (Bi/NAP1/027) of _C. difficile_ was found to be associated with high fluoroquinolone resistance, high toxin production and sporulation, and increased morbidity and mortality.

    Clostridium difficile has an increased predisposition to cause infection in patients with recent antibiotic use, age >65 years, immunocompromised, chemotherapy use, proton pump inhibitor use, and recent hospitalization. Community-acquired _C. difficile_ infection (CDI) is seen without any associated risk factors.

    1. **Diagnosis.** Testing stool for _C. difficile_ PCR, a highly sensitive DNA-based test (detects the presence of toxin-producing gene) is used widely. Presence of ≥3 loose watery stools in a 24-hour period with positive stool for _C. difficile_ PCR is diagnostic of CDI. Stool should not be tested in the absence of loose stools. Enzyme immunoassay (EIA) for toxins A and B is used at some centers but has a lower sensitivity. Stool culture alone for _C. difficile_ without toxin detection is not clinically useful. The presence of colonic pseudomembranes or characteristic plaques on colonoscopy is considered diagnostic, but these findings are present in no more than 50% of patients and require lower GI endoscopy for detection. "Screening" or surveillance for _C. difficile_ infection is not recommended because intestinal carriage (in the absence of diarrhea) is common and detection of carriage is not clinically meaningful.

    2. **Management.** Nosocomial diarrhea that is not attributable to hyperosmolar nutritional supplements or tube feeding preparations suggests the presence of symptomatic _C. difficile_ disease. Such patients should be placed in contact isolation, a test for _C. difficile_ toxin ordered, and empiric treatment considered.

        a. If the diarrhea is trivial and the offending antimicrobial agent can be stopped, resolution of diarrhea occurs in approximately 90% of patients without significant risk of relapse or recurrence.

        b. If the illness is mild (high fever, marked leukocytosis, and abdominal pain or tenderness are absent), then treatment with metronidazole is appropriate. Standard dose of metronidazole is 500 mg oral t.i.d. Metronidazole is avoided due to increased adverse effects of nausea and vomiting seen in patients with ongoing cancer chemotherapy. Vancomycin 125 mg q.i.d. for 10 to 14 days may be considered first-line treatment option in cancer patients.

        c. If the illness is severe (presence of high fever or abdominal pain or renal failure or high WBC >15,000 cells/μL), oral vancomycin, 125 mg q.i.d. for 10 to 14 days, is appropriate.

d. Patients with severe complicated CDI (peritonitis, ileus, toxic mega-colon, hemodynamic instability) should receive higher dose of oral or nasogastric vancomycin 500 mg q.i.d. with metronidazole 500 mg IV t.i.d. for 10 to 14 days. Rectal vancomycin may be given for patients with complete ileus.

e. Surgical consultation for consideration for colectomy is indicated with clinical evidence of progressive toxicity, radiographic evidence of progressive colonic dilation (toxic megacolon), or concern regarding loss of bowel wall integrity.

f. Approximately 25% of patients treated for *C. difficile* diarrhea with oral metronidazole or vancomycin have a relapse or recurrence of diarrhea. Generally, retreatment is effective, although multiple relapses are not uncommon and may require a tapering course of vancomycin over several weeks.

g. Oral fidaxomicin 200 mg b.i.d. for 10 days has been approved for treatment of *C. difficile*–associated diarrhea. Use of fidaxomicin is limited due to high cost, but the drug may be useful in recurrent infection.

h. Fecal microbiota transplant (FMT) is a currently widely used treatment option for recurrent/refractory CDI. Stool obtained from healthy donors is instilled via nasogastric tube or enema in patients with CDI has resulted in high success rate. The use of FMT is promising in patients with recurrent CDI and those who failed standard treatment. FMT is a safe, cost-effective treatment, pending guidelines update for CDI.

B. *Staphylococcus aureus*

Effective treatment of infection due to *S. aureus* has changed substantially in the past decade and likely will continue to change. MRSA is most common of all infections due to *S. aureus*. Agents to be considered for treatment of suspected or documented infections due to *S. aureus* include vancomycin, daptomycin, and linezolid.

1. Vancomycin. The greatest clinical experience for treatment of MRSA is with vancomycin; it is considered by most experts to be the drug of choice. However, progressively rising concentrations of vancomycin ("MIC creep") that are now required to treat MRSA infection have many experts concerned that this drug may eventually be lost as a first-line agent. Recommendations for treatment of serious MRSA infections include a target serum vancomycin trough level of 15 to 20 mcg/mL of blood.

2. Daptomycin also has good activity against MRSA and has been used with success. The drug is significantly bound by pulmonary surfactant; hence, daptomycin is not indicated for treatment of pneumonia. In addition, the vancomycin "MIC creep" noted above appears often to also be associated with a daptomycin MIC creep as well; the clinical significance of this finding is unclear but definitely of concern.

3. Linezolid has good activity against most gram-positive organisms, including MRSA. The major concerns about linezolid are its bacteriostatic nature and potential hematologic toxicity. The latter includes thrombocytopenia, anemia, and myelosuppression. Thrombocytopenia, the most concerning hematologic adverse effect, is thought to be an immune-mediated process that is particularly associated with linezolid therapy of >2 weeks duration.

4. Ceftaroline is a cephalosporin with activity against a variety of microorganisms, including MRSA. It was approved by the FDA for treatment of acute skin and soft tissue infections and community-acquired pneumonia due to susceptible organisms. Data to support ceftaroline's efficacy for infections in immunosuppressed patients are scant. In addition, it is unclear whether it will become another useful agent to treat most infections caused by MRSA (aside from skin/soft tissue infection).

C. **Vancomycin-resistant** *Enterococcus* **(VRE)** has become an important pathogen in many centers. The recommended empiric therapy for suspected VRE is either linezolid or daptomycin.

D. **Multidrug-resistant gram-negative bacteria (GNB)** are becoming increasingly common isolates and present a major clinical challenge. They are ESBL-producing organisms (the most common form of MDR GNB) and carbapenemase-producing organisms (a relatively uncommon form).

1. ESBL-producing GNB are considered to be resistant to penicillins (including piperacillin–tazobactam) and cephalosporins (including cefepime). Because there is not a single standardized clinical laboratory test for ESBL production, microbiology experts and the FDA have proposed a revision of laboratory susceptibility (minimal inhibitory concentration, MIC) interpretation. This should eliminate testing for ESBL and provide a more uniform interpretation of antimicrobial activity.

   In general, GNB that produce ESBLs are often resistant to other classes of antibiotics, such as aminoglycosides and fluoroquinolones. Most experts recommend use of a carbapenem (ertapenem or imipenem or meropenem) if the patient is clinically unstable or have cultures that are suspicious for resistant GNB because of the high incidence of ESBL production.

2. Carbapenemase-producing GNB infections are uncommon, but there is significant concern regarding widespread dissemination of these organisms. In general, most experts would consider adding either polymyxin B or colistin or tigecycline to the regimen if the patient is clinically unstable or if culture results are suspicious for a carbapenemase-producing GNB. Clinical data regarding the efficacy of these agents for treatment of infection in neutropenic patients are sparse. Infectious diseases consultation would be prudent in such situations.

3. Newer agents such as ceftolozane/tazobactam (activity against pseudomonas) and ceftazidime/avibactam (activity against *Klebsiella pneumoniae* carbapenemase) are good alternatives for intra-abdominal and complicated urinary tract infections to limit use of broad-spectrum carbapenem agents.

E. **Mycobacteria**

Active **tuberculosis** (TB) develops in 0.5% to 1% of patients with malignancies. Infection is predominantly pulmonary in 70%, is widely disseminated in 20%, and involves lymph nodes or other nonpulmonary sites in 10% of cases.

The incidence of **atypical *Mycobacterium* infection** (particularly with *M. kansasii* and *M. avium* complex [MAC]) is significantly higher in patients with cancer or AIDS than in the general population. *M. kansasii* infection has been associated with hairy cell leukemia. Resistance to classic antituberculosis drugs is not uncommon among atypical mycobacteria. A variety of other atypical mycobacteria is occasionally isolated from patients with malignancy.

1. **Pathogenesis.** Cutaneous anergy and treatment with corticosteroids, cytotoxic agents, or irradiation predispose to reactivation of quiescent *M. tuberculosis*. It is now appreciated, however, that some cases of tuberculosis in adults represent new acquisition of infection rather than reactivation.

2. **Resistant TB.** Immigration from high-prevalence countries, coinfection with HIV, and outbreaks in congregative facilities are primarily responsible for the increased incidence of TB cases during the past decade. Coincident

with the increase in TB, outbreaks of MDR TB have occurred. A history of antituberculous therapy is the strongest predictor of the presence of resistance.

3. **Diagnosis**
   a. Chest radiographic evidence of infiltrates in apical or posterior segments of the upper lobe or superior segment of the lower lobe is the most frequent manifestation of post-primary TB. Radiographic features may be confusing in immunosuppressed patients, however, in whom intrathoracic lymphadenopathy, pleural effusions, miliary infiltrates, or cavities may be lacking. Chest radiographs are normal in 10% to 15% of immunosuppressed patients with TB.
   b. The tuberculin skin test or QuantiFERON-TB Gold test or T-SPOT test can often be negative in immunocompromised patients with TB and may not be helpful in evaluating patients thought to have active TB. The diagnosis of TB can be established by visualizing the organism in stained sputum smears or culturing *M. tuberculosis* from sputum or from extrapulmonary sites. Expectorated sputum may be adequate for smears and culture. Aerosol-induced sputum is superior to expectorated sputum or gastric juice aspiration in patients who produce little sputum. Bronchoalveolar lavage or transbronchial biopsy may be required when other material is not diagnostic. After identification of positive AFB in sputum smear, DNA probe testing, if available, is helpful in rapid mycobacterial species identification. Mycobacterial cultures are, however, still required for antimicrobial susceptibility testing; recent methods (e.g., GeneXpert) are of promise.
   c. Effusions: Pleural fluid samples may yield the organism in up to 30% of cases, and percutaneous needle pleural biopsies (three biopsies in three locations) provide up to a 75% yield. Culture of pericardial fluid may be positive in up to 50% of cases, and pericardial biopsy yields 80% positive results on either histology or culture. Analysis of ascitic fluid findings is not helpful unless the fluid is concentrated; peritoneal biopsy is preferred.

4. **Management**
   a. **Latent TB**: A positive tuberculin skin test in immunocompromised patients is defined as cutoff ≥ 5 mm induration. Treatment includes isoniazid (INH) 300 mg/d for 9 months, rifampin 600 mg daily for 4 months, or isoniazid 900 mg/d with rifapentine 900 mg/d weekly for 12 weeks under directly observed therapy.
   b. **Active TB.** Because of increasing drug resistance, the U.S. Public Health Service has issued new guidelines for the initial treatment of TB. Until drug susceptibility data are available, patients with active TB should be treated with daily administration of isoniazid, rifampin, pyrazinamide, and ethambutol. After 2 months of therapy, the regimen for patients with drug-sensitive organisms should be changed to isoniazid and rifampin administered daily for an additional 4 months or until sputum cultures are negative for 3 months. Alternative regimens are recommended for patients who require directly observed therapy to ensure compliance.
   c. **MDR TB,** defined as resistance to at least isoniazid and rifampin, is exceedingly difficult to treat, and early diagnosis with individualized therapy is crucial. To interrupt the transmission of MDR TB, stringent isolation procedures and aggressive chemotherapy with a combination of drugs are essential.

  d. Mycobacterium avium complex (MAC): Distinguishing colonization from true infection is challenging. Therapy is often difficult to tolerate. Treatment of pulmonary MAC should include two to three antimicrobials containing macrolides either clarithromycin (1,000 mg) or azithromycin (500 mg) and ethambutol (25 mg/kg) and rifampin (600 mg/d) given three times weekly for 1 year. Therapy for disseminated MAC is clarithromycin (1,000 mg/d) or azithromycin (250 mg/d), with ethambutol (15 mg/kg/d), with or without rifabutin (150 to 350 mg/d) until reconstitution of the immune system occurs.

F. *Nocardia asteroides* complex

Several types of cell-mediated immune defects have been described in association with nocardiosis. About 20% of cases occur in patients receiving corticosteroids. In immunocompromised subjects, 75% of nocardiosis involves the lung.

Nocardiosis can be asymptomatic, heal spontaneously, or produce a lower lobe bronchopneumonia with cavities, abscesses, or empyema. Disseminated nocardiosis typically involves subcutaneous tissue, muscle, and brain. All patients with nocardiosis are recommended to have CT/MRI brain to rule out intracranial brain abscess.

  1. Diagnosis. Gram stain of sputum reveals gram-positive, beaded, branching filaments. Sputum should also be examined with modified Ziehl-Neelsen stain, because the organism is weakly acid-fast.

  2. Management. Currently due to rising antibiotic resistance, combination therapy is the recommended therapy for treatment of nocardiosis. Trimethoprim–sulfamethoxazole (trimethoprim component as 5 to 10 mg/kg/d in divided doses) remains the drug of choice. Other effective agents include carbapenems like imipenem or meropenem, amikacin, or third-generation cephalosporins (e.g., ceftriaxone). A combination of these agents is recommended. In patients with sulfa allergy, imipenem with amikacin is preferred. In patients with CNS nocardiosis, a minimum of 12 months of treatment or longer till end of immunosuppressive therapy is recommended.

G. *Listeria monocytogenes* may be confused with gram-positive cocci, *H. influenzae*, or diphtheroids on Gram stain of specimens. Infections are more common in patients with defects in cell-mediated immunity.

Listeria monocytogenes is a common cause of bacterial meningitis in patients with carcinoma, receiving corticosteroids or other immunosuppressive therapy, especially for lymphoma, or age >65 years. CNS infection with meningitis or meningoencephalitis or cerebritis or brain abscess accounts for 80% of cases. The mortality rate for CNS infections is 20% to 30%. Bacteremia or sepsis accounts for 20% of cases in adults. Pulmonary involvement is usually in the form of an empyema.

  1. Diagnosis
    a. Blood cultures are positive in 60% to 75% of patients with CNS infection. CSF cultures are usually positive in Listeria meningitis.
    b. In spinal fluid, either lymphocytes or polymorphonuclear neutrophils are predominant. Spinal fluid protein concentration ranges from normal to 100 mg/dL. Glucose levels are low in only half of the cases.

  2. Management
    Ampicillin, 200 mg/kg/d, is given IV in six divided doses. Most experts recommend adding gentamicin for the first week to ampicillin for synergy. Total duration of therapy is longer in immunocompromised patients, at least 3 weeks for meningitis and 6 weeks for brain abscess. In patients who cannot tolerate ampicillin, the best alternative appears to be sulfamethoxazole–trimethoprim.

H. *Legionella*

Legionnaires disease can affect normal and immunosuppressed hosts, especially patients receiving glucocorticoids. A delay in treatment is associated with high fatality rate. The disease typically produces lobar pulmonic consolidation evolving from patchy infiltrates. Features that suggest Legionnaires disease include nonproductive cough, pulmonary consolidation, and extra pulmonary processes including diarrhea, hyponatremia, and confusion.

1. **Diagnosis:**
   a. Detection of *Legionella* antigen in urine should be sought. This test only detects *Legionella pneumophila* serogroup 1; however, serogroup 1 organisms cause the most severe forms of disease in humans.
   b. Cultures of respiratory specimens on specialized media developed specifically for recovery of *Legionella* should be requested.
   c. Dieterle (silver) staining can be used to detect bacteria in tissue. Positive direct fluorescent antibody (DFA) examination of tissue strongly suggests Legionnaires disease.
   d. Antibody titers do not help in the diagnosis.

2. **Management**
   Respiratory fluoroquinolones such as levofloxacin 750 mg IV/PO daily is the drug of choice in immunocompromised patients with Legionnaires disease. Other alternatives include macrolides such as azithromycin 500 mg daily or doxycycline 100 mg b.i.d. A longer duration of therapy for 21 days is recommended in immunocompromised patients.

VI. FUNGAL INFECTIONS

The profoundly immunosuppressed host, particularly with prolonged neutropenia, is at risk for infection by a variety of fungi, many of which rarely cause infection in healthy hosts. For many fungal infections, specific laboratory identification may not be possible. Recovery of traditional "nonpathogenic" fungi from sterile fluids such as spinal fluid or blood or from biopsy cultures should raise the suspicion that such organisms in the immunocompromised host may be "opportunistic" pathogens.

Accurate diagnosis of fungal infection is a challenge. Serum galactomannan, serum beta-D-glucan and CT imaging have become helpful in diagnosing fungal etiology. PCR test remains investigational. In general, candidal infection occurs early in neutropenia, while mold infection occurs after 2nd week of neutropenia.

A. **Antifungal Agents**

The three major classes of antifungal agents that are useful in the patient with neutropenia and persistent fever are echinocandins, triazoles, and amphotericin B (AmB) preparations. Dosages are shown in Table 36-1.

1. **Echinocandins.** The echinocandins are the newest group of antifungal agents; those currently marketed are caspofungin (Cancidas), anidulafungin (Eraxis), and micafungin (Mycamine). Although the greatest clinical experience is with caspofungin, these three agents have remarkably similar antifungal activities and toxicities, so they can be used interchangeably. The echinocandins have excellent *in vitro* activity against most species of *Candida* (including fluconazole-resistant *C. glabrata*) and *Aspergillus*.

2. **Triazoles** are clinically useful antifungal agents that have substantially differing spectra of activity, adverse effects, and potential for drug–drug interactions. All are effective for treatment of infections caused by *Candida albicans*.

a. Fluconazole. Although highly effective against *C. albicans*, it has much less activity against some non–*Candida albicans* than do the newer triazoles. In the past, fluconazole had been considered an acceptable alternative to amphotericin B at institutions in which infections with certain *Candida* species (*C. krusei* and some isolates of *C. glabrata*) and molds (e.g., *Aspergillus* species) were relatively uncommon. The main value of fluconazole in neutropenic patients is for treatment of mucocutaneous *Candida* infection and systemic infection caused by *C. albicans* in patients, for whom broader-spectrum antifungal agents are not indicated.

b. Itraconazole has a broader spectrum of activity than fluconazole. Its main clinical utility is against the agents histoplasmosis and blastomycosis. It also has only modest activity against *Aspergillus*.

c. Voriconazole has an appreciably broader spectrum of activity than fluconazole or itraconazole and is active against most species of *Candida*, *Aspergillus*, and several less common fungi. It is the drug of choice today for invasive aspergillosis. It is the most useful of the triazoles for empiric and pathogen-specific treatment of fungal infection in neutropenic patients. The potential for drug–drug interactions is high with the use of voriconazole. The most common adverse reactions are visual disturbances that usually do not require discontinuation of therapy and skin reactions. IV voriconazole is solubilized in sulfobutylether-beta-cyclodextrin (SBECD), which accumulates with moderate renal dysfunction; it is recommended that the IV preparation not be used if the creatinine clearance is <50 mL/min. Bioavailability of oral voriconazole is excellent, and the oral preparation does not contain SBECD. In selected patients with appreciably impaired renal function, a change to oral therapy with voriconazole may be feasible.

d. Posaconazole appears useful as an agent for prophylaxis of infection in severely immunosuppressed patients, such as those with acute leukemia and stem cell transplant recipients. The drug effectively prevents both candidemia and aspergillosis.

e. Isavuconazole, recently released, is effective in aspergillosis and mucormycosis.

f. Of importance, a number of important drug–drug interactions involve voriconazole and to a lesser extent the other triazoles. Most of these interactions involve cytochrome P450 isoforms and may result in significantly increased or decreased concentrations of voriconazole or of the interacting drug, resulting in either potential toxicity or lack of efficacy, respectively.

3. **AmB preparations**

   a. Amphotericin B deoxycholate (AmBD, Fungizone) has been the gold standard for treatment of fungal infections, but there is reluctance to use it because of its nephrotoxicity and infusion-related adverse events. In neutropenic patients, this concern is heightened by the frequent concomitant use of nephrotoxic chemotherapeutic agents and antimicrobial agents. Hence, this preparation of amphotericin B is avoided in cancer patients.

   b. Lipid formulations of AmB have not been shown to be more effective than AmBD for treatment of fungal infections, but they are safer and much less likely to cause nephrotoxicity. Their major drawback has been greater cost. These lipid preparations include:

   (1) Amphotericin B lipid complex (ABLC, Abelcet)

   (2) Amphotericin B colloidal dispersion (ABCD, Amphotec)—not favored

(3) Liposomal amphotericin B (LAmB, AmBisome), which currently is the only U.S. Food and Drug Administration (FDA)-approved lipid formulation for empiric therapy for presumed fungal infections in febrile neutropenic patients

B. **Choice of Antifungal Agent:** Reasonably clear guidelines have been developed for antifungal therapy early in the course of neutropenia, largely because the greatest concern is for disseminated candidiasis. With prolonged broad-spectrum antibacterial therapy and empiric antifungal therapy, increasing opportunity and selective pressure tend to result in unusual infections. The availability of the newer triazoles and echinocandins has provided greater therapeutic options with reduced toxicity; it has also increased the risk of administration of an antifungal agent that is not active against the patient's present fungal pathogen. This makes microbiologic diagnosis of infection imperative and may require invasive procedures to procure biopsy material for culture and fungal staining.

1. **Principles.** The strategy for providing empiric antifungal therapy in cancer patients with neutropenia is based on the following principles:

   a. During the first several days of neutropenic fever, the most likely pathogens are bacteria; diagnostic approaches and empiric treatment, therefore, are not focused primarily on fungal pathogens.

   b. During the first 4 to 7 days of neutropenic fever, the fungal pathogens most likely to be encountered are *Candida* spp. and, much less frequently, *Aspergillus* spp. The echinocandins and newer triazoles have excellent *in vitro* activity against most *Candida* spp. and most *Aspergillus* spp., and they possess limited toxicity. Fluconazole is chosen if the target organism is only *Candida*; however if *Candida* and *Aspergillus* need to be targeted, then, among the azoles, voriconazole is the appropriate drug. Posaconazole has no FDA approval for therapy in such situations.

   c. As the duration of neutropenia and fever increases beyond 7 to 10 days, the likelihood of infection by a mold increases. This should prompt an aggressive search for occult infection and consideration of more aggressive antifungal therapy.

   d. AmBD and the lipid formulations of AmB possess the broadest spectrum of antifungal activity of all groups of antifungal agents. The echinocandins may lack the broader activity of AmB preparations and of the newer triazoles against genera of clinically important fungi that may cause infection later in neutropenia.

   e. Among the echinocandins, the greatest clinical experience is with caspofungin; however, micafungin and anidulafungin have similar clinical efficacies. It is important to note that echinocandins are not available as oral agents and are inactive against *Cryptococcus neoformans*, the endemic mycoses (e.g., *Coccidioides* spp., *Histoplasma capsulatum*), and many molds (e.g., *Fusarium* spp., *Scedosporium apiospermum*, Zygomycetes). Drug–drug interactions are generally less than those seen with triazoles.

   f. Among the triazoles, voriconazole may be a reasonable alternative to an echinocandin or AmB preparation. With voriconazole, attention must be paid to potential side effects and drug–drug interactions; also, it is recommended that the drug not be given intravenously, if at all possible, when the creatinine clearance is <50 mL/min to avoid accumulation of the diluent used to solubilize the drug. Of the other azoles, fluconazole and itraconazole are thought not to have a sufficiently broad spectrum of activity against all *Candida* spp.

2. **Recommendations**
   a. After 4 to 7 days of persistent fever and neutropenia despite antibiotics, initiate empirical antifungal treatment with a lipid formulation of amphotericin B *or* caspofungin *or* voriconazole.
   b. For patients already receiving antimold prophylaxis, consider switching to another class of antimold agents given intravenously because of potential selection of a resistant mold by the prophylactic agent. Antimold agents include:
      (1) Amphotericin (all preparations are active against many molds)
      (2) Echinocandins (anidulafungin, caspofungin, and micafungin have good *in vitro* activity against some molds, particularly the most common *Aspergillus* species, *A. fumigatus*).
      (3) Azoles. Voriconazole and posaconazole have differing but broad activity against molds. Voriconazole has broad *in vitro* activity against most clinical species of *Aspergillus*, including *A. fumigatus*. Posaconazole is active against *Candida*, *Aspergillus*, and *Mucor*. Fluconazole lacks clinically useful activity against molds.
   c. Renal concerns. With concerns regarding renal function (pre-existing impairment of renal function, concomitant use of nephrotoxic agents, or development of renal dysfunction during AmB administration), use of an echinocandin or voriconazole is frequently reasonable and appropriate. With substantial clinical deterioration that might be caused by fungal infection, the initiation of antifungal therapy with an AmB lipid preparation would be prudent.

C. **Candidiasis**
   The major risk factors for systemic candidiasis include treatment with immunosuppressive agents, neutropenia, antibiotics, gastrointestinal surgery, glucocorticoids, and parenteral hyperalimentation. Indwelling central venous catheters, IV drug abuse, and underlying diseases that produce defects in polymorphonuclear neutrophil function or cell-mediated immunity (e.g., leukemia, lymphoma, diabetes mellitus) also are associated with this infection. Vascular catheter-associated candidemia are the most common.
   1. **Clinical presentation.** Localized candidiasis can involve the skin, mouth, esophagus, rectum, or vagina. Disseminated candidiasis can present with fever alone, sepsis, endophthalmitis, skin nodules, renal disease, arthritis, or myositis. With dissemination, *C. albicans* and occasionally other *Candida* species may produce discrete, yellow–white retinal lesions of *Candida* endophthalmitis. Visceral involvement (hepatosplenic candidiasis) is another sequela of dissemination and typically becomes evident at the time of resolution of neutropenia.
   2. **Diagnosis**
      a. Cultures: Although studies have shown that blood cultures were positive in only 50% of patients with disseminated candidiasis at autopsy, the yield using modern culture method is higher. Growth of *Candida* in the laboratory allows for speciation; this may have implications for selection of therapeutic agents. Documentation of disseminated candidiasis may also avoid a continued search for causes of fever.
      b. Serology: Serum beta-D-glucan is a useful test. Mostly, a negative test has a high negative predictive value.
   3. **Management:** Infected foreign bodies, such as CVC, should be promptly removed.
      a. Prophylaxis: Topical agents such as nystatin or clotrimazole are not appropriate for prevention of systemic infection. The prophylactic use of

fluconazole (or other triazole antifungal agents) is appropriate, particularly in AML patients undergoing induction chemotherapy.

b. Systemic therapy: If a *Candida* species is isolated from a neutropenic patient, then treatment with an echinocandin is appropriate. When the isolate has been speciated or susceptibility testing has been done, changing to a triazole might be appropriate, depending on the species of *Candida* recovered, whether the patient is tolerating the echinocandin, and whether clinical stability has been achieved.

D. Cryptococcosis

Patients receiving corticosteroids and those with AIDS or Hodgkin lymphoma have the highest incidence of infection with *C. neoformans*.

Pulmonary infection can be asymptomatic. Chest radiographs reveal local bronchopneumonia, lobar involvement, or discrete nodules that may cavitate. CNS infection is the most common; it usually presents as insidious meningoencephalitis without evidence of infection outside the meninges. A variety of skin findings, ranging from maculopapular or nodular lesions to cellulitis, can be seen in disseminated infection.

1. Diagnosis

a. Culture: *C. neoformans*, an encapsulated yeast that replicates by budding, can easily be grown from blood, respiratory secretions, spinal fluid, and skin biopsies on common laboratory media.

b. Cerebrospinal fluid typically reveals an elevated opening pressure and lymphocytic pleocytosis in cryptococcal meningoencephalitis. A low glucose concentration is found in half of the cases. The India ink preparation is positive in approximately 40% of cases; because of low sensitivity, most laboratories no longer offer this test.

c. Serology: The presence of cryptococcal polysaccharide antigen in spinal fluid is diagnostic and is detected in cerebrospinal fluid in >90% of meningitis cases. The presence of cryptococcal antigen in serum documents infection, however, may not be a reliable tool for diagnosis. Antibody assays are not useful.

2. Management. The major difficulty the clinician faces with management of cryptococcal infection is determining whether meningeal infection exists. The greatest clinical experience with treatment of cryptococcal infection is that from HIV-infected patients; this experience heavily influences management algorithms. All **echinocandins lack** activity against *Cryptococcus*.

a. Meningitis or disseminated disease may be treated with AmBD, 0.7 mg/kg/d, with adjunctive flucytosine for 2 weeks. Amphotericin lipid preparations are preferred. This 2-week induction is followed by fluconazole given at a dose of 400 mg/d (after a 400-mg loading dose) either PO or IV. Opening pressure during LP must be assessed. Intracranial hypertension in the absence of intracranial mass lesions may require repeated LP to reduce intracranial pressure and ensure adequate perfusion of the brain.

b. Extrameningeal infection. Most patients with extrameningeal infection can be treated with fluconazole (400 to 800 mg/d), if meningeal infection has been excluded.

E. Aspergillosis

Infection usually occurs via inhalation of spores leading to infection of lung parenchyma or of the paranasal sinuses; dissemination usually occurs from the lung. Approximately 70% to 80% of isolates are *Aspergillus fumigatus*.

The typical presentation for pulmonary aspergillosis in immunosuppressed patients is fever and pulmonary nodules or infiltrates; as disease progresses, there may be infarction, hemoptysis, and gangrene from vascular invasion. Nearly one-third of patients have no radiologic abnormalities early in the disease.

Dissemination complicates pulmonary disease in 25% to 50% of cases. Various skin lesions, multiple abscesses, brain infarction, or GI ulceration with hemorrhage can result. Bone marrow recovery may lead to the liquefaction of pulmonary foci leading to hemoptysis. Potentially lethal erosion and bleeding may occur because of the vasculotropic nature of the infection.

1. **Diagnosis.** The "gold standard" for diagnosis is recovery of the organism by the laboratory from an appropriate clinical sample; this invariably involves culture of a biopsy specimen. *Aspergillus* species are infrequently recovered from tracheobronchial secretions and essentially never from blood cultures. The serum galactomannan assay, which detects a cell wall polysaccharide of *Aspergillus* species, is a good tool for diagnosis. The diagnosis of aspergillosis is often based on demonstration of septate, acutely branching hyphae in tissue. Other fungi (e.g., *Scedosporium apiospermum*, *Fusarium* species, *Penicillium* species), however, may not be distinguishable from *Aspergillus* in tissue section. Chest radiographic studies may reveal nodules, with or without cavitation, or pleural-based infiltrates. The presence of a "halo sign" (low attenuation surrounding a nodular lesion) on high-resolution CT may be seen in early pulmonary aspergillosis. Later, an "air-crescent" sign indicative of cavitation, with the return of neutrophils, may be noted. Similar radiographic findings may, however, be present with other vasculotropic organisms. Hence, the emphasis should be on biopsy and culture, whenever possible. Bronchoalveolar lavage fluid should be tested for galactomannan antigen. Presence of the antigen is highly suggestive of aspergillosis. With confirmation of infection difficult to achieve, frequently, clinical and radiologic criteria are used for diagnosis.

2. **Management**
   a. The greatest experience is with AmBD, given in a dose of 1.0 to 1.5 mg/kg/d; this dose regimen almost invariably results in significant renal dysfunction. The lipid preparations of AmB (ABLC and LAmB) are better tolerated and are usually given in a daily dose of at least 5 mg/kg/d.
   b. Voriconazole has FDA approval for treatment of invasive aspergillosis and has become a mainstay of treatment of invasive aspergillosis. Therapy should be initiated with two doses of 6 mg/kg given IV 12 hours apart, followed by 4 mg/kg every 12 hours. Patients who respond to this treatment can be switched to oral drugs at 7 days.
   c. Fluconazole is **inactive** against aspergillosis. Posaconazole is not FDA approved for therapy. Isavuconazole is an alternative agent to voriconazole.
   d. Caspofungin has FDA approval for treatment of aspergillosis in patients who cannot tolerate or who have failed other forms of therapy ("salvage therapy"). Micafungin or anidulafungin may be alternatively used.
   e. Recent data suggest the use of combination therapy for invasive aspergillosis with voriconazole and anidulafungin.
   f. Surgical resection of localized invasive pulmonary aspergillosis with a cavitating lesion may prevent hemoptysis and recurrence in selected patients. In leukemic patients, the achievement of complete remission combined with aggressive antifungal therapy has led to markedly increased cure rates for aspergillosis.

F. **Mucormycosis.** Members of the taxonomic class *Zygomycetes* are a complicated group of organisms. Infection has been recognized with increasing frequency in patients who have leukemia or lymphoma, glucocorticoid therapy, diabetes mellitus, malnutrition, burns, or undergone transplantation. Mortality is high.

The genera *Rhizopus, Absidia,* and *Mucor* produce similar pathologic and clinical manifestations because of neutrophil exudation, tissue necrosis, and vascular invasion that result in thrombosis and infarction.

Pneumonia can be associated with a dry cough or hemoptysis. Radiographs may show interstitial infiltrates, lobar consolidation, or cavitation.

Cerebral disease is usually secondary to pulmonary involvement and presents as brain infarcts or abscesses. Spinal fluid studies are not usually helpful. In contrast, rhinocerebral mucormycosis occurs most frequently in uncontrolled diabetes mellitus.

Disseminated disease can result in gastroenteritis, bowel perforation or hemorrhage, peritonitis, or abscess in any organ.

1. **Diagnosis:** *Zygomycetes* organisms have broad, nonseptate hyphae, often with right-angled branching in tissue specimens. The agents of zygomycosis may be difficult to recover by culture. Diagnosis is made by demonstrating the organism by culture or, more commonly, by special stains of tissue sections.

2. **Management:** A high dose of either AmBD or one of the AmB lipid formulations is recommended, although these drugs are largely adjunctive. Reversal of the predisposing condition and resection of infected tissue, if feasible, are the mainstays of therapy. Posaconazole appears to provide benefit following treatment with an AmB preparation. Isavuconazole is FDA approved for the treatment of mucormycosis.

G. **Pneumocystosis**

PJP, now considered a fungus, reactivates in patients with profound neutropenia or cell-mediated immune deficiency to cause pneumonia. Commonly affected patients are those receiving corticosteroids, lymphoma patients and stem cell recipients with graft versus host disease. Pneumonia is acute in onset and rapidly progressive, unlike in AIDS patients. Rapidly progressive hypoxemia with diffuse interstitial infiltrates should raise suspicion for PJP. Specific staining of the organism in induced sputum or bronchoalveolar lavage is helpful in diagnosis.

Trimethoprim–sulfamethoxazole remains the therapy of choice; use of steroids in non–HIV-infected patients is not proven to be of benefit. Routine prophylaxis with trimethoprim–sulfamethoxazole is appropriate in patients receiving corticosteroids (prednisone >20 mg/d for >3 weeks), particularly those with brain tumors.

H. **Other mycoses**

1. **Endemic mycoses:** *Histoplasma capsulatum, Coccidioides immitis, and Blastomyces dermatitidis* can readily be recovered from tissues and display typical (pathognomonic) histopathologies. These common human pathogens can present as opportunistic infections in patients who are immunocompromised, particularly in areas endemic for such organisms.

2. **Trichosporonosis:** *Trichosporon beigelii* refers to a group of fungi that cannot readily be distinguished without the use of molecular techniques. *Trichosporon beigelii* causes white piedra, an infection of hair shafts. It causes an emerging opportunistic mycosis that can be difficult to diagnose and has a high attributable mortality rate. Systemic infection has been most frequently described in neutropenic patients receiving chemotherapy.

   a. Cutaneous involvement occurs in about 30% of patients and frequently presents as purpuric papules and nodules with central necrosis or ulceration. Biopsy specimens of these lesions reveal dermal invasion by fungal elements. Culture is positive in >90% of cases.

    b. Resolution of disseminated infection appears to require resolution of neutropenia. The antifungal triazoles are most active. AmBD, liposomal AmB, and the echinocandins appear not to be very effective.

3. Scedosporiosis: Scedosporiosis is caused by the asexual form *Scedosporium apiospermum* (*Pseudallescheria boydii*); it is an increasingly common cause of opportunistic infection and may cause CNS disease and fungemia in patients with leukemia. Although infections are usually resistant to AmB, the triazoles may be effective, with voriconazole being preferred. Some species (e.g., *S. prolificans*) are resistant to all available drugs.

4. Fusariosis: Members of the genus *Fusarium* are ubiquitous fungi uncommonly associated with infection. Disseminated fusariosis typically occurs in neutropenic patients, carries a high mortality rate, and presents with fever and diffuse cutaneous macules, papules, and nodules. *Fusarium* species can be isolated from biopsy of skin lesions (hyphae are often observed on direct microscopy) or bronchial aspirates of lung lesions or from blood cultures. AmBD and AmB lipid formulations may eradicate this infection. Voriconazole is indicated for those with fusariosis who are intolerant of, or refractory to, other therapy. Some clinicians prefer a lipid preparation of AmB plus voriconazole since susceptibilities may vary.

5. Fungemic shock: As the use of empiric antibiotics for bacteria has increased, the likelihood has increased that fungi, particularly *Candida* species, can cause a septic shock-type picture, not unlike those due to bacteria.

VII. PARASITIC INFECTIONS
A. Toxoplasmosis

Parasites in general are rare causes of infections in febrile neutropenic patients. The main risk factors for toxoplasmosis are in patients with AIDS, bone marrow and solid organ transplant recipients, hematologic malignancy (Hodgkin disease) and pregnancy. The common manifestation of toxoplasmosis in immunocompromised population is disseminated or toxoplasma encephalitis due to reactivation of toxoplasma in seropositive individuals.

    Patients with symptomatic disease present with a low-grade febrile illness characterized by localized or generalized lymphadenopathy, hepatosplenomegaly, malaise, and fatigue. Any organ may become involved. Infection in patients with abnormal cellular immunity may mimic brain tumor or lymphoproliferative disorder.

1. Diagnosis

    a. Histology. Identification of trophozoites rather than cysts is important because cysts can persist for decades. Lymph node pathology is characteristic of toxoplasmosis. Immunohistochemical staining (IHC) is performed on tissue sample for visualization of organisms. The positive IHC result is suggestive of infection; however, negative result does not rule out disease. Culture is rarely used.

    b. Serology is widely used for diagnosis of the disease. IgM antibody is suggestive of recent infection. Many patients, however, develop symptomatic disease as a result of reactivation of a quiescent infection. In the latter instance, only IgG antibody will likely be detectable. If both IgM and IgG are negative, it suggests no recent or past infection, except in severely immunocompromised patients when serology is not reliable.

    c. PCR. Toxoplasma PCR of any body fluid such as blood, CSF, bronchoalveolar lavage, or brain tissue is highly specific for diagnosis of toxoplasmosis. This test is useful for early detection in blood/cerebrospinal fluid.

    d. Imaging. CT/MRI of the brain is utilized to detect multiple toxoplasma ring-enhancing lesions in the brain or brain calcifications. Differential diagnosis is CNS lymphoma; biopsy is required for confirmation.

   2. Management. Pyrimethamine (a folic acid antagonist) and a sulfa derivative are given in divided doses for 3 to 6 weeks. The development of hematologic toxicity often interrupts treatment. Leucovorin is also given to minimize marrow suppressive effects.

    a. Pyrimethamine is given as a loading dose of 200 mg PO followed by maintenance of 50 to 75 mg/d in association with leucovorin, 10 to 20 mg/d orally. Sulfadiazine, 1.0 to 1.5 g q.i.d., is given in conjunction with pyrimethamine.

    b. Another combination for acute disease is pyrimethamine (100 mg/d PO) and leucovorin plus clindamycin (1.2 g/d IV in divided doses).

    c. Atovaquone was FDA approved for use as combination agent with pyrimethamine or sulfadiazine for acute toxoplasma encephalitis among patients with sulfa allergy or pyrimethamine unavailability or allergy respectively.

    d. Adjuvant agents include corticosteroids in patients with significant brain edema or anticonvulsants in patients with seizures.

  B. Other parasitic infections such as strongyloidiasis, malaria, giardiasis, and babesiosis are less common in the United States. Management is the same as in nonimmunocompromised hosts.

Suggested Readings

Freifeld AG, et al. Clinical practice guidelines for the use of antimicrobial agents in neutropenic patients with cancer: 2010 update by the Infectious Diseases Society of America. *Clin Infect Dis* 2011;52:e56.

Maertens JA, et al. Isavuconazole versus voriconazole for primary treatment of invasive mould disease caused by Aspergillus and other filamentous fungi (SECURE): a phase 3, randomised-controlled, non-inferiority trial. *Lancet* 2016;387:760.

Marr KA, et al. Combination antifungal therapy for invasive aspergillosis: a randomized trial. *Ann Intern Med* 2015;162:81.

Marty FM, et al. Isavuconazole treatment for mucormycosis: a single-arm open-label trial and case-control analysis. *Lancet Infect Dis* 2016;16(7):828.

Mermel LA, et al. Clinical practice guidelines for the diagnosis and management of intravascular catheter-related infection: 2009 update by the Infectious Diseases Society of America. *Clin Infect Dis* 2009;49:1.

Pappas PG, et al. Clinical practice guidelines for the management of candidiasis: 2016 update by the Infectious Diseases Society of America. *Clin Infect Dis* 2016;62(4):e1.

Pfeiffer CD, et al. Diagnosis of invasive aspergillosis using a galactomannan assay: a meta-analysis. *Clin Infect Dis* 2006;42:1417.

Price TH, et al. Efficacy of transfusion with granulocytes from G-CSF/dexamethasone-treated donors in neutropenic patients with infection. *Blood* 2015;126:2153.

Smith TJ, et al. 2006 update of recommendations for use of white blood cell growth factors: an evidence-based clinical practice guideline. *J Clin Oncol* 2006;24:3187.

Walsh TJ. Treatment of aspergillosis: clinical practice guidelines of the Infectious Diseases Society of America. *Clin Infect Dis* 2008;46:327.

Wong GC, Abdul Halim NA, Tan BH. Antifungal prophylaxis with posaconazole is effective in preventing invasive fungal infections in acute myeloid leukemia patients during induction and salvage chemotherapy. *Clin Infect Dis* 2015;61:1351.

37

AIDS-Related Malignancies and Malignancies Related to Other Immunodeficiency States

Ronald T. Mitsuyasu and Mary Territo

AIDS-RELATED MALIGNANCIES

I. INTRODUCTION

Despite great advances in the treatment and survival of individuals infected with the human immunodeficiency virus (HIV), cancer is now one of the leading causes of death in patients with AIDS. In the era of highly active antiretroviral therapy (HAART), patients infected with HIV are living longer than ever, and HAART has greatly reduced the incidence of most of the AIDS-defining cancers, including Kaposi sarcoma (KS), non-Hodgkin lymphoma (NHL; including primary central nervous system [CNS] lymphoma), and invasive cervical carcinoma. Unfortunately, the incidence of other, non–AIDS-defining cancers (NADCs) has increased significantly, and the management of patients who develop malignancies in the setting of HIV remains very challenging.

II. AIDS-RELATED LYMPHOMA

A. Incidence

1. NHL remains one of the most common AIDS-defining conditions, occurring in approximately 16% of all new cases of AIDS. All age groups and all groups at risk for acquisition of HIV infection are equally likely to develop lymphoma.

2. The incidence of NHL generally tracks with the progressive loss of CD4 lymphocytes. With widespread use of HAART in various areas of the world, resulting in population-wide increases in CD4 cells, the incidence of lymphoma has declined. In this setting, the risk for lymphoma depends on the latest CD4 cell count and not the nadir count.

B. Pathology. Most AIDS-related lymphomas are B-cell tumors of high-grade pathologic type. About 60% of patients are diagnosed with immunoblastic, plasmablastic, or small noncleaved lymphoma; the latter may be Burkitt or Burkitt-like subtypes. Intermediate-grade, diffuse, large B-cell lymphomas, and many non-GCB type have been reported in 30% to 40%. HIV-infected patients also have an increased incidence of low-grade B-cell lymphoma and of various T-cell lymphomas, as well, although they are much less common.

Primary effusion lymphoma (PEL) has also been identified among HIV-infected patients who are also infected with human herpesvirus-8 (HHV-8). Patients present with malignant serous effusions, usually in the absence of specific mass lesions. Median survival time is in the range of 6 months.

C. **Clinical features.** About 80% of patients with newly diagnosed AIDS-related lymphoma present with systemic B symptoms, consisting of fever, drenching night sweats, and/or weight loss. About 60% to 90% of patients have advanced-stage disease, often presenting in extranodal sites. This occurrence is in sharp distinction to the general lymphoma population, of whom approximately 40% present with extranodal disease. The more common sites of initial extranodal disease include the CNS (about 30% prevalence at diagnosis), gastrointestinal (GI) tract (25%), bone marrow (20% to 33%), and liver (10%).

D. **Diagnosis and staging evaluation**

1. **Biopsy.** Immunophenotypic or genotypic studies are often helpful to confirm the monoclonal nature and the histologic subtype of the tumor.

2. **Computed tomography (CT) scans.** Staging evaluation should begin with CT scans of the chest, abdomen, and pelvis. Nearly two-thirds of patients with AIDS-related lymphoma have evidence of intra-abdominal lymphomatous disease, which most commonly involves the lymph nodes, GI tract, liver, kidney, and/or adrenal gland.

3. **Positron emission tomography (PET) scanning** is now commonly used in conjunction with CT scans and can detect more minimal disease activity and may be used posttreatment to differentiate residual active lymphoma from scar and fibrosis.

4. **Bone marrow** aspiration and biopsy should be performed.

5. **Lumbar puncture (LP).** LP should be performed routinely as part of the staging evaluation of patients with AIDS-related lymphoma. About 20% of HIV-infected patients are found to have leptomeningeal involvement even without CNS symptoms. It is now common practice to inject the first dose of methotrexate or cytarabine at the time of this initial staging LP in an attempt to prevent isolated CNS relapse. In the presence of active cerebrospinal fluid (CSF) involvement by lymphoma, abnormalities may be relatively minor, with median white cell count of often <10 cells/mL although elevated protein and decreased CSF glucose levels are very often present. Abnormal lymphoma cells are generally clearly recognizable upon cytologic, flow cytometric, or cytogenetic evaluation in those with active disease.

E. **Prognostic factors.** Decreased survival in AIDS-related lymphoma is associated with the following factors: CD4 cells <100/mL, Karnofsky performance status <70%, age >35 years, stage IV (especially leptomeningeal disease is present), elevated lactate dehydrogenase in serum, higher IPI scores (2 to 3), certain subsets of lymphoma (e.g., primary CNS lymphoma, PEL), and perhaps subtypes of diffuse large B-cell lymphoma (DLBCL; e.g., activated B-cell phenotype).

F. **Management**

1. **Use of full-dose chemotherapy regimens.** Before the availability of HAART, use of low-dose modifications of standard regimens was advocated because prospective clinical trials indicated that standard-dose regimens were associated with significantly increased toxicity. In the era of HAART, *these recommendations are no longer valid.*

   Studies using full-dose regimens, generally in conjunction with HAART, have shown better outcomes with full-dose and more dose-intensive regimens and with the combined use of rituximab. While responses and progression-free survival were improved with rituximab, especially when used concurrently with the EPOCH regimen, concerns about poorer outcomes due to infectious deaths have resulted in recommendations for greater use of prophylactic antibiotics and hematopoietic growth factors in this population, especially with CD4 <100 cells/mm^3.

2. **Antiretroviral therapy** may be used simultaneously with multiagent chemotherapy (currently accepted practice) or may be discontinued during chemotherapy administration and then restarted immediately. Pharmacokinetic studies have indicated no clinically significant interactions between HAART (including protease inhibitors [PIs]) and multiagent anti-lymphoma chemotherapy.

3. **Infusional chemotherapy: (R)-EPOCH.** A dose-adjusted EPOCH regimen has been used with excellent results, including those with Burkitt lymphoma. Three of the five drugs are given by continuous IV infusion (CIV). Cycles are repeated every 21 days for a total of six cycles. The specific dose-adjusted regimen for patients with AIDS is as follows:

Rituximab, 375 mg/m^2 IV on day 1 (in the R-EPOCH study)

Etoposide, 50 mg/m^2/d on days 1 through 4 by CIV

Doxorubicin, 10 mg/m^2/d on days 1 through 4 by CIV

Vincristine, 0.4 mg/m^2/d on days 1 through 4 by CIV (with no maximum dose)

Prednisone, 60 mg/m^2/d PO on days 1 through 5

Cyclophosphamide IV on day 5; 375 mg/m^2 if CD4 >100; 187 mg/m^2 if CD4 <100

   a. On subsequent cycles, if the nadir absolute neutrophil count (ANC) was >500 cells/mL, the dose of cyclophosphamide was adjusted in increments of 187 mg/m^2 to a maximum dose of 750 mg/m^2 IV.

   b. Granulocyte colony-stimulating factor was given at a dose of 5 mg/kg/d subcutaneously from day 6 until the ANC was >5,000 cells/mL after the nadir.

   c. Intrathecal methotrexate was given at a dose of 12 mg on days 1 and 5 for a minimum of 4 doses prophylactically or until CSF clear of malignant cells in those with active disease.

   d. Prophylaxis for *Pneumocystis pneumonia* was mandated, and prophylaxis against *Mycobacterium avium* was given to patients with CD4 cells <100/mL.

   e. **Results of EPOCH in AIDS-related lymphoma**

      (1) In the initial NCI trial, the overall complete remission rate was 74%, including 56% of patients with CD4 cells <100/mL and 87% of patients with CD4 cells >100/mL. With a median follow-up of 56 months, there were only two relapses, and the disease-free survival was 92%. Overall survival at 56 months was 60%, whereas the overall survival of patients with CD4 cells >100/mL at entry was 87%.

      (2) In a subsequent randomized trial, patients received the same dose-adjusted NCI EPOCH regimen with rituximab administered either concurrently on day 1 of each cycle or weekly for 6 weeks after completing EPOCH therapy. Response rate and 1-year disease-free survival were better in the concurrently treated group (RR: 82% vs. 75% and DFS: 78% vs. 68%).

G. **Primary CNS lymphoma** (PCNSL; see also Chapter 22, Section VIII.C in "Non-Hodgkin Lymphoma")

   1. **Clinical features.** Patients with PCNSL present with far-advanced HIV disease, with median CD4 cells of <50/mL and/or a history of AIDS before the lymphoma. Initial symptoms and signs include seizures, headache, or focal neurologic dysfunction. Isolated subtle changes in personality or behavior may also be seen.

   2. **Diagnosis.** Radiographic scanning reveals mass lesions in the brain, occurring at any site. These masses are likely to be relatively large (2 to 4 cm)

and relatively few in number (one to three). Ring enhancement may be seen. PET scans may help differentiate PCNSL from other space-occupying lesions within the brain of HIV-infected patients. Further, because AIDS-related PCNSL is essentially always associated with infection by EBV, determination of latent EBV proteins within the CSF may also be used to diagnose PCNSL. In the case of equivocal results and for definitive diagnosis, brain biopsy is required.

3. **Management.** High-dose methotrexate with leucovorin rescue is now considered the primary treatment modality for PCNSL in patient with or without AIDS. Radiation therapy (RT) is associated with complete remission in 20% to 50% of cases, but the median survival time is generally only 2 to 3 months. Although RT may not improve the duration of survival, the quality of life does improve, often dramatically. Use of HAART with antineoplastic therapy has been shown to improve survival.

III. HODGKIN LYMPHOMA

A. **Incidence.** Hodgkin lymphoma (HL) is not an AIDS-defining condition, although the incidence of HL has increased significantly in HIV-infected patients in the HAART era. This is likely due to the fact that the Reed-Sternberg cell (RS), the malignant cell of HL, requires the presence of CD4+ lymphocytes, which provide proliferation and survival signals to the malignant RS cells.

B. **Biology.** An association of HL with EBV has been suggested for years based on epidemiologic data in non-HIV patients where approximately half have presence of clonally integrated EBV within the RS cells. In the setting of HIV, EBV is almost universally present within the malignant RS cells.

C. **Clinical features.** Patients with underlying HIV infection have different clinical and pathologic manifestations of HL than those expected in patients without HIV disease.

1. **Sites of disease.** Most HIV-infected patients with HL have widespread extranodal disease at diagnosis, with about 80% to 90% presenting with stage III or IV disease. Systemic B symptoms are seen in about 80% to 90% of patients. Unusual extranodal sites of disease may be seen, including the anus, rectum, and CNS. Bone marrow is involved in approximately 50% to 60% at diagnosis and may be the only site of disease in patients with B symptoms, usually in the setting of peripheral cytopenias.

2. **Pathology.** Mixed cellularity and lymphocyte depletion subtypes of HL are prominent. Nodular sclerosis and lymphocyte predominant subtypes also occur in the setting of HIV infection.

D. **Management.** The ABVD regimen (see Appendix C-1) is used most frequently, along with hematopoietic growth factors. The BEACOPP regimen (see Appendix C-1), when used with concomitant HAART, has been associated with improvements in response rate and overall survival. Whether this improvement is due to the addition of HAART or to that specific regimen is not known, although HAART is probably the most important factor. A study of brentuximab vedotin with AVD in AIDS-associated HL is in progress in the United States and France.

IV. KAPOSI SARCOMA

A. **Incidence and epidemiology.** AIDS-related KS is seen in all HIV-risk groups worldwide, with most cases in the United States being in gay or bisexual men. With the advent of effective antiretroviral therapy (HAART), the incidence of KS has fallen dramatically in the United States and other resource-rich countries. This dramatic change in the incidence of disease, coincident with the marked decrease in HIV viral load and improvement in immune function associated with HAART, serves to emphasize the crucial role of immunity in the development and control of KS.

B. Pathogenesis: human herpesvirus-8 (HHV-8)

  1. HHV-8 is directly associated with all types of KS, including that associated with HIV, with organ transplantation, and with the classic KS seen in elderly men of Mediterranean descent.

  2. The virus is found at highest titer in saliva. The salivary transmission of HHV-8 infection would be consistent with the primary mode of transmission of other HHVs, such as EBV.

  3. HHV-8 infection is clearly required for development of KS, although the virus itself may not be sufficient for KS to emerge. About 2% to 10% of normal, healthy people in the United States have evidence of antibody to HHV-8, without clinical illness.

C. Pathogenesis. HIV infection induces an inflammatory cytokine response, with secretion of interleukin-6 (IL-6), IL-1, tumor necrosis factor-α, and others. These cytokines serve as growth factors for endothelial cells infected with HHV-8 and may also be operative in changing the morphology of these cells to the typical spindle cell, which characterizes the KS lesion. Further, secretion of angiogenic factors, such as basic fibroblast growth factor (bFGF), vascular endothelial growth factor (VEGF), and others, by HIV-1–infected mononuclear cells serves to induce the prominent proliferation of vascular tissue that characterizes the KS lesion. HHV-8 itself has genes that encode a viral IL-6 and other proteins that further contribute to the growth and dissemination of the tumor.

D. Clinical features

  1. Natural history of disease. Some patients experience slowly progressive disease over many years, whereas others have fulminant, rapidly advancing KS that quickly leads to death.

  2. Sites of involvement. The patient with KS usually presents with disease on the skin that may consist of nodular or irregular hyperpigmented lesions. The lesions are generally asymptomatic. Lymphedema may occur and can be profound occasionally even in the absence of visible skin lesions. Lymphadenopathy, sometimes in the absence of KS lesions on the skin, is also sometimes seen.

  Another common site of involvement is the oral cavity, which is sometimes associated with the presence of KS in the lower GI tract. Literally, any visceral organ may be involved, although CNS involvement is rare. KS in the lung is associated with a poor prognosis and has a higher mortality rate and usually mandates immediate chemotherapy.

E. Diagnosis and staging evaluation. An initial biopsy with pathologic confirmation should be obtained. The detection of HHV-8 genes in the tumor assists in the diagnosis. Routine staging is not necessary in the patient with KS. Assessment of visible disease on the skin and oral cavity, a baseline chest radiograph, and determination of the number of CD4 cells in blood should be performed. If the patient has symptoms suggestive of GI involvement (e.g., abdominal pain, weight loss, or diarrhea), endoscopy should be performed. With unexplained abnormalities on chest radiograph, bronchoscopy should be performed; the diagnosis of KS is usually made by visualization rather than biopsy due to the submucosal or parenchymal location of most pulmonary tumors.

F. Prognostic factors. Factors associated with poor prognosis include (1) history or presence of opportunistic infection; (2) presence of systemic B symptoms, consisting of fever, drenching night sweats, or weight loss in excess of 10% of the normal body weight; and (3) CD4 cells <200/mL.

G. **Management**

1. **HAART.** The initial treatment of patients with KS should be an effective antiretroviral regimen alone. In patients who have never taken HAART before, the overall response rate of KS to HAART alone is approximately 60% after 6 months of use (with complete remission in 11%) and increases to a 75% response rate at 24 months, with complete remissions seen in approximately 60%. If the KS does not regress despite a reduction in HIV viral load and an increase in CD4 cells, alternative treatment for KS may be considered. Due to possible effects of HIV PI on inhibition of matrix metalloproteinase (MMP-2) and down-regulation of bFGF and VEGF and their antiangiogenic effects, many clinicians tend to prefer using PI-containing HAART regimens in patients with HIV and KS.

2. **Antiherpetic therapy** with ganciclovir, cidofovir, foscarnet, and acyclovir has no proven function in the treatment of KS. Approaches to stimulating HHV-8 lytic gene expression with or without antiherpetic therapy are under investigation.

3. **Local therapy.** KS is a disseminated disease at the time of diagnosis in patients with AIDS, even though only localized disease may be clinically evident.

   Topical alitretinoin (9-*cis*-retinoic acid) is associated with a 30% to 50% response rate and has been licensed for use in cutaneous KS. Individual lesions may be injected with vincristine (0.1 mg) or vinblastine (0.1 mg), or with interferon-α (1 million U), although these modalities are painful and associated with the possibility of secondary infection. Such local injections are not advocated at this time.

   Local lesions may also be treated effectively with cryotherapy, laser, or surgical excision. Local radiation may be helpful for rapid control of bulky lesions or to control extensive lymphedema due to locally invasive tumors or extensive lymphadenopathy; however, great care must be taken to avoid undue local toxicity.

4. **Immune response modifiers.** Oral 9-*cis*-retinoic acid may be useful in the therapy of KS, working by means of its ability to down-regulate IL-6, which is a growth factor for KS. Interferon-α (1 to 2 million U/d) is also effective, especially when combined with antiretroviral agents. Additional biologic agents that aim to decrease either inflammatory cytokines or angiogenic factors have been studied, with preliminary evidence of some antitumor efficacy. These agents include rapamycin, bevacizumab, thalidomide, lenalidomide, and pomalidomide.

5. **Chemotherapy** is indicated for rapidly progressive disease, severe lymphedema, pulmonary involvement, and symptomatic visceral disease. Liposomal doxorubicin and liposomal daunorubicin are most commonly used as the first-line treatment. The use of these drugs is associated with the highest efficacy and least toxicity. Paclitaxel (100 or 135 mg/m^2 given IV every 2 to 3 weeks) is also highly effective. Other chemotherapeutic agents with some activity in KS include the vinca alkaloids (vincristine, vinblastine, and vinorelbine), bleomycin, and gemcitabine.

V. CERVICAL CANCER

A. **Incidence.** Cervical cancer is an AIDS-defining diagnosis. Women constitute one of the fastest growing groups of new AIDS cases in the United States.

The primary risk factor for HIV infection in these patients is heterosexual transmission, usually from a partner whose HIV status is unknown to the woman.

The precise incidence of cervical carcinoma, while increased statistically when compared with that in HIV uninfected women, is still very low in the United States and other countries in which routine Papanicolaou (Pap) or human papillomavirus (HPV) screening and ablative intervention are common. The incidence of the precursor lesions (cervical intraepithelial neoplasia [CIN] on biopsy or squamous intraepithelial lesions [SIL] on Pap smear) is unknown, although various large cohort studies of HIV-infected women have indicated a high prevalence of oncogenic HPV strains. HAART has been associated with spontaneous clearing of these precursor lesions. The incidence of invasive cervical carcinoma and of premalignant lesion increased in the era of HAART, most likely due to the increased patient and provider awareness and increased screening.

B. **Biologic factors**
   1. **Role of human papillomavirus (HPV)** (see Chapter 12). Lower CD4+ lymphocyte counts have been associated with greater prevalence of HPV infection among HIV-infected women.
   2. **Role of HPV vaccine.** An HPV vaccine against serotypes 6, 11, 16, and 18 has been licensed in the United States and is recommended for use in girls and boys from the age of 9 to 26 years for prevention of primary HPV infection. The vaccine has been remarkably effective in inducing immunity against HPV and in decreasing the risk of incident CIN/SIL. Safety and immunogenicity studies of the quadrivalent HPV vaccine have been completed in HIV+ men and HIV+ women, demonstrating good safety and immunogenicity in HPV subtype–negative individuals. Nonetheless, because most HIV-infected women have already been infected by multiple types of HPV, the actual effectiveness of this approach in preventing CIN or invasive cervical cancer will need to be established.

C. **Clinical features** of cervical cancer in the HIV-infected women are not different from those in uninfected women. Preliminary evidence suggests that HIV-infected women are more likely to have advanced-stage disease, high-grade pathologic type, and relapse after definitive therapy.

D. **Management.** Because of the aggressive nature of cervical carcinoma in HIV-infected women, it has become extremely important to diagnose such patients early, at the time of precancerous abnormalities on Pap smear or local biopsy. It is recommended that HIV-infected women undergo routine Pap testing every 12 months with evaluation of HPV status as well. Colposcopy and biopsy should be performed in the presence of positive HPV status or any abnormal Pap smear results, including atypia. After definitive ablative therapy for CIN II or III, about half of patients relapse within 1 to 2 years. Thus, continued monitoring and follow-up are required. Invasive cervical cancer is treated based on stage and concurrent conditions and is the same in HIV+ as in HIV- women.

VI. ANAL CARCINOMA

A. **Incidence.** Although not diagnostic of AIDS, the incidence of HPV-related anal carcinoma is known to be increased in homosexual men, even independent of HIV infection. In HIV+ men in the post-HAART era, the incidence of anal cancer has been estimated to be between 78 and 137 cases per 100,000 patient-years, which is as high as the incidence of cervical cancer in women in the pre-Pap screening era. As in HIV+ women, men with HIV have a greater likelihood of developing both premalignant dysplasia and malignant invasive anal lesions.

Anal HPV infection is also quite common in HIV-infected women and also in HIV-infected men without history of homosexual activity.

B. **Biologic factors.** As with cervical cancer, anal cancer is associated with prior infection by HPV, usually involving serotypes 16, 18, 31, 33, or 35. Most anal cancer in HIV+ men in the United States is due to serotypes 16 or 18. Cytologic abnormalities occur in nearly 40% of patients, especially those with CD4 counts <200 cells/mm^3.

C. **Clinical features.** Most individuals with anal dysplasia or cancer are completely asymptomatic. However, rectal pain, bleeding, discharge, and symptoms of obstruction or a mass lesion found on rectal exam are the most frequent presenting symptoms and signs. Patients with severe immunosuppression (i.e., CD4 <50/mm^3) may present with more advanced and more aggressive disease.

D. **Management.** Because of the high prevalence of HPV infection and the growing incidence of anal SIL (ASIL) and invasive anal cancer detected in HIV+ men and women, the screening of HIV+ individuals with either yearly anal Pap smears and/or direct visualization via high-resolution anoscopy (HRA) and biopsy is becoming a standard procedure in many HIV practices. Discovery of any grade ASIL on Pap smear or anal intraepithelial neoplasm (AIN) requires HRA and biopsy. For those with AIN II-III, ablative treatment with surgery, electrocautery, or infrared coagulation is generally performed. For these individuals as well as those with AIN I or ASUC, follow-up every 6 months is recommended.

Invasive anal cancer can be controlled effectively with high response rates with chemotherapy (e.g., mitomycin C or *cis*-platinum with 5-day fluorouracil) and concurrent RT. Patients with lower CD4 counts appear to have a greater likelihood of severe toxicities with treatment and may require colostomy and extensive resection for salvage therapy upon relapse.

VII. OTHER NON–AIDS-DEFINING MALIGNANCIES

A. **Incidence.** With improved HIV therapy, patients are living longer and are developing other cancers that are not AIDS defining. A large number of reports from around the world now show that other cancers including HL, anal cancer, lung cancer, liver cancer, head and neck cancers, nonmelanomatous skin cancers, Merkel cell carcinoma, germ cell tumors, squamous cell cancers of various organs, and leiomyosarcoma in pediatric patients are occurring with greater frequency in HIV-infected individuals. Rates of these NADC now suggest that these cancers are occurring at higher frequencies than the AIDS-defining cancers in the developed world. Interestingly, the rates of the more common tumors, such as breast, prostate, and colon cancers, do not appear to be higher in the HIV populations.

B. **Biologic factors.** The reason for this increase incidence of NADC is not completely understood, but greater longevity due to HAART coupled with continued immunosuppression is likely to play a significant role. In addition, more rapid immunologic aging due to continued immune activation by HIV, coinfection with other oncogenic viruses, and exposure to potential carcinogens also may be contributing. Even when controlled for the high rate of smoking in the HIV population, the relative risk for lung cancer in HIV appears to be at least twofold greater in the HIV+ than the general population. Induction of genetic instability or direct involvement of HIV in the expression of oncogenes or inhibition of tumor suppressor genes has also been suggested by several tumor models.

C. **Clinical features.** While systematic comparison studies have not yet been performed, individuals with HIV and NADC generally seem to present at a younger age, with more advanced-stage tumor at diagnosis and with a greater likelihood of relapse after definitive therapy.

D. Management. Treatment strategies have generally followed the same stage-adjusted approaches as used in individuals not infected with HIV. Appreciation of the greater likelihood and/or severity of drug toxicities, the potential for drug interactions between anticancer agents and drugs used in the management of HIV (especially with PI and cobicistat), and the need to provide supportive treatment and prophylactic antibiotics and growth factors need to be incorporated into the management of the HIV patient with malignancies.

Because of the higher risk of these cancers in people with HIV, a greater focus on screening and prevention of cancer should also be incorporated into the management. Thus, in addition to yearly cervical and anal Pap screening, administration of hepatitis and HPV vaccinations, use of sunscreen, and avoidance of sun overexposures should be recommended to HIV+ patients.

MALIGNANCIES RELATED TO ORGAN TRANSPLANTATION

Solid organ transplantation (SOT) has been an important therapeutic intervention. Patients after SOT are noted to have a 3- to 10-fold increased risk of development of de novo malignant neoplasms when compared with the general population. The need for ongoing immunosuppression is likely the major risk factor. The immunosuppression can lead to reduced cancer surveillance and promotion of oncogenic viruses. In addition, the immunosuppressive medications can have a direct effect on tumor cells.

In hematopoietic stem cell transplants (HSCT), solid tumors are seen at about twice the rate as in the normal population with rate rising to about threefold for patients followed longer than 15 years. In these patients, ongoing immune suppression is not usually needed except in ones with graft versus host disease (GVHD), but other risk factors such genetic predispositions and prior chemo/radiotherapy likely play a role.

A. Cutaneous malignancies are the most common of secondary cancers, with over half of transplanted patients developing a skin malignancy.

1. **Cutaneous squamous cell cancers** (SCC) are the most frequent, and their incidence increases over time after transplant. They tend to be multiple and of more aggressive behavior. Recipients of heart or lung transplants have a higher incidence compared to recipients of kidney or liver transplants. HSCT patients with GVHD requiring prolonged immunosuppression also have a higher incidence. The incidence is increased in smokers, fair skinned individuals, older age, and males. Calcineurin inhibitors and azathioprine have a higher association with SCC; the incidence appears to be lower when mTOR inhibitors are used. SCC are associated with human papilloma virus (HPV) in 80% of transplant-associated SCC cases (compared to 40% in immunocompetent cases).

2. **Basal cell carcinomas** are also more common in transplant recipients (about 4 times that of immunocompetent individuals), but they do not appear to be more aggressive.

3. **Kaposi sarcoma** is seen in about 6% of transplant patients and tends to occur within the first few years after transplant. Most cases are associated with HHV-8 reactivation.

4. **Merkel cell carcinomas** although rare are seen 5 to 10 times more commonly in transplant recipients.

5. **Malignant melanoma** is seen only slightly more commonly in transplant patients, but it appears to be more aggressive.

6. **Management.** Patients should be instructed on preventive measures such as the use of sunscreen and sun avoidance measures, and on smoking cessation, HPV vaccination can be considered. Routine full-body skin examinations should be undertaken posttransplantation, and patients should be instructed to report any unusual skin findings. For SSC, once one lesion is detected, the likelihood of additional multiple lesions increases, and examinations should be performed more frequently. Treatments of posttransplant skin tumors are generally similar to those recommended for immunocompetent patients (see Chapter 17). In addition, modification of immunosuppression to lowest doses necessary to maintain the graft and consideration of switching to an mTOR inhibitor such as sirolimus rather than cyclosporine, tacrolimus, or azathioprine may be undertaken. Patients needing chemotherapy leading to further infection risks should also be considered for prophylactic antimicrobial therapies.

B. **Lymphomas (Posttransplant Lymphoproliferative Diseases [PTLD]).**

1. **Histology.** PTLD are a heterogeneous group of lymphoid disorders occurring after transplantation. They range from indolent polymorphic hyperplasias to aggressive monomorphic neoplasms. The majority of cases (>80%) arise from B cells. The most common subtype is DLBCL, but Burkitt/Burkitt-like lymphoma and plasma cell myeloma are also seen. T-cell variants account for 10% to 15% of the cases and include peripheral T-cell lymphomas, gamma/delta T-cell lymphoma, and T-natural killer (NK) cell varieties. Hodgkin disease–like lymphoma is less common. Extranodal involvement including CNS involvement is commonly seen.

2. **Risk factors** for development of PTLD include type of organ transplanted, intensity of immunosuppression, age, viral infections (EBV), and time after transplant. The risk of DLBCL is 10 to 15 times higher in transplant patients than in the normal population. The incidence is highest (5% to 20%) in intestinal and multivisceral transplants, followed by lung and heart transplants (2% to 10%), and lower (1% to 5%) in renal and liver transplant patients. Differences likely relate to the degree of immunosuppression and donor lymphocyte content of the graft. The risk of developing PTLD is highest in the first year following transplant with about 90% of these tumors being EBV driven.

3. **Pathogenesis.** In SOT patients, PTLD is usually of recipient cell origin although rare cases of donor cell involvement have been reported.

   The early PTLDs, that is, within the first year after transplant, are most common in younger patients who are EBV seronegative prior to transplant (especially when the donor is EBV positive). PTLDs occurring after the first year are more likely to present similarly to lymphomas in immunocompetent hosts. Only about 50% of these late lymphomas are EBV related, and they are often associated c-myc translocations.

   In HSCT patients, PTLD is uncommon, but when present, it is usually seen in the first 6 months after transplant and is almost exclusively of donor cell origin. Late PTLD is rare in HSCT, but there is an increased incidence of HL in this group.

4. **Clinical presentation.** Fever and lymphadenopathy are the most common symptoms, but extranodal disease is frequent and may involve the allograft, so any unexplained symptoms should raise clinical suspicion, and surveillance should be undertaken in order to make an early diagnosis. CNS is involved in up to 30% of the patients and may be the only site of involvement.

5. **Workup.** PET-CT scanning of head, chest, abdomen, and pelvis is important for diagnosis and for monitoring of therapeutic response. MRI of the brain and spinal cord and spinal fluid examination should be performed for patients with CNS involvement. Excisional biopsy when possible or multiple core needle biopsies should be obtained to obtain adequate tissue for standard histology, immunophenotyping, flow cytometry, EBV status, and genetic analysis.

   Determination of EBV serology prior to transplant helps assess risk. Rising levels of EBV-DNA in the blood after transplant is a predictive risk factor for the onset of PTLD. Monitoring of these levels may allow for early treatment with reduction of immunosuppression and can help assess response to therapy.

6. **Treatment.**

   a. **Reduction of immunosuppression** should be undertaken with close monitoring to avoid loss of graft or flare of GVHD.

   b. **Rituximab** should be used for CD-20-positive PTLD including polymorphic and monomorphic DLBLC subtypes. A 2-year progression-free survival of >40% can be achieved with rituximab monotherapy in adults, but additional cytotoxic chemotherapy is required to cure PTLD in the majority of adult patients and for all patients with aggressive disease.

   c. **Chemotherapy.** Anthracycline-based chemotherapy (e.g., cyclophosphamide, doxorubicin, vincristine, prednisone [CHOP] see Chapter 22) in combination with rituximab or sequentially following an initial 3 to 4 week course of rituximab is useful in adult patients. In early onset pediatric patients, a low-dose regimen consisting of six cycles of therapy given every 3 weeks has resulted in a 63% CR rate. The first two cycles included cyclophosphamide (600 mg/m^2 intravenous) on day 1 of each cycle, prednisone (1 mg/kg orally twice a day) or methylprednisolone (0.8 mg/kg intravenous every 12 hours) on days 1 to 5 of each cycle, and rituximab (375 mg/m^2 intravenous) on days 1, 8, and 15 of each cycle for a total of 6 doses. Patients with more aggressive disease however require higher doses of chemotherapy.

   Treatment of CD20-negative PTLD should be similar to non-transplant patients (see Chapter 22). For PTLD, subjects with CNS lymphoma are treated with high-dose methotrexate-based therapy, concurrent rituximab therapy, and sequential high-dose cytarabine (see Chapter 22).

   d. **Other therapies.** Donor leukocyte infusions can be considered in HSCT and related solid organ donors but can be associated with increased GVHD or organ rejection. Adoptive immunotherapy using EBV-specific cytotoxic T cells has shown some promising results with low toxicity profile, but awaits improved product availability and further studies.

   e. **Side effects** of these treatments can be substantial for these patients. In addition to possible graft rejection secondary to immunosuppression reduction, there is a significant increase in infectious complications and possible hepatitis reactivation. IVIG can be considered both to replenish the drop in immunoglobulin levels seen with rituximab and for the possibility of providing anti-EBV antibodies for some patients. Prophylactic antimicrobials should also be considered, and early treatment of infectious symptoms is important.

C. **Other cancers.** Visceral cancers also occur at an increased rate after transplant; the risk increases with age and time after transplant. In addition to immuno-suppression, exposure history (i.e., smoking, drugs, hepatitis) and underlying disease all play a role in the tumor development. Renal transplant recipients have a 12-fold higher chance of developing solid tumors (especially urinary tract, GI, and gynecologic cancers). In liver transplant patients, the cumulative risks for development of noncutaneous malignancies at 5 and 15 years post-SOT are about 9% and 25%, respectively, with the risk being twice as high if patients were transplanted for alcoholic cirrhosis versus other indications. Heart transplant patients showed an incidence of malignancies of 16% at 5 years and 26% at 8 years after transplant (especially of squamous cell lip/anus tumors, and renal tumors). Lung transplant recipients also have an incidence of malignancies of 16% at 5 years and 26% at 8 years after transplant (especially lung, anus, and oral cancers).

Routine screening and surveillance for possible cancers are important for all transplant patients. Minimizing risk factors (i.e., sun exposure, smoking, alcohol consumption) and reduction of immunosuppression when possible should be undertaken.

Treatment of the cancers in these patients is similar to that in immuno-competent patients; however, care should be taken to appreciate the underlying infection risks and organ function when choosing therapies. Immune check-point inhibitors are commonly used as treatment of variety of malignancies in immunocompetent patients, but their benefit is immunocompromised patients has not been established, and it is associated with an increased risk of the allograft rejection.

MALIGNANCIES IN AUTOIMMUNE DISORDERS

A. **Introduction.** Immune dysregulation is a hallmark of autoimmune disorders. Immune dysregulation and therapy-related immunosuppression can inhibit cancer-related immune surveillance in these patients, likely leading to the increased development of malignant disorders.

B. **Autoimmune disorders**
1. **Rheumatoid arthritis** is associated with a twofold increased risk of lym-phoma/leukemia and a marked increase risk of lung and nonmelanoma skin cancers.
2. **Inflammatory bowel disease (IBD)** is associated with an increased risk of GI, liver, and renal cancers.
3. **Psoriasis** is associated with increased risk of nonmelanoma skin cancers.
4. **Systemic lupus** has an increased risk of lymphomas and renal cancers.

C. **Treatment and the risk of cancer.** Over the past few years, many novel immu-nosuppressive treatments have been developed for the treatment of autoimmune disorders such as rheumatoid arthritis, IBD, and psoriasis. These treatments have made a major impact on the responses in these disorders. Controversy remains with respect to whether these biologics carry an additional cancer risk for these patients. There does appear to be an increased risk of the develop-ment of lymphomas and skin cancers (especially squamous cell) with the use of these biologic agents, especially with combinations of TNF inhibitors with methotrexate or azathioprine. A significant increase in a rare type of lymphoma (hepatosplenic T-cell lymphomas) is seen in IBD patients treated with the combination of azathioprine plus a TNF inhibitor, so that alternative treatment approaches should be considered for these patients.

   D. **Treatment of cancers in the setting of autoimmune disorders** is similar to
      that for standard treatments of the cancer. However, care should be taken to
      appreciate the increased infection risk accompanying their underlying disor-
      der. Patients should be instructed on preventative measures such as the use
      of sunscreen and sun avoidance measures and on smoking cessation. Routine
      full-body skin examinations should be undertaken, and patients should be
      instructed to report any unusual skin findings. Lymphomas may occur in
      extranodal sites and may involve target organs of the underlying autoimmune
      disease (i.e., salivary glands in Sjögren) so that a high index of suspicion should
      trigger clinical evaluation.

Suggested Readings

AIDS-Related Malignancies

Barta SK, Xue X, Wang D, et al. Treatment factors affecting outcomes in HIV-associated non-
   Hodgkin lymphomas: a pooled analysis of 1546 patients. *Blood* 2013;122:3251.
Brickman C, Palefsky JM. Cancer in the HIV-infected host: epidemiology and pathogenesis in the
   antiretroviral era. *Curr HIV/AIDS Rep* 2015;12:288.
Carbone A, Vaccher E, Gioghini A, et al. Diagnosis and management of lymphomas and other
   cancers in HIV-infected patients. *Nat Rev Clin Oncol* 2014;11:223.
Coghill AE, Shiels MS, Suneja G, et al. Elevated cancer-specific mortality among HIV-infected
   patients in the United States. *J Clin Oncol* 2015;33:2376.
Gibson TM, Morton LM, Shiels MS, et al. Risk of non-Hodgkin lymphoma subtypes in HIV-
   infected people during the HAART era: a population-based study. *AIDS* 2014;28:2313.
Spano JP, Poizot-Martin I, Costagliola D, et al. Non-AIDS-related malignancies: expert consensus
   review and practical applications from the multidisciplinary CANCERVIH Working Group.
   Ann Oncol 2016;27:397.
Suneja G, Shiels MS, Angulo R, et al. Cancer treatment disparities on HIV-infected individuals in
   the United States. *J Clin Oncol* 2014;32:2344.

Malignancies Related to Other Immunodeficiency States

Chockalingam R, Downing C, Tyring SK. Cutaneous squamous cell carcinomas in organ transplant
   recipients. *J Clin Med* 2015;4:1229.
Dierickx D, Tousseyn T, Gheysens O. How I treat posttransplant lymphoproliferative disorders.
   Blood 2015;126:2274.
Gross TG, Orjuela MA, Perkins SL, et al. Low-dose chemotherapy and rituximab for post-transplant
   lymphoproliferative disease (PTLD): a children's oncology group report. *Am J Transplant*
   2012;12:3069.
San-Juan R, Comoli P, Caillard S, et al.; on behalf of the ESCMID Study Group of Infection in
   Compromised Hosts (ESGICH). Epstein Barr virus-related post-transplant lymphoproliferative
   disorder in solid organ transplant recipients. *Clin Microbiol Infect* 2014;20:109.

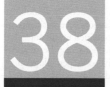

Hematopoietic Stem Cell Transplantation

Mary Territo

I. PRINCIPLES

A. **Hematopoietic stem cell transplantation** (HSCT) is an important treatment option for an increasing number of malignant and nonmalignant disorders. HSCT can be used in malignant diseases for the following situations:

1. To restore marrow function for the patient following the administration of very high doses (myeloablative/immunoablative) of chemotherapy with or without radiotherapy (CT/RT), which is given to kill tumor cells. This approach requires that:

   a. The tumor must have a steep dose–response curve so that escalating to high doses of drug results in increased tumor killing.

   b. The drugs that give that steep dose–response curve must have the bone marrow (BM) as their main dose-limiting toxicity.

   c. The types of tumors that can utilize this approach include primarily the hematologic malignancies (leukemias, lymphomas, myelomas, myelodysplasias) but also testicular and germ cell tumors, neuroblastoma, and selected other solid tumors.

2. To replace deficient or defective hematopoietic cells for diseases such as aplastic anemia and congenital hematologic, immunologic, and metabolic disorders

3. To effectively administer adoptive immunotherapy against tumor cells (the graft vs. tumor [GVT] effect)

B. **The choice of the type of transplant** that is performed and the type of conditioning therapy used will depend on the disease being treated, the clinical status of the patient, and the donor cells that are available.

C. **Outcomes of transplantation** depend on multiple factors including age of the patient, stage of disease, disease risk factors, prior therapies, comorbid conditions, and the type of conditioning therapy used. For allogeneic transplants, donor relationship, HLA matching, donor type, and cell dose are also important variables impacting outcome.

II. STEM CELL SOURCES

Hematopoietic stem cells (HSCs) normally reside primarily in the BM, but can be found in increased numbers in the blood during recovery from chemotherapy-induced cytopenias and can also be mobilized from the BM into the blood with agents such as granulocyte colony–stimulating factor (GCSF) or plerixafor. Umbilical cord blood (UCB) is a very rich source of HSCs that can also be used for transplantation.

A. **Bone marrow** (BM) is obtained through multiple marrow aspirations to a desired target dose of about 3×10^8 nucleated cells per kilogram of recipient weight (about 1 to 1.5 L for an adult). If needed, the collected cells can be processed to deplete red blood cells (RBCs) or plasma for ABO-incompatible transplants or to deplete specific lymphocyte populations.

B. **Peripheral blood stem cells** (PBSCs). Donors are first given GCSF to mobilize the HSC into the peripheral blood (for autologous donors, chemotherapy is frequently given prior to the GCSF). PBSCs are then obtained in the nucleated cell fraction of the blood by apheresis. Multiple collections may be required to reach the target dose (1 to 5 × 10⁶ CD34-positive cells per kilogram of patient weight). The cells can then be processed and cryopreserved for later use or directly infused intravenously into the patient. This product engrafts a little faster than BM, has a similar incidence of acute graft versus host disease (GVHD) as BM, but has a greater occurrence of chronic GVHD (CGVHD).

C. **Umbilical cord blood (UCB) cells** are obtained from the umbilical vein of the placenta after the umbilical cord has been severed from the newborn. This blood is very rich in HSC, and the lymphocytes are naive. This product requires less stringent HLA matching, results in less GVHD than either BM or PBSC, but is slower to engraft.

D. **Manipulation and graft engineering.** All of these stem cell sources can be manipulated in a variety of ways depending on the intent of the transplant. Types of manipulations include depletion of T cells or lymphocyte subsets, enrichment of CD34-positive cells, and stem cell expansion. HSCs and lymphocyte subpopulations are also being engineered to augment tumor killing, and infection control, or to replace genetic deficiencies.

III. TYPES OF HSCT

A. **Autologous transplant.** The patient's own cells are used as the HSC source. This approach is primarily used to permit the use of very high doses (myeloablative) of CT/RT to kill tumor cells and then provide subsequent autologous cells for marrow recovery. The advantage of this approach is that you do not have to search for an allogeneic donor and there is no GVHD. The disadvantage is that you may have residual tumor cells in the graft and there is no graft versus tumor effect from the graft.

B. **Allogeneic transplant.** The HSCs are obtained from someone other than the patient. The donor of the HSCs must be matched by HLA tissue typing with the patient. HLA typing is performed for the class I antigens (A, B, and C) and the class II DR antigens to identify properly matched donors. The advantage of allogeneic transplantation is that the product is free of tumor or abnormal cells. In addition to allowing recovery after the myeloablative CT/RT used for tumor control, allogeneic HSCs can be used to replace deficient or defective stem cells (as used for aplastic anemia or genetic disorders). Allogeneic transplantation also provides adoptive immunotherapy against tumor cells of the recipient (GVT effect). This GVT effect can be the major goal of the transplant and can sometimes allow for a reduction in the intensity of the conditioning therapy. The disadvantages of allogeneic transplantation are that you need to find an appropriately matched donor and that the patient is at risk for GVHD.

1. **Matched Related Sibling Donors (MSD):** The best donor is a sibling with the same two HLA haplotypes as the recipient (matched on both chromosomes for HLA-A, HLA-B, HLA-C, and HLA-DR; an "8 of 8 HLA match"). Identical twin (syngeneic) donors are the best donors immunologically (with essentially no risk of GVHD), but have a higher risk of relapse after transplant due to less GVT effect. Only about 30% of patients have an identifiable matched sibling donor so that alternative stem cell sources need to be considered for most patients. The choice of which alternative donor source to use depends on multiple factors including availability of the donors, urgency of the transplant, likelihood of relapse, need for additional cells post transplant, and transplant center experience.

2. **Matched Unrelated Adult donors (MUD):** There are large registries of individuals around the world who have volunteered to donate HSCs for unrelated patients in need of a transplant. Results with HLA-matched unrelated donors have been comparable to MSD transplants. Time to identify and collect the donor is variable and may be a factor for patients who need an urgent transplant. The chances of finding an appropriate unrelated donor for an individual patient depends on the specific HLA typing of the patient and varies significantly with different ethnic groups (about 90% for Caucasians, but only about 60% in Blacks).

3. **Partially Matched or Haploidentical Related Donors (Haplo):** Family members who are matched for only one HLA haplotype (4 of 8 HLA match) can be used as donors. Parents, children, or non-HLA identical siblings can be considered as donors thus improving the chances of finding a donor. The use of haplo-related donors requires additional strategies such as the use of posttransplant cyclophosphamide or graft manipulations to limit GVHD and allow for effective engraftment. These approaches may also limit the GVT effect.

4. **Unrelated Cord Blood Cells (UCB):** Many Cord Blood Banks store cord blood units for use in unrelated patients in need of transplant. The cells are relatively rapidly available if urgent transplant is needed; the cord blood cells require less stringent HLA compatibility, so 4 of 6 HLA-matched units (HLA-A, HLA-B, HLA-DR) can be used, allowing for improved chances of finding a donor. There appears to be less GVHD and less relapse with CB, but there is slower engraftment and immune reconstitution. Cell dose is limited and may necessitate using 2 cord blood units (double cord transplant) in larger individuals.

IV. CONDITIONING THERAPY

Patients receive a preparative regimen (conditioning) with high doses of CT/RT prior to the transplant. For allogeneic and autologous transplants, the therapy is aimed at getting the greatest tumor killing while ignoring the myeloablative toxicity of the agents, but doses are limited by toxicity to other organs. Choice of conditioning therapy for autologous transplants depends of the type of tumor and patient risk factors. For allogeneic transplants, the conditioning must also provide sufficient immune ablation, to prevent rejection of the foreign HSCs.

Myeloablative conditioning (MAC) regimens use maximally tolerated doses of chemotherapy with or without radiation therapy. These doses will not allow for autologous hematologic recovery and require subsequent infusion of the donor hematopoietic cells to provide for hematologic and immune recovery. Typical doses used in MAC include cyclophosphamide 200 mg/kg with either busulfan 16 mg/kg or total body irradiation (TBI) 10 Gy. Other agents such as melphalan, thiotepa, or etoposide can also be combined. MAC regimens have maximal direct tumor killing but can also have substantial nonhematologic toxicity, which may not be tolerated in patients with comorbidities or older age.

Reduced intensity conditioning (RIC) uses lower doses of conditioning that still may be myeloablative and allow for donor hematologic and immunologic engraftment. The most common regimens use fludarabine in combination with reduced doses of busulfan, cyclophosphamide, melphalan, or thiotepa or with reduced TBI (5 to 8 Gy). These transplants rely more on the graft versus tumor (GVT) effects than on the direct tumor killing of the regimen, and are associated with some increase in tumor relapse compared to MAC regimens.

The advantage is that they have decreased nonrelapse mortality so transplantation in patients with comorbidities or older age can be considered.

Nonmyeloablative conditioning (NMC) regimens use further reduction of doses with minimal cytopenias or toxicities and could allow for autologous cell recovery without the need for donor stem cells. They are primarily effective as immunosuppressive therapy and can result in full engraftment of allogeneic donor lymphohematopoietic cells. Examples of NMC regimens include TBI (1 to 2 Gy), total lymphoid radiation, antithymocyte globulin, or combinations of fludarabine (90 mg) and cyclophosphamide (1 to 2 G/m^2). They have primarily been used in low-grade lymphomas.

V. SUPPORTIVE CARE

A. Blood products. All blood products (*except the HSC*) should be irradiated with 1.5 Gy (to prevent transfusional GVHD) as soon as the conditioning regimen is initiated. **RBC transfusions** should be given to maintain the hematocrit at 27% (or higher if clinically indicated). For allogeneic transplants, when there is an ABO mismatch between patient and donor, the patient should be transfused with type O blood for all RBC transfusions starting at the time of admission. **Platelet transfusions.** Prophylactic platelet transfusions are usually given to keep platelets above 10,000/mL, but higher levels are needed if patients are febrile or having bleeding symptoms.

B. Specific supportive care measures. Patients should receive adequate hydration and antiemetic therapy throughout the preparative regimen. Allopurinol should be given for all patients with bulky tumors and stopped on day minus 1 or sooner depending on the original tumor burden and patient response. Because of poor oral intake along with antibiotic therapy, most patients require weekly vitamin K1 replacement. Menstruating females should be started on anovulatory agents prior to initiation of the conditioning regimen (i.e.: norethindrone 5 to 10 mg PO daily) and remain on it until the platelet count recovers to >50,000/mL. Depending on the clinical status and the underlying malignancy, GCSF or granulocyte–macrophage colony–stimulating factor can be given starting day plus 2 following transplantation.

C. Protective isolation and prophylaxis

1. **Protective isolation** should begin when the absolute neutrophil count is <500/mL. Hospital rooms should be equipped with air filtration units. Individuals entering the patient's room must perform good handwashing or gloving prior to entering the patient area. While in isolation, patients will wash daily with a microbicidal cleaning solution. Antibacterial, antifungal, and antiviral prophylaxis can be initiated at the beginning of the conditioning regimen.

2. ***Pneumocystis* prophylaxis.** All allogeneic transplant patients and patients receiving autologous transplants who have had extensive corticosteroid exposure should receive *Pneumocystis* prophylaxis. Start trimethoprim–sulfamethoxazole (Bactrim DS, one tablet PO every 8 hours) at the onset of the conditioning therapy and stop at day minus 1 before transplantation. Prophylaxis should be restarted after sustained neutrophil engraftment (Bactrim DS, one tab PO t.i.d. twice a week, with folinic acid 5 mg twice a week) and continued until day 100 after transplant or longer if the patient continues to require immunosuppression. Dapsone (50 to 100 mg PO daily), atovaquone (1,500 mg once daily), or pentamidine (aerosolized 300 mg or 4 mg/kg IV) monthly can be used as an alternative for patients with an allergy to sulfa.

3. **Cytomegalovirus (CMV) prophylaxis/prevention.** Patients who are CMV seronegative prior to transplant should receive only blood products that are CMV seronegative or leukoreduced. CMV-seropositive patients undergoing an allogeneic transplant can receive ganciclovir (6 mg/kg IV/d) starting at the onset of conditioning therapy and stopping at day minus 1 prior to the transplant. After allogeneic transplantation, the ganciclovir (6 mg/kg IVPB/d, 5 d/wk) can be restarted after sustained neutrophil engraftment and continued to day 100 for prophylaxis. Alternatively, after engraftment, patients can be monitored for viremia weekly with evaluation of blood CMV DNA to determine when preemptive treatment is needed.

D. **Prevention and suppression of GVHD.** Patients undergoing an allogeneic HSC transplant require immunosuppression treatment to prevent or suppress GVHD.

1. **Calcineurin inhibitors.** *Cyclosporine* (3 mg/kg/d) *or tacrolimus* (0.03 mg/kg/d) should be given to all allogeneic transplant recipients starting on day minus 2. Doses are adjusted to maintain therapeutic serum levels. Doses are also adjusted for renal failure.

2. **Posttransplant cyclophosphamide** (unmodified Haplo donor cells are infused on day 0, initially allowing alloreactive T cells to proliferate; cyclophosphamide 50 mg/kg/d is then given on days plus 3 and plus 4 post transplant for in vivo T-cell depletion) has been demonstrated to be an effective GVHD prophylaxis in Haplo transplants.

3. **Other agents** (corticosteroids, antithymocyte globulin [ATG, Thymoglobulin], mycophenolate, sirolimus, or methotrexate) can also be used depending on the GVHD risk of the transplant and patient status.

4. **T-cell and subset depletions.** GVHD is a T-cell–mediated process. Extensive depletion of T cells from the HSC graft can markedly reduce the incidence and severity of GVHD. Extensive T-cell depletion, however, is accompanied by an increased risk of graft failure, posttransplant lymphoproliferative disease, and an increased risk of tumor relapse so that disease-free survival is not improved. Programs using partial T-cell depletion or adding back of lymphocyte subpopulations at various times may be helpful.

VI. COMPLICATIONS OF HSCT

A. **GVHD** is a syndrome resulting from the reaction of immunocompetent donor cells against the tissues of an immunocompromised recipient. Recipient antigen presentation results in activation and proliferation of donor T lymphocytes. Thus, host-specific cytotoxic lymphocytes are generated that mediate tissue damage. During this process, cytokines are secreted and enhance tissue damage by recruiting nonspecific cytotoxic mechanisms (direct cytokine damage, natural killer cells, macrophages). Manipulations such as T-cell depletion of the graft, anti–T-lymphocyte agents, and antibodies to certain cytokines have been used to reduce GVHD. GVHD can be subclassified as acute GVHD (AGVHD), which usually occurs 2 to 8 weeks following allogeneic HSCT, and CGVHD, which usually occurs beyond the 8th week.

1. **Incidence.** The incidence of GVHD is influenced by a number of factors including the degree of histoincompatibility, patient age, intensity of conditioning regimen, type of GVHD prophylaxis, and stem cell source.

a. Grade II to IV AGVHD occurs in <30% of HLA-matched siblings but can be 60% to 90% with mismatched unrelated transplants. The incidence of grade III to IV AGVHD is about 35% for 7 of 8 HLA-mismatched adult donor transplants but only about 10% for mismatched UCB donor transplants.

b. CGVHD occurs in 25% to 60% of patients surviving >4 months post allogeneic transplant. About two-thirds of the patients who develop CGVHD had preceding AGVHD.

2. Diagnosis

a. AGVHD is manifested primarily by the involvement of the skin, liver, and gastrointestinal (GI) tract. Table 38-1 shows the grading system for AGVHD depending on the severity of organ involvement.

  (1) Usually, the onset of AGVHD is marked by a maculopapular rash on the head, palms, and soles that can subsequently spread and involve the entire body. Severe cases may go on to develop bullae or desquamation.

  (2) Bilirubin levels are elevated. Elevation of alkaline phosphatase can occur later; transaminase elevations may occur and can progress to liver failure.

  (3) The presence of secretory watery diarrhea, which can be quite severe, is characteristic of the GI involvement; paralytic ileus can occur. Persistent nausea and vomiting can be seen with upper GI involvement. Radiographically, bowel wall edema, sometimes with a "thumb-printing" appearance, can be demonstrated.

  (4) The clinical diagnosis of AGVHD is frequently confounded by the presence of chemotherapy-related toxicity, infection, allergic

TABLE 38-1	Staging and Grading of Acute Graft Versus Host Disease (GVHD)	
Organ	**Extent of Involvement**	**Stage**
Skin	Maculopapular rash <25% of body surface area	1
	Maculopapular rash 25%–50%	2
	Maculopapular rash >50%	3
	Rash >50% with desquamation, with or without bullae	4
Liver	Bilirubin 2–3 mg/dL	1
	Bilirubin 3.1–6 mg/dL	2
	Bilirubin 6.1–15 mg/dL	3
	Bilirubin >15 mg/dL	4
Gastrointestinal	Diarrhea >500 mL/d (>500 mL/m^2 for pediatrics)	1
	Diarrhea >1,000 mL/d (500–1,000 mL/m^2 for pediatrics)	2
	Diarrhea >1,500 mL/d (1,000–1,500 mL/m^2 for pediatrics)	3
	Diarrhea >1,500 mL/d and pain/ileus/ blood (>1,500 mL/m^2, blood or ileus for pediatrics)	4
Overall Grading of Acute GVHD		
Grade I	Rash involving >50% of body surface (skin stage 1–2); bilirubin levels >2 mg/dL; diarrhea >500 mL/d	
Grade II	Rash up to entire body surface (skin stage 1–3); bilirubin >3 mg/dL (liver stage 1); diarrhea >1,000 mL/d (intestine stage 1)	
Grade III	Skin stage 1–3; bilirubin >15 mg/dL (liver stage 2–3); diarrhea >1,500 mL/d (intestine stage 2–3)	
Grade IV	Any organ with stage IV involvement	

Adapted from Glucksberg H, Storb R, Fefer A, et al. Clinical manifestations of graft-versus-host disease in human recipients of marrow from HLA-matched sibling donors. *Transplantation* 1974;18:295.

reactions, or venoocclusive disease (VOD), which can mimic some of the findings of AGVHD.

   b. CGVHD is characterized by a chronic inflammatory process leading to fibrosis and collagen vascular disease–like syndromes. CGVHD can involve the skin, eyes, mouth, lungs, GI tract, liver, genitourinary tract, and musculoskeletal, immune, and hematopoietic systems. Disorders mimicking autoimmune processes such as arthritis, immune cytopenias, polymyositis, and sclerodermatous skin, GI, and lung changes can also be seen.

3. Treatment. All patients undergoing allogeneic HSCT receive prophylaxis (see Section V.D) to help prevent significant complications from GVHD. Development of GVHD post transplant also correlates with a graft versus tumor effect and may be beneficial.

   a. Patients with grade II to IV AGVHD are usually taking a calcineurin inhibitor when diagnosed. Doses are adjusted for subtherapeutic serum levels. Further T-cell suppression with agents such as corticosteroids, mycophenolate, and sirolimus can be instituted. Treatment with ATG, alemtuzumab, anti–interleukin-2 inhibitor (daclizumab), or anti-TNF inhibitors (etanercept) has also been used. Treatments aimed at specific organ problems, such as topical skin treatments, topical enteric steroids (budesonide), antiperistalsis (loperamide), antisecretory (octreotide), and bile acid (ursodiol) agents, can also be instituted.

   b. Treatment of CGVHD includes calcineurin inhibitors, corticosteroids, mycophenolate, sirolimus, and thalidomide. Other treatments that have also been used with occasional success include extracorporeal photochemotherapy (photopheresis with exposure of blood mononuclear cells to the photosensitizing compound PUVA [psoralen plus ultraviolet A] prior to reinfusion), mesenchymal stem cells, pentostatin, alemtuzumab (anti-CD52 antibody), or rituximab (anti-CD20 antibody).

     (1) CGVHD patients are at increased risk of infections and thus need prophylaxis and early treatment of infections, monitoring of immunoglobulin G (IgG) levels, and infusion of intravenous IgG (IVIG) for patients with significant hypoglobulinemia.

     (2) Supportive care measures include topical steroids, skin lubricants, eye drops, artificial saliva, and nystatin or acyclovir when indicated for oral or skin infections.

     (3) Patients with sclerodermatous GVHD and restricted range of motion can benefit from physical therapy.

     (4) All posttransplant patients should use sunscreen and avoid sun exposure.

B. Infections. Although many advances in antimicrobial therapies have improved the overall posttransplant survival, infectious complications remain among the most common causes of morbidity and mortality following allogeneic or autologous HSCT.

   1. Conditioning therapy results in severe neutropenia for prolonged periods (2 to 4 weeks and more), and patients are at high risk for infections. Gram-positive and gram-negative bacteria, as well as *Candida, Aspergillus,* and other fungal infections are common. Patients should receive treatment with broad-spectrum antibiotics and antimycotic agents either prophylactically after the transplant or therapeutically at the earliest signs of fever or infection.

   2. Viral infections and reactivation: Reactivation of herpes viral infections is common post transplantation, especially with intensive GVHD treatment, and following UCB transplants. CMV infection is particularly problematic after allogeneic transplantation. CMV infections usually occur after patients have engrafted. Treatment doses of ganciclovir (5 mg/kg IV every 12 hours for 3 weeks) should be used. Patients with CMV pneumonia should additionally receive IVIG (500 mg/kg every other day for 10 doses). Other antiviral agents including foscarnet, cidofovir, or valganciclovir can also be considered.

Infections with varicella zoster, adenovirus, respiratory syncytial virus, influenza, and other viruses posttransplant can be quite severe and are associated with a high rate of mortality. Treatment with acyclovir, oseltamivir, ribavirin, vidarabine, IVIG, or other agents should be instituted early. Epstein-Barr virus reactivation can be associated with posttransplant lymphoproliferative disease (see Chapter 36).

3. ***Pneumocystis jirovecii*** infections can be problematic posttransplant, and patients should receive prophylactic treatment with trimethoprim–sulfamethoxazole as discussed in Section V.C.2. Patients who develop *Pneumocystis* infections should be treated with therapeutic doses of trimethoprim–sulfamethoxazole (15 to 20 mg/kg/d [trimethoprim component] IV administered in three to four divided doses every 6 to 8 hours). Dapsone, atovaquone, or pentamidine can be used for patients with sulfa allergies.

4. **Infections with encapsulated bacteria** (*Pneumococcus, Meningococcus, Haemophilus*) can be seen late in the course (sometimes a year or more) after engraftment has been complete and is usually related to poor opsonization of the organisms. IVIG should be given if immunoglobulin levels are low. Patients should receive vaccination for these organisms (as well as other primary and booster vaccinations) once their prophylactic GVHD immunosuppressive drugs have been discontinued. Rapid treatment of symptomatic patients is important.

C. **Delayed immune reconstitution.** HSCT results in profound and protracted immune dysfunction. The type of transplantation, the conditioning regimen, and the presence of GVHD affect both the severity and the duration of immunodeficiency. After transplant, the entire immune system of the patient will be reconstituted with the donor cells. In addition to quantitative impairment of lymphocytes, loss of skin test reactivity, impaired proliferative responses, and reduced cytokine production by lymphocytes and macrophages can be seen and predispose the patient to infections and also to posttransplant lymphoproliferative syndromes. Antibody response can also be impaired and may result in poor response to vaccinations as well as susceptibility to pathogens. Replacement doses of IVIG should be considered for patients who fail to normalize their IgG level. The presence of GVHD and its treatments further delays immunologic recovery.

D. **Bleeding.** Patients are at risk of bleeding from thrombocytopenia until platelet engraftment occurs. Platelet engraftment usually lags behind neutrophil engraftment, but spontaneous platelet counts of >20,000/mL are attained by most patients by day 21 following autologous transplants and by day 28 following allogeneic transplants (but may require >40 days for UCB transplants). Hepatic abnormalities can also contribute.

E. **Nonmarrow organ toxicity.** The use of high doses of CT/RT for conditioning patients prior to transplant allows one to ignore the marrow toxicity of the agents, but does not eliminate the nonmarrow toxicities of these agents.

1. Toxicity to the lungs, kidneys, heart, liver, GI tract, endocrine glands, and central nervous system can be seen post transplant.
2. Infections, sepsis, tumor lysis, and other drug exposures can also add to the insult experienced by the nonmarrow organs after transplantation.
3. GVHD can also result in toxicity to target organs following allogeneic transplants.
4. **Venoocclusive disease of the liver**, also known as **hepatic sinusoidal obstruction syndrome** (VOD/SOS), probably results from injury to the sinusoidal endothelial cells and hepatocytes from the high-dose conditioning therapy (see Chapter 31.VII). VOD is usually seen within the first 1 to 2 months post transplant and is characterized by hepatomegaly with right upper quadrant pain, unexplained fluid retention, and jaundice. Mild VOD may occur in up to 60% of patients and can be reversible without treatment. When severe, however, VOD is associated with multiorgan failure and is frequently fatal.

Suggested Readings

Bacigalupo A, Ballen K, Rizzo D, et al. Defining the intensity of conditioning regimens: working definitions. *Biol Blood Marrow Transplant* 2009;15:1628.

Bejanyan N, Haddad H, Brunstein C. Alternative donor transplantation for acute myeloid leukemia. *J Clin Med* 2015;4:1240.

Cohn CS. Transfusion support issues in hematopoietic stem cell transplantation. *Cancer Control* 2015;22:52.

Gyurkocza B, Sandmaier BM. Conditioning regimens for hematopoietic cell transplantation: one size does not fit all. *Blood* 2014;124:344.

Hamadani M. Autologous hematopoietic cell transplantation: an update for clinicians. *Ann Med* 2014;46:619.

Isidori A, Clissa C, Loscocco F, et al. Advancement in high dose therapy and autologous stem cell rescue in lymphoma. *World J Stem Cells* 2015;7:1039.

Jamil MO, Mineishi S. State-of-the-art acute and chronic GVHD treatment. *Int J Hematol* 2015;101:452.

Laubach J, Garderet L, Mahindra A, et al. Management of relapsed multiple myeloma: recommendations of the International Myeloma Working Group. *Leukemia* 2016;30(5):1005–1017.

Nishihori T, Shaheen M, El-Asmar J, et al. Therapeutic strategies for cytomegalovirus in allogeneic hematopoietic cell transplantation. *Immunotherapy* 2015;7:1059.

Pintail SR, Champlin RE. Pushing the envelope—nonmyeloablative and reduced intensity preparative regimens for allogeneic hematopoietic transplantation. *Bone Marrow Transplant* 2015;50:1157.

Reddy NM, Perales MA. Stem cell transplantation in Hodgkin lymphoma. *Hematol Oncol Clin North Am* 2014;28:1097.

Richardson PG, Riches ML, Kernan NA, et al. Phase 3 trial of defibrotide for the treatment of severe veno-occlusive disease and multi-organ failure. *Blood* 2016;127(13):1658–1665.

Vyas P, Appelbaum FR, Craddock C. Allogeneic hematopoietic cell transplantation for acute myeloid leukemia. *Biol Blood Marrow Transplant* 2015;21:8.

Appendices

Appendix A

Glossary of Cytogenetic Nomenclature

Symbol	Definition	Example
p	**Short arm** of a chromosome (arm above centromere); a prefix number gives the number of the chromosome, and a suffix number refers to a particular band on the chromosome.	22p5 is the fifth band from the centromere on the short arm of chromosome 22.
q	**Long arm** of a chromosome (arm below centromere); numbering is the same as for **p**.	22q5 is the fifth band from the centromere on the long arm of chromosome 22.
t	**Translocation** of part of one chromosome to another. The first set of parentheses indicates the chromosomes involved, and the second set indicates the bands affected by the breakpoints on the respective chromosomes.	t(3;21)(q26;q22) is the translocation of material between the long arms of chromosomes 3 and 21 with breakpoints at band q26 for chromosome 3 and band q22 for chromosome 21.
ins	**Insertion** of extra material (e.g., portions of a chromosome) within a chromosome	ins(3;3)(q26;q21q26) is the insertion of band 26 to a position between bands 21 and 26 in the long arms of chromosome 3 (for different chromosomes being involved, the conventions for **t** are followed).
inv	**Inversion** (or turn in the opposite direction) of a portion of the chromosome	inv(3)(q21q26) is inversion of bands of 21 through 26 on the long arm of chromosome 3.
+ or −	**Before a chromosome**: addition (+) or loss (−) of a whole chromosome	+8 or −7 is an extra chromosome 8 or a missing chromosome 7 (see **del**).
+ or −	**After an arm**: additional material (+) or loss of material (−) in the designated arm of the specified chromosome	7q⁻ is missing material in the long arm of chromosome 7 (see **del**).
del	**Deletion** of all or part of a chromosome	del (7q) or del (7)(q22) is deletion of the long arm or of band 22 in the long arm of chromosome 7, respectively (see "+ or −").
der	**Derivative chromosome**: an abnormal chromosome resulting from structural rearrangement, generally of a balanced nature, involving two or more chromosomes	der(1;7)(q10;p10) (see **t, ins, inv**)
i	**Isochromosome**: a symmetric chromosome composed of duplicated long or short arm with associated centromere	i(17q) is chromosome 17 with duplicated long arms.
idic	**Isocentric**: symmetrical abnormal chromosome composed of the duplication of a total arm and its centromere with part of the adjacent other arm	idic(X)(q13)
dic	**Dicentric**: chromosome with two centromeres	
/	**Mosaicism: two populations of cells**	46,XX/47,XX,+8—some cells have a normal karyotype; some have an additional chromosome 8.

Tumor Identifiers and 2016 WHO Classification of Hematolymphoid Neoplasms

B1–B5: Maria E. Vergara-Lluri and Russell K. Brynes

B6: Mary Territo

Appendix B1 | Immunohistochemistry Diagnostic Algorithms

I. Immunohistochemistry Diagnostic Algorithm for Tumors of Uncertain Origin and/or Undifferentiated Neoplasms

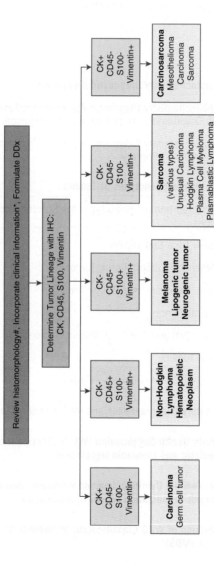

Review histomorphology#; Incorporate clinical information*; Formulate DDx

Determine Tumor Lineage with IHC:
CK, CD45, S100, Vimentin

CK+ CD45- S100- Vimentin-	CK- CD45+ S100- Vimentin+	CK- CD45- S100- Vimentin+	CK- CD45- S100- Vimentin+	CK+ CD45- S100- Vimentin+
Carcinoma Germ cell tumor	**Non-Hodgkin Lymphoma Hematopoietic Neoplasm**	**Melanoma Lipogenic tumor Neurogenic tumor**	**Sarcoma** (various types) Unusual Carcinoma Hodgkin Lymphoma Plasma Cell Myeloma Plasmablastic Lymphoma	**Carcinosarcoma** Mesothelioma Carcinoma Sarcoma

DDx, differential diagnosis; *Clinical information includes: age, sex, tumor location, prior malignancy;
#Histomorphology: spindle cell, epithelioid, small cell, pleomorphic. **Bolded** entities represent the most commonly
encountered diagnoses in these categories.

+, positive; −, negative; CK, cytokeratin; IHC, immunohistochemical stain.
See Appendix B2 and B3 for detailed evaluation.

II. **Immunohistochemistry Diagnostic Algorithm for Carcinoma/Tumor of Unknown Primary**

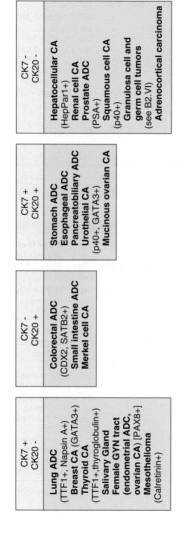

CK7 + CK20 -	CK7 - CK20 +	CK7 + CK20 +	CK7 - CK20 -
Lung ADC (TTF1+, Napsin A+) **Breast CA** (GATA3+) **Thyroid CA** (TTF1+, thyroglobulin+) **Salivary Gland** **Female GYN tract** **(endometrial ADC,** **ovarian CA)** [PAX8+] **Mesothelioma** (Calretinin+)	**Colorectal ADC** (CDX2, SATB2+) **Small intestine ADC** **Merkel cell CA**	**Stomach ADC** **Esophageal ADC** **Pancreatobiliary ADC** **Urothelial CA** (p40+, GATA3+) **Mucinous ovarian CA**	**Hepatocellular CA** (HepPar1+) **Renal cell CA** **Prostate ADC** (PSA+) **Squamous cell CA** (p40+) **Granulosa cell and** **germ cell tumors** (see B2.VI) **Adrenocortical carcinoma**

+, positive; −, negative; ADC, adenocarcinoma; CA, carcinoma, CK, cytokeratin; HepPar-1, hepatocyte paraffin-1;
PSA, prostate-specific antigen; TTF, thyroid transcription factor

See Appendix B2. VIII for expanded evaluation of carcinoma of unknown origin

I. Expected Immunophenotypes for Specific Malignant Cell Types

Cell Type	CK	Vim	CEA	S100	NET	CD45	EMA	Other Useful Positive Markers
Adenocarcinoma	+	0	+	–/+	0	0	+	B72.3, BerEP4, MOC-31; See VIII.
Lymphoma	0	+	0	0	0	+	0	See Appendix B4.
Melanoma	0	+	–/+	+	0	0	0	Mart1 (Melan-A), HMB-45, MiTF, SOX10, PNL2
Mesothelioma	+	+	0	0	0	0	+	Calretinin, CK5/6, WT1, D2-40, mesothelin
Neuroendocrine tumors	+/–	+/–	–/+	0	+	0	+	Carcinomas: punctate keratin
Sarcoma	0	+	0	Variable	0	0	0	See III.
Squamous cell carcinoma	+	+/–	+/–	0	0	0	+	CK5/6, p63, p40, SOX2, desmocollin-3
Urothelial cell carcinoma	+	0	+/–	0	0	0	+	GATA3, p63, S100P, CK5/6, CK903, CK20

II. Small Blue Cell Tumors

A. Small blue cell tumors in adults

Tumor	CK	EMA	CD99	S100	NET[a]	CD45	Des	Other Useful Positive Markers [Molecular/ Genetic Events]
Carcinoma	+	+	0	0	0	0	0	
Carcinoma, small cell	+/–[b]	+/–	0	0	+/–	0	0	TTF1+ in lung primary
Carcinoma, Merkel cell	+	+/–	–/+	0	+/–	0	0	CK20[b]
Desmoplastic small round cell tumor	+	+	–/+	0	–/+	0	+[b]	WT1 (N-terminus) [EWSR1–WT1 fusion]
Synovial sarcoma	+/–	+/–	+/–	–/+	0	0	0	TLE1 Monophasic: [SS18–SSX1, SS18–SSX2, or SS18–SSX4 fusion] Biphasic: [Predominantly SS18–SSX1 fusion]
Lymphoma	0	0	0	0	0	+	0	See Appendix B3
Melanoma	0	0	0	+	0	0	0	Mart1 (Melan-A), HMB-45, MiTF, SOX10, PNL2

[a]NET, neuroendocrine markers: synaptophysin, chromogranin, neuron-specific enolase, CD56.
[b]Punctate pattern/perinuclear dot like.

See footnote to all parts of Appendix B2 at the end of this section (B2.VIII.).

Appendix B2 **Expected Immunophenotypes of Tumors (*Continued*)**

B. Small blue cell tumors in children

Tumor	CK	EMA	CD99	S100	NET[a]	WT1	Musc[b]	Other Useful Positive Markers [Molecular/ Genetic Events]
Neuroblastoma	0	0	0	–/+	+	–	0	CD56, NSE, neuroblastoma
PNET/Ewing sarcoma	0	0	+	–/+	–/+	0	0	[*EWSR1* with multiple fusion partners: *FLI1, ERG, FEV, ETV1, E1AF, ZSG; FUS–ERG* fusion]
Rhabdomyo-sarcoma	0	0	–/+	0	0	+/–[c]	+	Alveolar: [*PAX3–FOXO1A* fusion *PAX7–FOXO1A* fusion *PAX3–NCOA1* fusion *PAX3–AFX* fusion] Embryonal: [Trisomies 2q, 8, and 20; loss of heterozy-gosity at 11p15]
Synovial sarcoma	+/–	+/–	+/–	–/+	0	0	0	TLE1 Monophasic: [*SS18–SSX1, SS18–SSX2,* or *SS18–SSX4* fusion] Biphasic: [Predominantly *SS18–SSX1* fusion]
Wilms tumor/ nephroblastoma	+	+	–/+	+/–	0	+	[d]	

[a]NET, neuroendocrine markers: synaptophysin, chromogranin, neuron-specific enolase, CD56.
[b]Muscle markers: desmin, MSA, MyoD1, myogenin.
[c]Cytoplasmic positivity.
[d]Blastemal component: desmin +.

See footnote to all parts of Appendix B2 at the end of this section (B2.VIII.).

Appendix B2 Expected Immunophenotypes of Tumors (*Continued*)

III. Mesenchymal/Soft Tissue Tumors

Tumor	CK	Vim	Des	SMA	CD34	S100	Others
Alveolar soft part sarcoma	0	–/+	Focal	–/+	0	–/+	TFE3 [*TFE3–ASPL* fusion]
Angiosarcoma	–/+	+	0	–/+	+	0	CD31, FLI1
Chordoma	+	+	0	0	0	+	EMA, HBME, brachyury
Clear cell sarcoma of tendon sheath/ melanoma of soft parts	0	+	0	0	0	+/–	SOX10, Melan-A, MiTF, HMB-45 [*EWSR1–ATF1* fusion; *EWSR1–CREB1* fusion]
Epithelioid sarcoma	+	+	0	–/+	+/–	0	EMA, CK and CD34 coexpression [loss of *INI1*]
Extraskeletal myxoid chondrosarcoma	0	+	0	0	0	+/–	[*EWS–NR4A3* fusion; *TAF2N–NR4A3* fusion; *TCF12–NR4A3* fusion]
Fibrosarcoma	0	+	0	0	0	0	Congenital infantile: [*ETV6–NTRK3* fusion]
Gastrointestinal stromal tumor (GIST)	0	+	0	–/+	+/–	0	CD117 (c kit), DOG1 [mutations in *c-KIT*, *PDGFRA*, etc.]
Granular cell tumor	0	+	0	0	0	+	Inh, CD68
Inflammatory myofibroblastic tumor	+/–	+	+/–	+/–	0	0	ALK+/–, actin with distinctive peripheral cytoplasmic accentuation [*TPM3–ALK* fusion; *TPM4–ALK* fusion; *CLTC–ALK* fusion; *RANB2–ALK* fusion]
Kaposi sarcoma	0	+	0	0	+	0	HHV8, CD31
Leiomyosarcoma	0	+	+/–	+	0	0	Caldesmon [complex with frequent deletion of 1p]
Liposarcoma	0	+	–/+	–/+	–/+	–/+	MDM2+, CDK4+ Well-differentiated: [ring form of chromosome 12; amplification of *MDM2*, *CDK4*, and others] Myxoid/round cell: [*TLS–DDIT3* fusion; *EWSR1–DDIT3* fusion] Pleomorphic: [complex]
Malignant peripheral nerve sheath tumor	0	+	0	0	–/+	Focal +/–	[Complex]
Rhabdoid tumor	+	+	–/+	–/+	0	+/–	[Deletion of 22q; *INI1* inactivation]
PEComas	0	+/–	+/–	+	–/+	–/+	Smooth muscle (SMA, desmin) and melanocytic (HMB-45, Melan-A, MiTF) differentiation [*TFE3* rearrangements or amplifications in a subset]
Pleomorphic high-grade sarcoma[a]	0	+	0	–/+	–/+	0	

See footnote to all parts of Appendix B2 at the end of this section (B2.VIII.).

Tumor	CK	Vim	Des	SMA	CD34	S100	Others
PNET/Ewing sarcoma	0	+	0	0	0	–/+	CD99, FLI1 [*EWSR1* with multiple fusion partners: *FLI1, ERG, FEV, ETV1, E1AF, ZSG; FUS–ERG* fusion]
Rhabdomyo-sarcoma	0	+	+	+/–	0	0	MyoD1 Alveolar: [*PAX3–FOXO1A* fusion *PAX7–FOXO1A* fusion *PAX3–NCOA1* fusion *PAX3–AFX* fusion] Embryonal: [Loss of heterozygosity at 11p15]
Solitary fibrous tumor	0	+	0	0	+	0	[*NAB2-STAT6* fusion]
Synovial sarcoma	+/–	+	0	0	0	–/+	CD99, TLE1 Monophasic: [*SS18–SSX1, SS18–SSX2,* or *SS18–SSX4* fusion] Biphasic: [Predominantly *SS18–SSX1* fusion]

[a]Pleomorphic high-grade sarcoma was previously designated malignant fibrous histiocytoma.

IV. Liver, Pancreas, and Biliary Tract

Carcinoma	CK7	CK20	S100P	CD5	CD10	CK19, CA19-9	AFP	HepPar-1, Arginase-1, Glypican-3
Cholangio-carcinoma	+	–/+	0	+	0	+	0	0
Hepatocellular	0	0	0	0	+[a]	0	+/–	+
Pancreas adenocarci-noma	+	–/+	+	–/+	0	+	0	0

[a]Canalicular pattern; same pattern seen with polyclonal CEA.

V. Neural Tumors

Tumor	CK	S100	Syn	GFAP	EMA	Others Positive Stains
Astrocytoma	+/–	+/–	0	+	+/–	
Chordoma	+	+	0	0	+	HBME, brachyury
Choroid plexus papilloma	+	+/–		+/–	–/+	Transthyretin
Craniopharyngioma	+	0	0	0	+/–	
Ependymoma	+/–	+/–	0	+	–/+	
Medulloblastoma	0	–/+	+	–/+	0	CD56, NSE
Meningioma	–/+	–/+	0	0	+	PR
Neuroblastoma	0	–/+	+/–	0	0	CD56, NSE
Neurofibroma	0	+	0	0	0	
Oligodendroglioma	0	+	0	–/+	0	Olig2
Paraganglioma	0	0[a]	+	–/+	0	
Schwannoma	0	+	0	+/–	0	

[a]Sustentacular cells surrounding the zellballen are S100+.

See footnote to all parts of Appendix B2 at the end of this section (B2.VIII.).

VI. Germ Cell and Sex Cord Stromal Tumors

Tumor	CK	PLAP	OCT4	SALL4	CD117	hCG	AFP	Other Useful Positive Markers
Choriocarcinoma	+	+/–	0	+/–	0	+	0	CD10
Embryonal carcinoma	+	+/–	+	+	0	0[a]	–/+	LIN28, NANOG, CD30, SOX2
Seminoma	–/+	+	+	+	+	0[a]	0	LIN28, D2-40
Sertoli and granulosa cell tumors[b]	–/+	0	0	0	0	0	0	SF-1, inhibin, calretinin, FOXL2
Leydig cell tumor	+/–	0	0	0	0	0	0	SF-1, inhibin, Melan-A, CD10, CD99, calretinin
Teratoma	+	–/+	0	–/+	0	0	0	
Yolk sac tumor	+	+/–	0	+	+/–	0	+/–	Glypican-3, LIN28

[a]Positive in syncytiotrophoblasts.
[b]Negative for EMA.

VII. Skin Tumors

Tumor	CK7	CK20	CK903[a]	EMA	BerEP4	S100	Others
Melanoma	0	0	0	0	0	+	Mart1 (Melan-A), HMB-45, MiTF, SOX10, PNL2
Basal cell carcinoma	–/+	0	+	0	+	0	
Squamous cell carcinoma	–/+	0	+	+	–/+	0	CK5/6, p63, p40, SOX2, desmocollin-3
Merkel cell carcinoma	0	+[b]	NA	+	+	0	NET[c]
Paget disease	+	–/+	+/–[d]	+	+/–	0	CEA, CAM5.2, GCDFP-15
Granular cell tumor	0/0		0	0	NA	+	Inhibin, CD68

[a]High-molecular-weight keratin.
[b]Paranuclear dot-like positivity.
[c]NET, neuroendocrine markers: synaptophysin, chromogranin, neuron-specific enolase, CD56.
[d]Positive in lobular neoplasia; negative in ductal neoplasia.

| Appendix B2 | Expected Immunophenotypes of Tumors (*Continued*) |

VIII. Carcinomas of Unknown Primary ("CUP")/Tumors of Unknown Origin

CK7	CK20	Carcinoma/Tumor of Unknown Origin	Additional Markers
+	0	GYN serous	PAX8+, ER+, WT1+
		GYN endometrioid	PAX8+, ER+, Vim+
		GYN mucinous	CDX2–
		Breast carcinoma	GATA3+, ER+, GCDFP+/–, MGB+/–
		GI, upper tract (e.g., stomach)	CDH17+, CDX2+/–
		Lung adenocarcinoma	TTF1+, napsin A, GATA3–, CDX2–
		Mesothelioma	Calretinin+, CK5/6+, WT1+, D2-40+, mesothelin; BerEP4–, CD15–, B72.3–, TTF1–, MOC-31
		Thyroid, follicular/papillary	PAX8+, TTF1+, Thyg+, Calc–
		Thyroid, medullary	TTF1+, Thyg–, Calc+, NET+, mCEA+
		Renal cell (chromophobe)	CD10–/+, CD117+; CAIX–, PAX2/8–
0	+	GI, lower tract (i.e., colorectal)	SATB2+, CDX2+, CDH17+
		Merkel cell	NET+, CK20 paranuclear dot+
+	+	Pancreatobiliary, ductal adenocarcinoma	MUC5AC+, CK17+, S100P+, Maspin +, IMP3+, CA 19–9+, mCEA+
		Urothelial cell	GATA3, UPII/UPIII, CK5/6+, p63+, CK903+, S100P+
0	0	Granulosa cell and germ cell tumors	See B2.VI
		Hepatocellular	HepPar1+, glypican-3+, arginase-1+, AFP+/–
		Prostate	PSA+, PSAP+, ERG, NKX3.1
		Small cell	NET+, pankeratin (punctate)+
		Squamous cell	CK5/6+, p63+, p40+, SOX2+, desmocollin-3+
		Renal cell (clear cell)	pVHL+, CAIX+, CD10+, RCC+, PAX2/8+, Kim-1
		Adrenocortical carcinoma	Mart1+, calretinin+, Inh-A+, SF-1+

Key to all parts of Appendix B2: +, positive in ≥90% of cases; – or 0, negative in ≥90% of cases; +/–, usually positive (positive in 40%–89% of cases); –/+, usually negative (positive in 11%–39% of cases); **AE1/AE3**, cytokeratin often referred to in literature as "pancytokeratin/pankeratin," although this does not detect all keratins; **AFP**, α-fetoprotein; **AMACR**, P504S α-methylacyl-CoA racemase; **CA**, cancer antigen; **CAIX**, carbonic anhydrase IX; **Calc**, calcitonin; **CD**, clusters of differentiation; **CD45**, leukocyte common antigen (LCA); **CDH17**, cadherin 17; **CEA**, carcinoembryonic antigen; **CK**, cytokeratins; **Des**, desmin; **DOG1**, discovered on GIST1; **DPC4**, SMAD family member 4; **ER**, estrogen receptor; **EMA**, epithelial membrane antigen; **FLI1**, friend leukemia virus integration 1; **GATA3**, GATA binding protein 3; **GCDFP-15**, gross cystic disease fluid protein-15; **GFAP**, glial fibrillary acid protein; **GYN**, gynecologic cancers; **hCG**, human chorionic gonadotropin; **HepPar-1**, hepatocyte paraffin 1; **HMB-45**, human melanoma black 45; **Inh**, inhibin; **IMP3**, insulin-like growth factor II messenger RNA binding protein 3; **LCA**, leukocyte common antigen (CD45); **mCEA**, monoclonal CEA; **Mart-1** (Melan-A), melanoma-associated antigen recognized by T cells 1; **Maspin**, mammary serine protease inhibitor; **MGB**, mammoglobin; **MiTF**, microphthalmia-associated transcription factor; **Musc**, muscle markers (Des, MSA, MyoD1); **MyoD1**, myogenic differentiation 1; **MSA**, muscle-specific actin; **NET**, neuroendocrine tumor markers (CD56, chromogranin, synaptophysin); **NSE**, neuron-specific enolase; **OCT4**, octamer transcription factor 4; **PSAP**, prostatic acid phosphatase; **PLAP**, placental alkaline phosphatase; **PNET**, primitive neuroectodermal tumor; **PR**, progesterone receptor; **PSA**, prostate-specific antigen; **pVHL**, von Hippel-Lindau tumor suppressor; **RCC**, renal cell carcinoma; **SALL4**, Sal-like 4 protein; **S100**, S100 protein; **S100P**, placental S100; **SMA**, smooth muscle actin; **Thyg**, thyroglobulin; **TTF-1**, thyroid transcription factor-1; **TFE3**, transcription factor-E3; **TLE1**, transducin-like enhancer of split 1; **Vim**, vimentin; **vWF**, von Willebrand factor (factor VIII–related antigen).

References: (1) Lin F, Liu H. Immunohistochemistry in undifferentiated neoplasm/tumor of uncertain origin. *Arch Pathol Lab Med* 2014;138;1583–1610; (2) Rekhtman N, Bishop JA, eds. *Quick Reference Handbook for Surgical Pathologists*. Berlin: Springer-Verlag, 2011; (3) PathIQ/ImmunoQuery. Amirsys. https://immunoquery.pathiq.com/PathIQ/Home.do (Last accessed on April 7, 2016); (4) CAP SoftTissue 3.1.2.0 protocol. Protocol for the examination of specimens from patients with tumors of soft tissue. http://www.cap.org/ShowProperty?nodePath=/UCMCon/Contribution%20Folders/WebContent/pdf/softtissue-13protocol-3120.pdf (Last accessed on April 7, 2016); (5) Society for Hematopathology, WHO Update, USCAP 2015 Presentations by Arber DA, Campo E, Jaffe ES, Harris NL. http://www.uscap.org/meetings/detail/2015-annual-meeting/sessions/1316 (Last accessed on April 8, 2016).

Appendix B3	Discriminatory Immunophenotypes for Lymphoid Neoplasms	
Cells or Neoplasm	**Positive**	**Negative**
B cells	CD19, 20[a], 22, 23, 45RA, 79a; PAX5 [a]Generally absent following anti-CD20 (rituximab) therapy	
B-Cell Neoplasms		
B-lymphoblastic leukemia/ lymphoma	CD10, 19, 79a, [CD20, 22, 34]; HLA-DR, PAX5, TdT	MPO
Chronic lymphocytic leukemia/ small lymphocytic lymphoma (CLL/SLL)	CD5, 19, 20[dim], 23, 38[b], 43, 49d, 200 [CD11c]; BCL2, LEF1, Zap-70[b] [[b]Defines a group with more aggressive disease]	CD10, FMC7
B-cell prolymphocytic leukemia	CD19, CD20, CD5, CD23 positive in 10%–30% of cases	
Lymphoplasmacytic lymphoma	CD19, 20, 22, 138, 200	CD5, 10
Follicular lymphomas (FL)	CD10, 19, 20, 22; BCL2, BCL6, LMO2, HGAL	CD5, 11c, 23, 43; MUM1
Primary cutaneous follicle center lymphoma	CD10, 19, 20, 22; BCL6	Igs, BCL2, MUM1
Marginal zone lymphomas (extranodal [MALT], splenic, nodal)	CD19, 20, 22, [CD11c, 43]	CD5, 10, 23, 103
Hairy cell leukemia (HCL)	CD11c, 19, 20, 22, 25, 103, 123; FMC7; TRAP; cyclin D1[weak]; Annexin A1; BRAF	CD5, 10, 23
HCL variant	CD11c, 19, 20, 103; FMC7; DBA-44, bright Igs	CD5, 10, 23, 25, Annexin A1, TRAP, BRAF, CD123
Mantle cell lymphoma (MCL)	CD5, 19, 20, 43; FMC7; cyclin D1, SOX11, BCL2	CD11c, 23, 25
Diffuse large B-cell lymphoma (DLBCL)	CD19, 20, 22, 79a, [CD10, BCL2, BCL6, MUM1, c-MYC]	CD10
DLBCL, NOS	Coexpression of MYC and BCL2 considered a prognostic marker ("double expressor" lymphoma) BCL2, MUM1, [BCL6]	
T-cell/histiocyte-rich LBCL	EBER [CD30, MUM1]	
Primary DLBCL of the CNS	EBER	
Primary cutaneous DLBCL, leg type	EBER	
EBV+ DLBCL, NOS* (formerly EBV+ DLBCL of the elderly)		
DLBCL associated with chronic inflammation		
Lymphomatoid granulomatosis		
Primary mediastinal large B-cell lymphoma	CD19, 20, 23, 30 (weak), 79a	Igs; CD5, 10
Intravascular large B-cell lymphoma	CD5 (many cases), 19, 20, 22, 79a,	CD10
ALK+ LBCL	ALK cytoplasmic, EMA, CD138, IgA, [CD45]	CD3, 20, 30, 79a
Plasmablastic lymphoma	CD30, 38, 138, 79a, MUM1, EMA, EBER [79a, IgG]	CD20, 45, PAX5, HHV8
HHV8+ DLBCL, NOS* (formerly LBCL arising in HHV8-associated multicentric Castleman disease)	IgM, Lambda, HHV8 [CD20, 38]	CD79a, 138, EBER
Primary effusion lymphoma	CD30, 38, 45, 138; EBER; HHV8; EMA	CD19, 20, 22, 79a; Igs, BCL6

Appendix B3	Discriminatory Immunophenotypes for Lymphoid Neoplasms (*Continued*)	
Cells or Neoplasm	**Positive**	**Negative**
Burkitt lymphoma (BL)	CD10, 19, 20, 22 [21]; BCL6, Ki 67 (100%), c-MYC, *MYC/Ig* rearrangement	CD5, 23, TdT, BCL2, MUM1
High-grade B-cell lymphoma, with *MYC* and *BCL2* and/or *BCL6* rearrangements* (formerly B-cell lymphoma, unclassifiable with features intermediate between DLBCL and BL, so-called double/triple hit lymphoma)	CD10, 19, 20, 22,79a, [BCL2], BCL6, Ki 67 (>80%), c-MYC	
B-cell lymphoma, unclassifiable, with features intermediate between DLBCL and classical Hodgkin lymphoma	CD15, 20, 30, 45, 79a; PAX5; OCT2; BOB.1	
Plasma cell neoplasms (MGUS, plasma cell myeloma, solitary plasmacytoma, etc.)	CD38, 43, 56, 79a,138 [CD117, cyclin D1] Cytoplasmic light/heavy chain	CD19, [CD20, 45]
T cells	CD1a, 2, 3, 4, 5, 7, 8, 43, 45RO	
NK cells	CD2, cytoplasmic 3, 7, 8, 11c, 16, 56, 57; TIA-1, granzyme B, [perforin]	
T/NK Cell Neoplasms		
T-lymphoblastic leukemia/lymphoma	CD2, 3, 5, 7, [CD1a, 4, 8, 10, 34, 99]; TdT	
Adult T-cell leukemia/lymphoma	CD2, 3, 4, 5, 25, [30]; HTLV-1	CD7, 8, 16, 56, 57; ALK
T-cell prolymphocytic leukemia	CD2, 3, 4, 5, 7, [CD8]; TCL1	CD1a, TdT, HLA-DR
T-cell large granular lymphocytic leukemia	CD2, 3, [5, 7], 8, 11c, 57; TIA-1	CD4
Chronic lymphoproliferative disorder of NK cells	CD3 cytoplasmic, 7, 11c, 16, 56, [2, 5, 7, 8, 57], TIA-1	CD3, 4
Aggressive NK cell leukemia	CD2, 3 cytoplasmic, 16, 56	CD57
Peripheral T-cell lymphoma, NOS	CD2, 3, 5 [CD4 >8]; loss of pan-T antigens common [CD5, 7]	CD10, CXCL13, PD-1
Anaplastic large cell lymphoma (ALCL), ALK positive	CD2, 4, 5, 25, 30, 43, [CD3, 45, 45RO]; ALK-1; TIA-1; EMA; loss of pan-T antigens common	CD7, 8; EBER
ALCL, ALK negative	CD2, 3, 4, 5, 43, [EMA, TIA-1]	CD8, ALK
Angioimmunoblastic T-cell lymphoma	CD3, 10, [CD2, 3, 5, 7], CD4 > CD8, BCL6, CXCL13, PD-1, EBER, CD20+ immunoblasts	Loss of pan-T antigens common
Follicular T-cell lymphoma *Nodal PTCL with TFH phenotype*	2 of 3 TFH-related antigens must be positive: CD279/PD-1, CD10, BCL6, CXCL13, ICOS, SAP, and CCR5	
Extranodal NK/T-cell lymphoma, nasal type	CD2, cytoplasmic CD3, 43, 45RO, 56; EBER; TIA-1; granzyme B	CD3 (surface), CD4, 5, 8
Hepatosplenic T-cell lymphoma	CD2, 3, 7, [56]; TIA-1, TCRγδ	CD4, 5, 8; TCRαβ (rarely +)
Enteropathy-associated T-cell lymphoma	CD2, 3, 7, 43, 103, [CD8, 30, 56]	CD4, 5
Monomorphic epitheliotropic intestinal TCL (MEITL)*	CD8, 56, MATK, TCR γδ (most)	
Subcutaneous panniculitis–like T-cell lymphoma	CD3, 8; TIA-1	CD4, 56

(*Continued*)

Appendix B3	Discriminatory Immunophenotypes for Lymphoid Neoplasms (*Continued*)	
Cells or Neoplasm	**Positive**	**Negative**
Mycosis fungoides Sézary syndrome	CD2, 3, 4, 5, 25[c], 45RO; TCRβ [[c]Defines a group with more aggressive disease]	CD7, 8, 26
Hodgkin Lymphoma (HL)		
L&H "popcorn" cells of "nodular lymphocyte predominant" type	CD20, 45, 79a, [EMA], PAX5, OCT2, BOB.1	CD15, 30
Reed-Sternberg cells of classical HL	CD15, 30, [20, 79a], PAX5, BCL6, Ki 67	CD45, EMA, ALK-1, OCT2, BOB.1

[X], occasionally positive. *Provisional entities are listed in italics.*

ALK-1, anaplastic lymphoma kinase [up-regulated by t(2;5) in ALCL]; **BCL**, breakpoint cluster location (**BCL2** is positive in MCL, most FL, CLL/SLL, and some DLBCL; **BCL6** is positive in FL and some DLBCL); **BOB.1**, positive in Reed-Sternberg cells of lymphocyte-predominant Hodgkin lymphoma; **CD**, clusters of differentiation; **CD45**, leukocyte common antigen (LCA); **CNS**, central nervous system; c**yclin D1**, (BCL1) is positive in MCL, some HCL, and plasma cell malignancies; **CXCL13**, C-X-C motif chemokine 13; **EBER**, EBV-encoded RNA; **EBV**, Epstein-Barr virus; **EMA**, epithelial membrane antigen; **FMC7**, B-cell surface antigen found on mantle cell lymphoma, follicular lymphoma, and HCL; **HHV8**, human herpes virus type 8; **HLA-DR**, human leukocyte antigen-DR; **HTLV-1**, human T-cell lymphotropic virus type I; **Igs**, immunoglobulins; **L&H**, lymphocytic and histiocytic; **MGUS**, monoclonal gammopathy of undermined significance; **MPO**, myeloperoxidase; **MUM1**, multiple myeloma oncogene 1; **NK**, natural killer; **OCT2**, positive in Reed-Sternberg cells of lymphocyte-predominant Hodgkin lymphoma; **Pax-5**, pan-B antigen positive in B-cell lymphomas and in lymphocyte-predominant and classical Hodgkin lymphomas; **PD-1**, programmed death-1; **TCL1**, T-cell leukemia lymphoma protein 1; **TCR**, T-cell receptor protein (TCRαβ recognizes αβ chains of the TCR; TCRγδ recognizes the γδ chains of the TCR); **TdT**, terminal deoxytransferase (positive in cortical thymic lymphoid cells and lymphoblastic neoplasms); **TIA-1**, T-cell intracellular antigen (found in cytotoxic T cell and NK cell cytoplasmic granules); **TRAP**, tartrate-resistant acid phosphatase.

*Changes from the 2008 classification.

Appendix B4	2016 World Health Organization (WHO) Classification of Hematopoietic and Lymphoid Neoplasms	

Neoplasms	%NHL	Variants [Synonyms] and Comments; Most Common Genetic and/or Molecular Abnormalities Detected; Selected Highlights of Changes in 2016 WHO Classification
Precursor Lymphoid Neoplasms (see Appendix B5—Acute Leukemias)		
Other Myeloid and Lymphoid Neoplasms		
Myeloid neoplasms with PDGFRB rearrangement		t(5;12)(q31~31;p13); ETV6–PDGFRB
Myeloid and lymphoid neoplasms with eosinophilia and abnormalities of PDGFRA		Cryptic del(4)(q12;q12); FIP1L1–PDGFRA
Myeloid and lymphoid neoplasms with FGFR1 abnormalities		FGFR1 rearrangements with different fusion partners. t(8;13)(p11;q12) ZNF198–FGFR1 most common
Mature B-Cell Neoplasms		
CLL/SLL[L]	7%	[CLL, SLL] Poor prognostic category: unmutated IgVH; 17p13 deletion/P53 mutation del13q14.3 Trisomy 12 NOTCH1, SF3B1, TP53, ATM, BIRC3— mutations of potential clinical relevance
Monoclonal B-cell lymphocytosis (MBL)*[L]		Must distinguish low-count from high-count MBL
B-cell prolymphocytic leukemia[M]	Rare	1% of lymphocytic leukemias
Splenic MZL[L]	<2%	[Splenic lymphoma with circulating villous lymphocytes] Loss of 7q21-32
Hairy cell leukemia[L] (HCL)	2%	BRAF V600E in 79%–100% HCL MAP2K1 mutations in most cases that use IGHV4-34 and lack BRAF mutation
Splenic B-cell lymphoma/ leukemia, unclassifiable Splenic diffuse red pulp small B-cell lymphoma Hairy cell leukemia variant	Rare	[Hairy cell leukemia variant, splenic diffuse red pulp small B-cell lymphoma] MAP2K1 in 50% HCL-v, in 50% HCLc IGHV4-34
Lymphoplasmacytic lymphoma[L] (LPL) Waldenström macroglobulinemia	1.2%	[Waldenström macroglobulinemia] MYD88 mutation in 90%–100% WM/LPL CXCR4 mutation in 25% WM resistance to ibrutinib
Monoclonal gammopathy of undetermined significance (MGUS), IgM*	—	[Benign monoclonal gammopathy] More closely related to LPL and other B-cell lymphomas than myeloma
μ Heavy-chain disease (HCD)	Rare	Mu HCD resembles CLL
γ Heavy-chain disease	Rare	Gamma HCD resembles LPL
α Heavy-chain disease	Rare	Alpha HCD considered variant of MALT lymphoma
Monoclonal gammopathy of undetermined significance (MGUS), IgG/A*		
Plasma cell myeloma (multiple myeloma)	10%–15% of hematopoietic neoplasms	Indolent, smoldering, nonsecretory; plasma cell leukemia

(Continued)

Appendix B4	2016 World Health Organization (WHO) Classification of Hematopoietic and Lymphoid Neoplasms (Continued)

Neoplasms	%NHL	Variants [Synonyms] and Comments; Most Common Genetic and/or Molecular Abnormalities Detected; Selected Highlights of Changes in 2016 WHO Classification
Solitary plasmacytoma of bone		
Extraosseous plasmacytoma		
Monoclonal immunoglobulin deposition diseases*		Primary amyloidosis Monoclonal light- and heavy-chain deposition diseases Plasma cell neoplasms associated with paraneoplastic syndromes, including POEMS syndrome; TEMPI syndrome (provisional)
Extranodal marginal zone lymphoma of mucosa-associated lymphoid tissue (MALT lymphoma)	7%–8%	[MALToma] t(11;18)(q21;q21); API2–MALT1 t(14;18)(q32;q21); IGH–MALT1 t(3;14)(p14.1;q32); FOXP1–IGH
Nodal marginal zone lymphoma[L] *Pediatric nodal marginal zone lymphoma*	1.6%	[Monocytoid B-cell lymphoma]
Follicular lymphoma[V] *In situ follicular neoplasia** *Duodenal-type follicular lymphoma*[*L]	20%	t(14;18)(q32;q21); IGH–BCL2 *CREBBP, KMT2D (MLL2), EZH2* mutations are common early events and potential therapeutic targets. Diffuse-appearing low-grade FL* is a group of localized inguinal masses that lack *BCL2* rearrangements and have 1p36 deletions.
Pediatric-type follicular lymphoma*[L] *Large B-cell lymphoma (LBCL) with IRF4 rearrangement**		Localized; variable morphology with indolent behavior New provisional entity distinguished from pediatric-type FL and other DLBCL Localized; usually involves Waldeyer ring and cervical lymph nodes
Primary cutaneous follicle center lymphoma		60% of B-cell PCL
Mantle cell lymphoma[M] *In situ mantle cell neoplasia**	3%–10%	Blastoid, pleomorphic, small cell, marginal zone-like variants t(11;14)(q13;q32); CCND1–IGH MCL subtypes: 1. Unmutated/minimally mutated IGHV, mostly SOX11+ 2. Mutated IGHV, mostly SOX11– (indolent leukemic nonnodal MCL with PB, BM and/or splenic involvement) – *TP53, NOTCH1, NOTCH2* mutations in a small proportion of cases of potential clinical importance – *CCND2* rearrangements in ~50% of cyclin D1-negative MCL
Diffuse large B-cell lymphoma, NOS[M] *Germinal center B-cell type** *Activated B-cell type** [genetic or immunophenotypic; cell of origin classification]	25%–30%	t(14;18)(q32;q21); *IGH–BCL2* Coexpression of MYC and BCL2 considered a prognostic marker ("double expressor" lymphoma)

Appendix B4	2016 World Health Organization (WHO) Classification of Hematopoietic and Lymphoid Neoplasms (*Continued*)	
Neoplasms	**%NHL**	**Variants [Synonyms] and Comments; Most Common Genetic and/or Molecular Abnormalities Detected; Selected Highlights of Changes in 2016 WHO Classification**
T-cell/histiocyte-rich LBCL[H]		<10% of all DLBCLs
Primary DLBCL of the CNS[M]	<1%	
Primary cutaneous DLBCL, leg type[M]		4% of PCL, 20% of B-cell PCL
EBV+ DLBCL, NOS*,[H] (formerly: EBV+ DLBCL of the elderly)		10% of DLBCL in Asia
EBV+ mucocutaneous ulcer*,[L]		Occurs in setting of immunosuppression
DLBCL associated with chronic inflammation		
Lymphomatoid granulomatosis[L,H]	Rare	
Primary mediastinal (thymic) LBCL[M]	2%–4%	[Mediastinal large cell lymphoma] *CIITA* mutations 9p24 amplicon (involving *JAK2, PD-L1, PD-L2*)
Intravascular LBCL[H]	Rare	
ALK-positive LBCL[H]	Rare	
Plasmablastic lymphoma[H]		*MYC* rearrangements common
Primary effusion lymphoma[H]		[Body cavity–based lymphoma] Includes "extracavitary" PEL vs. "solid" PEL
HHV8+ DLBCL, NOS* (formerly LBCL arising in HHV8-associated multicentric Castleman disease)		
Burkitt lymphoma[H]	2%	t(8;14)(q24;q32); *MYC–IGH* t(2;8)(p12;q24); *MYC–IGK* (uncommon) t(8;22)(q24;q11); *MYC–IGL* (uncommon) *TCF3* or *ID3* mutations in 70% of cases
Burkitt-like lymphoma with 11q aberrations*		Absence of MYC rearrangement; *ID3* mutation; 11q aberrations
High-grade B-cell lymphoma with *MYC* and *BCL2* and/or *BCL6* rearrangements*,[H] (formerly B-cell lymphoma, unclassifiable, between DLBCL and Burkitt lymphoma)		All LBCL with *MYC* and *BCL2* and/or *BCL6* rearrangements (so-called "double hit" lymphoma) except for cases that fulfill criteria for follicular or lymphoblastic lymphoma Specify DLBCL or B-cell lymphoma unclassifiable (BCLu) morphology
High-grade B-cell lymphoma, NOS*		BCLu morphology or other high-grade features without "double hit" rearrangements
B-cell lymphoma, unclassifiable, with features intermediate between DLBCL and classical Hodgkin lymphoma[M/H]		[CHL-DLBCL gray zone lymphoma] Two subtypes: (1) Mediastinal CHL-DLBCL gray zone (2) Nonmediastinal CHL-DLBCL gray zone
Mature T-Cell and NK-Cell Neoplasms		
T-cell prolymphocytic leukemia[H]	2%	Small cell, "cerebriform" cell; 2% of adult mature lymphocytic leukemias t(14;14)(q11;q32), inv14q(q11;q32); *TCRα-TCL1*

Appendix B4	2016 World Health Organization (WHO) Classification of Hematopoietic and Lymphoid Neoplasms (*Continued*)

Neoplasms	%NHL	Variants [Synonyms] and Comments; Most Common Genetic and/or Molecular Abnormalities Detected; Selected Highlights of Changes in 2016 WHO Classification
T-cell large granular lympho-cytic leukemia[L]	2%–3%	*STAT3* and *STAT5* mutations, latter associated with clinically more aggressive disease
Chronic lymphoproliferative disorder of NK cells[L]	—	[Chronic NK large granular lymphocyte leukemia; chronic NK cell lymphocytosis] *STAT3* mutations
Aggressive NK cell leukemia[H]	Rare	Asians
Systemic EBV+ T-cell lymphoma of childhood* (formerly "systemic EBV+ T-cell LPD" to emphasize aggressive clinical course)		
Hydroa vacciniforme-like lymphoproliferative disorder* (formerly Hydroa vaccin-iforme-like lymphoma)		
Adult T-cell leukemia/lymphoma[V] (HTLV-1)		Acute[H], lymphomatous[H], chronic[L], smoldering[L]
Extranodal NK/T-cell lymphoma, nasal type[V]		*STAT5B*, *STAT3* mutations
Enteropathy-associated T-cell lymphoma (EATL)[H]		Polymorphic Associated with celiac disease, primarily in those of northern European origin
Monomorphic epitheliotropic intestinal T-cell lymphoma* (formerly EATL II)		Monomorphic Not associated with celiac disease, primarily in Asians and Hispanics Gains of 8q24 involving *MYC* *STAT5B* mutations in all types of γδ T cell origin
Indolent T-cell lymphoprolifera-tive disorder of the GI tract[*,L]		
Hepatosplenic T-cell lymphoma[H]	<1%	Isochromosome 7q *STAT5B*, *STAT3* mutations
Subcutaneous panniculitis–like T-cell lymphoma[L, M]	<1%	
Mycosis fungoides (MF)[L]	—	Pagetoid reticulosis; folliculotropic MF; granulomatous slack skin; 50% of PCL
Sézary syndrome[M]	Rare	
Primary cutaneous CD30+ peripheral T-cell lymphoprolif-erative disorders[V]		
Lymphomatoid papulosis (LyP)[V]		LyP variants: Type A: mimics C-ALCL, scattered large cells Type B: mimics MF Type C: mimics C-ALCL, monotonous large cells Type D: mimics primary cutaneous CD8+ aggressive, epidermotropic cytotoxic TCL Type E: angioinvasive LyP with chromo-some 6p25 rearrangement
Primary cutaneous anaplastic large cell lymphoma (ALCL)		
Primary cutaneous γδ T-cell lymphoma		
Primary cutaneous CD8+ aggressive epidermotropic cytotoxic T-cell lymphoma[H]		

Appendix B4	2016 World Health Organization (WHO) Classification of Hematopoietic and Lymphoid Neoplasms (*Continued*)	

Neoplasms	%NHL	Variants [Synonyms] and Comments; Most Common Genetic and/or Molecular Abnormalities Detected; Selected Highlights of Changes in 2016 WHO Classification
Primary cutaneous acral CD8+ T-cell lymphoma[*,L]		
Primary cutaneous CD4-positive small/medium T-cell lymphoproliferative disorder[*,L] (formerly primary cutaneous CD4-positive small/medium T-cell lymphoma)		
Peripheral T-cell lymphoma, NOS[H]	4%	Lymphoepithelioid (Lennert lymphoma), T zone; 30% of peripheral T-cell lymphomas
Angioimmunoblastic T-cell lymphoma[H] (AITL)	1%–2%	*RHOA, IDH2* mutations
Follicular T-cell lymphoma (FTCL)		*TET2, IDH2, DNMT3, RHOA, CD28* mutations
Nodal peripheral T-cell lymphoma of T follicular helper (TFH) phenotype (umbrella category that includes AITL, FTCL, and other nodal PTCL with TFH phenotype)		*ITK–SYK* or *CTLA4–CD28* gene fusions
Anaplastic large cell lymphoma (ALCL), ALK-positive[L]	3%	t(2;5)(p23;q35); *NPM–ALK*
Anaplastic large cell lymphoma (ALCL), ALK-negative[M,*]		*DUSP22* and *IRF4* mutations in chromosome 6p25 (superior prognosis) *TP63* rearrangements (very aggressive)
Breast implant associated anaplastic large cell lymphoma[*]		
Hodgkin Lymphoma (HL)		
Nodular lymphocyte predominant HL		[Nodular L & H]
Classical HL (CHL)		
Nodular sclerosis CHL		
Mixed cellularity CHL		
Lymphocyte-rich CHL		
Lymphocyte-depleted CHL		
Posttransplant Lymphoproliferative Disorders (PTLD)		
Plasmacytic hyperplasia PTLD		
Infectious mononucleosis PTLD		
Florid follicular hyperplasia PTLD*		
Polymorphic PTLD		

(*Continued*)

Appendix B4	2016 World Health Organization (WHO) Classification of Hematopoietic and Lymphoid Neoplasms (*Continued*)

Neoplasms	%NHL	Variants [Synonyms] and Comments; Most Common Genetic and/or Molecular Abnormalities Detected; Selected Highlights of Changes in 2016 WHO Classification
Monomorphic PTLD (NK-/T- and B-cell types)		
Classical Hodgkin lymphoma PTLD		

Provisional entities are listed in italics.

Lymphoma grades reflecting clinical behavior: ᴸ, low; ᴹ, intermediate/high; ᴴ, high; ᵛ, variable.

ALK-1, anaplastic lymphoma kinase; **ALL**, acute lymphoblastic leukemia; **AIDS**, acquired immunodeficiency syndrome; **CLL/SLL**, chronic lymphocytic leukemia/small lymphocytic lymphoma; **HTLV-1**, human T-cell lymphotropic virus type I; **L&H**, lymphocytic and histiocytic; **NHL**, non-Hodgkin lymphoma; **NK**, natural killer; **NOS**, not otherwise specified; **PCL**, primary cutaneous lymphomas; **POEMS**, polyneuropathy, organomegaly, endocrinopathy, monoclonal gammopathy, and skin changes; **TEMPI**, telangiectasias, elevated EPO/erythrocytosis, monoclonal gammopathy (IgG MGUS), perinephric fluid collections, intrapulmonary shunting.

Information from (1) Swerdlow SH, Campo E, Harris NL, et al. *World Health Organization Classification of Tumours of Haematopoietic and Lymphoid Tissues.* Lyon, France: IARC Press, 2008; (2) Swerdlow SH, Campo E, Pileri SA, et al. The 2016 revision to the World Health Organization classification of lymphoid neoplasms. *Blood* 2016;127(20):2375–2390.

*Changes from the 2008 classification.

Appendix B5 — Acute Leukemias

Acute Leukemias: Cytology, Immunophenotype, and the 2016 World Health Organization (WHO) Classification

WHO Subtype of Acute Leukemia	Immature Cells	Recurrent Cytogenetic Abnormalities and Comments
AML with Recurrent Genetic Abnormalities		
Acute myeloid leukemia (AML) with t(8;21)(q22;q22); RUNX1–RUNX1T1	N: round, indented G: present AR: ++	t(8;21). Blasts and early promyelocytes predominate; secondary neutrophil granules present; thin, sharp ends in AR; splenomegaly; MS CD34, CD13, CD33dim, CD19, MPO+
Acute promyelocytic leukemia [APL] with PML–RARA* [formerly APL with t(15;17) (q22;q12); PML–RARA]	N: round, folded, twisted G: large AR: +++	t(15;17), t(11;17), and t(5;17) and variants; "faggot cells" (bundles of AR); DIC common CD13, CD33, CD117; MPO++, [CD2, CD4, CD56]; CD34–, CD14–, HLA-DR–
APL microgranular variant with PML–RARA	N: twisted, bilobed G: few AR: +	Submicroscopic-sized granules gives appearance of their paucity; MPO strongly +; easily mistaken for AMML CD2, CD4dim, CD13, CD33, CD34, CD117, MPO++; CD14–, HLA-DR–
AML with inv(16)(p13.1q22) or t(16;16)(p13.1;q22); CBFB–MYH11	N: reniform, folded G: variable AR: +/–	Myelomonocytic morphology; some eosinophil granules are darkly stained, MS. Suspect this if CD2+ and coexpressed with myeloid markers; CD10–, CD20– MPO+, NSE+
AML with t(9;11)(p22;q23); MLLT3–KMT2A* [formerly AML with t(9;11) (p22;q23); MLLT3–MLL]	N: round, reniform, folded G: Rare AR: –/+	Large cells, monoblastic, or myelomonocytic features MPO–, NSE+, associated with topoisomerase II inhibitor therapy; MS CD4, CD11b, CD11c, CD33, CD14, CD56. CD64, HLA-DR [CD34, CD117]; CD34–
AML with t(6;9)(p23;q34); DEK–NUP214		Increased basophils, ringed sideroblasts, multilineage dysplasia; AMML or AML with maturation common
AML with inv(3)(q21;q26.2) or t(3;3)(q21;q26.2); GATA2, MECOM* [formerly AML with inv(3)(q21;q26.2) or t(3;3)(q21;q26.2); RPN1–EVI1]		Multilineage dysplasia, normal or high platelet count, atypical bone marrow megakaryocytes
AML (megakaryoblastic) with t(1;22)(p13;q13); RBM15–MKL1		Small and large megakaryoblasts similar to AMegL, NOS. Fibrosis +/– CD33, CD34, CD31, CD41, CD61, CD64dim, CD117dim; CD13–, HLA-DR–
Provisional entity: AML with BCR/ABL1 fusion*		
AML with mutated NPM1		Myelomonocytic or monocytic features; NPM cytoplasmic protein+
AML with biallelic mutations of CEBPA* [AML with mutated CEBPA]		AML with maturation or (myelo)monocytic differentiation
Provisional entity: AML with mutated RUNX1*		

(Continued)

Appendix B5	Acute Leukemias (*Continued*)	
WHO Subtype of Acute Leukemia	**Immature Cells**	**Recurrent Cytogenetic Abnormalities and Comments**
AML with myelodysplasia-related changes		Dysplasia in at least 50% of cells of two marrow cell lines; abnormalities of chromosomes 5, 7, etc. [*Remove *de novo* cases with no MDS-related cytogenetic abnormalities if *NPM1* and *CEBPA^{dm}* mutated]
Therapy-related myeloid neoplasms		Present with AML, MDS, or mixed features (t-AML, t-MDS); MDS prodrome common
Alkylating agent related or radiation therapy related		Abnormalities of chromosomes 5 and 7
Topoisomerase II inhibitor related		Overt AML often monocytic without MDS phase common;11q23 [*MLL*] abnormalities
AML, NOS		
AML with minimal differentiation	N: round G: absent AR: −	Confused with ALL and AMegL; requires CD13+, CD33+, or CD117+ to confirm CD34+, CD38+; HLA-DR+; [CD7+, CD11b+, CD14+, CD64+, TdT+]; MPO−
AML without maturation	N: round to indented G: scarce AR: rare	Some cases confused with ALL CD13+, CD33+, CD34+, CD117+, HLA-DR+, MPO+
AML with maturation	N: round to reniform to PPH G: present AR: +	Cases with increased basophils are associated with t(6;9) and 12p abnormalities. CD13+, CD33+, CD34+, CD117+, MPO++, [CD7+], CD2−, CD19−, CD56−
Acute myelomonocytic leukemia (AMML)	N: round to reniform to folded G: present AR: +	Both granulocytic and monocytic differentiation; MS CD4+, CD11b+, CD11c+, CD13+, CD14+, CD33+, CD34+, CD56+, CD64+, CD15+, CD117+; HLA-DR+; MPO+; NSE+/++
Acute monoblastic and monocytic leukemia (AMoL)	N: large, round to reniform; large nucleoli G: present AR: −	Monoblastic composed of >80% monoblasts and promonocytes, MS CD4+, CD11b+, CD11c+, CD13+, CD14+, CD56+, CD64+, CD68+; [CD7+, CD34+, D117+]; MPO−; NSE++
Acute erythroid leukemias (AEL; erythroleukemia and pure erythroid leukemia)	N: round G: few AR: +	Erythroleukemia: ≥20% myeloblasts plus florid erythroid hyperplasia and dysplasia with bi- and multinucleated, vacuolated forms, and ring sideroblasts; important to distinguish from megaloblastic anemias, MDS with excess blasts-2. E-cadherin+, Hemoglobin A+, glycophorin ±, CD36+; CD71dim+; MPO±, NSE−

Appendix B5 | Acute Leukemias (*Continued*)

WHO Subtype of Acute Leukemia	Immature Cells	Recurrent Cytogenetic Abnormalities and Comments
Acute megakaryoblastic leukemia (AMegL)	N: round to indented G: scarce to numerous and fine AR: –	CD41+ and CD61+ (platelet glycoproteins); often with prominent marrow fibrosis CD41+ (GpIIb/IIIa), CD61+ (GpIIIa), CD36+; CD34–, CD45–, HLA-DR–, MPO–
Acute panmyelosis with myelofibrosis (APMF)	N: round to indented G: scarce to numerous AR: —	Distinguished from AMegL by panmyelosis. Blasts are MPO–, lysozyme–, CD34+, CD68+, and CD117+. CD41–, CD61–, von Willebrand factor–, glycophorin–, HbA– Presence of MDS-related cytogenetic abnormalities (e.g., deletion 5/5q–, deletion 7/7q–, etc.) excludes diagnosis of APMF

Myeloid Sarcoma
Myeloid Proliferations Related to Down Syndrome

Transient abnormal myelopoiesis (TAM)		Usually megakaryoblastic proliferation Occurs at birth or within days of birth → resolves in 1–2 mo Associated with *GATA1* mutations
Myeloid leukemia associated with Down syndrome		Usually megakaryoblastic proliferation Usually occurs in first 3 years of life with or without prior TAM and persists if not treated Associated with *GATA1* mutations
Blastic plasmacytoid dendritic cell neoplasm	N: round to oval G: scarce AR: —	Skin lesions common CD4+, CD56+, CD 123+ [CD43, CD45RA, weak TdT]

Acute Leukemias of Ambiguous Lineage

Acute undifferentiated leukemia	N: round G: – AR: –	Express no more than one lineage-associated marker; may be CD34, HLA-DR, or CD38+
Mixed-phenotype acute leukemia (MPAL)		Two or more immunophenotypically distinct populations—one myeloid and one B-ALL or T-ALL; or single population marking as B-ALL or T-ALL with MPO+
MPAL with t(9;22) (q34.1;q11.2); *BCR/ABL1*		Usually B and myeloid phenotype
MPAL with t(v;11q23) *KMT2A* rearranged* [formerly *MLL*]		Dimorphic blasts, often B lymphoblasts and monoblasts
MPAL, B/myeloid, NOS		Dimorphic B lymphoblasts and blasts with myeloid markers
MPAL, T/myeloid, NOS		Dimorphic T lymphoblasts and blasts with myeloid markers

Precursor Lymphoid Neoplasms

B-lymphoblastic leukemia/lymphoma, NOS	N: round to convoluted G: absent to rare AR: –	Homogeneous cell population (synonymous with ALL); blasts express myeloid and B- or T-cell markers; See Appendix C5. CD10+, CD19, CD79a, TdT, HLA-DR, PAX5+, MPO–, NSE–

(Continued)

Appendix B5 — Acute Leukemias (*Continued*)

WHO Subtype of Acute Leukemia	Immature Cells	Recurrent Cytogenetic Abnormalities and Comments
B-lymphoblastic leukemia/lymphoma with t(9;22)(q34.1;q11.2); *BCR/ABL1*		
B-lymphoblastic leukemia/lymphoma with t(v;11q23); *KMT2A* rearranged* [formerly *MLL*]		
B-lymphoblastic leukemia/lymphoma with t(12;21)(p13;q22); *ETV6–RUNX1*		
B-lymphoblastic leukemia/lymphoma with hyperdiploidy		
B-lymphoblastic leukemia/lymphoma with hypodiploidy		
B-lymphoblastic leukemia/lymphoma with t(5;14)(q31.1;q32.3); *IL3–IGH*		
B-lymphoblastic leukemia/lymphoma with t(1;19)(q23;p13.3); *TCF3–PBX1*		

Provisional entity:
B-lymphoblastic leukemia/lymphoma, *BCR-/ABL1*–like (i.e., "Philadelphia-like" B-ALL)*—similar gene expression signature to Ph+ ALL
Provisional entity: **B-lymphoblastic leukemia/lymphoma with *iAMP21***

T-lymphoblastic leukemia/ lymphoma	N: round to convoluted G: absent to rare AR: –	Homogeneous cell population (synonymous with T-cell ALL); see Appendix C5. CD2, CD3, CD5, CD7, TdT+; MPO– NSE–

Provisional entity: Early T-cell precursor lymphoblastic leukemia

Information from (1) Swerdlow SH, Campo E, Harris NL, et al. *World Health Organization Classification of Tumours of Haematopoietic and Lymphoid Tissues.* Lyon, France: IARC Press, 2008; (2) Arber DA, Orazi A, Hasserjian R, et al. The 2016 revision to the World Health Organization classification of myeloid neoplasms and acute leukemia. *Blood* 2016;127(20):2391–2405.

++, strongly positive; +, usually positive or present; ±, variable; –, usually negative, absent, or weak; N, nuclei; G, cytoplasmic granules; AR, Auer rods.

ALL, acute lymphoblastic leukemia; **DIC**, disseminated intravascular coagulation; **Gp**, platelet glycoprotein; **LYS**, lysozyme (muramidase); **MPO**, myeloperoxidase and Sudan black B; **MDS**, myelodysplastic syndrome; **MS**, myeloid sarcoma; **NPM**, nucleophosmin; **NOS**, not otherwise specified; **NSE**, nonspecific esterase; **PPH**, pseudo-Pelger-Huet anomaly; **TdT**, terminal deoxytransferase.

Note:
Panmyeloid antigens: CD13, CD33, and CD117.
Hematopoietic progenitor cell antigens: CD34, HLA-DR.
Monocytic antigens: CD11b, CD14 (also CD4, CD11c, CD56, CD64).
Increased lysozyme levels are measured in the serum and characterize mixed (AMML) or pure (AMoL) monocytic leukemias.
*Changes from the 2008 classification.

Appendix B6	**2016 Revision of WHO Classification of Myelodysplastic Syndromes (MDS)**[a]	

MDS Type [Proportion of Cases]	Peripheral Blood	Bone Marrow
MDS with single lineage dysplasia (MDS-SLD)* [10%–20%] (formerly RA)	Isolated anemia (normocytic/macrocytic), +/– neutropenia, or thrombocytopenia Blasts: <1%	Dysplasia in 1 line <10% in affected MCL RS: <15% [or <5%, if *SF3B1* mutation present] Blasts: <5%; AR: none No Auer rods
MDS with multilineage dysplasia (MDS-MLD)* [30%] (formerly RCMD)	1–3 cytopenias Blasts: <1%	Dysplasia in <10% in multiple MCL RS: <15% Blasts: <5%
MDS with RS* [3%–11%] (formerly RARS) MDS-RS-SLD: single lineage dysplasia* MDS-RS-MLD: multi-lineage dysplasia	<1% blasts 1–2 cytopenias 2–3 cytopenias	<5% Blasts, RS: >15% [or >5%, if *SF3B1* mutation present] No AR Erythroid hyperplasia and dysplasia only 1–3 dysplastic lines
MDS with isolated del (5q)	Anemia ww/o other cytopenias, ww/o thrombocytosis Blasts: <1%	Blasts: <5%; AR: none Hypolobated megakaryocytes and frequent erythroid hypoplasia Evidence of del(5q) alone, or with 1 additional abnormality except –7 or del(7q)

MDS with excess blasts (MDS-EB)* [40%]
    MDS-EB-1* (formerly RAEB-1)
    MDS-EB-2* (formerly RAEB-2)
	Cytopenias with dysplasia in 1–3 MCL
	Monocytes: <1,000/mL
	Blasts: 2%–4%
	Blasts: 5%–19%
		Dysplasia in 0–3 MCL; usually hypercellular
		
		Blasts: 5%–9%;
		AR: none
		Blasts: 10%–19%; or AR.
		AR: none or present

MDS, unclassifiable (MDS-U)[c]	1. MDS with 1% blasts in peripheral blood (<5% blasts in marrow, no AR) 2. MDS-SLD with pancytopenia (<1% blasts in blood, <5% in marrow, no AR) 3. Have a defining cytogenetic abnormality (<1% blasts in blood, <5% in marrow, <15% RS, no AR)	
Refractory cytopenias of childhood	Cytopenias in 1–3 lines. Usually dysplastic changes in >10% of neutrophils. Blasts: <2%	Dysplasia in >10% of cells in 1–3 MCL Blasts: <5% Micromegakaryocytes may be present

Provisional entities are listed in italics.

AR, Auer rods; **MCL**, marrow cell lineages; **Ph+**, Philadelphia chromosome or BCR/ABL fusion gene; **RA**, refractory anemia; **RCMD**, refractory anemia with multilineage dysplasia; **RS**, ringed sideroblasts (five or more iron granules encircling one-third or more of the nucleus); ±, with or without.

*Changes from the 2008 classification.

[a]Adapted from Arber DA, Orazi A, Hasserjian R, et al. The 2016 revision to the World Health Organization classification of myeloid neoplasms and acute leukemia. *Blood* 2016;127(20):2391–2405.

[b]See Chapter 26 Myelodysplastic Syndromes Section II for definitions of the various dysplasias.

[c]MD-SLD: refractory anemia (RA, by far the most predominant type), refractory neutropenia, or refractory thrombocytopenia. MDS-U should not be equated with "idiopathic cytopenias of undetermined significance."

Appendix C

Chemotherapy Regimens for Lymphomas

Lauren C. Pinter-Brown and Mary Territo

Appendix C1 Regimens for Hodgkin Lymphoma (HL)[a]

Regimen (Cycle Frequency)	Alkylating Agent	Plant Alkaloid	Anthracycline or Antibiotic	Corticosteroid	Others
I. Traditional first-line regimens for HL					
ABVD (28 d)		Vbl 6 [d 1 + 15]	Doxo 25 [d 1 + 15] Bleo 10 [d 1 + 15]		DTIC 375 [d 1 + 15]
MOPP (28 d)	Mechl 6 [d 1 + 8]	Vcr 1.4 [d 1 + 8]		Pred 40 PO [d 1→ 14]	Pcz 100 PO [d 1→ 14]
COPP (21 d)	Cyclo 400–650 [d 1 + 8]	Vcr 1.4[b] [d 1 + 8]		Pred 40 PO [d 1→14]	Pcz 100 PO [d 1→ 14]
MOPP–ABV hybrid (28 d)	Mechl 6 [d 1]	Vcr 1.4[b] [d 1] Vbl 6 [d 8]	Doxo 35 [d 8] Bleo 10 [d 8]	Pred 40 PO [d 1→ 14]	Pcz 100 PO [d 1→ 7]
II. Dose-intense regimens for HL					
Stanford V (28 d)	Mechl 6 [d 1 + 15]	Vbl 6 [d 1 + 5] Vcr 1.4[b] [d 8 + 22] Etop 60 [d 15]	Doxo 25 [d 1 + 15] Bleo 5 [d 8 + 22]	Pred 40 PO [every other day for three cycles]	
BEACOPP (21 d)	Cyclo 650 [d 1]	Etop 100 [d → 3] Vcr 1.4[b] [d 8]	Doxo 25 [d 1] Bleo 10 [d 8]	Pred 40 PO [d 1 → 14]	Pcz 100 PO [d 1 → 7]
BEACOPP escalated (21 d)	Cyclo 1,250 [d 1]	Etop 200 [d → 3] Vcr 1.4[b] [d 8]	Doxo 35 [d 1] Bleo 10 [d 8]	Pred 40 PO [d 1 → 14]	Pcz 100 PO [d 1 → 7]

Bleo, bleomycin (dose in units/m²); Chl, chlorambucil; Cyclo, cyclophosphamide; Doxo, doxorubicin (Adriamycin); DTIC, dacarbazine; Etop, etoposide; Mechl, mechlorethamine (nitrogen mustard); Pcz, procarbazine; Pred, prednisone; Vbl, vinblastine; Vcr, vincristine.
[a]Drugs and dosage in mg/m² (days given in cycle). All doses are given intravenously (IV) except when they are oral (PO), where indicated.
[b]Maximum, 2.0-mg dose.

Appendix C2 Regimens for Non-Hodgkin Lymphoma (NHL) [a]

Regimen (Cycle Frequency)	Alkylating Agent	Plant Alkaloid	Anthracycline or Antibiotic	Antimetabolite	Corticosteroid	Others (Consider Adding Rituximab to Regimen for all CD20 + NHL)
I. Low-grade NHL						
Chl and P (14–28 d)	Chl 16 PO [d 1 or d 1 → 5]				Pred 40 PO [d 1 → 5]	
CVP (21 d)	Cyclo 1,000 PO [d 1] or Cyclo 400 PO [d 1 → 5]	Vcr 1.4[b] [d 1]			Pred 100[c] PO [d 1 →5]	
BR (21–28 d)	Bendamustine 70–90 mg/m² IV [d 1 + 2]					Ritux 375 [d 1]
II. Intermediate–high-grade NHL						
CHOP (21 d)	Cyclo 750 [d 1]	Vcr 1.4[b] [d 1]	Doxo 50 [d 1]		Pred 100[c] PO [d 1 → 5]	
III. High-grade NHL (e.g., mantle cell lymphoma)						
CODOX-M/IVAC: Codox-M (2 cycles alternating with IVAC)	Cyclo 800 [d 1] Cyclo 200 [d 2 → 5]	Vcr 1.5 [d 1 + 8]	Doxo 40 [d 1]	Mtx 1,200 over 1 h, then 240/h × 23 h [d 10]	IT Cytar 70[c] [d 1 + 3] IT Mtx 12[c] [d 15]	Leuc[d] GCSF from d 13 until ANC >1,000
IVAC (2 cycles alternating with CODOX-M)	Ifos 1,500 over 1–2 h with mesna 360 over 1 h q3h [d 1 → 5]	Etop 60 [d 1 → 5]		Cytar 2,000 over 1–2 h q12h [d 1 + 2]	IT Mtx 12[c] [d 5]	GCSF from d 7 until ANC >1,000
R-HyperCVAD Course 1	Cyclo 300 q12h [d 1 → 3]	Vcr 2[c] [d 4 + 11]	Doxo 25/d CIV [d 4 + 5]		Dexa 40[c] PO [d 1 → 4 and d 11 → 14]	Ritux 375 [d 1 and 8] GCSF from d 6 until WBC >4,500
R-HyperCVAD Course 2				Mtx 200 bolus then 800 over 24 h [d 1]	Cytar 3,000[e] over 1 h q12h × 4 doses [2 + 3]	Leuc[f] Ritux 375 [d 1]

ANC, absolute neutrophil count per µL; Bleo, Bleomycin; CIV, 24 h continuous IV infusion; Chl, chlorambucil; Cyclo, cyclophosphamide; Cytar, cytarabine; Dexa, dexamethasone; Doxo, doxorubicin (Adriamycin); Etop, etoposide; GCSF, granulocyte colony-stimulating factor (5 mcg/kg SQ or IV daily); Ifos, ifosfamide; Leuc, leucovorin; Mtx, methotrexate; Pred, prednisone; Ritux, rituximab; Vcr, vincristine; WBC, white blood cell count per µL.

[a]Drugs and dosage in mg/m² (days given in cycle). All doses are given intravenously (IV) except when they are oral (PO) or intrathecal (IT), where indicated. Rituximab, 375 mg/m² weekly for 4 weeks, is frequently added to these regimens for CD20 positive NHLs.

[b]Maximum, 2.0-mg dose.

[c]Total dose (not per m²).

[d]Leucovorin 192 mg/m² given at 36 h after Mtx started and then 12 mg/m² q6h until serum Mtx level <10⁻⁸ M.

[e]Reduce cytarabine dosage to 1,000 mg/m² per dose for patients older than 60 years or with serum creatinine levels higher than 1.5 mg/dL.

[f]Leucovorin 50 mg PO given 24 h after Mtx is finished for 15 mg q6h × 8 doses (adjusted according to serum Mtx level).

Appendix C3	**Salvage Regimens for Hodgkin and Non-Hodgkin Lymphoma**[a]			
Regimen (Cycle Frequency)	**Alkylating Agent**	**Plant Alkaloid**	**Anthracycline/ Antibiotic**	**Others (Consider Adding Rituximab to Regimen for all CD20 + NHL)**
EPOCH (21 d) (can also be considered for initial therapy)	Cyclo 750 IV bolus [d 5]	Etop 50/d CIV [d 1 → 4] Vcr 0.4/d CIV [d 1 – 4]	Doxo 10/d CIV [d 1 → 4]	Prednisone 60/d PO [d 1 → 5] GCSF daily starting d 6 until ANC >10,000/μL Cotrimoxazole 2 tabs b.i.d. × 3 consecutive d/wk Doses modified according to CD4 count in AIDS (see Chapter 37, Section II.F.3)
ESHAP (21–28 d)	Cis 25/d CIV [d 1 → 4]	Etop 40 [d 1 → 4]		Cytarabine 2,000 over 2 h [d 5 × 1 dose] Solu-Medrol 500[b] [d 1 → 4]
IGEV (21 d)	Ifos 2,000 IV (infuse over 2 h) [d 1 → 4] + mesna	Vin 20 IV [d 1]		Gem 800 IV [d 1 + 4] Prednisone 100 mg PO [d 1→ 4]
DHAP (21–28 d)	Cis 100 CIV [d 1]			Cytarabine 2,000 q12h × 2 doses (+ prednisolone eye drops) Dexamethasone 40 mg/d PO [d 1→4]
ICE (21–28 d)	Ifos 5,000 CIV [d 2]	Etop 100 [d 1 → 3]		Carboplatin AUC = 5 [d 2] Mesna 5,000 CIV [d 2]
MINE (21–28 d)	Ifos 1,330 over 1 h [d 1 → 3]	Etop 65 [d 1 →3]	Nov 8 [d 1]	Mesna 1,330 IV over 1 h with Ifos [d 1 → 3] and 500[b] mg PO 4 h after Ifos ends
GDP (21 d)	Cis 75 IV [d 1]			Gem 1,000 IV [d 1 + 8] Dexamethasone 40 mg/d PO [d 1–4]
GemOx (14–21 d)	Ox 100 (d 1)			Gem 1,000 [d 1]

AIDS, acquired immunodeficiency syndrome; ANC, absolute neutrophil count per μL; AUC, area under the curve using Calvert formula; b.i.d., twice daily PO; Cis, cisplatin; CIV, by 24-h continuous intravenous infusion; Gem, gemcitabine; Vin, vinorelbine. Cyclo, cyclophosphamide; Doxo, doxorubicin; Etop, etoposide; GCSF, granulocyte colony-stimulating factor (filgrastim); Ifos, ifosfamide; Nov, Novantrone (mitoxantrone); Ox, oxaliplatin; Vin, Vinorelbine; Vcr, vincristine.
[a]Drugs and dosage in mg/m[2] (days given in cycle). All doses are intravenous (IV) bolus except when they are oral (PO) or CIV, where indicated. Rituximab, 375 mg/m[2] IV, is frequently added to these regimens for CD20-positive tumors.
[b]Total dose (not per m[2]).

Index

Note: Page numbers followed by t indicate table; those in *italics* indicate figure.